Psychiatric Nursing

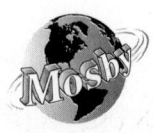

Visit our website at **www.mosby.com**

Psychiatric Nursing

THIRD EDITION

Norman L. Keltner, RN, EdD, CRNP
Associate Professor
School of Nursing
University of Alabama, Birmingham
Birmingham, Alabama

Lee Hilyard Schwecke, RN, MSN, EdD
Associate Professor
School of Nursing
Indiana University
Indianapolis, Indiana

Carol E. Bostrom, RN, MSN, CS
Clinical Assistant Professor
School of Nursing
Indiana University
Indianapolis, Indiana

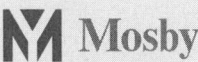

A Harcourt Health Sciences Company

St. Louis   London   Philadelphia   Sydney   Toronto

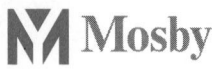

A Harcourt Health Sciences Company

Publisher: Sally Schrefer
Editor: Jeanne Allison
Associate Developmental Editor: Jeff Downing
Project Manager: Dana Peick
Production Editor: Dan Begley
Designer: Bill Drone
Manufacturing Manager: Karen Boehme

THIRD EDITION

www.mosby.com

Mosby, Inc.
11830 Westline Industrial Drive
St. Louis, Missouri 63146

Library of Congress Cataloging-in-Publication Data

Keltner, Norman L.
    Psychiatric nursing / Norman L. Keltner, Lee Hilyard Schwecke,
Carol E. Bostrom. — 3rd ed.
        p. cm.
    Includes bibliographical references and index.
    ISBN 0-323-00399-0
    1. Psychiatric nursing. 2. Psychotherapy. 3. Nurse and patient.
I. Schwecke, Lee Hilyard. II. Bostrom, Carol E. III. Title.
    [DNLM: 1. Psychiatric Nursing 2. Nurse-Patient Relations.
3. Psychotropic Drugs nurses' instruction. WY 160K29p 1999]
RC440.K36 1999
610.73'68—dc21
DNLM/DLC   98–38935

01 02 / 9 8 7 6 5 4 3

Contributors

Gary M. Carroll, BSN, MS, JD
Assistant Vice President, Risk Management
Protective Life Insurance Company
Birmingham, Alabama

Cathy S. Childers, RN, MSN
Clinical Care Coordinator, Psychiatry
University of Alabama Hospital
Birmingham, Alabama

Ruth Cox, RN, PhD
Assistant Professor
School of Nursing
University of Alabama, Birmingham
Birmingham, Alabama

Linda K. Hinkle, PhD
Clinical Psychologist
Developmental Associates
Indianapolis, Indiana

Bette R. Keltner, RN, PhD, FAAN
Assistant Vice-President for Medical
　Management
Honda of America
Marysville, Ohio

Bruce Payne Mericle, RN, MS
Assistant Professor
The College of New Jersey
School of Nursing
Ewing, New Jersey

Cleo Metcalf, RN, MSN, CNAA
Assistant Chief, Nursing Services
Veteran Affairs' Northern California System of
　Clinics
Pleasant Hill, California

Gordon I.G. Pugh, M.Div., M.Phil.
Substance Abuse Therapist
Chilton-Shelby Mental Health Center
Calera, Alabama
Instructor
Jefferson State Community College
Birmingham, Alabama

Renee Wilson Saul, MSN, CRNP
Adult Nurse Practitioner
University of Alabama Hospital
Birmingham, Alabama

Larry Scahill, MSN, PhD
Assistant Professor, Nursing and Child Psychiatry
Yale Child Studies Center
Yale School of Nursing
New Haven, Connecticut

Richard A. Sugerman, PhD
Professor of Anatomy
Western University of Health Sciences
Pomona, California

Kris L. Wang, RN, MSN, CS
Psychiatric Clinical Nurse Specialist
VAMC
Prescott, Arizona

Barbara Jones Warren, RN, PhD, CNS
Assistant Professor of Clinical Nursing
Ohio State University
College of Nursing
Clinical Research and Program Evaluation
The Ohio Department of Mental Health
Office of Program Evaluation & Research
Columbus, Ohio

Reviewers

Deanah Alexander, RN, MSN, CS
Instructor
Psychiatric Mental Health Nursing
West Texas A & M University
Canyon, Texas

Charla Mae Andrews, RNC, MS
Instructor
Spokane Community College
Staff Nurse
Sacred Heart Medical Center
Spokane, Washington

Andrea C. Bostrom, RN, PhD
Associate Professor
Kirkhof School of Nursing
Grand Valley State University
Allendale, Michigan

Mary B. Davies, RN, BSN
Psychiatric Nurse/Resource Nurse
Healthfront Educational Corporation
Melrose, Massachusetts

Patricia R. Dean, RN, MSN
Associate Professor
School of Nursing
Florida State University
Tallahassee, Florida

Susan Dewey-Hammer, RN, MN, CS
Associate Professor
Suffolk County Community College
Selden, New York
Nursing Education
Pilgrim Psychiatric Center
Brentwood, New York

Kathleen Shannon Dorcy, BSN, MN
Researcher
Fred Hutchinson Cancer Research Center
Seattle, Washington
Lecturer
University of Washington
Tacoma, Washington

Ginger W. Evans, RN, MS, MSN, CS
Assistant Professor
College of Nursing
University of Tennessee
Knoxville, Tennessee

Rauda Gelazis, RN, PhD, CS, CTN
Associate Professor
Ursuline College
Pepper Pike, Ohio

Rebecca Crews Gruener, RN, MSN
Associate Professor of Nursing
Louisiana State University
Alexandria, Louisiana

Brigitte Haagen, RN, DNS©, CS
Coordinator, Mental Health Nursing
School of Nursing
Pennsylvania State University
Hershey, Pennsylvania

Pamela F. Helms, RN, MN
Assistant Professor
School of Nursing
University of Mississippi
Jackson, Mississippi

Alice R. Kempe, RNCS, PhD
Associate Professor
Ursuline College
Pepper Pike, Ohio

Jeanne B. Kozlak, RN, MSN, CS
Professor of Mental Health Nursing
Humboldt State University
Arcata, California

Joyce A. Roberson, RN, PhD
Level Coordinator
University of Iowa
College of Nursing
Iowa City, Iowa

Anna Tichy, RN, MS, PhD
Professor, Administrative Studies in Nursing
College of Nursing
University of Illinois at Chicago
Chicago, Illinois

Jean H. Woods, RN, PhD, CS
Professor
Department of Nursing
Temple University College of Allied Health
    Professions
Philadelphia, Pennsylvania

Student Reviewer
Anna Buterbaugh
Kotzebue, Alaska

Preface

The first edition of this book, published in 1991, coincided with the dawning of the "decade of the brain." Quite frankly, when we wrote the prospectus for the book in late 1987, we had never heard of the decade of the brain—but we had anticipated it. From the beginning we emphasized the psychobiological nature of mental disorders and the need for psychiatric nurses to grapple with these concepts without letting go of their traditional emphasis on the nurse-patient relationship. These ideas were first presented in an article featured in Perspectives in Psychiatric Care entitled "Psychotherapeutic Management: A Model for Nursing Practice."

Alice R. Clarke, RN, MA, was the publisher/editor of *Perspectives* at that time, and her enthusiastic and rapid embrace of this concept launched what has followed. She understood the need for a change in thinking about psychiatric nursing practice and placed a high priority on publishing this conceptual piece. With this encouragement a prospectus for a book based on this model was developed and submitted to Mosby.

It is important for us (the authors) to remember and recapture our original zeal for bringing clarity to practice. In looking back, we may have overreacted to traditional psychodynamic approaches in our efforts to bring balance to practice. Today the pendulum has swung, and now nearly all psychiatric nursing textbooks use a psychobiological and psychopharmacological approach.

Our textbook was and is proactive and not reactive. Older psychiatric nursing textbooks (published before 1991) tended to be very lengthy (what one academician referred to as encyclopedic) and had little to say about psychobiological influences on mental disorders or psychopharmacology. Further, in an effort to emphasize mental health concepts these textbooks often avoided terms such as *schizophrenia*. This alone underscores the effect the decade of the brain has had on psychiatric nursing.

Thus we remain committed to our original notions about psychiatric nursing practice. We continue to propose the simple paradigm of interventions outlined in the psychotherapeutic management model, that is, the nurse, psychopharmacology, and environment all informed by an understanding of psychopathology. One size does not fit all!

So, while the idea is simple, implementation requires diligent study and much practice. The most obvious example is psychobiology. To utilize the psychotherapeutic management model one needs to have a basic appreciation of the psychobiological bases of mental disorders. Many students (and some of us ex-students) find this to be a very challenging area of study. However, a solid grounding in psychobiology raises one's level of practice. The same is true for psychopharmacology. It is simple to recite the three interventions in the model, but it is a complex undertaking to explore the parameters of psychotropic drugs. Patient care and patient safety are improved when nurses understand the drugs they administer.

We believe the straightforward approach to psychiatric nursing care presented in this textbook is an effective method of care and is readily learned by students. The model can be used almost immediately by new students; that is, the model directs students' attention toward the important issues of care. The more experienced student and the seasoned nurse can mine each intervention approach and the related psychopathological factors to gain a deeper understanding and to refine their care. "Psychotherapeutic management is 'real world' nursing. Mastery of the components—psychopharmacology, therapeutic nurse-patient communication, and milieu management—grounded in psychopathological concepts, is a challenging but achievable undertaking; one that will provide a model for productive psychiatric nursing and a distinct sense of professional achievement and role clarity for psychiatric nurses" (Keltner, 1985).

ORGANIZATION

The book is organized into eight units. The crucial units are those that flesh out the three psychotherapeutic management interventions (The Therapeutic Nurse-Patient Relationship [III], Psychopharmacology [IV], and Milieu Management [V]) and the unit on Psychopathology (VI). Other units support the model or touch on issues not directly addressed by it. In Unit One, chapters on the history of psychiatric care and psychobiology are presented. Unit Two deals with the continuum of care available to people with mental disorders. Unit Seven discusses somatic and behavior therapies, and Unit Eight addresses special populations in psychiatric nursing such as the elderly mentally ill and children with psychiatric problems.

FEATURES

With students in mind we have provided a number of tools to facilitate understanding and promote clinical competence. Many of these features are highlighted by a distinctive logo.

- Drug cards for 32 of the most commonly used psychotropic medications can be torn out for handy reference during clinicals.
- Student worksheets (tear outs) for each chapter are available to reinforce key concepts.
- Learning objectives point students to important concepts within each chapter.
- Key concepts are placed at the end of each chapter to recap important content.
- Study questions are located at the end of each chapter (with answers provided in the back) to help the student focus on important content and prepare for course examinations.
- Family issues boxes in selected chapters facilitate the student's awareness of the issues families must confront when a member suffers from mental illness.

- *Diagnostic and Statistical Manual of Mental Disorders* (ed 4, 1994) (DSM-IV) diagnostic criteria are extensively utilized to prepare the student for interdisciplinary discussions and professional journal literature related to psychiatric care.
- Clinical examples, concise vignettes drawn from the authors' own experience, are interspersed throughout the text to provide realistic illustrations of specific content.
- Case studies, detailed depictions of psychiatric disorders, are used in selected chapters to help the student conceptualize the development of effective nursing care strategies.
- Nursing care plans, based on the six steps of the nursing process, are carefully developed from the case studies.
- DSM-IV and related North American Nursing Diagnosis Association (NANDA) diagnoses are compared to help the student's understanding of their interrelatedness.
- Key nursing interventions are presented in Units Four (Psychopharmacology) and Six (Psychopathology).
- Critical thinking questions of a legal, ethical, or philosophical nature challenge students to stretch their awareness of psychiatric nursing beyond the content of this book.
- Key terms unique to any particular chapter are grouped into a box format for easy reference, thus facilitating the understanding of chapter content.
- Drug side effects and nursing interventions are provided in the section on psychopharmacology (Unit Four).
- All boxes and tables containing pharmacology content are highlighted for emphasis and accessibility.
- A glossary with current and usable definitions for over 350 key psychiatric terms is available for quick reference.

ANCILLARY PACKAGE

This edition features a revised ancillary package to supplement instruction that includes:
- Instructor's Resource Manual, consisting of
    Chapter summaries
    Chapter outlines
    Critical thinking questions for class discussion

Student worksheets
Transparency masters
Test bank with 750 test items in NCLEX
format
• Set of 50 2-color transparency acetates
• Computerized test bank in IBM and Macintosh
formats

As is true of all nursing text authors, our goal is to present accurate and meaningful information to the student without the distraction of sexist language.

Where possible, we have made every attempt to avoid the use of sexist pronouns by using plural nouns and pronouns or *his or her* rather than risk stigmatizing by gender. Sometimes, to avoid awkwardness of style, we have referred to the nurse as "she" and the patient as "he."

Norman L. Keltner
Lee Hilyard Schwecke
Carol E. Bostrom

Acknowledgments

In reviewing the preface, I was again reminded of Alice Clarke's sustained influence on this book. Without her early encouragement, support, and advice we would not have written the first edition. Of course, the companion textbooks, *Psychotropic Drugs* and *Psychobiological Foundations of Psychiatric Care,* would never have found the light of day either. So I want to acknowledge Alice Clarke and her pioneering work at *Perspectives in Psychiatric Care.* Though Alice gave us that first prompting, another person encouraged us as well. Linda Duncan, the nursing editor at Mosby in the late 80s, believed in this approach to psychiatric nursing education and promoted this idea to her publishing colleagues. Her assistant Jeff Burnham, who later assumed the nursing editor position, was every bit as enthusiastic about our ideas and will always be remembered for his sage advice. Today, a new team of editors has guided us through the ups and downs of writing the third edition: Jeanne Allison and Jeff Downing. Their skillful navigation of the process has made what could be a hair-pulling experience quite livable.

Writing an 800-page book is not easy. Long after the highs of creativity have passed, the reality of grinding out one more round of editing or proofing can test the best of writing teams. I have been blessed with two wonderful coauthors who have always been able to focus on the goal ahead and not be sidetracked by the minor setbacks along the way.

In the first edition I acknowledged all those nurses who were instrumental in my career development. Now, after 33 years in this profession I can still remember my first teachers at Stockton State Hospital and at Delta College. They were excellent role models and left lasting impressions on me. I suppose a teacher cannot hope for more than that. I will not name each person as I did in the first edition but remain grateful to and humbled by the influential people in my professional life.

Finally, as author I have the opportunity to dedicate this edition if I choose to do so. I want to dedicate this book to the following young people who have brought a great deal of joy into my life: Reba, Justin, Luke, Drew, Andy, Jeremy, Sam, Michael, and Jacob.

N.L.K.

A loving thank you to my children, Jason and Renee, for their patience and support throughout the development of this edition. A special thank you to my parents, Mildred and Lawrence Hilyard, who always believed in and encouraged me. I wish my mother had lived to see the book in print. However, my stepmother, Virginia, is certainly a welcome addition to the family and has cheered me on as well.

This book would not have been possible without the hundreds of patients and victims who are willing to share their pain, experiences, and successes. I also appreciate the students, faculty, colleagues, and hospital personnel who questioned and challenged the content in the second edition and offered input for this edition. Norm Keltner, Carol Bostrom, Sandy Wood, and Sharon Holmberg deserve special mention for their insights. Over time, the staff of the VA Hospital and Community Hospital North have helped me expand my knowledge and develop more effective intervention strategies.

Working for nineteen years as a volunteer with the Crisis Intervention Service, with Mary Hoffmann (former Coordinator) and the other volunteer Clinical Associates, always kept me in touch with the issues and needs of clients/patients.

Thank you to all who have touched my life and thereby influenced this book.

L.H.S.

My efforts in writing the third edition of this textbook are dedicated to the many individuals and families who have shared their struggle and their joy with me. Their hope is for knowledgeable nurses to understand, care, and advocate for them. I hope this textbook will assist nurses in achieving some of the art and science of psychiatric nursing, regardless of where they practice.

Thank you to Norman Keltner and Lee Schwecke for the honor of working with them. Thank you Norman and Lee for truly caring about those who suffer with mental illnesses and brain disorders.

C.E.B.

Contents

UNIT ONE

Introduction to Psychiatric Nursing, 1

1 **Introduction to Psychiatric Nursing, 3**

2 **Psychotherapeutic Management in the Continuum of Care, 19**

3 **Theoretical Models for Working with Psychiatric Patients, 26**

4 **Legal Issues, 44**

5 **Psychobiological Bases of Behavior, 64**

UNIT TWO

Continuum of Care, 85

6 **Continuum of Care, 86**

7 **Hospital-Based Care, 91**

8 **Community-Based Care, 96**

9 **Case Management, 101**

UNIT THREE

The Therapeutic Nurse-Patient Relationship, 113

10 **Communication, 114**

11 **The Nurse-Patient Relationship, 123**

12 **The Nursing Process, 136**

13 **Anxiety, Coping, and Crisis 147**

14 **Working with the Aggressive Patient, 157**

15 **Working with Groups of Patients, 171**

16 **Working with the Family, 181**

17 **Cultural Competence in Psychiatric Nursing: An Interlocking Paradigm Approach, 199**

UNIT FOUR

Psychopharmacology, 219

18 **Introduction to Psychotropic Drugs, 220**

19 **Antiparkinson Drugs, 229**

20 **Antipsychotic Drugs, 244**

21 **Antidepressant and Antimanic Drugs, 270**

22 **Antianxiety Drugs, 298**

UNIT FIVE

Milieu Management, 309

23 **Introduction to Milieu Management, 310**

24 **Developing the Therapeutic Environment, 320**

25 **Roles of the Psychiatric Nurse in the Therapeutic Milieu, 336**

UNIT SIX
Psychopathology, 343

26 Introduction to Psychopathology, 344
27 Schizophrenia and Other Psychoses, 350
28 Mood Disorders, 382
29 Anxiety-Related Disorders, 422
30 Cognitive Disorders, 451
31 Personality Disorders, 477
32 Sexual Disorders, 493
33 Substance-Related Disorders, 501
34 Dual Diagnosis, 543
35 Eating Disorders, 550

UNIT SEVEN
Special Therapies in Psychiatric Nursing, 569

36 Behavior Therapy, 570
37 Electroconvulsive and Other Somatic Therapies, 579

UNIT EIGHT
Special Populations in Psychiatric Nursing, 589

38 Victims of Violent Behavior, 590
39 Child and Adolescent Psychiatric Nursing, 616
40 Mental Illness in the Elderly, 638
41 Working with Patients with HIV Infection, 666

Appendixes

Appendix A: Diagnostic Criteria for Mental Disorders, 680
Appendix B: American Nurses Association Standards of Psychiatric-Mental Health Clinical Practice, 689
Appendix C: American Nurses Association Psychopharmacology Guidelines for Psychiatric Mental Health Nurses, 691
Appendix D: The Mini-Mental State Examination, 694
Appendix E: The Geriatric Depression Scale, 696
Appendix F: A Simple Method to Determine Tardive Dyskinesia Symptoms: AIMS Examination Procedure, 697
Appendix G: A Rating Scale for Extrapyramidal Side Effects, 699
Appendix H: Mental Health Systems Act Recommended Bill of Rights, 701
Appendix I: Controlled Substance Chart, 702

Glossary, 703
Answer Key to Study Questions, 715
Index, 721
Student Worksheets
Answer Key to Student Worksheets
Drug Cards

Detailed Contents

UNIT ONE

Introduction to Psychiatric Nursing, 1

1 **Introduction to Psychiatric Nursing, 3**
Benchmarks in Psychiatric History, 4
  Period of Enlightenment, 4
  Period of Scientific Study, 7
  Period of Psychotropic Drugs, 7
  Period of Community Mental Health, 8
Deinstitutionalization, 9
  Shifting the Cost of Mental Illness, 9
  Depopulation of State Hospitals, 9
  Community Effects, 11
Homelessness, 11
Evolution of Psychiatric Concerns, 13
Nursing Education, 13
Nursing Research, 14
Standards of Practice, 14
Certification of Competency, 14
Community-Based Care, 14
  Developing a Continuum of Care, 15

2 **Psychotherapeutic Management in the Continuum of Care, 19**
Psychotherapeutic Management, 19
Continuum of Care, 21
The Therapeutic Nurse-Patient Relationship, 22
Psychopharmacology, 23
Milieu Management, 23
Psychopathology, 24
Special Therapies, 24
Special Populations, 24

3 **Theoretical Models for Working with Psychiatric Patients, 26**
Psychoanalytical Model, 26
  Key Concepts, 26
  Therapist's Role, 30
  Relevance to Nursing Practice, 30
Developmental Model, 30
  Key Concepts, 30
  Relevance to Nursing Practice, 33
Interpersonal Model, 33
  Key Concepts, 33
  Therapist's Role, 36
  Relevance to Nursing Practice, 36

Cognitive-Behavioral Models, 36
  Key Concepts, 37
  Therapist's Role, 37
  Relevance to Nursing Practice, 37
Reality Therapy Model, 38
  Key Concepts, 38
  Therapist's Role, 38
  Relevance to Nursing Practice, 38
Stress Models, 39
  Key Concepts, 39
  Relevance to Nursing Practice, 41
Eclectic Approach, 41

4 **Legal Issues, 44**
Precedent-Setting Legal Milestones in Psychiatric Care, 46
  Historical Perspective, 46
Commitment Issues, 48
  Voluntary Commitment, 48
  Involuntary Commitment, 48
  Commitment of Incapacitated Persons, 51
Patient Rights, 52
  Suspension of Patient Rights, 52
  Right to Treatment with the Least Restrictive Alternative, 52
  Right to Confidentiality of Records, 53
  Right to Freedom from Restraints and Seclusion, 54
  Right to Give or Refuse Consent to Treatment, 55
  Living Wills and Health Care Directives, 56
Nursing Liability and Related Issues, 57
  Malpractice, 57
  Duty to Warn of Threatened Suicide or Harm to Others, 57
  Civil Remedies for Wrongful Involuntary Commitment, 60
  Documentation, 61

5 **Psychobiological Bases of Behavior, 64**
The Brain, 64
Neuroanatomy and Neurophysiology of the Brain, 65
  The Cerebrum, 65
  The Diencephalon, 72
  Brainstem and Cerebellum, 73
  Neurons and Neurotransmitters, 75
  Autonomic Nervous System, 77
  The Ventricular System, 77

Clinical Application, 79
  Schizophrenia, 79
  Mood Disorders, 79
  Anxiety Disorders, 81
  Dementias, 81
  AIDS/HIV Disease, 81
  Degenerative Diseases, 81
  Demyelinating Diseases, 81
  Anorexia Nervosa, 81
  Trauma, 82
  Chemical Dependency, 82
  Mitochondrial DNA Problems, 82

UNIT TWO

Continuum of Care, 85

6 **Continuum of Care, 86**
   Managed Care, 87
   Impact of Managed Care on the Continuum of Care, 89
   Decision Tree for Continuum of Care, 89
   Accessing the Continuum of Care, 89

7 **Hospital-Based Care, 91**
   Purposes of Psychiatric Hospital-Based Care, 91
   Types of Hospital-Based Care, 92
     Discharge Planning, 93
   Psychotherapeutic Management, 93

8 **Community-Based Care, 96**
   Outpatient Services, 96
     Subacute Care, 96
     Partial Programs, 97
     Outpatient Programs, 97
   Psychiatric Home Care, 97
   Community Outreach Programs, 98
   Residential Services, 98
     Self-help Groups, 98
   Influences on the Continuum of Care, 99
   Psychotherapeutic Management, 99

9 **Case Management, 101**
   Goals and Purposes of Case Management and Psychiatric
       Rehabilitation, 101
   History of Case Management, 102
   Nursing Process, 103
     Assessment, 104
     Outcome Identification/Planning, 104
     Implementation, 104
     Evaluation, 105
   Case Management, 105
     Clinical Pathways, 105
     Nurse Roles and Qualities, 105
     Preparation, 105
     Location, 107
   Components of Case Management, 107
     Psychiatric Rehabilitation, 107
     Resource Linkage, 108
     Consultation, 108
     Advocacy, 108
     Crisis Intervention, 109
     Home Care, 110
     Therapy, 110

UNIT THREE

The Therapeutic Nurse-Patient Relationship, 113

10 **Communication, 114**
    Categories of Communication, 114
      Written Communication, 115
      Speech and Behavior, 115
      Dynamics of Therapeutic Communication, 115
    Therapeutic Communication, 117
      Therapeutic vs. Social Communication, 117
      Therapeutic Use of Self, 117
    Therapeutic Communication Techniques, 118
    Common Interferences with Therapeutic
        Communication, 118
      Nurse's Fears and Feelings, 118
      Nurse's Lack of Knowledge and Insecurity, 121
      Inappropriate Responses, 121

11 **The Nurse-Patient Relationship, 123**
    Therapeutic Relationships, 123
      Brief Therapeutic Relationships, 124
      Social vs. Therapeutic Relationships, 124
      Collaboration, 124
    Being Therapeutic vs. Providing Therapy, 125
    Development of a Therapeutic Relationship, 125
      Stages of the Nurse-Patient Relationship, 125
    Interactions with Selected Behaviors, 131
      Violent Behavior, 132
      Hallucinations, 132
      Delusions, 132
      Conflicting Values, 132
      Incoherent Speech Patterns, 132
      Manipulation, 133
      Crying, 133
      Sexual Innuendos or Inappropriate Touch, 133
      Lack of Cooperation/Denial, 133
      Depressed Affect/Apathy/Psychomotor Retardation, 133
      Suspiciousness, 134
      Hyperactivity, 134
      Transference, 134

12 **The Nursing Process, 136**
    Nursing Process, 136
      Assessment, 136
      Nursing Diagnosis, 137
      Outcome Identification, 137
      Planning/Intervention, 138
      Evaluation, 141
    Written Patient Assessments, 144
      Intake Interview, 144
      Nursing Care Plans, 144
      Progress Notes, 144
      Discharge Summaries, 144
      Process Recordings, 144

13 **Anxiety, Coping, and Crisis 147**
    Commonly Perceived Stressors, 147
    Recurring Themes of Anxiety, 149
    General Etiology of Anxiety, 149
      Psychodynamic Theory, 149
      Interpersonal Theory, 149
      Biological Theory, 149

Levels of Anxiety, 150
Coping with Anxiety, 150
Relationship Between Anxiety and Illness, 153
Crisis, 153
  Individual Reactions, 153
  Strategies of Crisis Intervention, 153

14 **Working with the Aggressive Patient, 157**
Related Concepts, 158
  Aggression, 158
  Verbal Aggression, 158
  Passive Aggression and Passivity, 159
  Assertiveness, 160
Developmental View of Aggression, 160
Etiology of Aggression, 160
  Individual, Social-Psychological, and Sociocultural
    Models, 160
  Stress Models, 161
  Assault Cycle, 161
Assessing Key Variables of Aggression, 161
  The Nurse (Self-Assessment), 161
  The Environment (Milieu), 162
  The Patient, 162
Nursing Interventions in Anger and Nonviolent
  Aggression, 163
Nursing Interventions Based on the Assault Cycle,
  164
  Triggering Phase, 165
  Escalation Phase, 165
  Crisis Phase, 166
  Recovery and Depression Phase, 168
Staff Members as Victims of Assault, 168

15 **Working with Groups of Patients, 171**
Benefits of Groups, 172
  Therapeutic Factors, 172
Types of Groups, 172
  Support Groups, 173
  Activity Groups, 173
  Education or Problem Solving Groups, 173
  Therapy Groups, 174
  Self-Help or Special Problem Groups, 175
Group Leadership, 175
  Coleadership, 176
  The Physical Setting, 176
  Formal Groups, 176
  Interventions, 177

16 **Working with the Family, 181**
Historical Evolution of Working with the Family, 181
Familial Characteristics to be Assessed, 182
  Definition of Family, 182
  Family Tasks, 182
  Stages of Family Development, 182
  Functional/Healthy Family Characteristics, 183
  Problematic Family Characteristics, 183
Other Aspects to Be Assessed, 183
  Effects of Mental Illness on the Family, 183
  Reasons for Seeking Family Treatment, 187
  Family Reactions to Psychiatric Hospitalization, 188
Theoretical Basis for Family Assessment and
  Interactions, 188

Brief Family Nursing Interactions vs. Family
  Therapy, 188
Using Theories for Family Assessment and
  Interactions, 189
Skills for Working with the Family, 190
Application of the Nursing Process to the Family, 192

17 **Cultural Competence in Psychiatric Nursing: An
Interlocking Paradigm Approach, 199**
Culture and Psychiatric Nursing, 199
  The Importance of Culture, 201
Interlocking Paradigm of Cultural Competence, 201
  Nurse-Patient Interaction, 202
  The Theory Factor, 202
  The Philosophy Factor, 204
  The Cultural Competence Process Factor, 208
  The Assessment Factor, 213
Summary, 215

UNIT FOUR

Psychopharmacology, 219

18 **Introduction to Psychotropic Drugs, 220**
Nursing Responsibilities, 221
Neurotransmitters, 223
Blood-Brain Barrier, 225
Teaching Patients, 226

19 **Antiparkinson Drugs, 229**
Parkinson's Disease and Parkinsonism, 229
Neurotransmitters, 233
  Parkinson's Disease and Depression, 234
Dopaminergic Agents, 234
Anticholinergic Agents, 236
  Pharmacologic Effects (Desired Effects), 237
  Side Effects, 238
  Interactions with Other Anticholinergics, 240
  Nursing Implication for Anticholinergic Drugs, 240
  Selected Centrally Acting Anticholinergic Drugs, 241

20 **Antipsychotic Drugs, 244**
Historical Perspective, 244
Classification Systems, 245
Neurochemical Theory of Schizophrenia, 249
Pharmacological Effects (Desired Effects), 250
  CNS Effects, 250
  Psychiatric Symptoms Modified by Antipsychotic
    Drugs, 250
Pharmacokinetics, 251
Side Effects, 253
  PNS Effects, 253
  CNS EPSEs, 253
Nursing Implications, 257
  Therapeutic vs. Toxic Levels, 257
  Use in Pregnancy, 258
  Use in Elderly, 258
  Side Effects, 258
  Interactions, 258
  Teaching Patients, 260
Traditional Drugs by Chemical Class, 261
  Other Phenothiazines, 261
  Butyrophenone: Haloperidol, 262
  Thioxanthenes: Chlorprothixene and Thiothixene, 262

Dibenzoxazepine: Loxapine, 262
Dihydroindolone: Molindone, 262
Atypical Drugs by Chemical Class, 262
Dibenzodiazepine: Clozapine, 263
Benzisoxazole: Risperidone, 264
New Atypical Antipsychotics, 265
Olanzapine, 265
Quetiapine, 266
Sertindole, 266
Ziprasidone, 266

21 **Antidepressant and Antimanic Drugs, 270**
Antidepressants, 270
Historical Perspective, 270
Tricyclic Antidepressants, 273
Pharmacological Effects (Desired Effects), 274
Pharmacokinetics and Dosing, 275
Side Effects, 275
Suicide, 278
Interactions, 279
Nursing Implications, 279
Individual TCAs, 281
Novel Cyclic Antidepressants, 282
Selective Serotonin Reuptake Inhibitors, 284
Pharmacological Effect (Desired Effect), 284
Absorption, Distribution, Administration, 284
Side Effects, 284
Interactions, 284
Toxicity, 284
Use During Pregnancy, 285
Use in the Elderly, 285
Individual SSRIs, 285
Monoamine Oxidase Inhibitors (MAOIs), 286
Pharmacological Effects (Desired Effects), 286
Absorption, Distribution, Administration, 287
Side Effects, 287
Interactions, 287
Nursing Implications, 289
Irreversible MAOIs, 290
Reversible Inhibitor of MAO-A, 290
Antimanic Drugs, 290
Lithium, 290
Pharmacological Effects (Desired Effects), 291
Absorption, Distribution, Administration, 291
Side Effects, 291
Interactions, 292
Nursing Implications, 292
Alternatives to Lithium: Carbamazepine and Valproic
Acid, 294
Carbamazepine, 294
Valproic Acid, 294

22 **Antianxiety Drugs, 298**
Benzodiazepines, 300
Pharmacological Effect (Desired Effect), 300
Pharmacokinetics, 300
Side Effects, 301
Interactions, 302
Nursing Implications, 302
Specific Benzodiazepines, 304
Diazepam, 304
Alprazolam, 304

Chlordiazepoxide, 304
Clonazepam, 304
Clorazepate, 304
Lorazepam, 304
Oxazepam, 305
Other Antianxiety Agents, 305
Buspirone, 305
Propranolol, 305
Clomipramine, 305
Other Tricyclic Antidepressants, 305
Selective Serotonin Reuptake Inhibitors (SSRIs), 306

UNIT FIVE

Milieu Management, 309

23 **Introduction to Milieu Management, 310**
Historical Overview, 311
Therapeutic Milieu, 313
The Goal of Milieu Management, 314
Elements of the Effective Milieu, 315
Safety, 315
Structure, 315
Norms, 316
Limit Setting, 316
Balance, 316
Environmental Modification, 317
Roles of the Psychotherapeutic Manager, 317

24 **Developing the Therapeutic Environment, 320**
Safety, 322
Structure, 322
Community Meetings, 322
Constitution, 323
Step System, 323
Token Systems, 323
Activity Groups, 323
Social Skills Groups, 323
Living Skills Groups, 324
Street Skills Group, 324
Physical Exercise Groups, 324
Psychoeducational Programs, 325
Transition Groups, 325
Work Groups, 325
Nursing Students and Group Work, 326
Norms, 326
Nonviolence, 326
Physical and Emotional Security, 327
Personal Control, 327
Openness, 327
Feedback, 327
Respect for the Individual, 327
Privacy, 327
Acceptance, 327
Independence, 327
Individual Responsibility, 328
Limit Setting, 328
Self-Destructive Acts, 328
Physical Aggressiveness Toward Others, 328
Noncompliance, 329
Alcohol and Illicit Drugs, 329
Over-the-Counter Drugs, 329

Inappropriate Sexual Behaviors, 329
Smoking, 329
Elopement, 330
Rules for the Treatment Setting, 330
Balance, 330
    The Suicidal Patient, 331
    Religious Patients, 331
    The Assaultive Patient, 331
    The Dangerous Patient, 331
Environmental Modification, 331
    Physical Environment, 332
    Orientation Strategies, 332
    Schedule Modification, 332
Community-Based Milieu, 332

25 Roles of the Psychiatric Nurse in the Therapeutic Milieu, 336
Colleague Role, 337
    Psychiatrist, 337
    Psychologist, 337
    Psychiatric Social Worker, 337
    Pharmacist, 338
    Occupational Therapist, 338
    Recreational Therapist, 338
Team Leader Role, 338
Supervisor and Trainer Role, 339
    Supervision, 339
    Training, 339
Consultant Role, 340

UNIT SIX

Psychopathology, 343

26 Introduction to Psychopathology, 344
Behavior, 345
Etiology, 346
Psychotherapeutic Management, 346
The Nurse's Need to Understand Psychopathology, 347

27 Schizophrenia and Other Psychoses, 350
Schizophrenia, 350
DSM-IV Terminology and Criteria, 353
Behavior, 357
    Objective Signs, 358
    Subjective Symptoms, 359
Etiology, 362
    Biological Theories, 362
    Psychodynamic Theories of Schizophrenia, 365
    Vulnerability-Stress Model of Schizophrenia, 366
Special Issues Related to Schizophrenia, 367
    Families of Schizophrenics, 367
    Depression and Suicide in Schizophrenia, 368
    Relapse, 368
    Stress, 369
    Substance Abuse Among People with Schizophrenia, 369
    Work, 369
    Psychosis-induced Polydipsia, 369
The Continuum of Care for People with Schizophrenia, 370
Psychotherapeutic Management, 370
Other Psychotic Disorders, 374
    Schizoaffective Disorder, 374
    Delusional Disorder, 375

Brief Psychotic Disorder, 375
Schizophreniform Disorder, 376

28 Mood Disorders, 382
Depressive Disorders, 384
    Criteria and Symptoms of Major Depressive Disorder, 385
    Dysthymic Disorder, 388
    Behavior, 388
    Etiology of Depression, 390
    Assessment of Depression, 393
    Psychotherapeutic Management, 397
Bipolar Disorders, 404
    Description, 404
    DSM-IV Terminology and Criteria, 404
    Behavior, 406
    Etiology, 409
    Psychotherapeutic Management, 410
Suicide and Mood Disorders, 413
    The Impact of Guns on Suicidal Behavior, 415
    Suicide and the Elderly, 415
    Assessment of Suicidal Patients, 415
    Intervention, 416

29 Anxiety-Related Disorders, 422
Anxiety Disorders, 422
Generalized Anxiety Disorder, 423
    Psychotherapeutic Management, 424
Panic Disorder, 426
    Etiology, 426
    Psychotherapeutic Management, 427
Obsessive-Compulsive Disorder, 428
    Etiology, 430
    Psychotherapeutic Management, 431
Phobic Disorders, 432
    Etiology, 432
    Psychotherapeutic Management, 432
Acute Stress Disorder and Posttraumatic Stress Disorder, 433
    Neurochemical Basis of Acute Stress Disorder and Posttraumatic Stress Disorder, 435
    Psychotherapeutic Management, 436
Adjustment Disorders, 439
Somatoform Disorders, 440
Somatization Disorder, 441
Pain Disorder, 441
Hypochondriasis, 442
Conversion Disorder, 442
Psychotherapeutic Management, 443
Dissociative Disorders, 445
Dissociative Amnesia, 445
Dissociative Fugue, 446
Depersonalization, 446
Disassociative Identity Disorder, 447
Psychotherapeutic Management, 447

30 Cognitive Disorders, 451
DSM-IV Terminology and Criteria, 453
Delirium, 454
    Objective and Subjective Behavior, 454
    Etiology, 455
    Treatment, 455

Dementia, 456
   Objective and Subjective Behavior, 456
   Reversible Dementia, 458
   Nonreversible Dementia, 458
Alzheimer's Disease, 458
   Description and Incidence, 458
   Progression of the Disease, 462
   Etiology, 463
   Psychiatric Symptoms of AD, 464
   Treatment, 465
   Family Considerations, 465
Parkinson's Disease, 466
   Description and Incidence, 466
   Progression of the Disease, 467
   Etiology, 467
Diffuse Lewy Body Disease, 467
Huntington's Disease, 468
Pick's Disease, 468
Creutzfeldt-Jakob Disease, 468
Vascular or Multiinfarct Dementia, 469
Alcoholic Dementia, 469
Transient Ischemic Attacks, 469
Psychotherapeutic Management, 470

31 **Personality Disorders, 477**
General Etiology, 478
   Traditional Views, 478
   Contemporary Views, 478
Personality Disorder Clusters, 479
Cluster A: Odd/Eccentric, 479
Paranoid Personality Disorder, 479
   Unique Etiology, 480
Schizoid Personality Disorder, 480
Schizotypal Personality Disorder, 481
Psychotherapeutic Management, 481
Cluster B: Dramatic/Erratic, 482
Antisocial Personality Disorder, 482
   Unique Etiology, 482
   Psychotherapeutic Management, 482
Borderline Personality Disorder, 483
   Unique Etiology, 484
   Psychotherapeutic Management, 485
Narcissistic Personality Disorder, 486
   Unique Etiology, 486
Histrionic Personality Disorder, 487
Cluster C: Anxious/Fearful, 487
Dependent Personality Disorder, 487
Psychotherapeutic Management, 488
Avoidant Personality Disorder, 488
Obsessive-Compulsive Personality Disorder, 489

32 **Sexual Disorders, 493**
DSM-IV Criteria and Terminology, 493
Sexual Dysfunctions, 494
   Sexual Desire Disorders, 494
   Sexual Arousal Disorders, 494
   Orgasm Disorders, 495
   Sexual Pain Disorders, 495
Paraphilia, 495
   Pedophilia, 496
   Incest, 496
   Exibitionism, 496

Fetishism, 496
Frotteurism, 496
Sexual Masochism, 496
Sexual Sadism, 497
Voyeurism, 497
Gender Identity Disorder, 497
Psychotherapeutic Management, 498

33 **Substance-Related Disorders, 501**
A Brief Introduction to Substance-Related Disorders, 502
   Assessment Strategies for Chemical Dependency, 504
   Interview Approaches, 505
DSM-IV Criteria, 507
Abused Substances, 510
Alcohol Abuse, 510
   Etiological Theories, 511
   Pharmacokinetics of Alcohol, 511
   Physiological Effects, 512
   Nursing Issues, 514
Barbiturates—CNS Depressants, 516
   Metabolism, 518
   Physiological Effects, 518
   Nursing Issues, 518
Inhalants, 519
Opioids (Narcotics), 519
   Metabolism, 519
   Physiological Effects, 520
   Nursing Issues, 520
   Specific Drugs, 520
Stimulants, 521
   Cocaine, 522
   Amphetamines, 523
   Nursing Issues, 523
Hallucinogens, 524
   Mescaline (STP, DMT, MDA), 526
   Psilocybin, Psilocin, 526
   Marijuana, 526
   LSD (Lysergic Acid Diethylamide), 528
   PCP (Phencyclidine), 528
   Nursing Issues, 528
The Treatment of Substance Related Disorders, 529
Family Issues, 529
Treating the Chemically Dependent Person, 530
Diagnostic Tools for Chemical Dependency, 530
   Alcohol, 530
   Drugs, 530
Psychotherapeutic Management, 532
Other Interventions, 535
   Alcoholics Anonymous, 535
   Another Self-Help Support Group, 537
Evaluation, Relapse, and Follow-Up Care, 538
   Evaluation, 538
   Relapse, 538
   Follow-Up Care, 538

34 **Dual Diagnosis, 543**
Dual Diagnosis Defined, 543
Etiology, 544
Treatment Issues, 544
   Problems Affecting Program Development, 544
Psychotherapeutic Management, 546
Continuum of Care, 548

35 Eating Disorders, 550
  Anorexia Nervosa, 550
    DSM-IV Criteria, 550
    Behavior, 551
    Etiology, 553
    Psychotherapeutic Management, 555
  Bulimia Nervosa, 559
    DSM-IV Criteria, 559
    Behavior, 560
    Etiology, 561
    Bulimia and Depression, 562
    Psychotherapeutic Management, 563
  Eating Disorders in Males, 564
  Obesity, 566
  Binge-Eating Disorder, 566

UNIT SEVEN

Special Therapies in Psychiatric Nursing, 569

36 Behavior Therapy, 570
  Classical Conditioning, 570
  Operant Conditioning, 571
  Application of Behavior Therapy in Psychiatric Nursing
    Practice, 571
    Behavior Modification: Helping Patients Change
      Behavior, 572
    Respondent Conditioning: Helping Patients Cope with
      Disturbing Stimuli, 574
  Behavioral Intervention with the Nursing Process, 575
    Guidelines for Behavioral Nursing Intervention, 575

37 Electroconvulsive and Other Somatic Therapies, 579
  Electroconvulsive Therapy (ECT), 580
    Modern ECT, 580
    How ECT Works, 581
    Number of Treatments, 582
    Indications for ECT, 582
    Contraindications for ECT, 583
    Advantages of ECT, 583
    Disadvantages of ECT, 584
  Other Somatic Therapies, 584
    Insulin-Coma and Metrazol-Induced Convulsion
      Therapies, 585
    Psychosurgery, 585

UNIT EIGHT

Special Populations in Psychiatric Nursing, 589

38 Victims of Violent Behavior, 590
  Violation by Crime, 591
    Effects of Crime, 591
    Recovery from Trauma, 591
    Psychotherapeutic Management, 592
  Torture and Ritual Abuse, 592
    Nature of the Problem, 592
    Effects of Torture and Ritual Abuse, 593
    Recovery from Torture and Ritual Abuse, 594
    Psychotherapeutic Management, 594
  Rape and Sexual Assault, 594

    Nature of the Problem, 594
    Effects of Rape and Sexual Assault, 594
    Recovery from Rape and Sexual Assault, 595
    Rape Trauma Symptoms, 596
    Psychotherapeutic Management, 596
  Adult Survivors of Childhood Sexual Abuse, 597
    Nature of the Problem, 597
    Effects of Childhood Sexual Abuse on the Child, 598
    Effects of Childhood Sexual Abuse on the
      Adolescent, 598
    Effects of Childhood Sexual Abuse on the Adult, 598
    Recovery from Childhood Sexual Abuse, 601
    Psychotherapeutic Management, 601
  Victims of Partner Abuse, 604
    Nature of the Problem, 604
    Effects of Partner Abuse, 604
    Recovery from Partner Abuse, 608
    Psychotherapeutic Management, 609

39 Child and Adolescent Psychiatric Nursing, 616
  Scope of the Problem, 617
    Epidemiology of Child Psychiatric Disorders, 617
    Genetic Factors, 617
    Environmental Factors, 619
  Diagnostic Categories of Child Psychiatric Disorders, 619
  Developmental Disorders, 620
    Mental Retardation, 620
    Pervasive Developmental Disorders, 620
    Specific Developmental Disorders, 621
  Disruptive Behavior Disorders, 622
    Attention-Deficit Hyperactivity Disorder, 622
    Oppositional Defiant Disorder, 623
    Conduct Disorder, 623
  Internalizing Disorders, 624
    Anxiety Disorders, 624
    Mood Disorders, 625
  Tic Disorders, 626
  Psychotic Disorders, 626
  Elimination Disorders, 626
  Enuresis, 626
  Encopresis, 627
  Treatment, 627
  Case Example #1, 627
  Treatment Settings, 627
  Psychopharmacology, 628
    Stimulants, 629
    Tricyclic Antidepressants, 629
    Selective Serotonin Reuptake Inhibitors (SSRIs), 630
    Traditional Antipsychotics, 630
    Atypical Antipsychotics, 631
    Alpha-2 Agonists, 632
  Cognitive Behavioral Therapy, 632
    Cognitive Behavioral Therapy in ADHD, 632
    Cognitive Behavioral Therapy in OCD, 633

40 Mental Illness in the Elderly, 638
  Continuum of Care, 640
    Social Support, 640
    Community Support, 640
    Local Alternatives to Formal Mental Health Care, 641
    OBRA-87 and Nursing Homes, 641
    Current and Future Trends, 642

Barriers to Mental Health Care for the Elderly, 642
    Ageism, 642
    Attitudes, 642
    Finances, 642
    Inadequate Detection of Mental Illness and
        Treatment, 643
Psychiatric Disorders in the Elderly, 643
Depression, 643
    Incidence, 643
    Presentation, 643
    Electroconvulsive Therapy, 644
    Suicide, 645
Bipolar Disorder, 646
Psychotic Disorders, 646
    Paranoid Thinking, 648
Anxiety Disorders, 648
Substance Abuse, 649
    Alcohol Abuse and Dependence, 649
    Drug Abuse, 651
    Factors Complicating Drug-Taking by the Elderly, 652
Assessment of the Elderly Mentally Ill, 652
Psychosocial Assessment, 652
Physical Assessment, 653
Psychotherapeutic Management, 654

41   **Working with Patients with HIV Infection, 666**
Overview of HIV Infection, 667
    Causes of HIV Infection, 667
    Opportunistic Illnesses, 668
    HIV Infection Transmission, 668
    Populations at Risk, 669
    AIDS Diagnosis, 670
    HIV Tests, 670
    Incidence and Distribution, 672
    Risk Behavior Prevention, 672

Neuropsychiatric Aspects of HIV Infection, 674
    Stress Related to Having AIDS, 674
    Neuropsychiatric Complications Related to HIV Brain
        Infection or Opportunistic Illness, 674
    Neuropsychiatric Complications Related
        to Treatment, 676
    Management, 677

Appendixes

    Appendix A: Diagnostic Criteria for Mental Disorders
        (DSM-IV), 680
    Appendix B: American Nurses Association Standards of
        Psychiatric Mental Health Clinical Practice, 689
    Appendix C: American Nurses Association
        Psychopharmacology Guidelines for Psychiatric Mental
        Health Nurses, 691
    Appendix D: The Mini-Mental State Examination, 694
    Appendix E: The Geriatric Depression Scale, 696
    Appendix F: A Simple Method to Determine Tardive
        Dyskinesia Symptoms: AIMS Examination Procedure,
        697
    Appendix G: A Rating Scale for Extrapyramidal Side Effects,
        699
    Appendix H: Mental Health Systems Act Recommended Bill
        of Rights, 701
    Appendix I: Controlled Substance Chart, 702

Glossary, 703

Answer Key to Study Questions, 715

Index, 721

Student Worksheets

Answer Key to Student Worksheets

Drug Cards

Introduction to Psychiatric Nursing

CHAPTER 1

Introduction to Psychiatric Nursing

NORMAN L. KELTNER

LEARNING OBJECTIVES

After reading this chapter you should be able to:
- Describe the enormity of mental health concerns in both human and financial contexts.
- Explain the history of psychiatry as a foundation for current psychiatric nursing practice.
- Identify the significant changes that occurred during the period of the Enlightenment.
- Relate the contributions of early scientists to the current understanding of mental illness.
- Explain the impact of psychotropic drugs on psychiatric care.
- Analyze the immediate and long-term effects of the community mental health movement.
- Describe the trends in psychiatric nursing over the past 50 years that have led to today's psychiatric nursing environment.
- Identify the specific strengths that enable psychiatric nurses to become effective in the new continuum of care.

"Some people's illnesses are so severe that they will always need **asylum.** A continuum of care is needed: from total freedom to total hospitalization, reflecting the diverse needs of mentally ill people." (Mona Wasow, MSW and mother of a mentally ill adult [1993])

Recent epidemiological evidence indicates that 5.7% of American adults over the age of 18 have a serious mental disorder in any 12-month period (News and Notes, 1996). When the full spectrum of mental and emotional disorders is incorporated, studies reveal that approximately 25% of

Americans are affected by mental and addictive disorders each year (Narrow, et al, 1993; News, 1997; Regier, et al, 1993). Table 1-1 provides a breakdown by diagnosis of the disorders prevalent at any time in our society. The pervasiveness of these maladies implies a great need for psychiatric professionals, including nurses, today and in the foreseeable future.

The magnitude of psychiatric and mental health complaints generates a good news–bad news scenario. First, the bad news. The extent and range of

KEY TERMS

Asylum 1. A place of safety or sanctuary; a refuge 2. An institution for the care of the mentally ill; often associated with mistreatment and callousness

Community mental health The application of the principles of psychiatric care to communities and groups of people. The goals of this effort are to maintain mental health, to prevent mental illness when possible, and if treatment is indicated, to treat individuals in close proximity to their support systems.

Continuum of care Levels of care through which an individual can move depending upon his/her needs at a given point in time.

Deinstitutionalization A shift in the location of treatment from large public hospitals to community settings

Homelessness Individuals or whole families who may live exclusively on the streets or who may make use of community shelters, halfway houses, cheap hotels, or board-and-care homes

Psychotropic drugs Medications used in the treatment of mental disorders

Table 1-1   12-Month Prevalence Rate of Mental Disorders in the United States

Diagnosis	Percentage of Population over 17 Years of Age	Number of Persons
Anxiety disorders	12.6	20,034,000
Phobia disorders*	10.9	17,331,000
Mood disorders	9.5	15,143,000
Alcohol disorders	7.4	11,766,000
Major depression†	5.0	7,950,000
Drug disorders	3.1	4,929,000
Cognitive impairment	2.7	4,293,000
Obsessive-compulsive disorder	2.1	3,339,000
Antisocial disorder	1.5	2,385,000
Panic disorders*	1.3	2,067,000
Bipolar disorder†	1.2	1,908,000
Schizophrenia	1.1	1,749,000
Somatization	0.2	365,000

From Regier DA, et al: The de facto U.S. mental and addictive disorders service system: epidemiologic catchment area prospective 1-year prevalence rates of disorders and services, *Arch Gen Psychiatry* 50:85, 1993.
*Also calculated in anxiety statistics.
†Also calculated in mood disorders statistics.

conditions generate a tremendous cost to our economy. Table 1-2 captures the costs of brain disorders in the United States, including both direct costs (e.g., medications) and indirect costs (e.g., lost wages, etc.). These costs are equivalent to 15% of the average American worker's paycheck. The good news is that we are getting better at treating the more serious disorders. Table 1-3 provides a summary of National Institute of Mental Health findings regarding treatment success.

Table 1-2   Cost of Brain Disorders in the United States

Psychiatric disorders	$136,000,000,000
Alcohol abuse	$ 90,000,000,000
Drug abuse	$ 71,000,000,000
Dementia	$113,000,000,000
Mental retardation	$ 35,000,000,000
Total	**$445,000,000,000**

National Foundation for Brain Disorders: *The cost of disorders of the brain,* Washington, DC, 1992, The Foundation.

Table 1-3   Success of Treatment for Selected Mental Disorders

Disorder	Treatment Success Rate*
Panic disorder	80%
Bipolar disorder	80%
Major depression	60%
Schizophrenia	60%
Obsessive compulsive disorder	60%

From: A Journal of Psychosocial Nursing summarization of National Institutes of Mental Health data, *J Psychosoc Nurs Ment Health Serv* 35(6):5, 1997.
*Treatment success is defined as improvement in symptomatology and includes patients who experience full remission of symptoms and those who experience a partial response.

BENCHMARKS IN PSYCHIATRIC HISTORY

"And a certain woman . . . had suffered many things of many physicians, and had spent all that she had, and was nothing bettered, but rather grew worse." (Mark 5: 25, 26 King James Version [1611])

The modern era of psychiatric care can be traced from events that occurred in England and France near the end of the eighteenth century, a time referred to as *the Enlightenment.* Before this time the mentally ill were often regarded as no better than wild animals.

Rosenblatt (1984) writes of the ABCs of community response during this time: assistance, banishment, and confinement. **Assistance,** the least restrictive approach, provided food and money and often enabled the family to maintain its integrity as a unit. **Banishment** occurred in some communities, particularly when the deranged were strangers. Banishment led to wandering bands of "lunatics . . . living no one cared how, and dying no one cared where" (Rosenblatt, 1984). The infamous "Ship of Fools"—boatloads of the mentally disordered cast out to sea to find their "right minds"—occurred during this period. In America during colonial times, wandering bands without shelter or food drifted from village to village, occasionally finding acceptance, but more often encountering rejection and hostility.

Confinement was the most restrictive method of coping with the mentally ill, who were often chained. The old and the young, men and women, the insane, criminals, and paupers were indiscriminately mixed. The mentally ill were thought to be immune to normal biological stressors such as cold, heat, and hunger, and they suffered accordingly (Foucault, 1967). Patients were placed on display for the amusement of their caretakers and the paying public. For example, until 1770, a small fee was charged of visitors of St. Mary of Bethlem Hospital (Bedlam) in England. At Bedlam treatments such as bleeding; bathing; vomiting and purging; and forced feedings were common "therapeutic" interventions (McMillon, 1997). At Bicétrè in France, the attendants served as "ringmasters," using whips to "encourage" their patients to perform (Rosenblatt, 1984). These warehouses for the tormented discouraged outside intrusion and attracted employees who were at the bottom levels of society both socially and morally.

As the late 1700s approached, a day of enlightenment dawned: the establishment of the asylum. Four different periods stand out as benchmarks in the evolution of modern psychiatric care: the late eighteenth century, the late nineteenth century, the 1950s, and the 1960s (Table 1-4). During each of these four periods, the way of thinking about the mentally ill underwent significant changes, due predominantly to certain individuals or specific events. Following each period, events occurred consequentially that were important in their own right, but the inspirational sources of these events can be traced to the aforementioned benchmarks.

Period of Enlightenment

"To consider madness incurable . . . is constantly refuted by the most authentic facts" (Philippe Pinel, December 11, 1794 [cited in Weiner, 1992])

The modern era of psychiatric care began with two men, Philippe Pinel in France and William Tuke in England. In 1793 Pinel became the superintendent of the French institution, Bicétrè (for men), and later the Salpêtrière (for women). He was dismayed by the conditions he found and wrote of the patients, "They were abandoned to the incompetence of a callous director and to the cold brutality of servants who opposed a premeditated force of their own to impetuous acts of a blind and seemingly automatic violence" (Weiner, 1992). Soon after assuming

TABLE 1-4 Benchmark Periods in Psychiatric History

Period	Key People or Developments	Significant Change in thinking	Result(s)
Enlightenment ~1790s>	Pinel (1745-1826)—unchained the mentally ill (1793) Tuke (1732-1822)—established the York Retreat	The insane were no longer treated as less than human. Human dignity was upheld.	The asylum movement developed.
Scientific study ~1870s>	Freud (1856-1939)—emphasized the importance of early life experiences in shaping mental health Kraepelin (1856-1926)—developed classification of mental illness Bleuler (1857-1939)—was optimistic about treatment	Humans could be studied, and that study held promise for treating and curing mental health problems.	The study of the mind and treatment approaches to psychiatric conditions flourished. The "Decade of the Brain" can be traced back to Kraepelin's thinking.
Psychotropic drugs ~1950s>	1949—lithium 1950—chlorpromazine 1952—Monoamine oxidase inhibitors (MAOIs) 1957—haloperidol 1958—Tricyclic antidepressants (TCAs) 1960—benzodiazepines	Some mental disorders are caused by chemical imbalances. If the chemical problem could be found through research, then a chemical cure could be found as well. Also, people would no longer need to be confined.	A destigmatizing of mental illness occurred. Parents and others were not to blame. The term *least restrictive environment* evolved from this discovery.
Community mental health ~1960s>	Community Mental Health Centers Act (1963)	Individuals do not need to be hospitalized away from family and community. People have the right to be treated in their own community.	Advantage: Intervention in familiar surroundings has helped many people and is less expensive. Disadvantage: Homelessness is linked to deinstitutionalization, and many people "slip through the cracks" of the system.

leadership and motivated by scientific considerations, Pinel unchained the shackled, clothed the naked, fed the hungry, and abolished the whips and other instruments of cruel treatment. Simultaneously in England, William Tuke was planning a private facility that would ensure moral treatment for the mentally ill after he had witnessed the deplorable conditions in public facilities. In 1796, based upon Quaker teachings, the York Retreat opened for patients providing "a place in which the unhappy might obtain refuge—a quiet haven in which the shattered bark might find a means of reparation or safety" (Gollaher, 1995). Pinel and Tuke were responsible for this first benchmark of modern psychiatric care.

Asylum

The concept of the asylum developed from the humane efforts of Pinel and Tuke. The term *asylum* can mean protection, social support, or sanctuary from the stresses of life. A touring Chinese gymnast pleading for asylum is a good example of this definition. Today, however, the term asylum most often provokes an image of mistreatment and neglect. It was the first definition that motivated Pinel, Tuke, and other like-minded individuals. Understanding that the mentally ill decompensated under stress, these individuals sought to provide an environment relatively free from stressors. Their language is inappropriate today–"madness," "lunacy," "insanity," "idiocy," "feeblemindedness"–but these were the accepted terms of their day. These early reformers were driven by a desire to improve the lot of abandoned, mentally ill persons and to provide asylum or sanctuary. An editorial in an 1803 issue of the *Alienest and Neurologist* made the following comment: "We owe the harmless lunatic a duty to save him from perpetual lunacy if we can. To leave him wholly to himself, even though he hurts no one, is not always kind. Such a course endangers incurable chronicity, and this is cruel to him" (Geller, 1992).

Dorothea Dix (1802-1887) was the first major reformer in the United States. She was instrumental in developing the concept of asylum and played a direct role in opening 32 state hospitals. Her efforts are invariably described as a crusade. Several years before launching her crusade she visited Tuke's York Retreat. Undoubtedly her impressions of Tuke's moral treatment influenced her concerns for the pain and suffering she had witnessed in her native land. Dix came to believe the greater citizenry, as represented by the government, had an obligation to their mentally ill brothers and sisters. She proposed to alleviate suffering with adequate shelter, nutritious food, and warm clothing. In Gollaher's (1995) exhaustive biography of Dix he quotes from one of her *Memorials*, the documents she wrote to expose the terrible plight of the insane. From her *Massachusetts Memorial* he notes:

"*Concord:* A woman from the [Worcester] hospital in a cage in the almshouse. In the jail several, decently cared for in general but not properly placed in a prison. Violent, noisy, unmanageable most of the time.

Lincoln: A woman in a cage.

Medford: One idiotic subject chained, and one in a close stall for 17 years . . .

Granville: One often closely confined: now losing the use of his limbs from want of exercise."

Though Dix is rightfully credited with being the first reformer with a nationwide perspective, other more regional sanctuaries had been established be-

fore her crusade. The first asylum in the United States was the Eastern Lunatic Asylum in Williamsburg, Virginia, founded in 1773. Others followed, such as the Frankford Asylum near Philadelphia (1813), the Bloomingdale Asylum in New York (1818), and the Hartford Retreat in Connecticut (1824). The Philadelphia and New York asylums were established under Quaker influence and thus can be traced to Tuke (Rosenblatt, 1984).

The period of Enlightenment was short-lived. Within 100 years of the establishment of the first asylum, the reformers were being assailed as misusers and abusers of their charges. State hospitals were beset with problems. The first definition of asylum (sanctuary) had materialized in the form of hospitals that were set apart from cities, usually in a rural setting, but those once sought-after characteristics would come to be viewed as liabilities. Patients were *isolated:* geographically, from family, and from follow-up care. While reformers were still focusing on asylum (i.e., sanctuary), the world was beginning to focus on treatment, and the term *asylum* had assumed a pejorative connotation (e.g., the "insane asylum").

Today there is a renewed interest in asylum as a place of rest and restoration (Munetz, Peterson, Vandershie, 1996). This concept can be considered in terms of the four P's: parents, professionals, patients, and the public. Each has a stake in the discussion of asylum. Mona Wasow, a professional social worker (MSW) and the parent of a mentally ill adult, writes persuasively for the need of asylum: "Some people's illnesses are so severe that they will always need asylum. A **continuum of care** is needed: from total freedom to total hospitalization, reflecting the diverse needs of mentally ill people" (Wasow, 1993).

The origin of psychiatric nursing

The official history of psychiatric nursing began approximately 100 years ago. Linda Richards, the first American psychiatric nurse, was a graduate of the New England Hospital for Women. She spent much of her professional career developing nursing care in psychiatric hospitals and also directed a school of psychiatric nursing in 1880 at the McLean Psychiatric Asylum in Waverly, Massachusetts. Because of her efforts more than 30 asylums had developed schools for nurses by 1890.

■ Critical Thinking Questions

1 Which of the two definitions of "asylum" do you believe is more prevalent in psychiatric nursing today?
2. What are some negative outcomes of deinstitutionalization that you have witnessed or have been personally involved with?

Period of Scientific Study

The shift in focus from sanctuary to treatment is linked to the second benchmark in psychiatric care, personified by Sigmund Freud (1856-1939). Toward the last third of the nineteenth century, a number of scientists devoted themselves to understanding the mind and mental illness. The fruits of their labor held great promise, some of which is still unfulfilled. Nonetheless, the efforts forever changed the world's view: Mental illness need not be suffered (however humanely patients were treated) but could be alleviated. In a sense, psychiatric care was popularized.

Early scientists

Although Freud had the greatest impact on the world's view of mental illness, he neither thought nor worked in a vacuum. Other men and women had tremendous impact on this new enthusiastic and optimistic approach to mental illness. Emil Kraepelin (1856-1926) made tremendous contributions to the classification of mental disorders. He was a true scientist whose descriptions of schizophrenia are classic and valuable reading. Eugene Bleuler (1857-1939) coined the term *schizophrenia* and added a note of optimism to its treatment. Still others, many of whom were colleagues or disciples of Freud, made significant contributions to the emerging field of psychiatry.

Freud's contributions still influence psychiatric care. Although for a number of years it was popular to belittle his accomplishments, doing so belied an understanding of the underpinnings of most current psychotherapies. To paraphrase a statement made by Sir Isaac Newton (1642-1727): If we see far today, it is because we stand on the shoulders of giants.

Freud described human behavior in psychological terms. He developed a theory of motivation, established the usefulness of talking (catharsis), explained the importance of dreams, and proposed to unlock the hidden parts of the mind. He introduced terms that are now daily fare, such as *psychoanalysis, id, ego, superego,* and *free association.* Freud was able to do this because he felt free to study human beings as he might study any animal. Darwin's work gave him permission to view humans in this context. From Freud's study evolved the work of others, many of whom studied with Freud. Alfred Adler, Carl Jung, Ernest Jones, Otto Rank, Helene Deutsch, Karen Horney, and Anna Freud (Freud's daughter) all made significant and, in most cases, lasting contributions to the field of dynamic psychiatry.

Freud's inspiration, however, reached far beyond those with whom he worked personally. Society in general is indebted to him, even if there has been disagreement with his ideas. Freud challenged society to look at human beings objectively. He fostered a milieu of thinking about the mind and mental disorders. Many theories were ripples of the arguments he put forth, including psychodynamic and behavioral theories (Watson, Wolpe, Skinner), somatic (electroconvulsive therapy, 1937; psychosurgery, 1935), and biological theories. (The selected theories of Freud, as well as other theorists' models of behavior, are presented in more detail in Chapter 3.) Unit Three builds on these concepts and is devoted to the implementation of strategies for working with psychiatric patients.

Period of Psychotropic Drugs

From this milieu of theory and scientific thought came the third benchmark, which began around 1950 with the discovery of psychotropic drugs (Ayds, 1991). Chlorpromazine (Thorazine), an antipsychotic drug, and lithium, an antimanic agent, were introduced first and imipramine (Tofranil), an antidepressant, was introduced a few years later. The impact of these drugs has been powerful. Patients who seemed beyond reach became less agitated and experienced a reduction in psychotic thinking. Depressed patients regained normal feelings. Hospital stays were shortened and hospital environments improved because there was less noise and less agitation. Many employees of state hospitals describe the confusion and hostility as deafening and "crazy" before the advent of psychotropic drugs. One such employee stated that he had to fight his way on the unit in the morning and fight his way off at night. It was widely believed that psychotropic drugs were truly miracle drugs. However, though psychotropic drugs allow many patients to be treated in less restrictive environments, many ethical, moral, and legal questions have arisen with this treatment modality (Trudeau, 1993). Unit Four is devoted to an understanding of the role of psychotropic drugs in the treatment of mental disorders.

Period of Community Mental Health

It is inaccurate to conceptualize one benchmark period ending entirely before the next one began. Trends overlap as advocates of one view struggle while more dynamic forces emerge elsewhere. As the various treatment approaches were being developed in the milieu derived from Freud's theories, criticism grew and the state hospital system continued its plunge into "psychiatric Siberia." The popular movie *The Snake Pit* portrayed a mindless, ineffective, and at times cruel system of care. In an even more devastating exposé, the book *The Shame of the States,* by Albert Deutsch (1948), vividly revealed with words and photographs the deplorable conditions in several large state hospitals around the country.

Legislators were watching, reading, and listening; legislation was passed that would change the approach to psychiatric care. In 1946 President Truman signed the National Mental Health Act, enabling the establishment of the National Institute of Mental Health (1949). In 1947 the Hill-Burton Act legislated funds to build general hospitals to include psychiatric units. This began the effort to intervene early and shorten the length of hospitalization for psychiatric patients.

In 1961 the Joint Commission on Mental Illness and Health (1961), appointed by President Kennedy, published a report entitled "Action for Mental Health." The report urged increased support for the state hospital system in recognition of the need for improved treatment of the mentally ill population. Supporters of this document were drowned out by opponents of the state hospital system. In fact, the more outspoken critics of the existing system pronounced it the *cause* of mental illness.

Instead of increasing monetary support for the state hospital system, a convergence of forces set the stage for this fourth benchmark period in psychiatric

history: the public's declining confidence in the state hospital system, the failure of various treatment approaches to eradicate mental illness, the legislative climate that had begun in the 1940s, a new emphasis on the civil rights of the mentally ill, and the new-found faith in psychotropic drugs. These factors led to the enactment of the Community Mental Health Centers (CMHC) Act in 1963 virtually destroying the state hospital system. A deliberate shift was made from institutional to extrainstitutional care. The goal was *deinstitutionalization* of the state hospital system population. The aforementioned problem of geographical isolation was addressed with community treatment centers and community living arrangements (e.g., halfway houses). Isolation from family was addressed by keeping the mentally disordered closer to family. Isolation from follow-up care was remedied because various levels of care were available locally.

Eventually community mental health programs were built to meet the needs of all persons living within the boundaries of a geographic catchment area. These programs had the following goals:
- Emergency care
- 24-hour inpatient care
- Partial hospitalization care
- Outpatient care
- Consultation and education for the population served by the center
- Screening services

Effect on nursing

The community mental health movement broadened the scope of psychiatric nursing. No longer did the psychiatric nurse simply work in the hospital or inpatient setting. A whole range of opportunities became available to the psychiatric nurse, from working with the chronically mentally ill to working with the "worried well," and from concentrating on individual treatment issues to focusing on broader social issues affecting mental health as well.

This professional evolution of care had both positive and negative effects. On the positive side, it gave nurses a better understanding of all humanity and broadened their professional vision of what psychiatric nursing could offer to society. Mental health care was no longer a concern reserved for a few severely ill souls, but was a legitimate concern for all people. A negative effect was the resultant confusion about mental illness. The criteria for defining mental illness became less rigid and resulted in more and more "problems" being claimed as legitimate concerns of mental health professionals. George Will (1996) scorned this softening of standards when he cited the criteria for oppositional defiant disorder, e.g., often loses temper, often deliberately annoys people, or spiteful or vindictive. Will notes, "If you are just slightly offensive, your right will not kick in. But if you are seriously insufferable to colleagues at work, you have a right not to be fired, and you are entitled to have your employer make reasonable accommodations for your 'disability.'"

As the public and public leaders became confused about what was or was not a mental health problem, the scope of community mental health concerns grew even wider. Inevitably the status of inpatient psychiatric nursing suffered as newer, more-visible roles with less-disabled patients became available to nurses.

DEINSTITUTIONALIZATION

"The practice, over the past four decades, of releasing people with severe mental illnesses from institutions has been one of the largest social experiments in 20th century America." (E. Fuller Torrey, 1997)

Deinstitutionalization refers to the depopulating of state mental hospitals. State hospitals reached their peak census in 1955 and then slowly began the process of trimming their census rolls. It is important to understand that the impetus for deinstitutionalization began as early as 1955. The roots of this process began with the growing concerns about asylum and were nurtured by some of the events previously discussed. A more subtle factor was psychiatry's and psychiatric nursing's growing disillusionment with the chronically mentally ill and an embracing of the "worried well."

These factors clearly laid the groundwork for deinstitutionalization; however, it was federal actions that fully detonated the process. First, as discussed above, was the CMHC Act. The second federal action was legislation that provided mentally disabled persons with an income while they were living in the community. This legislation was named Aid to the Dis-

abled (ATD), now called Supplemental Security Income (SSI) and Social Security Disability Insurance (SSDI). The number of persons with mental disorders receiving these benefits grew dramatically. Between 1986 and 1991 the number of workers with a mental disorder receiving SSDI increased by 48%, while the number of persons with mental disorders receiving SSI increased by 81% (News and Notes, 1993). A total of approximately 1.2 million persons receive SSI or SSDI for a mental disorder, not including those who are disabled by primary mental retardation or addiction (Ries and Dyck, 1997). Particularly controversial was the awarding of benefits to individuals with addictive disorders who often used these government funds to purchase more abused substances. Public concern and journalistic exposés led to termination of these benefits by Public Law 104-121 as of January 1997 (Rosenheck, 1997).

Shifting the Cost of Mental Illness

State governments soon found ATD, even when supplemented by the state, to be less costly than public hospitalization because the federal government was paying for SSI, Medicare, Medicaid, etc. The federal share grew from 2% in 1963 to 62% by 1994 (Torrey, 1997). State financial incentives to effectively treat the serious mentally ill declined in tandem with greater federal involvement.

Perhaps the final event in the deinstitutionalization movement was the change in commitment laws. Out of concern for the civil rights of mental patients, involuntary commitment to the state hospital became difficult (Rosenheck, 1997). The state had to demonstrate that the "accused" were a clear danger to themselves or to others. These sweeping changes were reactions to years of injustice wherein persons said to be mentally ill could be detained and involuntarily committed, with little recourse, for long periods of time. (Rosenhan's classic study [1973] [Box 1-1] illustrates how difficult it was for a "sane" person to be discharged from a mental hospital.) The stage was set for rapid depopulation of state hospitals.

Depopulation of State Hospitals

"State hospitals have functioned in different yet questionable ways throughout their history. Their current role of

Box 1-1 On Being Sane in Insane Places

Rosenhan wondered whether the "sane" could be distinguished from the "insane." He selected eight pseudopatients (people who pretended to be mentally ill) and instructed them to attempt to gain admission to public mental hospitals. The task was much easier than anyone had anticipated. Twelve hospitals in five states were used. The pseudopatient group consisted of a graduate student in psychology, three psychologists (including Rosenhan himself), a pediatrician, a psychiatrist, a painter, and a housewife. Three were women and five were men. No one in the hospital knew of the deception.

The pseudopatients were trained to do the following:
1. Call the hospital and make an appointment.
2. Upon arriving at the hospital they were to tell the psychiatrist they had been hearing voices.
3. Upon being asked to describe the voices all were to say they were not sure but did remember the words "empty," "hollow," and "thud."
4. Other than giving this false information and false information about their names, occupations, and employers, they were from that point forward to be truthful and "normal."
5. Immediately upon admission the pseudopatients were instructed to cease simulating abnormal behavior and to behave "normally."
6. When asked how they were doing the pseudopatients were trained to respond "fine" and to inform the staff that they were no longer experiencing problems.

Despite behaving normally, none of the pseudopatients were discovered by the staff. However, about 25% of the other patients made comments about the pseudopatients' "sanity" and a few even guessed that the pseudopatients were doing some kind of undercover work. Rosenhan noted a reluctance by the staff to see mental health in their patients. He stated, "Having once been labeled schizophrenic, there is nothing the pseudopatients can do to overcome the tag." Pseudopatient histories were written to support their diagnosis. In other words, psychiatrists saw problems that had never existed.

The pseudopatients were also asked to write down their observations. At first, elaborate precautions were followed to avoid detection. However, they were soon jotting down observations in front of the staff. The pseudopatients had discovered that no one was paying any attention to them.

Another part of the experiment was to determine how much time was spent with patients. This was difficult to measure so a proxy behavior was substituted: time the nurses spent outside of the nurses' station. Nursing attendants had the highest percentage of time outside the station: 11.3%. Rosenhan found it impossible to measure RN time outside of the nurses' station because it occurred so infrequently. Psychiatrists were even worse. They hid behind closed office doors; at least the patients were able to *see* the nurses. Rosenhan concluded, "Those with the most power have least to do with patients, and those with the least power are most involved with them."

Rosenhan decries the powerlessness and the depersonalization experienced by the pseudopatients. He remembered how he was frequently awakened in the hospital where he was admitted: "Come on you m----f----s, out of bed."

The pseudopatients were hospitalized on average for 19 days before they were deemed well enough for discharge. The range of stays was from 7 to 52 days.

From Rosenhan DL: On being sane in insane places, *Science* 179:250, 1973.

providing a revolving-door pattern of care to a considerable population is rooted in a contemporary shift in ideology. This role for state hospitals appears to make no more sense than did their earlier role as neglected and neglectful asylums, and it should be reevaluated." (Jeffery L. Geller, 1992)

The state hospital population reached its peak in 1955 with 558,922 patients. By 1992 the state hospital population had dropped to 70,000 patients (Torrey, 1997). This represents a drop of over 85%. Even more dramatic, the 558,922 patients in 1955 represented 0.3% of the U.S. population while the 70,000 in 1997 represent less than 0.03%. Torrey (1997) asserts 900,000 people would be in state hospitals today if the same proportions were used. Thus over 800,000 individuals are living outside such institutions that one could infer would have been hospitalized years ago. Table 1-5 provides insights into where these people may be living.

The general rate of reduction nationally was 1% to 2% per year from 1955 to 1965, and about 5% per year between 1965 and 1975 as the federal events of 1963 began to be felt (Morrissey, Witkin, and Bethel, 1986; Wallsten, 1992). This decline has resulted in the closing of more than 50 state hospitals since 1970 (Frank, 1989). Those patients who remain hospitalized require a high level of care, have few social relationships, and are psychotic. For the most part, they are involuntarily detained young men who are acutely ill and dangerous (Dorwart, 1988).

Revolving-door effect

Although deinstitutionalization has slowed in the last few years, its effect on public mental hospitals is still profound. *Recidivism,* a term traditionally used to describe repeat criminal offenders, is now being used to describe the "revolving-door" effect of persons recycling through public mental hospitals. Though an 80% reduction in beds has been achieved, there has been a 90% increase in admissions (Appleby, et al, 1993). This is due to high rates of recidivism. Saunders (1997) describes one case of a woman who over 18 years had 27 hospital admissions at a cost of $636,000. Geller (1992) points out that not since the asylum at Williamsburg opened in 1773 has it been more difficult to be admitted to and retained in a state hospital than it is today. Torrey (1997) captures the feelings of many professionals in the title of an article, "The Release of the Mentally Ill from Institutions: A Well-Intentioned Disaster." Due to population growth and other factors, a slight reversal of this trend is projected for the future (Goldsmith et al, 1993).

Community Effects

The effects of deinstitutionalization are felt also in community agencies. For example, emergency room use by acutely disturbed persons has increased dramatically in the absence of the previous system (400%-500% in some cities).

Emergency psychiatric services are sagging from the load they carry. General hospital psychiatric units are overwhelmed at times with a continuous flow of patients being admitted, discharged, or being observed for 23 hours (to avoid a full and costly admission). The mission of these hospitals has expanded as they have had to grapple with the new realities of health care. Many believe the typical patient is different as well. Compared to the patients of the 1960s and 1970s, today's patients are more aggressive. According to Ries (1997), about 4% to 8% of patients seen in psychiatric emergency rooms are

Table 1-5	Where Individuals with SMI Live	

Location	Numbers (Approximate)
Nursing homes	1,000,000
Prison	150,000
State hospitals	70,000*
Homeless	200,000+†
Home with families, group or board/care homes, or on their own	50%

National Institutes of Mental Health: *Mental health statistics,* Rockville, Md, 1993, Office of Consumer, Family, and Public Information, Center for Mental Health Services.
Torrey EF: The release of the mentally ill from institutions: a well-intentioned disaster, *The Chronicle of Higher Education* 43(40):B4, 1997.
*See Depopulation of State Hospitals, p. 9.
†See Homelessness, below

armed with weapons. Further, approximately 1000 homicides are committed each year by severely mentally ill (SMI) individuals who are not receiving adequate care (Torrey, 1997). Lastly, 10% to 15% of persons in state prisons have SMI (Lamb, Weinberger, 1998).

Though the foregoing is negative, there have been many positive community effects too. Bachrach (1993), a critic of deinstitutionalization, notes the following, ". . . it would be misleading to suggest that deinstitutionalization has been an unqualified failure. . . . I must also acknowledge the positive legacy of this policy. The legacy consists of our heightened awareness of the humanity and the needs of mentally ill individuals."

HOMELESSNESS

"People who are homeless and mentally ill have complex needs and require a broad array of resources, such as housing, mental health and substance abuse treatment, health care, and income support and entitlement." (Frances Randolph, et al, 1997)

Lamb (1988) believes that homelessness can be directly linked to deinstitutionalization. However, Bachrach (1992) states that, even after extensive study, the extent of mental illness among the homeless, the services they need, and the impact of deinstitutionalization are not clear to researchers. Homelessness is not new, but it clearly receives more media attention today than it did 20 years ago. The reason for increased media focus is the real growth in this population. Twenty years ago (when homeless people were not making headlines) the most popular view held that homeless people (mostly white men) were skid-row bums, alcoholics, and hobos who chose to be homeless. The current view has altered that perception considerably. It is now believed that the homeless are people (men, women, and children [families]) who have been displaced by social policies over which they have no control. Twenty-five percent of the homeless are children and another 25% are employed full- or part-time (Wallsten, 1992). Furthermore, a much greater percentage of the homeless are from minority groups, and they are much poorer than the homeless of 30 years ago.

The estimates of the dimension of the "problem" range from 200,000 to more than 3 million on any given day. Perhaps the best estimate comes from the Federal Task Force on Homelessness and Severe Mental Illness (FTFHSMI) (1992) which estimates that 600,000 people are literally living and sleeping on the streets on a given night.

Estimates concerning the prevalence of mental illness among this population also vary. The consensus of opinion, however, is that 25% to 50% of adult homeless persons have a psychosis and that 33% to 50% suffer from alcohol or drug abuse. Haugland, Siegel, and Hopper (1997) suggest about 10% to 20% have a dual diagnosis.

Those who are homeless and mentally ill present a challenge to our mental health system and to our political system. They are usually single or divorced and have a very weak social support system. The homeless SMI are found in parks, airport terminals, soup kitchens, jails, and general hospitals, often presenting a troubling spector (FTFHSMI, 1992). Furthermore, the economic windfall experienced by some Americans in recent years has not filtered down to the streets. Many homeless mentally ill persons have become bold in their efforts to survive, assaulting the sensitivities of passersby. From aggressive panhandling to embarrassing public elimination of bodily wastes, societal standards are being affronted. While much of this alienating behavior is required for survival on the "mean" streets, it is behavior that offends mainstream America. The

dilemma is real and mental health professionals are searching for answers.

One approach to this issue is the federally funded Access to Community Care and Effective Services and Supports (ACCESS), which began in 1993. The goals of ACCESS are to improve access to comprehensive services across the **continuum of care** by improving efficiency and reducing duplication and cost (Randolph, et al, 1997).

As mentioned earlier, homeless people may live exclusively on the streets (the so-called street people), or they may make use of community shelters, half-way houses, or board-and-care homes. A possible third group are those who are able to stay for short periods in cheap hotels, sometimes referred to as "psychiatric ghettos," between nights in less accommodating surroundings. Still another significant group moves between homeless shelters, rehabilitation programs, jails, and prisons (Haughland, et al, 1997).

Homelessness is an end product of chronic mental illness and probably exacerbates it as well. Stated another way, many chronically ill persons end up on the streets because of their inability to succeed in a competitive society and, once they are on the streets, the stresses of homeless life compound their mental health problems. They are in a no-win situation. Hypothesizing that such a situation might exist, Winkleby and White (1992) studied 1399 homeless adults in California and found that although 45.6 percent reported no impairment when they first became homeless, most eventually developed addictive and psychiatric disorders over time. As with many societal problems, some groups seem to fare worse than others. Racial and ethnic minorities are overrepresented among the homeless (FTFHSMI, 1992). As Carter (1986) points out, "The rush to depopulate state mental institutions resulted in the dumping of many socially unskilled and economically deprived black chronic patients on poverty-ridden black communities. . . . Society's preoccupation with protecting the mentally ill from the abuses of mental health professionals has contributed to the misuse of the criminal justice system to control socially unacceptable behavior." Carter believes that black people, who rely heavily on public psychiatric institutions, have been inordinately affected.

Most SMI are not homeless so it is important to recognize the differences between the homeless SMI and the nonhomeless SMI in developing preventative strategies. SMI individuals who are homeless tend to have the following characteristics when compared to their nonhomeless counterparts (FTFHSMI, 1992):

- Earlier age of onset
- Co-occuring personality disorder
- Alcohol/drug abuse disorder
- Physical illness (acquired immunodeficiency syndrome [AIDS] or tuberculosis [TB])
- History of being violent and aggressive during childhood

Proponents of deinstitutionalization argue that these problems are not inherently a part of depopulating state hospitals but have resulted because the money has not followed the patient out of the hospital. Inpatient psychiatric treatment still accounts for a majority of mental health dollars in the United States, so, proponents argue, community mental health has never been given the financial base to realize its promise. Critics, on the other hand, point to the homeless and the disproportionate effect felt by some minority groups as evidence of a need for change. Homelessness is more than a lack of shelter, they maintain, it is a lack of support systems that were available in the public mental hospital system.

EVOLUTION OF PSYCHIATRIC CARE CONCERNS

Psychiatry in general lost interest in the SMI as a result of the influx of psychoanalysts in the 1930s and 1940s (Miller, 1984). As Freud himself had discovered, his analytic approach was most helpful to persons with less-severe problems and was not particularly helpful to psychotic patients. It is human nature to seek out what one does well and to avoid what one does not do well. Thus, as more and more psychiatrists and psychiatric nurses were influenced by Freudian thinking, there was a natural withdrawal from the SMI and a refocusing on persons more amenable to treatment. Public mental hospitals lost prestige as did the physicians and nurses working in them. Within the psychiatric nursing fraternity, staff nurses were not as highly valued as those working in the therapist role. As participants in a self-fulfilling prophecy, the devalued inpatient psychiatric nurses in public hospitals, in many cases, became what they were perceived to be.

The mainstream of psychiatry and psychiatric nursing turned from chronically disturbed patients to individuals with *lowered self-esteem, those who were striving to reach their potential, those who had not developed the ability to trust, and the existentially unhappy* (Detre, 1987). Psychiatry changed its focus from one extreme of the psychiatric care continuum (the SMI) to the other (the worried well) over a few decades. Social issues started to emerge as legitimate professional concerns. Psychiatry and psychiatric nursing became interested in issues such as poverty, racism, alternate life-styles, and sexism at the professional level. It is the perception of some clinicians that this process of enlightenment and social relevance further distanced the mainstream of psychiatric care from those most in need of that care.

■ Critical Thinking Question

It has been stated that the fields of psychiatry and psychiatric nursing lost interest in the SMI and became more interested in working with the "worried well." Do you believe this is still true in psychiatric nursing? Support your answer.

NURSING EDUCATION

The first psychiatric nursing textbook was written by Harriet Bailey in 1920. The title of the book, *Nursing Mental Diseases,* reflects the appropriate terminology of the day. An important distinction about psychiatric nursing is that it was not brought into the greater nursing fold until the 1940s. Because psychiatric nurses were trained in state hospitals, they could work only in state hospitals. In 1937 the National League for Nursing (then called the National League for Nursing Education) recommended that psychiatric nursing be made a part of the curriculum of general nursing programs. As the views of the major theorists (such as Sullivan with his "interpersonal psychiatry" and Maxwell Jones with his "therapeutic milieu") became prominent, the role of psychiatric nurses grew.

As psychiatric nursing developed, others recognized its contribution to psychiatric care. Psychiatric nursing was one of four professional groups (along with psychiatry, psychology, and social work) given money for training in the 1946 National Mental Health Act. These monies enabled more nurses to be trained in basic psychiatric nursing (undergraduate) and spurred specialization at the advanced level (graduate).

The views of two important figures in psychiatric nursing in the 1950s shaped and gave direction to psychiatric nursing practice and contributed to a professional climate. Hildegarde Peplau (1952, 1959) developed a model for psychiatric nursing practice. Her book, *Interpersonal Relations in Nursing,* influences practice to this day. Her approach, heavily influenced by Harry Stack Sullivan, emphasizes the interpersonal dimension of practice. She also wrote a history of psychiatric nursing that carefully traced the unfolding of the profession. Peplau may be the single most important historical figure in psychiatric nursing.

Another influential figure was June Mellow (1953, 1967, 1986). Mellow viewed nursing therapy as taking place in an "experiential-action medium" in which nurses and patients share the factors in the environment. Her approach focuses on psychosocial needs and patient strengths. As Peplau, Mellow, and others began to articulate what psychiatric nurses do, the profession experienced another surge forward in its quest for professional accountability.

NURSING RESEARCH

One effect of the CMHC Act in 1963 was a broadened scope of psychiatric nursing practice and a consequential increased responsibility for improving practice. Research is now an integral part of practice. This research is communicated in journals dedicated exclusively to psychiatric nursing: *Perspectives in Psychiatric Nursing* (1963), *Journal of Psychosocial Nursing* (1963), *Archives of Psychiatric Nursing* (1987), and *Journal of the American Psychiatric Nurses Association* (1995). Perhaps one of the most pressing areas of inquiry for psychiatric nursing as we approach the twenty-first century is the effects of SMI on families (Saunders, 1997).

STANDARDS OF PRACTICE

In 1973 standards of care were developed by the American Nurses Association's (ANA) division of psychiatric and mental health practice. These standards were revised in 1982. A two-part docu-

ment was published in 1994 entitled "Statement on Psychiatric-Mental Health Clinical Nursing Practice and Standards of Psychiatric-Mental Health Clinical Practice." The revised standards reflect the current state of knowledge and incorporate a wider range of professional practice. These standards of care apply to all settings where nurses practice psychiatric nursing. Some standards are specifically applicable to advanced practitioners; for example, clinical specialists.

CERTIFICATION OF COMPETENCY

One of the more important developments in the evolution of psychiatric nursing was the decision by the ANA (1988) to provide certification for nurses who meet established criteria. This step represented a major milestone. In effect, the ANA endorsed the certified nurse as being competent at certain levels. Certification is available at both the generalist and clinical specialist levels.

Psychiatric nurses have evolved from caretakers to clinical specialists, from custodians to psychotherapists, from asylum-educated to doctorally prepared practitioners. The professional vision of the role of psychiatric nurses and their contributions to the care of the mentally ill has changed dramatically in the past 100 years. As it nears the end of the "decade of the brain," nursing continues to adapt to the changing needs and expectations of society.

Extremes in professional thinking are beginning to be resolved. Although some nurses still focus their interventions on the "worried well," SMI now have loud and persuasive advocates among the nursing community who are determined to redirect resources toward this traditionally underserved group.

COMMUNITY-BASED CARE

The future of psychiatric care and psychiatric nursing will be linked to continuing efforts to prevent mental health problems and to more effectively treat existing disorders. Because of economic realities much of that effort will be community based as part of a continuum of care. Nurses will need to continue to train for roles in the community while reestablishing a leadership role in inpatient services. An agenda for mental health has been established in the document

"Healthy People 2000" (1990), developed by the U.S. Department of Health and Human Services. Box 1-2 outlines mental health objectives from that document.

Developing a Continuum of Care

In the early 1960s mental health activists were successful in passing federal legislation that dramatically reshaped the way mental health services were delivered in this country. Converging forces related to these changes have been discussed above.

Specific problems associated with community mental health (CMH) were the liberalization of commitment laws, which allowed SMI patients to go untreated, and restrictive confidentiality rulings, which made discussing the difficult issues of treatment with family members a legal concern. As newspaper editorials, grass-roots mental health organizations, and families have clamored about the obvious unmet needs of the SMI, the mental health and legal communities have rallied to respond. This insistence has culminated in thoughtful and deliberate dialogue among mental health professionals with the objective to make the mental health system work.

In order to make it work, a seamless continuum of care must be developed that coordinates the activities of diverse treatment sources and facilitates movement between and among its entities. Until that time many patients will slip through the cracks of the system as bureaucratic misfunction and corporate self-interest drain energies away from programs. Box 1-3 suggests how the system is changing to develop this seamless continuum of care.

Role for nursing in the continuum of care

CMH nursing has been around for a number of years. In 1982 the ANA defined the CMH nurse's role in the continuum of care as follows: "The nurse participates with other members of the community in assessing, planning, implementing, and evaluating mental health services and community services that include the promotion of the **continuum** of primary, secondary, and tertiary prevention of mental illness."

Nursing has an opportunity to assert itself at this point in psychiatric history because so many

---

Box 1-2 Healthy People 2000 Mental Health Objectives

Health status objectives are to reduce the following:
1. All suicides from 11.7 per 100,000 to 10.5 per 100,000
2. Injurious teenage suicide attempts by 15%
3. Child and adolescent mental disorders from 12% to 10%
4. The number of mentally disordered adults in the community from 12.6% to 10.7%.
5. Negative effects of stress in adults from 42.6% to 35%

Risk reduction objectives are to increase the following:
1. Use of community resources to at least 30% of adults with severe mental illness (baseline: 15%)
2. Treatment for people with major depression to at least 45% of that population (baseline: 31%)
3. Percentage of adults with emotional problems who seek help to at least 20% of that population (baseline: 11.1%)

Services and protection objectives are to accomplish the following:
1. Decrease suicide among jail inmates
2. Reduce workplace stress
3. Establish mutual help clearinghouses in at least 25 states
4. Increase the number of primary care providers who routinely assess children and adults for emotional needs by 75% and 50%, respectively

---

Department of Health and Human Services: *Healthy people 2000*, Washington, DC, 1990, DHHS.

Box 1-3 Systemic Changes

In the new health care reality, community mental health must move rapidly away from some practices and toward new ways of conceptualizing the system.

Away from symptom stabilization
Toward recovery and reintegration

Away from a view that professionals have all the answers
Toward involving consumers and family members more

Away from medication management
Toward holistic thinking (e.g., stabilizing housing, medical health, finances)

values traditionally emphasized by psychiatric nursing fit with the concept of a continuum of care. For instance:

- Viewing the patient as a whole person
- Working with families
- Treating patients in their own homes
- Developing a relationship over time
- Educating patients about medications
- Assessing the environment for safety, hygiene, and supports

All of these traditional nursing activities position nurses to excel in the world of psychiatric care. Only time will tell if the profession is up to the challenges ahead and able to take advantage of its natural "fit" with today's health care realities.

Critical Thinking Question

Many large numbers referring to both people and money have been discussed in this chapter. To help sensitize you to these numbers, consider the following. Calculate the weeks, months, or years equivalent to 1 million, 1 billion, and 1 trillion seconds. Review the numbers referred to in the chapter with this concept in mind.

Key Concepts

1. Understanding the principles of psychiatric nursing is important because about 25% of the population is affected by mental health problems.
2. Modern psychiatry can be traced through four benchmark periods: Enlightenment, scientific study, psychotropic drugs, and community mental health.
3. Historically, the mentally ill were banished and confined, but the period of Enlightenment ushered in an era in which the mentally ill were treated humanely.
4. The asylum movement (providing sanctuary from the hostile world) grew out of the humane emphasis of the period of Enlightenment and resulted in the development of state hospital systems.
5. During the period of scientific study men such as Freud, Kraepelin, and Bleuler studied human beings objectively; this resulted in both psychodynamic and biological understandings of mental disorders.
6. During the period of psychotropic drugs, antipsychotic drugs (chlorpromazine [Thorazine] in the early 1950s), antidepressant drugs (imipramine [Tofranil] in the late 1950s), and other drugs were developed and greatly contributed to the treatment of specific mental disorders.
7. The period of community mental health began as a result of several converging factors including:

- hostility towards state hospitals
- psychotropic drugs
- civil rights
- financial incentives

8. Deinstitutionalization, changing the locus of treatment from large public hospitals to the community, is a product of the community mental health movement.
9. In 1955 over one-half million patients were in state hospitals: by 1997 about 70,000 were in these hospitals.
10. A high percentage of the nation's homeless have a diagnosable mental disorder. Critics of deinstitutionalization place some of the blame for homelessness on the community mental health movement.
11. Psychiatric care and psychiatric nursing have evolved during this century. At one time, psychiatric nursing was closely associated with the care of the SMI but, like medicine, became professionally interested in the worried well. Today, many are challenging psychiatric nurses to return to caring for those most in need.
12. The first psychiatric nursing textbook was written in 1920 by Harriet Bailey, but it is Hildegarde Peplau's book, *Interpersonal Relations in Nursing,* that has most influenced psychiatric nursing.
13. Community mental health nurses have a major role in the continuum of care due to their specific training in caring, comprehensive services, patient education, and case management.

Study Questions

(Answer key is in the back of the book.)

1. Approximately what percentage of Americans over the age of 18 are personally affected by mental or addictive disorders each year?
   a. 10%
   b. 15%
   c. 25%
   d. 40%
2. The cost of disorders of the brain is very high. Which of the following is closest to the total cost (both direct and indirect) of these disorders (in billions of dollars)?
   a. 100
   b. 200
   c. 300
   d. 400
3. What are the ABCs of the pre-Enlightenment era? *assistance banishment confinement*
4. Who were the two men most responsible for the period of Enlightenment? *Tuke & Pinnel*
5. The first state hospitals established by Dorothea Dix were meant to be:
   a. Asylums

b. Treatment centers

c. Places of confinement

6. The forces behind deinstitutionalization started gaining momentum during what period?

   a. 1940s and 1950s

   b. 1960s

   c. 1970s

   d. 1980s

7. Which of the following are part of the convergence of forces that created the groundswell for deinstitutionalization?

   a. Opponents of state hospitals

   b. Confidence in psychotropic drugs

   c. New emphasis on civil rights

   d. Economic forces; e.g., ATD and SSI

   e. All of the above

8. The decline of interest in inpatient psychiatric nursing may be attributed to which of the following?

   a. Community mental health centers and consequent outpatient care

   b. The advent of newer roles for psychiatric nurses

   c. Both of the above

9. The chief result of the scientific study era was:

   a. The asylum

   b. Objective study of psychiatric disorders

   c. Community mental health movement

   d. Homelessness

10. The psychiatrist who has had the most influence on modern psychotherapy is:

   a. Bleuler

   b. Freud

   c. Kraepelin

   d. Skinner

11. The number of patients in state hospitals today is approximately:

   a. 70,000

   b. 200,000

   c. 300,000

   d. 400,000

12. The best estimate of the number of homeless people who sleep on the streets on a given night comes from the Federal Task Force on Homelessness and Severe Mental Illness. It estimates:

   a. 200,000

   b. 400,000

   c. 600,000

   d. 800,000

REFERENCES

American Nurses Association: *Certification catalog,* Kansas City, 1988, The Association.

American Nurses Association: *Standards of psychiatric and mental health nursing practice,* Kansas City, 1982, The Association.

Appleby L, et al: Length of stay and recidivism in schizophrenia: a study of public psychiatric hospital patients, *Am J Psychiatry* 150:72, 1993.

Ayds FJ: The early history of modern psychopharmacology, *Neuropsychopharmacology* 5(2):71, 1991.

Bachrach LL: What we know about homelessness among mentally ill persons: an analytical review and commentary, *Hosp Community Psychiatry* 43(5):453, 1992.

Bachrach LL: The biopsychosocial legacy of deinstitutionalization, *Hosp Community Psychiatry* 44(6):523, 1993.

Bell CC: The new community psychiatry in 2000 A.D., *Hosp Community Psychiatry* 44(9):815, 1993.

Carter JH: Deinstitutionalization of black patients: an apocalypse now, *Hosp Community Psychiatry* 37:78, 1986.

Cohen CI and Thompson KS: Homeless mentally ill or mentally ill homeless? *Am J Psychiatry* 149:816, 1992.

Department of Health and Human Services: *Healthy people 2000,* Washington, 1990, DHHS.

Detre T: The future of psychiatry, *Am J Psychiatry* 144:621, 1987.

Deutsch A: *The shame of the states,* New York, 1948, Harcourt Brace.

Dorwart RA: A ten-year followup study of the effects of deinstitutionalization, *Hosp Community Psychiatry* 39:287, 1988.

Federal Task Force on Homelessness and Severe Mental Illness: *Outcasts on Main Street,* Washington, DC, 1992, Interagency Council on Homeless.

Foucault M: *Madness and Civilization* (translated from the French), New York, 1967, New American Library.

Frank RG: The mentally indigent mentally ill: approaches to financing, *Hosp Community Psychiatry* 40:9, 1989.

Geller JL: A historical perspective on the role of state hospitals viewed from the era of the "revolving door," *Am J Psychiatry* 149:1526, 1992.

Goldsmith HF, et al: Projections of inpatient admissions to specialty mental health organizations: 1990-2010, *Hosp Community Psychiatry* 44:478, 1993.

Goldstein JN and Horgan CM: Inpatient and outpatient psychiatric services: substitutes or complements, *Hosp Community Psychiatry* 37:433, 1988.

Gollaher D: *Voice for the mad: the life of Dorothea Dix,* New York Press, 1995, The Free Press, pp. 143-144.

Haugland G, et al: Mental illness among homeless individuals in a suburban county, *Psychiatric Services* 48(4):504, 1997.

Howie the Harp: Taking a new approach to independent living, *Hosp Community Psychiatry* 44:413, 1993.

Joint Commission on Mental Illness and Health: *Action for mental health: final report,* New York, 1961, Basic Books.

Lamb HR: Deinstitutionalization at the crossroads, *Hosp Community Psychiatry* 39:941, 1988.

Lamb HR: Is it time for a moratorium on deinstitutionalization? *Hosp Community Psychiatry* 43(7):669, 1992.

Lamb HR, Weinberger LE: Persons with severe mental illness in jails and prisons: a review, *Psychiatric Services* 49:483, 1998.

McMillan I: Insight into Bedlam: one hospital's history. Journal of Psychosocial Nursing, 35(6):28, 1997.

Mellow J: *An exploratory study of nursing therapy with two persons with psychoses* (master of science thesis), Boston, 1953, Boston University.

Mellow J: A personal perspective of nursing therapy, *Hosp Community Psychiatry* 37:182, 1986.

Miller RD: Public mental hospital work: pros and cons for psychiatrists, *Hosp Community Psychiatry* 35:928, 1984.

Morrissey JP, Witkin MJ, and Bethel HE: *Trends by state in the capacity and volume of inpatient services, state and county mental hospitals, United States, 1976-1980,* Series CN10, Pub ADM 86-146, Rockville, Md, 1986, National Institute of Mental Health.

Munetz MR, Peterson GA, and Vandershie PW: SAFER houses for patients who need asylum. *Psychiatric Services* 47(2):117, 1996.

Narrows WE, et al: Use of services by persons with mental and addictive disorders: findings from the NIMH epidemiologic catchment area program, *Arch Gen Psychiatry* 50:95, 1993.

National Foundation for Brain Disorders: *The cost of disorders of the brain,* Washington, DC, 1992, The Foundation.

News: Key messages of mental health month, *J Psycho Nurs Ment Health Serv* 35(5):9, 1997.

News and Notes: Dramatic rise reported in number of persons with mental disorders on SSDI and SSI rolls, *Hosp Community Psychiatry* 44:505, 1993.

News and Notes: Prevalence of serious mental illness among American adults estimated at 5.7 percent in 12-month period, *Psychiatric Services* 47(5):546, 1996.

Pearlmutter DR: Recent trends and issues in psychiatric-mental health nursing, *Hosp Community Psychiatry* 36:56, 1985.

Pelletier LR: Nurse-psychotherapists: whom do they treat? *Hosp Community Psychiatry* 35:1149, 1984.

Peplau H: *Interpersonal relations in nursing,* New York, 1952, GP Putnam's Sons.

Peplau H: Principles of psychiatric nursing. In Arieti S, editor: *American handbook of psychiatry,* vol 2, New York, 1959, Basic Books.

Randolph F, et al: Creating integrated service systems for homeless persons with mental illness: the ACCESS program. *Psychiatric Services* 48(3):369, 1997.

Regier DA, et al: One-month prevalence of mental disorders in the United States, *Arch Gen Psychiatry* 45:977, 1988.

Regier DA, et al: The de facto U.S. mental and addictive disorders service system: epidemiologic catchment area prospective 1-year prevalence rates of disorders and services, *Arch Gen Psychiatry* 50:85, 1993.

Ries R: Advantages of separating the triage function from the emergency service. Psychiatric Services, 48(6):755, 1997.

Ries RK and Dyck DG: Representative payee practices of community mental health centers in Washington state, *Psychiatric Services* 48(6):811, 1997.

Rosenblatt A: Concepts of the asylum in the care of the mentally ill, *Hosp Community Psychiatry* 35:244, 1984.

Rosenheck R: Disability payments and chemical dependence: conflicting values and uncertain effects, *Psychiatric Services* 48(6):789, 1997.

Rosenhan DL: On being sane in insane places, *Science* 179:250, 1973.

Saunders J: Symbolic interactionism for families living with severe mental illness. *J Psychosoc Nurs Ment Health Serv* 35(6):8, 1997.

Torrey EF: The release of the mentally ill from institutions: a well-intentioned disaster, *The Chronicle of Higher Education* 43(40):B4, 1997.

Trudeau ME: Informed consent: the patient's right to decide, *J Psychosoc Nurs Ment Health Serv* 31(6):9, 1993.

Wallsten SM: A portrait of homelessness, *J Psychosoc Nurs Ment Health Serv* 30(9):20, 1992.

Wasow M: The need for asylum revisited, *Hosp Community Psychiatry,* 44(3):207, 1993.

Weiner DB: Philippe Pinel's "Memoir on Madness" of December 11, 1794: a fundamental text of modern psychiatry, *Am J Psychiatry* 149(6):725, 1992.

Will G: Disabilities act protects obnoxious behavior on job, *The Birmingham News,* p. A5, April 4, 1996.

Winkleby MA and White R: Homeless adults without apparent medical and psychiatric impairment: onset of morbidity over time, *Hosp Community Psychiatry* 43(10):1017, 1992.

CHAPTER 2

Psychotherapeutic Management in the Continuum of Care

NORMAN L. KELTNER
LEE H. SCHWECKE

LEARNING OBJECTIVES

After reading this chapter you should be able to:
- Describe the components of psychotherapeutic management.
- Explain how the balancing of psychotherapeutic management components combine to form a powerful therapeutic model of care.

- Recognize the relationship between the continuum of care and the psychotherapeutic management model.

PSYCHOTHERAPEUTIC MANAGEMENT

Psychiatric nursing is in search of care delivery models that are not only effective for patient care but can also capitalize on the uniqueness of the discipline. Psychotherapeutic management proposes a "real-world" approach to psychiatric nursing care—an approach that recognizes the interdependence of the mental health professions but also exploits the strengths of psychiatric nursing. It answers the question: What do psychiatric nurses do that is different from other mental health professionals, particularly social workers, psychologists, marriage and family counselors, and other therapists? In 1979 Koldjeski wrote: "Psychiatric nurses must clearly demonstrate the exact nature of their practice and must differentiate their practice from the practice of other nonmedical mental health personnel." Following Koldjeski's prescription, psychotherapeutic management was proposed as a model to clarify and distinguish the role of the psychiatric nurse (Keltner, 1985). There are five basic categories into which psychiatric treatment can be divided: the use of words

KEY TERMS

Behavior therapy   A therapeutic approach that helps patients modify behavior by modifying or changing old patterns of behavior

Continuum of care   Levels of care through which an individual can move depending upon his/her needs at a given point in time

Milieu   Environment or setting

Psychopathology   The systematic study of mental disorders

Psychotherapeutic management   A model for nursing care that balances the three primary intervention modes used by psychiatric nurses: the therapeutic nurse-patient relationship, psychopharmacology, and milieu management

Psychotropic drugs   Medication used in the treatment of mental disorders

Somatic therapy   A therapeutic approach that uses physiological or physical interventions to effect behavioral changes; for example, electroconvulsive therapy is a somatic treatment

Therapy   The means, usually with words, to cure or manage the course of a mental disorder. Nurses who practice psychotherapy are trained in a specific therapy model; for example, psychoanalysis and cognitive therapy.

Therapeutic   Refers to the communication of respect, a desire to help, and understanding to another person. Understanding includes knowledge of mental mechanisms, coping strategies, and stressors. Active listening is a crucial component of being therapeutic.

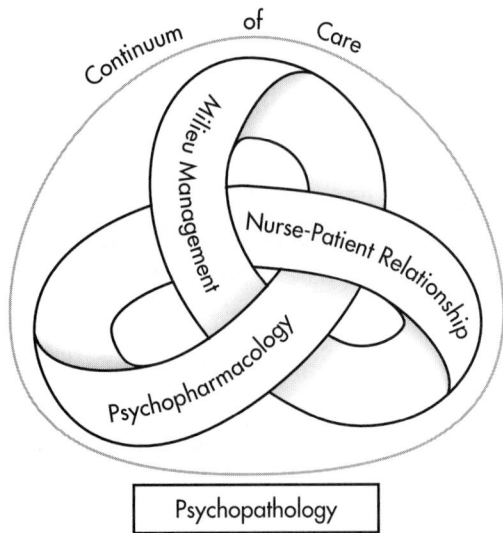

FIGURE 2-1   Psychotherapeutic management in the continuum of care.

(which encompass all forms of psychotherapy), the use of drugs, the use of the environment, somatic therapies, and behavioral conditioning. Psychotherapeutic management emphasizes three of these categories: the psychotherapeutic nurse-patient relationship (words), psychopharmacology (drugs), and milieu management (environment), all of which must be supported by a sound understanding of psychopathology (Figure 2-1).

The application of psychopathology and the knowledgeable use of psychotherapeutic management skill extends beyond inpatient settings into a variety of care settings, such as outpatient programs, residential services, and home care. The needs of the individual and the setting in which care is delivered will influence the degree to which each of the components of psychotherapeutic management is utilized within the continuum of care (Figure 2-2).

For example, persons with schizophrenia in an inpatient setting profit most when a therapeutic nurse-patient relationship, psychopharmacology, and a well-managed milieu are available. When one component is missing from the equation, treatment is compromised. Ordinarily, when psychotropic drugs and a well-managed milieu are subtracted from this equation, patients will decompensate into a pretreatment state. Likewise, if drugs and therapeutic communication are available (perhaps the latter from only a few motivated staff members), but the overall environment is poorly managed, patients are left to fend for themselves and are drained of internal resources needed for healing. When inpatients receive only drug therapy but are denied therapeutic interaction opportunities in a well-managed milieu, there is a return to the inadequacies of custodial care. In other words, all the components of the psychotherapeutic management equation must be

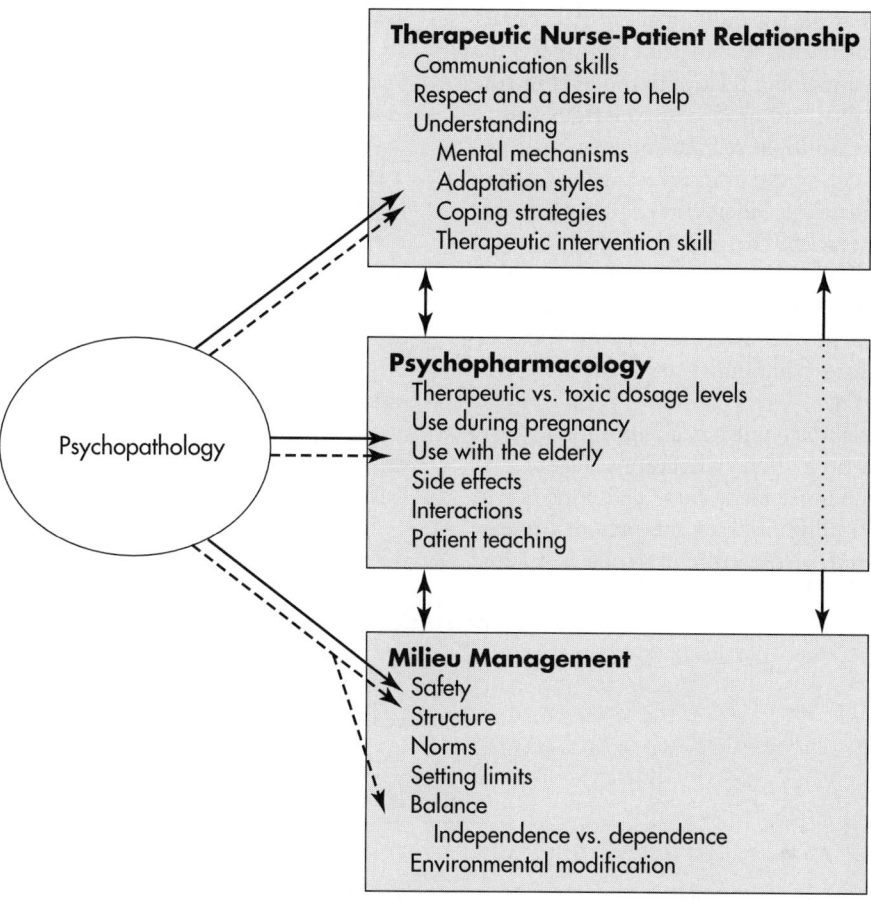

FIGURE 2-2 Psychotherapeutic management model.

present if patients are to fully realize the benefits of effective nursing intervention. However, one component may take precedence at a given point in time. For example, an individual with schizophrenia has missed his last appointment for his injection of haloperidol decanoate (Haldol). The nurse's priority might be to make a home visit to administer the injection. The psychopharmacology component is a priority at this time, but the nurse-patient relationship and milieu aspects are not ignored. Psychotherapeutic management endeavors to bring balance to practice and, with balance, role clarification, thus providing a valuable approach in both inpatient and outpatient settings.

Psychotherapeutic management owes a debt to the concepts of Mellow's experiential-action model (1967), which echoes the sentiments of Billings when she compared the view of psychiatric nursing from a psychosocial perspective to the realities of today.

Billings (1993) stated, "Caring is still nursing's cornerstone but it goes far beyond an innocent feeling and a sensitive act. Today my caring is based on an evolution of understanding. It is an informed decision-making process that has a theoretical and scientific base."

CONTINUUM OF CARE

Unit Two deals with the continuum of care within which the psychotherapeutic management approach is implemented. It includes providing services based on the needs of the individual. The services span the continuum from health promotion through prevention, treatment, and rehabilitation. These services can be provided in a variety of settings. An important aspect of the continuum of care is that the individuals can be guided through treatment or services as their needs change. The individual's initial contact with the mental health system should involve the process of assessment and referral to the least restrictive, most effective, and most cost-conscious source of services. The multiple services may or may not involve the nurse as the primary caregiver. Other disciplines or care providers may be responsible for a particular service. The psychotherapeutic management model has relevance in a variety of care settings and could be adapted by the nurse to any level of care. In Unit Two, the chapters focus on hospital-based care, community-based care, and case management.

How the patient is guided to an appropriate level of care is based on a series of decisions (Figure 2-3). Traditionally, the nurse made these decisions as part of discharge planning prior to the patient's release from the hospital. Given current trends in mental health care, the decisions may be made by the nurse or other professionals during the "risk assessment phase."

THE THERAPEUTIC NURSE-PATIENT RELATIONSHIP

It is crucial for the student of psychiatric nursing to differentiate *therapy* from *being therapeutic*. The authors propose that the art of therapy is the domain of graduate-level psychiatric nurses and that the art of being therapeutic is the domain of undergraduate-level psychiatric nurses. Therefore, when you finish this course, you will not be a therapist but you can learn to be therapeutic.

Unit Three is devoted to this first dimension of psychotherapeutic management. The different

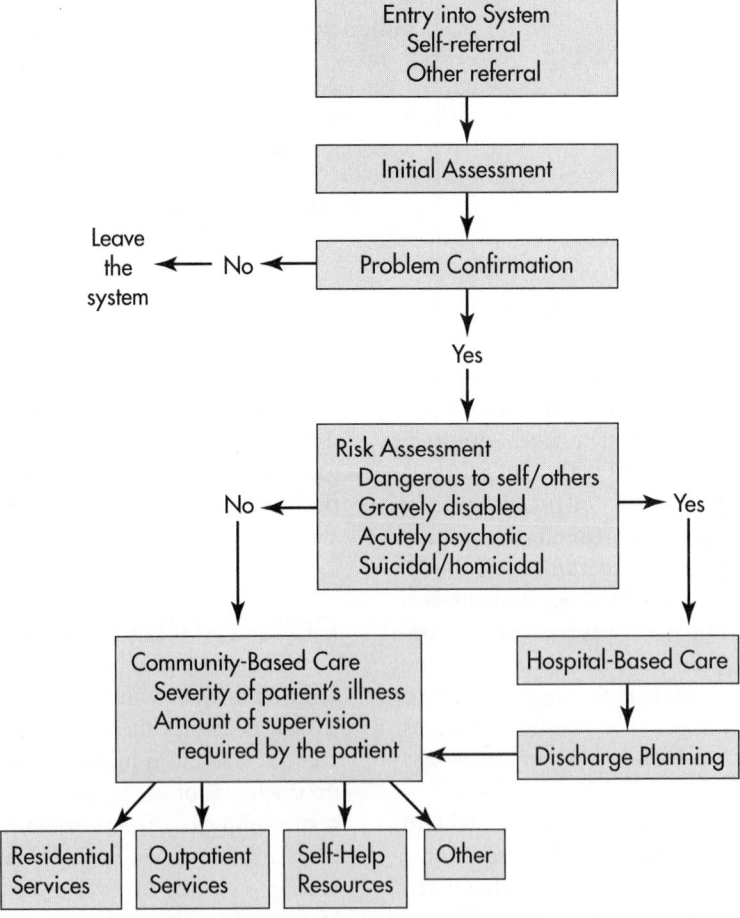

FIGURE 2-3 Decision tree for continuum of care.

emphases placed on words and the wide range of styles within the domain of words are discussed, specifically general communication skills, (Chapter 10), the nature of the nurse-patient relationship (Chapter 11), nursing process (Chapter 12), anxiety and coping (Chapter 13), working with the aggressive patient (Chapter 14), working with groups of patients (Chapter 15), working with the families of patients (Chapter 16), and working with patients from different cultures (Chapter 17).

PSYCHOPHARMACOLOGY

Unit Four is devoted to the contribution of psychotropic drugs to psychiatric nursing, the responsibilities of the nurse, and essential information about these drugs. Psychopharmacology is an important dimension in psychotherapeutic management as psychotropic drugs have enabled millions of persons to live more fulfilling lives. It must be noted that drug intervention is neither always desirable nor appropriate. However, when drug therapy is indicated, patients typically respond more rapidly than they would without drugs.

The nurse who uses the nursing process model is able to assess the patients' responses to medication, plan to respond to side effects should they occur, implement those plans, and evaluate for desired results (Jaretz, Flowers, and Millsap, 1992). The nurse's pivotal role, especially in an inpatient setting, allows intervention before serious drug-related problems occur. In addition, the nurse dispenses medications and makes decisions regarding as needed (prn) medications. Because about one-half of all psychotropic drug orders are written on a prn basis (Blair, 1990), the nurse makes decisions related directly to the pharmacological treatment of patients. For these and other reasons it is important for the nurse to have immediate access to information about psychotropic drugs.

Concerns frequently voiced by patients include what to do about a missed dose (Zind, Furlong, and Stebbins, 1992), the relationship between dosage and the severity of the psychiatric problem ("If I take twice as much as Joe, does that mean that my problem is twice as severe?"), and whether or not it is permissible to drink alcohol while taking medications. Questions regarding dosage requirements are really questions about pharmacokinetics and

how individuals absorb, distribute, metabolize, and eliminate drugs differently from one another. Older people handle drugs differently than younger people (Keltner and Folks, 1993), and people of some racial groups metabolize drugs at different rates than people of other groups (Keltner and Folks, 1992). Consumption of alcohol is almost always contraindicated when a psychiatric patient is taking a psychotropic drug. The nurse should build a psychopharmacologic knowledge base to become better equipped to help patients answer these and other questions. Unit Four expands on these ideas and provides separate chapters on antiparkinson, antipsychotic, antidepressant and antimanic, and antianxiety drugs.

MILIEU MANAGEMENT

Milieu management is a proactive approach to care that forges therapeutic benefits from patients' surroundings whether in the home, hospital, or outpatient setting. There are six environmental elements nurses must consider in creating a therapeutic milieu: safety, structure, norms, limit setting, balance, and environmental modification. These elements overlap; for example, safety is a component of all the other dimensions of milieu.

Nurses are the primary shapers of the milieu. Kyes and Hofling (1974) stated, "The interpersonal environment in which a patient lives may be therapeutic or nontherapeutic depending almost entirely on the interest and ability of the [nursing] staff." To this the authors add that the nurse is critical in guiding other staff into being therapeutic. Because human beings are incapable of *not* interacting with their environment, it behooves nurses to make those interactions therapeutic.

Nurses are the consistent force in the milieu. In managing the milieu, nurses serve multiple roles. They work with patients individually, lead groups, participate in community meetings, coordinate medical care with physicians and other departments, make discharge arrangements, and work with families. In addition, nurses provide leadership in interdisciplinary team meetings and are the professionals who most often implement team decisions (Keltner, 1985). Chapters 23, 24, and 25 cover the subject of milieu management in greater detail.

■ **Critical Thinking Question**

Using the telephone book for your city, make a list of the mental health services available in your area.

PSYCHOPATHOLOGY

Unit Six on psychopathology provides the foundation on which the three components of psychotherapeutic management rest. It facilitates therapeutic communication in the nurse-patient relationship and lays the groundwork for an understanding of psychopharmacology and milieu management. Unit Six includes information on the major mental disorders. Schizophrenia, mood disorders, anxiety-related disorders, cognitive disorders, personality disorders, sexual disorders, substance-related disorders, dual diagnosis, and eating disorders are considered in separate chapters of this text.

SPECIAL THERAPIES

Unit Seven on special therapies includes a chapter on behavioral therapy and one on electroconvulsive therapy. Behavior therapy includes all forms of behavior conditioning such as desensitization and reciprocal inhibition. Electroconvulsive therapy and behavioral therapies are important dimensions of psychiatric care and are effective treatments, but do not have the universal clinical applications of the other categories of psychiatric treatment and thus are not emphasized in this text.

SPECIAL POPULATIONS

Special populations in psychiatric nursing include victims of violence, child and adolescent psychiatric patients, the elderly mentally ill, and patients who have human immunodeficiency virus (HIV) disease.

■ **Critical Thinking Question**

Based on your clinical setting, evaluate the components of the psychotherapeutic management model that you have observed.

Key Concepts

1. Psychotherapeutic management is a model of care that clarifies the nature of psychiatric nursing and differentiates psychiatric nursing practice from the practice of other disciplines.
2. In the continuum of care, the individual is guided to services based on specific needs at a given point in time.
3. The components of psychotherapeutic management include a therapeutic nurse-patient relationship, psychopharmacology, and milieu management supported by a basic understanding of psychopathology.
4. The *therapeutic nurse-patient relationship* emphasizes the importance for the nurse to understand basic principles of therapeutic communication.
5. Being therapeutic is different from providing therapy in that therapeutic interactions should occur during every patient contact, whereas therapy indicates a more formal and structured interaction.
6. *Psychopharmacologic* understanding is important because nurses administer medication, make decisions about prn medication, and evaluate for therapeutic and adverse responses to medication.
7. Because human beings are incapable of not interacting with their environment, *milieu management* is an important nursing consideration. Nurses are uniquely responsible for developing patients' environment.
8. An understanding of *psychopathology* facilitates the nurse-patient relationship, lays the groundwork for understanding psychopharmacology, and provides a theoretical structure for milieu management.

Study Questions

(Answer key is in the back of the book.)
1. Which of the following are included in psychotherapeutic management?
   a. A therapeutic nurse-patient relationship
   b. Appropriate use of psychotropic drugs
   c. A well-managed milieu
   d. All of the above
2. What is the underlying foundation for the components of psychotherapeutic management?
   a. Knowledge of drugs
   b. Knowledge of psychopathology
   c. Knowledge of therapeutic skills
   d. Knowledge of milieu management
3. Which of the components of psychotherapeutic management is most important according to the authors?
   a. A therapeutic nurse-patient relationship
   b. Appropriate use of psychotropic drugs
   c. A well-managed milieu
   d. All are important functions of the psychiatric nurse

4. In making referrals in the continuum of care, which of the following concepts is most important to consider?
   a. Therapeutic communication
   b. Least restrictive setting
   c. Diagnosis
   d. Family participation

REFERENCES

Billings CV: Psychiatric-mental health nursing professional progress notes, *Arch Psychiatr Nurs* 7(3):174, 1993.

Blair DT: Risk management for extrapyramidal symptoms, *Quality Assurance Rev Bull* 17:116, 1990.

Jaretz N, Flowers E, and Millsap L: Clozapine: nursing care considerations, *Perspect Psychiatr Care* 28(3): 19, 1992.

Keltner NL: Psychotherapeutic management: a model for nursing practice, *Perspect Psychiatr Care* 23:125, 1985.

Keltner NL and Folks DG: Culture as a variable in drug therapy, *Perspect Psychiatr Care* 28(1):33, 1992.

Keltner NL and Folks DG: Pharmacokinetics and pharmacology: application to the geropsychiatric patient, *Perspect Psychiatr Care* 29(1):34, 1993.

Koldjeski D: Mental health and psychiatric nursing and primary health care: issues and prospects. Proceedings of the fourth national conference in graduate education in psychiatric and mental health nursing, Kansas City, Mo, 1979, American Nurses Association.

Kraus JB: Managing costs and managing care: managing to make our systems humane, *Archives of Psychiatric Nursing* 9(6):309, 1995.

Kyes J and Hofling C: *Basic psychiatric concepts in nursing,* ed 3, Philadelphia, 1974, JB Lippincott.

Lefkowitz PM: The continuum of care in a general hospital, *General Hospital Psychiatry* 17:260, 1995.

Mellow J: Evolution of nursing therapy through research, *Psychiatr Opinion* 4:15, 1967.

Schreter RK: Essential skills for managed behavioral care, *Psychiatric Services* 48(5):653, 1997.

Zind R, Furlong C, and Stebbins M: Educating patients about missed medication doses, *J Psychosoc Nurs Ment Health Serv* 30(7):10, 1992.

CHAPTER 3

Theoretical Models for Working with Psychiatric Patients

LEE H. SCHWECKE
CAROL E. BOSTROM

LEARNING OBJECTIVES

After reading this chapter you should be able to:
- Compare and contrast major theoretical models that contribute to the understanding of psychiatric patients and their behaviors.

- Identify key concepts of the major theoretical models.
- Describe the relevance of each theoretical model to psychiatric nursing practice.

The following theoretical models of human behavior have been selected for discussion in this chapter because they provide basic concepts for working with psychiatric patients: psychoanalytical, developmental, interpersonal, cognitive-behavioral, reality therapy, and stress models. These models are summarized in Table 3-1 and in Table 3-5 throughout the chapter.

PSYCHOANALYTICAL MODEL

The psychoanalytical model (Freud, 1936; Brill, 1938; Freud and Strachey, 1960) is a theory of the personality that originated with Sigmund Freud and emphasizes unconscious processes or psychodynamic factors as the basis for motivation and behavior. Freud believed that the personality is formed in early childhood and that knowledge of how an individual's drives, instincts, psychic energy or libido, and psychosexual attitude are formed during the first 6 years of life is crucial to an understanding of the personality.

Key Concepts

Personality processes

The personality consists of three processes, the id, the ego, and the superego, that function as a whole

KEY TERMS

Id Personality process that wants to experience only pleasure, is impulsive, and without morals

Ego Personality process that focuses on reality while striving to meet the needs of the id. The ego experiences anxiety and uses defense mechanisms for protection.

Superego Personality process that is concerned with right and wrong; the conscience. It provides the ego with an inner control to help cope with the id.

Consciousness State of awareness

Unconscious Memories, conflicts, experiences, and material cannot be recalled at will and are said to be repressed

Preconscious Memories that can be recalled to consciousness with some effort

Transference Unconscious emotional reaction to a current situation that is actually based on previous experiences

Free association In a therapeutic context, saying anything that comes to mind

Euphoria Complete lack of tension, an exaggerated sense of well being or happiness

Terror State of extreme tension

Satisfaction Relaxation of the tension of physiological needs

Interpersonal security Relaxation of the tension of anxiety

Irrational beliefs Beliefs that are not logical but influence feelings and behaviors

Primary appraisal Judgment an individual makes about an event

Secondary appraisal Evaluation an individual makes about potential actions to be taken

Reappraisal Appraisal made after new or additional information has been received

---

to bring about behavior. When these processes function in harmony, the individual experiences stability. When disharmony occurs, the individual is in conflict. The individual is all *id* at birth, wanting to experience only pleasure. This instinctual drive is known as the *pleasure principle*. Seeking pleasure involves *primary process thinking*, which enables the individual to strive for pleasure through the use of fantasies and images. The id is compulsive and without morals. The *ego* controls id impulses and mediates between the id and reality.

The ego focuses on the *reality principle* and strives to meet the demands of the id while maintaining the well-being of the individual by distinguishing fantasy from environmental reality. *Secondary process thinking* comprises rational, logical thinking and intelligence. The ego is the part of the personality that experiences anxiety and uses defense mechanisms for protection. Heredity, environmental factors, and maturation influence the formation of the ego.

The *superego* is concerned with right and wrong; that is, the conscience. It provides the ego with an inner control to help cope with the id. The superego is formed from the internalization of what parents teach their children about right and wrong through rewards and punishments. Self-esteem is affected by the perception of one's actions as good or right.

Guilt and inferiority are experienced if the individual cannot live up to parental standards. Inner conflict results when the id, the ego, and the superego are striving for different goals.

Consciousness

Freud's concepts of the levels of consciousness are central in understanding problems of the personality and behavior. *Consciousness*, or material within an individual's awareness, is only one small part of the mind. The *unconscious* is a larger area and consists of memories, conflicts, experiences, and material that have been repressed and cannot be recalled at will. *Preconscious* material refers to memories that can be recalled to consciousness with some effort. Freud believed that uncovering unconscious material generates an understanding of behavior that enables individuals to make choices about behavior and thus improve mental health. Insight into the meaning of symptoms and behaviors facilitates change.

Defense mechanisms

The ego usually copes with anxiety by rational means. When anxiety is too painful, the individual copes by using defense mechanisms to protect the

TABLE 3-1   Therapeutic Models

Model	Assumptions	Goals/Approaches	Dialogue
Psychoanalytical (Freud)	Individuals are motivated by unconscious desires and conflicts. Personality is developed by early childhood. Illness results from childhood conflicts and ego defenses inadequate to cope with anxiety. Change is a process of *insight*.	Insight into unconscious conflicts and processes. Personality reconstruction. Use of free association, dream analysis, and analyses of transference and resistance	Patient: All women hate me. Immediate response: Tell me about one woman you are having trouble with. *Insight*-oriented response: Tell me about your relationship with your mother.
Developmental (Erikson)	Biological, psychological, social, and environmental factors influence personality development throughout the life cycle. *Growth* involves resolution of critical tasks at each of the eight developmental stages. Lack of resolution of tasks results in incomplete development and difficulties in relationships. Change involves reexperiencing and resolving developmental crises. Change is a process of *growth*.	Mastery of developmental tasks through achievement of insight; continued development through death. Analysis of developmental issues, fears, and barriers to *growth* to achieve insight. Facilitation of mastery of developmental tasks with support and problem solving	Patient: I can't do anything right. Help me. Immediate response: I hear your doubt in yourself. But I did see you make a positive decision this morning. *Growth*-oriented response: I can help you look at ways to develop your self-confidence.
Interpersonal (Sullivan, Peplau)	Interpersonal relationships and anxiety facilitate development of the self system. Development occurs in stages with changing types of relationships. Faulty patterns of relating interfere with security and maturity. Security operations protect against anxiety and interfere with learning. Change is a process of *reeducation*.	Development of satisfactory relationships and maturity. Relative freedom from the interference of anxiety. Learning effective interpersonal skills. Examination of current interpersonal difficulties. Use of therapist-patient relationships as a vehicle for analyzing interpersonal processes and testing new skills. Consensual validation, validation, reality testing, and reflecting positive appraisals	Patient: I can't sit still. I'm too nervous. Immediate response: Let's take a walk for a few minutes. *Reeducation* response: Let's talk about what kind of things make you nervous and what you can do about them.

Model	Assumptions	Goals/Interventions	Clinical Example
Cognitive-Behavioral (Beck, Ellis)	An individual has value simply because he exists. Individuals have potential for *rational* and irrational thinking. Irrational beliefs produce irrational emotions and behaviors. Change involves changing beliefs in order to change feelings and behaviors. Change is a process of *rational* thinking.	Substitution of *rational* beliefs for irrational ones. Elimination of self-defeating behaviors. Increased responsibility for feelings, behaviors, and change. Challenging of irrational beliefs. Cognitive homework. Role playing and testing out new behaviors.	Patient: My wife makes me so angry. Immediate response: What did your wife do that you chose to get angry about? Cognitive-behavioral response: What is self-defeating about the statement you just made?
Reality Therapy (Glasser)	An individual's most basic psychological needs are to be loved (to be involved) and to feel worthwhile (to have respect from self and others). Meeting these needs must be done responsibly and within the context of reality. Responsibility is fulfilling one's own needs without interfering with others fulfilling their needs. Illness results from irresponsible behavior. Change is a process of *relearning*.	Facing reality and developing standards for behaving responsibly. Greater maturity, conscientiousness, and responsibility. Being accountable for one's behaviors. Being open, warm, honest, authentic, and accepting of the patient as a person. Becoming deeply involved with the patient. Focusing on current behaviors and consequences. Confronting irresponsible behaviors. Assisting with relearning of responsible behaviors.	Patient: The stupid doctor revoked my weekend pass. Immediate response: What did you do that showed you were not ready for a pass? Relearning response: What behaviors do you think will be necessary before you will be given a pass?
Stress (Selye, Lazarus)	A stress is any positive or negative occurrence or emotion requiring a response. Stress produces physiological and psychological responses. Inadequate handling of stress can lead to physical and/or mental illness. Change is a process of *problem solving*.	Developing effective coping mechanisms. Reduction of bodily tensions. Increasing resources and social supports. Stress management. Biofeedback. Relaxation training.	Patient: I'm so tense I can't sleep. Immediate response: I have a relaxation exercise I can show you. Problem-solving approach: You've said you're worried about seeing your family tomorrow. Let's talk about what you might say to them.

ego and to diminish anxiety. When these mechanisms are used excessively individuals are unable to face reality and do not solve their problems. Defense mechanisms are primarily unconscious behaviors; however, some are within voluntary control. Some common defense mechanisms are described in Table 3-2.

Painful feelings connected with childhood conflicts are often repressed. Later in life as similar conflicts are once again experienced, repression fails and these feelings emerge, causing anxiety and discomfort. Freud defined three kinds of anxiety that form the basis of many mental illnesses. Reality anxiety stems from an external real threat. Neurotic anxiety deals with the fear that instincts will cause one to do something to invite punishment such as being promiscuous. Moral anxiety deals with guilt that is experienced if one acts contrary to the conscience such as stealing money from a friend.

Goals of psychoanalysis

The goals of Freudian psychoanalytical therapy are to bring the unconscious into consciousness so that individuals can work through the past and understand their past and present behavior. By overcoming repression and resistance to exploring feelings and thoughts, childhood experiences can be analyzed. Uncovering the causes of current behaviors leads to insight. Only then will individuals be able to decrease their self-defeating behaviors and improve their mental health.

Therapist's Role

The therapist uses free association (letting the patient say everything that comes to mind) so that repressed material can be identified and interpreted for patients. Dream analysis helps patients uncover the meaning of dreams, which also increases awareness about present behavior. Patients' inconsistencies and resistance to therapy are confronted. Transference that occurs in the relationship is used to encourage working through feelings that would otherwise remain unconscious.

Relevance to Nursing Practice

In brief therapeutic encounters the nurse must recognize and understand maladaptive defense mechanisms used by patients. The nurse carefully points out these mechanisms and works with patients to decrease these behaviors and increase adaptive ones. In long-term relationships patients can be assisted with learning to think, feel, and behave according to their own individual values, beliefs, and needs—not according to someone else's. Patients may also need assistance with accepting their desires and drives as normal human phenomena for which they need not feel guilt or shame and with choosing acceptable ways of expressing their desires and drives.

DEVELOPMENTAL MODEL

Erik Erikson (Erikson, 1963; Erikson, 1968) built upon Freud's psychoanalytic model by including psychosocial and environmental influences along with the Freudian psychosexual concepts. His developmental model spans the total life cycle from birth to death. He believed that each of his eight stages of development afforded opportunities for growth, even up to the acceptance of one's own death.

Key Concepts

Each stage of development is an emotional crisis involving positive and negative experiences. Growth or mastery of critical tasks is the result of having more positive than negative experiences. Nonmastery of tasks inhibits movement to the next stage. Erikson believed that the drive of humans to live and grow is opposed by a drive to return to comfortable earlier states, even the one before birth; therefore, he saw regression as a possibility.

Implied but not clearly described in Erikson's model is the concept of partial mastery of critical tasks in development. The degree of mastery of each stage is related to the degree of maturity attained by the adult. Deficits in development carried from one stage to the next progressively interfere with functioning until the individual is no longer capable of growing without emotionally returning to an earlier stage in order to resolve the crisis. For example, a person may develop enough trust in others to engage in superficial relationships but may not be able to develop intimacy with a spouse. Another person may have enough initiative to accept a job but lacks the industry to stay with it. An environmental or social tragedy can shake the early foundations of

Table 3-2 Defense Mechanisms

Defense Mechanism	Definition	Common Example	Patient Example
Repression	Unconscious and involuntary forgetting of painful ideas, events, and conflicts	A car accident victim is unable to remember details of the impact, but was aware at the time.	Mrs. Young, a victim of incest, does not know why she has always hated her uncle.
Denial	Unconscious refusal to admit an unacceptable idea or behavior	A student refuses to admit that she is flunking a course despite an F on the first exam.	Mr. Davis, who is alcohol dependent, states that he can control his drinking.
Suppression	Voluntary exclusion from awareness, anxiety-producing feelings, ideas, and situations	A student states, "I cannot think about my wedding tonight. I have to study."	Michelle states to the nurse that she is not ready to talk about her recent divorce.
Rationalization	Attempts to make or prove that one's feelings or behaviors are justifiable	A student states, "I got a C on the test because the teacher asked poor questions."	Mr. Jones, a paranoid schizophrenic, states that he cannot go to work because he is afraid of his co-workers instead of admitting that he is mentally ill.
Intellectualization	Using only logical explanations without feelings or an affective component	A wife states to her husband that a dented car fender is much better than a completely wrecked car and garage door.	Mrs. Mann talks about her son's death and bout with cancer as being mercifully short without showing any signs of sadness.
Identification	A conscious or unconscious attempt to model oneself after a respected person	When a little girl dresses up like her mother to play house, she tries to talk and act like her mother.	Sheila states to the nurse, "When I get out of the hospital, I want to be a nurse just like you."
Introjection	Unconsciously incorporating wishes, values, and attitudes of others as if they were your own	While her mother is gone, a young girl disciplines her brother just like her mother would.	Without realizing it, a patient talks and acts like his therapist, analyzing other patients.
Compensation	Covering up for a weakness by overemphasizing or making up a desirable trait	An academically weak high school student becomes a star in the school play.	A schizophrenic patient who is unable to talk to other patients becomes known for his expressive poetry.
Reaction formation	A conscious behavior that is the exact opposite of an unconscious feeling	An older brother who dislikes his younger brother sends him gifts for every holiday.	Miss Marla, who unconsciously hates her mother, continuously tells staff how wonderful her mother is.
Sublimation	Channeling instinctual drives into acceptable activities	An adolescent arrested once for stealing later opens a business installing security systems in banks.	A former perpetrator of incest who fears relapse initiates a local chapter of Parents United.

Continued.

Table 3-2   Defense Mechanisms—cont'd

Defense Mechanism	Definition	Common Example	Patient Example
Displacement	Discharging pent-up feelings to a less threatening object	A husband comes home and yells at his wife after a bad day at work.	Mrs. Faust screams at another patient after being told by her psychiatrist that she cannot have a weekend pass.
Projection	Blaming someone else for one's difficulties or placing one's unethical desires on someone else	A teenager comes home late from a date and states that her friend did not bring her home on time.	Katrina states that she used marijuana while on pass because her boyfriend made her smoke it.
Conversion	The unconscious expression of intrapsychic conflict symbolically through physical symptoms	A student awakens with a migraine the morning of a final examination and feels too ill to take it. She does not realize that 1 hour of cramming left her unprepared.	Mr. Jenson suddenly develops impotence after his wife discovers he is having an affair with his secretary.
Undoing	Doing something to counteract or make up for a transgression or wrongdoing	After spanking her son, a mother bakes his favorite cookies.	After eating another patient's cookies, Mrs. Donnelly apologizes to the patients, cleans the refrigerator, and labels everyone's snack with their names.
Dissociation	The unconscious separation of painful feelings and emotions from an unacceptable idea, situation, or object	A young wife talks about her husband's extensive gambling debts as if they were nothing to be concerned about.	A patient recalls that when she was sexually molested as a child, she felt as if she were outside of her body watching what was happening without feeling anything.
Regression	Return to an earlier and more comfortable developmental level	A 6-year-old wets the bed at night since the birth of his baby sister.	Mr. Hivey has isolated himself in his room and has lain in a fetal position since his admission.

development, such as when divorce from a spouse threatens the individual's sense of trust in others and results in self-doubt.

Mastery of the critical tasks of each stage occurs more easily when it is chronologically appropriate. Overcoming delayed or incomplete development is difficult but possible.

Relevance to Nursing Practice

Most psychiatric patients demonstrate developmental delays or only partial mastery of the developmental stages preceding the stage expected for their chronological age. The nurse conducts an assessment of the patients' level of functioning through the interpretation of verbal and nonverbal behaviors and identifies the degree of mastery of each stage up to the patient's chronological age. The behavioral manifestations of problems are clues to issues to be addressed in working with the patient. Although Erikson focused on the polarity of each developmental stage (e.g., trust-mistrust), as if the "positive" pole were the desirable task to be accomplished, it is now recognized that the extremes of either pole produce problems in functioning. For example, being overly trusting can result in being repeatedly taken advantage of by others. Adult manifestations of Erikson's stages are listed in Table 3-3. Nursing interventions with specific developmental issues are discussed in Chapter 11 on the nurse-patient relationship and in the chapters on specific disorders.

INTERPERSONAL MODEL

Harry Stack Sullivan (1953) developed a comprehensive examination of interpersonal relationships called the *interpersonal theory of psychiatry*. He considered the healthy person as a social being with the ability to live effectively in relationships with others. Mental illness was viewed as any degree of lack of awareness of the processes in interpersonal relationships. Relationships were viewed as the source of anxiety, maladaptive behaviors, and personality formation.

Key Concepts

Sullivan conceived of the personality as an energy system in which the main goal is to reduce tension.

He identified three types of tension: the *tension of needs* (stemming from the physiochemical requirements of life), the *tension of anxiety* (stemming from interpersonal situations), and the *tension of need for sleep*. Theoretically, a person could vary from a state of complete lack of tension (euphoria) to a state of terror as a result of extreme tension, but Sullivan doubted that the pure extremes existed for very long after birth. The relaxation of the tension of needs is experienced as *satisfaction*, and the relaxation of the tension of anxiety is experienced as *interpersonal security* (Sullivan, 1953).

Self-system

Sullivan labeled the personality a "self-system" that develops relatively enduring patterns for avoiding or minimizing anxiety during interpersonal encounters and the meeting of biological needs. He believed that anxiety can be communicated empathically from one person to another. Anxiety activates behaviors that reduce it and helps individuals to differentiate among experiences (a process of learning). Severe anxiety (or panic) does not convey information and produces confusion, even to the point of amnesia (Sullivan, 1953). Less severe anxiety informs the individual of the different situations that cause and relieve tension. As the self-system is developing in infancy, it is initially organized into the "good me" when needs are satisfied, the "bad me" when needs are unmet and anxiety persists, and "not me" when anxiety is severe and information is not completely integrated into the personality on a conscious level.

As the infant moves to early childhood and develops language, the separate personifications of the self as good and bad begin to fuse into a sense of a whole individual with different behaviors in different situations. However, feedback from others (reflected appraisals) continues to shape the child's self-concept in positive and negative ways.

Since infants are unable to avoid "bad" caregivers or anxiety-producing situations, mechanisms called *security operations* develop to protect them from anxiety. In *somnolent detachment*, sleep is used to avoid the anxiety. *Apathy* is an emotional detachment or numbing, even though the experiences are remembered. *Selective inattention* is a process of tuning out details associated with anxiety-producing situations. *Dissociation* prevents situations from integrating into

Table 3-3   Adult Manifestations of Erikson's Stages of Development

Life Stage	Adult Behaviors Reflecting Mastery	Adult Behaviors Reflecting Developmental Problems
I. Trust vs. mistrust (0 to 18 months)	Realistic trust of self and others Confidence in others Optimism and hope Shares openly with others Relates to others effectively	Suspiciousness/testing of others Fear of criticism and affection Dissatisfaction and hostility Projection of blame and feelings Withdrawal from others *or* Overly trusting of others Naive and gullible Shares too quickly and easily
II. Autonomy vs. shame and doubt (18 months to 3 years)	Self-control and willpower Realistic self-concept and self-esteem Pride and a sense of goodwill Simple cooperativeness Generosity tempered by withholding Delayed gratification when necessary	Self-doubt/self-conciousness Dependence on others for approval Feeling of being exposed/attacked Sense of being out of control of the self and one's life Obsessive-compulsive behaviors *or* Excessive independence or defiance, grandiosity Denial of problems Unwillingness to ask for help Impulsiveness/inability to wait Reckless disregard for safety of self and others
III. Initiative vs. guilt (3 to 5 years)	An adequate conscience Initiative balanced with restraint Appropriate social behaviors Curiosity and exploration Healthy competitiveness Sense of direction Original and purposeful activities	Excessive guilt/embarrassment Passivity and apathy Avoidance of activities/pleasures Rumination and self-pity Assuming a role as victim/self-punishment Reluctance to show emotions Underachievement of potential *or* Lack of follow-through on plans Little sense of guilt for actions Excessive expression of emotion Labile emotions Excessive competitiveness/showing off
IV. Industry vs. inferiority (6 to 12 years)	Sense of competence Completion of projects Pleasure in effort and effectiveness Ability to cooperate and compromise Identification with admired others Joy of involvement in the world and with others Balance of work and play	Feeling unworthy and inadequate Poor work history (quitting, being fired, lack of promotions, absenteeism, lack of productivity) Inadequate problem-solving skills Manipulation of others/violation of others' rights Lack of friends of the same sex *or* Overly high-achieving/perfectionistic Reluctance to try new things for fear of failing

Stage	Adaptive Behaviors	Maladaptive Behaviors
V. Identity vs. role diffusion (12 to 18 or 20 years)	Confident sense of self Emotional stability Commitment to career planning and realistic long-term goals Sense of having a place in society Establishing relationship with the opposite sex Fidelity to friends Development of personal values Testing out adult roles	Feeling unable to gain love or affection unless totally successful Being a workaholic Lack of or giving up of goals, beliefs, values, productive roles Feelings of confusion, indecision, and alienation Vacillation between dependence and independence Superficial, short-term relationships with the opposite sex *or* Dramatic overconfidence Acting-out behaviors (including alcohol and drug use) Flamboyant display of sex role behaviors
VI. Intimacy vs. isolation (18 to 25 or 30 years)	Ability to give and receive love Commitments and mutuality with others Collaboration in work and affiliations Sacrificing for others Responsible sexual behaviors	Persistent aloneness/isolation Emotional distance in all relationships Prejudices against others Lack of established vocation; many career changes Seeking of intimacy through casual sexual encounters *or* Possessiveness and jealousy Dependency of parents and/or partner Abusiveness toward loved ones Inability to try new things socially or vocationally (staying in routine/mundane job and activities)
VII. Generative life-style vs. stagnation or self-absorption (30 to 65 years)	Productive, constructive, creative activity Personal and professional growth Parental and societal responsibilities	Self-centeredness/self-indulgence Exaggerated concern for appearance and possessions Lack of interest in the welfare of others Lack of civic and professional activities/responsibilities Loss of interest in marriage and/or extramarital affairs *or* Too many professional or community activities to the detriment of the family or self
VIII. Integrity vs. despair (65 years to death)	Feelings of self-acceptance Sense of dignity, worth, and importance Adaptation to life according to limitations Valuing one's life Sharing of wisdom Exploration of philosophy of life and death	Sense of helplessness, hopelessness, worthlessness, uselessness, and/or meaninglessness Withdrawal and loneliness Regression Focusing on past mistakes, failures, and dissatisfactions Feeling too old to start over Suicidal ideas or apathy Inability to occupy self with satisfying activities (hobbies, volunteer work, social events) *or* Inability to reduce activities Overtaxing strength and abilities Feeling indispensable Denial of death as inevitable

Developed by L. Schwecke and S. Wood, Indiana University. Revised 1997.

conscious awareness. Another operation to reduce anxiety is to convert it to anger. The powerlessness experienced with anxiety is exchanged for a temporary feeling of power associated with anger directed outwardly.

While these security operations protect against anxiety, they also interfere with the learning that normally occurs in interpersonal interactions (the socialization processes). For example, a child may use selective inattention to "tune out" a mother's suggestion about a more effective way to express anger. *Focal awareness,* or the ability to grasp the details and meanings of situations and the behaviors of others, is necessary for adequate learning. *Consensual validation* is a process of verifying the accuracy of perceptions and meanings of events with others involved in those situations.

Personality development

Sullivan's model includes a sequence of personality development focusing on tools or behaviors needed to accomplish developmental tasks. In infancy (birth to 1½ years), for example, crying is a tool used to establish contact with others so that children can learn to count on others. In childhood (1½ to 6 years), language assists with learning to delay the gratification of needs. In the juvenile period (6 to 9 years), competition, compromise, and cooperation are tools for developing relationships with peers. In preadolescence (9 to 12 years), collaboration and the capacity for love assist in the development of a "chum" relationship with a person of the same sex. These same tools, with sexual desire, facilitate learning to establish relationships with members of the opposite sex in early adolescence (12 to 14 years). The independence developed in early adolescence moves toward interdependence in late adolescence (14 to 21 years), and individuals learn to form lasting sexual relationships (Sullivan, 1953). Sullivan's development model did not describe changes beyond late adolescence.

Therapist's Role

For Sullivan the focus of therapy is on patients' current interpersonal relationships and experiences. The goal of the therapy is to develop mature and satisfactory relationships *relatively* free from anxiety. The therapist-patient relationship is a vehicle for analyzing the patient's interpersonal processes and testing out new skills in relating (Grinspoon, 1993). The therapist takes an active role as a "participant observer" in experiencing patients' interpersonal problems. Although the focus of therapy is on patients' here-and-now problems, distortions created by past experiences, especially "not me" experiences, are often revealed. The therapist helps correct these distortions with clear communications, consensual validation, and presentation of reality. In challenging a negative self-image, the therapist presents appraisals of patients as worthwhile, respectable individuals with rights, dignity, and valuable abilities. The focus of sessions is often on loneliness, fear of rejection, clarification of emotions and their causes, use of anxiety for learning about the self and others, management of interpersonal frustrations, and development of self-respect.

Relevance to Nursing Practice

Hildegard Peplau (1952, 1963) played a significant role in applying Sullivan's concepts to nursing practice. Peplau saw a major goal of nursing as helping patients to reduce their anxiety and convert it to constructive action. She elaborated on and applied to nursing Sullivan's concept of degrees of anxiety ("pure" euphoria, mild anxiety, moderate anxiety, severe anxiety, panic, terror states, and "pure" anxiety [Peplau, 1963]). Peplau described the effects of mild anxiety through panic levels on perception and learning (Chapter 13). She saw the nurse's role as helping patients decrease insecurity and improve functioning through interpersonal relationships that can be seen as microcosms of the way patients function in other relationships (Thompson, 1986). Specific applications of Sullivan's work as proposed by Peplau are presented in Chapter 11.

COGNITIVE-BEHAVIORAL MODELS

Aaron Beck's cognitive therapy (1967) and Albert Ellis's rational-emotive therapy (RET) (1973) models focus on thinking and behaving rather than on the expression of feelings. These models use a cognitive approach based on individual abilities to think, judge, decide, analyze, and do. Unlike Freud, who saw symptoms of disturbance as having been produced by childhood experiences, Ellis and Beck view individuals' present perceptions, thoughts, assumptions, beliefs, values, attitudes, and philosophies as needing modification or change (Beck, 1976; Ellis, 1973). Even distorted thinking learned from others in childhood can be unlearned. Individuals should value themselves simply because they exist and should not judge themselves by how they perform or by how they are rated by themselves and others.

Key Concepts

Beck and Ellis believe that individuals think both rationally and irrationally and that it is the *irrational beliefs* or *automatic thoughts* that cause problems because self-defeating behaviors are maintained. They also believe that individuals are capable of understanding their limitations and can change their values and beliefs while challenging their self-defeating behaviors. Emotional disturbances are produced by the repetition of irrational thoughts that keep dysfunctional behaviors operant. Individuals who blame themselves and others, and think and feel that something is "bad," maintain emotional disturbance. RET teaches individuals to stop blaming themselves and to accept themselves as they are with flaws and imperfections. Anxiety can be avoided by learning to change inappropriate emotions and self-defeating behaviors. RET attacks problems from a cognitive, emotive, and behavioral standpoint by using the A-B-C theory of personality. *A* is the *activating event; B* is the *belief about A;* and *C* is the *emotional reaction. A* (event) does not cause *C* (emotions); rather *B* (our irrational beliefs about *A*), causes *C*. Intervention, then, is aimed at *B* (our irrational beliefs) and is called *D*, or disputing and changing irrational beliefs (Ellis, 1973). Similarly, Beck proposed examining the distorted perceptions, erroneous beliefs, self deceptions and blind spots that lead to "excessive, inappropriate emotional reactions" to events or stimuli (Beck, 1976). Reality testing and problem solving are aimed at correcting faulty cognitions and processes so that the individual develops "more realistic appraisals of himself and his world" (Beck, 1976).

According to Ellis (1973) and Beck (1976), the following are some irrational beliefs and inappropriate rules for living that most individuals subscribe to:

- That one should feel loved and approved by everyone
- That one must be totally competent in order to be considered worthwhile

- That people have little ability to change or to control their feelings
- That influences of the past should definitely determine feelings in the present
- That rejection or unfair treatment has catastrophic consequences
- That it is terrible to be mediocre and unpopular
- That one is disliked when there is a disagreement with another
- That one should never make mistakes
- That people who are obnoxious should be judged as rotten or bad
- That it is easier to be passive in life than to confront difficulties and responsibilities
- That life is awful if problems are not solved with the "right" or precise solution

Therapist's Role

The patient-therapist relationship is viewed as a collaborative effort to achieve goals for improved self esteem, coping, relationships, and life-styles (Beck, 1976). Because patients have many irrational "should's," "ought's," and "must's," the therapist challenges these beliefs actively and directly. The therapist demonstrates how illogical their thinking is. Humor often is used to confront the patient's irrational thinking. The therapist explains how to replace irrational thinking with rational thinking to reduce dysfunctional feelings and behaviors. The process of therapy focuses on the present. Patients learn to take responsibility for their ideas and behaviors and work to eliminate disturbing behaviors. The therapist accepts patients as they are and does not allow patients to rate or condemn themselves. Homework assignments are given to focus on skill development and positive statements and behaviors. New, positive self-statements are encouraged to enable patients to begin to think, feel, and behave differently. Role-playing and modeling are also employed.

Relevance to Nursing Practice

Nurses help patients to change irrational beliefs and to reduce stress and anxiety through effective problem solving. Patients have many self-deprecating or negative feelings about themselves that the nurse can dispute by pointing out specific positive behaviors. Awareness of these qualities or aspects can facilitate patients' beliefs that they are worthwhile and have valuable characteristics. Self-blame and guilt can be reduced, and patients can feel better about themselves. Patients who project blame can be shown that they alone are responsible for their behaviors. For example, alcoholics are very skillful at blaming others for their problems when, in fact, they alone are responsible for continuing to drink and for the problems that result from drinking.

Other patients who continually function according to "should's," "must's," and "ought's" can be taught to act according to their personal wants and beliefs. They need not condemn themselves for being their own persons. Their anxiety and hostile feelings toward themselves and others can be eliminated if they can achieve feelings of comfort about themselves.

REALITY THERAPY MODEL

William Glasser (1965) developed reality therapy because he believed patients and delinquents share the common characteristic of denying "the reality of the world around them" instead of fulfilling their needs responsibly within the context of reality and society. He defined responsibility as "the ability to fulfill one's needs, and to do so in a way that does not deprive others of the ability to fulfill their needs" (Glasser, 1965). Glasser recognized that he could not change patients' histories or past relationship problems but that he could help them change current behaviors so that their futures could improve. He found that an improved sense of responsibility leads to improved mental health.

Key Concepts

According to Glasser (1965), all individuals continually strive to meet their needs. The two major psychological needs are to love and be loved (to have relatedness) and to feel worthwhile (to have respect from the self and others). Implied in these needs are the needs for identity and involvement. Children develop a positive identity by being involved with others who teach right, wrong, and a sense of responsibility while conveying to children that they are worthwhile. Children then learn to be comfortable with and enjoy being around others.

Unfortunately, individuals do not always strive to meet their needs responsibly. There may be an "incapacity or failure at the interpersonal level of functioning" (Glasser, 1965). Glasser believed that illness results from behaving irresponsibly rather than the reverse and that anger, fear, depression, and anxiety are also the result of irresponsible behavior in relationships. Common forms of irresponsible behavior are violations of one's morals, values, or standards; misinforming others about oneself or one's needs (being dishonest); shunning others because of fear of rejection; lying to oneself by rationalizing and excusing one's own behavior; not accepting the consequences of one's behavior; blaming others for problems; and, eventually, losing contact with reality (by denying it). Suicide and denial are major ways of avoiding reality and responsibility. Short-term pleasures such as those derived from alcohol and drugs also interfere with long-term satisfaction and happiness.

Therapist's Role

The goal of reality therapy is to help patients face reality and then to develop responsible behavior patterns so their needs for love and worth can be met. Directing patients "toward greater maturity, conscientiousness, and responsibility" improves their potential for long-term happiness and pleasure (Glasser, 1965). Glasser emphasized the need for the therapist's authenticity, openness, honesty, responsibility, and deep involvement with patients. Initially patients need warmth and uncritical acceptance as worthwhile persons who are cared about even though their irresponsible behaviors, and the excuses for those behaviors, are not accepted. The unrealistic and irresponsible behaviors are actively confronted, even disciplined, while the patients as human beings and their positive behaviors are supported. Patients repeatedly evaluate whether or not their actions are getting the desired results and whether or not others are hurt in the process. Patients are asked to choose more effective behaviors and to design specific, realistic plans to try those behaviors. Plans that are not successful are revised until accountability and responsibility are achieved.

Relevance to Nursing Practice

Psychiatric nurses are regularly involved in helping patients to identify reality and what interferes with effectively meeting their needs. Reality testing is a common nursing intervention. Nurses are routinely responsible for explaining the rules of the program or unit and for outlining expected, appropriate, and inappropriate behaviors. The milieu of the program or unit is normally designed to foster improvements in independence and responsibility, which are rewarded with increases in privileges and freedom. Setting limits on unacceptable (irresponsible) behaviors benefits patients in the long term.

Even without labeling behaviors as irresponsible, nurses are accustomed to helping patients examine the consequences of specific behaviors, especially in current relationships. Supportive confrontation encourages patients to make their own decisions about changes, choose their own solutions, and test out new behaviors. This type of relearning process is described in Chapter 11 on the nurse-patient relationship.

STRESS MODELS

Stress theories provide nurses with a framework for understanding how stress affects individuals and their responses. The ability to adapt to stress leads to conflict resolution, whereas the inability to adapt effectively may result in physiological or mental disorders, or even death.

Key Concepts

Selye's stress-adaptation theory

Selye defined stress as wear and tear on the body. He developed a framework, the stress-adaptation theory, to explain the physiological response to stress (Selye, 1956). Selye viewed stressors as any positive or negative occurrence, or any emotion requiring a response. Interaction with the environment and others inevitably produces stress. The type of response elicited depends on individual perception of the stressor. However, Selye discovered that by objectively measuring structural and chemical changes in the body, many individuals demonstrate the same symptoms regardless of the stressor. These changes became known as the general adaptation syndrome (GAS) and occur in three stages: alarm, resistance, and exhaustion. Selye did not elaborate on psychosocial changes, but his three stages can be correlated with the levels of anxiety (Chap-

ter 13). The three stages of GAS are summarized in Table 3-4.

In this text psychosocial changes are emphasized because sleep and weight disturbances are primarily the only physical changes that nurses can assess and evaluate.

Alarm reaction

The impingement of any kind of stressor on individuals activates the preparation for "fight or flight." Individuals experience an increase in alertness in order to focus on the immediate task or threat, and to mobilize resources and defenses to concentrate on the particular stressor. The levels of anxiety experienced are mild (1+) to moderate (2+). Learning and problem solving can occur. If the stressor continues, or is not adaptively or effectively resolved, individuals experience the next stage.

Stage of resistance

In this stage individuals strive to adapt to stress. For adaptation to occur, the use of coping and defense mechanisms is increased. Problem solving and learning are difficult but can be accomplished with assistance. Psychosomatic symptoms begin to develop. The levels of anxiety experienced are moderate (2+) to severe (3+). If individuals are overwhelmed by the stressor, they experience the next stage.

Stage of exhaustion

Exhaustion results from stress that lasts too long or is overwhelming, or may result from the individual's total inability to cope. Anxiety is experienced at the severe (3+) to panic (4+) levels. Defenses are exaggerated and dysfunctional, and the personality becomes disorganized, thinking illogical, and decision making ineffective. Delusions and hallucinations can occur with sensory misperception and a greatly reduced orientation to reality. Individuals may become violent, suicidal, or may be completely immobilized. In case of immobilization, a severe level of anxiety may occur though individuals may not appear to be visibly anxious. Death may occur if exhaustion continues without intervention.

Lazarus's interactional theory

In contrast to Selye's emphasis on the physiologic effects of stress, Lazarus (1966) focuses on the psychological aspects. He views psychological stress as "a

Table 3-4 **The Stress Adaptation Syndrome**

Stage	Physical Changes	Psychosocial Changes
Stage I: Alarm reaction Mobilization of the body's defensive forces and activation of the "fight-or-flight" mechanism	Release of norepinephrine and epinephrine causing vasoconstriction, increased blood pressure, and increased rate and force of cardiac contraction Increased hormone levels Enlargement of adrenal cortex Marked loss of body weight Shrinkage of the thymus, spleen, and lymph nodes Irritation of the gastric mucosa	Increased level of alertness Increased level of anxiety Task-oriented, defense-oriented, inefficient, or maladaptive behavior may occur
Stage II: Stage of resistance Optimal adaptation to stress within the person's capabilities	Hormone levels readjust Reduction in activity and size of adrenal cortex Lymph nodes return to normal size Weight returns to normal	Increased and intensified use of coping mechanisms Tendency to rely on defense-oriented behavior
Stage III: Stage of exhaustion Loss of ability to resist stress because of depletion of body resources	Decreased immune response with suppression of T cells and atrophy of thymus Depletion of adrenal glands and hormone production Weight loss Enlargement of lymph nodes and dysfunction of lymphatic system If exposure to the stressor continues, cardiac failure, renal failure, or death may occur	Defense-oriented behaviors become exaggerated Disorganization of thinking Disorganization of personality Sensory stimuli may be misperceived with appearance of illusion Reality contact may be reduced with appearance of delusions or hallucinations If exposure to the stressor continues, stupor or violence may occur

From Kneisl CR and Ames SW: *Adult health nursing: a biopsychosocial approach,* Menlo Park, Calif., 1986, Addison-Wesley.

relationship between the person and the environment that is appraised by the person as taxing or exceeding his or her resources and endangering his or her well-being" (Lazarus and Folkman, 1984). Lazarus believes that the basis of coping is not due to anxiety per se but to the appraisal of threat. "Anxiety is the response to threat" (Lazarus, 1966). The significance of the threat or what it means to the individual is of primary importance. Stressors are perceived differently by different individuals. For one person an event may be viewed as a challenge; for another it may be viewed as a severe threat or problem. This personal evaluation of a stressor or event is based on cognitive appraisal.

There are three kinds of cognitive appraisal. *Primary appraisal* refers to the judgment individuals make about a particular event: What does it mean personally? What are its effects? *Secondary appraisal* is the individual's evaluation of how to respond to an event. Possible strategies or solutions, as well as resources and supports, are examined. *Reappraisal* is simply appraisal made after new or additional information has been received.

Numerous personal and environmental factors influence appraisal: commitments, beliefs, values, feelings, emotions, and views of what is important. A seemingly appropriate solution may not be useful because it conflicts with individual values and beliefs. For example, a passive wife may be unable to be assertive and confrontive with her husband because she was taught and believes that women should be quiet and submissive to their husbands.

Stressful events often create demands with which individuals cannot effectively cope. Sometimes personal resources or social supports are not adequate. Preferred methods of coping may be ineffective in resolving the problem and actually lead to or result in more problems. Ineffective coping and the creation of additional problems result in additional stress and lead to physical illness, mental illness, or both.

Critical Thinking Questions

1. How can an understanding of the theoretical models assist you in working with psychiatric patients?
2. Which concepts and strategies derived from each of the theoretical models have you observed being used with patients?

Relevance to Nursing Practice

Stress theories provide a framework for the nurse to assess the effects of stress on patients and their coping processes. To assist patients with developing adaptive or effective coping methods, nurses must help patients to identify and evaluate palliative, maladaptive, and dysfunctional behaviors so that patients are aware of the consequences of their behavior. Palliative mechanisms decrease the emotions without solving the problems. Maladaptive mechanisms do not manage the emotions sufficiently and do not solve the problems. Dysfunctional mechanisms create new or additional problems. (For additional explanation, see Chapter 13).

Patients' appraisal of stressors or problems include what the stressors mean to them, what resources or supports they have to help them cope, and how their beliefs and values influence that coping. In considering what stressors mean to patients, the nurse can facilitate cognitive restructuring or problem solving by helping patients to choose adaptive and appropriate coping behaviors. At times the nurse will need to help initiate, encourage, and motivate patients to use adaptive behaviors. Together, the patient and the nurse can then evaluate the ef-

fectiveness of strategies used. When patients exhibit behaviors found in Selye's stage of exhaustion or are primarily using dysfunctional coping, the nurse is able to assess patients' inability to take constructive action; it may be necessary for the nurse to make decisions on behalf of patients. After patients gain some control over their behavior, they can benefit from stress management (Mandarino and Brown, 1992), problem solving, relaxation training, and biofeedback (Hahn, et al., 1993), depending on which method is needed.

ECLECTIC APPROACH

Most psychiatric nurses adopt an eclectic approach with the theoretical models presented in this chapter. They pick concepts from various models that best explain a patient's behaviors, problems, and needs. Each model uses different terms to explain similar phenomenon. Table 3-5 shows how each theoretical model would describe the patient's verbal and nonverbal behaviors.

Critical Thinking Question

You are working with a patient who is recently divorced, afraid of making decisions, and suicidal. Which combination of concepts from the various theorists would you use in planning your nursing interventions?

Key Concepts

1. Concepts from various theoretical models provide frameworks for understanding patients' behaviors and problems.
2. Extensive use of defense mechanisms and maladaptive coping behaviors are assessed and understood by the nurse as inhibitors of healthy or adaptive responses. The nurse then helps patients to develop adaptive coping responses or behaviors.
3. Unresolved developmental issues interfere with patients' ability to solve problems and meet their own needs. Therefore these issues must be addressed in the nurse-patient relationship.
4. Peplau used Sullivan's concepts of anxiety as a critical part of her framework in the nurse-patient relationship.
5. According to the cognitive-behavioral model, stress and anxiety can be reduced by replacing irrational beliefs with rational ones.

Table 3-5 Comparison of Theoretical Models

Patient Situation: Kim is a 28-year-old legal assistant, married, with no children. Her husband, Tony, is a 29-year-old lawyer who has told Kim that he is having an affair with Jamie and wants a divorce. Kim is talking to the nurse in her doctor's office and reveals the following behaviors:

Patient Verbal and Nonverbal Behaviors	Psychoanalytic	Developmental	Interpersonal	Cognitive-Behavioral	Reality	Stress
Initially, Kim expresses much hostility toward Tony for having an affair and accuses Jamie of causing the divorce.	• Projection of blame • Denial of her own role in the divorce • Ego anxiety	**Stage I** • Hostility • Projection of blame	• Difficulty maintaining a lasting sexual relationship • Tension of anxiety • Converting anxiety to anger	• Stimulus of divorce a) Irrational belief of blaming others b) Excess emotion of hostility	• Denying own responsibility for the divorce • Being dishonest with self and others • Anger at others	**Stage I** • Preparation for "fight" • Increased anxiety • Defense-oriented behaviors (denial, projection) **Stage II** • Intensified use of defensive coping behaviors (negativity, withdrawal)
Kim says that there is nothing left to her life and that all she does at home is cry and sleep.	• Superego guilt • Regression • Ego defense	**Stage I** • Dissatisfaction • Withdrawal	• Apathy • Crying—wishing for contact with others • Somnolent detachment	• Irrational belief about life being "awful"	• Feeling unloved • Loss of self-respect • Depression	
Kim describes not wanting to be seen by her friends, but at the same time wishing that others would tell her that she is still attractive.	• Superego guilt • Ego anxiety • Id desire	**Stage II** • Self-consciousness • Dependence on others for approval • Self-doubt	• Lack of self-respect • Need for positive reflected appraisals • Need for interpersonal security	• "Assumption" of possible rejection • Negative self-rating • Need to feel loved and approved of	• Fear of rejection • Loss of self-respect • Need to be loved • Need to feel worthwhile	**Stage I** • Activation of "flight" • Increased anxiety • Defense-oriented coping (withdrawal)
While showing no emotion, Kim then says that she just wants the divorce to be over so she can get on with her life. "If Tony can have sex with someone else, so can I."	• Intellectualization • Rationalization • Id impulse (pleasure principle)	**Stage III** • Reluctance to show emotion **Stage II** • Inability to wait • Impulsiveness • Disregard for safety of self	• Need for interpersonal security • Lack of delayed gratification • Tension of needs—sexual desire	• "Unrealistic appraisal" of divorce processes • Potential for self-defeating behaviors • Need to be loved	• Seeking involvement • Need to be loved • Irresponsibly violating one's morals	**Stage II** • Defense-oriented behaviors (rationalization) • Intensified inappropriate coping (revenge)
When the office nurse suggests to Kim that counseling could help her through the divorce, Kim says that she does not need counseling.	• Denial	**Stage II** • Denial of problems • Unwilling to ask for help	• Selective inattention to needs	• Self-defeating belief • Self-defeating behavior	• Being dishonest about needs • Lying to oneself	**Stage I** • Inefficient coping (denial) • Activation of "flight" mechanism

6. Facing reality and self-responsibility are major goals of reality therapy.
7. Stress models explain many of the physiological and psychological responses to stress and are a basis for stress-reduction strategies.

Study Questions

(Answer key is in the back of the book.)

Match the examples with the most appropriate defense mechanism.

1. __b__ "I told you that I do not want to talk about my boss now; maybe tomorrow."
2. __e__ "I do not have my list of goals because my pen ran out of ink."
3. __c__ Despite knowing about her husband's affair, the patient states, "My husband is such a good man. I love him."

    a. Denial
    b. Suppression
    c. Reaction formation
    d. Repression
    e. Rationalization

4. Mr. Lawrence tells the nurse that he has had three factory jobs in the last 8 months because he was too slow for the assembly line and his co-workers would not help him. He feels alone. He is having difficulty now with his ceramics project. With which developmental stage is Mr. Lawrence struggling?
   a. Autonomy vs. shame and doubt
   b. Initiative vs. guilt
   c. Industry vs. inferiority
   d. Intimacy vs. isolation
5. A new patient has had multiple stressors for a long time. You expect this patient to be in the stage of exhaustion (GAS) and show which behaviors?
   a. Personality disorganization, immobilization, suicide
   b. Increased alertness, mild anxiety, mobilization of resources
   c. Problem solving with assistance, somatic complaints
   d. Task-oriented behaviors, weight returns to normal
6. Using principles of cognitive behavioral therapy and reality therapy, the nurse working with patients would:
   a. Explain that irrational beliefs do not produce feelings of anxiety or hostility
   b. Encourage patients to shift blame to others when possible
   c. Support patients' denial so that grief is lessened
   d. Teach patients that they are responsible for themselves and for making appropriate choices.

REFERENCES

Beck AT: *Depression: chemical, experimental and theoretical aspects,* New York, 1967, Noeber Medical Division, Harper & Row.

Beck AT: *Cognitive therapies and the emotional disorders,* New York, 1976, International Universities Press.

Brill AA, editor: *The basic writings of Sigmund Freud,* New York, 1938, Random House.

Ellis A: *Humanistic psychotherapy: the rational-emotive approach,* New York, 1973, The Julian Press.

Erikson EH: *Childhood and society,* New York, 1963, WW Norton.

Erikson EH: *Identity: youth and crisis,* New York, 1968, WW Norton.

Freud S and Strachey J, editors: *The ego and the id,* New York, 1960, WW Norton.

Freud S: *The problem of anxiety,* New York, 1936, WW Norton.

Glasser W: *Reality therapy: a new approach to psychiatry,* New York, 1965, Harper & Row.

Grinspoon L: Interpersonal therapy, *Harvard MH Letter* 10(4):1, 1993.

Hahn YB, et al: The effect of thermal biofeedback and progressive muscle relaxation training in reducing blood pressure of patients with essential hypertension, *Image* 25(3):204, 1993.

Kneisl CR and Ames SW: *Adult health nursing: a biopsychosocial approach,* Menlo Park, Calif, 1986, Addison-Wesley.

Lazarus RS: *Psychological stress and the coping process,* St. Louis, 1966, McGraw-Hill.

Lazarus RS and Folkman S: *Stress, appraisal, and coping,* New York, 1984, Springer.

Mandarino MA and Brown MC: A practical, step-by-step approach to stress management for women, *Nurse Pract* 17(7):18, 1992.

Peplau HE: *Interpersonal relations in nursing,* New York, 1952, GP Putnam's Sons.

Peplau HE: A working definition of anxiety. In Burd SF and Marshall MA, editors: *Some clinical approaches to psychiatric nursing,* Toronto, 1963, Macmillan.

Selye H: *The stress life,* St. Louis, 1956, McGraw-Hill.

Sullivan HS: *Interpersonal theory of psychiatry,* New York, 1953, WW Norton.

Thompson L: Peplau's theory: an application to short-term therapy. *J Psychosoc Nurs Ment Health Serv* 24(8):26, 1986.

CHAPTER 4

Legal Issues

GARY M. CARROLL
NORMAN L. KELTNER *

LEARNING OBJECTIVES

After reading this chapter you should be able to:
- Identify landmark court rulings and their impact on psychiatric care.
- Distinguish the three categories of commitment.
- Define and apply the concept of *least restrictive alternative.*
- Define and apply the concept of *confidentiality.*
- Define and apply the concept of *freedom from restraint and seclusion.*
- Define and apply the concept of *the right to treatment and the right to refuse treatment.*

- Articulate the competing interests of individual rights and the state's interest in maintaining the health and safety of its citizens.
- Describe the liability of the nurse in issues such as wrongful commitment, duty to warn, and master-servant rule.
- Define the terms that apply to legal issues involved in health care.

Note to the student:

As a nurse, you must successfully navigate through a host of physical and psychological manifestations of illness as you arrive at the most appropriate course of intervention for your patients. This knowledge base is provided as a basic foundation in the nursing education process. Since nursing is about patient care, only a modicum of attention is given to legal issues in most nursing curricula. Legal issues, however, have now come to the forefront of public attention. The media, including some of the

most popular movies and television shows, revolve around legal issues and those who practice or are affected by them. Controversial cases such as those of the Oklahoma City bombing dominate the media. The general public as a result, has become far more sophisticated and aware of legal issues. Nurses who practice psychiatric nursing encounter special legal issues and concerns. In addition to achieving successful interventions, they must also apply the legal knowledge necessary to insure that the rights of the patient and society are safeguarded. In some cases, the correct intervention may be one dictated by law. This chapter reviews some of these issues, provides answers for others, and gives you the basis for safe, legal practice.

---

*This is a revision of a chapter originally written by Patricia Nord and Dorothy Dick Meyer.

KEY TERMS

Assault An act intended by the defendant to create a reasonable apprehension of harmful or offensive contact to another without consent.

Battery The harmful or offensive touching of another, the clothes of another, or anything else attached to another without consent.

Civil law This part of the legal system is concerned with the legal rights and duties of private persons. Civil lawsuits can recapture monetary loss from professionals who have been guilty of false imprisonment, defamation of character, assault and battery, or negligence.

Conservator One appointed by a court to manage the affairs of a person found to be incompetent and unable to manage his or her own affairs appropriately.

Gravely disabled Persons who are unable to provide food, clothing, or shelter for themselves because of a mental illness.

Informed consent Providing patients with information about specific treatments (including benefits, side effects, and possible risks) to enable them to make competent and voluntary decisions.

Involuntary commitment A commitment status in which a person who has the legal capacity to consent to mental health treatment refuses to do so and is involuntarily detained for treatment by the state. Three categories of involuntary commitment are: evaluation and emergency care, certification for observation and treatment, and extended or indeterminate care.

Least restrictive alternative/environment An environment that provides the necessary treatment requirements in the least restrictive setting possible. For example, a hospital setting is more restrictive than a board-and-care setting. If the board-and-care setting provides the necessary treatment requirements for a person, then that environment would represent the least restrictive alternative.

Liable Found responsible and answerable by law and compellable to make restitution or satisfaction.

Limited or Special Power of Attorney A power of attorney is a written document in which one person, the principal, authorizes another person, the attorney in fact, to act on the principal's behalf. In a limited power of attorney, the attorney in fact is granted only those powers specifically defined in the document.

Malpractice Negligence by a professional. Malpractice is a civil action that can be brought against a nurse who has breached a standard of care that a reasonably prudent nurse would meet.

Master-Servant Rule As applied to the employer-employee relationship, this rule holds the employer is responsible for the acts of employees as long as they are acting within the scope of their employment or authority.

Negligence The failure to do that which a reasonably prudent and careful person would do under the circumstances, or the doing of that which a reasonable and prudent person would not do.

Probable cause Sufficient, credible facts that would induce a reasonably intelligent and prudent person to believe that a cause of action exists.

Restraint Any method of physically restraining a person's freedom of movement, physical activity, or normal access to his or her body.

Seclusion The involuntary confinement of a person alone in a room where the person is physically prevented from leaving.

Standard of care The degree of skill, care, and diligence by members of the nursing profession, practicing in the same or a similar locality (Eskreis, 1998)

Voluntary commitment A commitment status in which patients or a conservator/guardian requests treatment and signs an application for that treatment. These persons are free to sign themselves out of the hospital also.

"If a madman suddenly experiences an unexpected attack and arms himself with a log, a stick, or a rock, the director-always mindful of his maxim to control the insane without ever permitting that they be hurt-would present himself in the most determined and threatening manner but without carrying any kind of weapon, so as to avoid additional vexation. He speaks with a thundering voice and walks closer toward the maniac in order to catch his eye. At the same time the servants converge on him at a given signal, from behind or sideways, each seizing one of the madman's limbs, an arm, a thigh, or a leg. Thus they carry him to his cell while thwarting his efforts and chain him if he is very dangerous or merely lock him up. That is how one dominates agitated madmen while respecting human rights." (Philippe Pinel, 1794 [cited in Weiner, 1992])

The evolution of humane treatment of mentally ill persons roughly parallels advances made in the jurisprudence system. It has been a slow process moving cautiously from viewing the mentally ill as demonic or weak-willed to viewing them as individuals with legitimate health care problems. Governmental systems thoughtfully attempt to achieve balance; that is, societies through the ages and up to the present time have grappled with balancing the rights of the individual against the rights of society at large. While most people are aware of the difficulty in reaching this goal in criminal cases, they are less aware of the struggle for such a balance in psychiatric care.

This chapter focuses on the laws that attempt to balance the basic rights of the individual against the interests of society in being protected from persons who, because of mental disorder, present a threat of harm to self, others, or the environment. The fundamental rights accorded each individual are derived from:

1. Amendments to the Constitution of the United States
2. Constitutions of the individual states
3. Precedent-setting legal cases.

The interests of society are weighed against individual rights such as the freedom from unreasonable search and seizure, the right to privacy, and the freedom of choice and self-determination.

This chapter is organized around the four categories of legal issues of particular concern to psychiatric nurses. These four categories are the following:

1. Precedent-setting legal milestones in psychiatric care
2. Commitment issues
3. Patient rights
4. Nursing liability and related issues

Additionally, the nursing implications of selected legal issues will be presented throughout the chapter to help the student understand the significant nursing tasks to be considered within the legal context.

PRECEDENT-SETTING LEGAL MILESTONES IN PSYCHIATRIC CARE

Society has not always been concerned with the individual rights of mentally ill persons. In fact, it can be argued that in no other area of nursing practice have patients been so deprived of personal rights, freedom of choice, and dignity. The student is encouraged to review Chapter 1 to appreciate the impetus for the humane care and legal protection of mentally ill persons today. Because the evolution of psychiatric legal thought parallels the evolution of psychiatric treatment presented in Chapter 1, historical information presented there will not be repeated.

Many rulings have influenced the current legal view of mental illness. Those presented below, although they in no way form an exhaustive list of major court decisions, do reflect decisions that have shaped the mental health treatment system and are part of an ongoing process to accomplish the following legislative objectives:

- To end inappropriate, indefinite, and involuntary commitment of mentally ill persons
- To provide prompt evaluation and treatment of mentally ill persons
- To guarantee and protect public safety
- To safeguard individual rights through judicial review
- To provide individualized treatment, supervision, and placement services through a conservatorship or guardianship program for gravely disabled persons
- To encourage the full use of all existing agencies, professional personnel, and public funds to accomplish these objectives and to prevent duplication of services and unnecessary expenditures

Historical Perspective

Ten landmark historical rulings have had a significant precedent-setting influence on our mental health treatment system

1. The *M'Naghten rule (1843)* states that persons who do not understand the nature and implications of murderous actions because of insanity cannot be held legally accountable for murder. This ruling was based on the case of Daniel M'Naghten, a Scotsman who felt persecuted by the ruling political party and attempted to kill the prime minister. Although he failed to kill the prime minister, he did shoot the prime minister's secretary. He was ruled *not guilty by reason of insanity* and was committed to an asylum. This case has provided a basis for legal decisions in American courts since 1851.
2. *Rouse v. Cameron 373 F2d 451 (DC Cir 1966)* was a case in which a man who pleaded not guilty by reason of insanity to the charge of illegally carrying a dangerous weapon was committed to a mental institution. After 4 years in the institution, the man argued that he was not receiving treatment (and therefore could not

improve enough to be discharged). The court ruled that he had the *right to treatment.*

3. *Griswold v. Connecticut (1965) 381 U.S. 479* was the case in which the United States Supreme Court first recognized that a *right of personal privacy* exists under the Constitution of the United States. The case addressed the issue of the state of Connecticut's right to prohibit the giving of birth control information to married couples. A majority of the Court held that the Ninth Amendment supports the creation of "peripheral rights" not expressly mentioned in the Bill of Rights, including the right of privacy. Subsequent cases that involved various aspects of treatment for mental disorders utilized this ruling.

4. *Wyatt v. Stickney 344 F Supp 373 (MD Ala 1972)* was another case involving *right to treatment.* In this case the entire mental health system of Alabama was sued for an inadequate treatment program. The court ruled that the Alabama mental health system must do the following at each institution:
   - Stop the use of patients for hospital labor needs
   - Ensure a humane environment
   - Develop and maintain minimum staffing standards
   - Establish institutional human rights committees
   - Provide the least restrictive environment for each patient

5. *Rogers v. Okin 478 F Supp (D Mass 1979)* was a case in which patients at Boston State Hospital sought the *right to refuse treatment.* The ruling prohibited the hospital from forcing nonviolent patients to take medications against their will. The court based its decision on the constitutional *right to privacy.* Furthermore, this decision required patients or their guardians to give informed consent before drug treatment could begin. This case has significant implications for nurses who are tempted to "force" patients to take medications for "their own good."

6. *Whitree v. State of New York (1968) 290 NYS 2nd 486* was a case in which the plaintiff, Whitree, successfully sued the State of New York. Whitree was awarded $300,000 for damages incurred in his 14 years of hospitalization. The court ruled that he did not receive treatment

and that, had he received adequate treatment, he could have been discharged 12 years earlier.

7. *Rennie v. Klein (3rd Cir 1983) 720 F2d 266* was a case in which a man claimed his rights were violated by the hospital when he was forced to take psychotropic medications. He won the *right to refuse treatment* based on *the right to privacy.* The ruling contained several significant statements concerning patient rights. The essence of these statements is the legal obligation of mental health professionals to obtain informed consent before administering psychotropic medications.

8. *Meier v. Ross General Hospital (1968) 69 Cal 2nd 420* was the case that established the *duty to warn of threatened suicide.* A physician was found liable for the death of his patient who committed suicide by jumping headfirst through an open window of his room. Prior to admission the patient had attempted suicide by slashing his wrists. The physician was deemed liable for not protecting the patient from his own actions (not warning).

9. *Tarasoff v. The Regents of the University of California (1976), 17 Cal 3rd 425* expanded further the liability of mental health professionals. The court established a *duty to warn of threats of harm to others.* In this case a patient confided to the therapist that he intended to kill an unnamed but readily identifiable girl when she returned from spending the summer in Brazil. The therapist notified campus police and requested their assistance in confining the man. The officers took the patient into custody but released him because he appeared rational. Shortly after her return from Brazil, Tatiana Tarasoff was killed by the man, Prosenjit Poddar on October 27, 1969. Her parents successfully sued the University of California, claiming that the therapist had a duty to warn their daughter of Poddar's threats. More recent cases have expanded and amplified this Tarasoff decision.

10. *Jackson v. Indiana 406 US 715 (1972)* and *Foucha v. Louisiana 60 USLW 4359 (1992).* Justice White of the Supreme Court wrote, "Due process . . . requires that the nature of the commitment bear some reasonable relation to the purpose for which the individual is committed." Patients like Jackson and Foucha were hospitalized presumably because they

were both mentally ill and dangerous. This ruling recognized that persons who are no longer mentally ill no longer require hospitalization; and because other categories of criminal behavior do not require individuals to prove themselves no longer dangerous, neither can such rigid criteria be used for the criminally insane (Appelbaum, 1993). More recent rulings indicate that sexual predator's (Megan's law) are exceptions.

COMMITMENT ISSUES

The decision to become a patient in a psychiatric facility is important. Patients must admit to themselves and to others that self-management is no longer a viable option for emotional stability. The paradox for individuals who require inpatient care is that the process of becoming a patient can itself cause anxiety and may be depressing. The psychiatric nurse should be consistently aware of this and the trust that it implies. Due to these and other considerations the American Psychiatric Association (APA) has developed guidelines to protect the rights of individuals thought to need inpatient care (News and Notes, 1992b). Box 4-1 contains these APA guidelines.

Box 4-1   APA Guidelines to Prevent Unnecessary Admissions to Psychiatric Hospitals

1. All admissions, voluntary or involuntary, must be clinically justified by the admitting psychiatrist.
2. Persons may be admitted to inpatient programs only after face-to-face evaluations have been made by a psychiatrist or other physician who determines the necessity of admission. In cases where a nonpsychiatrist physician admits a patient, the patient should be seen by a psychiatrist within 24 hours.
3. When a patient is admitted by a nonphysician, the admitting psychiatrist may order by telephone whatever measures may be needed for the safety of the patient. The face-to-face interview should occur as soon as possible but no later than 24 hours after time of admission.

Adapted from News and Notes, APA board approves new guidelines for hospital admission, *Hospital and Community Psychiatry,* 43(11):1156, 1992b.

All states have commitment procedures for the treatment of persons suffering from a diagnosable mental disorder. There are basically three types of commitments for psychiatric care: voluntary, involuntary, and the commitment of gravely disabled persons. (See the Key Terms box for the definition of these terms.)

Voluntary Commitment

The vast majority of persons with a mental health problem seek help voluntarily. Specific procedures vary from hospital to hospital and from state to state, but basically persons or their therapists request admission and the patient signs the appropriate documents, including consent to treatment. When persons are ready to leave the treatment setting, they sign themselves out. Most states have a grace period that allows professional staff the time and opportunity to assess patients before they leave voluntarily. Voluntary patients who want to sign themselves out can be placed on an involuntary commitment status by the court when the staff's assessment indicates a need for further treatment.

Involuntary Commitment

Mental illness is *not* equivalent to incompetence (Trudeau, 1993). Involuntary treatment means that an individual who has the legal capacity to consent to mental health treatment refuses to do so. In every state, persons considered *dangerous to self or others* because of a mental disorder can be involuntarily treated for that mental disorder. In about half the states there is a third criterion, *gravely disabled,* that is also cause for involuntary treatment. There are three common categories of involuntary treatment: evaluation and emergency care, certification for observation and treatment, and extended or indeterminate care. Not surprisingly, involuntary treatment is the area of psychiatric care where most legal issues develop. Although involuntary commitment usually implies inpatient care, it can also be applied to outpatient treatment, for example, DUI (driving under the influence) groups.

Evaluation and emergency care

Individuals who meet any one of the above three criteria can be detained involuntarily for evaluation and emergency treatment in most states. An authorized person such as a police officer signs documents to place persons under involuntary care. The length of the involuntary status varies from state to state; 72 hours or so is about average.

Nursing implications

Since the length of this involuntary treatment period is prescribed by law, the staff must scrupulously adhere to legal time constraints. The nursing staff must be absolutely aware of when the emergency treatment period is over and prepare the patient for discharge at that time. Patients may be asked to remain voluntarily in the facility and if they refuse, they may be asked to sign out *against medical advice* (AMA). The following clinical ex-ample provides a realistic vignette for involuntary detention.

CLINICAL EXAMPLE

Bill Wexler is a 52-year-old man who was informed that his job of 30 years was being eliminated. Although it was part of a larger downsizing effort, Mr. Wexler was deeply and personally affected. Within a week, he began to decompensate. He stopped bathing and wore the same suit every day. He showed up for work 2 weeks after being terminated not having bathed or shaved for a week and went to his usual work space. The space was occupied by a new employee and Mr. Wexler demanded he move out of his space or he would throw him out. Efforts by other employees who knew Mr. Wexler were unsuccessful in trying to calm him. He began shouting that he was going to kill everyone in human resources and that he had a gun in the car and was going to get it. Security and the police were called and were successful in restraining Mr. Wexler after a brief struggle. Mr. Wexler was taken to the county emergency department and involuntarily committed for 72 hours.

On the other hand, Hegner (1996) describes the liability involved when involuntary commitment is unwarranted.

CLINICAL EXAMPLE

In McCobe v. City of Lynn, a federal court ruled that a psychiatrist was liable for the death of an elderly woman who was to be involuntarily committed. Ms. Zinger, a holocaust survivor with eviction from her home imminent, was thought to be incapable of caring for herself. The police went to her home and when Ms. Zinger refused to open her door the police broke it down. In the struggle that ensued Ms. Zinger suffered myocardial infarction (MI) and died.

Certification for observation and treatment

Each state has laws that provide for the certification for observation and involuntary treatment of mental illness, laws that differ from state to state. These state laws authorize a qualified expert to determine if a person has a treatable mental disorder. A mental disorder can be defined as a condition that substantially impairs a person's thoughts, perception of reality, emotional process, judgment, or behavior. In most states a qualified expert may be a physician, a psychiatrist, a master's prepared nurse or social worker, or a psychologist. The student should note that the APA guidelines set forth in Box 4-1 indicate that if a nonpsychiatrist certifies a patient for observation and treatment, then that patient should be seen face-to-face by a psychiatrist within 24 hours. Figure 4-1 illustrates the certification procedure.

A treatable mental disorder indicates that the problem is amenable to and can improve with treatment. For example, someone who is hearing voices telling her to kill herself meets this criterion, whereas someone who is simply angry and threatening to kill someone does not.

During the certification process a complaint or a *probable cause* statement is written, indicating that the person is a danger to self or others, or is gravely disabled. The probable cause statement is required by the Fourth Amendment of the Constitution of the United States that prohibits "search and seizure of a person without probable cause." In this context, probable cause means that known facts would lead an ordinary person to believe that the person detained is mentally disordered and is a danger to self or others, or is gravely disabled. The probable cause hearing is not held to determine if the person is mentally ill, but whether or not there is just cause to keep the person for treatment against his or her will.

If it is determined that probable cause exists, persons can be detained for observation and treatment. Such persons must be informed of their rights upon

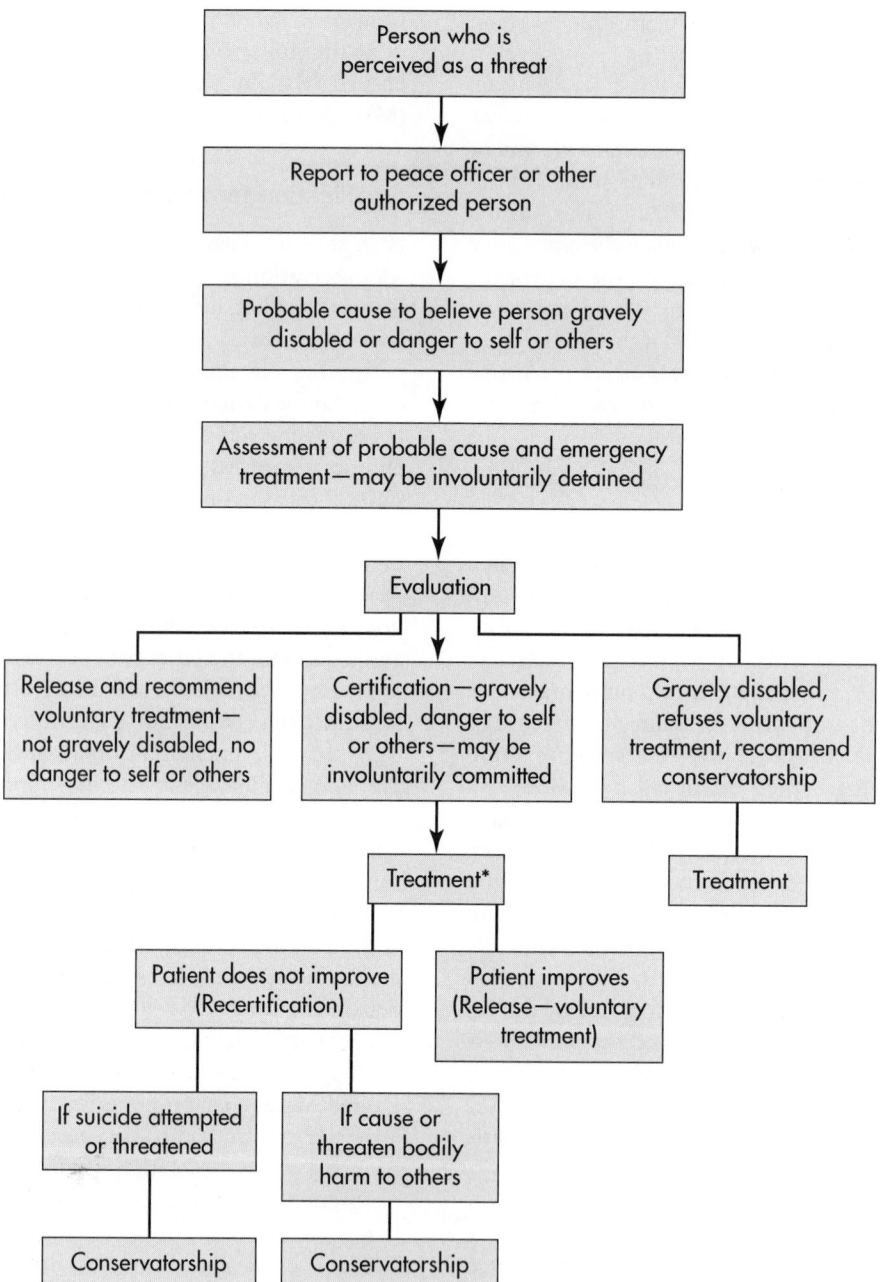

*The individual can be involuntarily committed but cannot be forced to accept treatment, e.g., medication, group therapy.

FIGURE 4-1 Flow chart for certification procedure.

being certified for this level of involuntary care. The length of the observation and treatment periods varies from state to state.

Nursing implications

Persons must be released if there is no legal basis for continued commitment. The hospital staff may suggest voluntary admission and, if it is refused, may require patients to sign out AMA. The nurse is often responsible for assuring AMA forms are signed and an opportunity for follow-up care is offered.

Extended or indeterminate commitment

Extended or indeterminate commitment is reserved for persons who need prolonged psychiatric care but refuse to seek such help voluntarily. Typically, extended hospitalizations last from 60 to 180 days. Indeterminate hospitalization can last much longer. Most states require that patients who have been recommended for an extended or indeterminate commitment be brought before a hearing officer. This system of checks and balances decreases the possibility of persons being "railroaded" into a mental hospital and assures persons of full legal protection.

Commitment of Incapacitated Persons

In most states there is a procedure for establishing a conservator or guardian for gravely disabled persons (the conservatees). The legal system in the United States maintains that while a person may be undergoing severe mental and emotional upheaval (in the clinical example of Mr. Wexler), that person is nonetheless recognized as competent before the law. The person who is identified as being gravely disabled, on the other hand, is viewed by the legal system as incompetent.

Gravely disabled is defined as the inability to provide food, clothing, and shelter for oneself because of a mental illness. This does not mean that all people living on the streets are gravely disabled nor that they should be hospitalized for "their own good." Judge David Bazelon addressed this concept in 1966: "Deprivations of liberty solely because of dangers to the ill persons themselves should not go beyond what is necessary for their protection" (Munetz and Geller, 1993). However, persons with money in their pockets who cannot negotiate arrangements for food or shelter are gravely disabled.

The appointment of a conservator or guardian is a serious legal matter, and full legal protection is provided for persons being evaluated for conservatee status. Proposed conservatees are entitled to representation by a private attorney or a court-appointed public defender to challenge conservatorship. An appointed conservator or guardian may be given broad powers, including the right to order the conservatee to receive psychiatric treatment. Although technically patients might receive treatment against their will, there is a legal distinction between this kind of commitment and an involuntary commitment. That distinction is based on the premise that the conservator now speaks *for* the patient; hence, the treatment is not involuntary.

Conservatorship should not be viewed as a nontherapeutic legal maneuver; when used skillfully, conservatorship can be a powerful therapeutic tool. Lamb and Weinberger (1993) cite instances in which patients, by relinquishing some of their freedom, were able to avoid hospitalization and maintain much of their independence and community standing. Nonetheless, being placed under conservatorship is an extreme legal step. Conservators exercise external controls over individuals who lack internal controls, and all factors must be considered before such action is taken. Conservators are legally obligated to act in the best interest of their conservatees.

Nursing implications

Because conservators speak for conservatees, the nurse must gain consent from conservators for decisions that are otherwise made by patients themselves. For instance, a newspaper reporter may want to interview patients about hospital living conditions. Other patients may agree or refuse to participate on their own, but the conservatee needs permission from the conservator. A nurse who forgets to gain conservator approval may face legal consequences.

CLINICAL EXAMPLE

Ms. Park, a 73-year-old woman, is found by a social worker to be living in a filthy, roach-infested, older home. The Department of Human Services is called by a neighbor who has not seen Ms. Park in several months. The neighbor explains that no one answers the door when she rings the doorbell. Ms. Park lived there for years with her husband. Since he died 5 years ago, Ms. Park has lived alone. The stench of cats and cat feces is almost unbearable. Ms. Park is emaciated, incoherent, and paranoid. The social worker decides to initiate involuntary commitment for Ms. Park in order to evaluate her mental and physical condition and need for a conservatorship hearing.

■ Critical Thinking Questions

Some states have a category of commitment called "gravely disabled" while other states do not. Obviously there are two firmly held views about this type of commitment. Does the state you live in have this commitment category? Do you find the arguments more compelling for or against this commitment category?

PATIENT RIGHTS

Box 4-2 contains a list of rights that patients should be afforded even if they are being treated involuntarily. The specific rights vary somewhat from state to state, but all are derived from a bill of rights established in 1980 by the federal Mental Health Systems Act. This congressional action recommended to state governing bodies a set of basic patient rights

---

Box 4-2 Most Commonly Adopted Patient Rights

1. Right to treatment using the least restrictive alternative/environment
2. Right to confidentiality of records
3. Right to freedom from restraints and seclusion
4. Right to give or refuse consent to treatment
5. Right to access to personal belongings
6. Right to daily exercise
7. Right to have visitors
8. Right to use of writing materials and uncensored mail
9. Right to use of telephone
10. Right to access courts and attorneys
11. Right to employment compensation
12. Right to be informed of rights
13. Right to refuse electroconvulsive therapy or psychosurgery

---

that most states either fully or partially support. A proposed bill amending and expanding the Patient Bill of Rights was formally unveiled in Washington in February 1997. The bill has the support of a large number of professional associations including the American Psychiatric Nurses Association. A copy of the proposed bill is included on pages 58-59. A list of patient rights should be prominently displayed for all to see and should also be explained to every patient on admission.

Suspension of Patient Rights

Occasionally it is necessary to suspend rights for the protection of patients or of others and for therapeutic purposes. For instance, no units have unlimited telephone privileges because it could be nontherapeutic to do so.

Nursing implications

Suspension of a patient's rights requires the nurse to clearly document that allowing the patient to continue to exercise the specific right could result in harm to the patient or to others. For example, a suicidal patient's right to access to personal belongings may be suspended because it is felt that he might attempt to harm himself with those objects. The nurse must document the concern and the suspension of this right in the nurse's notes.

Right to Treatment with the Least Restrictive Alternative

The concept of the least restrictive alternative/environment is central to the ideology of the deinstitutionalization movement (Munetz and Geller, 1993). Persons with mental health problems have the right to treatment of those problems in the least restrictive environment using the least restrictive means (i.e., without restraints and seclusion unless necessary.) This "right" has emerged from court decisions previously mentioned and was articulated by President Carter's Commission on Mental Health in 1978. The stated objective was to maintain ". . . the greatest degree of freedom, self-determination, autonomy, dignity, and integrity of body, mind, and spirit for the individual while he or she participates in treatment or receives services." Specifically, patients who are held against their will should not be detained without treatment, as occurred in the *Whitree v. State of New York* case described earlier.

Nursing implications

The nurse does not typically decide which treatment setting the patient will enter. However, the nurse has treatment responsibilities and can be held liable if the patient does not receive adequate treatment. The following clinical example illustrates the issue of the right to treatment using the least restrictive alternative.

CLINICAL EXAMPLE

Joe Kelly is a 53-year-old Vietnam veteran who suffers from posttraumatic stress syndrome characterized by periods of flashbacks and depression. After a flashback he is often confused and wanders about for days looking for friends he lost in the war. He poses no obvious danger to others or himself. His family is deceased, and he lives alone. When picked up by the police for loitering and evaluated by the social worker, he insists on going home. His case, however, is heard before the court, which rules he does not need commitment to a psychiatric unit, but does need a temporary structured environment. The social worker finds a halfway house with the veterans hospital, and Mr. Kelly agrees to temporary placement.

Right to Confidentiality of Records

Patient information is privileged material and should be treated confidentially. Both voluntary and involuntary patients are granted this legal consideration. Following this procedure is not always as easy as it might appear; hence, professional judgment is required. The guidelines in Box 4-3 provide a framework for mandatory confidentiality.

As straightforward as these guidelines are, they do not cover every situation or address exceptions. Jones (1993) points out that the rule of confidentiality is not absolute. She uses the obvious example of a patient at risk for self-harm. Keeping this kind of information confidential would constitute professional malpractice.

Based on a U.S. Supreme Court ruling in *Jaffe v. Redmond,* the therapist-patient relationship is viewed as privileged and the therapist need not divulge the content of therapy sessions even in a court of law (Applebaum, 1996).

Nursing implications

The nurse should document in the nursing notes all confidential information that is released, including the date and circumstances under which disclosure was made, the names of the individuals or agencies receiving the disclosure and their relationships to the patient, and the specific information disclosed.

In order to release information about patients a consent form must first be signed. Most states provide legal redress for patients should a nurse willfully disclose confidential information without the proper signature. The confidentiality of the patient's records should not be confused with the doctrine of privileged communication. Under this doctrine a psychiatrist is not obliged to reveal the contents of sessions with the patient. This privilege is based on the understanding of the need for trust between physicians and patients. Most states do not include nurses under this provision.

The therapeutic modality of group therapy, which is often led by nurses, is particularly vulnerable to violations of confidentiality. The group leader should always address this issue when starting a group or when a new member is introduced to the group. Eighty-two percent of group leaders surveyed in one study recognized the risk of breach

---

Box 4-3 Tips for Monitoring

1. Keep all patient records secure.
2. Carefully consider the content of all written entries.
3. Release information only with written consent.
4. Disguise clinical material when it is used for educational purposes.
5. Share information only with those who need to know, not with friends or in public areas.
6. Guard written material taken outside the clinical area.
7. Do not access written or electronic information out of curiosity.
8. Fax transmissions may be prohibited to unsecured areas where a receipt error is a possibility.
9. Know to whom you are talking when relating patient information over the phone; "family" may be a reporter, boss, or insurance attorney.

of confidentiality in the group setting (Applebaum and Greer, 1993). It is incumbent upon nurses leading group sessions to mention the limitations to confidentiality that exist in the group format. Of course, once such a proclamation is made, there may be the potential for less forthrightness by group members concerning their thoughts, feelings, and behaviors.

CLINICAL EXAMPLE

Students frequently find themselves in the following situation: After developing a relationship with a patient, the student may hear, "I want to tell you something, but I don't want anyone else to know." What should you say? Is it a breach of the patient's right to confidentiality to tell others or to chart? The student must let the patient know that anything said within the context of the nurse-patient relationship will be shared with other team members if appropriate.

■ Critical Thinking Question

Confidentiality is stressed in nursing school but it may be violated. What should you do when one of your classmates is discussing a patient inappropriately? Is it a violation of confidentiality to discuss patients by name in a clinical conference?

Right to Freedom from Restraints and Seclusion

Restraint and seclusion have been used to manage out-of-control psychiatric patients for thousands of years. Pinel is perhaps best known for unshackling the mentally ill in France (see Chapter 1). Historically, restraint and seclusion have been used to prevent patients from hurting themselves or others, to prevent damage to the physical environment, or to decrease countertherapeutic stimulation (Betemps, Buncher, and Oden, 1992). In some states only injury to the self or to another warrants restraint and seclusion (News and Notes, 1992a). Over the years, as respect for the rights of the mentally ill has evolved, the use of restraint and seclusion decreased; that is, until recently. Outlaw and Lowery (1992) point out that in recent times, use of these control techniques has started to increase. They hypothesize that the increase is linked to a growth in the number of violent patients being hospitalized–patients who

in previous years would have been confined in the criminal justice system. However, Outlaw and Lowry recognize that other variables may explain the current rise in usage of these techniques.

Outlaw and Lowery (1992) also note nonnursing professionals are more reluctant than nurses to utilize restraint and seclusion. This is particularly interesting given the fact that most other professionals have greater flexibility of their work schedule (that is, they can leave the unit) than nurses.

The proper procedure for dealing with harmful behavior is to first try to calm patients verbally. When it is determined that verbal and psychopharmacological interventions are not adequate to stem the aggressiveness, seclusion or seclusion with restraint may be required. Seclusion is defined as the process of isolating a person in a room where the person is physically prevented from leaving. Restraint, typically, means controlling a person's physical activity by mechanical devices such as leather restraints, but can also include bedrails. Evidence suggests that patients do not perceive this experience positively; up to 50% of patients state that it was either unnecessary or not helpful (cited in Norris and Kennedy, 1992). Nurses and patients tend to value seclusion differently. Tooke and Brown (1992) recommend that nurses bridge this gap in understanding by taking the time to talk with patients who are in seclusion and by debriefing patients after the seclusion experience.

Nursing implications

The use of seclusion and restraint continues to be both a legal and an ethical problem for nurses (Craig, Ray, and Hix, 1989). Because it is unlawful to seclude or restrain a person without justification, the nurse must have a physician's order and carefully document the following:
1. Type of restraint
2. Reason for restraint
3. Length of time of restraint; for example, "4-point leather restraint STAT for assaultive behavior until calm"
4. Observations to maintain safety

In a 1992 ruling a U.S. district judge reaffirmed and strengthened some of the elements of the *Wyatt v. Stickney* case of 25 years ago. Under this ruling a patient in restraint and seclusion must be checked every 15 minutes and bathed every 24 hours. The maximum length of time for this restrictive mechanism is 8 hours under the original order. In emergency situations a nurse can approve a seclusion or restraint order when no physician is available. A physician must see the patient within 4 hours (News and Notes, 1992a).

◼ Critical Thinking Question

Some psychiatric professionals believe the courts have gone too far in protecting the rights of patients and have actually set up barriers to effective mental health care. What do you think?

CLINICAL EXAMPLE

Kim Young is a 28-year-old Korean national married to an American serviceman who is currently assigned overseas. Mrs. Young is extremely well versed in the American culture and language, as well as exceptionally bright and talented. Mrs. Young performed endless hours of volunteer work within her community and church. She was viewed as a person with boundless energy who never seemed to stop. Her volunteer hours continued to increase, and she began to preach in local bars and taverns. Her language became incoherent at times and English and Korean were often mixed in the same sentence. When the owner of a local tavern called the police after she refused to leave, she began to curse him and tried to hit him with a beer bottle. The police were able to restrain her, and she was involuntarily committed to a psychiatric unit. When approached by the staff, she would spit, curse, and try to strike them. Four-point physical restraint was ordered. Mrs. Young required seclusion and restraint thereafter on several occasions for her aggressive behavior. The nursing progress record (Box 4-4) and the restraint and seclusion nursing notes provide a record of her behavior and the nursing responses to that behavior.

After making the decision to place Mrs. Young in restraint and seclusion, the nursing staff must then make sure that they have complied with a checklist for seclusion and restraints similar to the following:

1. Documentation of justification   Yes   No   NA
2. Alternative considered and   Yes   No   NA
   attempted
3. Physician's order   Yes   No   NA
4. Type of restraints   Yes   No   NA
5. Duration   Yes   No   NA
6. Checked by staff every   Yes   No   NA
   15 minutes
7. Checked by RN every
   2 hours for continued need   Yes   No   NA
8. Fluids offered every hour   Yes   No   NA
9. Limbs exercised every 2 hours   Yes   No   NA
10. Toileting and meals offered   Yes   No   NA

Right to Give or Refuse Consent to Treatment

The final patient right to be explored is the right to give or refuse consent to treatment. Court rulings mentioned previously provide legal precedents, and *Rogers v. Okin* provided the foundation for a patient's right to refuse treatment. Based on this and other constitutional arguments, New York State's highest court, the court of appeals, handed down a decision in 1986 that held in nonemergency situations, involuntary patients cannot be forced to take psychotropic medications. The decision, referred to as *Rivers v. Katz,* has led to diminished quality of care and has resulted in increased patient and staff injuries, according to a study by Ciccone et al (1993).

The right of voluntary patients to refuse treatment has been recognized for a long time. If

---

Box 4-4   Nursing Progress Record

Time	Format
0210	Pt has continued to pace hallway, dayroom, and her room. At 0045 was asking for sleep meds. Pt stated the best way to get well was walking.
0315	Pt refuses to go to room and try to rest. Pacing dayroom and at times kneeling as if in prayer.
0430	Pt asleep on top of bed, naked with door open.
0830	Pt refusing medication. Appears very agitated.
0930	Pt very agitated, tearing up another patient's magazine and throwing into trash. Placed in seclusion.
1030	Escalation of agitation. When staff went into room to check on Mrs. Young she swung at staff and attempted to bite the nurse. Placed in 4-point restraint by 4 female and 2 male staff members. Pt stated that she was being "raped" and that "Christ lives in me." Haldol 5 mg IM and Cogentin 2 mg IM given.

voluntary patients believe the treatment they are receiving is helpful, they can accept it; if they believe it is not helpful, they can refuse it. Involuntary patients, on the other hand, have not always been understood to have the same right to refuse treatment. In the case of medications, many involuntary patients through the years have been forced to take medications against their will. Legally it is now recognized that involuntarily admitted patients do not lose their right to give informed consent to the administration of psychotropic drugs. The key issue is whether or not patients have the capacity to give informed consent to the administration of these drugs. The court made the determination regarding drugs but does not respond to issues of need or alternative treatments. Once the court decides that a person is not competent to understand the need for treatment, medications can then be imposed upon that person. How this decision is implemented varies from state to state.

In cases of a psychiatric emergency, medications can be given without consent to prevent harm to the patient or to others.

Nursing implications

Nurses administer medications to patients. Because it is not uncommon for patients to refuse medications and for nurses to coax those patients into taking medications, nurses must be sure that coaxing does not escalate to the point of forcing medications on a patient. It is also not always clear what constitutes a psychiatric emergency. Nurses may be liable should their interpretation of a psychiatric emergency differ from that of another professional or from that of a judge. The following clinical example illustrates the dilemma associated with a patient refusing medication.

CLINICAL EXAMPLE

Joyce Zimmerman is a 44-year-old female with an admitting diagnosis of bipolar illness. This is her sixteenth admission to the county hospital psychiatric unit. The staff know Ms. Zimmerman well, having treated her during many prior periods of manic behavior. Historically, Ms. Zimmerman is angry, assaultive, and refuses medications. She says nasty things to staff and is particularly rude to Hispanic and black staff members. Although all staff recognize that she is mentally ill, her remarks are so biting

at times that some staff have difficulty maintaining a professional posture. Although no one has ever been seriously hurt by Ms. Zimmerman, her attempts to slap and choke people have both patients and staff on edge. The physician has ordered lithium carbonate 300 mg tid and chlorpromazine 50 mg IM q4h prn for assaultive behavior. Ms. Zimmerman has refused the lithium and the nursing staff continues to give chlorpromazine when her behavior justifies doing so. The consensus of the nursing and medical staff is that Ms. Zimmerman will not improve until she starts taking lithium on a regular basis, yet her illness is instrumental in her refusal of that medication. The staff requests a court hearing to evaluate Ms. Zimmerman's competency and the need for the appointment of a guardian. (In an emergency the nursing staff is permitted to medicate assaultive patients without consent. However, the staff is not permitted to medicate patients against their will at other times even when that behavior [e.g., hallucinations, extreme withdrawn behavior] indicates a need for pharmacological intervention.)

At the hearing the physician testifies concerning her evaluation of the patient, nursing documentation is reviewed, and Ms. Zimmerman appears with a court-appointed representative. During the proceedings Ms. Zimmerman states that she has been sodomized by a black technician on the unit and that she knows President Clinton personally. Furthermore, she makes various grandiose claims that substantiate the truth of the medical and nursing staff testimony. The court appoints a guardian for Ms. Zimmerman. The guardian agrees with the staff's assessment that Ms. Zimmerman should take the psychotropic medications prescribed by the physician and, should she refuse to do so, the nursing staff is to administer those drugs to her.

One week after the court order, Ms. Zimmerman is joking with the staff, taking medications voluntarily, and anticipating her return to the board-and-care facility where she lives.

Living Wills and Health Care Directives

A majority of states have recognized the rights of individuals to choose the type of medical treatment they receive in the event of a life-threatening medical condition. This is accomplished through use of living wills and health care directives. The U.S. Congress passed the Patient Self-Determination Act in 1991, which provided that all health care facilities that serve Medicare or Medicaid patients must provide each of their adult patients with written information regarding their right to make decisions about their medical care. These instructions must be consistent with the laws of each state. The patients are also made aware of the right to execute a living will or durable power of attorney. The living will and health care directive list specific actions that the patient may choose to implement or not implement under the aforementioned life-threatening medical condition. Some examples are mechanical ventilator support or artificial nutrition. A durable power of attorney is a written document in which one person, the principal, authorizes another person, the attorney in fact, to act on the principal's behalf IN THE EVENT the principal becomes unable to act on his or her own behalf secondary to a physical or mental disability. The disability causes this type of power of attorney to spring into existence.

Nursing implications

Nurses should be aware of the patient's right to make health care directives, living wills, and a durable power of attorney. The health care provider should have policies and procedure in place to assure that all patients are afforded the opportunity to exercise these rights. The nurse must ensure that:
1. Proper documentation in the medical record either contains the properly executed forms or a signed waiver that the patient does not wish to exercise his or her right to execute these forms.
2. That the attorney in fact chosen by the patient must be consulted before making decisions regarding the patient.
3. That decisions regarding treatment in patients who have executed health care directives can still be complex and must be addressed through a team approach headed by the primary physician with family support.

NURSING LIABILITY AND RELATED ISSUES

Malpractice

The psychiatric nurse is responsible for many significant decisions in the care of psychiatric patients. Lapses in attention to specific legal issues related to nursing practice can result in liability suits against

the nurse and the nurse's employer. Areas of concern that can lead to lawsuits include inappropriate dissemination of confidential information, illegal confinement, failure to obtain consent for medication and other treatments, inadequate treatment, medications errors, and the duty to warn of threatened suicide or harm to others. Malpractice is a civil action that can be brought against a nurse who has breached a professional standard of care (Beck, Rawlins, and Williams, 1988). A malpractice case rests on establishing the failure to adhere to the standard of care of nurses in the community once the nurse-patient relationship is initiated. The standard of care is the care a reasonably prudent nurse would give. These issues are potential sources of malpractice suits against the nurse, and legal rulings have, in many cases, established parameters of appropriate professional behavior to which the nurse will be compared.

Duty to Warn of Threatened Suicide or Harm to Others

Before the Tarasoff ruling, mental health professionals had no legal duty to warn of threatened suicide or harm to others. In 1976 the California Supreme Court issued the Tarasoff ruling, which stated that failure to warn, coupled with subsequent injury to the threatened person, exposed the mental health professional to civil damages for malpractice. Though a number of clinicians have speculated that warning a potential victim may compromise the relationship with the patient, available evidence cannot support them (Binder and McNeil, 1996). Based upon this and other rulings the mental health professional must balance a duty to protect confidentiality with a responsibility to warn society of possible danger.

Nursing implications

A nurse who is aware of a patient's intention to cause harm to the self or others must communicate that information to other professionals and take steps to protect the potential recipient of harm. Documentation in the patient's record is crucial to the effective communication of this information. The nurse who fails to take prudent action can be held liable. One of the authors spoke with the patient represented in the following vignette. This is an example in which a spurned suitor became emotionally unstable and

Principles for the Provision of Mental Health and Substance Abuse Treatment Services

A Bill of Rights

Our commitment is to provide quality mental health and substance abuse services to all individuals without regard to race, color, religion, national origin, gender, age, sexual orientation, or disabilities.

Right to Know

Benefits

Individuals have the right to be provided information from the purchasing entity (such as employer or union or public purchaser) and the insurance/third party payer describing the nature and extent of their mental health and substance abuse treatment benefits. This information should include details on procedures to obtain access to services, on utilization management procedures, and on appeal rights. The information should be presented clearly in writing with language that the individual can understand.

Professional Expertise

Individuals have the right to receive full information from the potential treating professional about that professional's knowledge, skills, preparation, experience, and credentials. Individuals have the right to be informed about the options available for treatment interventions and the effectiveness of the recommended treatment.

Contractual Limitations

Individuals have the right to be informed by the treating professional of any arrangements, restrictions, and/or covenants established between third party payer and the treating professional that could interfere with or influence treatment recommendations. Individuals have the right to be informed of the nature of information that may be disclosed for the purposes of paying benefits.

Appeals and Grievances

Individuals have the right to receive information about the methods they can use to submit complaints or grievances regarding provision of care by the treating professional to that profession's regulatory board and to the professional association.

Individuals have the right to be provided information about the procedures they can use to appeal benefit utilization decisions to the third party payer systems, to the employer or purchasing entity, and to external regulatory entities.

Confidentiality

Individuals have the right to be guaranteed the protection of the confidentiality of their relationship with their mental health and substance abuse professional, except when laws or ethics dictate otherwise. Any disclosure to another party will be time limited and made with the full written, informed consent of the individuals. Individuals shall not be required to disclose confidential, privileged or other than: diagnosis, prognosis, type of treatment, time and length of treatment, and cost.

Entities receiving information for the purposes of benefits determination, public agencies receiving information for health care planning, or any other organization with legitimate right to information will maintain clinical information in confidence with the same rigor and be subject to the same penalties for violation as is the direct provider of care.

Information technology will be used for transmission, storage, or data management only with methodologies that remove individual identifying information and assure the protection of the individual's privacy. Information should not be transferred, sold or otherwise utilized.

Choice

Individuals have the right to choose any duly licensed/certified professional for mental health and substance abuse services. Individuals have the right to receive full information regarding the education and training of professionals, treatment options (including risks and benefits), and cost implications to make an informed choice regarding the selection of care deemed appropriate by individual and professional.

Determination of Treatment

Recommendations regarding mental health and substance abuse treatment shall be made only by a duly licensed/certified professional in conjunction with the individual and his or her family as appropriate. Treatment decisions should not be made by third party payers. The individual has the right to make final decisions regarding treatment.

Parity

Individuals have the right to receive benefits for mental health and substance abuse treatment on the same basis as they do for any other illnesses, with the same provisions, co-payments, lifetime benefits, and catastrophic coverage in both insurance and self-funded/self-insured health plans.

Discrimination

Individuals who use mental health and substance abuse benefits shall not be penalized when seeking other health insurance or disability, life or any other insurance benefit.

Benefit Usage

The individual is entitled to the entire scope of the benefits within the benefit plan that will address his or her clinical needs.

Benefit Design

Whenever both federal and state law and/or regulations are applicable, the professional and all payers shall use whichever affords the individual the greatest level of protection and access.

Treatment Review

To assure that treatment review processes are fair and valid, individuals have the right to be guaranteed that any review of their mental health and substance abuse treatment shall involve a professional having the training, credentials and licensure required to provide the treatment in the jurisdiction in which it will be provided. The reviewer should have no financial interest in the decision and is subject to the section on confidentiality.

Accountability

Treating professionals may be held accountable and liable to individuals for any injury caused by gross incompetence or negligence on the part of the professional. The treating professional has the obligation to advocate for and document necessity of care and to advise the individual of options if payment authorization is denied. Payers and other third parties may be held accountable and liable to individuals for any injury caused by gross incompetence or negligence or by their clinically unjustified decisions.

American Psychological Association	American Psychiatric Association
American Association for Marriage and Family Therapy	American Counseling Association
American Family Therapy Academy	American Nurses Association
American Psychiatric Nurses Association	National Association of Social Workers

National Federation of Societies for Clinical Social Work

Participating Groups:
American Association for Marriage and Family Therapy (membership: 25,000)
American Counseling Association (membership: 56,000)
American Family Therapy Academy (membership: 1,000)
American Nurses Association (membership: 180,000)
American Psychological Association (membership: 142,000)
American Psychiatric Association (membership: 42,000)
American Psychiatric Nurses Association (membership: 3,000)
National Association of Social Workers (membership: 155,000)
National Federation of Societies for Clinical Social Work (membership: 11,000)

Supporting Groups:
National Mental Health Association
American Group Psychotherapy Association
American Psychoanalytic Association
National Association of Alcoholism and Drug Abuse Counselors
National Depressive and Manic Depressive Association

Source: Valentine NM: The patient's bill of rights–APNA collaborating with colleagues and consumers across the nation to manage the transition to managed care, *J of Amer Psychiatric Nurses Assoc* 3(4):18A, 1997.

threatened his ex-girlfriend. This is not only a fairly common occurrence, it often falls under the auspices of the mental health department to distinguish psychiatric aspects from criminal aspects.

CLINICAL EXAMPLE

Bud Hollman is a 36-year-old man with a past history of mental illness that was successfully treated. He has maintained a steady job for the past 12 years. He has a history of abusing his wife over the past 7 years. His wife of 10 years has made a decision to divorce Mr. Hollman and end the abuse. She is currently in a safe house for abused women. Mr. Hollman is obsessed with his wife and with finding her. He has gone to the homes of several friends and relatives searching for her. He is unsuccessful in finding her and becomes progressively more agitated. He becomes delusional, convinced that the only reason she could leave is because she is possessed. When he doesn't find her at her place of employment, he tells her fellow employees she has been demon possessed and if he finds her he will kill her. The police are called, and he is arrested. He is involuntarily committed for 72-hour evaluation and found to suffer from a psychosis manifested by delusions. He specifically tells the therapist of his wife's demonic possession and his plans to remove the demon. Upon review, the police and Mrs. Hollman are warned of his threats.

■ Critical Thinking Question

"Not guilty by reason of insanity" is a phrase that evokes passion in many people. Jeffrey Dahmer, the cannabilist murderer, did not say that he didn't do it. He said he was not guilty because he did not know what he was doing. His lawyers said he was not guilty "by reason of insanity." What do you think about this concept? Do you believe this legal defense is used often? Is it reasonable to have such protection under the law?

Civil Remedies for Wrongful Involuntary Commitment

Persons who are wrongfully committed to a psychiatric facility have several types of civil suits they can file against medical health professionals:

- False imprisonment: lack of probable cause, confining patients so that they have no way of escape, inappropriate use of restraint and seclusion, not allowing voluntary patients to leave when they are ready. A psychiatric facility should have a policy defining the parameters of confinement, and the nurse must follow those policy guidelines.
- Assault and battery: force used in unlawful detention, inappropriately forceful restraint (battery), telling patients you are going to force them to take medication (assault).
- Professional negligence: absence of measures to prevent harm to patients and failure to maintain the standard of care of nurses in the community.

Understanding the concept of the master-servant rule is vital to both clinical nurses and supervisors. Simply put, an employer is responsible for the acts of his or her employee as long as the employee is acting within the scope and authority of his or her employment. A nurse who exceeds his or her clinical boundaries or fails to act as a reasonable and prudent nurse would in the same or similar circumstances incurs liability to his or her employer. It is just as critical to understand that unlicensed assistive personnel who exceed their clinical boundaries or authority and are under the direction or supervision of a nurse will cause liability to be incurred upon the nurse.

Nursing implications

With the recent push to lower health care costs, there has been a significant increase in the utilization of unlicensed assistive personnel (UAPs). More nurses are finding themselves with job responsibilities that include delegating certain tasks to UAPs. When a nurse delegates, the authority to carry out the act on behalf of the nurse is conveyed to the assistant; however, the nurse remains accountable for the consequences of the act and for the adequate supervision of the assistant. When delegating, the nurse at a minimum should:

1. Know and follow the local hospital procedures in order to stay within his or her scope and authority.
2. Assure that assistive personnel assigned to you have been fully trained and are qualified to carry out the tasks they are expected to perform.

3. Know the limitations and responsibilities of nursing practice of his or her state.

CLINICAL EXAMPLE

Clara Meyers, a 40-year-old woman with a history of recent depression with sleep deprivation and suicidal ideation is admitted to your unit, is sedated, and placed on suicide precautions. The nurse assigns a new nursing assistant to check on the patient every 15 minutes for the entire shift. The nursing assistant, having checked the patient every 15 minutes for 2 hours and finding her asleep, decides that every 30 minutes is sufficient. The nurse who delegated this task was unaware that the new assistant had only general nursing assistant training and had never oriented on a psychiatric unit. During the 30-minute time period when the patient was left alone, she managed to get out of bed and go to the bathroom, where she fell and fractured her pelvis. In the subsequent lawsuit the nurse was identified as being liable for the UAP's poor decision that resulted in the fall.

Documentation

The nursing staff is responsible for completing a variety of forms that document the progress of patients and serve as legal records of the treatments they received. Nursing notes, restraint and seclusion forms, medication records, and physician order sheets are only a few of the forms required. Careful attention to these records promotes communication among staff, enhances treatment, diminishes treatment errors (e.g., medication errors), and reduces liability claims. Because the psychiatric nurse has the most patient contact and because of the unique contributions of nursing to psychiatric care, the nurse is in a position to positively influence the legal issues confronting those involved in that care today.

Key Concepts

1. The understanding of the rights of mentally ill persons has evolved over the centuries. Today, based upon several precedent-setting legal decisions, protection of the mentally ill from unreasonable hospitalization has been established.
2. These landmark cases triggered several states to legislate the end of inappropriate, indefinite, and involuntary commitment to mental hospitals.
3. There are three categories of commitment:
   a. Voluntary commitment: the person requests hospitalization
   b. Involuntary commitment: a person with the legal capacity to consent refuses to do so and is treated against his or her will
   c. Commitment of an incapacitated person: the treatment of a person who does not have the legal capacity to consent to treatment
4. There are three forms of involuntary commitment:
   a. For brief evaluation and emergency care
   b. For an intermediate certification for observation and treatment
   c. For a longer, extended or indeterminate commitment
5. Patients under psychiatric care have many rights guaranteed by the Constitution of the United States and the constitutions of individual states. These rights are derived from the following basic rights:
   a. The freedom from unreasonable search and seizure
   b. The right to privacy
   c. The right to freedom of choice and self-determination
6. Seclusion and restraint are special procedures for coping with assaultive and dangerous patients so that these patients can be isolated or mechanically restrained to prevent injury to the patient, other patients, or to staff.
7. Patients, even involuntarily admitted patients, must give informed consent before they are given psychotropic drugs and retain the right to refuse medication. Except for emergency situations, involuntarily admitted patients cannot be given medication against their will without judicial approval.
8. Psychiatric patients have the right to be treated in the least restrictive alternative/environment. In other words, if persons can receive appropriate care close to home in a community agency, they cannot be forced to go to a public mental hospital far away from family and friends.
9. Psychiatric patients have the right to confidential treatment of all information about themselves. Nurses and others can be held legally liable for discussing patients' situations outside of the professional context.
10. Psychiatric patients have the right to be free from restraint and seclusion. Patients cannot be arbitrarily placed in these freedom-limiting situations without justification.
11. All psychiatric patients have the right to treatment. This simply means that persons cannot be involuntarily committed to a psychiatric institution and then refused the benefit of therapeutic opportunities available at that facility.

12. Psychiatric nurses are at legal risk for civil action if they are guilty of false imprisonment, assault and battery, or negligent harm.
13. Mental health professionals have a duty to warn the potential victim of a psychiatric patient should that patient, in the course of treatment, reveal an intent to harm another person.

Study Questions

(Answer key is in the back of the book.)

1. The fundamental rights of individuals are derived from which of the following:
   a. Amendments to the Constitution of the United States
   b. Precedent-setting legal decisions
   c. Constitutions of individual states
   d. All the above

2. The individual right "freedom from unreasonable search and seizure" directly applies to:
   a. Right to treatment in the least restrictive environment
   b. Right to confidentiality of records
   c. Right to access courts and attorneys
   d. Right to have visitors

3. *Wyatt v. Stickney* was a court case that considered the issue of:
   a. Exemption from guilt by reason of insanity
   b. Right to treatment
   c. Right to personal privacy
   d. Right to refuse treatment

4. *Tarasoff v. The Regents of the University of California* was a court case that considered the issue of:
   a. The right to refuse treatment
   b. The duty to warn of threatened suicide
   c. The duty to warn of threatened harm to self or others
   d. The right to treatment

5. Individuals can be treated involuntarily if they are:
   1. Dangerous to self
   2. Dangerous to others
   3. Gravely disabled
   4. Convinced that they are Jesus Christ
      a. All of the above
      b. Only 1 and 2 above in about half of states
      c. 1, 2, 3 above in most states
      d. 1, 2, and 4

6. Margaret Jones is an elderly woman found wandering in the city park. She is disheveled, dirty, and not making much sense when she speaks. She is bothering people trying to enjoy themselves and, after several complaints, the police pick her up and bring her to the county hospital emergency department. Physical exam reveals a malnourished, dehydrated elderly female with either a delirium or a delirium superimposed upon a more chronic problem. She is admitted to the geriatric psychiatric floor. Ms. Jones tells everyone to leave her alone. Which of the following commitment categories best fits Ms. Jones' situation?
   a. Voluntary
   b. Involuntary
   c. Gravely disabled

7. Ms. Jones refuses to take any medication. She states that she does not need it. If this response continues, which of the following legal courses might be taken?
   a. Force her to take the medications
   b. Start conservatorship proceedings
   c. Allow her to refuse medication based upon her right to refuse treatment

8. The delirium clears after Ms. Jones has received intravenous (IV) fluids and a nutritious diet. It is evident to the staff that Ms. Jones has significant problems even when in relatively good physical health. The social worker starts to evaluate posthospital placement. A primary legal concern is:
   a. To ensure that Ms. Jones receives treatment
   b. To ensure that Ms. Jones' right to confidentiality is not violated
   c. To consider her right to the least restrictive alternative/environment
   d. To ensure that the appropriate people are warned of her impending discharge

9. Which of the following rights can be suspended with good cause?
   a. The right to treatment in the least restrictive environment
   b. The right to freedom from restraint and seclusion
   c. The right to confidentiality of records
   d. The right to warn others of danger

See answer key for rationale to this somewhat tricky question.

REFERENCES

Appelbaum PS: *Foucha v. Louisiana:* when must the state release insanity acquittees? *Hosp Community Psychiatry* 44(1):9, 1993.

Appelbaum PS and Greer A: Confidentiality in group therapy, *Hosp Community Psychiatry* 44(4):311, 1993.

Beck CK, Rawlins RP, and Williams SR: *Mental health-psychiatric nursing,* St. Louis, 1988, Mosby.

Betemps EJ, Buncher CR, and Oden M: Length of time spent in seclusion and restraint by patients at 82 VA medical centers, *Hosp Community Psychiatry,* 43(9):912, 1992.

Binder RL and McNeil DE: Application of the Tarasoff ruling and its affect on the victim and the therapeutic relationship. *Psychiatric Service* 47(11):1212, 1996.

Ciccone JR, et al: Medication refusal and judicial activism: a reexamination of the effects of the Rivers decision, *Hosp Community Psychiatry* 44(6):555, 1993.

Colorado Society of Clinical Specialists in Psychiatric Nursing: Ethical guidelines for confidentiality, *J Psychosoc Nurs Ment Health Serv* 28:43, 1990.

Eskreis TR: Seven common legal pitfalls in nursing, *AJN* 98:34, 1998.

Hegner RE: Managed care carveouts for mental health and substance abuse, *J of Amer Psychiatric Nurses Assoc* 2:63, 1996.

Hughes DH: Implications of recent court rulings for Crisis and Psychiatric Emergency Services, *Psychiatric Services* 47(12):1332, 1996.

Jones SL: More on confidentiality, *Arch Psychiatr Nurs* 7(3):123, 1993.

Klerman GL: The psychiatric patient's right to effective treatment: implications of *Osheroff v. Chestnut Lodge*, *Am J Psychiatry* 147:409, 1990.

Lamb HR and Weinberger LE: Therapeutic use of conservatorship in the treatment of gravely disabled psychiatric patients, *Hosp Community Psychiatry* 44(2):147, 1993.

Munetz MR and Geller JL: The least restrictive alternative in the postinstitutional era, *Hosp Community Psychiatry* 44(10):967, 1993.

News and Notes: Recent court ruling in Alabama's Wyatt case modifies 20-year-old patient care standards, *Hosp Community Psychiatry,* 43(8):851, 1992a.

News and Notes: APA board approves new guidelines for hospital admission, *Hosp Community Psychiatry* 43(11):1156, 1992b.

Norris MK and Kennedy CW: The view from within: how patients perceive the seclusion process, *J Psychosoc Nurs Ment Health Serv* 30(3):7, 1992.

Outlaw FH and Lowery BJ: Seclusion: the nursing challenge, *J Psychosoc Nurs Ment Health Serv* 30(4):13, 1992.

President's Commission on Mental Health: *Report to the President,* Washington, 1978, US Government Printing Office.

Tooke SK and Brown JS: Perceptions of seclusion: comparing patient and staff reactions, *J Psychosoc Nurs Ment Health Serv* 30(8):23, 1992.

Trudeau ME: Informed consent: the patient's right to decide, *J Psychosoc Nurs Ment Health Serv* 31(6):9, 1993.

Weiner DB: Philippe Pinel's "Memoir on Madness" of December 11, 1794: a fundamental text of modern psychiatry, *Am J Psychiatry* 149(6):725, 1992.

CHAPTER 5

Psychobiological Bases of Behavior

RICHARD A. SUGERMAN

LEARNING OBJECTIVES

After reading this chapter you should be able to:
- Describe the importance of the psychiatric nurse's understanding of brain biology.
- Identify and describe gross neuroanatomical structures.
- Discuss the significance and role of five specific neurotransmitters in normal brain function.
- Identify the role of five specific neurotransmitters in schizophrenia, depression, anxiety, and dementia.

- Differentiate the functions of the sympathetic and parasympathetic nervous systems.
- Describe the function of the extrapyramidal system and its significance for movement disorders.
- Discuss key psychobiological assessment issues for the psychiatric nurse.

THE BRAIN

The central nervous system (CNS) is composed of the brain and the spinal cord. The brain can be further divided into the cerebrum, the brainstem, and the cerebellum. The brain weighs only approximately 3 to 4 lb but contains 100 billion neurons, roughly the same number of stars that are in the Milky Way. The brain is incredibly complex, and there is much about the brain that science does not know. What is known, however, is that many mental disorders that were formerly thought to be caused by psychosocial stressors and/or traumatic early life

experiences are the result of altered or disordered brain biology. The National Foundation for Brain Research (1992) estimates that, at the present time, there are well over 650 brain disorders that affect approximately 50 million Americans.

The 1990s were declared the "decade of the brain," and psychiatric nursing is working diligently to become a full participant in mental health care as this century comes to a close. Psychiatric nursing has been influenced primarily by the dominant ideas of the last century: the ideas of Freud, Bleuler, and Jung that supposed mental disorders originated from psychodynamic causes. Chapter 1 addresses the

KEY TERMS

Axons   The long processes from the neuronal cell body that transmit impulses away from the cell

Basal ganglia   Large subcortical nuclei, including the caudate nucleus, putamen, and globus pallidus, that are responsible for modulating voluntary movement

Cerebral cortex   The narrow ribbon of gray matter that lies on the surface of the cerebrum. The gray matter lies "on top of" the white matter. The reverse is true in the spinal cord

Coma   Depressed consciousness wherein even extreme stimulation of the reticular activating system does not cause a response

Contralateral   The opposite side of the body

Corpus callosum   The major connecting and communicating pathway between the hemispheres

Dendrites   The many projections from the neuron that transmit impulses to the cell body

Diencephalon   The thalamus, hypothalamus, epithalamus, and metathalamus

Extrapyramidal   Outside the pyramidal system; the extrapyramidal system modulates and supports voluntary movement

Gray matter   Composed of the cell bodies and dendrites of neurons

Gyri   The convolutions of gray matter on the cerebrum

Ipsilateral   The same side of the body

Lesion   Injury to tissue

Medially   Toward the midline

Meninges   The outer lining of the CNS composed of the dura mater, arachnoid, and pia mater

Neuron   Nerve cell

Olfactory   Pertaining to the sense of smell

Pyramidal system   The motor system for voluntary movement

Sulcus   A groove separating gyri. Deep sulci are referred to as *fissures*

White matter   Composed of myelinated neuronal axons

historically significant benchmarks in psychiatry, including those associated with the roots of psychobiology. It also discusses the development of two distinct views of mental illness, nature (biological causation) vs. nurture (psychodynamic causation), and psychiatric nursing's attraction to the latter.

Those discussions are not repeated in this chapter, but it is important to note that psychiatric nursing is now fully integrating biological concepts, and, consequently, practicing holistically. In order for psychiatric nurses to do this, an understanding of basic neuroanatomy and neurophysiology is a prerequisite. The objective of this chapter is to make a balanced presentation of biological information so that the student can coherently engage the rest of this book, can participate in interdisciplinary discussions, and can read the psychiatric literature with understanding.

Understanding psychobiological concepts enables the nurse to better assess patients' behaviors and plan appropriate nursing interventions. Nursing diagnoses will become more specific and evaluation more refined as this knowledge base is more completely incorporated into nursing practice.

NEUROANATOMY AND NEUROPHYSIOLOGY OF THE BRAIN

The nervous system is divided into the CNS and the peripheral nervous system (PNS). The CNS can be further divided into the cerebrum, the brainstem, and the cerebellum. Other discussions critical to a basic understanding of the biological parameters of mental illness include neurons and neurotransmitters, the autonomic nervous system, and the ventricular system. Each is discussed separately in this chapter.

The Cerebrum

The cerebrum is divided into two cerebral hemispheres, which includes the diencephala, and constitutes the bulk of the nervous system. The hemispheres are composed of a multitude of nervous system pathways, the cerebral cortex, certain limbic structures, and the basal ganglia. The hemispheres are interconnected by the corpus callosum. These are explained in the following section.

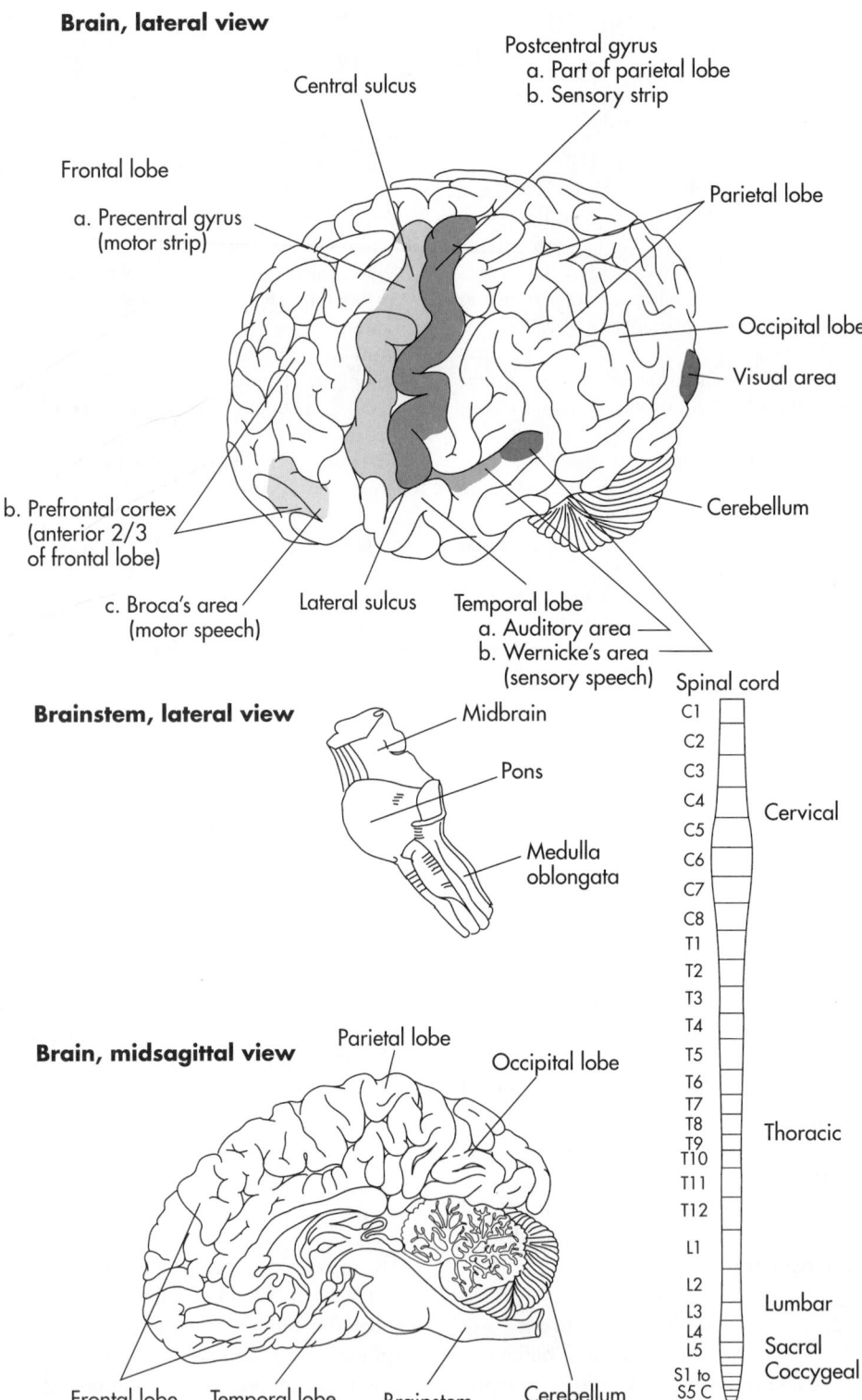

Brain, lateral view

Central sulcus

Postcentral gyrus
a. Part of parietal lobe
b. Sensory strip

Parietal lobe

Frontal lobe

a. Precentral gyrus
(motor strip)

Occipital lobe

Visual area

b. Prefrontal cortex
(anterior 2/3
of frontal lobe)

Cerebellum

c. Broca's area
(motor speech)

Lateral sulcus

Temporal lobe
a. Auditory area
b. Wernicke's area
(sensory speech)

Brainstem, lateral view

Midbrain

Pons

Medulla
oblongata

Spinal cord

C1
C2
C3
C4
C5   Cervical
C6
C7
C8
T1
T2
T3
T4
T5
T6
T7
T8
T9   Thoracic
T10
T11
T12

L1

L2
L3   Lumbar
L4
L5   Sacral
S1 to   Coccygeal
S5 C

Brain, midsagittal view

Parietal lobe

Occipital lobe

Frontal lobe   Temporal lobe   Brainstem   Cerebellum

FIGURE 5-1 Expanded view of the central nervous system showing the major components. Components are not to scale. (From Sugerman RA, Edmundson MJ, and Robinson S: *Human anatomy*, Edina, 1979, Burgess.)

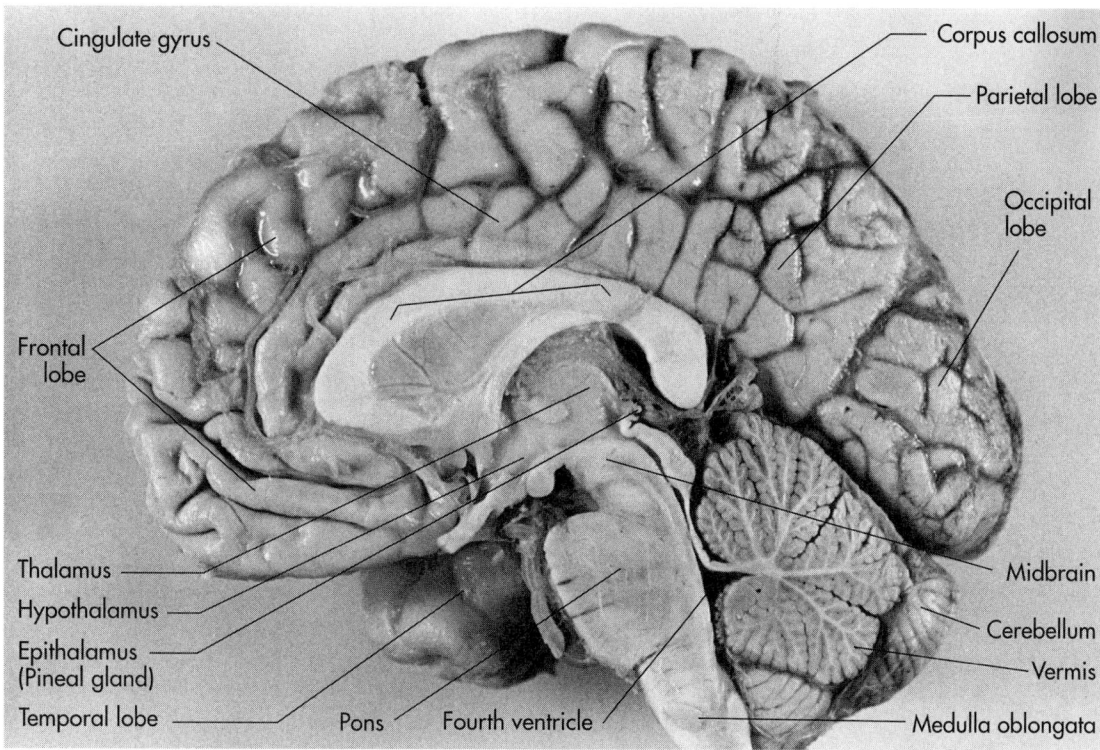

FIGURE 5-2 Midline view of right hemisphere with anatomical sites labeled. (Photograph by Berto Tarin, Multimedia Department, Western University of Health Sciences.)

Nervous system pathways

Some specialized neurons in the cerebral cortex transmit information by way of pathways throughout the CNS. A pathway is a bundle of these communicating neurons. In the CNS, a neuronal pathway (a bundle of neurons) can be called a *tract,* a *fasciculus,* a *peduncle,* or a *lemniscus.* (In neuroanatomy, a single anatomical entity can have several names.) In the PNS, a neuronal pathway is called a *nerve.* Hence, it is easy to recognize that cranial "nerve" III (CN III) is part of the PNS.

A number of large CNS pathways are readily apparent structures within white areas of the brain (white matter). For example, major pathways include the corpus callosum (Figures 5-2, 5-3), the internal capsule in each hemisphere (Figures 5-3, 5-4), and the corona radiata (Figures 5-3, 5-4). Although there has been much public interest in differences between the right brain (visual-spatial, experiential tasks) and the left brain (language, mathematics, reasoning), many scientists now have a greater appreciation for the interrelatedness of the two hemispheres. The corpus callosum connects the two hemispheres and is the communication pathway between them. If the corpus callosum is severed, a split brain syndrome develops. The internal capsule and the corona radiata are pathways through which motor and sensory information is passed; for example, motor impulses from the motor cortex (precentral gyrus) to the foot pass through these pathways. In addition to these large pathways, there are many smaller tracts interconnecting the four lobes of the cerebral cortex.

Cerebral cortex

The cerebral cortex is the outermost part of the brain and is composed of gray matter. The gray matter, actually tan in color, does the work of the brain. Gray matter consists of neuronal cell bodies, dendrites, and synapses and is not myelinated (myelinated axons compose the white matter). The cerebral

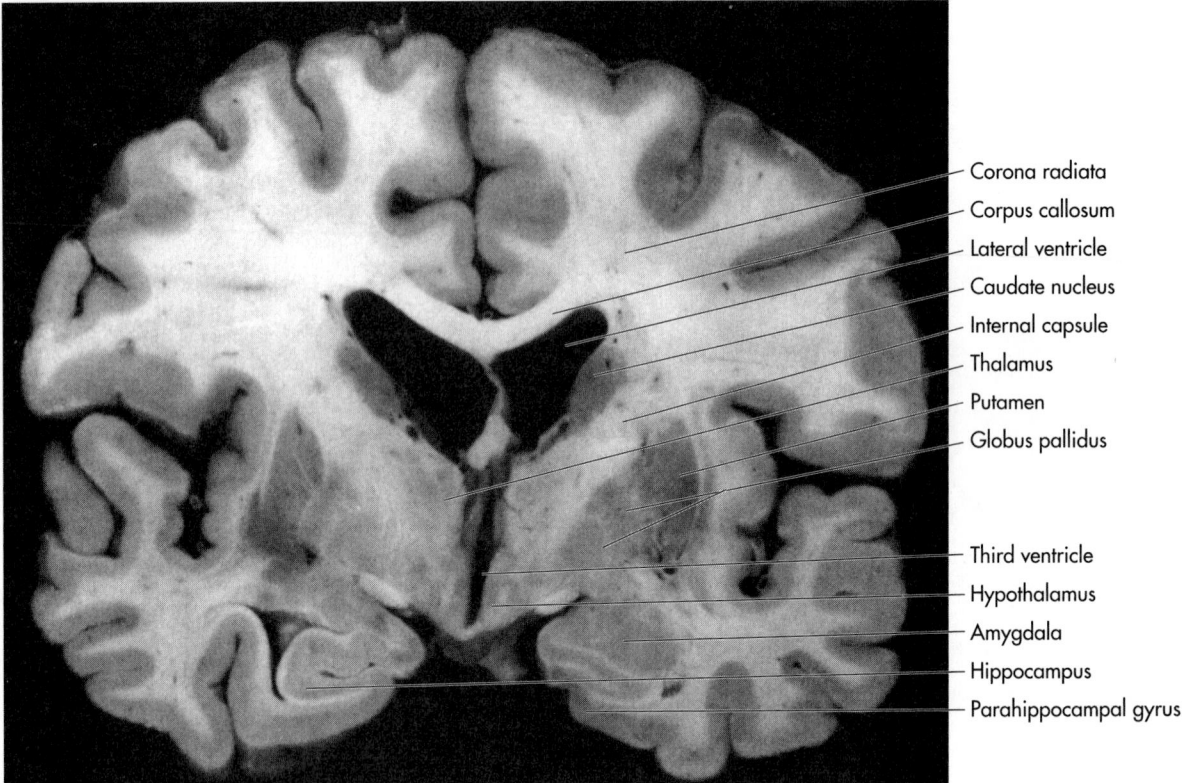

FIGURE 5-3 Coronal section of the cerebrum at the level of the hypothalamus. (Courtesy Richard E. Powers, MD, UAB Brain Resource Program.)

cortex is divided into four lobes: the frontal, temporal, parietal, and occipital lobes (Figures 5-1, 5-2). Upon visual examination of the brain, one is struck by the raised areas, or convolutions, and the grooves between those areas. Convoluted gray matter is referred to as a *gyrus* (or plural, *gyri*) and a groove between two gyri is called a *sulcus* (or plural, *sulci*). A deep sulcus is referred to as a *fissure.*

The net effect of this convoluted configuration is that it provides more gray matter to perform the work of the brain. This principle can be visualized by considering the coastline of Norway. If Norway did not have the fjords, its coastline would be rather small (i.e., about 1600 miles). However, due to the fjords, the actual coastline of Norway is extraordinary for a country of its size (i.e., about 12,500 miles). The gyri and sulci of the cerebral cortex are the "fjords" of the brain. The indentations provide for a much larger "coastline" of "working" gray matter than would be true if the brain's surface

were smooth. The four lobes of the cerebral cortex are divided by three sulci.

The frontal lobes

The frontal lobes are divided into a *motor cortex* (also called the *motor strip*), the *premotor cortex,* and the *prefrontal areas.* The motor cortex lies just rostral to (in front of) the central sulcus (Figure 5-1), which separates the frontal and parietal lobes. Because it lies in front of the central sulcus, the motor strip is also called the *precentral gyrus.* The motor cortex controls voluntary motor activity and the pathway (Figure 5-4) from this area descends through the corona radiata, the internal capsule, crosses in the caudal brainstem, and synapses in the spinal cord. From the spinal cord spinal nerves branch out into the periphery to cause muscle movement. This system of voluntary movement is referred to as the *pyramidal system* or the *corticospinal tract.* The term *pyramidal* is used because many of the neurons in

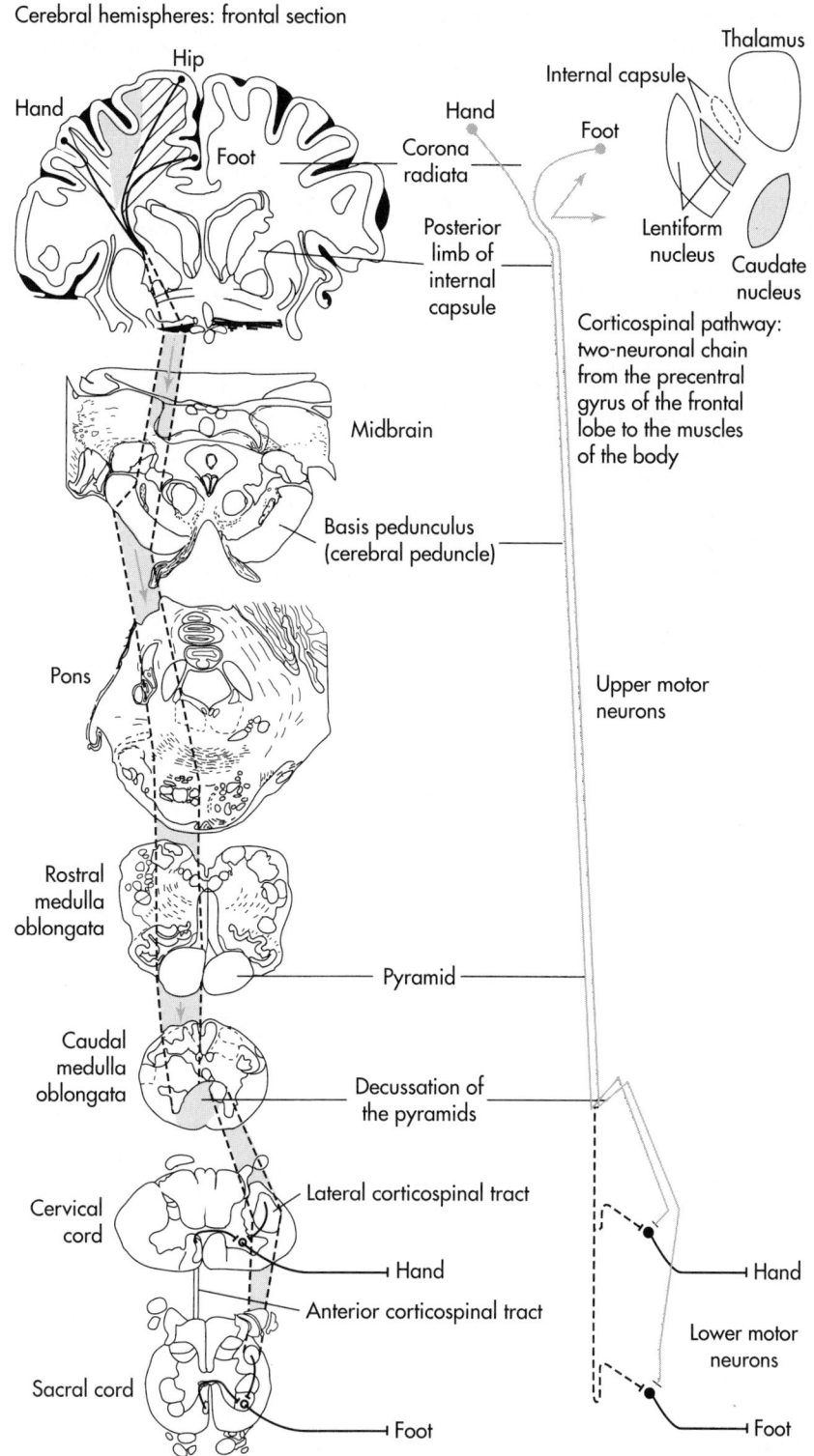

FIGURE 5-4   Distribution of the corticospinal tract. *Left*, actual representation; *Right*, schematic representation.

this tract pass through the pyramids of the lower (or caudal) brainstem (medulla oblongata). The extrapyramidal system lies outside the pyramids.

CLINICAL EXAMPLE

Think about wiggling your right big toe. Now wiggle it. What is not known is how we translate a thought into a muscle movement. What is known is that this voluntary movement is a two-neuron system; that is, there are neurons from the motor cortex that descend as described previously and synapse with spinal neurons. The spinal neurons project as a spinal nerve from the spinal cord and descend to the toe. The neurons from the motor cortex to the spinal cord are called *upper motor neurons* (Figure 5-4). The neurons that project from the spinal cord down to the toe are *lower motor neurons*. Whether a disease is an upper motor neuron disease (e.g., stroke) or a lower motor neuron disease (e.g., polio) is clinically

significant. If you are a tall person, the single neurons to your big toe may be over 3 feet long.

The premotor area is associated with movement patterns for voluntary motor activity (Haines, 1997) and with inhibiting lower motor neurons from overreacting to stimuli (Liebman, 1991). This area is not under conscious control. It is from the premotor cortex and extrapyramidal system that many movement disorders arise, including those associated with psychotropic drug use. Both the motor cortex and the premotor cortex are organized systematically (Kandel, Schwartz, and Jessell, 1991). This is referred to as *somatotropic organization,* meaning simply that the area of the motor strip that controls a certain part of the body is relatively specific. This biological reality has been visually depicted as a little man or, more commonly, an homunculus (Figure 5-5). Perhaps a word picture can best describe this specific pattern of voluntary motor localization. Think of a

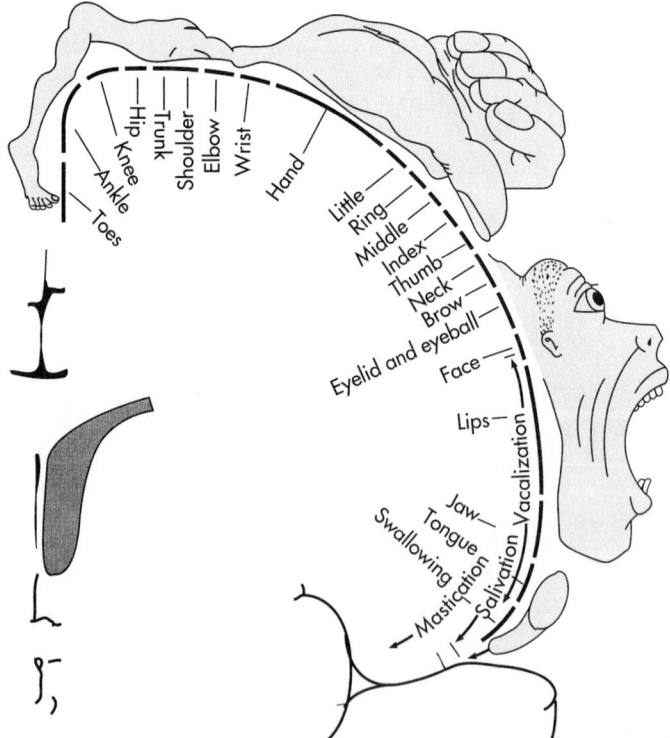

FIGURE 5-5 Homunculus of the precentral gyrus. This is a frontal section depicting the relative amount of cortex subserved in controlling the motor functions of various body areas. (From Penfield W and Rasmussen T: *The cerebral cortex of man,* New York, 1950, Macmillan.)

child hanging on the monkey bars with her head down and her feet hanging over the bar. Think of the top of the hemisphere as the bar, with the head hanging down laterally and the feet hanging down between the hemispheres. The area of the motor strip where the head is located controls head movements, the area where the feet are hanging controls feet movements, and so on.

A health professional can give a physical examination to a person with a neurological lesion, i.e., stroke, gunshot wound, etc. and, utilizing a knowledge of the corticospinal tract and homunculus (Figures 5-4, 5-5), can often predict the site of cortical lesions in the CNS. Knowing the brainstem location of the cranial nuclei allows you to localize subcortical lesions.

The prefrontal area of the cerebral cortex is responsible for thought, goal-oriented behavior, and inhibition. The frontal poles are the seat of the personality, and injuries here result in personality changes.

The temporal lobes

The temporal lobes lie under (or caudal to) the *lateral sulci* (the *lateral fissures of Sylvius*). The temporal lobes are divided into a primary auditory receptive area, secondary auditory association areas, and visual association areas (Westmoreland, et al, 1994). Aphasias, both visual and auditory, are caused by damage to the temporal lobe. Individuals with visual aphasia cannot recognize words in print that they once understood; the words are as unrecognizable as printed Russian would be to most people. Persons with auditory aphasia hear sounds but cannot associate the sounds with meaning.

The parietal lobes

The parietal lobes are posterior to the central sulcus. They are primarily sensory-association areas, and there is a sensory strip (the postcentral gyrus) that corresponds to the homunculus of the motor strip. The sensory areas interpret sensations. Behind this area are the association areas of the parietal lobes.

The occipital lobes

The occipital lobes are divided into visual receptive areas and visual association areas. The primary function of the occipital lobes is vision.

Limbic system

The limbic lobe forms the central core of the limbic system and is composed of the septal area, cingulate gyrus, and parahippocampal gyrus. The *limbic system* is a broad term, referring to the limbic lobe and the structures that function with it: the frontal cortex, hypothalamus, amygdala, hippocampus, numerous tracts, brainstem nuclei, and the autonomic system. The limbic system controls the four Fs (feeding, fighting, fleeing, and fornicating), memory, and emotions/motivation. The emotions/motivation component includes the "feelings" about people, institutions, and life that affect behavior. For example, "feelings" help to determine if an act is right or wrong, good or bad, and whether or not a particular act will be performed. Most authors refer to these "feelings" as *visceral aspects of behavior*.

Limbic olfactory function

The first pathway discussed is the olfactory pathway, which is concerned with odor detection, feeding, and feeling pleasure. This chapter does not discuss odor detection beyond how it relates to limbic functions. It is important to note how significant smell is to emotion. Big department stores have recognized for years that having a perfume display sells more than just perfume.

Olfactory information is picked up by receptor neurons in the nasal cavity and transmitted to the olfactory bulbs, which are located directly under the surface of the frontal lobes. The olfactory bulbs project axons that synapse in the parahippocampal gyrus and a subdivision of the amygdala (Figure 5-3). Olfaction is the only sensory information not relayed through the thalamus.

Pleasure/feeding functions

The septal area connects neuronally with the hypothalamus, which is involved in several aspects of feeding (e.g., the feeding and satiety centers). Experimentally, researchers can electrically stimulate or lesion (destroy) these areas and affect whether an animal overeats or stops eating.

Electrical stimulation of the reward pathway can cause animals and people to feel pleasure. Rats will press a bar repeatedly so that they can receive electrical stimulation to this pathway. The dopaminergic neurons projecting from the ventral tegmental area

(VTA) are of particular importance. These neurons project to the cortical and limbic areas, especially the nucleus accumbens. Recently investigators have hypothesized that cocaine and many other drugs may produce their effects by increasing the action of dopamine in the nucleus accumbens. The nucleus accumbens is said to be one of the brain's key pleasure centers. The nucleus accumbens is located just inferior and lateral to the septal area.

Fight or flight limbic function

The fight or flight pathway is composed of three major areas: amygdala, hypothalamus, and midbrain. Electrical stimulation of these areas elicits rage behavior or flight. Bilateral lesioning (destroying) of the amygdala and hypothalamus can have a calming effect.

Memory limbic function

The limbic system is crucial to memory. The amygdala and the hippocampus, located deep in the temporal lobe, are key structures in the transfer of information from short-term to long-term memory (Boss and Stowe, 1986). The complex process by which memories are made and stored is known as the *Papez circuit*. Discussion of the Papez circuit is beyond the scope of this book; however, it is important to recognize that lesions along this circuit cause memory problems. For example, bilateral lesions of the hippocampus nuclei related to the anoxia that is associated with near drownings and lesions of the mamillary bodies related to thiamine deficiencies in alcoholics (i.e., Korsakoff's psychosis) cause memory problems. Often these individuals maintain long-term memory, but they cannot "make" new memories.

Amnestic states, amnestic dementias, punch-drunk syndrome, herpes encephalitis, and Alzheimer's disease all involve dysfunction of the hippocampi and possibly other limbic structures (Boss and Stowe, 1986).

Basal ganglia

The basal ganglia (Figure 5-3) are made up of three major nuclei: the caudate nucleus, the putamen, and the globus pallidus. These structures are also involved in motor functions. The putamen and globus pallidus together are referred to as the lentiform nucleus (lense shaped). The basal ganglia or extrapyramidal system interrelates motor activity between the cerebral cortex, thalamus, basal ganglia, substantia nigra, subthalamic nucleus, red nucleus, reticular formation, and brainstem nuclei. The extrapyramidal system complements the pyramidal system. The pyramidal (or corticospinal) tract transmits commands for voluntary movement, and the extrapyramidal system modulates those movements and maintains appropriate muscle tone and adjusts posture.

The extrapyramidal system balances excitatory and inhibitory neurons that have different neurotransmitters. Dopamine is the primary inhibitory neurotransmitter, and acetylcholine is the primary excitatory neurotransmitter. Gamma-aminobutyric acid (GABA) is another important inhibitory neurotransmitter in this system.

The extrapyramidal system affects the contralateral side (other side) of the body. (A basal ganglia stroke affects the opposite side of the body.) Because this system maintains muscle tone and posture, movements are most noticeable during rest. For instance, Parkinson's disease, an extrapyramidal disorder, manifests with a resting tremor. These unwanted movements diminish with concentration and with intentional movement, and are absent during sleep.

In general, then, the pyramidal tract or corticospinal tract *controls* precise, voluntary movements; the basal ganglia, in conjunction with the cerebellum, *stabilize* motor movements. Lesions of the basal ganglia result in abnormal motor movements, such as those seen in Parkinson's disease (due to decreased dopamine bioavailability) and Huntington's disease (due to alterations in GABA and the cholinergic system). All of the basal ganglia areas receive, integrate, and transmit motor information.

The Diencephalon

The diencephalon (Figures 5-2, 5-3) is made up of the thalamus, hypothalamus, epithalamus (including the pineal gland), and subthalamus. Although all of the nuclei of the diencephalon are important, only a brief review of the thalamus and the hypothalamus is provided in this text. The thalamus is the major sensory/basal ganglia relay nuclear area to and from the cerebral cortex. All sensory pathways, except the olfactory pathways, synapse in the thalamus (Barr and Kiernan 1993). Sensory fibers ascend to and synapse in the thalamus and are then relayed to the cerebral cortex via the internal capsule (Goldberg, 1990). The hypothalamus maintains homeostasis and is the controller of the autonomic nervous system. The hypothalamus (Barr and Kiernan, 1993) is a tiny structure lying below the thalamus. It modulates such visceral functions as body temperature regulation, gastrointestinal activity, and cardiovascular functions. In addition, it serves as a chemoreceptor by "sampling" cerebrospinal fluid and blood. The hypothalamus controls and influences functions such as food and water intake and endocrine secretion. The hypothalamus has two modes of affecting the pituitary gland. The first mode is by the production of releasing and inhibiting factors that pass into the pituitary portal system, such as thyrotropin-releasing hormone or prolactin-inhibiting factor. These factors are transmitted to the anterior pituitary, where they cause the release or inhibition of anterior pituitary hormones into the blood. The second mode is by the direct projection of hypothalamic neurons upon the posterior pituitary, where the neurons directly release their hormones (such as oxytocin) into the pituitary blood supply. Lesions of the subthalamic nucleus can result in hemiballismus (Box 5-1).

Brainstem and Cerebellum

The brainstem, cerebellum, and spinal cord reside beneath the cerebrum (Figure 5-1). The *brainstem* is a collective term for the midbrain, pons, and medulla oblongata. The cerebellum is an expansive area attached to the posterior surface of the pons and resembles its Latin name, *little brain.* The most caudal portion of the CNS is the spinal cord.

Midbrain

The midbrain (Figure 5-6) represents the continuation of the CNS below the cerebrum. It is about 1.5 cm long and is relatively narrow. The red nuclei and substantia nigra are large structures in the midbrain that can be distinguished easily on gross examination. The red nuclei in freshly cut brains are large, reddish, round balls; the substantia nigra, as its name implies, is black. The black coloration is due to melanin pigment found in neurons within the substantia nigra. It is from these dark cells that most of the brain dopamine is synthesized. In Parkinson's disease, these cells are depigmented and thus produce less dopamine. Dopamine deficiency causes the extrapyramidal motor disorders associated with parkinsonism.

Pons

Pons literally means bridge, and it does form a bridge between the midbrain and the medulla oblongata. It is a bulbous area approximately 2.5 cm long that lies between the midbrain and the medulla oblongata and is anterior to the cerebellum. Some pathway fibers descending from the cerebrum pass through

Box 5-1 Differences Between Basal Ganglia and Cerebellar Movement Disorders

General Difference:

Cerebellar dysfunction: awkwardness of intentional movement

Basal ganglia dysfunction: meaningless, unintentional movement that occurs unexpectedly

Cerebellar disorders:

1. Ataxia: awkwardness of posture and gait; incoordination; overshooting the goal when reaching for an object; inability to perform rapid, alternating movements, such as finger tapping; awkward use of speech muscles, resulting in irregularly spaced sounds
2. Decreased tendon reflexes on affected side
3. Asthenia: muscles tire easily
4. Intention tremor: noticed when intending to do something, such as reaching for a pencil
5. Nystagmus

Basal ganglia disorders:

1. Parkinsonism: rigidity, bradykinesia, resting tremor, masklike face, shuffling gait
2. Chorea: sudden, jerky, and purposeless movements (e.g., Huntington's disease, Sydenham's chorea)
3. Athetosis: slow, writhing, snakelike movements, especially of fingers and wrists
4. Hemiballismus: a sudden, wild flailing of one arm

Adapted from Goldberg S: *Clinical neuroanatomy,* Miami, 1990, MedMaster.

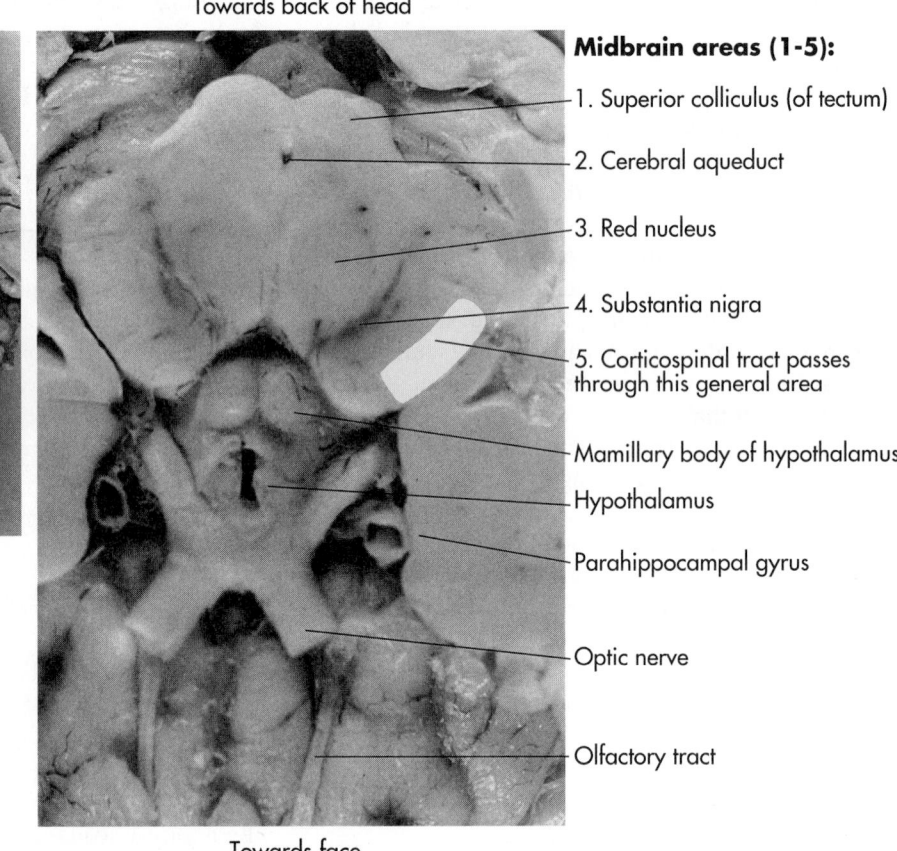

Towards back of head

Midbrain areas (1-5):

1. Superior colliculus (of tectum)
2. Cerebral aqueduct
3. Red nucleus
4. Substantia nigra
5. Corticospinal tract passes through this general area

Mamillary body of hypothalamus

Hypothalamus

Parahippocampal gyrus

Optic nerve

Olfactory tract

A

B

Towards face

FIGURE 5-6 A, Brain sectioned transversely through the midbrain and parahippocampal gyri. **B,** Enlargement of the area through the midbrain. (Photographs by Berto Tarin, Multimedia Department, Western University of Health Sciences.)

the midbrain and terminate in the pons. The pontine nuclei project motor and posture information to the cerebellum.

Medulla oblongata

The medulla oblongata is about 3 cm long and narrows until it becomes continuous with the cervical spinal cord. Many cerebral cortex motor fibers that are in the midbrain and travel through the pons continue their descent on the anterior surface of the medulla oblongata; these fibers collectively form pyramidal shaped bulges known as the *pyramids*. The decussation of the pyramids—that is, the crossing over of the lateral corticospinal motor pathway contralaterally (to the opposite side)—takes place at the lower end of the medulla oblongata (Figure 5-4). This crossing over is the reason that a right brain stroke results in left-side impairment. The medulla oblongata is responsible for many important functions, including respiration, regulation of blood pressure, partial regulation of heart rate, vomiting, and swallowing.

Reticular formation

A multineural pathway called the *reticular formation* resides within the brainstem. This pathway comprises a series of large nuclei, beginning within the midbrain, and extending through the pons and the medulla oblongata. The reticular formation may be thought of as a primitive brain buried deep within the brainstem. Input from most sensory pathways passes into the reticular formation, where it is integrated and then projected to areas such as the thalamus and hypothalamus. The reticular formation affects motor, sensory, and visceral functions.

The reticular activating system (RAS) is part of the reticular formation. It serves as a screening device that allows individuals to "tune out" some stimuli and attend to other stimuli. The ability to tune out is fortunate; otherwise, studying or even sleeping in some environments would not be possible. The RAS allows us to fall asleep. The RAS is activated by sensory stimuli, pain, movement, feedback from the cortex, muscle tone, and sympathomimetic drugs (stimulants). Any of these help a person to remain awake. Due to its many synapses, the RAS can be depressed easily. If a disruption occurs in the RAS and a person cannot sleep, psychosis can occur. Once it is "turned off," however, coma results. Some people have had their RAS deactivated, and no one knows how to reactivate it.

Cerebellum

The cerebellum (Figures 5-1, 5-2) consists of two hemispheres separated by a central portion called the *vermis*. The cerebellar hemispheres and most of the vermis simultaneously receive sensory input from muscles and joints and receive motor signals from the cerebral cortex indicating how muscles are to be directed. Most of the cerebellum then communicates with the cerebral cortex through the thalamus to coordinate the final motor activity. Writing with a pen, reading a book, shooting a basketball, or climbing a mountain are all possible because of a functioning cerebellum. Most of the cerebellum functions in coordinating muscle synergy and activity, but it does *not* initiate movement. The second function of the cerebellum is the maintenance of equilibrium. Differences between movement disorders associated with cerebellar dysfunction and movement disorders associated with basal ganglia dysfunction are found in Box 5-1.

Cerebellar dysfunction can produce intention tremors that are on the same side of the body as the lesion. Unlike the basal ganglia resting tremors, which occur at rest, intention tremors occur when a person is asked to try to touch something, like their own nose or a doctor's moving finger. These people have tremors when they try to concentrate on moving a limb.

Neurons and Neurotransmitters

Neurons are the basic subunit of the nervous system, and there are *100 billion* of them in the brain. The neuron is composed of a cell body with a large nucleus. It is the cell body and dendrites of the neuron that makes up the gray matter of the cortex and the brain nuclei. Neurons transmit information by sending action potentials, or waves of electrical depolarization, down their processes to other neurons. There are two processes projecting from the cell body: *dendrites* and *axons*. The dendrites receive impulses from other neurons and transmit those impulses to the cell body. Axons carry impulses away from the cell body to another neuron, muscle, or gland. Each neuron usually projects only one axon. As mentioned previously, some axons are up to 3 feet long, but microscopically thin. It should be clearly noted that a single axon can synapse with thousands of dendrites, and the dendrites of one neuron can receive impulses from the axons of thousands of other neurons (Haines, 1997). The brain is extremely complex, and knowledge of this intricate wiring schematic continues to develop.

There are basically three types of neurons: sensory neurons (or afferent neurons) that send messages to the CNS, motor neurons (or efferent neurons) that send messages from the CNS to the periphery, and association neurons (or interneurons) that lie between sensory and motor neurons. The vast majority of CNS neurons are association neurons. Most impulses (action potentials) travel from one neuron to another by sending a chemical called a *neurotransmitter* across a 20 nm space (the synapse), which separates these cells, to evoke the next action potential. It is in or around the synapse that many drugs have their site of action in the nervous system.

Neurotransmitters have been divided into four major groups or systems: cholinergic, monoamines, neuropeptides, and amino acids. Table 5-1 is a summary of the four major groups of neurotransmitters. Specific examples for each group, where these specific transmitters can be found concentrated in the brain, and major pathways in the brain that utilize these neurotransmitters are found in this table.

TABLE 5-1 **Classification of Neurotransmitters and Pathways**

Neurotransmitter	Chemical Transmitter	Location Found	Major Pathways
Cholinergic systems	ACh	Myoneural junctions, post-ganglionic neurons, autonomic ganglia, parasympathetic postganglionic neurons	Basal nucleus of Meynert to cerebral cortex, septal area (rostral to hypothalamus) to hippocampus
Monoamine systems	Catecholamines		
	Dopamine		Nigrostriatal (substantia nigra to putamen) Mesolimbic Mesocortical Tuberoinfundibular
	Norepinephrine	Locus ceruleus	Locus ceruleus (in midbrain) to thalamus, cerebral cortex, cerebellum, and spinal cord; lateral midbrain to hypothalamus and basal forebrain
	Epinephrine		Central tegmental tract
	Indolamine		
	Serotonin	Raphe nuclei	Central brainstem nuclei up to forebrain and down to spinal cord
Neuropeptides	Enkephalins	Spinal cord, hypothalamus, midbrain	
	Endorphins	Spinal cord, hypothalamus, midbrain	
	Substance P	Spinal cord, hypothalamus, and many other places	
	Somatostatin, VIP, CCK, ACTH, neurotensin, angiotensin II, and others		
Amino acids	GABA	Many neurons, indicating ubiquitous distribution	
	Glycine	Spinal cord, brainstem, and many other CNS areas	
	Glutamate	Widely distributed in the CNS	
	Aspartate	Hippocampus, dorsal root ganglion	

ACh, Acetylcholine; *ACTH,* adrenocorticotropic hormone; *CCK,* cholecystokinin; *CNS,* central nervous system; *GABA,* gamma-aminobutyric acid; *VIP,* vasoactive intestinal polypeptide. (From Keltner NL and Folks DG: *Psychotropic drugs,* St. Louis, 1997, Mosby.) This table presents a simplified summary of many of the better known neurotransmitters and, in general, where they are produced and released in the nervous system.

Neurotransmitters are thought to play major roles in some mental disorders (Table 5-2).

■ Critical Thinking Question

Explain why mature neurons do not give rise to brain tumors.

Autonomic Nervous System

The autonomic nervous system (Figure 5-7) is divided into the parasympathetic (craniosacral) and the sympathetic (thoracolumbar) nervous systems. The parasympathetic nervous system, which is a cholinergic system, conserves energy and is divided into cranial and sacral portions. The cranial part has neuronal components within the oculomotor (CN III), facial (CN VII), glossopharyngeal (CN IX), and vagus (CN X) cranial nerves; the sacral part is composed of neuronal elements located in the second through fourth sacral spinal cord areas. Parasympathetic neurons are of particular interest to psychiatric nurses because so many psychotropic drugs have anticholinergic properties. Anticholinergic drugs block the function of these nerves; for example, CN III affects pupil and ciliary body constriction, CN VII affects tearing and salivation, CN IX affects salivation, and CN X affects the vagus nerve (e.g., the heart and GI tract). Thus anticholinergic effects on these nerves cause pupil dilation, decreased lacrimation, dry mouth, tachycardia, and a slowed GI system respectively.

The sympathetic nervous system expends energy and forms a continuous column running from the first thoracic to the third lumbar spinal cord areas. Although sympathetic neuron cell bodies are confined within portions of the thoracic and lumbar spinal cord, sympathetic neurons innervate effector organs throughout the body.

Both the sympathetic and the parasympathetic systems contain two neurons between the spinal cord and the effector organs. The first neuronal cell body is in the cord, and its myelinated axon extends outward to synapse with another neuron. The first neuron in the system is referred to as the *pregan-*

Table 5-2 Neurotransmitters and Related Mental Disorders*

Neurotransmitter	Mental Disorder
Increase in ($\uparrow$) dopamine	Schizophrenia
Decrease in ($\downarrow$) norepinephrine	Depression
Decrease in ($\downarrow$) serotonin	Depression
Decrease in ($\downarrow$) acetylcholine	Alzheimer's disease
Decrease in ($\downarrow$) GABA	Anxiety

*This is a simplified explanation. A more refined explanation will be offered in appropriate chapters.

glionic neuron; the second is the *postganglionic neuron.* Preganglionic neurons secrete acetylcholine as their neurotransmitter (Figure 5-7). The postganglionic neurons send their unmyelinated axons to their effector organs: smooth muscle, cardiac muscle, or glands. In general, the parasympathetic postganglionic neurons secrete acetylcholine, and the sympathetic postganglionic neurons secrete norepinephrine as their neurotransmitters.

The hypothalamus has both sympathetic and parasympathetic functions and is considered the highest autonomic center in the CNS. It can drive both systems selectively (Figure 5-7).

The Ventricular System

The brain "floats" in approximately 140 cc of cerebrospinal fluid (CSF); however, the CNS produces about 800 cc per day. CSF circulates around the brain in the subarachnoid space and inside ventricles in the brain (Figure 5-8). The brain is covered by three connective tissue layers called *meninges.* The subarachnoid space is a narrow space between the middle meningeal layer, the arachnoid, and the innermost layer, the pia mater, that adheres to the brain. The thick outer layer, the dura mater, attaches to the inner surface of many bones of the skull. The ventricles form four spaces within the brain (Figures 5-3, 5-8). There is one large ventricle in each cerebral hemisphere, and small third and fourth ventricles are located, respectively, in the midbrain and between the pons and the cerebellum. The fourth ventricle communicates with the subarachnoid space

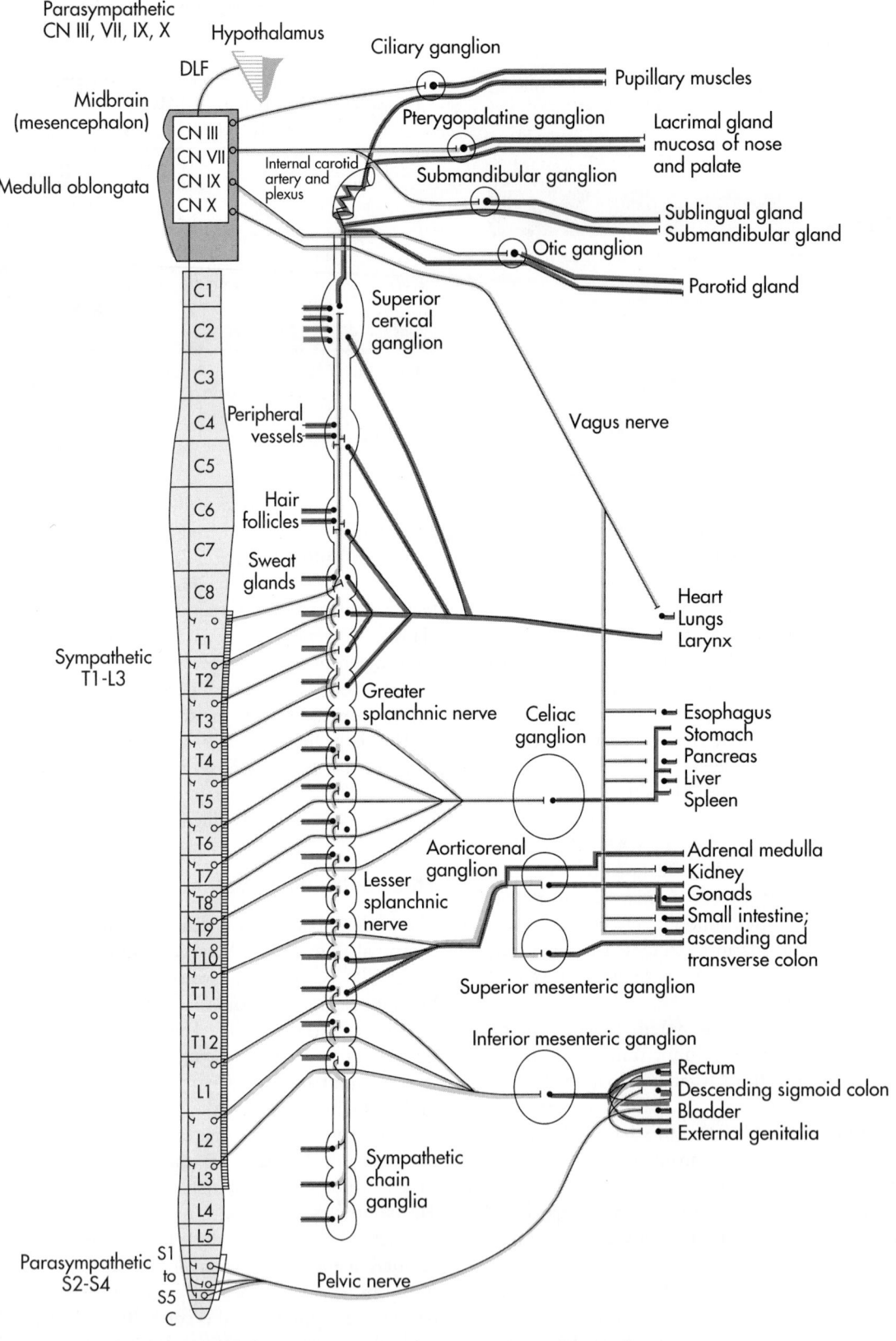

FIGURE 5-7 Diagram of the entire autonomic nervous system. Preganglionic neurons are represented as **green** lines, and the postganglionic neurons are represented as **grey** lines. The dorsal longitudinal fasciculus *(DLF)* interconnects the hypothalamus with parasympathetic and sympathetic autonomic neurons down to the sacral spinal cord level.

and, eventually, the CSF in the subarachnoid space enters the vascular system through arachnoid villi that protrude into the superior sagittal sinus on the superior surface of the brain (Figure 5-8). If for some reason the arachnoid villi are compromised, such as from a head trauma or meningitis, the CSF builds up quickly.

Enlargement of the ventricles takes place primarily due to blockage of the CSF outflow within or from the brain, from overproduction of CSF (which can cause ventricular expansion), and from brain atrophy due to the death of large numbers of cortical neurons, or from developmental problems. The first two problems are causes of hydrocephalus while brain atrophy (neurodegeneration) is commonly found in chronic alcoholics and patients with Alzheimer's disease. Neurodevelopmental problems resulting in ventricular variance is thought to be associated with schizophrenia (Crow, 1997; Roberts, Leigh, and Weinberger, 1993). In the case of neurodegeneration, creation of new space results in the enlargement of the ventricles to fill the void.

CLINICAL APPLICATION

As is stressed throughout this textbook, many mental disorders have biological bases. A brief overview of those biological influences is presented here, but the major discussion of these issues is found in the respective disorder chapter. This approach is in concert with the authors' view that the biological context of mental disorders is intricately linked to symptoms and behaviors and is part of a holistic approach to understanding psychiatric patients. To place most of the specific discussion of the psychobiological parameters of mental disorders in a separate chapter titled "psychobiology" reinforces the mindset that this etiological view is just one of many from which the student can select. The authors believe differently. Thus, the student is urged to use this chapter to review brain anatomy and physiology, and to apply that information to other chapters.

Schizophrenia

Several psychobiological influences on schizophrenia have been proposed. First, researchers have noted that in many people with schizophrenia, an increase in ventricular size is apparent. As noted previously, ventricles enlarge for one of four reasons. In schizophrenia, increased ventricle size is most likely related to neurodevelopmental reasons; that is, the brain around the ventricles has failed to develop and the ventricles are enlarged to fill the empty space. This phenomenon is referred to as an increase in *ventricular brain ratios* (VBRs). Furthermore, in many individuals with schizophrenia, a decrease in the gray matter of the cortex and major subcortical nuclei is evident.

Other biological differences found in people with schizophrenia include a decrease in cerebral blood flow (CBF), particularly in the prefrontal areas of the cortex. The term used to describe this is *hypofrontality*. New imaging technology that tracks blood flow and glucose metabolism has substantiated this physiological change. These brain changes result in a decline in frontal cognitive functions such as organizing, planning, learning, problem solving, and critical thinking.

By far the most celebrated and widely known biological theory for schizophrenia is the dopamine hypothesis. According to this theory, schizophrenia is caused by alterations of dopamine in the brain. Chapter 27 provides an elaboration of this theory and of the biologically related genetic theory of schizophrenia. Antipsychotics are discussed in Chapter 20.

■ Critical Thinking Question

It has been detected in some patients with schizophrenia that a decrease in blood flow occurs in the dorsolateral prefrontal area. If that were true, what kind of symptoms might you expect to see?

Mood Disorders

Mood disorders are also thought to have a biological basis. Decreased amounts of norepinephrine and serotonin, two important brain neurotransmitters, are thought to play a role in depression (Table 5-2). It seems that there is an overall deficiency in these neurotransmitters, and psychopharmacological treatment is based on restoring

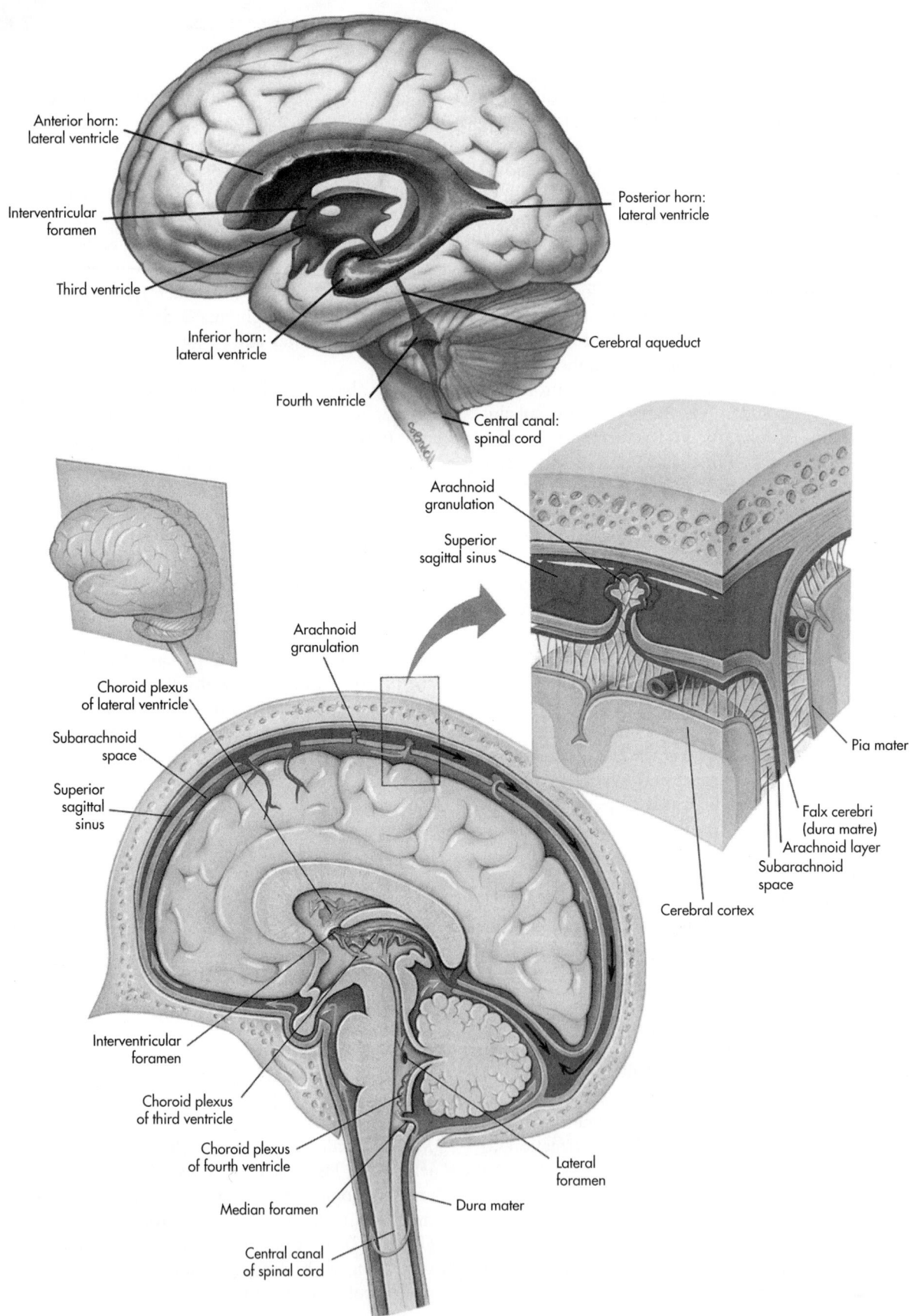

FIGURE 5-8 For legend see opposite page.

them to optimum levels. More recent findings suggest that other neurotransmitters may also be factors in depression. For instance, some researchers find evidence for the involvement of acetylcholine, dopamine, and GABA.

Chapter 28 will present a discussion of these neurotransmitters as well as the roles of receptor, thyroid, hypothalamic, and pituitary function in depression.

Anxiety Disorders

Anxiety disorders appear to have a biological basis as well. It is known that drugs that activate GABA receptors, an inhibitory effect, can calm anxious patients. Other neurotransmitters, such as norepinephrine, dopamine, and serotonin, may also have roles in anxiety. Certainly, stimulation of the sympathetic system, which is accomplished by epinephrine, norepinephrine, and dopamine (Table 5-1), causes an anxietylike reaction. Anxiety disorders are discussed in Chapter 29.

Dementias

Dementias are directly related to brain pathology. Alzheimer's disease (AD), the leading cause of dementia in the United States, is caused by brain atrophy, which manifests microscopically as neurofibrillary tangles and amyloid plaques. Patients with AD tend to have enlarged ventricles, narrowing of the cortical ribbon (gray matter), widening of the sulci, and decreases in the width of the gyri. Further, a loss of cholinergic pathways is found in AD and contributes to memory problems. Persons affected with AD forget facts, how to use words, and how to use common objects. AD and other dementias are discussed in Chapter 30.

AIDS/HIV Disease

Acquired immunodeficiency syndrome (AIDS) dementia is caused by a direct assault on the brain by the human immunodeficiency virus (HIV). It attacks the brain in two ways: it weakens and destroys T4 lymphocytes, which are part of the body's natural defense, exposing the brain to other pathogens; and the HIV directly attacks the neuronal cell bodies and white matter of the brain. Because of the attack on white matter, AIDS can sometimes be mistaken for multiple sclerosis. AIDS dementia is discussed in Chapter 41.

Degenerative Diseases

Parkinson's disease is an example of a degenerative disease that affects both motor function and emotional stability. In parkinsonism, microscopic examination of the basal ganglia, specifically the caudate nucleus and the globus pallidus, reveals degenerative changes. The most significant change, however, is the deterioration of the substantia nigra, the chief synthesizing site of dopamine in the brain. The decreased availability of dopamine in the extrapyramidal system leads to tremor, bradykinesia, and rigidity. Parkinsonism is discussed in Chapter 19 and Chapter 30.

Demyelinating Diseases

Multiple sclerosis is an example of a demyelinating disease. In this disorder, the myelin, but not the cell bodies or axons, breaks down. This degeneration of myelin causes a variety of problems, including loss of sensation, muscle weakness, fatigue, double vision, and tingling in the extremities. People with multiple sclerosis also experience psychological symptoms, no doubt related to demyelinization that occurs in the brain.

Anorexia Nervosa

Anorexia nervosa, a disorder characterized by the refusal to eat, appears to be associated with hypothalamic dysfunction. Anorexia nervosa is discussed in Chapter 35.

FIGURE 5-8 Cerebrospinal Fluid Circulation. The green arrows represent the route of the CSF. The black arrows represent the route of blood flow. CSF is produced in the ventricles, exits the fourth ventricle, and returns to the venous circulation in the superior sagittal sinus. The inset depicts the arachnoid granulations in the superior sagittal sinus, where the CSF enters the circulation. (Modified from Seeley RR, Stephens TD, and Tate P: *Anatomy and physiology*, ed 3, St. Louis, 1995, Mosby.)

Trauma

Individuals who have experienced CNS trauma can experience brain insults that are similar to those found in dementia or parkinsonism. Victims of automobile accidents or gunshots, as well as boxers, can exhibit symptoms based on the nature of the injury. Persons with an injury to the temporal lobe may experience memory loss or aphasia. Persons with a prefrontal lobe injury may experience personality changes or psychosis. Dementia pugilistica (punch-drunk syndrome), a dementing syndrome with the same molecular pathology as AD, can result from repeated blows to the head; for example, in the sport of boxing (Roberts, Leigh, and Weinberger, 1993).

Chemical Dependency

The biological pathways that might be responsible for the control that addictive substances have on people are just beginning to be understood. Current research suggests that a small nucleus in the basal ganglia (specifically, the nucleus accumbens) may be an important part of the addiction puzzle. Fischback (1992) suggests that such studies may help us better understand mechanisms for motivation.

Mitochondrial DNA Problems

Most people are familiar with a large number of genetic diseases that affect the psychological health of individuals, such as Huntington's disease. Many other diseases have been credited with genetic predispositions like that of AD. These problems have their genesis in the DNA of the chromosomes in each cell of our bodies. In 1988 scientists found that the DNA of mitochondria, the powerhouses of our body, can mutate and give rise to physical and psychological problems (Wallace, 1997). These mutant mitochondria have been implicated in AD, MELAS (mitochondrial encephalopathy, lactic acidosis, and strokelike episodes), diabetes mellitus, etc. Unlike chromosomes, mitochondria are passed only by the mother in the ovum. There are a variety of mutant mitochondria that can result in a number of diseases. The mechanism is that the mutant mitochondria, which fail to properly produce the energy that cells need to function, increase in number over time and damage particular cells and body organs.

Critical Thinking Question

From what you have read in this chapter, defend Kraepelin's view of schizophrenia as a dementia.

Key Concepts

1. The brain is a complex organ composed of 100 billion neurons, and changes in its anatomy or physiology affect behavior. Holistic nursing care requires an understanding of the impact of brain dysfunction on behavior.
2. Many mental disorders that were formerly thought to have a psychological etiology are now known to be influenced by brain dysfunction.
3. The nervous system is divided into the central nervous system (CNS) and the peripheral nervous system (PNS).
4. The CNS is divided into the brain and the spinal cord.
5. The nervous pathways in the brain are composed of myelinated axons (white matter) that connect and communicate between brain nuclei (gray matter).
6. The cerebral cortex is the outer layer of gray matter of the brain. Gray matter consists of neuronal cell bodies and is responsible for the work of the brain.
7. The two major neurotransmitters in the extrapyramidal system are dopamine (inhibitory) and acetylcholine (excitatory).
8. The pyramidal motor system controls precise movement; the extrapyramidal motor system stabilizes motor movement.
9. The reticular activating system is concerned with degrees of consciousness. Sensory stimuli received in this system are forwarded to the thalamus. The more it is stimulated, the greater the level of alertness.
10. Neurons are the basic subunit of the nervous system. The neuron consists of a cell body, *dendrites* that send information to the cell body, and a process called an *axon* that transmits impulses away from the cell body.
11. Impulses travel from one neuron to another by sending a chemical called a *neurotransmitter* across a microscopic gap called a *synapse*.
12. The dopamine hypothesis postulates that schizophrenia is caused by increased levels of brain dopamine. Treatment is aimed at reducing those levels through the use of antipsychotic drugs. This broad view of causation is refined in Chapter 27.
13. The neurotransmitter theory of depression states that depression is related to decreased levels of norepi-

nephrine and/or serotonin. This broad view of causation is refined in Chapter 28.

14. Anxiety disorders are likely related to alterations in GABA levels.

15. Dementias, specifically Alzheimer's disease, are related to brain atrophy manifested by microscopic changes in the cortical neurons, neuronal tangles, and amyloid plaques. A deficiency in the neurotransmitter acetylcholine occurs as well.

Study Questions

(Answer key is in the back of the book.)

1. Schizophrenia may be best thought of as:
   a. A neurodegenerative problem
   b. A neurodevelopmental problem
   c. Overproduction of CSF
   d. Decreased serotonin production
2. Cranial nerve XII is part of the:
   a. Central nervous system
   b. Parasympathetic nervous system
   c. Peripheral nervous system
   d. Sympathetic nervous system
3. The connecting white matter between the two cerebral hemispheres is the:
   a. Corticospinal tract
   b. Corpus callosum
   c. Extrapyramidal system
   d. Internal capsule
4. The white matter of the brain is:
   a. Myelinated dendrites
   b. Myelinated axons
   c. Cell bodies
   d. Corona radiata
5. The thin outer layer of gray matter is called the:
   a. Cerebral cortex
   b. Basal ganglia
   c. Diencephalon
   d. Frontal lobe
6. Why is the brain configured with many gyri and sulci? *gives brain more gray matter coastline*
7. The area of the brain associated with voluntary movement is referred to as:
   a. The precentral gyrus
   b. The motor cortex
   c. The corticospinal pathway
   d. The pyramidal system
   e. All of the above
8. The area of the brain associated with thought, goal-directed activity, and inhibitions is known as the:
   a. Parietal lobe
   b. Satiety center

   c. Prefrontal area
   d. Hypothalamus
9. The system associated with the four Fs, emotions/motivation, and memory is the:
   a. Cortex
   b. Limbic system
   c. Thalamus
   d. Hypothalamus
10. When the Papez circuit is lesioned somewhere along its intricate path, which of the following occurs?
    a. The thirst mechanism is compromised
    b. Memory is compromised
    c. Fight or flight is compromised
11. The Babinski response is a reflex. Does it occur with an upper motor neuron disorder, such as a stroke, or with a lower motor neuron disorder, such as polio?

Match the following movement disorder with the correct site of dysfunction.

   a = Basal ganglia disorder
   b = Cerebellar disorder
12. Awkwardness of gait   b
13. Intention tremor   b
14. Parkinsonism   a
15. Chorea   a

Match the following change in neurotransmitter bioavailability with the disorder it is thought to precipitate.

   a = Increased dopamine
   b = Decreased dopamine
   c = Decreased norepinephrine
   d = Decreased serotonin
   e = Decreased GABA
   f = Increased norepinephrine
16. Depression   c, d
17. Schizophrenia   a
18. Parkinsonism   b

REFERENCES

Barr ML and Kiernan JA: *The human nervous system: an anatomical viewpoint,* ed 6, Philadelphia, 1993, Lippincott.

Boss BJ and Stowe K: Neuroanatomy *J of Neuroscience Nursing* 18(4):214, 1986.

Collins RC: *Neurology,* Philadelphia, 1997, WB Saunders.

Crow TJ: Schizophrenia as failure of hemisphere dominance for language, *TINS* 20:339, 1997.

Fischback GD: Mind and brain, *Sci Am* 267(3):48, 1992.

Goldberg S: *Clinical neuroanatomy,* Miami, 1990, MedMaster.

Haines DE: *Fundamental Neuroscience,* New York, 1997, Churchill Livingstone.

Heath RG: Pleasure and brain activity in man, *J Nerv Ment Dis* 154:3, 1972.

Kandel ER, Schwartz JH, and Jessell TM: *Principles of neural science,* ed 3, New York, 1991, Elsevier.

Liebman M: *Neuroanatomy made easy and understandable,* ed 4, Gaithersburg, Md, 1991, Aspen.

National Foundation for Brain Research: *The cost of disorders of the brain,* Washington, DC, 1992, The Foundation.

Roberts GW, Leigh PN, and Weinberger BR: *Neuropsychiatric disorders,* London, 1993, Mosby-Europe.

Wallace DC: Mitochondrial DNA in aging and disease, *Sci Am* 277(2):40, 1997.

Westmoreland BF, et al: *Medical Neurosciences,* ed 3, New York, 1994, Little, Brown & Co.

Continuum of Care

CHAPTER 6

Continuum of Care

CAROL E. BOSTROM
LEE H. SCHWECKE

LEARNING OBJECTIVES

After reading this chapter you should be able to:
- Comprehend the concept of the continuum of care.
- Understand services necessary for prevention and treatment of mental disorders.
- Identify the impact of managed care on the continuum of care.
- Explain the importance of assessment in making decisions about referrals to various levels of care.

KEY TERMS

Continuum of care Levels of care through which an individual can move depending upon his or her needs at a given point in time.

Managed care A system of entities that arranges the relationships between payers, providers, and consumers; monitors and influences the behavior of the mental health providers and the outcomes of care; and reimburses for services.

With the current trends in health care, mental health and psychiatric care are now evolving into a broader continuum of services. This unit provides an overview of the continuum of care including chapters on hospital-based care, community-based care, and case management.

Nursing has a long history of involvement in health promotion, primary prevention, treatment, and rehabilitation. The challenge for psychiatric nursing involves the use of traditional knowledge and skills in nontraditional settings and programs. As reimbursement models, including managed care, influence type and duration of services, nurses are struggling to provide quality care in a holistic framework. For psychiatric nursing, short, crisis-oriented inpatient stays produce a demand for more intensive outpatient services. The continuum of care provides consumers a wide range of treatment modalities to assist the individual in achieving his or her optimal level of functioning.

One model that includes prevention is the Mental Health Intervention Spectrum developed by the Committee on Prevention of Mental Disorders of the Institute of Medicine (Institute of Medicine, 1994). This model describes a spectrum of interventions for mental disorders, including prevention, treatment, and maintenance. Box 6-1 provides examples of each level of intervention.

Ideally, psychiatric mental health services should cover all areas within the spectrum. However, in

86

Box 6-1 **The Mental Health Spectrum for Mental Disorders**		
Interventions	**Goal**	**Examples**
Universal prevention	Promoting the health of individuals and groups who are identified as not being at risk for any of the mental disorders	Stress management classes, self-esteem workshops, wellness programs
Selective prevention	Programs for individuals and groups who are at risk for developing mental disorders due to psychological, economic, and environmental factors	School breakfast and lunch programs, children of divorce groups, grief groups, depression screening programs
Indicated prevention	Early identification of individuals having a biological predisposition for or early symptoms of a mental disorder	Children of the mentally ill, employee assistance programs, walk-in clinics, crisis services, shelters
Treatment interventions	Diagnosing and treating of individuals with mental disorders	Hospital-based care, community-based care, home care
Maintenance interventions	Decreasing disability and preventing relapse of individuals and groups with mental disorders	Self-help groups, psychoeducational groups, vocational rehabilitation, special skill training

Adapted from Institute of Medicine: *Reducing risks for mental disorders,* Washington, DC, National Academy Press, 1994.

reality, the focus is on treatment and maintenance activities. There is an effort to integrate these treatment and maintenance services into a seamless continuum of care so that an individual can move smoothly among services (Haber and Billings, 1995). The role of the nurse and other professionals is to assess the individual's current level of functioning in order to direct the person to the appropriate resources that will enhance quality of life and decrease fragmentation of care. Coordination of services for the individual necessitates multidisciplinary collaboration. *Multidisciplinary* has been expanded to include not only professional staff but also nonprofessionals, consumers, family, and a variety of nonpsychiatric resources such as representatives from Medicare, Medicaid, nursing homes, group homes, medical clinics, etc.

MANAGED CARE

During the 1980s, the high cost of health care became a major focus nationally. Models of care delivery, treatment approaches, and professional roles began to evolve to meet the demand to reduce costs. Today, managed care is one model of reimbursement that has assumed prominence.

Managed care is a system of entities that provides for reimbursement for services. Managed care ar-

ranges the relationships between payers, providers, and consumers to monitor and influence the behavior of mental health providers and the outcomes of care. Health maintenance organizations, independent practice associations, and preferred provider organizations are examples of managed care. In the private sector managed care is restricted to designated providers (Cuffel, et al, 1996). In the public mental health system, managed care is influencing care delivery through HMOs and community mental health centers (McFarland, 1996).

Confusion sometimes exists between the terms *case management* and *care manager.* *Case management* involves the coordination of and access to care. The *care manager* monitors and controls utilization of services on behalf of payers for managed care in the private sector (Cuffel, et al, 1996).

Managed care as well as private insurance has progressively dictated shorter lengths of hospital stay, types of treatment, and even which medications may be prescribed. As a result, psychiatric treatment must be cost-effective, problem oriented, outcome based, and occur in the least restrictive setting. The goal is to help the individual achieve an optimal level of functioning in the least amount of time. Schreter (1997) describes this as the "principle of parsimony," which "holds that each patient should receive the least intensive, least expensive treatment at

Box 6-2 Impact of Managed Care on the Continuum of Care

Positive

New innovative treatment modalities
New levels of services within the community
Reduced costs
More efficient use of treatment strategies
Outcome-based treatment
Improvement in coordination of services
Incentives for health promotion and prevention services

Negative

Inadequate reimbursement for some services such as hospital-based care
Shifting of some consumers to nonmental health services such as social services and the legal system
Competition of providers for clients and resources
Inconsistencies in reimbursement for services
Fragmentation of services
Downsizing of psychiatric facilities and staff
Difficulties in complying with guidelines and procedures of a variety of reimbursement plans
Lack of parity for mental health services

Adapted from Lefkovitz PM: The continuum of care in a general hospital setting, *Gen Hosp Psychiatry* 17:260, 1995; Schreter RK: Essential skills for managed behavioral health care, *Psychiatr Serv* 48(5):653, 1997; and Worley NK: *Mental health nursing in the community*, St. Louis, 1997, Mosby Year Book.

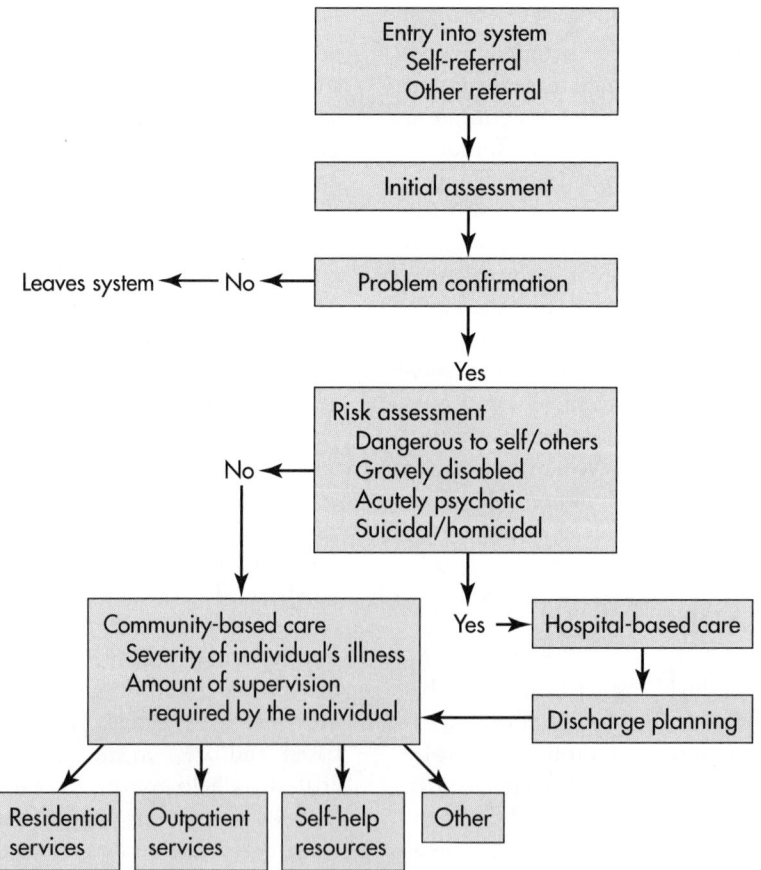

FIGURE 6-1 Decision tree for continuum of care

the lowest level of care that will permit a return to health and function."

Some consumers and caregivers have questions as to whether managed care is sufficiently meeting their needs. There is an increase in tendency to restrict the types of services that will be reimbursed. For example, in many instances academic testing for children and adolescents is not reimbursed even though clinicians consider it an essential part of comprehensive assessment (Schreter, 1997). Other examples are the restriction or limits on the number of home visits and how long an individual may participate in an evening therapy program. One reason for these restrictions is that funds were not shifted from inpatient to outpatient and community services as originally expected (McFarland, 1996).

■ Critical Thinking Question

Based on your interactions with patients, identify what would facilitate quality care in terms of accessibility, availability, and acceptability.

IMPACT OF MANAGED CARE ON THE CONTINUUM OF CARE

The overall impact of managed care on the continuum of care has been a dramatic reduction in inpatient lengths of stay and an inadequate range of community-based services. More specific examples of the impact on the continuum of care are listed in Box 6-2. Hospitals are now used primarily for acute and emergency situations such as dangerous to self and/or others, inability to meet self-care needs, extensive or intensive evaluation, treatment of overdose or suicide attempt, combinations of medical and psychiatric problems, and management of acute detoxification or toxicity (Hendryx and Rohland, 1997). Other services or care will be needed for those who do not meet the criteria for inpatient care.

DECISION TREE FOR CONTINUUM OF CARE

In order to match the needs of individuals with appropriate services, comprehensive assessment is required. The decision to hospitalize an individual is only one aspect of deciding on the most appropriate referral for mental health problems (Figure 6-1). When inpatient psychiatric treatment is not deemed appropriate, a determination must be made about the level of care required. Such decision-making incorporates assessment of severity of symptoms, level of functioning, intensity of supervision needed (e.g., safety), and type of treatment required in order to promote optimal level of functioning. For example:

1. An individual with thoughts of suicide but without a plan might be managed effectively by attending a day treatment program 5 days a week for several weeks,
2. An individual with a history of medication noncompliance who needs a place to live might be appropriately placed in a group home with 24-hour-a-day supervision, and
3. An individual with alcoholism who has completed acute detoxification might need referral to a self-help group such as Alcoholics Anonymous and outpatient counseling.

For any of these individuals additional referrals along the continuum of care may be made if their needs change.

ACCESSING THE CONTINUUM OF CARE

An individual may be referred to mental health services at the suggestion of a family physician; minister, priest, or rabbi; police; family; friends; or staff from the health clinic, emergency room, crisis service, or employee assistance program, to name a few. Self-referral is also a means by which individuals gain entry into the mental health system.

The individual and the care provider develop specific problem-oriented goals and/or outcomes based on subjective (i.e., self) reports and objective data. Several problems exist with measuring and evaluating outcomes. Problems with subjective reports include (1) an individual's denial of the need for further treatment may result in the premature termination of treatment and (2) individuals may have a tendency to overestimate their ability to function (Olsen, 1995). Because self-reports may be unreliable, more objective measures of outcomes are being established, such as compliance with medication and treatment, job attendance, and community living skills. Clinician and staff reports of achievement of outcomes are used but may lack a complete understanding of the individual's inner feelings and experiences. The achievement of specific outcomes is critical for the issue of reimbursement by payers and for determining quality of care. Ethical issues also demand that treatment results in outcomes that benefit the individual (Olsen, 1995). The 5 As of quality along the continuum of care have been identified by Schreter (1997):

1. Availability
2. Accessibility
3. Acceptability
4. Accountability
5. Appropriateness

By continually monitoring for and valuing these indicators, a seamless continuum of care can be developed.

Critical Thinking Question

Identify resources in your local community that offer services for the prevention and treatment of mental health problems.

Key Concepts

1. Emerging trends in health care are impacting the practice of psychiatric nursing.
2. The range of services is rapidly evolving to meet the needs of individuals with mental health problems.
3. Managed care has a major influence on the continuum of care.
4. The goal of managed care is to foster functioning and health by providing the least expensive, least restrictive, and least intensive treatment.
5. Assessment of the individual's needs and the level of supervision the individual requires determines referral to hospital-based or community-based care.
6. Appropriate and specific outcome-based care is critical to optimizing the individual's level of functioning as well as reimbursement.

Study Questions

(Answer key is in the back of the book.)

1. Which of the following activities of the nursing process is most critical in utilization of the continuum of care?
   a. Assessment
   b. Planning
   c. Intervention
   d. Evaluation
2. Which of the following statements would least likely be considered a goal of managed care?
   a. Fostering functioning and health
   b. Encouraging the least expensive and least intensive treatment
   c. Influencing the behavior of mental health providers
   d. Developing restrictive environments for care
3. A concern about the impact of managed care is reflected in which of the following statements?
   a. Managed care is more interested in cure than care
   b. Services provided by managed care may be insufficient in meeting an individual's needs
   c. Innovative treatment programs are being discouraged
   d. Managed care interferes with outcome-based care

REFERENCES

Cuffel BJ, et al: Managed care in the public mental health system, *Community Ment Health J* 32(2):109, 1996.

Haber J and Billings CV: Primary mental health care: a model for psychiatric-mental health nursing, *J Am Psychiatr Nurses Assoc* 1(5):154, 1995.

Hendryx MS and Rohland BM: Psychiatric hospitalization decision making by community mental health center staff, *Community Ment Health J* 33(1):163, 1997.

Institute of Medicine: *Reducing risks for mental disorders,* Washington, DC, 1994, National Academy Press.

Lefkovitz PM: The continuum of care in a general hospital setting, *Gen Hosp Psychiatry* 17:260, 1995.

McFarland BH: Ending the millennium: commentary on "HMOs and the seriously mentally ill—a view from the trenches," *Community Ment Health J* 32(3):219, 1996.

Olsen DP: Ethical cautions in the use of outcomes for resource allocation in the managed care environment of mental health, *Arch Psychiatr Nurs* 9(4):173, 1995.

Schreter RK: Essential skills for managed behavioral health care, *Psychiatr Serv* 48(5):653, 1997.

CHAPTER 7

Hospital-Based Care

CAROL E. BOSTROM
LEE H. SCHWECKE

LEARNING OBJECTIVES

After reading this chapter you should be able to:
- Describe the impact of length of stay on hospital-based care.
- List the purposes of hospital-based care.
- Understand the types of care that may be available in hospitals.

- Comprehend the importance of discharge planning in hospital-based care.
- Identify the role of the nurse in implementing the psychotherapeutic management model in hospital-based care.

As a result of deinstitutionalization in the 1960s and 1970s (see Chapter 1), the inpatient care of the mentally ill shifted away from large state hospitals to smaller, private facilities and psychiatric units within general hospitals located more in the "community." This planned reduction in state hospital beds has been reinforced as managed care and reimbursement issues have decreased the number of hospital beds for individuals with psychiatric disorders in all facilities. The length of stay (LOS) for each hospitalized individual has also decreased. State institutions usually hospitalized patients for long periods of time, even up to a year or more. At the present time, the length of stay is more likely to be 1 to 3 months in state hospitals but much shorter in the more community-based acute care inpatient programs. For about 10% to 20% of the seriously mentally ill and the severely disabled, state institutions or long-term care is appropriate (Torrey, 1995). For these individuals, long-term hospitalization is the least restrictive

environment in which they can function. Historically patients admitted to acute care units often stayed 4 to 6 weeks. Today length of stay in the units is typically 3 to 5 days. As reimbursement decreased, hospital-based care, including medical, surgical, and other specialties, changed in the following areas: purpose and goals of hospitalization, implementation of care, staffing patterns, increased acuity of patients, and increased importance of discharge planning. Hospitals were the point of entry into the health care system, whereas now the point of entry can be anywhere along the continuum of care.

PURPOSES OF PSYCHIATRIC HOSPITAL-BASED CARE

The highest priority for admission to hospital-based care is safety for self and others. This includes individuals who are actively suicidal, self-mutilating, or threatening others with harm. Individuals who have attempted suicide are often transferred to a psychiatric unit when medically stable. Hospitalization provides 24-hour supervision in a safe environment (Hughes and Ashby, 1996).

Other individuals who require hospitalization are those at risk for accidental harm, that is, those who are gravely disabled (see Chapter 4). For example, individuals who are acutely psychotic or those who are confused and disoriented may not function well enough to meet their basic needs for food, clothing, shelter, medical care, and/or physical safety. In addition to safety and protection, hospitalization provides thorough medical and psychiatric evaluation to identify the underlying cause of their symptoms.

Another group that may be admitted are individuals who are experiencing toxic reactions to medications or other substances and those who need medical intervention when withdrawal from substances could produce life-threatening conditions. Some individuals may be admitted because their medical illness produces or complicates a psychiatric disorder or for medication evaluation.

The goals of hospital-based care are to assist individuals with attaining a safe level of functioning and/or stabilization and to provide referrals for aftercare (Hughes and Ashby, 1996). Attempts are made to interact with family or support systems to determine their problems and needs as well as their role in assisting the individual after discharge.

TYPES OF HOSPITAL-BASED CARE

Inpatient units vary from hospital to hospital and from community to community. For example, a small hospital may have only one closed (i.e., locked) inpatient unit that accepts all patients with all diagnoses. A larger hospital may offer more options for specialized care. Some common specialty care areas are described in Table 7-1.

Table 7-1   Types of Programming

Age-Based Programming	Examples of Major Target Issues	Examples of Typical Groups
Child	Family issues, developmental issues, peer relationships, academic issues, behavior management, life stresses, coping strategies	Feelings expression, self-esteem, storytelling, family education groups
Adolescent	Same as above plus intimate relationships, sexuality, substance abuse	Self-esteem, conflict management, anger management, educational groups
Adult	Same as above plus acceptance of illness and medication compliance; social, occupational, and financial problem solving	Self-esteem, stress management, educational, activity groups
Older adult	Same as above plus aging processes, death and dying, retirement adjustment, disabilities/chronic illnesses, assistance in living issues	Spirituality, grief and loss, reminiscence, educational groups
Diagnosis-Based Programming		
Acute and/or nonpsychotic	Insight into illness and life situations, problem solving, interpersonal relationships	Same as adult above plus problem solving group
Chronic and/or psychotic	Symptom management, medication compliance, social skills, community living skills, vocational assessment	Same as adult above but on a more concrete level plus social skills, community living skills, educational groups
Addictions	Dynamics of addiction, effects of addictions	Same as adult above plus self-help groups

An important type of inpatient service is the psychiatric intensive care unit (PICU). The PICU typically has 8 to 10 beds with more safety precautions and more staff in order to handle high-risk behaviors such as suicide, assault, and escape. Seclusion and restraints may be used more often on this type of unit. The purpose of the PICU is symptom and behavior control. Group activities may or may not occur. If group activities occur, the focus is typically reality or activity based.

Discharge Planning

Hospital-based care utilizes multidisciplinary treatment conferences and discharge planning to insure holistic care. Team members collaborate and coordinate inpatient care and determine aftercare services within the continuum of care based on the individual's needs. The team may include the psychiatrist, nurse, social worker, dietician, pharmacist, activity therapist, and chaplain. Consults occur as needed with other services such as physical therapy, neurology, internal medicine, and representatives from aftercare services. The individual has the opportunity to meet with any or all team members. The multidisciplinary team uses a decision tree in its discharge planning process. (See Chapter 6 for discussion of a decision tree.)

Psychotherapeutic Management

Nurse-Patient Relationship. Nurses are the only members of the multidisciplinary team who provide 24-hour care during the hospital stay. Individuals admitted to psychiatric units today are more acutely ill than in the past and exhibit severe psychopathology. With the aforementioned shorter LOS "Nurses must establish a therapeutic alliance, assess priority needs, and administer care in a matter of days" (Hughes and Ashby, 1996). Often the nurse begins to intervene while the individual is being admitted to the unit because of behaviors that are dangerous to self or others. No matter how sick the individual or what behaviors are being exhibited, the individual needs to quickly know the nurse is caring, empathetic, supportive, and helpful. The nurse may need to set limits on behaviors but at the same time convey respect and maintain the dignity of the individual (Coker, et al, 1997).

Once the individual is safe and more able to control his or her behavior, further assessment occurs. The nursing assessment must be very direct, specific, and comprehensive. It is important to gather information from as many sources as possible, such as family, significant others, old charts/records, and professionals in outpatient services with whom the individual may have had contact.

Discharge planning has always been an important nursing role. With decreased LOS, discharge planning has become even more critical. Discharge planning begins at admission and is incorporated into the multidisciplinary treatment plan. For some individuals, discharge planning may be relatively simple, such as "return home with outpatient follow-up." For others, the discharge plan may be very complex and involve a number of community services along the continuum of care such as housing, medicine clinic, dental service, outpatient counseling, and a self-help group for the family. Although the nurse may not directly arrange for all of these services, the nurse coordinates this activity. As much as possible, it is important to include the individual and the family/significant others in multidisciplinary conferences so that they are participating in the development and implementation of goals, including those for aftercare (Bartol, Moon, and Linton, 1994). For more information about the nurse-patient relationship, see Chapter 11.

■ Critical Thinking Question

You are admitting a 15-year-old boy to an inpatient unit because of alcohol and marijuana abuse, sexual promiscuity, and failing grades. These behaviors developed over the last 3 months after his father was diagnosed with terminal cancer. Describe the types of programming that would be most appropriate.

Psychopharmacology. The nurse is instrumental in obtaining the medication history: past and current medications and dosages, medication allergies, the individual's perspective on medication effectiveness, problems with side effects, and present and past compliance. An important role includes monitoring the effectiveness of medication, the presence of side effects, and educating the individual and family about the medication and side effects. The nurse must carefully assess the need for as-needed (prn) medication so that problem behaviors and symptoms can be alleviated as quickly as possible. The nurse emphasizes the importance of medication compliance in symptom management and control with the individual and family. (For specific information on medications, see Chapters 18 to 22.)

Milieu Management. Traditionally, hospital-based care emphasized milieu therapy (see Chapter 23). Today the milieu or inpatient environment is still therapeutic and supportive in order to encourage a return to adequate functioning in the community. The emphasis of milieu activities is on helping the individual cope with immediate needs and with stressors and problems in his or her home or living environment. "The inpatient stay should help the patient adapt to his or her external social environment, not the inpatient milieu" (Johnson, 1997). Because of short-term stays, there is a need for structured milieus to include groups that are problem focused, goal oriented, and relevant to the needs of the individuals. Box 7-1 provides a sample daily schedule. The nurse assists the individual in applying information obtained in educational groups to his or her own situation. The nurse teaches the individual how to solve prob-lems rather than focusing on resolving all problems before discharge. With these skills hopefully the individual can continue to problem solve after discharge. Homework assignments, journal writing, and educational handouts provide even more structure in the milieu.

■ Critical Thinking Question

Discuss the roles of the nurse in a multidisciplinary team in a setting in which you have had experience.

▶ Key Concepts

1. The majority of hospital-based care is now short-term, focusing on crisis intervention and safety.
2. The overarching goals of hospital-based care are provision of safety and discharge planning.
3. The type of hospital-based care available to individuals varies according to the size of the hospital and the community.
4. Discharge planning begins at the time of admission and varies in complexity.
5. The psychotherapeutic management model is the most relevant approach to short-term hospitalization.

Box 7-1	**Sample of an Inpatient Daily Schedule***
7:00 AM	Wake up and morning care
8:00	Breakfast
9:00	Goal-setting group
10:00	Stress management group
11:00	Exercise group
12:00 PM	Lunch
1:00	Medication education group
2:00	Self-esteem group
3:00	Addictions group
4:00	Free time
5:00	Dinner
6:00	Family education group
7:00	Visiting
9:00	Relaxation group
10:00	Free time
10:30	Bedtime

*All groups last 45 minutes. Interactions with staff are expected between groups and/or during free time.

▶ Study Questions

(Answer key is in the back of the book.)
1. Which of the following purposes of hospital-based care is most critical?
   a. Referrals to outpatient services
   b. Medication education and compliance
   c. Family education and support
   d. Safety for the individual and others
2. Which of the following would be a unique and important target issue in programming for older adults?
   a. Medication education
   b. Coping strategies
   c. Death and dying
   d. Interpersonal relationships
3. Which of the goals of hospital-based care is least important to achieve by discharge?
   a. Resolving the majority of the individual's problems
   b. Referrals for appropriate aftercare

c. Medication evaluation

d. Return to safe level of functioning

4. The individual is brought to the inpatient unit because she was wandering on the interstate in her nightgown. She has a history of prior admissions for psychotic episodes and medication noncompliance. She tells the nurse she just wants to go home. Which of the following would be the nurse's initial response?

a. "You cannot go home until your doctor says you can."

b. "I know you want to go home but right now we are very concerned about keeping you safe."

c. "First, we need to get you back on your medicine."

d. "Since it is the middle of the night, you have to stay until morning."

REFERENCES

Bartol GM, Moon E, and Linton M: Nursing assistance for families of patients, *J Psychosoc Nurs Ment Health Serv* 32(12):27, 1994.

Coker M, et al: Implementation of total quality management after reconfiguration of services on a general hospital unit, *Psychiatr Serv* 48(2):231, 1997.

Hughes KH, and Ashby C: Essential components of the short-term psychiatric unit, *Perspect Psychiatr Care* 32(1): 20, 1996.

Johnson DR: Toward parsimony in the inpatient community meeting on a short-term unit, *Psychiatr Serv* 48(1): 93, 1997.

Torrey EF: *Surviving schizophrenia: a manual for families, consumers, and providers,* ed 3, New York, 1995, Harper Collins.

CHAPTER 8

Community-Based Care

CAROL E. BOSTROM
LEE H. SCHWECKE

With the shift from hospital-based to community-based care, the range of community service is expanding. This chapter provides an overview of the types of services available within the continuum of care outside the hospital setting. Nurses have a potential role in any of the services because of their psychotherapeutic management skills, knowledge of psychopathology, and their ability to adapt the use of the nursing process to any setting. Another valuable asset nursing brings to the health care system is its involvement with reimbursement systems and budget restrictions. Recent trends (e.g., economic realities and patients' rights) in health care have fostered the goal of providing the most effective care in the least restrictive setting at the lowest possible cost (Schreter, 1997).

OUTPATIENT SERVICES

Subacute Care

When inpatient hospitalization is not needed, individuals may be referred to outpatient services according to their needs, the amount of supervision that is appropriate, and which services will be reimbursed. The most restrictive service after inpatient hospitalization is subacute care. This is appropriate when an individual requires 24-hour supervision but less intensive and less extensive services than the hospital provides (Lefkovitz, 1995). Individuals are provided with beds, meals, medications, groups, and activities. Subacute care allows the individual autonomy and independence in choosing which activities and groups will be attended and which outside activities are appropriate, such as seeking employment and housing and/or applying for school or training.

CLINICAL EXAMPLE

Tiffany, a 23-year-old woman with borderline personality disorder and anorexia, describes herself as being in crisis because her boyfriend has left her. She has not been sleeping or eating for the past 3 days and has superficial cuts on both wrists. After the cuts were cared for in the emergency room, she was taken to a subacute unit. She received care for 4 days. Upon admission to the unit, she agreed to sign a "no harm contract." She received wound care, an evaluation of her nutritional status, and assistance with sleeping using relaxation tapes. She attended groups that focused on coping with anger and self-esteem issues. One evening she attended a survivors of incest group in the community, which she had been previously attending. Upon discharge, Tiffany was referred back to her counselor at the neighborhood mental health clinic.

Partial Programs

Individuals who need some supervision, structured activities, and ongoing treatment may benefit from partial programs. Partial programs vary in length from 4 to 8 hours per day and 1 to 5 days per week (Lefkovitz, 1995). Programming can occur during the day, evening, and night. Depending on the community, these programs may provide treatment for specific populations based on age (child, adolescent, adult, older adult) or type of problem (addictions or chronic mental illness).

CLINICAL EXAMPLE

John, a 52-year-old man with severe depression due to the unexpected death of his wife, is discharged from the hospital but unable to return to work. He attends a partial program for 2 weeks that meets from 10:00 AM to 3:00 PM Monday through Friday. He attends groups focused on exercise, spirituality, coping with losses, and self-esteem issues. There is an opportunity for socialization with program members during lunch.

Outpatient Programs

Traditionally, outpatient treatment has occurred in mental health clinics and private offices. The person providing counseling may be a psychiatrist, psychologist, social worker, clinical nurse specialist, nurse, or other professional. The number of visits per week or month varies according to the individual's needs. The typical pattern for an individual with a chronic mental illness may be a visit once a month with a counselor or case manager and periodic appointments with a psychiatrist for medication review. During these counseling visits, an assessment of needs

for additional services is made to determine if the individual needs more intense or a different type of service.

CLINICAL EXAMPLE

Larry, a 31-year-old man with the diagnosis of chronic undifferentiated schizophrenia, attends a Community Support program. He meets with his case manager every other week after he receives his haloperidol decanoate (Haldol Decanoate) injection from the nurse, who assesses for medication effectiveness and side effect management. He also participates in "social club," which offers lunch and social activities twice a week. The psychiatrist meets with him every 3 months for medication evaluation.

PSYCHIATRIC HOME CARE

Psychiatric home care services are available for the homebound because their illness or disability inhibits their leaving home to obtain services elsewhere. It is a growing industry due to "earlier hospital discharge, the need for alternatives to institutional care, and broader third party payment coverage" (Morris, 1996). Home visits may occur in conjunction with other community-based services such as case management (see Chapter 9). Home care often serves individuals with severe and persistent mental illnesses and those with a combination of psychiatric and medical illnesses. Home care may be provided by traditional public and private home care agencies that have added psychiatric home services. Many psychiatric hospitals and community mental health centers have instituted their own home care programs.

CLINICAL EXAMPLE

Joe, an 80-year-old man with Alzheimer's disease, lives at home with his wife. The nurse assesses his mental status and level of functioning. Assistance is given to the wife in implementing safety measures in the home because of Joe's wandering behavior. The nurse assists with arranging respite care so that the wife can go shopping and attend a weekly caregivers support group.

COMMUNITY OUTREACH PROGRAMS

Outreach services have developed to reach individuals in areas where there is a lack of traditional medical and social services such as individuals in rural areas (Worley and Sloop, 1996). There are other programs that attempt to reach individuals who have had poor success with community-based services, such as the homeless or transient groups (e.g., migrant workers and their families). Mobile programs in various cities that serve the needs of mentally ill individuals on the street, under bridges, in parks, in missions, and at lunch programs exemplify outreach service (Morse, et al, 1996). Some programs arrange for physician and nurse volunteers to operate a neighborhood clinic once or twice weekly to serve homeless individuals with medical and/or psychiatric needs.

RESIDENTIAL SERVICES

Residential services are available to individuals who need temporary or long-term housing. Most states have long-term care facilities for individuals needing prolonged 24-hour-a-day supervision. Length of stay may be 3 to 6 months or longer. *Extended care facilities* (e.g., nursing homes) are available for those people requiring 24-hour-a-day supervision and medical nursing care. This level of care is often required for individuals with severe developmental disabilities, dementia, or acute and chronic medical illnesses.

Group homes may provide temporary or permanent housing for individuals with chronic mental disorders. Depending on the needs of the residents, staff may be present for 24 hours a day or less. Some provide group therapy and structured activities, while others may provide just meals, a bed, and laundry facilities.

Traditionally, halfway houses were available for individuals with chemical dependency. Residents were expected to seek employment and participate in cooking and cleaning chores. Residents also attended self-help groups that met on site, such as Alcoholics Anonymous. Some halfway houses may now be open to individuals with other problems.

Apartment living programs provide varying degrees of supervision and programming. Staff may be on site on a daily basis offering groups and activities or may visit periodically to ensure medication compliance.

CLINICAL EXAMPLE

Lois, a 63-year-old-woman with the diagnosis of bipolar disorder–manic, had been living with her son until her behaviors became unmanageable due to medication noncompliance. Because of her need for more supervision, she was placed in an apartment living program. A nurse visits her 3 times a week to monitor medication compliance. The nurse also assists her with keeping outpatient appointments.

Foster care and *boarding homes* are generally staffed by nonprofessionals but with professional supervision offered on an outpatient basis. Shelters provide room and board to the homeless. Some may provide services for specific populations such as victims of violence or those with addictions.

Self-help Groups

Self-help groups are another source of support on the continuum of care. Self-help group meetings are conducted by members, not professionals, and can occur on a weekly basis. Box 8-1 provides examples of types of self-help groups.

In providing holistic care, the nurse or other professional may assist the individual in linking with

Box 8-1 **Self-Help Groups**	
Type of Group	**Examples**
Addiction based	Alcoholics Anonymous
	Narcotics Anonymous
	Overeaters Anonymous
Survivor based	Survivors of Suicide
	Incest Survivors Anonymous
	Adult Children of Alcoholics
Disorder based	Eating disorders
	Bipolar disorder
	Families/caregivers support groups
	National Alliance for the Mentally Ill
Loss based	Grief, divorce, bereavement support groups
Medically based (chronic or terminal illness)	Lupus, cancer, chronic fatigue, AIDS support groups
Prevention based	Parenting, tough love support groups

other community resources. Besides linking, the nurse may need to advocate and negotiate for services (Worley, 1997). The following are examples of some of these services (Bartol, Moon, and Linton, 1994; Guarnaccia and Parra, 1996; Schreter, 1997):

    medical clinics
    dental services
    financial services
    vocational services
    transportation
    housing
    Medicare/Medicaid
    legal/justice system
    church-related programs
    employee assistance programs

■ Critical Thinking Question

Choose a patient with whom you are currently working. Given the services available on the continuum of care in the patient's community, which levels of care would be beneficial to the patient?

INFLUENCES ON THE CONTINUUM OF CARE

The U.S. Congress and state legislatures are immersed in debates on health care reform. Governments, health care providers, and consumers are interested in improving health care coverage and accessibility to care. However, controversy exists about how to implement health care reform and who will pay for it (Washington Focus, 1993). As the debates continue to be unresolved, managed care has emerged as a systemized approach to contain health care costs. Managed care has provided an impetus to develop community-based services and to decrease services in inpatient settings. However, community-based services are struggling to keep up with the increasing demand for a full range of services and reimbursement is insufficient (Lefkovitz, 1995). Funding for developing new programs is inadequate as well.

The result for those with mental health problems has been a lack of availability of or accessibility to services they need. The lack of coordination of services among the levels of care sometimes results in fragmentation of services to the individual. For those

with chronic mental illness, community agencies have not fully developed services nor are they delivering services efficiently and effectively (McFarland, 1996). Mental health consumers and their families are concerned about the lack of services and the lack of reimbursement for services that are needed by the mentally ill family member (Guarnaccia and Parra, 1996). It is unknown whether managed care will continue to be the funding mechanism model behind reimbursement along the continuum of care or if another system will emerge.

■ Critical Thinking Question

What levels of care are needed to adequately address the health care concerns of the mentally ill in your community?

▶ Psychotherapeutic Management

Psychiatric nursing advocates for the inclusion of nurses as members of the multidisciplinary team in any of the settings described in this chapter. Psychiatric nurses offer valuable contributions to community-based care because of their ability to adapt the nursing process and the psychotherapeutic management model of care to any setting.

Nurse-Patient Relationship. Developing a nurse-patient relationship in the community is challenging due to the decreased contact and time spent with the individual. Establishing rapport and trust quickly is critical to effectively and efficiently implement the nursing process. Individuals are more likely to maintain contact with the nurse over time if they feel valued and respected, as well as feeling satisfied with their care. The nurse also uses the principles of developing the nurse-patient relationship in working with caregivers and family members. Developing collaborative relationships with other professionals is crucial for maintaining the continuum of care.

Psychopharmacology. In community-based settings, it becomes more critical for the individual and caregiver/family to have knowledge about medications and to know the importance of taking them as prescribed. Noncompliance with medication is the major cause of relapse and rehospitalization.

The nurse has a major role in teaching about medication effects, side effects, side effect management, and the relationship between medication and symptom management. The nurse must be astute in recognizing early signs of both side effects and noncompliance in order to intervene quickly. To miss the first can result in unnecessary patient discomfort (or worse). To miss the second can lead to poor symptom management.

Milieu Management. In community-based care the principles of milieu management are adapted in assessing agencies, programs, and private homes. After assessing the individual's needs, the nurse is responsible for determining which services in the continuum of care would best meet the individual's needs in the least restrictive setting. Naturally, the nurse has less direct control and influence over environments in the community than in inpatient settings. Further economic factors affecting the health care system, individuals, and families may put constraints on environmental modifications and the type of care that can be accomplished. What this means is the nurse adapts care based upon limitations of the environment and availability of resources.

■ Critical Thinking Question

If you were to write a letter to your local congressman, what would you say about the status of mental health care in your community?

▼ Key Concepts

1. Community-based services are evolving to meet the needs of individuals and families in the continuum of care.
2. The continuum of care includes inpatient hospitalization, outpatient services, residential care, self-help, and other resources.
3. Nursing process and the psychotherapeutic management approach can be adapted in any setting along the continuum of care.

▼ Study Questions

(Answer key is in the back of the book.)
1. The patient has been hospitalized for 3 days after a suicide attempt. Suicidal ideation is still present but the patient no longer has a specific plan. Lack of appetite and disturbance in sleep are present. The patient lives alone, has no support system, and insurance will not cover further hospitalization. Which of the following levels of care would be most appropriate?
   a. Community outreach program
   b. Weekly outpatient counseling
   c. Subacute care
   d. Further inpatient hospitalization
2. Of all of the recent influences on the continuum of care, which of the following has had the most impact?
   a. Managed care
   b. Chronic mental illness
   c. Caregiver concerns
   d. Acceptability of care
3. In community-based care, which of the following would interfere with the nurse-patient relationship?
   a. Rapport
   b. Time
   c. Setting
   d. Medications

REFERENCES

Bartol GM, Moon E, and Linton M: Nursing assistance for families of patients, *J Psychosoc Nurs Ment Health Serv* 32(12):27, 1994.

Guarnaccia PJ and Parra P: Ethnicity, social status and families' experiences of caring for a mentally ill family member, *Community Mental Health J* 32(3):243, 1996.

Lefkovitz PM: The continuum of care in a general hospital setting, *Gen Hosp Psychiatry* 17:260, 1995.

McFarland BH: Ending the millennium: commentary on "HMOs and the seriously mentally ill—a view from the trenches," *Community Ment Health J* 32(3):219, 1996.

Morris M: Patients' perceptions of psychiatric home care, *Arch Psychiatr Nurs* 10(3):176, 1996.

Morse GA, et al: Outreach to homeless mentally ill people: conceptual and clinical considerations, *Community Ment Health J* 32(3):261, 1996.

Schreter RK: Essential skills for managed behavioral health care, *Psychiatr Serv* 48(5):653, 1997.

Washington Focus: Health care reform proposals compared, *Nurs Health Care* 14(9):455, 1993.

Worley NK: *Mental health nursing in the community,* St. Louis, 1997, Mosby-Year Book.

Worley NK and Sloop T: Psychiatric nursing in a rural outreach program, *Perspect Psychiatr Care* 32(2):10, 1996.

CHAPTER 9

Case Management

KRIS L. WANG

LEARNING OBJECTIVES

After reading this chapter you should be able to:
- Identify the goals of case management.
- Define the concepts of case management.
- Identify the nurse's roles in case management.
- Recognize the importance of case management across the continuum of care.
- Understand the various approaches to case management.
- Identify the utilization of clinical/critical pathways.
- Apply the nursing process to patients receiving case management services.

This chapter addresses issues of case management in psychiatric/mental health nursing. Elements of case management are resource linkage, consultation, advocacy, psychiatric rehabilitation, crisis intervention, home care, and therapy. The efficient use of the nursing process is the foundation of case management.

GOALS AND PURPOSES OF CASE MANAGEMENT AND PSYCHIATRIC REHABILITATION

Case management is "a collaborative process which assesses, plans, implements, coordinates, monitors, and evaluates options and services to meet an individual's health needs through communication and available resources to promote quality cost-effective outcomes" (Case Management Society of America, 1995). In addition to individuals, case management is also applied to families and groups receiving treatment across a continuum of care. The overall objectives of case management are to increase continuity of care, to insure access to care, and to provide cost-effective care (American Nurses Association [ANA], 1994).

Although these services can be utilized for many persons with varying degrees of mental illness, they are implemented primarily in the mental health field for those with chronic conditions. Case management and psychiatric rehabilitation often are used together to help prevent patients from "falling through the cracks." Psychiatric rehabilitation (also known as psychosocial rehabilitation) is a component of case management in which patients receive care in the least restrictive setting that enables them to be successful in their environment (Anthony,

KEY TERMS

Case management a collaborative process for meeting health needs through utilization of a variety of services in a cost-effective manner

Psychiatric rehabilitation promotion of the patient's highest level of functioning in the least restrictive environment

Advocacy negotiating with others to develop, improve, and provide services for a patient

---

Box 9-1 Goals and Purposes of Case Management and Psychiatric Rehabilitation

Hope
Increased quality of life
Participation in treatment
Competency
Empowerment
Decreased readmissions to inpatient units
Increased social, vocational, and emotional functioning

Decreased burden on caregivers
Independence and growth
Community involvement
Adaptation to or recovery from mental illness
Satisfaction with environment
Continuous treatment
Cost-effective treatment

1992). Case management in conjunction with psychiatric rehabilitation reduces psychiatric symptoms and promotes higher levels of functioning (Macias, et al, 1994). As an example, a patient may have difficulty participating in treatment because she lacks the knowledge, skills, or income to ride the bus to her appointments. The case manager coordinates the patient's care so that she can learn, practice, or be directed to the appropriate resources that will assist her with acquiring the necessary skills to ride the bus and get to her appointments. The case manager incorporates a cost-effective approach in the coordination of these services. Patients whose needs are met more often experience success in their chosen environment while avoiding relapse and rehospitalization. As patient needs change, the case manager works with other care providers to ensure continuity of care. The goals and purposes of case management and psychiatric rehabilitation, which are ultimately the outcomes for patients receiving these services, are presented in Box 9-1.

HISTORY OF CASE MANAGEMENT

Many similarities exist between case management and psychiatric rehabilitation.

The goals of psychiatric rehabilitation generally can be met with intensive case management. For example, in Los Angeles, the Village Integrated Services Agency is a psychiatric rehabilitation program utilizing nurses as case managers to facilitate optimal functioning for patients (Thompson and Strand, 1994).

Case management and psychiatric rehabilitation have their roots in the era of deinstitutionalization (see Chapter 1). The purpose of deinstitutionalization was to provide community-based treatment for those with chronic mental illness. Unfortunately, many patients did not receive the care and support they required. A lack of coordinated care, increased acuity at discharge, decreased lengths of inpatient stays, emphasis on decreasing costs, deficiencies in housing and residential settings, a lack of support systems, continued chronicity, and the "revolving door syndrome" have caused many patients to be rehospitalized or to become homeless (ANA, 1994; Pittman, 1989).

Case management and psychiatric rehabilitation expanded in an attempt to meet the needs of this deinstitutionalized population. The development of case management and psychiatric rehabilitation has been impeded by boundary or "turf" issues among the disciplines (primarily between psychiatry and other care providers). *Psychiatric* does not mean *psychiatry;* therefore disciplines must work together in an integrated manner to provide services across boundaries (Bachrach, 1992). Case management began in the 1970s with the National Institute for Mental Health's development of community support programs/services. Comprehensive and coordinated support services were developed, with case management emerging as the means to assure that services were provided (Worley, 1991). Some examples of case management models include the following:

1. *Full support model:* emphasizes the provision of support of patients, clinical management, and coping skills education

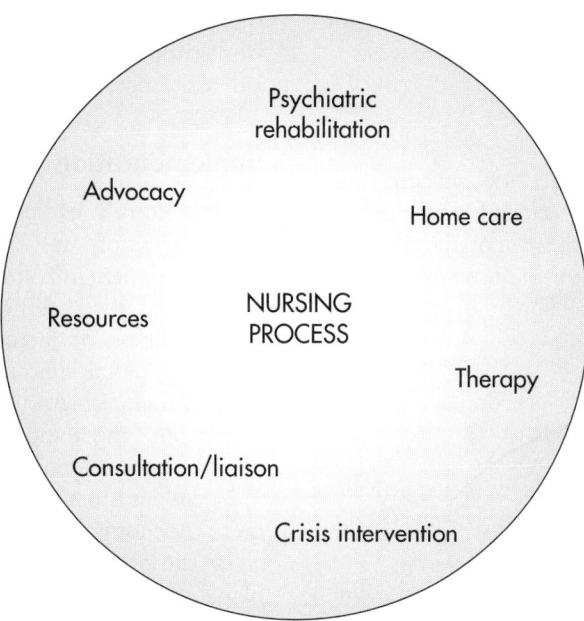

FIGURE 9-1   Case management components.

2. *Personal strengths model:* assumes that those living successfully have the resources necessary to develop and use their skills, and that behavior is directly related to available resources

3. *Rehabilitation model:* helps patients to become satisfied and functional to the fullest extent in their chosen environments with the least amount of professional intervention

4. *Expanded broker model:* involves assessing, planning, linking, and advocating for and with patients (Solomon, 1992)

5. *Intensive case management (assertive case management) model:* involves outreach to patients in their natural settings with high staff/patient ratios.

Intensive case management is more costly and labor intensive than other models; it is usually implemented for those with high rehospitalization rates, emergency room visits, and/or greatest difficulty in community adjustment (Firn, 1997; Worley, 1997). Morse, et al (1997) found intensive case management to be superior to expanded broker model in those with serious mental illness who are also at risk of homelessness. Scott and Dixon (1995) also report that intensive case management programs have been demonstrated to reduce hospitalization rates.

Lapierre and Padgett (1992) propose the implementation of the ANA Standards of Psychiatric and Mental Health Nursing Practice as a guide for nurses who perform case management services. The use of nurse case managers can vary by preparation and setting. Jambunathan and Van Dongen (1995) report in a pilot study that the use of nurse case management for those with nonchronic mental illness in an outpatient setting resulted in more nursing than psychiatric care and decreased hospital length of stay. A program described by Atkinson (1996) reports that psychiatric clinical nurse specialists in intensive case management roles promote patient entry into treatment at more appropriate and less costly levels of care for those with serious mental illness.

NURSING PROCESS

The nursing process is the foundation of case management. Effective use of the nursing process in the areas of psychiatric rehabilitation, crisis intervention, therapy, home care, consultation/liaison, resource linkage, and advocacy provide case management services for psychiatric patients (Figure 9-1). The nurse is skilled in synthesizing these components in an understandable and useful manner for patients.

Assessment

A comprehensive assessment of variables contributing to and interfering with successful rehabilitation and functioning is crucial to the case management of psychiatric patients. The following are typical areas to be assessed (Dunn, 1993; Forchuk, et al, 1989; Hellwig, 1993; Kanter, 1989):

Functional level	Motivation
Medication compliance	Strengths
Social supports	Housing
Family involvement	Mastery of the activities
Medical needs/limitations	of daily living (ADL)
Skills	Resources
Cognitive	Financial
Vocational	Environmental
Social	Transportation
Problem solving	Leisure time usage
Spiritual needs/concerns	Self-esteem
Coping abilities	Educational level

CLINICAL EXAMPLE

The nurse assesses Mary in her first appointment at the mental health clinic after a recent hospitalization. Mary complains that she has little to do during the day and that she does not have enough money to buy groceries toward the end of the month. Mary also is disturbed about her increased hand tremors. The nurse learns that Mary enjoys reading and has a library card. The needs assessed by the nurse include ineffective use of leisure time, limited financial resources, and bothersome hand tremors.

Outcome Identification/Planning

The nurse plans and prioritizes the appropriate care based on comprehensive assessment and nursing diagnoses. In the previous clinical example, the nurse prioritizes Mary's needs. The hand tremors need to be addressed first, followed by Mary's ineffective use of leisure time and her financial needs. The nurse's plan includes 1) consultation with the psychiatrist regarding Mary's hand tremors; 2) working with Mary in structuring and using her leisure time in a healthful manner, such as using

the library; and 3) linking Mary with the social worker for further exploration of financial resources and assistance.

Implementation

Many factors must be considered when prioritizing interventions and the nurse must take a holistic approach when implementing those interventions. This means recognizing and addressing the interconnectedness of factors in a patient's life, e.g., physical, mental, emotional, spiritual, environmental, and financial. Another factor to consider is that by encouraging temporary dependency and compliance the nurse enhances the prospect for greater independent functioning by the patient later in treatment (Anthony, Cohen, and Cohen, 1984).

In the above example, the nurse initiates the plan by building rapport and trust in order to establish the therapeutic relationship with Mary. The nurse arranges for psychiatrist evaluation before she leaves. An adjustment is made in Mary's haloperidol (Haldol), and she is given a prescription for benztropine (Cogentin) 1 mg bid prn. The nurse teaches Mary about the purpose and side effects of benztropine. During this discussion, Mary reports that she has insufficient funds to purchase both the benztropine and groceries. The nurse discusses the financial situation with Mary and discovers enough money for a 2-week supply of benztropine. The nurse then consults with the pharmacy to ensure that Mary can purchase a 2-week supply now and fill the remainder of the prescription at the beginning of the following month. The nurse then assesses Mary's transportation situation. Since the pharmacy is not on Mary's bus line and since the cold weather prohibits walking, the nurse and Mary engage in problem solving. Mary agrees to call her sister before she leaves the clinic to obtain a ride to the pharmacy in the morning. The nurse also encourages Mary to ask her sister to stop by the library and check out two books. Mary verbalizes agreement with this plan and feels it will be beneficial.

The nurse links Mary with the social worker by making an appointment for her in 2 weeks to discuss her financial situation. The nurse also evaluates Mary's areas of interest and develops with her a daily schedule based on these interests and routine daily living tasks (e.g., going to the library, reading, cooking, cleaning, and bathing). This degree of nurse involvement increases Mary's dependence temporarily, but has the potential for progressive independence in the future.

Evaluation

Evaluation is an ongoing process. Each intervention and overall patient status must be continually evaluated. Patients have changing needs, issues, and concerns. The nurse must be attuned to these changes during all interactions with patients. Responses to medication, including effectiveness and side effects, must be evaluated in an ongoing manner. For example, before Mary leaves the mental health clinic, the nurse evaluates the following:

* Mary's understanding of the medication changes, the desired responses, and the potential side effects
* Mary's plan for purchasing the benztropine
* The purpose, date, and time of the appointment with the social worker
* The purpose and understanding of using the library and the written schedule of daily activities

CASE MANAGEMENT

Case management utilizes the nursing process as its foundation to meet the goals outlined in Box 9-1. Benefits of case management include the following (ANA, 1994; Bigelow and Young, 1991; Wilbur and Arns, 1998):

* Increased cost-effectiveness
* Increased continuity of care
* Decreased readmissions

Clinical Pathways

Working tools of case management that nurses may use are *clinical* or *critical pathways* (also known as care paths and Care Maps—see Figure 9-2). These pathways are interdisciplinary written plans and timetables for patients' care that outline treatments, outcomes, lengths of stay, and discharge plans (ANA, 1994).

The clinical pathway focuses on interdisciplinary interventions and outcomes. It needs to be user friendly. Clinical pathways are most common in an inpa-

tient setting and often include the following categories: consults, tests, medications, diet, interventions, activities/milieu/recreation therapy, psychosocial therapy, teaching, and discharge planning (Smith, 1997). Nurses report that these clinical pathways guide patient care, increase nurse satisfaction, decrease patient anxiety, and enhance teaching (Mosher, et al, 1992). The nurse case manager utilizes the clinical pathway to plan, implement, evaluate, and adjust interventions during patients' treatments (Giuliano and Poirier, 1991). These pathways become part of the quality improvement process by decreasing costs and improving outcomes. Continuous quality improvement and total quality management offer benefits such as restructuring health care, improving outcomes, increasing team effectiveness, enhancing communication, managing costs, and educating students, nurses, patients, and families (Lapierre, Padgett, and Malone, 1994).

Nurse Roles and Qualities

The nurse may assume multiple roles, such as teacher, counselor, advocate, and coordinator. The nurse must also possess key qualities to be effective, including warmth, sensitivity, creativity, empathy, and patience. These qualities facilitate independent living and enhance the quality of life.

Preparation

Multiple disciplines, such as nursing, social work, and psychology, provide case management services (Worley, 1991). Nursing's advantage in providing case management services is related to additional training and skills in the areas of illness detection, physical assessment, medication administration, and managing side effects (Firn, 1997; Mound, et al, 1991; Pittman, 1989).

The level of preparation required for providers has been a topic of debate. In psychiatric nursing, the master's prepared clinical specialist is preferred for providing case management services (Maurin, 1990). This is largely because the clinical specialist can provide therapy in addition to fulfilling the other roles of the case manager. Worley, Drago, and Hadley (1990) propose a model of case management in which the clinical specialist acts as consultant and supervisor, and the nurse practitioner provides primary care for chronically mentally ill

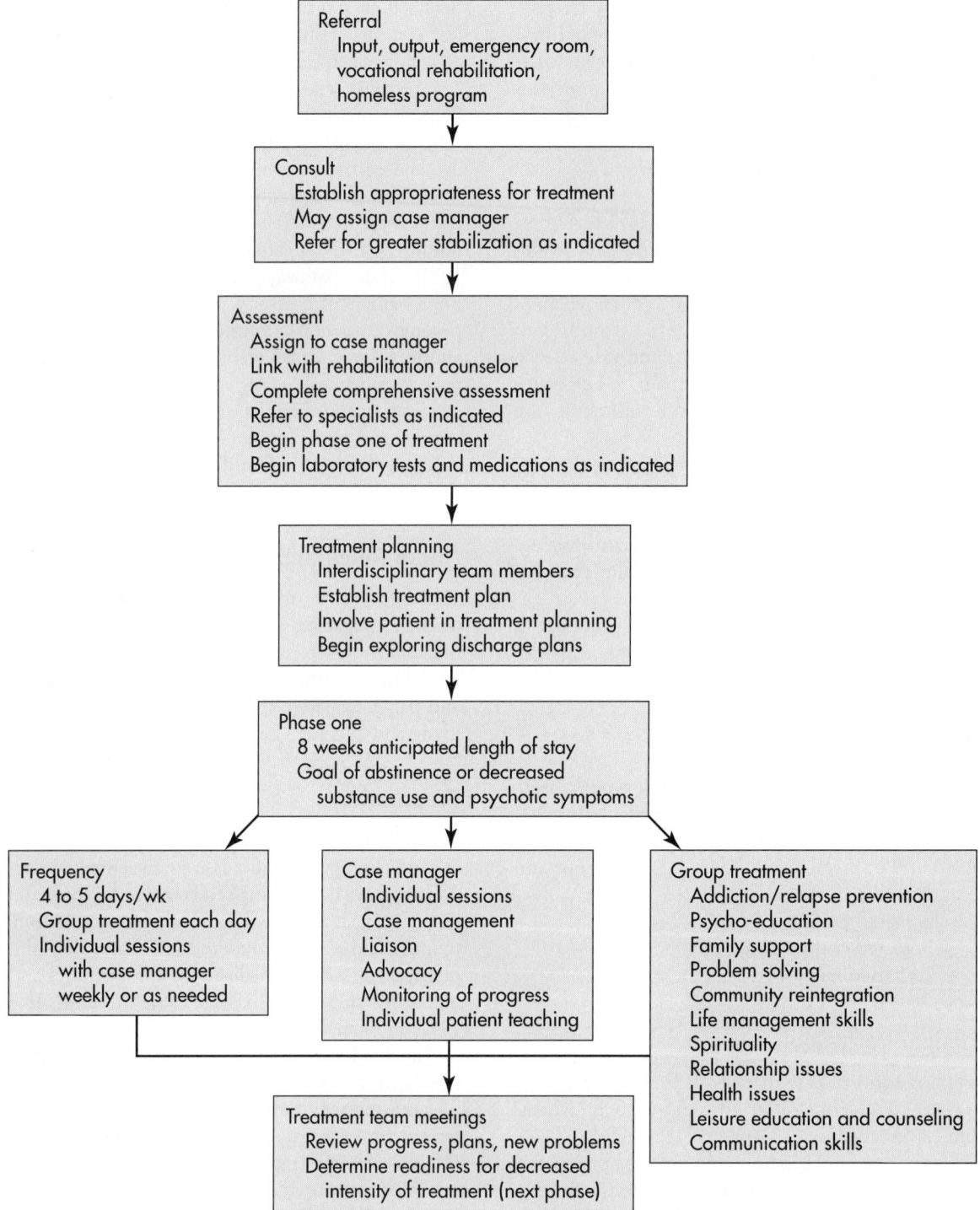

FIGURE 9-2 Clinical pathway.

patients. Other nurses can provide many of the additional components of case management in areas such as educating patients, linking them with resources, or advocating on their behalf. When therapy is indicated, patients are referred to the clinical specialist. It is important to note that with health care reform, alternatives are being explored; for example, the advance practice registered nurse (APRN) provides the care or supervises other care providers in a primary care model. The APRN is a registered nurse who is prepared at least at the master's degree level and who is nationally certified (ANA, 1994).

Location

Case management services can be provided in a variety of settings. Ideally, case management occurs over an extended period across treatment settings, and the case manager remains actively involved in treatment to enhance continuity of care regardless of where the patient is receiving services on the continuum of care.

■ Critical Thinking Question

Marie is being discharged after a 9-month hospitalization at a long-term psychiatric facility. Much of her treatment has included psychiatric rehabilitation techniques. She is going to live with a cousin, 600 miles away. What is your approach to case management?

COMPONENTS OF CASE MANAGEMENT

The nursing process is the foundation of case management. Case management includes the components of psychiatric rehabilitation, resource linkage, consultation, advocacy, crisis intervention, home care, and therapy (see Figure 9-3). Nursing can provide all facets of case management, including psychiatric rehabilitation.

Psychiatric Rehabilitation

Psychiatric rehabilitation helps individuals with psychiatric disabilities become satisfied and successful in their environments with the least amount of pro-

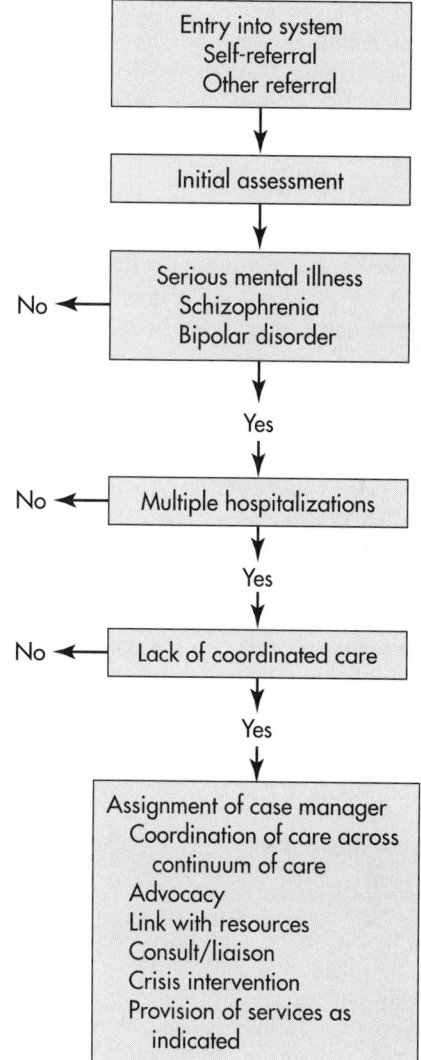

FIGURE 9-3 Decision tree for case management appropriateness.

fessional assistance (Anthony, 1992). It is further defined as helping individuals with mental illness function at the highest level possible within their limitations (Mound, et al, 1991). The principles of psychiatric rehabilitation have their roots in physical rehabilitation, and these principles address patients' illnesses, disabilities, and disadvantages (Anthony, 1992). For example, a patient's illness is schizophrenia that includes hallucinations; the disability from the illness is difficulty maintaining concentration on tasks; and the disadvantage is discrimination against individuals with mental illness. Thompson and Strand (1994) note that psychiatric rehabilitation models are becoming more oriented toward wellness, ability, and functional level.

Resource Linkage

Linking the chronically mentally ill with needed resources is another crucial element in case management. Patients may need assistance with food stamps, housing, job training, supported education, finances, or transportation.

Patients may also need assistance in managing their personal resources and time. For example, a patient's only transportation to appointments is the bus. He knows where to catch the bus but does not feel comfortable riding on it. He feels anxious and becomes paranoid about the activity itself and about the other people riding with him. The case manager goes with the patient on his first bus ride and helps him use anxiety-reducing techniques and reality testing. Over time, his comfort level increases.

Consultation

Consultation is an important role in case management. The nurse negotiates compromises between patients and their families or significant others, the community, the treatment team, and treatment facilities. The nurse may also function as a liaison between patients and multiple treatment providers (Hellwig, 1993).

■ Critical Thinking Question

Barry has chronic paranoid schizophrenia, hypertension, and kidney disease. He has a limited income and will be moving into a new, low-cost residence after his discharge from the hospital. What does your case management approach include?

Advocacy

The nurse is an advocate on behalf of patients in areas such as decreasing the stigma of mental illness and helping others to understand the limitations of

*C*ase *S*tudy

Joe, 39 years old, was discharged recently from an inpatient psychiatric unit with a diagnosis of chronic paranoid schizophrenia. He was referred to a partial hospitalization program because of his level of acuity and the need to make the transition back into the community. His medications include fluphenazine decanoate (Prolixin Decanoate) 37.5 mg IM q2 weeks and benztropine mesylate (Cogentin) 1 mg PO bid. Joe's primary therapist is a psychiatric APRN in the partial hospitalization program. The APRN determines that Joe has limited social skills, unproductive use of leisure time, a poor work history, a desire to live independently of his parents, and elevated liver function. The APRN builds a therapeutic relationship with Joe, provides therapy to enhance his social skills, and supervises the student nurse who works with Joe in order to structure and use his leisure time in a healthful manner. The APRN also does the following:
• Consults with the vocational rehabilitation specialist
• Schedules an evaluation for supported employment
• Consults with the psychiatrist about the implications of the elevated liver function studies and appropriate Prolixin Decanoate dosage

• Refers Joe to an internal medicine physician for further evaluation of the elevated liver function studies

The APRN educates and supports Joe during this process and serves as a liaison between Joe and the two physicians. The APRN monitors Joe's response to the Prolixin.

Joe also receives education and support from the groups and his peers in the partial hospitalization program. The APRN recommends that Joe remain with his parents because of the stressors he is currently experiencing. Joe agrees that, after a period of stabilization, he will pursue independent living with the assistance of his therapist and through linkage with the appropriate resources. After treatment in the partial hospitalization program, Joe reports increased self-esteem, knowledge of his illness and medications, empowerment, and quality of life. The initial dependence upon the pro-gram leads to greater independence, and Joe now lives independently and works in the supported work program.

*C*are *P*lan

NAME: Joe Smith _____   **ADMISSION DATE:** _____

DSM-IV DIAGNOSIS: Chronic paranoid schizophrenia _____

ASSESSMENT: **Areas of strength:** motivation, family support, sufficient income
Problems: impulsive; poor work history, social skills and use of leisure time; elevated liver function studies

DIAGNOSIS: Self-esteem disturbance related to poor social skills and inability to work successfully, as evidenced by withdrawal and poor use of leisure time

OUTCOMES: **Short-term goals:**   Date met
 • Short-term goals: Patient will interact with his peers in the program at least three times a day.   _____
 • Patient will verbalize activities he enjoys to structure his leisure time.   _____
 Long-term goals:
 • Patient will report increased self-esteem.   _____
 • Patient will become actively involved in the supported work program.   _____
 • Patient will demonstrate productive and healthful use of leisure.   _____

PLANNING/ INTERVENTIONS: **Nurse-patient relationship:** Establish trust, build rapport, and provide support and encouragement
Psychopharmacology: Teach the patient about his medications and respective side effects; teach the meaning and implications of the elevated liver function studies and medication decrease; monitor the response to medications, side effects, and changes in liver function studies; and teach the importance of medication compliance.
Milieu management: Actively engage the patient in the milieu of the partial hospitalization program; provide ongoing safety in the environment; and monitor response in the milieu of the program and with other patients.

EVALUATION: Patient is socializing with his peers, responding well to the reduced dosage of Prolixin with decreasing liver functions, is punctual, and receives positive comments about his work. Patient reports increased self-esteem and has more quality in his life.

REFERRALS: Patient will have an evaluation for the supported work program in one month.

---

those who are mentally ill. Advocacy for the best interests of patients sometimes conflicts with what patients desire.

For example, it is not in the best interest of a young patient with schizophrenia to drink beer with his buddies even though this is his only social activity. The nurse would discourage the use of alcohol and explore more beneficial social activities. For the patient who wants to explore the use of modalities such as healing touch (Hoover-Kramer, 1994), massage therapy, and vitamin supplementation, the nurse may advocate for education regarding "complementary" modalities that are appropriate in combination with "traditional" modalities.

Crisis Intervention

The nurse must be alert to signs of relapse and decompensation. Patients experience a variety of stressors that may evolve into a crisis. The nurse must intervene quickly to prevent further decompensation since individuals with chronic mental illness often are unable to cope with stress effectively. A seemingly small event, such as receiving a request for updated information from an agency, can precipitate a crisis.

Other situations that could potentiate relapse include change in living arrangements, the onset of physical illness, and environmental stressors (e.g., loud noises) (Hunter and Storat, 1994). Nurses can help patients to avoid or manage crisis situations by teaching them how to monitor relapse indicators (Hamera, et al, 1992) and effectively use coping or problem-solving skills.

Home Care

Many patients with chronic mental illness are homebound. *Homebound* refers not only to a patient's home, but also to nursing homes, halfway houses, prisons, shelters, and homelessness. Psychiatric home care is a cost-effective alternative to inpatient hospitalization. In psychiatric home care, the nurse often functions as a case manager. Many of the issues already described, such as linking resources and advocacy, apply in the home care setting (Hellwig, 1993).

■ Critical Thinking Question

Ron is a homeless patient who avoids taking his medications because he believes "the pills are poisoned." You have had one previous interaction with Ron, and you are not sure if he trusts you. You assess that Ron's paranoia prevents him from seeking assistance at a local shelter. What are your interventions to engage Ron in treatment?

Therapy

The case manager may need to provide individual therapy and must have the appropriate training and experience to do so. If the case manager is not prepared to conduct therapy, other therapeutic interventions can be implemented, while the patient is referred for formal therapy elsewhere.

▣ Key Concepts

1. The foundation of case management is the nursing process. The components of case management are psychiatric rehabilitation, resource linkage, consultation, advocacy, crisis intervention, home care, and therapy.
2. The nurse assumes multiple roles in prioritizing patient care, such as teacher, counselor, advocate, and coordinator.
3. Case management can be provided in various treatment settings along the continuum of care.
4. Multiple levels of care providers may assist in case management.
5. Critical or clinical pathways are integrated into an overall quality improvement plan to evaluate and adjust patient care.

▣ Study Questions

(Answer key is in the back of the book.)
1. Important benefits of case management include the following:
   a. Increased continuity of care
   b. Assisting patients to be successful in their environments
   c. Increased cost-effectiveness
   d. Ensured access to care
   e. All of the above
2. The key factor in the development of case management and psychiatric rehabilitation was deinstitutionalization
3. Goals of case management include which of the following? (Circle all that apply.)
   a. Increased quality of life
   b. Increased function
   c. Empowerment and participation in treatment
   d. Cure of mental illness
   e. Increased community involvement
4. Which of the following is the foundation of case management?
   a. Psychiatric rehabilitation
   b. The nursing process
   c. Resources
   d. Consultation/liaison
5. Critical or clinical pathways:
   a. Guide patient care
   b. Outline treatment, length of stay, and discharge plans

c. Increase patient satisfaction
d. a and b
6. A holistic approach means _____ *working toward interconnectedness of peace between the mind, body & spirit*
7. Case management can take place in which settings?
   a. Inpatient unit
   b. Clinic
   c. Prison
   d. Home
   e. Streets
   f. All of the above

REFERENCES

American Nurses Association: A statement on psychiatric–mental health clinical nursing practice and standards of psychiatric–mental health clinical nursing practice, Kansas City, Mo, The Association, 1994.

Anthony WA: Psychiatric rehabilitation: key issues and future policy, *Health Aff (Millwood):*164, 1992.

Anthony WA, Cohen MR, and Cohen BF: Psychiatric rehabilitation. In Talbott JA, editor: *The chronic mental patient: five years later,* Orlando, Fla, 1984, Grune & Stratton.

Atkinson, M: Psychiatric clinical nurse specialists as intensive case managers for the seriously mentally ill, *Semin Nurse Managers* 4(2):1130, 1996.

Bachrach LL: Psychosocial rehabilitation and psychiatry in the care of long-term patients, *Am J Psychiatry* 149(11): 1455, 1992.

Bigelow DA and Young DJ: Effectiveness of a case management program, *Community Health J* 27(2):115, 1991.

Case Management Society of America: *Standards of practice,* Little Rock, Ark, 1995, The Society.

Dunn J K: Medical skills and knowledge: how necessary are they of psychiatric nurses? *J Psychosoc Nurs Ment Health Serv* 31(12):25, 1993.

Firn S, editor: Developing nursing skills in an intensive case management service, *J Psychiatr Ment Health Nurs* 4:159, 1997.

Forchuk C, et al: Incorporating Peplau's theory and case management, *J Psychosoc Nurs Ment Health Serv* 27(2):35, 1989.

Giuliano K and Poirier C: Nursing case management: critical pathways to desirable outcomes, *Nurs Management* 22(3):52, 1991.

Hamera E, et al: Symptom monitoring in schizophrenia: potential for enhancing self-care, *Arch Psychiatr Nurs* 6(6):324, 1992.

Hellwig K: Psychiatric home care nursing: managing patients in the community setting, *J Psychosoc Nurs Ment Health Serv* 31(12):21, 1993.

Hoover-Kramer D., *Healing touch for health care professionals,* Albany, NY, 1996, Delmar Publishers.

Hunter E and Storat B: Psychosocial triggers of relapse in persons with chronic mental illness: a pilot study, *Issues Ment Health Nurs* 15:67, 1994.

Jambunathan J and Van Dongen C: Use of RN case management and costs and utilization of outpatient mental health services: a pilot study, *Issues Ment Health Nurs* 16:407, 1995.

Kanter J: Clinical case management: definition, principles, components, *Hosp Community Psychiatry* 40(4): 361, 1989.

Lapierre E and Padgett J, editors: What does a nurse need to know and do to maintain an effective level of case management? *J Psychosoc Nurs Ment Health Serv* 30(3): 35, 1992.

Lapierre E, Padgett J, and Malone J, editors: What are the implications of continuous quality improvement and total quality management for education and psychiatric nursing practice? *J Psychosoc Nurs Ment Health Serv* 32(2):43, 1994.

Macias C, et al: The role of case management within a community support system: partnership with psychosocial rehabilitation, *Community Ment Health J* 30(4): 1323, 1994.

Maurin JT: Case management: caring for psychiatric clients, *J Psychosoc Nurs Ment Health Serv* 28(7):7, 1990.

Morse G, et al: The experimental comparison of three types of case management for homeless mentally ill persons, *Psychiatr Serv* 48(4):497, 1997.

Mosher C, et al: Upgrading practice with critical pathways, *Am J Nurs* 41, 1992.

Mound B, et al: The expanded role of nurse case managers, *J Psychosoc Nurs Ment Health Serv* 29(6):18, 1991.

Palmer-Erbs V: Psychiatric rehabilitation: a breath of fresh air in a turbulent health care environment, *J Psychosoc Nurs Ment Health Serv* 34(9):16, 1996.

Palmer-Erbs V and Unger K: An innovation in psychiatric rehabilitation programming–supported education, *J Psychosoc Nurs Ment Health Serv* 35(1):16, 1997.

Pittman DC: Nursing case management: holistic care for the deinstitutionalized chronically mentally ill, *J Psychosoc Nurs Ment Health Serv* 27(11):23, 1989.

Scott J and Dixon L: Assertive community treatment and case management for schizophrenia, *Schizophrenia Bulletin* 21(4):657, 1995.

Smith G: Critical pathway and patient and family teaching protocol for major depression, *Nurs Care Management* 2(1):23, 1997.

Solomon P: The efficacy of case management services for severely mentally disabled clients, *Community Ment Health J* 28(3):163, 1992.

Thompson J and Strand K: Psychiatric nursing in a psychosocial setting, *J Psychosoc Nurs Ment Health Serv* 32(2):25, 1994.

Wilbur S and Arns P: Psychosocial rehabilitation nurses: taking our place on the multidisciplinary team, *J Psychosoc Nursing* 36(4):33, 1998.

Worley N: Mental health: advisor to the team, *Nurs Times* 87(33):38, 1991.

Worley NK: *Mental health nursing in the community,* St. Louis, 1997, Mosby.

Worley NK, Drago L, and Hadley T: Improving the physical health–mental health interface for the chronically mentally ill: could nurse case managers make a difference? *Arch Psychiatr Nurs* 4(2):108, 1990.

The Therapeutic Nurse-Patient Relationship

CHAPTER 10

Communication

BETTE R. KELTNER

LEARNING OBJECTIVES

After reading this chapter you should be able to:
- Understand major influences on communication.
- Distinguish between social and therapeutic communication.
- Identify goals of therapeutic communication.

- Discuss critical therapeutic communication issues.
- Describe a variety of techniques that facilitate patient-centered communication.
- State common interferences with therapeutic communication.

Most communication is a two-way process between two or more individuals. In nursing this process is focused on patients' needs and problems. Professional or therapeutic communication is one of the means by which the nursing process is implemented in order to achieve quality patient care. In psychiatric nursing, therapeutic communication is one of the most important tools used by nurses to assist patients. It is the means for building trust, developing therapeutic relationships, providing support and comfort, encouraging growth and change, and implementing patient education.

Nurses as health care professionals rely on verbal, written, and electronic (computer) communication for sharing information, analyzing data, collaborating with other disciplines, and delivering services. Consequently nursing requires a sound foundation in effective communication concepts and skills. For nurses who work with psychiatric patients (patients with alterations in thinking and behavior) the chal-

lenge of communicating is even greater. In psychiatric nursing the goal is not only to understand patients and ensure that they understand you, but also to teach patients more effective communication skills for interaction with mainstream society.

CATEGORIES OF COMMUNICATION

Communication is an interaction between two or more persons involving the exchange of information between a sender and a receiver. The product of communication is the message, to be interpreted by the receiver. Words (verbal or written) and behaviors (nonverbal) are the primary channels for communication. The evolution of human communication has resulted in sophisticated technology, including ever-improving computerized communication capabilities (Modai and Rabinowitz, 1993).

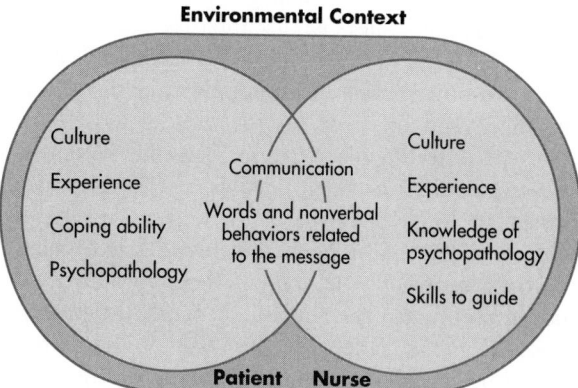

FIGURE 10-1   Essential and influencing variables of the therapeutic communication environment.

Written Communication

Since written material is a primary means of acquiring and sharing information, mastery of language skills is imperative. All professions require some form of written reports, instructions, or sharing of findings and ideas. Vocabulary, grammar, and organization of ideas are critical skills.

Speech and Behavior

In addition to sound, oral communication includes the mannerisms that modify the message. The timbre and tone of the voice have meaning. The rate and emphasis of speech affect the message. Body language can enhance or change the meaning of words. It is important for verbal and nonverbal communication to be congruent (Farran and Keane-Hagerty, 1989). Behaviors can negate a verbal message; for example, a patient is not likely to (nor should) believe a nurse who says, "Yes, I will help you," with a frown and an angry tone of voice.

Dynamics of Therapeutic Communication

Therapeutic communication requires attention to multiple, interacting factors. At the core of communications are the words and nonverbal behaviors that relate to patients' health needs and are exchanged between patients and the nurse. Figure 10-1 illustrates key dimensions of participants in communication that should be understood. It is important to view the patient and the nurse as a whole operating within an environmental context. Communication is influenced by the individual's personal experiences, gender, culture, values, and beliefs; by the purpose of the interaction; and by the physical and emotional context of the interaction. It is important to communicate on patients' levels (according to their vocabulary, educational backgrounds, and the effects of their illnesses) without using a patronizing or condescending manner.

Interpretation of communication

Interpretation of a message is filtered through an individual's knowledge, experience, and biases. Some aspects of communication are more commonly understood than others. Words generally are understood more precisely than behaviors. Anyone who has studied a foreign language, however, appreciates that nuances are often lost in translation because of the limitations of words. It is important to have a broad knowledge of the effects of cultures if the nurse is to interpret accurately and respond appropriately to patient communications. Only the patients, however, can ultimately clarify and validate the meaning of their messages (Ingram, 1991). For example, only the patient can explain whether a lack of eye contact is a cultural trait (in some cultures, eye contact with a stranger is considered to be rude) or is a reflection of the patient's low self-esteem. See Chapter 17 for cultural considerations in psychiatric nursing.

Patient communications often convey indirect messages or underlying themes about content, mood, or interaction issues. For example, a patient may spend 30 minutes describing his divorce of 3 years ago, two other broken relationships since then, having been laid off from his job, having to sell his house, and feeling like a failure. The underlying *content theme* might be interpreted as a series of major losses. As he describes all of these losses, he might convey anger and/or guilt. These *mood themes* would be congruent with the content theme. Feelings do not always match the content theme. If the patient was laughing as he described his losses, his happiness would be considered an incongruent mood theme.

Assessing for *interaction themes* involves examining the ways the patients relate to family, friends, other patients, and the staff. A patient might call the crisis center each time her roommate is out of town to complain about nervousness and loneliness. When her roommate returns, the patient is once again comfortable. The interaction theme could be assessed as one of dependency. The patient who plays one staff member against another and seeks attention by complaining about all the other patients might be showing an interaction theme of manipulation. Themes are frequently the source of nursing diagnoses upon which care plans are based.

Environmental considerations

The environment can facilitate or impede therapeutic communication. Factors such as noise level, privacy, type of furniture, space, and temperature can all affect the quality of communication.

Proxemics refers to the way people perceive and use environmental, social, and personal space in interactions. Typically boundaries of personal space for public and social communication are more distant than those for intimate or therapeutic communication. However, the amount of space needed between the patient and the nurse will be affected also by illness and emotional factors such as suspiciousness, anxiety, perceptual distortions, aggressiveness, the genders of the two parties, and personal comfort. Generally patients are more comfortable when the nurse is at their eye level rather than standing over them. Face-to-face contact may not be as effective as sitting at a slight angle to patients so that they may look away more easily (Dee, 1991). Some patients may require the presence of a table or an empty chair between themselves and the nurse in order to feel safe enough to talk.

Physical considerations

Patients with certain physical problems may experience communication difficulties. For example, sensory limitations, developmental disabilities, speech impediments, pain, and physical deformities can all interfere with clear communication. Patients with certain sensory limitations such as hearing loss may have compromised communication necessitating compensatory measures such as slow face-to-face speech for lip-reading. Developmental disabilities may seriously limit the ability of patients to comprehend and remember. Simple sentences with a single main idea may have to be repeated several times. Speech impediments or other problems may interfere with understanding patients' messages. Asking for repetition, clarification, and validation are important, but this can increase a patient's frustration if overdone. Having patients write their answers is an alternative if they are able to read and write. Physical pain often interferes with patients' abilities to think clearly and concentrate, and may affect the sense of priority in problems to be addressed. Physical deformities and injuries, especially facial ones, may inhibit the ability to talk and may interfere with the nurse's ability to concentrate on other problems.

Kinesic considerations

Kinesics is the study of body movements. *Body language* is the popular term that emphasizes the meaning of facial expressions, eye movements, gestures, and mannerisms. Awareness of the cultural meanings of nonverbal and verbal communication facilitates a positive therapeutic alliance with patients (Siantz, 1991). A variety of body language is used to indicate an individual's feelings. Avoiding prolonged eye contact is often used to disengage or ignore communication. Crossing the arms over the chest occurs many times when a person feels defensive (however, this also occurs when a person is cold). It is important that the nurse be sensitive to these cues and interpret them in a global context of therapeutic communication. If the message seems inconsistent or confusing, exploring the meaning of body language may be useful. For example, the nurse might say,

"Many times when people back away from someone, it is because they are afraid. Is there something that makes you fearful?"

Body language may communicate feelings or merely reflect a habit. Nurses must become aware of their own "body habits" and consider positive and negative meanings associated with these behaviors (Dee, 1991). Behaviors that communicate caring, confidence, and calmness should be cultivated. Sensitivity to and understanding of kinesics are important in interpreting messages from a patient but should be viewed as cues rather than as diagnostic tools. Again, validating the meaning of the patient's behavior *with the patient* is crucial (Dee, 1991).

■ Critical Thinking Question

Ann Williams has multiple facial injuries, has both eyes patched, is breathing with a ventilator, and has been sedated. In what ways would you modify your techniques to facilitate communication with her?

THERAPEUTIC COMMUNICATION

Therapeutic vs. Social Communication

Therapeutic communication occurs with the purpose of helping patients. Social communication involves equal disclosure of personal information and intimacy, and both parties enjoy equal opportunities for spontaneity. Therapeutic communication focuses on the patient but is planned and directed by the professional. In social exchanges both participants seek to have personal needs met, whereas the needs of the patient are the focus of therapeutic communication. Therapeutic communication relies on patients' disclosures of personal and sometimes painful feelings with the professional at a calculated emotional distance—near enough to be involved but objective enough to be helpful. In a social relationship a friend may share feelings of anger and aggression toward a mutual friend with the expectation that the feelings will be kept confidential. In therapeutic communication it must be understood that while confidentiality will be respected outside the treatment setting, a professional is obligated to share information within the treatment team. The nurse is a patient's advocate, *not* a patient's friend (see Chapter 11).

Therapeutic Use of Self

In psychiatric nursing the nurse, using verbal and nonverbal communication, is the primary therapeutic agent with psychiatric patients (as compared with treatment procedures and physical interventions used by a medical-surgical nurse). The nurse's communication is a major vehicle for helping patients achieve productive emotional and behavioral outcomes. Use of self, use of medications, and use of the environments are the major components of psychotherapeutic management (see Chapter 2).

Therapeutic listening is an important component of the therapeutic use of self with patients and is crucial for getting to know patients as individuals, their needs, and concerns. It has been described as being composed of the following attributes (Kemper, 1992):

Being actively alert
"Hearing" with all the senses
Using eye contact
Having an attending posture
Ensuring concentration
Being patient
Having an openness to receive information
Offering empathy and support
Asking questions

Assimilating verbal and nonverbal information
Organizing, synthesizing, and interpreting information
Validating and clarifying information
Responding verbally and nonverbally to encourage patients to continue
Summarizing important points
Giving feedback appropriately

■ Critical Thinking Question

Select 3 or 4 of the above behaviors and "communicate" with a friend. What difference did you see in how your friend responds?

Therapeutic use of the self requires the *sensitivity* to recognize important cues and make decisions about the priority of these cues. *Objectivity* is the process of remaining open to as many aspects of patients, their problems, and potential solutions as possible. Nurses must not allow their own issues and biases to color interactions with patients and should avoid being "swept away" by patients' emotions and perceptions.

Communicating *empathy* is an essential skill of the nurse. Empathy is the emotional and ". . . intellectual ability to identify and understand another person's feelings and perspective from an objective stance" (Morse, 1992). It verbally and nonverbally conveys caring, compassion, and concern for patients, but the nurse does not experience patients' feelings. Empathy helps patients to be more accepting of their feelings and express them more readily. (See Chapter 11 for more detail about empathy.)

Being therapeutic includes being *genuine* and *sincere* as conveyed by congruent verbal and nonverbal behaviors, authenticity, and honesty (without total self-disclosure by the nurse). Patients need to feel respected, valued, and accepted by the nurse, even if all of their behaviors are not tolerated. A nurse should not evaluate patients' beliefs, feelings, and behaviors as right or wrong; rather, the nurse helps patients themselves to evaluate the effects or consequences of these aspects. However, the nurse must also set limits on destructive behaviors to protect the integrity and dignity of patients, as well as the safety and rights of others.

Touching is a complex issue. The meaning of touch varies widely between cultures, individuals, and patients with different diagnoses. Touching a patient's hand or shoulder, or giving a light hug can convey caring, empathy, support, and acceptance. It can also be viewed, however, as a violation of personal space or privacy, or it may be misinterpreted as a sexual gesture or an aggressive move. Therefore the use of touch with patients must be approached with caution. Patients' behaviors can give clues to the ability to tolerate and benefit from touch. For example, a patient who is not able to sit close to the nurse is less likely to want to be touched. A patient who is quite trusting of the nurse is more likely to accept it. A patient who is sexually preoccupied could misinterpret any type of touch. With many patients (especially those who have been sexually or physically abused), it is appropriate to ask about giving a gentle hug: "Could you use a hug right now?" or "Would a hug help you feel better?"

THERAPEUTIC COMMUNICATION TECHNIQUES

Therapeutic techniques are a means of helping patients toward productive goals but are not goals in themselves. The communication techniques presented in Box 10-1 are arranged according to the steps of the nursing process that they tend to facilitate. Some techniques may be versatile enough to be used in more than one step. Interactions with patients do not involve using all of these techniques sequentially. It is common to move back and forth between the steps of assessment,

nursing diagnosis, and planning before reaching implementation and evaluation. Even during the implementation step, the nurse may realize that more analysis is needed and return to the step of nursing diagnosis. Many nurse-patient interactions do not use the complete nursing process in a single session, but they always involve using therapeutic techniques. At times interactions have primarily a social or recreational focus instead of a problem-solving process, but these may still be beneficial to the patient. Every encounter with a patient can be therapeutic with or without full use of the nursing process (see Chapters 11 and 12).

> ### ▣ Critical Thinking Question
>
> Jack Riley was admitted with chronic paranoid schizophrenia. His only contact for years has been with his parents. Explain how various social and recreational activities could be therapeutic for him.

COMMON INTERFERENCES WITH THERAPEUTIC COMMUNICATION

In the same manner that therapeutic communication guides the patient toward goals, certain messages and behaviors interfere with reaching goals. Some behaviors occur frequently because of nervous mannerisms or are the result of social expectations in the therapeutic situation. The nurse must recognize and overcome any habitual communication problems that could interfere with effective therapeutic communication.

Nurse's Fears and Feelings

Since therapeutic communication involves the use of self, many personal feelings are naturally evoked and can be disturbing. It is not unusual for a nurse to feel fear when communicating with individuals who are experiencing severe psychic or physical distress. Fear compromises therapeutic communication. The nurse may have concerns such as, "Could this be me someday?" or "My brother does this sometimes; does that mean he's crazy?" or "What if this patient gets angry with me?" Therapeutic communication relies on coming to terms with such questions. Individuals become patients because of serious difficulties in functioning, not because of an occasional dysfunctional behavior. The nurse should avoid personalizing what patients

Box 10-1   Therapeutic Techniques to Facilitate the Nursing Process in Psychiatric Nursing

Assessment

Techniques fostering description

Offering self: making self available and showing interest and concern

"I'll sit with you awhile."
"I'll stay with you."

Active listening: paying close attention to verbal and nonverbal communications, patterns of thinking, feelings, and behaviors

Face the patient; maintain eye contact; be open, alert, and patient; respond appropriately

Silence: planned absence of verbal remarks to allow patients to think and say more

Maintain eye contact; convey interest and concern in facial expressions

Empathy: recognizing and acknowledging patients' feelings

"I can hear how painful it is for you to talk about this."

Questioning: using open-ended questions to achieve relevance and depth in discussion

"Who?" "What?" "Where?" "When?" "What did you say?" "What happened? Tell me about it."

General leads: using neutral expressions to encourage patients to continue talking

"Go on, I'm listening." "I hear what you are saying."

Restating: repeating the exact words of patients to remind them of what they said; to let them know they are heard

"You say you are going home soon." "Your mother wasn't happy to see you?"

Verbalizing the implied: rephrasing patients' words to highlight an underlying message

Patient: "There is nothing to do at home." Nurse: "It sounds as if you might be bored at home."

Clarification: asking patients to restate, elaborate, or give examples of ideas or feelings

"What do you mean by 'feeling sick inside'?" "Give me an example of feeling 'lost.'"

Nursing Diagnosis

Techniques fostering analysis and conclusions

Making observations: commenting on what is seen or heard to encourage discussion

"You seem restless." "I noticed you had trouble making a decision about . . ."

Presenting reality: offering a view of what is real and what is not without arguing with the patient

"I know the voices are real to you, but I don't hear them." "I don't see it the same way."

Encouraging description of perceptions: asking for patients' views of their situations

"What do you think is happening to you right now?" "What do you think is your main problem?"

Voicing doubt: expressing uncertainty about the reality of patients' perceptions and conclusions

"Is that the only way to interpret it?" "What other conclusion could there be?"

Placing an event in time or sequence: asking for relationships among events

"When did you do this?" "Then what happened?" "What led up to . . . ?" "What is the connection between . . . ?"

Encouraging comparisons: asking for similarities and differences among feelings, behaviors, and events

"How does this compare to the last time?" "What is different about your feelings today?"

Identifying themes: asking patients to identify recurrent patterns in thoughts, feelings, and behaviors

"So what do you do each time you argue with your wife?" "What feeling do you get when you see your father?"

Summarizing: reviewing main points and conclusions

"Let's see, so far you have said . . ."

Techniques fostering interpretation of meaning and importance

Focusing: pursuing a topic until its meaning or importance is clear

"Explain more about . . ." "What bothers you about . . . ?" "What happens when you feel this way?"

Interpreting: providing a view of the meaning or importance of something

"It sounds as if this is very important to you." "You seem to get in trouble when you . . ."

Encouraging evaluation: asking for patients' views of the meaning or importance of something

"So what does all this mean to you?" "How serious is this for you?" "How important is it to change this behavior?"

Continued

| Box 10-1 | Therapeutic Techniques to Facilitate the Nursing Process in Psychiatric Nursing—cont'd |

Planning

Techniques fostering problem solving and decisions

Suggesting collaboration: offering to help patients solve problems

Encouraging goal setting: asking patients to decide on the type of change needed

Giving information: providing information that will help patients make better choices

Encouraging consideration of options: asking patients to consider the pros and cons of possible options

Encouraging decisions: asking patients to make a choice among options

Encouraging the formulation of a plan: probing for step-by-step actions that will be needed

"I can help you understand this better." "Let's see if we can find an answer."

"What do you think needs to change?" "What do you want to do differently?"

"I can tell you about your medicines." "There are self-help groups available."

"What would be the advantage of trying . . ." "What might happen if you tried . . ."

"Which is the best alternative for you?" "What would work best?"

"What exactly will it take to carry out your plan?" "What else do you need to do?"

Implementation

Techniques fostering the completion of plans

Testing out new behaviors:

1. *Rehearsing:* requesting a verbal description of what will be said or done
2. *Role playing:* practicing behaviors; the nurse plays a particular role

Supportive confrontation: acknowledging the difficulty in changing, but pushing for action

Limit setting: discouraging nonproductive feelings and behaviors, and encouraging productive ones

Feedback: pointing out specific behaviors and giving impressions of reactions

"Tell me exactly what you will say to your wife on Friday."

"I'll play your wife. What do you want to say to me?"

"I know this isn't easy to do, but I think you can do it." "It's hard but give it a try."

"You're slipping into your aggressive tone again. Try it again . . ." "That is a negative comment about yourself. Tell me something positive about yourself."

"I thought you conveyed anger when you said . . ." "When you said . . . I felt . . ."

Evaluation

Encouraging evaluation: asking patients to evaluate their actions and the outcomes

Reinforcement: giving feedback on positive behaviors

Repeating steps of the nursing process if needed: using the steps of the nursing process to get a description of what happened, the degree of success, and ideas for change

"How well did it work when you tried . . ." "What was your husband's reaction?"

"This new approach worked for you. Keep it up."

"What would help you do even better next time?" "If things didn't go well, what do you want to do differently this time?"

---

say and do. Patients who abruptly end a conversation with a nurse are more likely responding to their own thoughts or anxieties than to something the nurse said. It is important that nurses understand their personal values, biases, and vulnerabilities. Nurses can benefit not only from analyzing the technique and content of interactions with patients, but also from analyzing their own feelings and reactions. (See Chapter 14 for further discussion on self-awareness.)

Sometimes a nurse is afraid of harming patients by saying the "wrong thing." Patients do not fall apart or act out because of a nurse's single mistake if the nurse's overall attitude is positive and helpful; however, patients are sensitive to malicious intent and rejection. A mistake can actually become a therapeutic encounter because the nurse becomes a role model for how to admit and apologize for an error. Many people including pychiatric patients have trouble doing this with individuals who are significant to them. In many situations, a sincere apology, if warranted, can strengthen the relationship.

Another concern is *invasion of privacy*. Psychiatric nurses investigate intensely personal areas of patients' lives, such as values, beliefs, feelings, intimate relationships, and sexuality. The focus may also be on legally sensitive areas such as incest, partner abuse, and drug use. Although these are areas that patients need to address, they are not easy to discuss. The nurse enhances patients' abilities to be open and honest by explaining the need to know about a sensitive area, by asking questions in a kind and matter-of-fact manner, by conveying empathy, and by reiterating a desire to help.

Nurse's Lack of Knowledge and Insecurity

A lack of knowledge about psychiatric illnesses, defense mechanisms, medication responses, and the dynamics of behaviors and relationships causes insecurity and diminishes patients' confidence in the nurse. Patients usually are accepting, however, when the nurse is honest about not knowing an answer if the nurse is willing to find out.

In an attempt to achieve a sense of security, the nurse may assume a parental type of role toward the patient. Emrich (1989) reports that many staff-patient interactions are parental, maintain illness, and are disconfirming. Parental responses can be caused by remarks that are *consistently* nurturing, critical, or condescending. Nurses sometimes exhibit one of these three patterns in order to decrease the feelings of insecurity in themselves but it is important to avoid these responses.

Inappropriate Responses

The nurse's response to messages should be based on assessment and knowledge of the situation, as well as the dynamics of patients' illnesses and problems, but nurses may not always interact effectively. A nurse may withdraw from patients who are angrily cursing instead of discussing the behavior. Nurses may get caught up in the unfounded fears and accusations of paranoid patients and thereby reinforce the symptoms. It is often difficult to distinguish between fact and distortion in what patients say, so the nurse must avoid premature conclusions. For example, staff members do not believe a patient who says he wrote

the theme song for a popular play. The patient finally brings in his original handwritten sheet music and the list of credits from the play's manuscript for the staff to see. It sometimes helps to get information from family members to validate information or to wait until medications help clear delusional thinking.

Nurses may be preoccupied with what they want to say next instead of listening to patients. Overuse of one or two therapeutic skills, such as reflecting or restating, can stagnate communications if there is not movement toward analyzing and problem solving. Problem solving can also be impeded by giving advice to patients instead of helping them to evaluate and choose their own solutions. False reassurances ("Everything will be all right" or "Things are bound to get better") are basically promises that the nurse cannot keep. Box 10-2 lists other responses and behaviors that are generally ineffective or inappropriate. Mistakes by the nurse can generally be corrected, explanations can be given, and damage to the relationship can be reversed. Patients usually evaluate nurses by an overall attitude of caring and concern rather than by a single inappropriate response.

Critical Thinking Question

Describe strategies you would use to be the patient's advocate rather than the patient's friend.

Box 10-2 Ineffective Responses and Behaviors

Not listening	Talking too much
Looking too busy	Not paying attention
Seeming uncomfortable with silence	Laughing nervously
Being opinionated	Smiling inappropriately
Avoiding sensitive topics	Showing disapproval
Arguing	Belittling feelings
Changing the subject	Minimizing problems
Being superficial	Being defensive
Having a closed posture	Focusing on personal problems of the nurse
Ignoring the patient	
Making false promises	Using cliches
Making sarcastic remarks	Making flippant remarks
	Lying/being insincere

▼ Key Concepts

1. Therapeutic techniques are skills to help people but are not goals in themselves.
2. Therapeutic communication occurs with a plan and a purpose, whereas social communication involves equal levels of intimacy, sharing, and the opportunity for spontaneity.
3. Therapeutic communication differs from social communication because it focuses on patients rather than on a give-and-take experience.
4. Goals of psychiatric nursing are to understand patients, to assure patients understand the nurse, and to teach more effective communication skills.
5. Listening is a therapeutic communication technique that requires careful concentration in order to guide the conversation toward a goal.
6. Nurses are responsible for therapeutic communication and must recognize communication interferences they may be causing.
7. Some common interferences to therapeutic communication are fear, lack of knowledge and insecurity, and inappropriate responses (see Box 10-2).

▼ Study Questions

(Answer key is in the back of the book.)
1. Therapeutic communication:
   a. Involves intimacy and spontaneity between patients and nurses.
   b. Resembles the give-and-take of social communication.
   c. Is structured with a plan and a purpose.
   d. Is dominated by the nurse.
2. One goal of therapeutic communication is to:
   a. Assist patients with learning communication skills.
   b. Allow the nurse to express feelings.
   c. Become the patient's friend.
   d. Develop consistent communication techniques.
3. Encouraging a description of perception is reflected in which of the following statements?
   a. "What do you mean by 'feeling alienated'?"
   b. "I know what you mean."
   c. "It sounds as if you have been depressed."
   d. "What do you think is happening in your marriage?"
4. Listening is an aspect of therapeutic communication that
   a. Encourages patients to guide the interview.
   b. Allows the nurse to interpret and validate data.
   c. Is easy for most people to do.
   d. Reflects what patients say.
5. Which of the following reflects a common interference in nurse-patient communications?
   a. Discussing fears about patients with a colleague.
   b. Validating patient information with the family.
   c. Admitting and apologizing to a patient for a mistake.
   d. Avoiding issues that are uncomfortable for patients.

REFERENCES

Davis DD and Kurtz P: Assessing interaction patterns of students, *Nurse Educator* 16(5):9, 1991.

Dee V: Professionally speaking (on culturally specific body language), *J Psychosoc Nurs Ment Health Serv* 29(11):40, 1991.

Emrich K: Helping or hurting? Interacting in the psychiatric milieu, *J Psychosoc Nurs Ment Health Serv* 27(12):26, 1989.

Farran CJ and Keane-Hagerty E: Communicating effectively with dementia patients, *J Psychosoc Nurs Ment Health Serv* 27(5):13, 1989.

Ingram CA: Professionally speaking (on culturally specific body language), *J Psychosoc Nurs Ment Health Serv* 29(11):41, 1991.

Kane G: Computers and psychiatric clients, *J Psychosoc Nurs Ment Health Serv* 27(3):12, 1989.

Kemper BJ: Therapeutic listening: developing the concept, *J Psychosoc Nurs Ment Health Serv* 30(7):21, 1992.

Modai I and Rabinowitz J: Why and how to establish a computerized system for psychiatric case records, *Hosp Community Psychiatry* 44(11):1091, 1993.

Morse JM: Exploring empathy: a conceptual fit for nursing practice? *Image J Nurs Sch* 24(4):273, 1992.

Siantz ML: Professionally speaking (on culturally specific body language), *J Psychosoc Nurs Ment Health Serv* 29(11):38, 1991.

CHAPTER 11

The Nurse-Patient Relationship

LEE H. SCHWECKE

LEARNING OBJECTIVES

After reading this chapter you should be able to:
- Describe what it means to be therapeutic.
- Describe the stages of a therapeutic nurse-patient relationship.

- Identify the major tasks of each stage of the nurse-patient relationship.
- Recognize verbal strategies in interacting with patients.

Hildegard Peplau defined nursing as "a significant, therapeutic, interpersonal process. . . . Nursing is an educative instrument, a maturing force, that aims to promote forward movement of personality in the direction of creative, constructive, productive, personal, and community living" (Peplau, 1952). The nurse's relationship with patients consists of a series of goal-directed interactions. The nurse uses verbal and nonverbal communications to convey a willingness to listen, a genuine respect, a desire to help, and an understanding of patients as individuals with problems and needs. The nursing process (see Chapter 12) is the tool with which the nurse assesses patients' problems, elicits patient input, selects interventions, and evaluates the effectiveness of care. In psychiatric nursing, the nursing process is grounded

in the knowledge of the nature of therapeutic relationships, psychopharmacology and milieu management, all based on an understanding of concepts and processes of psychopathology. Developing the nurse-patient relationship is the first, and often the most pivotal, step in effective psychotherapeutic management (see Chapter 2).

THERAPEUTIC RELATIONSHIPS

Many factors influence the relationship between the nurse and the patient, and various therapeutic activities can be used within the relationship to facilitate successful patient outcomes. No theoretical

KEY TERMS

Empathy   objective understanding of how patients feel or how they see their situations, "putting yourself in their shoes"

Hallucination   false sensory perception not related to external stimuli; for example, seeing things that are not there

Delusion   false belief not consistent with the individual's intelligence and culture and not amenable to reason; for example, the belief that one's body is inhabited by aliens

Psychomotor retardation   markedly slowed speech and body movements

Transference   unconscious emotional reaction to a current situation that is actually based on previous experiences

---

model is effective with every patient, in every situation, or with every kind of problem. Even patients with the same psychiatric diagnosis will have somewhat different manifestations of symptoms depending on their history, current life situation, and emerging needs. Everyone, including patients, are unique, worthwhile, holistic individuals struggling with internal needs and external realities. The nurse should approach each patient individually by tailoring selected strategies to each patient's problems and needs.

Brief Therapeutic Relationships

Brief therapeutic relationships are not as formalized as therapy but are planned, patient-centered, and goal-directed. The nurse purposefully and carefully guides conversations with patients toward the exploration of problems, issues, and needs. The nurse then selects therapeutic strategies to facilitate awareness, decisions, changes, and/or comfort. Concern, compassion, and interest are demonstrated while maintaining an objectivity that patients may lack. The nurse may share some personal data such as age, marital status, or title, but should rarely disclose personal problems. Occasionally a brief self-disclosure may help patients to clarify specific issues, to feel less vulnerable, or to feel more "normal" (Simon, 1997) ("When I feel depressed, it's usually because I'm angry and not expressing it for some reason. What kinds of things do you get angry about?" or "Sometimes I'm afraid to tell my husband something because I don't know how he will react. What is hard for you to talk to your wife about?") Therapeutic self-disclosure facilitates comfort, honesty,

openness, and risk taking, but never burdens patients with the nurse's problems.

Social vs. Therapeutic Relationships

The nurse-patient relationship is not a social relationship (see Chapter 10). A social relationship involves companionship, mutual support, intimacy, and equal disclosure of personal information. Although a nurse may relate informally with patients, the maintenance of objectivity and goal-directedness is crucial. Patients, especially those with a history of unsatisfying relationships, may misinterpret the nurse's interest and concern. Patients often ask (or wish to ask) the nurse to be a friend or to go out on a date. When this occurs, it is necessary to remind the patient of the nurse's role and to take the opportunity to discuss the need for friendship, love, and support; for example, "I realize you would like to date. As a nurse I can help you find ways to form friendships that can offer you emotional support."

Collaboration

The nursing axiom of involving patients in their own care has relevance in psychiatric nursing. Patients have a right to make decisions about their care. When patients recognize their problems and needs, desire to change, and ask for assistance, the nurse is able to work with them on goals and plans. Collaboration generally produces more effective and enduring change than coercion or simple compliance (Mason, Breen, and Whipple, 1994). Unfortunately, there are instances when this is not possible, such as when patients have an obvious disturbance in their thought processes (as with severe hallucinations or delusions). They may be incapable of collaborating with the nurse in their care until these problems subside. At times the only goal a patient will agree to is "to get out of the hospital." Even this goal, however, provides an opening for discussion of behavioral changes necessary before discharge can occur. Patients with chronic illnesses may be able to agree to only small changes. Unless the nurse is patient, flexible, and realistic, the patient may feel overwhelmed.

CLINICAL EXAMPLE

Jason Schmidy had four admissions in 3 years with a diagnosis of paranoid schizophrenia. During each admission, he has achieved new small goals. Initially he was so suspicious that he talked only to his sister and refused medications "because they were poison." At the end of his second admission, he talked with staff members and agreed to monthly injections of a long-acting antipsychotic medication. During the third admission he related that he enjoyed helping a neighbor in his garden. At Mr. Schmidy's last discharge, he expressed interest in attending a self-help group for chronically ill patients.

BEING THERAPEUTIC VS. PROVIDING THERAPY

The nurse's basic education provides the knowledge and skills for being therapeutic in encounters with patients; training as a psychotherapist is not required. Psychotherapists receive specialized training that is often focused on a particular therapeutic model that attempts to explain the causes of mental illness and offers specialized techniques for achieving desired outcomes. Psychotherapists are interested in formalized, ongoing sessions that have a specified time, place, and length. They are selective in their choice of patients and are restrictive in the sense that they have rules for conducting sessions.

In contrast, nurses who engage in therapeutic activities, especially in an inpatient setting or outpatient program, recognize that each encounter with patients is part of an overall therapeutic picture: a therapeutic milieu. Patients discuss real problems and practical solutions, and practice skills needed in real life situations to enhance their functioning in the real community. Brief encounters offer an opportunity for patients to process feelings and thoughts as they occur. Validation and feedback are available quickly. Many patients are unable to tolerate intense, ongoing therapy but can benefit from consistent therapeutic encounters with nurses, even if their hospitalization lasts only a few days or when attendance at an outpatient program is sporadic.

Informal or recreational encounters with patients (card games, craft classes, holiday parties) may be spontaneous but must be therapeutic. For example, the nurse might observe inappropriate social behaviors or lack of social skills. It is appropriate for the nurse to then help the patient develop appropriate social and verbal skills, to test reality, and to solicit feedback and support for new behaviors. These informal activities also help patients to reduce anxiety and body tension, to develop a sense of competence, and to take risks. Informal encounters are also opportunities for the nurse to demonstrate ways of handling situations: "Well, we didn't win this hand, but I'm enjoying the game anyway." "I've made that mistake before too. I can show you how to correct it." "Everyone has a right to his or her opinion. I'll listen to yours and then you can hear mine."

DEVELOPMENT OF A THERAPEUTIC RELATIONSHIP

Stages of the Nurse-Patient Relationship

When psychiatric care was provided primarily in long-term hospitals, Peplau believed that the nurse and the patient begin as strangers and move in stages to become collaborators in problem solving (Forchuk, 1992). The stages in the nurse-patient relationship have been given various names by various authors, but Peplau's concepts remain valid (Morrison, et al, 1996). In the *stage of orientation*, patients feel needs and seek help. The nurse helps patients to understand their problems and to accept the help that is available. The nurse actively works to foster trust and to develop the relationship. In the *identification and exploration stage*, or *working stage*, there is clarification of perceptions and expectations about the relationship. There is further definition of problems and identification of tentative solutions. Patients become more motivated to take advantage of available resources to resolve problems. Patients may test the nurse and may fluctuate between dependence and independence. Peplau believed the *resolution stage,* or *termination,* needs close attention to avoid destroying the benefits gained thus far from the relationship. Focus is on the growth that occurred and on helping the patient to develop self-responsibility for setting new goals. The entire relationship is seen as promoting growth and as a learning experience for the nurse and for patients (Peplau, 1952).

Therapeutic relationships vary in depth, length, and focus. A brief therapeutic encounter may last only a few minutes, focusing on patients' *immediate needs, current feelings,* or *observed behaviors.* In a long-term hospitalization or program, the relationship may last 1 to 3 months with regular meetings that focus on underlying causes of behaviors, developmental issues, or long-term problems. In an acute-care setting or outpatient program, patients relate to many nurses and staff members each day. In this situation, progress in the nurse-patient relationship is the responsibility of every nurse with whom the patient has contact. One nurse admits the patient to the unit or program and begins the relationship. Another nurse may discharge the patient and complete termination. Shift reports, care plans, and/or progress notes help each nurse to work with the patient toward the same goals.

In this era of brief hospitalization and time-limited outpatient care, the phases of the nurse-patient relationship are not a sequence of processes but a matter of different emphases or goals. The nurse concentrates on nursing approaches of a particular phase depending on the status and needs of individual patients. For example, the orientation phase approaches have priority if the patient is very suspicious, because there is a need to develop trust with the patient. For the patient with good insight and motivation, the working phase approaches are most important because they concentrate on problem solving and change. If the patient is to be seen for only a few days, the termination phase approaches are critical because of the need for formalizing plans for follow-up care and referrals to other services along the continuum of care (see Chapter 6). Moving in and out of the three phases may depend on the patient's ability to cope with various issues. The patient may be ready to work on divorce issues but may not be able to process incest issues until more trust is established.

The knowledge and skills of the nurse also may affect which processes are emphasized. Less experienced nurses sometimes stay focused on orientation activities rather than facilitating working interventions. Nurses in short-term settings/programs tend to move quickly and concentrate on the working and termination phase interventions.

Orientation stage

The orientation stage involves nurses learning about patients and their initial concerns and needs. It also involves patients learning about the role of the nurse. Patients are informed of the general purpose of talking with the nurses. The initial purpose may be stated as broadly as "identifying a problem you want to work on," "helping you figure out what has been happening to you lately," or "getting to know what has been bothering you." Once the problems become more evident, the nurse collaborates with patients to define more specific areas to pursue; for example, learning to be assertive or processing feelings about a divorce. It is important that patients know that nurses cannot solve problems or make decisions for their patients. Rather, nurses help patients to look at realistic options so they can make their own decisions.

In a longer-term outpatient relationship between the patient and the nurse, arrangements are made for when to meet, how long, and how often. This might be for 30 to 60 minutes once a week in a clinic or office or in the patient's home. In brief encounters in an outpatient setting or on an inpatient unit, nurses should be aware of the need for privacy and might suggest moving to an uncrowded area to talk. It helps patients to know how much time the nurse can spend with them (usually 30 minutes or less) and that the relationship will end at the time of discharge or transfer to another level of care in the continuum of care.

Building trust

Regardless of the formality or length of the relationship, each nurse actively encourages patients to feel comfortable in the relationship. An effective connection is based on the patients and the nurse getting to know one another. The nurse cares about the patient, and the patient trusts the nurse (Heifner, 1993). Trustworthiness is built when the nurse is honest regarding intentions, is consistent, and keeps promises. Warmth, interest, and concern are conveyed with words and congruent body language. Clear, specific communications decrease confusion and suspiciousness. Confidentiality is explained in terms of patient information being shared *only* with the immediate unit or program staff and not with anyone outside of the treatment setting. (See Chapter 4 for legal issues related to confidentiality.)

Many patients are afraid or unable to approach the nurses, so reaching out and initiating conversations is important. Quiet, withdrawn patients often are overlooked because they cannot ask for assistance. An offer to listen and help conveys to patients that they are worthwhile individuals who are respected. Initially the nurse is nonconfrontational by not openly challenging what the patient says. Such a challenge would interfere with trust and with data collection. (Supportive confrontation is discussed in the working stage.)

Beginning assessment

The initial sessions, including intake interviews, provide an opportunity to begin an assessment of patients' needs, coping strategies, defense mechanisms, and adaptation styles. Patients' recurring thoughts, feelings, and behaviors are clues to problem areas. It is important to assess the degree of a patient's awareness of problems and the ability and motivation to change. Although assessment is ongoing and progresses over time, tentative goals are based on the most immediate needs or problems; for example, suicidal or homicidal thoughts, hallucinations, self-mutilation, or acting out. (For many facilities and programs, the initial care plan must be written within 24 hours of admission.)

There are many opportunities between interviews to observe patients and their behaviors, e.g., during activities, meals, free time with other patients, and at medication times. The family may contribute information as well. Assessment tools may be used, such as a depression scale or personality test.

Management of emotions

At the time of admission to a unit or a program, patients typically experience painful emotions such as fear, grief, anger, ambivalence, confusion, shame, embarrassment, or guilt. They are often afraid of losing control of themselves or of being viewed as weak for expressing their feelings. A way to keep feelings from escalating is to talk about them directly. Because patients are likely to try to conceal or minimize feelings, the nurse must be alert to indirect references, nonverbal cues, and voice tones. The nurse can then identify the feeling and ask for validation: "I'm getting the impression that you are angry. What are you feeling right now?"

In order to cope effectively with feelings, especially anger, it is helpful to remember that the feeling is created not by the nurse but by some situation or significant person in the patient's life. A patient may displace anger onto the nurse at first. If supportively confronted about the anger, however, the patient is more likely to recognize the real source of his or her emotions. Patients need to understand that feelings are natural but that the way they are expressed can cause a problem. Belittling or minimizing a patient's emotions is inappropriate, as is false reassurance; for example, saying, "Everything will be all right." In fact, patients may feel worse for a while as they begin to face their problems and feelings; thus such reassurance is dishonest as well as inappropriate.

Empathy is an objective understanding of how patients feel or see their situations. Conveying empathy is a way of helping patients deal with emotional pain. Empathy comes from actively listening to patients' perspectives about their experiences. (Wilt, et al, 1995) Empathy can also convey a hope for improvement: "I hear how painful this is for you and would like to try to help you deal with the situation in a productive way." Sympathy, by contrast, is when the nurse feels the same feelings as the patient, and objectivity is lost. Sympathy often leads to comforting, reassuring, or pitying patients. The outcome for patients is a sense of "poor me, I have a right to stay this way."

Once patients are able to talk directly about emotions, the focus can be on coping more effectively with them. In the orientation stage it is not possible to resolve the problem that created the feelings, but it is possible to temporarily reduce the feelings to a tolerable level by using palliative coping mechanisms (see Chapter 13). Explaining the experiences and feelings to an empathic listener helps, but if ventilation intensifies the feelings, it may be necessary to distract patients from that topic for a while. Adequate rest and nutrition reduce the impact of tension on the body. Physical exercise, meditation, imagery, and relaxation techniques also alleviate some of the tension patients may feel (Bradshaw, 1993). Although palliative mechanisms are less desirable than adaptive ones in the long run, the goal at this stage is to prevent loss of control or total retreat from pain.

Providing support

Support, like empathy, begins in the orientation stage and continues throughout the relationships between the nurse and patients. Support confirms patients' worth and rights as human beings and includes the nurse avoiding value judgments of patients (as bad, stupid, crazy, lazy), even if patients have made poor choices. This acknowledges that no one is perfect, that making mistakes is human, and that learning from mistakes is beneficial. Support focuses realistically and concretely on patients' abilities and strengths; for example, the nurse would not say, "You're a good person," but rather, "I'm glad you were able to share your ideas with the others in group today." Patients need recognition of their healthy actions and feelings. Patients' dependence is tolerated until they are capable of being more independent, but any independent actions are pointed out. Support includes realistic hope and promises, such as "I don't have an answer right now, but I will work with you to find one."

Providing structure

A major strategy in the orientation stage is to provide structure for patients. If patients lose control of their thoughts, feelings, or behaviors, the nurse has the responsibility for taking temporary control. This may mean offering a prn medication; directing patients to a quieter, less stimulating place; or staying with patients at a comfortable distance. If these measures are not effective, seclusion or restraints may be indicated (see Chapter 14). However, providing structure also includes decreasing the withdrawal and isolation of quiet, nonparticipating patients. Spending time with these patients, even in silence, is important. The nurse can also suggest activities such as watching television or taking a walk with the patient. A major facet of providing structure is *limit setting* (see also Chapter 24). It is in the best interest of patients to decrease or stop dysfunctional behaviors. The nurse accepts patients as human beings while discouraging self-defeating behaviors. Patients' rights

and self-esteem need protection but so do those of others who are around the patients. Limit setting involves pointing out behaviors and their negative effect, and suggesting alternative behaviors. For example, if a patient is self-deprecating, the nurse points out the negative comments and how they affect the patient's self-esteem, then suggests that the patient identify something positive about himself or herself.

Behaviors that typically require immediate intervention are verbal and physical aggression, self-destructive behaviors, setting fires, noncompliance with rules and medications, alcohol or drug use, manipulation of others, inappropriate touching of others, indecent exposure, attempts to leave the hospital without permission, and failure to eat or sleep. Continuous rumination over painful feelings or disturbed thought processes is nonproductive and self-perpetuating. The nurse listens to the content and the process of negative feelings or thoughts long enough to understand the messages or themes conveyed, but then begins to distract the patient with more productive topics. Limit setting is a kind but firm strategy: "I know you are angry right now, but I'm having trouble understanding the situation because of all the swearing; please stop" or "I realize these thoughts are really important to you, but there are other areas I need to know about so I can help you."

The transition from the orientation stage to the working stage is not smooth or firmly defined. Patients' anxiety may increase when they are working on issues, and they may return to more superficial matters for a while. Some patients with chronic illnesses or multiple hospitalizations may need a prolonged orientation stage because of their difficulty in forming relationships (Forchuk, 1992).

▪ Critical Thinking Question

John Slider is suspicious, denying his illness, and hyperactive. What combination of nursing interventions would you use in working with him?

Working stage

When patients are ready, the work toward behavioral change can begin. However, change may not be the goal for some patients, especially the chronically ill. Instead, stabilization with medications, reduction of symptoms, and development of supportive relationships are valid goals. For patients with chronic schizophrenia in particular, the ability to relate to someone is an important goal. Some patients may be hospitalized several times before they are able to accept the painful fact that they have a chronic illness and need ongoing treatment (McIntosh, 1991). For most patients there is enough awareness, motivation, and trust in the nurses to begin to explore problems, to identify possible solutions, and to test out new behaviors.

The process of learning

Changing behavior is difficult. Peplau (1963) identified the process of learning as necessary for change. (See Chapter 10 for therapeutic techniques that facilitate learning.)

The first step, *observation,* is a prerequisite because without awareness of a problem there is no motivation to change. The nurse learns how well patients understand their problems by asking for in-depth, detailed descriptions of situations, thoughts, feelings, and behaviors. The *analysis* step is then necessary to encourage accuracy in patients' conclusions about their problems. It is one thing for a patient to describe the type and sequence of arguments she has with her husband; it is another process to conclude that she is afraid of losing control over her husband. Even when patients are able to identify problems accurately, they may not automatically decide their behavior is worth changing. The *interpretation* step leads to a decision that change is necessary and appropriate.

Problem solving is the crux of the *planning* step. Patients are guided in decisions about change, in developing and considering alternative solutions, and in formulating a method for carrying out the plan. The nurse does not give advice but helps patients solve their own problems. The nurse encourages short-term, realistic, and achievable daily goals.

The *testing-out* step involves trying the new behavior or solution in a safe environment first (e.g., with the nurse) and then in a real situation. The nurse asks patients to rehearse what they will say and do in an upcoming situation: "Tell me what you will say to your daughter this weekend." Practice allows the patient to get feedback and modify the plan. Role-playing is another way of practicing behaviors. The nurse plays the role of persons with whom patients are having difficulty, and assesses for

communication and behavior patterns. This approach helps patients handle situations more effectively.

The objectives of the step of *evaluation* are to assess the success of new behaviors or solutions to problems and to determine whether modification or a different approach is needed. The nurse gives feedback in a constructive manner and helps patients learn to ask for and use feedback appropriately. Effective behaviors are more likely to continue if their benefits are discussed and reinforcement is given. Destructive behaviors are more likely to be identified if patients are taught to evaluate the effects of their actions on themselves and others.

In-depth data collection

Nurses facilitate awareness, analysis, and interpretation through in-depth (but selective) exploration of issues and by identifying priority issues. Patients may be overwhelmed by focusing on too many problems at once. The nurse helps patients make sense out of their confusion by directing the data collection and focusing on manageable and changeable issues. It is frustrating, both to patients and to the nurse, to spend time and energy exploring an unchangeable problem; for example, rehashing what the patient *could have* done to prevent the divorce instead of focusing on what he *can do* now to adjust to being single. In-depth data collection increases the nurse's knowledge of patients' needs, problems, and factors that can enhance or interfere with treatment. Nursing interventions can then be more individualized, and utilize the patient's abilities and strengths (Mason, Breen, and Whipple, 1994). Assessments include estimating what can and cannot be accomplished during the expected length of care and identifying the types of referrals likely to be needed at the next level of treatment within the continuum of care.

Reality testing and cognitive restructuring

Reality testing is an important strategy in the analysis, interpretation, and planning steps. It helps patients see reality more clearly and objectively where there may have been distortions or inaccuracies in the past. Reality testing is not a matter of arguing a point of view but of presenting one so the patient can consider another option. It is constructive, not destructive, feedback: "I know the voices seem real to you, but I don't hear any" or "You make it sound as if all men are alike, and I don't see it that way."

The goal of reality testing is cognitive restructuring: helping patients cope with negative thoughts and beliefs and see other viewpoints that will help them come to more realistic conclusions. (San Blise, 1995). Patients might need to redefine how they interpret a situation, or they may need to change their perception of another person's behavior. They might need to give up an irrational belief in favor of a more rational one; for example, changing from "I have to be perfect" to "It's OK to make mistakes; I can learn from them." It could also mean giving up an unrealistic goal for a more appropriate one. The redefinition might involve discovering that sadness is concealing anger.

Writing/journaling

It is often useful to have patients write down their thoughts and feelings each day. This can be a release for emotions and can facilitate a more objective analysis of issues (McGihon, 1996). The nurse asks patients to write a "homework assignment" between sessions; for example, making a list of their positive qualities and strengths. Patients might also write "letters" (that are *not* sent) to others with whom they are having problems. In some instances a letter may be reworked several times and the message eventually shared with the person to whom the patient is writing.

Supportive confrontation

Supportive confrontation is similar to reality testing but has a broader focus than specific perceptions, interpretations, or feelings. It is aimed at contradictions, discrepancies, responsibility, accountability, independence, and behavioral change. It combines support with encouragement for constructive, productive action. The support acknowledges fears, pain, ambivalence, and the difficult process of change, while the confrontation includes hope and confidence that an action is possible.

"Giving up alcohol is a scary idea, but by participating in this program, you can get the information and support needed to do it."

"I hear your ambivalence, but taking the risk has much to offer."

"We all like to be taken care of once in a while, but making our own decisions helps our self-esteem."

Supportive confrontation challenges patients to meet their own needs appropriately and to be accountable for their own feelings, behaviors, and decisions. Confrontation without support is generally perceived as an attack and is nonproductive. It is avoided because it is often what the patient has experienced from others at home, school, or work.

Promoting change

In addition to problem solving and supportive confrontation, several other important strategies facilitate change as well. One strategy is to change the balance of the risk/benefit ratio because all change has a risk of failure. For example, with change there may be the loss of a comfortable habit, rejection, or even creation of new problems. The potential benefits might be growth, self-satisfaction, improved relationships, and a healthier self-esteem. For all of us, change is more likely to occur if the risks are low and the potential for benefits is high. The nurse can help decrease risks by discussing ways to overcome them. Short-term and long-term benefits also need to be discussed. Change is difficult but several time-tested approaches increase the likelihood for success. For example:

1. Carefully considered, rational decisions are more likely to result in healthy changes than decisions that are hasty and emotional.
2. Patient-initiated change (with specific plans and actions) tends to be more successful than change imposed by others.
3. Practicing or rehearsing changes with the nurse builds confidence for trying new behaviors with others and increases success.
4. Support and acceptance of change by patients' friends and families help.
5. Support groups can reinforce new behaviors.
6. Patients are more likely to change when they are ready and motivated.
7. Pushing for change too quickly is frustrating for all concerned.

Teaching new skills

The desire to change is not sufficient; one must know how to change. For example, patients cannot change from being passive to being assertive if they do not know what assertion is or sounds like. Skills that a nurse takes for granted may not have been learned by some patients. Common skills that patients need to learn are relaxation; stress, conflict, and anger management techniques; assertiveness; problem-solving processes; symptom management; coping skills; stress reduction; and communication, social, and community living skills (Blair and Ramones, 1997). At times skill training must begin at a basic, concrete level. One patient's first exercise was to approach another patient and *read* from his 3 × 5 inch card: "Hi, my name is Bill, and I'm from Greenfield. What's your name?" Skills are taught in small steps with frequent intermittent opportunities for practice and feedback. Again, homework assignments can be used; for example, the nurse might suggest that between sessions the patient practice a particular skill and report the results at the next session.

Termination stage

In acute inpatient settings and outpatient programs, the "work" and changes are rarely completed. Patients are discharged or transferred to another level of care, and nurses change units or jobs. However, there are strategies that facilitate a healthy closure of the relationship for both the patient and the nurse. If all the nurses involved with the patient are not available to discuss termination, the one assigned to discharge or transfer the patient can implement the strategies.

Evaluation/summary of progress

The nurse guides discussions to help patients identify *for themselves* the specific changes in thoughts, feelings, and behaviors that have occurred. Even small steps toward long-term goals are discussed. It is important to reinforce the changes in and strengths of patients. Areas or issues that need more work are outlined, cautioning patients not to try to change everything at once. Patients are encouraged to set priorities for these issues and to establish reasonable time frames for action.

Synthesizing what has occurred. Synthesizing focuses on the more indirect outcomes of the nurse-patient relationship, such as more open communications or more appropriate expression of feelings. As a result of the relationship, patients often feel more comfortable with initiating interactions, making requests, and expressing opinions, even if these behaviors were not discussed during the nurse-patient encounters. Increased participation and socialization need to be recognized as well. As the nurse points out the accrued benefits of the relationship, patients are encouraged to form other relationships with future counselors and new friends.

Referrals. For the problems that need continuing attention after discharge, referrals to appropriate resources are finalized (see Chapter 8). The resources provide support, foster treatment compliance, and promote continued growth. It is helpful for patients to receive written discharge instructions that list medications, dosages, and times, as well as phone numbers, addresses, dates, and times of appointments and self-help meetings.

Discussion of Termination. Regardless of the length, frequency of contact, or intensity of the nurse-patient relationship, it is important to discuss the participants' reactions to it. Feelings may be positive, ambivalent, or negative and may vary in degree. Superficial relationships are likely to produce mild reactions. However, the relationship may mean more to the patient than it does to the nurse; therefore the loss of contact with the nurse may be significant to the patient. Patients may experience anger or fear about losing the support and acceptance provided by the nurse. Some patients may avoid any discussion of termination. Even so, the nurse should attempt to "make it official" by saying "good-bye" and stating his or her feelings about the relationship, for example, "I'm glad I had a chance to work with you." The nurse serves as a role model for the patient who is at the time unable to discuss termination. The feelings of the nurse are important and open to discussion (but not to the point of burdening the patient with the nurse's issues). Nurses may feel as if they are abandoning the patient, especially if building trust was difficult for the patient.

■ Critical Thinking Question

Describe exactly what you will say to patients about your role and the role of the other nurses in the treatment of patients.

INTERACTIONS WITH SELECTED BEHAVIORS

Certain problem behaviors, such as anger and withdrawal, have already been discussed under the stages of the nurse-patient relationship. The purpose of this section is to discuss interventions with selected behaviors that are appropriate in brief encounters with patients. Longer-term interventions are discussed in the chapters dealing with psychiatric disorders.

Violent Behavior

Fear of violent behavior and of being injured is a concern with the few patients who do not respond to the verbal diffusing of anger or who feel extremely threatened by staff members (usually because of internal thought disturbances). The following are a few precautions to take for protection:

- Stay out of striking distance (this also reduces the threat to the patient).
- Do not touch patients without approval.
- Change the topic temporarily if a patient's behavior is escalating.
- Suggest "time out" for the patient in a quiet area with fewer stimuli.
- Sit by the door (with the door open) until the patient is calmer.
- Do not go into a room alone with a patient who is not in control of his or her behavior.
- Leave temporarily if the patient is agitated and asking to be left alone.
- Call for staff assistance if the patient is losing control.

Chapter 14 focuses on working with aggressive patients.

Hallucinations

The initial approach with patients who appear to be listening to or talking with "voices" is to comment on their behavior: "You look as if you are listening to something. What do you hear?" If the patient acknowledges hearing something the nurse cannot hear, the nurse can say, "I don't hear anything. Tell me what you hear." The early assessment of hallucinations is based on the content of messages. It is presumed that hallucinatory content reveals the dynamics of the patient's illness and typically revolves around themes of powerlessness, hatred, guilt, or loneliness. Once the content is known, there is no need to focus on the hallucinations; doing so could reinforce them: "I know the voices are important to you, but let's talk about your loneliness right now." The exception is with hallucinations that command patients to harm themselves or others or to do other destructive acts. Then it is important to contract

with patients not to act on the commands they hear and to tell the staff.

Delusions

The initial approach with respect to delusions is clarification of meanings, for example, "Who do you think is trying to hurt you?" or "Tell me about this power you think you have." Similar to hallucinations, delusions are not discussed once the meanings are clarified. Arguing with a patient about delusions is ineffective, inappropriate, and may strengthen the patients' belief in them (Jensen & Kane, 1996). The underlying themes reflected in the delusions are more appropriately addressed in interventions such as helping the patient, who says she is a queen, to feel important in realistic ways. Careful monitoring is needed if the delusions could lead patients to harm themselves or others; for example, a patient does not want to eat because he believes all the food is poisoned.

Conflicting Values

Occasionally nurses and patients encounter conflicts with their beliefs or values. Both can state their views in a discussion, but arguing is inappropriate. A better approach is to help patients examine the effects or outcomes of their beliefs on their lives, relationships, and happiness. For example, a patient may believe she has the right to drink as much and as often as she wants to because it is legal. Supportive confrontation can help her look at the effects of drinking on her marriage, job, health, and economic status.

It is not necessary to agree with every patient's beliefs, values, or behaviors to be an effective nurse. It is important for nurses to be aware of their own stance on issues and to understand patients' points of view *as the patients see it*. There is usually no need for patients to change a belief or a behavior that is not causing problems for them or for others around them. Beliefs and behaviors that have positive effects need reinforcement.

Incoherent Speech Patterns

Disturbed thought processes are sometimes evident in speech; when this occurs, the approach is to try to clarify the meanings of the communications. However, severely ill patients may be unable to be more clear, and repeated questions will only increase anxiety. Medications often clear the thought disturbances within a week. Until then, the nurse spends frequent, brief time with these patients (without pressuring or frustrating them), offers support, and builds trust.

Manipulation

Common manipulations are a means to gain attention, sympathy ("poor me"), control, and dependence (for others to take responsibility). Manipulation often is not recognized until it has already "worked." The nurse may then experience anger or embarrassment. The initial approach is to address what is happening (or has happened): "I'm getting the feeling you would like me to tell you what to do. What scares you about this decision?" or "You are experiencing a lot of pain and would like me to relieve it for you. Let's talk about what *you* can do to relieve it." Limit setting is useful with manipulative patients. A power struggle with the patient is useless. Helping patients to directly express their needs to others is more productive.

Crying

Unless crying is a manipulative gesture or is prolonged and unproductive, it should be allowed and even encouraged, verbally and nonverbally. By saying, "It's OK to cry" or quietly offering a tissue, the nurse gives patients permission to cry and relieve tension. Privacy should be provided. The nurse should be as quiet and unobtrusive as possible until the crying has ceased. Then the patient is offered an opportunity to talk about what precipitated the tears.

Sexual Innuendos or Inappropriate Touch

Patients generally stop these behaviors when asked to and are reminded that they are inappropriate. The nurse then discusses the underlying need. If the behaviors continue, limit setting can be stronger: "I want to talk to you but not if you continue to touch me. If you don't stop, I will have to leave and come back later." It may also help to pair sexually acting-out patients who have poor impulse control with staff members of the same sex until these patients are further along in treatment. This strategy may not be effective with homosexual patients.

Lack of Cooperation/Denial

There are many reasons patients might not cooperate with the nurse in working toward treatment goals. A common reason is severe disturbances in thought processes (hallucinations, delusions, disorientation, and confusion) that interfere with patients' understanding of what the problems are and what changes are needed. With some patients, the disturbances are less evident, but there is lack of insight into or denial of any problems and the need for treatment. In fact, such patients may be angry about being "forced" into treatment. Occasionally a patient may admit to the need for help but disagree with the type of treatment offered. Others may be afraid of changing even though they realize their behaviors are nonproductive or harmful. Listening, clarifying, and verbalizing what has been implied are appropriate for identifying the underlying causes of a lack of cooperation. Then, as possible, the causes, fears, and outcomes of patients' behaviors are discussed directly. "What are you afraid will happen if you have to give up alcohol as a way of avoiding your problem?" Trust is often an issue for these patients, so measures to increase trust and a great deal of patience from the nurse will be needed.

Depressed Affect/Apathy/ Psychomotor Retardation

When patients express sadness, helplessness, hopelessness, lack of energy, and/or a negative attitude about everything, the nurse sometimes experiences sadness, helplessness, sympathy, or frustration. Patience, frequent contact, and empathy are more appropriate. Even when patients know what needs to change, they do not always have the energy to accomplish much very quickly. The nurse acknowledges feelings but discourages rumination: "You are so focused on your sadness that you are just stuck. Come take a walk with me for a few minutes." Personal hygiene, nutrition, and a gradual increase in activities are encouraged. Major decisions are postponed until emotions subside and thinking is more logical.

Suspiciousness

When patients are suspicious, they may be afraid of everyone, everything, and every interaction around them. It is therefore important to communicate clearly, simply, and congruently. Misinterpretations by patients are clarified, but arguments over differences in opinion are avoided. Rationales or explanations for rules, activities, occurrences, noises, and requests are offered regularly. Patients' participation is encouraged but not forced in order to avoid increasing their fears.

Hyperactivity

Excessive physical and emotional activity in patients is upsetting to the staff, to other patients, and often to the hyperactive patients themselves. Even unintentionally, patients may harm themselves or others (see the previous discussion of violence). These patients need to be in a quiet area with minimal auditory and visual stimulation. Physical activity such as walking or using a stationary bicycle may help to drain excess energy. The nurse must remain calm, speak slowly and softly, and respect patients' personal space. Directions are given in a kind, simple, but firm manner. Occasionally a prn medication is needed.

Transference

Transference involves the unconscious emotional reaction patients have in a current situation that is really based on previous, even childhood, relationships and experiences (Smith, et al, 1997). For example, a patient perceives the nurse as acting the way his mother did, regardless of how the nurse is really acting (Miles and Morse, 1995). Transference may explain feelings patients exhibit that do not fit in the current context of a situation or that are out of proportion to the situation. The main issue of transference is the wish to be taken care of and to have needs met (Schroder, 1985). Transference may be severe in the form of delusions or may be subtle, as in stereotyping all males as aggressive and all females as submissive. Transference can be positive if patients view the nurse as helpful and caring. Negative transference is more difficult to deal with because of unpleasant emotions such as anger and fear that interfere with treatment (Miles and Morse, 1995).

Nurses may experience transference reactions with patients, co-workers, and doctors. Guilt or anger about not helping a particular patient or anger toward a demanding patient may be an unconscious transference response (Schroder, 1985). Countertransference (reactions based on the nurse's past experiences) (Smith, et al, 1997) may occur in response to a patient's transference after the nurse-patient relationship is established. For example, when a patient criticizes the nurse, the nurse may relive feelings that were experienced in childhood when the nurse was criticized in class by a teacher. These feelings will interfere with the nurse's ability to be therapeutic. A reaction might lead to the nurse becoming sympathetic and unable to confront the patient appropriately. Another reaction could lead to avoidance or rejection of the patient. In either case, the nurse's behavior is not therapeutic.

The first intervention is to recognize the transference or countertransference. This is difficult because of the unconscious processes involved. Co-workers are more likely to recognize the phenomenon initially and give feedback to the nurse about it. Once the reaction is recognized, the nurse can seek assistance in examining the countertransference issues (Smith, et al, 1997). Nurses need to examine their feelings, reactions, and behaviors before they will be able to interact more appropriately with patients. The transference reactions of patients also must be examined gently but directly. Nurses must be open and clear about their genuine reactions when patients misperceive behavior. Nurses should also state what they can and cannot do to meet patients' needs. Limit setting is useful when patients act inappropriately toward the nurse. Redirection of needs to more appropriate persons can also be a helpful intervention; for example, "I can't be your girlfriend, but let's talk about making new friends at home."

Key Concepts

1. To be therapeutic the nurse uses verbal and nonverbal communications to convey a willingness to listen, genuine respect, a desire to help, and an understanding of the patient as a person with unique problems and needs.

2. The nurse-patient relationship is a series of goal-directed interactions focused on the patient's thoughts, feelings, behaviors, and potential solutions to problems.
3. The nursing process is a tool with which the nurse assesses each patient's problems, selects and carries out specific interventions, and evaluates the effectiveness of care.
4. Each stage of the nurse-patient relationship (orientation, working, termination) involves specific tasks that are used according to the needs and problems of each patient.
5. Issues and patient behaviors that interfere with the progress of the nurse-patient relationship need to be addressed by the nurse.

Study Questions

(Answer key is in the back of the book.)
1. The nurse-patient relationship is:
   a. Based on a single theoretical model that explains the dynamics of the patient's needs.
   b. Conducted by a nurse psychotherapist who offers specialized techniques for specialized problems.
   c. Based on a foundation of companionship, mutual support, and interest.
   d. A series of goal-directed interactions conveying respect and a willingness to help the patient.

Match the stage of the nurse-patient relationship with the appropriate description.
2. ___C___ Exploring problems, identifying solutions, testing new behavior
3. ___b___ Facilitating trust, defining tentative goals, collecting information
4. ___d___ Discussing feelings about the relationship, identifying community resources

   a. Preparation
   b. Orientation
   c. Working
   d. Termination

5. Issues and patient behaviors that interfere with progress in the nurse-patient relationship are:
   a. Generally ignored until the patient is more stable.
   b. Usually not significant enough to address directly.
   c. Usually assessed and then a specific intervention is designed.
   d. Generally not charted because of the need for confidentiality.

REFERENCES

Blair DT and Ramones VA: Education as psychiatric intervention: the cognitive-behavioral context, *J Psychosoc Nurs Ment Health Serv* 35(12):29, 1997.

Bradshaw WH: Coping-skills training versus a problem-solving approach with schizophrenia patients, *Hosp Community Psychiatry* 44(11):1102, 1993.

Forchuk C: The orientation phase of the nurse-client relationship: how long does it take? *Perspect Psychiatr Care* 28(4):7, 1992.

Heifner C: Positive connectedness in the psychiatric nurse-patient relationship, *Arch Psychiatr Nurs* 7(1):11, 1993.

Jensen LH and Kane CF: Cognitive theory applied to the treatment of delusions of schizophrenia, *Arch Psychiatr Nurs* 10(6):338, 1996.

Mason WH, Breen RY, and Whipple WR. Solution-focused therapy and inpatient psychiatric nursing, *J Psychiatr Nurs* 32(10):46, 1994.

McGihon, N: Writing as a therapeutic modality, *J Psychosoc Nurs Ment Health Serv* 34(6):31, 1996.

McIntosh D: Supportive therapy: the other therapy, *Perspect Psychiatr Care* 27(4):26, 1991.

Miles M and Morse J: Using the concepts of transference and countertransference in the consultation process, *J Am Psychiatr Nurses Assoc* 1(2):42, 1995.

Morrison EG, et al: Work roles of staff nurses in psychiatric settings, *Nurs Sci Q* 9(1):17, 1996.

Peplau HE: *Interpersonal relations in nursing,* New York, 1952, GP Putnam's Sons.

Peplau HE: A working definition of anxiety. In Burd SE and Marshall MA, editors: Some clinical approaches to psychiatric nursing, Toronto, 1963, Macmillan.

San Blise ML: Radical positive reframing, *J Psychosoc Nurs Ment Health Serv* 33(12):18, 1995.

Schroder PJ: Recognizing transference and countertransference, *J Psychosoc Nurs Ment Health Serv* 23(2):21, 1985.

Simon RL: Boundaries in psychotherapy: a safe place to heal, *Harvard Mental Health Letter* 13(12):4, 1997.

Smith LL et al: Nurse-patient boundaries: crossing the line, *Am J Nurs* 97(12):26, 1997.

Wilt DL, et al: Teaching with entertainment films: an empathetic focus, *J Psychosoc Nurs Ment Health Serv* 33(6):5, 1995.

The Nursing Process

LEE H. SCHWECKE

After reading this chapter you should be able to:
• Relate the nursing process to psychiatric nursing practice.
• Identify the components of an initial holistic patient assessment.

• Describe the importance of writing a specific nursing diagnosis and care plan.
• Recognize components of written patient assessments.

NURSING PROCESS

The use of the nursing process (Figure 12-1) has the same goal in psychiatric nursing as in other areas of nursing: "patient-centered, goal-directed action" (Van Servellen, 1982). Care is adapted to patients' unique needs. Individualized care begins with a detailed assessment.

Assessment

Assessment starts upon admission to a unit or program with an intake interview that includes an evaluation of mental status (Box 12-1). Information obtained by the multidisciplinary team (nurse, psychiatrist, psychologist, social worker, pharmacist, etc.) is used by all staff to expand on and confirm the initial patient assessment and to minimize the patient repeating information. Results from laboratory tests, physical examinations, x-ray examinations, and psychological testing are other sources of data. It is important to include patient self-assessments, such as the "Geriatric Depression Scale" (see Appendix E), and patient perceptions of personal strengths, support systems, and resources (Mason, Breen, and Whipple, 1994).

Some patients are too ill to participate in or complete the assessment interview. In such cases, objective data, such as patient behaviors and reports by their family members, are utilized. In some instances, information from staff in the outpatient setting attended by the patient will be available. During the initial assessment, behaviors can be described without knowing or identifying their causes; for example, anxiety level, degree of withdrawal, thought disturbances reflected in speech, voice tone, and/or general appearance. Causes and dynamics can be elicited later to form a better basis for a treatment plan.

Even when the initial assessment is complete, each encounter with a patient involves a continuing assessment that may or may not be congruent with

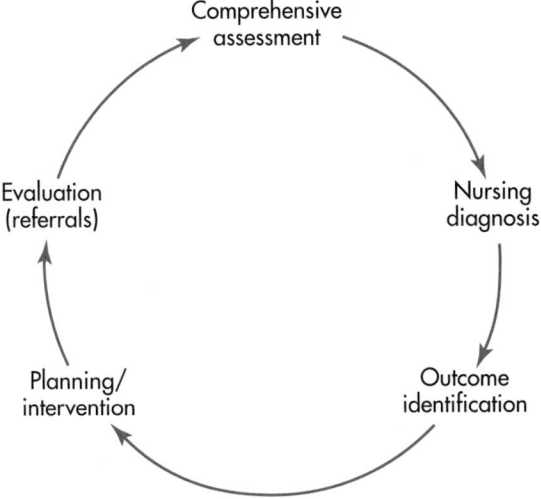

FIGURE 12-1   Nursing process.

the initial assessment. No one acts or feels the same way 24 hours a day, 7 days a week. The ongoing assessment often involves an investigation of what a patient is saying or doing at the moment: "You have been sitting alone for a while. What have you been thinking about?" or "You mentioned being worried; what about?" When the nurse decides to investigate a patient's specific behavior, it is valuable to explore the following:

- The context or situation that precipitated the behavior
- What the patient was thinking at the time
- What the patient was feeling then and now
- Whether the behavior makes sense in that context
- Whether the behavior was adaptive or dysfunctional
- How this episode fits with the total picture of the patient
- Whether a change is needed

Nursing Diagnosis

Nursing diagnoses are the identification of patients' problems based on conclusions about the dynamics of verbalizations and behaviors. Emergency behaviors (e.g., suicidal/homicidal ideas or attempts, aggression, destructive behaviors, risk of escape) are given priority in establishing nursing diagnoses and in negotiating "no harm contracts" with patients.

Regardless of the format or style of nursing diagnosis in a particular setting, the diagnosis should be specific and point to a desired outcome for the patient. In this text the North American Nursing Diagnosis Association (NANDA) diagnoses are used because they are the most widely accepted and commonly used nursing diagnoses. NANDA diagnoses suggest a statement that has three components:

1. Potential or actual problems
2. Contributing or etiological factor
3. Defining characteristic or behavioral outcome

The statement is typically written as follows: (Problem) related to (contributing factor) as evidenced by (behavioral outcome); for example, "Anxiety related to marital problems as evidenced by decreased concentration."

Actual or potential problems are identified from the list approved by NANDA (Box 12-2). Contributing/etiological factors can include stressors, losses, past experiences, developmental issues, environmental circumstances, relationship issues, and self-perceptions. Defining characteristics or behavioral outcomes are the verbal and nonverbal cues that reflect the actual or potential patient problems. These dysfunctional behaviors or cues are the focus of the nursing interventions—behaviors that it would be helpful to change. Being specific in describing the dysfunctional behaviors/cues is useful in giving direction for selecting desirable/adaptive behaviors identified in the desired patient outcomes (Snyder, Egan, and Nojima, 1996).

Outcome Identification

A goal specifies an adaptive behavior to replace a dysfunctional one. It is unrealistic to expect patients to change a negative self-image to a positive one during a short inpatient stay or outpatient program. A more realistic behavioral goal would be to ask patients to write a list of their strengths, abilities, or positive qualities. This goal is achievable and measurable. Short-term goals are those achievable in perhaps 4 to 6 days for hospitalized patients and perhaps a little longer for patients in other settings. Long-term goals relate to issues that require follow-up counseling after discharge to another type of service within the continuum of care. For example, a patient's short-term goal may be to identify her fears about relationships with men. The longer-term goal is to practice ways of responding to potential dating

Box 12-1   Initial Patient Assessment

Demographic data: full name, sex, age, date of birth, address, marital status, family members' names and ages.

Admission data: date and time of admission, type of admission (voluntary or committed).

Reason for admission: current problems as perceived by the patient. These include stressors, difficulty with coping, developmental issues, "emergency behaviors" (suicidal or homicidal ideas/attempts, aggression, destructive behaviors, risk of escape), and family history.

Previous psychiatric history: dates, inpatient/outpatient, reasons for and types of treatment and their effectiveness, current medications, compliance, current medical problems and medications.

Drug and alcohol use/abuse: amount, frequency, duration of past and present use of legal/illegal substances, date and time of last use.

Disturbances in patterns of daily living: sleep, intake, elimination, sexual activity, work, leisure, self-care, and hygiene.

Culture/spirituality: ethnicity, beliefs, practices, religious preference.

Support systems: amount of contact, nature/quality of relationships, and availability of support.

Mental Status Examination

General appearance: type and condition of clothing, cleanliness, physical condition, and posture.

Behaviors during the interview:
Expression of anger: covert, overt, verbal, or physical.
Degree of cooperation, resistance, or evasiveness.
Social skills: positive/unpleasant habits, shyness, withdrawal.

Amount/type of motor activity: psychomotor retardation, agitation, restlessness, tics, tremors, hypervigilance, lack of activity.

Speech patterns: amount, rate, volume, pressure, mutism, slurring, or stuttering.

Degree of concentration and attention span.

Orientation: to time, place, and person; and level of consciousness.

Memory: recent/remote, amnesia, blackouts, confabulation.

Thought clarity: coherence, confusion, vagueness.

Thought processes reflected in speech: blocking, circumstantiality, loose associations, flight of ideas, perseveration, tangential ideas, ambivalence, neologisms, or "word salad."

Thought content: helplessness, hopelessness, worthlessness, guilt, suicidal ideas/plans, homicidal ideas/plans, suspiciousness, phobias, obsessions, compulsions, preoccupations, antisocial attitudes, blaming of others, poverty of content, or denial.

Hallucinations: visual, auditory, or other.

Delusions: of reference, influence, persecution, grandeur, religious, or somatic.

Intellectual functioning: use of language and knowledge, abstract vs. concrete thinking (proverbs), or calculations (serial sevens), educational level.

Affect/mood: anxiety level; elevated or depressed mood; labile, blunted or flat affect; or inappropriate affect; specific feelings expressed.

Insight: degree of awareness of problems and their causes.

Judgment: soundness of problem solving and decisions.

Motivation: degree of motivation for treatment.

---

situations that would decrease her fears and enable her to handle such situations.

In establishing goals/outcomes *with* a patient (Mason, Breen, and Whipple, 1994), it is crucial to understand what problems the patient wants to address and what goals the patient wants to achieve. Patient desires and motivation play a major role in attaining outcomes (Stolte, 1997). Patient support systems and resources may also facilitate outcome achievement (Jones, et al, 1997).

Planning/Intervention

Nursing staff on units or in programs often develop standardized care plans with expected outcomes for certain types of patient problems. These care plans may focus on psychiatric diagnoses (e.g., major depression) or more specific problems (for example, self mutilation). Standardized care plans may be called clinical pathways, critical pathways, or multidisciplinary care plans. (See Chapter 9 for an example.) Regardless of the name, the general purpose is to provide guidelines for desired patient outcomes and related nursing interventions within specific time constraints. For example, a patient who has *suicidal ideations* (problem) would be expected to *sign a "no harm contract"* (outcome) *within 24 hours* (time constraint) and to *verbalize an absence of suicidal ideation* (outcome) by *day 3 of admission* (time constraint). Related nursing interventions would include

Box 12-2   NANDA-Approved Nursing Diagnoses

Adjustment, impaired
Anxiety
Body image disturbance
Caregiver role strain
Caregiver role strain, risk for
Communication, impaired verbal
Community coping, ineffective
Confusion, acute
Confusion, chronic
Constipation
Coping, defensive
Coping, family: potential for growth
Coping, ineffective family: compromised
Coping, ineffective family: disabling
Coping, ineffective individual
Decisional conflict (specify)
Denial, ineffective
Diversional activity deficit
Family processes, altered: alcoholism
Family processes, altered
Fatigue
Fear
Grieving, anticipatory
Grieving, dysfunctional
Growth and development, altered
Health maintenance, altered
Health-seeking behaviors (specify)
Home maintenance management, impaired
Hopelessness
Injury, risk for
Knowledge deficit (specify)
Loneliness, risk for
Management of the therapeutic regimen, families: ineffective
Management of the therapeutic regimen, individuals: ineffective

From North American Nursing Diagnosis Association: *NANDA nursing diagnoses: definitions and classifications, 1997-1998,* Philadelphia, 1997. The Association.

(1) contract with the patient for safety and (2) assess for suicidal ideation every shift.

Given the current managed care climate, a goal of standardized care plans is to expedite treatment activities to achieve patient outcomes more cost effectively (i.e., more quickly). However, it is also important to remember that each patient is an individual even if some of her or his problems "fit" into a standardized plan. A patient's unique problems and needs must not be ignored when formulating the plan of care.

Psychiatric nursing interventions involve few "hands-on" activities other than monitoring vital signs and giving medications. Instead, the focus is on the verbal strategies discussed in this chapter and in Chapter 10 that are used to guide patients in solving problems for themselves and in achieving outcomes (Snyder, et al, 1996). **Psychiatric**

Box 12-3 Initial Nursing Assessment (Intake Form)

Name: Anita Jarvis   Sex: Female   Age: 46
Date of birth: 6/27/52   Marital status: Separated, married 26 years

Names of family members: Relationship: Age:
  David Jarvis   Son   24
  Beth Samuels   Daughter   23
  Brian Jarvis   Husband   48

Date and time of admission:

Type of admission: Voluntary, brought by son

Reason for current admission: Husband left approximately 1 week ago. Patient has felt fatigued and spends most of the day in bed. Son found his mother yesterday and called the crisis clinic. Patient was seen today, and admission was recommended. Patient admits to suicidal thoughts but has no plan. She presently wishes she were dead. Patient is afraid to live alone.

Previous psychiatric history: None, no medications.

Current medical problems: None, no medications.

Disturbances in patterns of daily living:
  Sleep: In bed 14 to 16 hours a day but sleeps only 3 to 4 hours a night.
  Intake and elimination: Has not cooked a meal in 1 week but has eaten a little every day—mostly snack foods. Had a small BM yesterday. No problem with voiding.
Sexual: Decreased frequency and pleasure progressively over the last year because of marital problems.
Leisure: No activities, except TV, in last 1 to 2 months. Used to enjoy mah jong, temple sisterhood activities, and travel.
Self-care: Patient says she is normally a good housekeeper and takes good care of herself. In last 2 weeks she has not cleaned house or done laundry. Last shower was 4 days ago.
Work: Patient called in sick 8 days ago. Previously had a good work record as an elementary school teacher.
Culture/spirituality: Conservative Jewish. Kosher dietary practices, requests to light sabbath candles. Desires visits with rabbi.
Support systems: Progressive decline in socializing during last 6 months. No phone calls or visits with adult children in last 2 weeks, until yesterday when son arrived. Limited support except for children. Patient states she used to have a close friend (seen a month ago) but is afraid she has alienated her. Is not close to parents or younger brother, all of whom live out of state.

Mental Status Examination

General appearance: Dressed appropriately for season; clothes are clean but unpressed. Hair is unwashed and uncombed. Slouched shoulders. Pale. Blank expression.

Behaviors during interview:
  Anger: Covert anger is evident but not expressed.
  Cooperation/resistance/evasiveness: Slow to respond but cooperative.
  Social skills: Withdrawn, no unpleasant habits, reduced socialization.
  Motor activity: Slowed, crying at times, no tics or tremors noted.
  Speech patterns: Amount is reduced with slowed rate and soft tone.
  Concentration/attention span: Decreased concentration, easily distracted by stimuli, slight shortening of attention span.
Orientation: Aware of person, place, and time; responsive.
Memory:
  Remote: Complete with good detail.
  Recent: Difficulty organizing sequence but mostly complete except for last week.
Thought clarity: Clear, coherent.
Thought processes: No disturbances except ambivalence about divorce.
Thought content: Expressing helplessness, hopelessness, and suicidal thoughts without a plan. Fears being alone.
Hallucinations: None reported or evident.
Delusions: None reported or evident.
Intellectual functioning: College education evident in vocabulary. Calculations and proverbs were not done. Abstract thinking evident in discussion of love and fidelity.
Affect: Blunted with depressed mood. Anxiety level is moderate. Guilt and covert anger expressed.
Insight: Aware of problems in facing divorce but not yet able to describe factors leading to separation.
Judgment: No impairment until past 2 weeks when she became unable to make decisions, take action, or seek support.
Motivation for treatment: Wants help with depression, tiredness, and handling divorce. Is unable to state what type of help she needs.

Box 12-4   Progress Note Components

Subjective content (S): what the patient says about his or her own thoughts, feelings, behaviors, and problems.

Objective data (O): the nurse's observations or measurements, such as the patient's appearance, nonverbal behaviors, and vital signs.

Analysis or conclusions (A): the nurse's impressions of what the patient is experiencing or demonstrating in behavioral or descriptive terms (not medical diagnoses). Defenses, mood, and issues are identified. Depressed mood and paranoid ideas can be discussed but "depression" and "paranoia" are not listed as illnesses. Conclusions about changes (regression or progression) in the patient and medication responses are described.

Plans (P): what the nurses or other team members can do to intervene with the problems described in the progress note.

Sample Progress Note

Date and time

46-year-old white female voluntarily admitted to 3N, accompanied by son. Initial nursing assessment is complete.

S: Patient states she has been tired and in bed most of the day since husband left her a week ago. States she is unsure of what led to the separation and cannot face living alone. Has thoughts of suicide but no plan. "I still wish I were dead." Describes decrease in socialization and support. Saw one friend a month ago. Did not contact children about separation and is not close to family of origin. Verbalizes that she doesn't know what to do about impending divorce and her future alone.

O: Exhibits blunted, depressed affect, limited eye contact, slowed motor activity and speech. Cries occasionally. A "no suicide contract" was signed and placed in chart.

A: Patient cannot describe her feelings, but guilt, helplessness, and hopelessness are evident. Anger is barely evident at this point. Suicidal but lacks energy to plan. Support is available but not perceived as such.

P: 1. Approach and sit with patient frequently.
   2. Encourage verbalization of feelings as tolerated in small doses.
   3. Monitor energy level and suicidal ideation.
   4. Initiate medications as ordered.
   5. Encourage attendance at group meetings.

---

nurses are primarily facilitators and educators. Solving problems and changing behaviors are never quite as easy as they sound. Patients may need help with developing specific/concrete plans for reaching their goals. For example, a patient may set a goal of finding a new apartment but needs assistance in locating rental options and in evaluating the pros and cons of each apartment option.

Evaluation

The more realistic and measurable the goals, the greater the likelihood patients and nurses will have a sense of progress (Mason, Breen, and Whipple, 1994). A major problem arises with evaluating care in psychiatric nursing when too much change is expected too soon. When the patient and/or nurse become aware of a lack of progress toward goals, evaluation should lead to reassessment. Using the nursing process leads to reformulation of the nursing diagnoses and the establishment of more realistic or appropriate outcomes (Barrell, Merwin, and Poster,

1997). This is especially true in short-term settings, where patients are discharged before "all their problems are solved." Even when short-term goals are met, patients have other unsolved problems. If the short-term goals were related to learning better skills (for example, communication, problem solving, and social skills), patients are able to continue to progress after discharge.

Evaluating patient progress is important in determining patient referrals to other levels of care and supervision within the continuum of care (see Chapter 6). In addition to evaluating the progress of patients, nurses evaluate the quality of their interventions and their professional behaviors.

■ Critical Thinking Question

For the patient in this chapter (see Box 12-5 and Care Plan), identify two additional nursing diagnoses, two short-term goals, two long-term goals, and two nursing interventions.

Box 12-5   Sample Process Recording

(Nurse introduces himself and leads the way to office, walking slowly but slightly ahead of the patient. The patient follows without looking at the nurse. In the office the nurse sits in a chair at a desk and opens a folder of papers. The patient sits in chair at side of desk, holding her purse with both hands on her lap.)

| Nurse | | Patient | | Analysis | |
Verbal	Nonverbal	Verbal	Nonverbal	Themes	Therapeutic Techniques
What do you prefer to be called, Mrs. Jarvis or Anita?	Has pen in hand. Other hand flat on desk. Looking at patient.	(pause) Anita.	Looking at the floor.		Questioning, active listening
Anita, we will be better able to help you if we know more about you. What has happened in your life recently?	(same as above)	(pause) I couldn't get out of bed. (pause) I was so tired.	Turns head slightly, still looking at floor. No smile or frown.	Content—describes fatigue and effects. Mood—sadness. Interaction—opening up with nurse.	Giving information, questioning
How long were you feeling so tired?	Writing and looking at patient.	I don't know. (pause) A week, I guess.	(same as above)	Content—unsure of time frames, marital separation, possible divorce. Mood—sadness, guilt. Interaction—conflict with husband, more trusting of the nurse.	Placing event in time or sequence, active listening
What happened a week ago?	Leans toward patient. Moves tissue box.	(pause) My husband (pause) left. That he was fed up. (pause) That he wanted a divorce.	Tears in eyes. Tries to open purse.		Focusing
I can see this is difficult for you to talk about. (pause) What did he say when he left?	Looking at patient. Both arms on lap.		Nods head. Raises eyes slightly, still not looking at nurse. Starts to cry. Gets tissue. Sobs occasionally.		Empathy, use of silence, questioning
What did you say to him?	Leans slightly toward patient. One arm on lap. Other on arm of chair.	I don't know. I don't remember. (pause) Maybe I asked him to stay.	Crying quietly.	Content—difficulty describing situations, short-term memory disturbance. Mood—sadness and guilt. Interaction—abandonment, loneliness.	Focusing, active listening
Then what happened?	(same as above)	It's all a blur, I think I cried all day.	(same as above)		Focusing

Nurse (verbal)	Nurse (nonverbal)	Patient (verbal)	Patient (nonverbal)	Analysis	Technique
Whom did you talk to?	(same as above)	No one. (pause) My kids are married and gone. I just stayed in bed.	Same but crying less often.	Content—did not ask for help, avoidance of divorce issue. Mood—sadness. Interaction—perceived lack of support.	Focusing
When you were feeling so tired, did you have thoughts of killing yourself?	(same as above)	(pause) I was so scared of being alone. I thought I'd rather be dead.	Looks at nurse for the first time. Both hands in lap.	Content—aware of fears, suicidal ideation but no plan, difficulty with problem solving. Mood—sadness, depression. Interaction—abandonment, lack of support, open with nurse.	Questioning
How did you think about killing yourself?	(same as above)	I couldn't think of anything. I didn't know what to do.	Looks at floor again. Fumbling in purse.		Focusing
Are you still thinking about suicide?	Hands patient a tissue.	Not really. But (pause) I still wish I were dead. I don't know what to do.	Blows nose and then puts hands in lap. Looks at nurse.	Content—minimizing suicidal ideation but ambivalent, helplessness. Mood—sadness. Interaction—asking for help.	Focusing
While you are here, we are going to help you consider some options about what to do so you won't feel so alone and scared. (pause)	Leans forward. Looking at patient. Both hands on lap.	(silence)	Looking at floor. Crying has stopped. Looks at nurse.		Suggesting collaboration, verbalizing the implied, active listening
It will help us if I ask you some questions.	Turns back to papers, ready to write.	OK.	Looking at nurse.		Giving information

WRITTEN PATIENT ASSESSMENTS

Intake Interview

Each psychiatric hospital, unit, clinic, and program has its own version of an intake or nursing assessment form, which usually includes a mental status assessment. Box 12-3 provides a sample initial patient assessment. Physiological systems and medical problems are reviewed to identify the need for medical orders, special nursing care, or diets. Allergies, if any, are listed as well. Current medications with dosages, frequency, and time of last dose are important for obvious reasons. The potential for withdrawal from medications or other drugs is a risk to be noted. Since most facilities use an intake form or checklist, the results of the interview do not have to be written in a narrative form. Summarization of the critical content as an admission note to be included in the progress notes may be expected.

Nursing Care Plans

The initial care plan may be updated at any time but begins with one or two behavior-oriented problems to be addressed immediately; for example, suicide, aggression, self-mutilation, escape, withdrawal or isolation, delusions, hallucinations, impulsive or compulsive acts, suspiciousness, uncooperativeness, or altered thought processes. Updated care plans are often developed by a treatment team during weekly meetings that may include the psychiatrist, nurses, social worker, psychologist, pharmacist, activity therapists, and nutritionist. Care plans generally include patient problems, patient strengths, goals, nursing diagnoses and interventions, patient education, discharge criteria, and referrals. See the sample nursing care plan at the end of this chapter.

Progress Notes

The style of charting progress notes varies in each setting, but the components are basically the same: what the patient says and the nurse's observations, analyses, and plans. Charting is an important way to communicate with team members so that care is consistent and directed toward goals. Charting is also a way of evaluating the effectiveness of treatment plans (Poster, Dee, and Randell, 1997) and progress toward patient outcomes. Box 12-4 details the components

of a progress note and provides a sample progress note based on the patient referred to in the initial nursing assessment and the nursing care plan.

Discharge Summaries

Many facilities and programs expect nurses to participate in writing discharge summaries or transfer summaries and discharge instructions that will be given to patients. Summaries usually identify outcomes achieved by the patient and outcomes that still need to be addressed. The following information is included in the discharge summary and in the patient discharge instructions: medications (including dosage and times), follow-up appointments (with dates and times), and other services along the continuum of care.

Process Recordings

Peplau (1968) used process recordings in her writings to show applications of concepts and examples of interventions. She emphasized the use of communication skills as the means to help patients learn and solve problems. Process recordings are a tool for the nurse, particularly for the student nurse, to learn about working effectively with patients.

This method provides a means of assessing and analyzing communication skills, identifying patient themes, and evaluating the effectiveness of interventions. Audiotape or videotape recordings are more accurate but are not possible in most settings or with many patients. Written process recordings may begin with notes taken during the interview or may be done totally by recall afterward. A process recording is a record of an encounter with a patient that is as verbatim as possible. It generally includes the nonverbal behaviors of the nurse and the patient, as well as the verbal interaction. Analysis of content, mood, and interaction themes may be included next to each written statement or may be summarized at the end of the process recording (see Chapter 10). The process recording may be analyzed by the nurse or shared with a colleague who can give constructive feedback on problem areas and strategies for improvement. The recording is a *learning* tool, not an end in itself, that can be used periodically for professional growth. A sample process recording is presented on this chapter's patient in Box 12-5.

Care Plan

NAME: Anita Jarvis   **ADMISSION DATE:** _____

DSM-IV DIAGNOSIS: Major Depression

ASSESSMENT:	**Areas of strength:** Has family who cares; had good work record; asking for help; thinking abstractly.
	Problems: Unable to get out of bed and care for self; suicidal thoughts but no plan; decreased socialization and support; impending divorce.

DIAGNOSES:
- Potential for self-directed violence related to impending divorce as evidenced by a wish to be dead.
- Moderate anxiety related to fear of living alone as evidenced by expressed helplessness.
- Hopelessness related to lowered self-esteem as evidenced by not caring for self.

OUTCOMES:

Short-term goals: Date met
- Patient will verbalize that she is no longer suicidal.   _____
- Patient will verbally express guilt and anger at husband and situation. _____
- Patient will phone friend, employer, and children for assistance.   _____

Long-term goals:
- Patient will decide where to live after discharge.   _____
- Patient will verbalize confidence in ability to support self.   _____
- Patient will describe resources available to her.   _____

**PLANNING/
INTERVENTIONS:** **Nurse-patient relationship:** Initiate suicide precautions as a nursing measure; monitor energy level and suicidal ideas; offer support as feelings are expressed; reinforce strengths; compile list of resources.

Psychopharmacology: Fluoxetine 20 mg PO q. AM.

Mileu management: Encourage patient to stay out of room; request patient attendance at grief/loss, self-esteem, assertiveness, problem-solving, and recreational groups.

EVALUATION: Patient will stay with daughter after discharge; patient called employer and requested extended sick leave.

REFERRALS: Patient made appointment for outpatient counseling; patient has information on divorce recovery group.

■ Critical Thinking Question

What are your fears of writing and analyzing a process recording after a conversation with your patient? What are the benefits of this method?

💬 Key Concepts

1. Nursing process (a systematic approach to treatment) is relevant in psychiatric nursing practice.
2. Nursing process is a tool with which the nurse assesses each patient's problems, selects and carries out specific nursing interventions, and evaluates the effectiveness of these interventions on patient outcomes.
3. The initial patient assessment is holistic and includes data from all members of the multidisciplinary team.

4. Written patient assessments, care plans, and progress notes provide an important means of ensuring consistency and continuity of care.

5. Evaluation of patient progress is a foundation for discharge planning and for referrals to other services within the continuum of care.

6. Process recordings are a learning tool to facilitate professional growth.

Study Questions

1. When nursing interventions are being planned, the nursing diagnoses are:
   a. Based on what the patient says are issues that need work.
   b. Specific problems that point to a desired patient outcome.
   c. Specific behavioral goals the patient needs to address.
   d. Specific nursing activities needed to assist the patient.

2. In the afternoon after a patient was admitted, the patient is overheard yelling to someone on the phone. The patient had not shown signs of aggression previously. The nurse decides to investigate this patient behavior. Which of the following would be most important to explore first?
   a. How the patient could be less aggressive.
   b. What goal the patient wants to accomplish now.
   c. The context or situation that precipitated the aggression.
   d. What the patient will do in the next phone call.

3. Which of the following is the most appropriate nursing diagnosis?
   a. Depression related to loss of wife as evidenced by suicidal ideation.
   b. Suicidal ideation related to depression as evidenced by a wish to be dead.
   c. Loss of support related to wife's death as evidenced by grieving.
   d. Dysfunctional grieving related to loss of wife as evidenced by suicidal ideation.

4. A patient who has been making cuts on her wrist when she is angry is admitted to the unit. Which is the most appropriate initial outcome or goal?
   a. Patient will tell the nurse when she is feeling angry.
   b. Patient will verbalize that she no longer wants to harm herself.
   c. Patient will sign a contract stating she agrees not to harm herself.
   d. Patient agrees that she will not threaten the safety of herself or others.

5. During an interview with the nurse, the patient states, "I might as well die. No one cares about me anymore. My suicide would show them." Which of the following best describes the themes in this interaction?
   a. Content—hopelessness, suicidal ideation, revenge. Mood—anger. Interaction—open, frank.
   b. Content—revenge, suicidal plan. Mood—sadness. Interaction—withdrawal.
   c. Content—loneliness, hopelessness. Mood—depressed. Interaction—feels alone.
   d. Content—suicidal, lonely. Mood—anger. Interaction—resistant to help.

REFERENCES

Barrell LM, Merwin EI, and Poster EC: Patient outcomes used by advanced practice psychiatric nurses to evaluate effectiveness of practice, *Archives of Psychiatric Nursing* 11(4):184, 1997.

Jones KR, et al: Policy issues associated with analyzing outcomes of care, *Image J Nurs Sch* 29(3):261, 1997.

Mason WH, Breen RY, and Whipple WR: Solution-focused therapy and inpatient psychiatric nursing, *J Psychosoc Nurs Ment Health Serv* 32(10):46, 1994.

Peplau HE: Psychotherapeutic strategies, *Perspect Psychiatr Care* 6(6):264, 1968.

Poster EC, Dee V, and Randell BP: The Johnson Behavioral Systems Model as a framework for patient outcome evaluated, *J Am Psychiatr Nurses Assoc* 3(3):73, 1997.

Snyder M, Egan EC, and Nojima Y: Defining nursing interventions, *Image J Nurs Sch* 28(3):137, 1996.

Stolte KM: Wellness nursing diagnoses: accentuating the positive, *Am J Nurs* 97(7):16B, 1997.

Van Servellen G: The concept of individualized care in nursing practice, *Nurs Health Care* 3(9):482, 1982.

CHAPTER 13

Anxiety, Coping, and Crisis

LEE H. SCHWECKE

LEARNING OBJECTIVES

After reading this chapter you should be able to:
- Explain the relationships between anxiety and neuro-chemical and physiological responses to anxiety.
- Explain the relationships among anxiety, coping, and crisis.
- Identify common stressors that are likely to cause anxiety.
- Distinguish symptoms reflective of each of four levels of anxiety.

- Match appropriate nursing interventions to each level of anxiety.
- Describe criteria for evaluating coping mechanisms.
- Identify differences among adaptive, palliative, maladaptive, and dysfunctional coping mechanisms.
- Describe characteristics of and effects of crisis situations.
- Outline major crisis intervention goals and strategies.

Anxiety in response to stress is inevitable in everyday life. How individuals cope with anxiety and stress is important in understanding how well the individuals are functioning in their personal, social, and occupational roles. All of the theoretical models for working with psychiatric patients described in Chapter 3 address stress, anxiety, and coping either directly or indirectly. For nurses in any setting, including nonpsychiatric ones, it is crucial to understand *what* anxiety is, *where* it comes from, *why* it is difficult to deal with, and *how* individuals normally cope with it (Figure 13-1).

COMMONLY PERCEIVED STRESSORS

The stressor that precipitates anxiety is whatever the individual perceives as a danger, a loss, or a threat to his safety and security (Beck and Clark, 1997). The way in which individuals perceive an event depends on their background, needs, desires, self-concept, resources, knowledge, skills, personality traits, and maturity. For example, a skilled athlete might perceive a competitive event as an exciting challenge with a high probability of success. A less skilled athlete

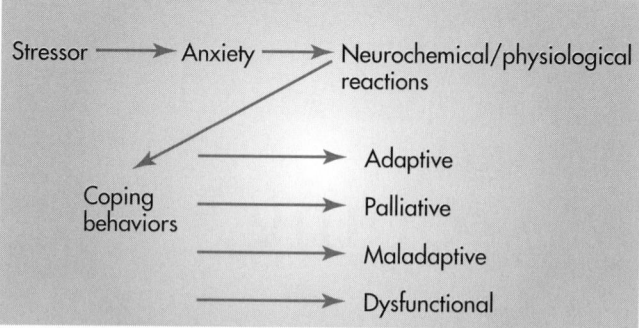

FIGURE 13-1 Process of anxiety.

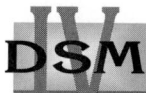 **NANDA Diagnoses Related to Anxiety, Coping, and Crisis**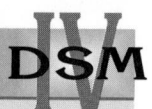

NANDA*
Adjustment, impaired
Anxiety
Breathing pattern, ineffective
Communication, impaired verbal
Coping, ineffective family
Coping, ineffective individual
Decisional conflict
Fear
Injury, risk for
Post-trauma response

Powerlessness
Role performance, altered
Self-esteem disturbance
Sensory/perceptual alteration
Sleep pattern disturbance
Social interaction, impaired
Social isolation
Spiritual distress
Thought processes, altered
Violence, risk for, self-directed or directed at others

*From North American Nursing Diagnosis Association: *NANDA nursing diagnoses: definitions and classifications, 1997-1998,* Philadelphia, 1997, The Association.

might perceive the same event as an overwhelming test with a high probability of failure. Each athlete, on the basis of his or her perception of the situation, will have different emotional and physical responses (i.e., different level of anxiety), of course.

There are commonalities among perceptions of what constitutes a threat, loss, or danger. Individuals typically feel anxious when they perceive a loss of or threat to the following:

1. Health or the ability to perform and function
2. Self-esteem or self-respect
3. Self-control
4. Control or power over one's life
5. Status or prestige
6. Resources (emotional, physical, financial, spiritual, social, and cultural)

7. Loved ones
8. Freedom or independence
9. Needs, goals, desires, and expectations

Some threats or losses are external and visible to observers (objective); others are internal and less evident to observers (subjective). The perception of a threat or loss may not seem "valid" to others; perceptions can be inaccurate, misinterpreted, exaggerated, or unjustified. For example, your best friend turns down your invitation to dinner, saying she has to visit her grandmother who is ill. She has always been honest with you, but you mistakenly begin to doubt if she really cares about you anymore.

Stressors may also be classified as maturational or situational. Maturational stressors are those experiences that are expected as a part of normal processes of growth and development for most of the individuals in a given society (see Chapter 3). For example in the United States, most individuals start school, leave school, develop relationships, become employed, support families, lose loved ones, and prepare for their own deaths. To varying degrees, these stressors can be anticipated and plans made.

Situational stressors are less predictable, and specific actions are taken only when the threat is eminent or the event has occurred. General precautions may be possible. For example, most individuals recognize that acute illnesses and accidents can happen, so they purchase health, life, and/or car insurance; but, they do not know exactly when, where, or how serious the illness or accident will be. Natural and man-made disasters, such as tornadoes, earthquakes, terrorist attacks, and explosions, fall into this category. Some situational stressors have early warning signs that an individual may ignore until the threat is more eminent or obvious, such as divorce, layoffs from work, and chronic illnesses.

RECURRING THEMES OF ANXIETY

Anxiety as a concept and process has been studied, defined, and described by many respected authors: Peplau, 1952; Sullivan, 1953; Lazarus, 1966; Levitt, 1967; Beck and Clark, 1997; and Aguilera, 1998. Anxiety is described as:

- A subjective experience that can be detected only by the objective behaviors that result from it
- Emotional pain
- Apprehension, fearfulness, or a sense of powerlessness due to a threat that is less visible or definable than fear, which has a visible object or trigger
- A warning sign of a perceived danger or threat
- An emotional response that triggers behaviors (automatic relief behaviors) aimed at eliminating it
- Alerting an individual to prepare for self-defense
- Occurring in degrees
- "Contagious": communicated from one person to another
- Part of a process, not an isolated phenomenon

GENERAL ETIOLOGY OF ANXIETY

Psychodynamic Theory

Freud viewed the ego as the part of the personality that develops defenses to help individuals to control or cope with anxiety (see Chapter 3). The need to control anxiety stems from conflicts between the id (instincts) and the superego (conscience) (Freud, 1936). Repression of feelings connected with early conflicts occurs.

Later in life, as conflicts are once again experienced, the defenses fail, and these feelings emerge, causing anxiety and discomfort. Freud viewed unrealistic or "neurotic" anxiety as the fear that instincts will cause one to do something that will result in punishment (Freud, 1936).

Interpersonal Theory

Sullivan (1953) considered interpersonal relations and the socialization process important to how individuals feel about themselves. Sullivan saw individuals striving for security and relief from anxiety to protect their self-systems. In childhood, individuals take on the values of their parents and family to receive approval and to feel good about themselves. Later in life, a threat to the self is based on how individuals perceive the danger or threat and on how they were taught to handle conflict early in life. Because children are dependent on others' for feelings of self-worth, they strive to gain approval in order to feel secure. The sense of self is based on others evaluations. Issues of dependency, control, security, and the related conflicts form the basis of how anxiety is handled. Parent-child conflicts change form as the child matures, but the issues remain the same. For example, a 2 year old who is resisting getting dressed is trying to take control of his/her life to a small degree, but dependency and security needs prevail. Years later, when the adolescent feels less dependent and more secure, the resistance to parental control becomes more obvious and usually culminates in moving out of the home.

Biological Theory

Selye (1956) found that the effects of stress can be seen by the objective measurement of structural and clinical changes in the body. He called these changes the *general adaptation syndrome* (see Chapter 3). More recent research on the effects of anxiety and the resulting neurochemical reactions has centered on the hypothalamic-pituitary-adrenal axis, the hypothalamic-pituitary-gonadal axis, and the limbic system–reward pathway (Putnam and Trickett, 1993). Major neurochemical changes identified include the following (Aguilera, 1998; Charney, et al, 1993; Putnam and Trickett, 1993; van der Kolk and Saporta, 1991):

- Increased regional norepinephrine turnover in the locus ceruleus, limbic regions, and cerebral cortex
- Increased corticotropin-releasing factor (CRF)
- Increased adrenocorticotropin (ACTH) and corticosterone levels
- Increased dopamine release and metabolism in the prefrontal cortex and nucleus accumbens
- Increased endogenous opiate release
- Increased glucocorticoid levels
- Increased thyrotropin-releasing hormone (TRH)
- Increased thyroid-stimulating hormone (TSH)
- Increased peripheral sympathetic nervous system activity

Anxiety-related responses are critical for surviving and tolerating dangerous situations. Rapid behavioral reactions are facilitated by the increased noradrenergic and dopaminergic system activity (leading to central nervous system [CNS] hyperarousal and hypervigilance). Tolerating fear and pain associated with serious injuries is enhanced by increased release of the endogenous opiates (allowing emotional blunting and physical analgesia). Increased physical activity is facilitated by increased cortisol levels (resulting in metabolic activation) (Charney, et al, 1993). However, the effectiveness of these responses fade as the individual is exposed to the stressor. If the "threshold set point" for anxiety is changed, the individual becomes more sensitive to subsequent stressors that more easily reactivate the anxiety-related response (Mackey, 1992). This is discussed in relation to acute stress disorder (ASD) and posttraumatic stress disorder (PTSD) in Chapter 29.

LEVELS OF ANXIETY

To assess how patients are responding to the feeling of anxiety generated by a stressor, the nurse should ask about patients' perceptions of and reactions to it (subjective). Another way of assessing the severity of responses to a stressor is to observe behaviors (objective). Table 13-1 describes the psychomotor, emotional, and cognitive symptoms of four levels of anxiety, as well as the nursing interventions for each level.

Even a moderate level of anxiety (+2) is uncomfortable and difficult to tolerate. As anxiety increases, there is a drive to relieve it as soon as possible. Selye's stress model included in Chapter 3 identifies stages of responses that result from the feeling of anxiety. More specific neurochemical and physiological reactions were described earlier in this chapter. Long-lasting high levels of anxiety (+3 and +4) are so physically and emotionally draining that an individual will do almost anything to escape the pain, such as becoming ill (physically or emotionally) or even committing suicide in rare instances. Fortunately, there are many less debilitating and more productive ways to cope with anxiety.

COPING WITH ANXIETY

Methods of coping with anxiety and the resulting neurochemical and physiological reactions can be divided into four categories, according to the degree of effectiveness in decreasing anxiety or eliminating the source of anxiety as described in Table 13-2.

Although *effectiveness* is the primary criterion for evaluating a coping method, *outcomes* also need to be considered. Sometimes coping reduces the anxiety and solves the problem, but, at the same time, creates other significant problems. Stealing class notes from a friend may result in both an examination score of A and permanent damage to the friendship. *Duration* and *frequency* of coping methods need to be considered as well. Prolonged late-night studying may yield an A, but it may result in reduced resistance to a virus and an episode of the flu. Excessive studying may lead to a poorly balanced life of work, love, and play. Thus a coping method must be examined for its primary effectiveness and for its consequences on the patient's well-being and relationships.

A major role of psychiatric nurses is helping patients to learn or regain more effective coping strategies and to give up less effective or destructive strategies including most of the defense mechanisms (Reed, 1996). To accomplish this, it is important to

TABLE 13-1 Levels of Anxiety

Level of Anxiety and Interventions	Symptoms		
	Psychomotor	Emotional	Cognitive
Mild +1			
Discuss source of anxiety (steps of learning)	Preparation of body for constructive action	Occasional slight irritability	Alertness
Problem solving	Slight muscle tension	Feeling challenged	Awareness of surroundings
Accept anxiety as natural; tolerate and benefit from it	Slight fidgeting	Confident	Concentration
	Energetic		Accurate perceptions
	Good eye contact	(Use of adaptive coping mechanisms)	Attentiveness
			Logical reasoning and problem solving
Moderate +2			
Decrease anxiety—ventilation, crying, exercise	Preparation of body for protective action	Feeling uncomfortable, on edge, keyed up	Difficulty in concentrating
Refocus attention. Relate feelings and behaviors to anxiety. Then use problem solving. Oral medication if needed	Moderate muscle tension	Motivated to decrease anxiety	Easily distracted, can focus with assistance
	Increased blood pressure, pulse, and respirations	Increased irritability	Circumstantiality
	Startle reflex	Decreased confidence	Tangentiality
	Slight perspiration		Loose associations
	Difficulty sitting still	(Use of palliative coping mechanisms)	Narrowed perceptions
	Repeated fidgeting		Decreased span of attention
	Periodic slow pacing		Misperception of stimuli
	Increased rate of speech		Tuning out of stimuli
	Sporadic eye contact		Problem solving and reasoning with effort or assistance
Severe +3			
Decrease anxiety, stimuli, and pressure	Preparation of body for "flight or fight"	Extreme discomfort	Distorted perceptions
Use kind, firm, simple directions. Use time out (seclusion). Intramuscular medications if needed	Extreme muscle tension	Feeling of dread	Difficulty focusing even with assistance
	Increased perspiration	Hypersensitivity	Flight of ideas
	Continuous and rapid pacing	Defensiveness with threats and demands	Ineffective reasoning and problem solving
	Reflex responses		Disorientation
	Loud and/or rapid speech	(Use of maladaptive coping mechanisms)	Delusions and hallucinations if prolonged
	Poor eye contact		Suicidal/homicidal ideations if prolonged
	Somatic symptoms		
	Sleep disturbance		
Panic +4			
Guide firmly or physically take control. Intramuscular medication. Restraints if needed	Actual flight, fight, or immobilization	Feeling overwhelmed and out of control	Disorganized perceptions
	Suicide attempts or violence	Rage	Disorganized or irrational reasoning and problem solving
	Depletion of body resources	Desperation	Neologisms
	Eyes fixed	Feeling totally drained	Clang associations
	Hysterical or mute		Word salad
	Incoherent	(Use of dysfunctional coping mechanisms)	Out of contact with reality
			Personality disorganization

Adapted from Longo D and Williams R: *Clinical practice in psychosocial nursing: assessment and intervention,* New York, 1986, Appleton-Century-Crofts; Peplau HE: *Interpersonal relations in nursing,* New York, 1952, GP Putnam's Sons; Selye H: *The stress of life,* New York, 1956, McGraw-Hill; Sullivan HS: *The psychiatric interview,* New York, 1954, WW Norton.

TABLE 13-2   **Coping with Anxiety**

Type of Coping	Description	Common Use	Patient Example
Adaptive	Solves the problem that is causing the anxiety, so the anxiety is decreased. The patient is objective, rational, and productive.	Anxiety about an upcoming exam is reduced by studying effectively and passing the exam with a grade of A.	Anxiety about being discharged from the hospital is handled by writing down medications, dates and times of follow-up appointments, and self-help meetings in a calendar. The patient keeps appointments and attends two self-help meetings; takes medications and returns to work.
Palliative	Temporarily decreases the anxiety but does not solve the problem, so the anxiety eventually returns. Temporary relief allows the patient to return to problem solving.	Anxiety about the exam is temporarily reduced by jogging for half an hour. Effective studying is then possible and a grade of A is still achievable.	Anxiety about being discharged is handled by watching television in the evening. In the morning, the patient takes the discharge instructions written by the nurse and puts them in his pocket. He keeps his first follow-up appointment and attends one self-help meeting. He takes his medications and is able to return to work.
Maladaptive	Unsuccessful attempts to decrease the anxiety without attempting to solve the problem. The anxiety remains.	Anxiety about the exam is first ignored by going to a movie and then handled by frantically cramming for a few hours. A passing grade of C is obtained.	Anxiety about the discharge is handled by saying that he can remember all the appointments and meetings, and that the directions for the medications will be on the bottles. He misses the meetings and his appointment, but makes another appointment when called. He takes his AM and PM medication but forgets the noon dose all week. He goes to work but complains of being anxious all day.
Dysfunctional	Is not successful in reducing anxiety or solving the problem. Even minimal functioning becomes difficult, and new problems begin to develop.	Anxiety about the exam is first ignored by going out drinking with friends and then escaped by "passing out" for the night. A grade of F results and the course has to be repeated.	Anxiety about the discharge is handled by ignoring the nurse and starting an argument with another patient. When asked to take a "time out," the patient leaves the hospital without being discharged, and his bill is not paid by insurance. He does not get his prescriptions and is brought back to the hospital in 3 weeks.

identify which strategies the patient knows and is using, knows but is not using, and does not know. Nurses often assume that patients know more about adaptive coping than they really do. The most common coping techniques taught and/or encouraged are:

- Problem solving
- Assertiveness
- Positive self-talk
- Stress and anger management
- Skills needed for:
  - Communications
  - Relationships
  - Conflict resolution
  - Community living

Coping strategies take time to learn and use consistently. In a short-term hospitalization or program, nurses begin the education process, but this should be continued in an aftercare program. New skills need ongoing reinforcement until they become "habits."

■ **Critical Thinking Question**

Identify symptoms of each level of anxiety you have experienced at different times. Match these with various coping mechanisms you have used to deal with the anxiety levels.

RELATIONSHIP BETWEEN ANXIETY AND ILLNESS

Individuals feel increasing pain and discomfort as anxiety escalates from moderate to severe, and then panic levels. To feel better, these individuals use behaviors and defense mechanisms to protect themselves. These behaviors are individualized. For instance, biological and genetic endowment influence reactions to stress. An individual is born with unique personality traits, predispositions, and physiological and neurological systems. If long-term palliative, maladaptive, or dysfunctional coping behaviors are employed, an anxiety-related disorder, a physiological health problem, or even a psychosis may develop.

CRISIS

Any "stressful event or hazardous situation" has the potential for precipitating a crisis (Lindemann, 1956). It may be a "minor" event or situation at the end of a series of stressors that becomes more than the individual can handle (i.e., the proverbial "straw that breaks the camel's back"). A crisis differs from stress in that a crisis results in a period of severe disorganization due to the failure of individuals' usual coping mechanisms and/or the lack of usual resources. The feeling of being totally out of control of one's life and being unable to function on a daily basis is extremely disturbing and motivates patients to escape the pain (Caplan, 1961).

Individual Reactions

Anxiety generally rises to a severe or panic level during a crisis (see Table 13-1). Individuals feel a sense of overwhelming helplessness and hopelessness when nothing seems to be working. They may feel immobilized and either give up or keep trying the same, ineffective coping methods. An individual in a crisis state needs and is generally receptive to help. During the period of disorganization there is a natural tendency to depend on others for guidance and assistance. (Trust is less of an issue at this time.) The right kind of help at the right time generally enables individuals to overcome the problem, regain equilibrium, and return to normal. It is common for individuals to learn new coping skills, develop new or improved relationships with others, and begin functioning better than they did before the crisis occurred. This is the reason crisis is said to have growth-promoting potential (Aguilera, 1998).

The disorganization period of a crisis is so distressing that it usually cannot be tolerated emotionally or physically for more than 4 to 6 weeks. If the right kind of help is not available and the crisis is not successfully resolved in that time period, the individual in crisis is likely to become exhausted and physically ill, adopt dysfunctional coping patterns that manage the intense feelings without solving the problems (that is, become emotionally ill), become violent, or attempt suicide to escape the pain. Dysfunctional patterns of coping tend to persist unless the individual seeks intensive counseling for a prolonged period of time. It takes less time and is more effective to intervene *during* the crisis to prevent the development of dysfunctional coping patterns than to intervene after the crisis has occurred.

■ **Critical Thinking Question**

You are seeing a patient in an obstetrician's office. She complains of anxiety and lack of sleep for 2 weeks. Write a list of questions you would use to assess her stressors, level of anxiety, and coping mechanisms utilized, and the type of intervention needed.

Strategies of Crisis Intervention

Crisis intervention is appropriate any time a crisis occurs for an individual in any setting. Strategies of crisis intervention are directed toward the immediate cause of the anxiety and are aimed at bolstering emotional security and reestablishing equilibrium, rather than focusing on underlying issues and long-term resolutions (Aguilera, 1998). See Table 13-3 for a comparison of crisis intervention and stress counseling. Crisis strategies begin with identifying when the crisis began, in response to what stressor or series of stressors, and how the individual's life is being affected as a result. The strengths, coping skills, resources, and support systems of the individual are assessed (Aguilera, 1998). Management of emotion and support are valuable parts of crisis intervention to prevent further decompensation, violence, or a suicide attempt. (See Chapter 11, Chapter 14, and Chapter 28.) Identification of irrational thought processes and supportive confrontation aid in moving individuals to immediate decisions and actions to relieve immediate problems and the accompanying sense of helplessness. Alternative ways of coping are explored (Aguilera, 1998). Individuals may need kind but firm directions and assistance in finding and using external resources when they are feeling overwhelmed and immobilized.

Working with an individual in crisis is demanding and intense for a short period of time, usually a few days to a few weeks. Therefore it is essential to involve other staff members and individuals' significant others who can be there to help. These significant others are taught to help and to find resources if they lack knowledge. As the crisis subsides, support persons and community resources are important for continued assistance, especially since the risk of suicide can persist for 2 to 3 months after the crisis has abated. This period is valuable for counseling aimed at learning or reinforcing adaptive coping strategies. With the trend of shorter hospital stays and patients being managed primarily in outpatient treatment settings, hospitalization is primarily for crisis intervention. Patients are admitted only when they are unable to function (to meet their basic needs for food, clothing, and shelter) or are at risk of harming themselves or others. In these situations, the nurse uses crisis intervention strategies

Table 13-3   Crisis/Suicide Intervention Stress Counseling

	Crisis/Suicide Intervention	Stress Counseling
Major focus	Immediate action	Promoting growth
	Prevention of more decompensation	Developing insight
	Prevention of suicide/harm to others	New coping
	Resolution of crisis	
	Restoration of functioning	
Content of sessions	Survival, safety, security	Stressors
	Immediate action needed by client	Feelings
	External resources needed	Coping
	Emotion management	Internal resources
	Immediate goals	Short and long goals
Counselor-client relationships	Intense and continuous over a short time period (hours-days)	Moderately intense and at regular intervals (1 hr/week for 1-20 sessions)
	Then 1-6 sessions for follow-up	
Role of counselor	Supportive with confrontation	Varies according to philosophy and style
	Active, directive	Facilitate problem solving
	Gives commands if needed	Teach adaptive coping strategies
	Suggest adaptive coping strategies	
Significant others	Involved as soon as possible for continuous support, then sporadic follow-up	May or may not become involved in counseling or used for support
	Taught how to help and resources available	
Other agencies	For rescue, longer term follow-up and/or a new support system	May or may not be used

Adapted from Admi H: Stress intervention: a model of stress inoculation training, *J Psychosoc Nurs* 35(8):37, 1997; Aguilera DC: *Crisis intervention: theory and methodology*, ed 8, St. Louis, 1998, Mosby.

focused on providing physical safety, emotional security, and stabilization so the patient can be discharged as soon as possible. Although patients may be in crisis for 4 to 6 weeks, they are not hospitalized that long. Therefore the nurse ideally collaborates with and makes referrals to an outpatient treatment facility or to other community resources.

Crisis intervention can be offered in a variety of ways. There can be walk-in crisis units/teams within a mental health center or mobile crisis teams who see individuals in their homes, in community clinics, or in emergency departments of hospitals (Liefland, et al, 1997). Many communities and mental health centers offer 24-hour telephone crisis (or hot) lines. Mobile disaster teams are often sent to areas experiencing natural or man-made tragedies, such as earthquakes, tornadoes, or bombing of a building.

Key Concepts

1. A stressor is whatever an individual perceives as a threat, loss, or danger.
2. Anxiety has been described in a variety of ways and can generate a variety of responses.
3. Based on Peplau's model, four levels of anxiety have been identified: mild, moderate, severe, and panic.
4. Nursing interventions vary according to the level of anxiety being experienced by the patient.
5. It is crucial to evaluate patients' adaptive, palliative, maladaptive, and dysfunctional coping mechanisms.
6. A crisis results in a period of severe disorganization due to the failure of individuals' usual coping mechanisms and/or the lack of their usual resources.
7. Crisis intervention strategies concentrate on the immediate precipitant, physical safety, and emotional security.

Study Questions

(Answer key is in the back of the book.)

1. An individual's definition of an event as a stressor is influenced by which of the following:
   a. How much anxiety is experienced
   b. The individual's self-concept, skills, and resources
   c. Whether the stressor is internal or external
   d. The accuracy of the individual's interpretation of stimuli
2. The characteristics of anxiety have been defined in a variety of ways. Which of the following is *not* one of the characteristics?
   a. Part of a process instead of an isolated phenomenon
   b. A warning sign of perceived danger or threat
   c. A sense of powerlessness in the face of a less visible threat
   d. A subjective experience of physical pain

Match the appropriate nursing intervention with the symptoms of each level of anxiety

3. ___c___ Discuss problem-solving strategies for resolving the anxiety
4. ___b___ Decrease stimuli and pressure. Use time out.
5. ___a___ Guide firmly. Use intramuscular (IM) medication.

   a. Feeling out of control and desperate; irrational reasoning
   b. Defensiveness with threats and demands; distorted perceptions
   c. Irritability and fidgeting; alertness and slight muscle tension

6. Pam is being evaluated in an emergency room for chest pain, elevated blood pressure, and headaches. All test results are negative. Then Pam reports a series of recent stressors. She describes trying to manage her stressors by taking pain pills with alcohol, so she can "just go to sleep and forget it." She admits her strategies are not working. "I wake up, and the problems are still there, and I can't even make it to work on time." The nurse assesses Pam's coping as:
   a. Maladaptive
   b. Palliative
   c. Dysfunctional
   d. Adaptive
7. Dan Jackson was admitted to the unit a week ago with complaints of fatigue, the inability to get out of bed, and low self-esteem. During a phone call to his wife, he begins screaming, "Don't leave me, I need you!" He then throws all of his clothes into his suitcase and says repeatedly, "Home . . . Jane . . . she can't . . ." Your assessment and immediate intervention is:
   a. The patient is in crisis. Allow him to cry and talk about what has happened. Tell him he cannot leave the unit.
   b. The patient is angry. Encourage him to discuss his feelings and what he will do during this weekend's pass.
   c. The patient is afraid of divorce. Encourage him to discuss ways to reconcile with his wife while on pass.
   d. The patient is out of control due to stress. Let him cry for a few minutes and then teach him assertiveness skills.

REFERENCES

Aguilera DC: *Crisis intervention: theory and methodology,* ed 8, St. Louis, 1998, Mosby.

Beck AT and Clark DA: An information processing model of anxiety: automatic and strategic processing, *Behav Res Ther* 35(1):49, 1997.

Caplan G: *An approach to community mental health,* New York, 1961, Grune & Stratton.

Charney DS, et al: Psychobiologic mechanisms of post-traumatic stress disorder, *Arch Gen Psychiatry* 50(4):294, 1993.

Freud S: The problem of anxiety, New York, 1936, WW Norton.

Lazarus RS: *Psychological stress and the coping process,* St. Louis, 1966, McGraw-Hill.

Levitt E: The psychology of anxiety, Indianapolis, 1967, Bobbs-Merrill.

Liefland L, et al: A crisis intervention program: staff go the extra mile for client improvement, *J Psychol Nurs* 35(2):32, 1997.

Lindemann E: The meaning of crisis in the individual and family, *Teachers College Record* 57:310, 1956.

Mackey T: Factors associated with long-term depressive symptoms of sexual assault victims, *Arch Psychiatr Nurs* 6(1):10, 1992.

Peplau HE: *Interpersonal relations in nursing,* New York, 1952, GP Putnam's Sons.

Putnam FW and Trickett PK: Child sexual abuse: a model of chronic trauma, *Psychiatry* 56:82, 1993.

Reed PG: Transforming practice knowledge into nursing knowledge—a revisionist analysis of Peplau, *Image* 28(1): 29, 1996.

Selye H: *The stress life,* St. Louis, 1956, McGraw-Hill.

Sullivan HS: Interpersonal theory of psychiatry, New York, 1953, WW Norton.

van der Kolk BA and Saporta J: The biological response to psychic trauma: mechanisms and treatment of intrusion and numbing, *Anxiety Res* 4:199, 1991.

CHAPTER 14

Working with the Aggressive Patient

LEE H. SCHWECKE

LEARNING OBJECTIVES

After reading this chapter you should be able to:
- Describe the differences between anger, aggression, passive aggression, and assertiveness.
- Recognize the developmental, individual, and stress models of aggression.
- Describe the five stages of the assault cycle.
- Explain the verbal nursing interventions for anger and nonviolent aggression.

- Match the external control interventions with the escalation and crisis phases of the assault cycle.
- Describe the nursing care of patients in seclusion and restraints.
- Explain the functions needed to support a staff victim of patient assault.

Anger is a normal human emotion that is crucial for individual growth and is a factor present in all relationships. When handled appropriately and expressed assertively (directly, without violating the rights of the self or others), it is a positive creative force that leads to problem solving and productive change. When channeled inappropriately and expressed as verbal aggression (verbal attacks on others) or physical aggression, it is a destructive and potentially life-threatening force. Physical aggression is also called *assault, battery,* or *violence*. Anger may be expressed indirectly as passive aggression (for example, sarcasm or pouting) or may be passively internalized and lead to unpleasant emotional and physical problems.

The focus of this chapter is on the individual patient's expressions of anger with the nursing staff and with other patients in inpatient or outpatient psychiatric settings. However, it is important for nurses to recognize that anger and aggression occur in any setting, including emergency rooms, medical and surgical units, nursing homes, community-health settings, and clinics. (Carroll, 1996; Carroll and Sheverbush, 1996; Whitney, Jacobson, and Gawrys, 1996) Aggressive behaviors that occur in nonpsychiatric settings are usually unexpected and very disturbing. Nonpsychiatric staff may be unfamiliar with anticipating, preventing, and managing aggression (Whitney, Jacobson, and Gawrys, 1996). Psychiatric nursing staff are normally trained in assessing and

KEY TERMS

Anger Normal emotional response to the perception of a frustration of desires or a threat to one's needs

Assault Legally defined as any behavior that physically or verbally presents an immediate threat of physical injury to another individual

Battery Inflicting physical injury on another individual

Passive aggression Anger expressed indirectly through subtle and evasive ways

Assertiveness Direct expression of feelings and needs in a way that respects the rights of others and the self

Seclusion Process of placing a patient alone in a specially designed room for protection and closer observation

Restraint Physical control of a patient to prevent injury to the patient, staff, and other patients

defusing anger and in safe management of aggressive behaviors.

RELATED CONCEPTS

Aggression

Everyone experiences feelings of anger, but aggressive displays of anger are considered socially inappropriate and are discouraged in our society. When adults in American culture aggressively express their anger toward someone, the recipient generally responds with fear, frustration, and avoidance of that person, if possible. The recipient may also feel helpless, guilty, defensive, or angry. At times, the recipient of anger may retaliate, seek revenge, or hold a grudge.

In its early stages, anger is healthy when it is expressed verbally and assertively to the person perceived as causing the anger. Visible angry behaviors span a continuum from mild irritation and arguing, to verbal or physical abuse of the self or others, to uncontrolled violence (Table 14-1).

Externally expressed anger may lead to assault. The legal definition of assault is any behavior that is physically or verbally aggressive and presents an immediate threat of physical injury to a person. Carrying out the threat of injury is defined as battery and includes actions such as hitting, kicking, pulling hair, throwing a chair, biting, and scratching, but does not include verbal abuse.

Nurses have the right, professionally and legally, to use physical restraint to prevent patients from injuring themselves and others. Nursing interventions are based on the principle of the least restrictive al-

ternative (Morales and Duphone, 1995). (See discussion in Chapter 4.) This principle means that the nurse will set limits in a "humane and least restrictive manner" (such as talking and oral medications) to assure the safety and security of patients and others. Physical restraint cannot be used unless there is eminent danger of physical injury.

In psychiatric settings, assault is never tolerated, but norms usually allow controlled physical aggression, such as using a punching bag or foam bats. If a patient hits a staff member, the staff member is not allowed to strike back. However, the patient may be restricted with seclusion or restraint without legal consequences in most states. Nurses need to be familiar with regulations that govern the use of seclusion and restraints in their own state. A patient may be allowed (while being carefully monitored) to hit a pillow but would be stopped from damaging furniture.

Verbal Aggression

Verbal anger may be shown assertively or aggressively (Table 14-1). Most of the research findings in this area indicate that verbally aggressive attacks on others tend to have a repetitive pattern and are among the major warning signs of assault and battery (Maier, 1996). Verbal aggression tends to provoke unproductive counterreactions that seldom result in constructive solutions to problems. (Reactions tend to be the same as the recipient's reactions to physical aggression described above.)

Social norms influence the degree and amount of verbal aggression that are tolerated. At a sporting event, fans are allowed to scream, swear, and be

TABLE 14-1   **Expressions of Anger**

Turned Outward		Turned Inward	
Overt Anger	**Passive Aggression**	**Subjective**	**Objective**
Verbalization of anger	Impatience	Feeling upset	Crying
Irritation	Pouting	Tension	Self-destructive behavior
Pacing with agitation	Sulking	Unhappiness	Self-mutilation
Swearing	Frustration	Feeling hurt	Substance abuse
Hostility	Tense facial expressions	Disappointment	Suicide
Contempt	Pessimism	Guilt	
Clenched fists	Annoyance	Feelings of inferiority	
Insulting remarks	Resentment	Low self-esteem	
Intimidation	Jealousy	Sense of failure	
Bragging about violent acts	Bitterness	Humiliation	
Provoking behaviors	Complaining	Somatic symptoms	
Sadistic acts	Deceptive sweetness	Feeling harassed	
Maliciousness	Unreasonableness	Envy	
Verbal abuse	Intolerance	Feeling violated	
Temper tantrums	Resistance	Feeling alienated	
Violation of others' rights	Cynicism	Feeling demoralized	
Screaming	Stubbornness	Feeling depressed	
Deviance	Intentional forgetting	Resignation	
Rage	Noncompliance	Powerlessness	
Argumentativeness	Procrastination	Helplessness	
Overt defiance	Antagonism	Hopelessness	
Threats: words or weapons	Belittling remarks	Desperation	
Damage to property	Sarcasm	Apathy	
Assault	Fault finding		
Rape	Manipulation		
Homicide	Power struggles		
	Unfair teasing		
	Sabotage of others		
	Domination		

verbally abusive, especially toward referees and umpires. The same behaviors toward an employer are not tolerated. A brother may verbally pick on his sister, but he stops the same behavior of a neighbor child toward his sister. In psychiatric settings, the quiet mumbling or swearing by a patient with schizophrenia or an organic brain syndrome might be ignored. The louder swearing of a patient who is in contact with reality is not tolerated, especially if directed toward a patient who is unable to respond assertively. If two relatively competent patients are arguing, staff members might not intervene, except with brief suggestions, to allow patients the positive experience of conflict resolution. If one of those patients is less competent, staff members might stop the argument as soon as it begins.

Passive Aggression and Passivity

Passive-aggressive individuals express their anger indirectly and undermine others in a variety of subtle, evasive ways (see Table 14-1). They tend to deny the anger and its source, even when confronted about their behaviors, because they are afraid of rejection or punishment. It is difficult to discuss issues and maintain a quality relationship with passive-aggressive persons. They are often inefficient in accomplishing tasks and frustrate those around them.

Passive individuals turn their anger inward (Table 14-1), may be unaware of their underlying anger, and see themselves as good, kind, congenial, and helpful. They replace their anger with fear and indirectly damage, destroy, or avoid relationships and intimacy. They are unable to say "no" and feel that others take advantage of them. Passive persons waste energy by setting up and repeating nonassertive situations and seldom achieve their goals. They show signs of distress through low self-esteem, depression, substance abuse, physical illnesses, and suicide attempts.

Assertiveness

One of the widely accepted methods for replacing aggressive, passive-aggressive, and passive behaviors is healthy assertiveness—the direct expression of feelings and needs in a way that respects the rights of others and the self. Assertive individuals use their energy constructively to achieve goals and build productive relationships. Assertiveness training is aimed at teaching individuals the behavioral skills needed to interact successfully with others. Training employs a variety of behavior-modification techniques, such as relaxation training, homework assignments, and role-playing with feedback.

DEVELOPMENTAL VIEW OF AGGRESSION

Frequently, hostile individuals are described as being in "a rage"—a primitive, irrational, infantile response. Diffuse rage reactions are present in an infant's loud, uncontrollable crying and screaming, profuse perspiration, difficulty in breathing (sometimes turning "blue"), and flailing of arms and legs. Children move from infantile rage to more focused "temper tantrums." With the progression of impulse control and the maturing of coordination, children learn to focus unpleasant feelings on persons, objects, or situations perceived to be responsible for their anger. By the early school-age years, or even earlier, children hit one another quite frequently (Smith, 1981).

Normally preadolescents learn to restrict hitting each other and translate aggressive impulses to competitive sports, character assassinations, slander, sarcasm, practical jokes, and destructive gossip. By adolescence, fighting is controlled and purposeful.

Group cooperation is emphasized in competitive, aggressive activities, accounting for the tendency of teenage groups to deteriorate pathologically to gangs or cults (Smith, 1981).

As age increases, the ability to control impulses tends to increase, except in criminals and psychiatric patients with certain diagnoses (described later in the chapter). Between the ages of 22 and 45 years, most expressions of aggression and fighting occur within the family, taking the form of spouse, elder, and child abuse. After the age of 45 years, people seem to stop fighting until around the age of 70, when aging may result in diminished impulse control and cognitive impairment, and expressions of aggression again emerge as a problem (Smith, 1981).

■ Critical Thinking Question

In American culture, aggression toward family members often decreases after age 45 until age 70. What factors do you think contribute to this temporary decrease in aggression?

ETIOLOGY OF AGGRESSION

Individual, Social-Psychological, and Sociocultural Models

Individual models explain violence as a quality of being human and use biologically based explanations of aggression (Ollendick, 1996). Research continues to focus on the areas of the limbic system, the frontal lobe, and the temporal lobe. The neurotransmitters—serotonin, gamma-aminobutyric acid (GABA), and dopamine—influence the expression or suppression of aggressive behaviors (Harper-Jaques and Reimer, 1992). (See Chapter 5). Common problems related to aggression include*:
- Bifrontal head injuries, damage to the frontal cortex
- Damage to hippocampus, amygdala, and/or limbic system
- Temporal lobe dysfunctions
- Alzheimer's disease
- Multiinfarct dementia

---

*Charney et al., 1993; Harper-Jaques and Reimer, 1992; Ollendick, 1996; Putnam and Trickett, 1993; Whitney, Jacobson & Gawrys, 1996)

- Decreased serotonin, GABA, and/or acetylcholine
- Increased dopamine and/or norepinephrine
- Imbalances in hormone levels
- Alcohol/drug use or abuse
- Alcohol/drug withdrawal
- Nutritional deficiencies: tryptophan, thiamine, niacin, and/or lecithin

Social-psychological models focus on the interaction of individuals with their social environment and locate the source of violence in interpersonal needs and frustrations (Gil, 1996; Ollendick, 1996). *Sociocultural models* focus on social structures, norms, values, institutional organizations, and systems operations to explain individual violence (Gil, 1996; Ollendick, 1996).

Stress Models

Stress models provide a useful framework for the nurse to understand and intervene when intense emotional reactions, such as aggression, anxiety, panic, fear, and phobic attacks occur. Stress-driven aggression involves a chain of responses due to neurophysiological actions and reactions known as general adaptation syndrome (GAS), which is explained in chapter 3.

Assault Cycle

Smith's stress model (1981) includes the assault cycle with five stages of a predictable pattern or chain of aggressive responses to emotional or physical stress (Figure 14-1). Patients who are repeatedly assaultive exhibit behavior patterns that are ritualistic, stereotypical, and automatic. As the acuity of the aggressive response increases, there is a comparable decrease in patients' problem-solving abilities, creativity, spontaneity, and behavioral op-

tions. Interventions in each stage of the cycle are discussed later in the chapter. The five-phase assault cycle adapted from Smith (1981) includes the following:

1. *Triggering phase:* the stress-producing event occurs, initiating the stress responses.
2. *Escalation phase:* responses represent escalating behaviors that indicate a movement toward the loss of control.
3. *Crisis phase:* a period of emotional and physical crisis in which loss of control occurs.
4. *Recovery phase:* a period of "cooling down" in which the person slows down and returns to normal responses.
5. *Postcrisis depression phase:* a period in which the person attempts reconciliation with others.

ASSESSING KEY VARIABLES OF AGGRESSION

The Nurse (Self-Assessment)

Working with psychiatric patients who may "act out" requires nurses to be aware of their own aggressive impulses, how they deal with their anger, and how they channel it into constructive, productive actions. It is important that nurses know how they respond to patients showing anger, anxiety, fear, panic, and assaultive behaviors. Nurses cannot defuse patients' anger or aggression when nurses themselves are in a similar state, and their anger may actually intensify the patients' emotions. Neither are nurses effective if they withdraw from hostile patients (Corrigan, Yudofsky, and Silver, 1993).

When patients become aggressive, nurses may experience frustration, a feeling of professional inadequacy, or a sense of failure. They may become overly controlling and stimulate power struggles with patients.

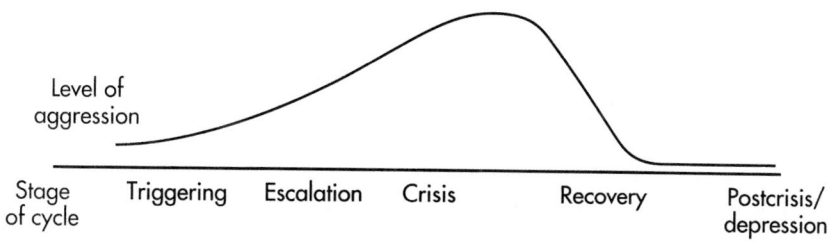

FIGURE 14-1 Assault cycle.

Some nurses believe their participation in physical control of acting-out patients damages the chances of developing or continuing a therapeutic relationship; in most cases, however, just the opposite is true. If patients' behaviors are viewed as a form of communication, then escalating anger should alert the staff to the fact that patients' inner controls are failing and that assistance is needed to regain impulse control. Nurses have the opportunity to convey to patients that help is available to regain control and deal more constructively with the stresses in the environment that caused the initial problems and hospitalization.

The Environment (Milieu)

Variables in the milieu of a facility may contribute to the development and escalation of aggression: (1) an environment with excessive stimuli; (2) overcrowding and lack of sufficient space; (3) lack of resources for energy-draining activities, such as exercise equipment and sports areas; (4) patients' perceived lack of control of life and freedom (Joseph-Kinselman, et al, 1994); and (5) boredom due to lack of structured and unstructured diversionary activities, such as movies, games, cards, crafts, television, and therapeutic and recreational reading materials (Corrigan, Yudofsky, and Silver, 1993; Joseph-Kinselman, et al, 1994).

Staff may need to guide patients in selections of appropriate activities. For example, watching television violence, including sexual aggression, may increase aggressiveness in some patients (Waite, Hillbrand, and Foster, 1992). Staffing needs to be sufficient for monitoring patients and supervising activities (Poster, 1996). Tolerance of a degree of pacing and smoking may reduce tension, but an excess of these activities may disturb other patients. Nurses can be instrumental in helping patients learn assertiveness, social skills, and coping behaviors (Corrigan, Yudofsky, and Silver, 1993).

The biases and attitudes of the staff, as well as the philosophies and policies of a facility, affect both the milieu and patients' behaviors. An overly controlled environment, such as excessive or unfair restriction of rights and privileges, may lead to aggression and rebellion. Reasonable yet flexible rules reduce the risk of power and control issues between staff and patients. Policies and rules can contribute to the structure, predictability, and consistency of the milieu.

The Patient

There are specific times when patients are more likely to become aggressive or assaultive: at admission, at change of shifts, at mealtimes, at visiting hours, during the evening, in elevators, during transportation to outside areas, and during periods of change. Hospitalization is a stress-producing situation that may escalate patients' anger, anxiety, and symptoms (Joseph-Kinselman, et al, 1994). For example, paranoid patients may see the nursing staff as part of a plot to restrict them, while compulsive patients may become more stereotyped and rigid when they cannot repeat compulsive behavior.

Many aspects of admission are threatening and can undermine what little impulse control patients have left. The admission process unavoidably involves focusing on emotionally charged issues, explaining rules and policies, personal searches, the removal or restriction of personal items, physical examinations, and meeting unfamiliar professionals and patients (Joseph-Kinselman, et al, 1994). Nurses need to be sensitive to these stresses and integrate patients slowly into the unit. When patients have a history of assault or are currently agitated, it is important to delay all but essential procedures and to decrease the stimuli and stress as much as possible.

Patients may be disruptive to each other, especially those who are hyperactive, intrusive, openly sexual, manipulative, threatening, or exhibiting bizarre behaviors. Staff members are responsible not only for helping these patients control their behaviors, but also for helping the other patients learn assertive responses for handling such situations.

Change is especially unnerving for patients who have great dependency needs and shaky impulse control. Even positive changes in a patient's status may be experienced as a loss of support, care, and protection; for example, when a patient is transferred to a less restrictive unit or discharged back to the community. All physical moves, status changes, and changes in treatment, such as medications, should be carefully explained in advance. Rapid changes cause the most anxiety, and the nurse needs to convey support and confidence that the patient has the coping skills to deal with the event. Acting-out behavior is one way patients have of telling the staff that change is highly threatening. Fear of change may be the reason patients do not ask for more freedom, such as passes. Requests for more freedom may be a way of testing the staff.

Patients' admitting diagnoses and coexisting medical conditions may provide clues to potential aggression. Patients with a diagnosis of schizophrenia (especially paranoid), mania, substance abuse disorder, or an organic brain disorder have a higher incidence of aggression after admission. Patients with antisocial, passive-aggressive, and borderline traits may also have aggressive tendencies (Kennedy, 1993; Tardiff, et al, 1997a; Tardiff, et al, 1997b). As described earlier, brain injury and brain dysfunction are medical problems especially associated with aggressive outbursts. Patients who suffer from intellectual or neurological impairments that limit their abilities to communicate with or understand others are at high risk of assault.

Factors in patients' backgrounds that are particularly relevant in the assessment of aggression potential are a history of family (or cultural) violence, abuse, or gross disorganization (Ollendick, 1996). Other indicators are histories of truancy, setting fires, impulsivity, previous assaults, and destruction of property. A particularly relevant indicator is a specific threat of violence made approximately 2 weeks before admission. This indicator is also related to a likelihood of being violent after discharge (Tardiff, et al, 1997a).

Documentation in progress notes should include patients' habitual coping patterns and personal eccentricities. Specific examples of communications alerting staff to potential triggers of aggression include "thinks all female nurses are going to be mean to him, like his mother"; "abuses men as his father abused him"; "gets upset whenever the female doctor is here"; "is terrified whenever men are around." Other information includes the times and places patients seem to be especially vulnerable, such as when a parent visits, in large groups, when alone with a staff member of the opposite sex, or when in the bathroom.

NURSING INTERVENTIONS IN ANGER AND NONVIOLENT AGGRESSION

Three factors to consider in intervening with anger and nonviolent (or verbal) aggression are the *source* and the *target* of the patient's anger, and the *likelihood of escalation*. For example, a patient may be angry about a situation/person outside the psychiatric setting but is directing her anger inward as depression or suicidal ideation. Another patient, angry at a situa-

tion/person outside, might show his anger as passive aggression and aim it at no one in particular. A third patient might express anger openly and loudly. In these instances, the anger is likely to be defused by talking about it directly each time it is apparent.

In other situations there is a greater possibility that the patient will lose control of the anger. For example, a patient may be angry at a situation/person in the treatment setting; angry about an outside situation but displacing it onto the staff; threatening suicide with an available object; or responding to internal stimuli, such as hallucinations, delusions, or physiological disruptions.

Nursing interventions in both escalating and nonescalating anger begin with an assessment *at a safe distance*. Chapter 11, on the nurse-patient relationship, describes normal precautions to take with any patient in a potentially unpredictable situation; for example, the nurse stays between the patient and an exit without blocking the exit and uses body language that is the least threatening to the patient (Maier, 1996). Warmth and empathy are essential, but there may also be a need for firm limit setting to help patients contain their behavior at a safe level: "I want to talk, but put the ashtray down first" or "Stay here. I don't want you to leave the room."

If patients are less verbal, less direct, or overly controlling of their anger, the nurse needs to take an active, supportive, and directive role in facilitating ventilation and then problem solving. Initially the nurse may have to point out specific behaviors and ask patients to explain the situation; for example, "I hear a lot of sarcastic remarks. What happened during your phone call?" or "You look so down right now. What are you thinking about?" Getting a full description of situations, thoughts, and feelings requires thorough questioning and patience. Patients who turn anger inward should also be asked if they are thinking about suicide.

The process of asking patients to describe their thoughts, feelings, and situations allows them to ventilate and diffuse some of the emotion. As the anger subsides, problem solving can focus on more effective ways of handling situations and feelings. It can be helpful to ask patients to assess their own potential for acting on anger. "How likely are you to try to hurt your wife when you are angry?" "How serious are you about killing yourself?" The nurse may "contract" with patients to approach the staff and talk about their feelings each time they feel angry (Morrison, 1992).

If the anger does not gradually diffuse during the assessment and ventilation process, or if patients begin to become irrational and out of control, interventions based on the assault cycle become necessary.

NURSING INTERVENTIONS BASED ON THE ASSAULT CYCLE

The goal of all interventions based on the assault cycle (Table 14-2) is to strengthen patients' control of feelings and impulses. Nurses should document that attempts to use less restrictive measures (talking and oral prn medications if ordered) were employed before the more restrictive interventions of seclusion and restraints are used. Nurses should strive to achieve a balance between giving the least restrictive care and the restriction of rights in order to protect patients and others, while still providing quality care (Trudeau, 1993).

Patients' responses at each stress level and to each progressively restrictive intervention should be documented. Except in rapidly escalating situations, verbal strategies should be tried before using physical interventions. Although interventions with patients who are potentially assaultive are unpleasant for nurses, studies show that many patients appreciate

Table 14-2 Interventions Based on the Assault Cycle

Phase	Behaviors	Nursing Interventions
Triggering phase	Muscle tension, changes in voice quality, readiness to retaliate, tapping of fingers, pacing, repeated verbalizations, noncompliance, restlessness, irritability, anxiety, suspiciousness, perspiration, tremors, glaring, changes in breathing	Convey empathic support Encourage ventilation Use clear, calm, simple statements Ask patient to maintain control Facilitate problem solving by discussing alternative solutions If needed, ask the patient to go to a quiet area Offer safe tension reduction If needed, offer oral prn's
Escalation phase	Pale or flushed face, screaming, anger, swearing, agitation, hypersensitivity, threats, demands, tautness, loss of reasoning ability, provocative behaviors, clenched fists	Take charge with calm, firm directions Direct patient to a quiet room for "time out" Give oral prn's if ordered Ask the staff to be on stand-by at a distance Prepare for a "show of determination" to take control
Crisis phase	Loss of self-control, fighting, hitting, rage, kicking, scratching, throwing things	Use involuntary seclusion, restraints, and/or intramuscular (IM) prn's if ordered Initiate intensive nursing care
Recovery phase	Accusations, recriminations, lowering of voice, decreased body tension, change in conversational content, more normal responses, relaxation	Continue intensive nursing care Process the incident with the staff and other patients Assess patient/staff injuries Evaluate patient's progress toward self-control
Postcrisis depression phase	Crying, apologies, reconciliatory interactions, repression of assaultive feelings (which may later appear as hostility, passive aggression)	Process incident with patient Discuss alternative solutions to the situation and feelings Progressively reduce the degree of restraint and seclusion Facilitate reentry to unit

Adapted from Maier, GJ, Managing threatening behavior: The role of talk up and talk down. *J Psychosoc Nurs Ment Health Serv* 34(6):25, 1996; Smith P: Empirically based models for viewing the dynamics of violence. In Babich K, editor: *Assessing patient violence in the health care setting*, Boulder, Colo, 1981, Western Interstate Commission for Higher Education; Stevenson S: Heading off violence with verbal de-escalation, *J Psychosoc Nurs Ment Health Serv* 29(9):6, 1991.

and want the staff to provide the external controls that are lacking and needed, such as seclusion. Calm, positive approaches convey to patients that they are expected to cope, and this attitude supports healthy functioning.

Triggering Phase

In the triggering phase, patients' responses are non-violent and present no danger to others. The behavior reflects patients' usual coping and defense mechanisms. It is important to know how patients perceive the nurse and the environment during the triggering phase, and how likely it is that patients will act on these perceptions.

If a patient's stressor is another individual in the immediate environment, the two can be separated and two nurses can talk with each patient individually in order to promote safe ventilation of emotions.

To facilitate ventilation of anger, emphasis is on being supportive by using an empathic, nondirective, yet concerned technique. The nurse speaks softly in calm, clear, simple statements, avoiding any challenge to the patient (Maier, 1996). Aggressive, confrontational, or threatening approaches at this time usually result in escalation. While ventilation is encouraged, patients are reminded to stay in control of themselves and to use relaxation techniques (Maier, 1996). Patients' loss of control is socially embarrassing for them and counterproductive, leaving them with feelings of vulnerability and loss of autonomy. To protect the dignity of patients and the rights and safety of others, patients can be asked to move to a quieter area or other patients may be asked to leave (Maier, 1996).

When the anger subsides, a problem solving approach can begin to identify alternative solutions. If, however, the ventilation has not been successful, it is important to offer patients alternatives that allow them to express threatening emotions safely, while helping them regain control. Popular approaches with some empirical support include exercise, punching pillows, tearing up telephone books, pounding clay, or walking up and down the hall. Calming medications can also be given if ordered (Maier, 1996; Morales and Duphone, 1995).

CLINICAL EXAMPLE

John Henderson has been a patient on the unit for 3 days. While talking to his wife on the phone, he becomes upset and raises his voice to her. The nurse calmly suggests that he tell his wife that he will continue their conversation later. He hangs up the phone and starts pacing in the hallway. The nurse says, "Tell me what you are upset about." For 15 minutes he describes the phone conversation in detail, expresses anger toward his wife, and says he is afraid she will divorce him. As he visibly calms down, the nurse asks, "What would be most helpful in handling the situation with your wife?"

Escalation Phase

When tension-reduction strategies fail and patients become irrational (for example, begin to swear, scream, and threaten), the nurse must take control of the situation. For example, at a safe distance, the nurse calls the patient by name and states in a calm, firm manner that the patient's behaviors indicate a loss of control. The nurse does not threaten punishment, but offers help by taking charge on behalf of the patient, who is unable to do so at the time. The nurse avoids sudden movements and loud tones to prevent giving the appearance of an attack (Maier, 1996).

If the patient has orders for prn antianxiety or antipsychotic medications, an oral dose can be offered early in the escalation phase. If the oral dose is refused, or if the escalation is rapid, an intramuscular (IM) medication may be necessary, and the nurse may require help from other staff members. Among the oral antianxiety medications, lorazepam (Ativan) and alprazolam (Xanax) are often the drugs of choice because they take effect rapidly and have relatively few side effects. They may occasionally lower a patient's inhibitions and aggravate behaviors. Lorazepam may be given IM. Among the antipsychotic medications, the high-potency ones—haloperidol (Haldol) and fluphenazine (Prolixin)—have less sedating qualities, but help to decrease agitation (Corrigan, Yudofsky, and Silver, 1993; Grinspoon, 1991).

Given the principle of the least restrictive alternative, a time out in a quiet room is offered first by the nurse in a kind but firm manner. If this measure is ineffective, then more restrictive measures may be instituted when the patient actually begins to lose control (Cashin, 1996). Other staff members may be called to be on standby, but should try initially to remain out of the patient's view. When patients are potentially violent, their physical proximity to others is perceived as being much closer than it actually is, and they may feel threatened (Maier, 1996).

CLINICAL EXAMPLE

For the second time this shift, John Henderson is talking by phone with his wife. He is now shouting, making threats, and demanding that she come to the hospital *now*. The nurse again asks him to end the call and talk about what is happening. As he describes this call, he gets more agitated and yells that he wants to go home immediately. The nurse calmly and firmly says, "I can hear how angry you are. (Pause.) You cannot go home now. (Pause.) I want you to go to your room and I will bring you an Ativan." Mr. Henderson does not respond immediately, but he stops yelling. The nurse says, "Please go to your room. I will get the Ativan." He goes to his room and slams the door. The nurse alerts other staff members to what she is planning to do for Mr. Henderson. She asks them to stay outside of his room until she can assess if "time out" is going to be helpful for him and if he is willing to take the medication.

The nurse who has been talking with the patient decides whether the patient is able to respond to directions in a reasonable time. If the patient does not respond to directions for self-control or to move to a quiet, safe place, the nurse then asks for staff assistance for a stronger "show of determination" to take control. This involves having four to six staff members within sight of the patient, but at a greater distance from the patient than the primary nurse, so they do *not* appear ready to attack the patient. Often, when the patient becomes aware of the other staff members and is informed that the staff *will* take control if the patient does not comply with directions, the patient is able to gain reasonable composure, to cooperate with the nurse's request, and will often take the medications and go to the quieter room. If not, the patient is usually close to entering the crisis phase.

Crisis Phase

The crisis phase is reached when the patient is approaching an attack on the environment, the self, other patients, or the staff. Verbal limits are ineffec-

tive and external control by the staff is essential. In such emergency or crisis situations, immediate seclusion, restraint, and/or the administration of "stat" medications become necessary. The patient has the right to refuse medications, but staff may give it in the presence of a *significant* physical threat to others (Trudeau, 1993). These actions should be supported by emergency protocols that have been approved by the physicians and hospital, and the actions should be carefully and thoroughly documented in the patient's records.

Psychiatric emergencies must be dealt with in coordinated and organized ways, and it is important that the staff have the opportunity to role-play their approach in advance of a crisis. All staff members need to master self-protection techniques against such behaviors as kicking, hitting, and biting. Facilities usually provide aggression-management programs for staff members who are required to periodically update these skills similarly to other emergency skills, such as cardiopulmonary resuscitation. Staff members who are well trained in preventing and managing aggression are less likely to be victims of patient assaults (Rosenthal et al, 1992).

Seclusion

Seclusion is the process of placing the patient alone in a specially designed, lockable room that is equipped with a security window or a camera for observation. Nurses usually make the decision to initiate and terminate the seclusion of patients according to the established protocols and are almost always involved in the care of patients during seclusion. The principle of seclusion is *containment:* restricting persons so they do not hurt themselves or others, decreasing stimulation, and increasing intensive nursing care. Agitation and disruptive or inappropriate sexual behaviors are the major reasons for seclusion (Tooke and Brown, 1992). Seclusion may be viewed as a preventative strategy to *avoid* aggressive assaults, as well as a responsive action. "Time out," closer supervision, quiet interactions, and medication are therapeutically effective when used appropriately for brief periods.

The degree of seclusion depends on the patient's current status. The patient who is able to choose "time out" voluntarily, especially if that patient is already taking regular medicine, may stay voluntarily in his or her room without a locked door. This degree of seclusion may be relatively brief. The less co-operative patient may be escorted by two staff members, without bodily contact, to a seclusion room that contains only a bed (bolted to the floor) and a mattress. This kind of room decreases stimuli, protects the patient from injury, prevents destruction of property, and provides for the patient's privacy. The security window or camera allows observation of the patient, and the door, lockable from the outside, keeps the patient from leaving the room. Dangerous articles (for example, belts, sharp objects such as pens and keys, shoes, and eyeglasses) are taken away from the patient.

Restraint

The staff must take immediate action when assaults occur. Six to eight staff members (including hospital security officers if there are insufficient unit staff available) are needed to *safely* control a patient and assure there will be no injuries to the staff, the patient, or to other patients on the unit. It is important not to underestimate the number of staff needed because of the size, age, or sex of the patient. Some agencies include patients' previous athletic interests and accomplishments, such as weight lifting and black belts, on the admission form.

Details of restraint procedures are not described here, but a general outline is presented. To prepare for control of a patient, staff members remove their own glasses, rings, earrings, pens, watches, keys, and anything else that could cause injury to the patient or to the staff. Furniture and objects that can be used as weapons are removed from the area. One staff member becomes the team leader to organize and direct the planned, coordinated approach, while a different staff member continues talking with the patient. At least one staff member gets the other patients to a safe place and stays with them.

The team approaches the patient calmly, in a show of force or determination, to take control. The patient is told that the team is there to help, will not hurt the patient, and will not allow the patient to hurt anyone. Two team members approach from each side and take control of the patient's arms. Simultaneously, three other staff members quickly take control of the patient's legs and head so the patient can be carried to the room, or held on the floor until a bed is brought to the patient. Physical contact is protective and defensive, not aggressive. One staff

member brings the restraint cuffs, opens doors, and moves obstacles. A nurse prepares the IM medication (or calls to get an order if there is not a routine prn order). Once in the seclusion room, the patient is usually placed on the bed on his or her back. Four or more staff members hold the patient's extremities and head securely without hyperextending any joints. Wrist and ankle restraints, often made of leather lined with sheepskin, are applied to all four extremities and buckled to the frame of the bed. The patient's arms are tied in a position at the side, not above the head. The restraints are tight enough to inhibit slipping out of them, but not tight enough to interfere with circulation. A waist restraint, a restraint between the ankles, and/or a restraint blanket are applied only if the patient is at risk of injury because of fighting the restraints. Before staff members leave, the patient is checked for injuries and observed for the ability to move safely in the restraints. Medications may be administered at this time. As soon as possible, an order to restrain the patient is obtained, if it was not obtained prior to the restraint.

■ Critical Thinking Question

A visitor to the unit begins to hit a patient. How would you handle this situation?

Care of patients in seclusion or restraints

When a patient is placed in seclusion or restraints, intensive nursing care is instituted. The patient is to be free of all belongings, all things that could cause harm, and all objects that the patient could use to harm others. The patient is monitored closely, at least every 15 minutes; the nurse announces himself or herself and the purpose of the visit. Other patients are not allowed to be near a restrained patient. The patient's mental status, response to and side effects of medications, hydration, nutrition, elimination, range of motion, vital signs, and hygiene are monitored. Immediate attention to any injuries resulting from the incident or from the restraints is critical and requires documentation. Every 1 to 2 hours, with two staff members present, the restraints are removed one at a time, for 10 minutes each, to allow range of motion. Change of position and skin care are also important. Stimuli are reduced by restricting visitors, phone calls, and diversional materials such as radios and magazines; however, frequent staff contact decreases the patient's sense of isolation and loneliness (Norris and Kennedy, 1992).

Recovery and Depression Phase

In this phase, patients are assured that they are not being punished while in seclusion and that they will be allowed back in the milieu as soon as possible. Patients need to be assisted in relaxing, sleeping, and benefiting from these phases of cooling down and reconciliation. The time patients are in restraints or seclusion should be a supportive, restorative time. Otherwise, patients may remain afraid, frustrated, and angry, possibly leading to future aggression.

Once patients are calm and in control, they are encouraged to discuss what happened when they lost control and alternatives for handling similar situations in the future (Tooke and Brown, 1992).

Patients are ready to be released from restraints when they show signs of self-control, decreased anxiety and agitation, stabilization of mood, increased attention span, reality orientation, and judgment. They may be kept in the seclusion room a brief time to assess the reaction to release from the restraints. Patients need assistance to reenter the unit with as little fear and embarrassment as possible (Norris and Kennedy, 1992). The nurse should make efforts to help other patients accept these patients back into the unit.

Immediately after a patient is secluded and restrained, the staff should meet, ensure that there were no staff injuries, evaluate how they handled the situation, and give each other mutual support and feedback. Feelings and attitudes are discussed, along with suggestions for improved use of procedures. These debriefing meetings provide the unit staff with ongoing, in-service opportunities to monitor their reactions as well as augment their skills. Careful documentation of patients' behaviors before, during, and after these incidents, and a rationale for physical control interventions, seclusion, and restraint are essential legal protections for the staff. Documentation may be recorded as "incident reports" and should be written after all concerned have calmed down. Staff perceptions are compared for accuracy. Documentation is descriptive, sequential, organized, and specific about what was seen, heard, and felt; what was said and by whom; who was notified; and what actions were taken and are to be taken. The request for and granting of a physician's order for seclusion and restraint are also recorded. Other patients' reactions to restraint and seclusion situations should be openly discussed and explored in a special meeting. Patients need the opportunity to share their concerns, reactions, and fears of losing control. It is important to tell the other patients that staff members are providing control and care until the patient who has lost control regains it.

■ Critical Thinking Question

Why is it important for other patients to share their opinions and reactions to the seclusion and restraint of another patient?

STAFF MEMBERS AS VICTIMS OF ASSAULT

Most incidents of patient outbursts of anger do not result in restraint procedures, but when they do, the process is always a difficult one for the staff and for the patient. The staff and the patient are understandably drained physically and emotionally. The process of debriefing and recovery is complicated if a staff person has been injured.

Being injured by a patient is similar emotionally to being a victim of crime (Chapter 38). Such an occurrence can destroy the staff member's sense of trust in others and sense of control of his or her life and can result in a loss of self-esteem (Cooper, 1995). The staff member often expresses feelings of being vulnerable, irritable, depressed, and anxious; experiences grief and symptoms of posttraumatic stress disorder (PTSD); and is afraid of the patient who caused the injury (Cooper, 1995). The assault may be minimized, and feelings may even be denied, if emotional support and debriefing are not provided after the medical examination and treatment are completed. If the injured staff member is away from work for a period of time, the rest of the unit staff may not realize that their emotions have subsided much more than those of their injured colleague. To ensure that the staff victim achieves emotional resolution of the incident, some facilities have developed a formalized process of follow-up. A peer support program that understands the dynamics of assault and the common responses of victims is important. Supportive interventions should be available to the injured person (Cooper, 1995; Poster, 1996; Whitney, Jacobson, and Gowrys, 1996). The needs of the victim determine the frequency and number of meetings. A counselor may facilitate meetings between the victim and staff, and between the victim and the assaultive patient, to facilitate the victim's return to work (Lanza, 1992). Victims are encouraged to share their feelings with family or significant others. The goal of this process is to facilitate emotional resolution, help the person remain productive, and decrease the chance of resignation (Morrison, 1992; Poster, 1996; Whitney, Jacobson, and Gowrys, 1996). There is current debate about whether staff assaulted by patients can or should take legal action against the patient (Poster, 1996).

Key Concepts

1. Anger is a normal human emotion that may be expressed assertively, passively, passive-aggressively, and aggressively.
2. Verbal and physical aggression, especially assault and battery, require safe, immediate interventions based on the principle of the least restrictive alternative.
3. The individual, social-psychological, and stress models of aggression offer explanations for the development of aggression.
4. Factors regarding the nurse, the environment, and the patient affect the development and expression of anger.
5. The assault cycle describes the predictable phases of aggression: triggering, escalation, crisis, recovery, and depression.
6. Nursing interventions with anger and nonviolent aggression concentrate on ventilation to defuse the anger and then on problem solving to identify ways of appropriately handling the causes of the anger.
7. Tension reduction, medications, physical control, seclusion, or restraints become necessary in the escalation and crisis phases of the assault cycle.
8. Patients in seclusion and restraints require intensive physical and emotional nursing care.
9. Staff members who are injured by a patient may require assistance in recovering.

Study Questions

(Answer key is in the back of the book.)
1. Which of the following statements about anger is most accurate?
   a. Open displays of anger should be discouraged.
   b. Verbalization of anger is detrimental to relationships.
   c. Anger is a normal response to frustration of desires and needs.
   d. Suppression of anger helps to decrease the potential for violence.
2. Which of the following is the major guide in dealing with overt aggression?
   a. American Nurses Association standards for nursing
   b. Social norms defining assault and battery
   c. Hospital protocols for seclusion and restraint
   d. Principle of the least restrictive alternative
3. In a staff in-service program on aggression management, you would emphasize which of the following?
   a. Verbal aggression is a safe alternative to physical aggression.
   b. Assertiveness allows for expression of anger while protecting the rights of the self and others.
   c. Passive-aggressive individuals turn their anger inward.
   d. Passive individuals rarely cause trouble for themselves or others.

Match the phase of the assault cycle with the most appropriate nursing intervention.

4. _____ Escalation phase
5. _____ Recovery phase
6. _____ Triggering phase

a. Encourage ventilation of feelings and ask for a description of the situation
b. Offer prn medications and time out in a quiet room
c. Staff control by use of seclusion and restraints
d. Debriefing among staff and with other patients

References

Carroll V: Violence in the workplace: we are the missing link, *Am J Nurs* 96(12):80, 1996.

Carroll V and Sheverbush J: KNSA violence assessment in hospitals provides bases fraction, *Am Nurse,* p 18, Sept 1996.

Cashin A: Seclusion: the quest to determine effectiveness, *J Psychosoc Nurs Ment Health Serv* 34(11):17, 1996.

Charney DS, et al: Psychobiological mechanisms of posttraumatic stress disorder, *Arch Gen Psychiatry* 50(4):294, 1993.

Cooper C: Patient suicide and assault: their impact on psychiatric hospital staff, *J Psychosoc Nurs Ment Health Serv* 33(6):26, 1995.

Corrigan PW, Yudofsky SC, and Silver JM: Pharmacological and behavioral treatments for aggressive psychiatric inpatients, *Hosp Community Psychiatry* 44(2):125, 1993.

Gil DC: Preventing violence in a structurally violent society: mission impossible, *Am J Orthopsychiatry* 66(1):77, 1996.

Grinspoon L, editor: Violence and violent patients: part II, *Harvard Mental Health Letter* 8(1):1, 1991.

Harper-Jaques S and Reimer M: Aggressive behavior and the brain: a different perspective for the mental health nurse, *Arch Psychiatr Nurs* 6(5):312, 1992.

Joseph-Kinselman A, et al: Clients' perceptions of involuntary hospitalization, *J Psychosoc Nurs Ment Health Serv* 32(2):28, 1994.

Kennedy MC: Relationship between psychiatric diagnosis and patient aggression, *Issues Mental Health Nurs* 14: 263, 1993.

Lanza ML: Nurses as patient assault victims: an update, synthesis, and recommendations, *Arch Psychiatr Nurs* 6(3):163, 1992.

Maier GJ: Managing threatening behavior: the role of talk up and talk down, *J Psychosoc Nurs Ment Health Serv* 34(6):25, 1996.

Morales E and Duphone PL: Least restrictive measures: alternatives to four-point restraints and seclusion, *J Psychosoc Nurs Ment Health Serv* 33(10):13, 1995.

Morrison EF: Answers, professionally speaking, *J Psychosoc Nurs Ment Health Serv* 30(7):41, 1992.

Myers S: Seclusion: a last resort measure, *Perspect Psychiatr Care* 26(3):24, 1990.

Norris MK and Kennedy CW: The view from within: how patients perceive the seclusion process, *J Psychosoc Nurs Ment Health Serv* 30(3):7, 1992.

Ollendick TH: Violence in youth: where do we go from here? behavior therapy's approach, *Behav Ther* 27:485, 1996.

Poster EC: A multinational study of psychiatric nursing staffs' beliefs and concerns about work safety and patient assault, *Arch Psychiatr Nurs* 10(6):365, 1996.

Putnam FW and Trickett PK: Child sexual abuse: a model of chronic trauma, *Psychiatry* 56(2):82, 1993.

Rosenthal TL, et al: Hospital violence: site, severity and nurses' preventive training, *Issues Ment Health Nurs* 13: 349, 1992.

Smith P: Empirically based models for viewing the dynamics of violence. In Babich K, editor: *Assessing patient violence in the health care setting,* Boulder, Colo, 1981, Western Interstate Commission for Higher Education.

Tardiff K, et al: A prospective study of violence by psychiatric patients after discharge, *Psychiatr Serv* 48(5):678, 1997a.

Tardiff K, et al: Violence by patients admitted to a private psychiatric hospital, *Am J Psychiatry* 154(1):88, 1997b.

Tooke SK and Brown JS: Perceptions of seclusion: comparing patient and staff reactions, *J Psychosoc Nurs Ment Health Serv* 30(8):23, 1992.

Trudeau ME: Informed consent: the patient's right to decide, *J Psychosoc Nurs Ment Health Serv* 31(6):9, 1993.

Waite BM, Hillbrand M, and Foster HG: Reduction of behavior after removal of music television, *Hosp Community Psychiatry* 43(2):173, 1992.

Whitney GA, Jacobson GA, and Gawrys MT: The impact of violence in the health care setting upon nursing education, *J Nurs Educ* 35(5):211, 1996.

CHAPTER 15

Working with Groups of Patients

CAROL E. BOSTROM

LEARNING OBJECTIVES

After reading this chapter you should be able to:
- Describe specific therapeutic benefits of groups.
- Identify the major purpose of each type of group.
- Explain the value of coleadership of groups.
- Recognize qualities the nurse leader of groups should have.
- Identify intervention strategies for specific group situations.

Working with groups of patients is an integral component of both inpatient and outpatient psychiatric care. Nursing has 24-hour accountability for patient care on the inpatient psychiatric unit and is responsible for leading patient groups. This responsibility dictates economical use of nursing personnel; hence, working with groups of patients addresses manpower concerns while providing a proven therapeutic intervention. Similarly, working with groups in the community or outpatient arena has increased because of brief inpatient psychiatric hospitalization and the demand of managed care for the least expensive, most effective care.

Patients with mental illnesses face problems in their daily living like anyone else, but with the complication of symptoms of mental illness. Even though mental illness interferes with the way patients are able to cope with their problems, conflicts, and interpersonal relationships, patients have the capacity to learn how to cope and negotiate life's problems. Groups deal with current "here and now" issues and stressors whether patients are in or out of the hospital. Patients gain awareness and knowledge about their behaviors and how those behaviors impede communication and coping. They become aware of alternatives that help them make better decisions and choices. On inpatient units and in community settings numerous educational and skill-development groups are led by nurses. Nurses also lead groups for patients' families in order to teach them about mental illness and to help them cope with the mentally ill family member. This chapter is dedicated to answering two questions:

1. Given a patient population that has serious interpersonal and cognitive disturbances, how does group work benefit the individual?
2. What can the nurse realistically expect to accomplish through informal and formal group work with patients?

Since inpatient groups typically have short-term, goal-oriented sessions and are composed of acutely ill patients, nurses need relevant information for developing group strategies. Benefits of groups, types of groups, and leadership of groups are addressed to provide this information. Because working effectively with groups of patients is inextricably related to milieu management, the nurse is encouraged to read the chapters on milieu.

BENEFITS OF GROUPS

Following are some of the benefits that patients receive from any group experience:

- Patients gain knowledge about how to *relate* to and *communicate* with others (Yalom, 1995).

Box 15-1 Yalom's Therapeutic Factors

- **Instillation of hope:** Patients receive hope from observing others who have benefited from the group experience.
- **Universality:** Patients experience relief in knowing that they are not alone and unique but that others experience similar problems, feelings, and concerns.
- **Imparting of information:** Patients learn or are provided with information about areas related to their needs.
- **Altruism:** Patients experience themselves as helpful or useful to others.
- **Corrective recapitulation of primary family group:** Patients review previous dysfunctional family patterns and learn that those past patterns can be changed to effectively meet their present needs.
- **Development of socializing techniques:** Patients are taught appropriate social skills.
- **Imitative behavior:** Patients selectively model healthy behaviors of the leader and other group members.
- **Catharsis:** Patients not only are allowed to express feelings but learn how to express them appropriately.
- **Existential factors:** Patients share feelings about "ultimate concerns" of existence, like death or isolation, and learn to accept that there exists a limit to their control of these issues.
- **Cohesiveness:** Patients experience feelings of being accepted, valued, and part of a group experience.
- **Interpersonal learning:** Patients learn how their behaviors affect others and try out more appropriate ways of relating in the supportive atmosphere of the group.

From Yalom I: *The theory and practice of group psychotherapy,* ed 4, New York, 1995, Basic Books.

- Patients gain *acceptance, reassurance,* and *support* from their peers and the group leader.
- Patients gain *feelings of hopefulness* and a *sense of power* regarding their ability to help themselves and each other.
- Patients are provided with the opportunity to *test out new behaviors* with others during their treatment.
- Patients can *share their feelings,* problems, concerns, and ideas with others in a safe and structured environment.
- Patients' strengths that can *enhance self-esteem* are affirmed and further developed.
- Patients experience a *sense of importance* and an increased *sense of worth.*

These benefits may occur at different times for individual patients and in different group situations. Each group, depending on its goal or purpose, may focus on one particular outcome. For example, an activity group for art may focus on acceptance so that no matter what the patients paint, they will be accepted and praised for their work.

Therapeutic Factors

Dr. Irvin Yalom has described 11 "therapeutic factors" that help patients regardless of the therapeutic group (Box 15-1). Patients experience certain factors or benefits, depending on the type of group they participate in and what the patients as individuals deem to be beneficial and important to them. The meaning of these therapeutic factors and their significance to patients are important for the nurse to understand. The nurse who understands the ways groups help patients will be more likely to initiate, lead, and participate in informal and formal groups. Nurses do not make therapeutic factors happen, but they facilitate the development and occurrence of these factors for patients.

TYPES OF GROUPS

Making the inpatient group a positive, beneficial experience for patients is of primary importance (Yalom, 1995). Patients need to feel they have gained something for themselves during their hospitalization. A positive inpatient group experience favorably predisposes patients to seek treatment on an outpatient basis. After discharge, follow-up care in the community is where the majority of ongoing treatment occurs (Hughes and Ashby, 1996).

Numerous types of groups can be offered in both inpatient and outpatient settings: support, activity, education or problem solving, and therapy (Van Servellen, 1983). Self-help or special-problem groups and multiple-family or couple groups are also available in some treatment settings.

Support Groups

The very nature of nursing implies support. The nurse supports patients in therapeutic interactions. Support means accepting, empathizing, and showing concern while listening and talking with patients. The nurse focuses on responding to patients' needs. The nurse's presence, interest, and encouragement facilitate the expression of patients' feelings and concerns. The nurse is then instrumental in helping patients cope with their feelings and situations. Support is useful in many types of group situations.

The support group is a maintenance group. Its purpose is to reinforce or maintain the existing strengths and behaviors of patients rather than to confront or change behaviors or defenses. Patients in a support group can be acutely or chronically ill. They may need much reassurance and emotional support during their hospitalization. These patients also need to reduce their anxiety to mild or moderate levels.

The reality-orientation group is an example of a support group frequently found in inpatient settings. Patients who exhibit confusion and short attention spans due to psychopathology benefit from this type of group. The nurse must provide an atmosphere of safety and security because these patients may be frightened, unsure, anxious, uncomfortable, and isolated. The reality-orientation group can assist patients with decreasing isolation and increasing self-esteem. Focusing on the here and now provides a framework with structure, social support, and reality testing. The nurse as leader of this group facilitates orientation to time; person and place; rules and routines of the unit; and behavioral expectations, including some limit setting. Feeling valued, respected, and important as human beings is a feeling these patients may not have experienced in a while.

Activity Groups

Activity groups use a variety of techniques to facilitate patient communication and interaction (Van Servellen, 1983). For example, some groups may use art or music to motivate patients to interact and to promote socialization. Withdrawn, depressed, and regressed patients benefit from these groups because they have experienced isolation and lack interpersonal relationships. The general goals of these groups are to help patients increase self-esteem, openness, and the expression of feelings while decreasing isolation. When interpersonal communication increases, focus on the activity per se decreases. The activity is a vehicle or means to facilitate self-expression and patient interaction. Table 15-1 describes two types of activity groups.

Education or Problem Solving Groups

Nurses working in inpatient and outpatient settings lead groups to teach patients and their families a variety of content and skills. Typical groups deal with medication, dynamics and management of illness, problem solving, stress management, social

Table 15-1   Activity Groups

Type	Purpose/Nurse's Role	Examples
Recreation	Provide opportunity for fun and relieve tension. Patients experience sense of participation, acceptance, and accomplishment.	Indoor/outdoor sports, field trips, exercise groups, and games.
Creative expression	Facilitate expression of feelings, communication with others, and socialization. Allow for creativity, self-expression, and praise for accomplishments.	Arts and crafts, activities of daily living, art, poetry, music, dance, and pet therapy.

Table 15-2 **Education Groups**

Type	Purpose/Nurse's Role	Examples
Psychoeducation	Teach patients/families content related to dynamics of illness, symptoms of illness, signs of relapse, management of illness, and dealing with crises.	Addiction processes, coping with symptoms, management of moods, causes and treatments of illnesses, relapse prevention, community resources.
Medication	Dispense medications. Assess symptoms and side effects. Explain type and purpose of medication, dosage, therapeutic effects and side effects. Support adherence to medication regimens and to prevent relapse.	Groups based on category of medications (e.g., antipsychotics vs. antidepressants, intramuscular vs. oral).
Problem solving	Help to identify and describe current problems; discuss and develop solutions and their effects; and decide on an alternative method and how to try it. Evaluation and choosing another method are also part of the process.	Milieu issues, conflict resolution, job concerns, relationship issues, discharge planning.
Stress management	Teach and facilitate adaptive coping behaviors.	Life-style balance and management, relaxation training, tension-reduction strategies, and anger management.
Social skills	Teach, develop, and practice skills to enhance interactions with others. Focus on realistic, day-to-day patient needs.	Assertiveness training, handling social interactions (e.g., meeting new people, going on interviews, and negotiating the return of a purchase).

skills, interpersonal skills, and relapse prevention. The reduction in inpatient hospitalization has increased the need for patients to learn skills to manage their illnesses and their lives in the community.

Table 15-2 shows an example of a model that can be used in a community mental health center for groups of patients with similar education needs (Elmore and Young, 1996). This model offers a series of sessions that vary in length but typically include an hour for content presentation followed by an hour of discussion. An example could be a six-session module for patients with bipolar disorder or an eight-session module for patients with schizophrenia. The sessions could focus on issues related to medication. The nurse's expertise, empathy, and support help patients to learn that they can successfully take care of their illnesses and themselves.

Nurses also provide psychoeducational programs for families of the mentally ill. Families prefer content on "future course of the illness, medication benefits and side effects, and how to manage crisis situations with patients" (Ascher-Svanum, et al, 1997).

Families benefit not only from the information they receive in groups but also from groups that provide a high level of support. The benefits families receive from group participation are similar to the patient benefits discussed earlier. In addition, families experience less anger and improved relationships with family members as they learn new family communication skills. They also learn about available sources and how to recognize competent professional care (Heller, et al, 1997).

Therapy Groups

Therapy groups help patients to develop an understanding of and insight into their feelings, behaviors, and roles in relationships. Some groups assist patients in changing behaviors and developing healthier responses to others. Patients must want to develop awareness of their problems and be motivated and willing to change in order for therapy groups to be most beneficial. Table 15-3 lists examples of therapy groups.

Table 15-3   Therapy Groups

Type	Purpose/Nurse's Role	Examples
Insight-oriented	Facilitate an understanding of how individuals affect and are affected by others. Assists in examining role relationship issues. Helps in developing healthier ways to handle feelings and respond to others.	Process groups, survivors groups, self-esteem groups.
Psychodrama	Intense emotional release and insight are achieved through acting out intrapersonal and interpersonal conflicts. Helps patients to improvise their roles in specific situations or a script/play can be used. Support and discussion after the drama are provided by the therapist, nurse, and other patients.	Psychodrama, but may be called by other names.
Sociodrama	Focuses on solutions and insight into role communication. Specific social roles are reenacted. Feedback is given and alternative methods of communication are role-played. (Examples of roles are parent-child, worker-boss, and teacher-student.)	Sociodrama is also considered a form of psychodrama.

Self-Help or Special Problem Groups

Problem-centered groups

Numerous groups focus on helping persons with special problems; for example, child abuse, anorexia and bulimia, and diabetes. These groups are homogeneous, meaning that all group members share the same problem. Members feel accepted and understood by the group and therefore feel more free to share concerns and ask questions. Information is shared along with personal feelings and difficulties. Members assist each other with helpful strategies. They do not feel alone or isolated but learn that others with the same problem or need are coping effectively. The nurse who leads special problem groups is interested, knowledgeable, and skilled in working with the specific problem area and the specific type of patient (Van Servellen, 1983).

Traditional self-help groups

Traditional self-help groups are also homogeneous but are not professionally organized and led. Self-help groups are organized and led by group members who share a problem. Self-help is based on the belief that an individual with a problem can only be truly understood and helped by others who have the same problem. Millions of people participate in hundreds of self-help groups. In some groups, such as Alcoholics Anonymous, individual 24-hour support is available. Members of self-help groups understand each other's life-styles and needs, help each other solve problems and cope with stress, and confront each other about alcoholic behaviors.

Professionals may be invited to a self-help group for a specific purpose, such as providing an educational program. Nurses commonly refer individuals to self-help groups and need to be knowledgeable about the self-help groups in their area. Interested individuals can call their local mental health organization for information about the availability of groups such as the Alliance for the Mentally Ill, Recovery Incorporated, and Incest Survivors Anonymous.

■ Critical Thinking Question

A patient is very depressed and almost mute. Which combination of groups would you encourage this patient to attend?

GROUP LEADERSHIP

Group leadership functions range from the informal to the formal. The inpatient psychiatric nurse may engage in spontaneous, informal interactions with a group of patients in a card game or may participate formally in a planned, structured group session in a special setting. An informal card game provides the nurse with an opportunity for therapeutic interpersonal interaction, socialization, and role-modeling behavior. Another example might be responding to medication questions that come up in small informal groups; the nurse reinforces compliance with medication and may alleviate anxiety or concerns. Such informal, spontaneous interventions with groups of patients occur repeatedly during the course of a day on an inpatient unit.

Although degrees of formality and types of patients vary, the nurse invariably uses group leadership skills to meet patients' needs in the therapeutic milieu. As managers and providers of patient care (24 hours a day), nurses intervene with groups of patients. Consequently, nurses need to utilize communication skills to interact with groups of patients (described later).

Nurses on inpatient units should be aware of factors that influence the clinical setting. Short-stay inpatient hospitalization affects group work in many ways. For example, short hospitalizations create a rapid turnover of patients in groups, and it is unrealistic to expect a high level of trust and cohesion to develop. Also patients may have an assortment of serious illnesses. The nurse must quickly assess the mental status of patients to determine how soon they can enter groups or if they can tolerate a group at all. The nurse will also assess the appropriate placement of patients in specific groups based on the level of functioning and the ability to tolerate particular groups. Charting patient progress in the group is an important nursing responsibility for both therapeutic and legal reasons.

Similarly, in outpatient care and in the community factors work against group effectiveness. For example, patients may be limited to a specific number of visits because of payment providers or participation in day treatment or in substance-related programs may be limited to a specific number of days during the course of a year. These factors dilute the therapeutic potential of outpatient group work.

Confidentiality must be explained to group participants; that is, they must understand that what is said or takes place in the group must stay in the group. However, what is stated in group sessions may be shared with staff members or the treatment team since they are all responsible for patient care. Of course, information shared in the group should not leave the unit or care facility. In reality, group confidentiality can be very difficult to ensure particularly until trust and cohesion are developed.

Coleadership

An important factor to consider about group leadership, particularly on the inpatient unit, is that nurses have days off and may rotate shifts. Therefore, the presence of a coleader can lend consistency to the group and directly support its structure and purpose. Coleaders can complement each other and learn from each other. They collaborate and share responsibility for the group. If the group is large, charting and communicating information to other staff members can be expedited. In addition, one leader may observe something in the group that the other nurse may not see. Coleadership provides patients with examples of how to relate to another person with respect. A coleader may be a professional from another discipline, and it may sometimes help to have a man and a woman as coleaders. In the community, the nurse may be the only leader of education groups for patients and families.

The Physical Setting

Physical arrangements are important considerations in creating an atmosphere conducive to group work. It is often difficult to find adequate space or a private room, but this is important to ensure privacy and a quiet atmosphere. Adequate lighting, comfortable temperature, seating, and equipment also contribute to successful group function. Forming a circle of chairs allows patients to see each other and indicates an expectation that patients will relate to leaders and to each other. Chairs in rows may be appropriate for a didactic group. A blackboard, a dry marker board, a projector, or a VCR may be necessary. Handouts or printed materials may be used for patients and families.

Formal Groups

Nurse leaders must be active, structured, and empathetic. Because of time constraints, leaders cannot afford to be nondirective or to allow the group to be free floating. The nurse must be goal-directed and focus on the here and now in each inpatient or outpatient group session. The nurse assesses the needs of the patients and formulates a realistic goal for that session. Each session should be treated as a separate entity with the patient feeling that something positive was attained during group (Yalom, 1995). The formal group should meet for about an hour. The leader succinctly states the group's purpose at the beginning of the session, and most of the session is spent on the work to be accomplished. Patients generally prefer leaders who provide the group "with an active structure" (Yalom, 1995). The final 5 to 10 minutes is used to summarize and close the session. The summary should have a positive focus and include what the patients have learned or gained from the group. The leader gives positive feedback to the group on how well they have done during the session.

Patients are expected to arrive at the group session on time. Depending on the patient's level of functioning, the group leader may gather the members of the group and walk with them into the room. No smoking or refreshments are permitted during group sessions. Patients remain for the entire group session if possible. The group leader may permit patients to pace or leave the room and then return when they are able. The inability to sit still for a period of time may be due to anxiety or to drug side effects (usually, akathisia). The decision to exclude patients from the group should be made carefully. The nurse may exclude patients who are acutely manic, disoriented, too psychotic to benefit from group therapy, or those who will disrupt the group. Patients who are hostile and verbally threatening are also not appropriate candidates for group therapy.

Interventions

Basic interventions for groups are based on facilitative communication techniques (see Chapter 10). Nurses use these skills with patients individually and with groups. Nurses who facilitate group interactions on a therapeutic level enable patients to share feelings and problems. Some basic communication skills useful for nurse leaders are found in Table 15-4. These skills are not unique to the group

Table 15-4   Communication Skills: Eliciting, Qualifying, and Clarifying Communication

Techniques of the Leader(s)	Group Member Response	Outcome
1. **Giving information:** "My purpose in offering this group experience is . . ."	**Further validates** his assumptions: "How is this going to happen?"	Leader(s) and member(s) enter into a dialogue in which member(s) get more information to make decisions and build trust in group experience.
2. **Seeking clarification:** "Did you say you were upset with John because he said that?"	**May try to restate** his thoughts or feelings: "Yes, I guess I was upset."	Member becomes aware that he was not clear and learns to identify thoughts and feelings more precisely, at the same time taking responsibility for them.
3. **Encouraging description and exploration** (delving further into communication or experiences): "How did you feel when Joann said that to you?"	**Elaborates** on his message: "I was angry."	Member deals in greater depth with an experience in the group and again takes responsibility for his reactions. (This example also places events in time or in sequence lending further perspective to group events.)
4. **Presenting reality:** "Would other members think Joann was unstable if they interviewed her for a job? You don't appear shaky to me."	**Listens and considers** other possibilities.	Member compares perception of self with others' perceptions of him.
5. **Seeking consensual validation** (seeking mutual understanding of what is being communicated): "Did I understand you to say that you feel better now than you did last week?"	**Further clarification:** "Well, yes, I'm better than last week but not as good as I'd like to be."	Group and leader(s) learn how member views his progress and in which way they should receive his evaluation of himself.

From Van Servellen G: *Group and family therapy*, St. Louis, 1983, Mosby.   *Continued*

Table 15-4 **Communication Skills: Eliciting, Qualifying, and Clarifying Communication—cont'd**

Techniques of the Leader(s)	Group Member Response	Outcome
6. **Focusing** (identifying a single topic to concentrate on): "Maybe we could identify one problem you have and talk more about that."	**Channels thinking:** Members may think of the most puzzling problem they have.	Group and leader(s) identify specific topics they can resolve before the meeting ends. They increase their understanding of one problem before jumping to others.
7. **Encouraging comparison** (asking members to compare and contrast their experiences with others in the group): "How did the rest of the group handle this problem?"	**Group members share their experiences** as they relate to the topic.	Leader(s) and members gain greater insight into their commonalities and differences and learn from one another alternative ways of responding to problems.
8. **Making observations:** "You look more comfortable now, John, than you did at the beginning of the meeting."	**Group members have something to respond to:** "I feel more at ease now."	Group members and leader(s) place attention on significant events and can elaborate on their meanings.
or	or	
"The group has been silent for the last 5 minutes."	"I think we are quiet because we are bored."	
9. **Giving recognition or acknowledging:** "John, you are new to the group. Perhaps we can introduce ourselves."	**Feels acknowledged and included:** "Yes, I'm John, and I came here because . . ."	Members view specific instances as important and the leaders reinforce the behavior or event they choose to notice; in this case, the desire to come to group.
10. **Accepting** (not necessarily agreeing with but receiving communication with openness): "Yes, I hear you say that you don't know if you want to be in the group or not."	**Feels heard and understood** without fear or attack.	Members learn that even "nonacceptable" attitudes can be talked about and perhaps any thought is not so horrible that they cannot share it.
11. **Encouraging evaluation** (asking the group as a whole or individual members to judge their experiences): "When Marilyn gives you support do you feel better?"	**Members reflect** on progress made: "Not exactly, because I don't know if I can trust her to be honest."	The criteria for success become clearer to members and new directions may be formulated as a result of the discussion.
or	or	
"How did we do in helping Joann with her problem?"	"It was hard. I'd like to know from her."	
12. **Summarizing** (encapsulating in a few sentences what has occurred): "The group discussed several issues and problems today–they were . . ."	**Members recall** significant points and close off consideration of new or extraneous topics.	Members and leader(s) place events in perspective, identifying salient points of a group session. Such a summary can lead to a better understanding of group process.

setting; they are skills nurses use on a daily basis. These general interventions are therapeutic regardless of the type of group. The use of positive feedback helps patients in their attempt to use new skills. For example, in an attempt to use a particular assertiveness skill, the patient goes off on a tangent. The nurse can say, "You have done well, Mr. J. When you gave us the example of saying to your boss, 'I need to talk with you about my work schedule,' you used an excellent example of 'I' statements." The nurse chooses to repeat the portion of Mr. J.'s statement that is realistic and is a correct example of an "I" statement for emphasis and clarity. As a result the patient feels a sense of accomplishment and increased self-esteem.

Dominant patient

The dominant patient monopolizes the entire group session to the extent that other patients may feel that they do not have the opportunity to participate. The nurse employs gatekeeping functions to offer all patients the opportunity to contribute to the group. For example, the nurse can say, "Miss B., you are doing well in contributing to our session today, but I would like to hear what others are thinking about at this time." This intervention can forestall monopolization of the group by a single patient without putting her down so that others have the opportunity to express themselves. The other patients in the group may be unable to handle this patient or may be too afraid. If the group leader is afraid or cannot control the patient, the integrity of the group is compromised.

Uninvolved patient

The uninvolved patient presents another challenge to the nurse leader. The patient may be quiet because of anxiety or fear. As patients become more comfortable in the group, their ability to participate verbally increases (Van Servellen, 1983). Chronic schizophrenics find it difficult and threatening to relate in group sessions. The nurse can say, "It is hard to talk about ourselves in group, but I know that everyone here has something to share that can help someone else." The nurse recognizes that patients are mistrustful and anxious but relates the message that each individual is important and capable of helping another.

Patients who are uninvolved in the group may believe themselves to be at a higher level of functioning than the other members. They may feel they are not as sick as the others, do not belong in group, and will not benefit from it. The nurse leader may give attention to such members by giving them a job to perform for the group; for example, recording suggestions (Pollack, 1991). Respect and recognition by the nurse is therapeutic for these patients because they will feel they can contribute to group.

Critical Thinking Question

During a group session on problem solving, a patient states, "I learn more by listening." How and why would you involve this patient in the group discussion?

Hostile patient

Hostility may mask a patient's fear, self-anger, or unresolved anger toward others. To help this patient appropriately verbalize what the anger is all about, the nurse can say, "Mrs. R., you sound angry today. What happened?" Or "Tell us about it." The nurse directly confronts the patient in a supportive manner and attempts to help the patient deal with her feelings. Allowing nonverbal or verbal hostility to continue jeopardizes the progress of the group session. Unchecked hostility causes discomfort and uneasiness, and impairs the ability of other patients to attend to the group's work. Patients may also mistakenly interpret anger as being directed toward them.

These group interventions will help the nurse develop as a group leader. Patients quickly recognize the group leader's empathy, understanding, and respect for each patient as caring behaviors. Even though some patients make only minimal progress toward their individual treatment goals, they can increase their feelings of worth as human beings by interacting with the nurse who possesses these traits.

Critical Thinking Question

A member of the group states, "This group is a waste of time. I don't get anything out of it." Which communication skills would you use in this situation?

Key Concepts

1. The psychiatric nurse interacts and intervenes with patients and families in informal groups as well as in formal structured sessions in inpatient and community settings.
2. Patients benefit from group experiences by gaining acceptance, hopefulness, and support from others. Through mutual sharing of feelings and problems, patients learn how their communication methods and behaviors interfere with relationships. Their strengths are reinforced and built upon.

3. Families of the mentally ill benefit from the information and support they receive in a group.
4. Nurse leaders must be active, empathetic, goal-directed, and deal with the here and now in each group session.
5. Various types of groups exist in inpatient and outpatient settings to benefit the acutely and chronically ill. Typical types are support, remotivation, education and problem solving, therapy, and self-help or special problem groups. Support and educational groups exist for families of the mentally ill.
6. Nurses use facilitative communication techniques and role-modeling behaviors as group leaders.
7. The nurse leader intervenes therapeutically with dominating, uninvolved, and hostile patients.

Study Questions

(Answer key is in the back of the book.)

1. The leadership functions of the psychiatric nurse are:
   a. Observed only in formal, planned, and structured group meetings.
   b. Seldom demonstrated on an inpatient unit.
   c. Inherent in the role of a psychotherapeutic manager.
   d. Utilized only in an outpatient setting.
2. Which of the following statements best describes how patients benefit from groups?
   a. Patients gain support from the group leader only.
   b. Patients can test out new behaviors when discharged.
   c. Patients' feelings of powerlessness are not addressed.
   d. Patients learn how their behaviors affect others.

Match each of the following groups with its appropriate description.

3. _____ Support group   a. Helps patients to cope and negotiate problems in living
4. _____ Activity group
5. _____ Education or problem-solving group   b. Reinforces patients' strengths and behaviors
   c. Facilitates communication and interaction among group members

6. A patient has been monopolizing the group for the past 10 minutes about how her doctor has treated her unfairly. The most appropriate response to this patient is:
   a. "You are taking up too much of the group's time."
   b. To say nothing and let the patient continue.
   c. "I think patients in this group are getting bored with this discussion."
   d. "You are doing well in contributing to our session today, but I would like to hear what others are thinking."

REFERENCES

Ascher-Svanum H, et al: Educational needs of families of mentally ill adults, *Psychiatr Serv* 48(8):1072, 1997.

Elmore J and Young D: Modular group therapy in a community mental health center, *Psychiatr Serv* 47(12):1390, 1996.

Heller T, et al: Benefits of support groups for families of adults with severe mental illness, *Am J Orthopsychiatry* 67(2):187, 1997.

Hughes K and Ashby C: Essential components of the short-term psychiatric unit, *Perspect Psychiatr Care* 32(1): 20, 1996.

Pollack L: Problem-solving group therapy: two inpatient models based on level of functioning, *Issues Ment Health Nurs* 12:65, 1991.

Van Servellen G: *Group and family therapy,* St. Louis, 1983, Mosby.

Yalom I: *The theory and practice of group psychotherapy,* ed 4, New York, 1995, Basic Books.

CHAPTER 16

Working with the Family

RUTH P. COX

LEARNING OBJECTIVES

After reading this chapter you should be able to:
- Discuss the benefits and problems associated with including families in the care of psychiatric inpatients.
- Define the term *family* and describe common family compositions.
- List the factors to assess when working with families.
- Describe the effects of mental illness on families.

- Describe useful theoretical approaches to working with families.
- Describe the principles for therapeutic interactions with families.
- Describe the skills necessary for working with families.
- Identify the issues that commonly arise when families visit inpatient units.

The family has been the unit of socialization of all cultures throughout the generations. It is the institution for procreation; child rearing; physical and emotional care, love, and affection; maintenance of self-esteem; and the transference of cultural values and beliefs (Reinhard, 1994). An individual's hopes, attitudes, and aspirations are influenced by the early years with the family. Over the past four decades, treatment has shifted from the individual as a single unit to viewing the individual within the context of the family system. Today, nurses work with patients *and* their families to solve mental health problems.

This chapter presents characteristics of families, the effects of mental illness on families, major family theories, and issues of working with families on inpatient units. The emphasis in this chapter is

the understanding and assessment of families as a basis for brief therapeutic interactions, family conferences, education, support, and referrals.

HISTORICAL EVOLUTION OF WORKING WITH THE FAMILY

The first half of the twentieth century was dominated by the psychoanalytical view that therapy should focus only on the individual. Families typically were seen as the cause of mental illness and were alienated by mental health professionals. With the growing knowledge of neurochemical bases of mental illnesses (Grinspoon, 1993a) and less emphasis on psychoanalytical theory, attitudes of professionals toward families have improved. At the same time, it has become clear that many psychiatric patients struggle with issues arising from dysfunctional families and that these issues are appropriately addressed within a family context rather than in isolation.

Deinstitutionalization of state hospitals and insufficient services for outpatient care have increased the responsibilities of families for care of the mentally ill. The National Alliance for the Mentally Ill (NAMI) and other groups have appropriately advocated for the rights of patients and their families, including the need for information on the effectiveness of various services and treatments, the risks and benefits of treatments, and the relationship of costs to the benefits of services (Hatfield, 1990; Grinspoon, 1992a).

FAMILIAL CHARACTERISTICS TO BE ASSESSED

Definition of Family

A *family* is usually defined as two or more persons who reside together; share economic resources; are related by birth, marriage, or adoption; and/or who have a commitment to each other over time (F. Walsh, 1993). Even family pets may be considered "members of the family" (Cox, 1993). Table 16-1 provides definitions of the various types of families.

Individuals may move in and out of various "families" in a lifetime. For example, a woman may leave her family of origin to live with a roommate prior to marrying and creating a nuclear family. A divorce may lead the woman and her baby to move back in with her family of origin for a short time. She may then move out on her own as a single parent and later remarry, forming a blended family. Patients may have unresolved issues related to any or all of the "families" in which they have been involved.

Family Tasks

As a group, families have certain tasks that must be accomplished and that directly or indirectly contribute to the mental health or mental illness of family members. Duvall and Miller (1985) described eight basic tasks of the family as follows:
1. Physical maintenance and safety
2. Allocation of resources: meeting family needs and costs; apportioning materials, facilities, space, and authority
3. Division of labor
4. Socialization of family members
5. Reproduction and release of family members
6. Maintenance of order, authority, and decision making
7. Placement of members into the larger society (school, church, organizations, work, politics)
8. Maintenance of motivation and morale; encouragement and affection; meeting personal and family crises; refining a philosophy of life and family loyalty through rituals

Stages of Family Development

Family tasks may be carried out in different ways or with difficulty, depending on the stage of family development (Duvall and Miller, 1985):
1. Beginning families (married couple)
2. Early childbearing families (oldest child age 30 months)
3. Families with preschool children (oldest child age 2 to 5 years)

Table 16-1 Family Compositions

Type	Definition
1. Nuclear	Two-generational; married couple with children by birth or adoption
2. Nuclear dyad	A married couple who are childless or whose children are not living at home
3. Extended	A nuclear family and other relatives, whether by birth, adoption, or marriage
4. Alternative	Adults of a single generation or a combination of adults and children who live together without the social sanction of marriage (e.g., communal arrangement or roommates who are heterosexual or homosexual)
5. Single parent	One adult left alone with children due to death, separation, divorce, or abandonment; single adult with adopted child
6. Blended/step	Remarriage in which a parent, stepparent, children, and/or stepchildren live together

4. Families with schoolchildren (oldest child age 6 to 13 years)
5. Families with teenagers (oldest child age 13 to 20 years)
6. Launching center families (children leaving home)
7. Families of middle years (empty nest through retirement)
8. Families in retirement and old age (retirement until the death of both spouses)

It is important to know the stage of family development in order to assess whether or not the tasks for that stage are being accomplished appropriately (McGoldrick, Heiman, and Carter, 1993). A family may experience different stages at the same time. For example, a blended family, involved with children leaving home, may reenter the school-age stage when the couple blends into one family. Families who cope with several stages at once may need extra support to successfully negotiate the changes.

Functional/Healthy Family Characteristics

The ability to cope with constant life changes and stress stems from skills learned in the family. Characteristics have been identified that affect the development of competent, healthy individuals who are able to maintain a mentally healthy life-style (Beavers, 1977; Kelly, 1978). Table 16-2 specifies healthy family characteristics. The way individuals apply the skills learned in the family to manage life changes determines relative mental wellness. If individuals leave the family with healthy communication, high self-esteem, few unresolved issues, and a hopefulness about the world, their relationships have greater potential to be healthy. If individuals prematurely or suddenly leave their family in an effort to deal with unresolved family conflict, or leave at the appropriate time but with unresolved issues (incest or abuse), future relationships may be adversely affected. Relationships with and within the family also may be adversely affected.

Problematic Family Characteristics

Families with difficulties often produce individuals with inadequate relationship skills, mental health problems, behavior disorders, troubled relationships, or psychiatric disorders (Beavers, 1977; Kelly,

1978). Table 16-3 lists characteristics of families with problems.

Individuals who come from unhealthy families, or who leave their family of origin with unresolved issues and carry these issues and problems into a new family, may seek out a person with whom they can work through these unresolved issues or past relationship problems (Dicks, 1967; Scharff and Scharff, 1991; Grinspoon, 1993b). For example, adult children from alcoholic family systems may transport the unresolved problems and the same difficult relationship patterns from their family of origin into their new family. Survivors of incest and other abuse in the family of origin often experience marital problems in their new family. In assessing a family, the nurse must discern whether the problem lies only within the present family, is part of an unresolved issue from the family of origin, or is a combination of both.

OTHER ASPECTS TO BE ASSESSED

Effects of Mental Illness on the Family

Mental illness is a particularly traumatic stressor that can precipitate a family crisis or decompensation (Hatfield, 1990). Stress models (see Chapter 3) and crisis models (see Chapter 13) can be useful in evaluating a family's unique responses to a mentally ill member, family members' perspectives of what it is like to live with this situation, and their ability to cope with it. It is helpful to get together family members and others who have concerns about the patient in order to gather information about the situation. Typical effects encountered by families with a mentally ill member are described in Box 16-1 on page 186. Additionally, families may have to deal with other institutions outside of the family, such as schools, law officers, court officials, community agencies, and religious/spiritual organizations. The effects on families or their individual members must be assessed. (Hatfield and Letley, 1993).

In addition to these effects of mental illness, families must learn to cope with patients' behaviors and problems. Some of the most common difficulties that families report are as follows (Hatfield, 1990; Hellwig, 1993; Reinhard, 1994):

- The patient's conflict between dependence and independence
- Side effects of medication

Table 16-2   Healthy Family Characteristics and Components

Characteristic	Component
1. Open-system orientation	Events have multiple causes
	Need for each other and other people
	Flexible and open
2. Boundaries	Well defined, but open boundaries
	Appropriate touching
	Family members interact face to face
	Privacy is provided for members in the household
	Links to society: work, school, church, friends, community
3. Contextual clarity	Clear generational lines
	Strong parental coalition
	Maintenance of marital relationship
	Communication is clear, honest, direct, specific, and congruent
4. Power	Maintained in the parental dyad
	Delegated to children as appropriate
	Roles clearly defined: members know and agree on the performance of activities
	Not defined by gender
	Well defined and respected rules
5. Encouragement of autonomy	Acceptance of differences
	Encouragement to express ideas that differ from family's
	Members' idiosyncrasies are tolerated with good humor
6. Affective	Members have empathy, warmth, and caring for each other
	Feelings are attended to
	Level of conflict is low
	Resolution of conflict occurs without loss of self-esteem
	High self-esteem of members
7. Negotiation and task performance	Led by parents at family meetings
	Input from all members
	Parents make final decisions
	Little conflict
	No significant deviance in school or work performance, or in relationships with others
8. Transcendent values	Expect, prepare for, and recover from loss
	Hopeful, positive outlook
	Altruism
	Concern for the environment
9. Health measures	Healthful diet
	Nonuse of alcohol and drugs
	Regular exercise and recreation
	Absence of dangerous activities
	No significant health problems

Adapted from Beavers W: *Psychotherapy and growth: a family systems perspective,* New York, 1977, Brunner/Mazel; Kelly A: *Evaluating and improving family health: the holistic health handbook,* Berkeley, Calif, 1978, And/Or Press.

Table 16-3   Problematic Family Characteristics and Components

Characteristic	Component
1. Open-system orientation	Absent: members need others for certain circumstances
	Believe there are specific causes for events and search for answers
	Strive to do well
	Family may appear rigid or disordered
2. Boundaries	May appear clear, but when under pressure, members turn inward and solidify boundaries, or problems spill into the environment
	Intrasystem interaction is restricted and distancing may be prevalent
	Links to society may be present, but disrupt under pressure
	May appear rigid with few links to society
	Interpersonal boundaries may be diffuse with the whole family responding to outside input
	Links to society may be tentative and mistrustful, with limited input from larger society
3. Contextual clarity	Parental coalition present, but weak and ineffective as undermined by other coalitions
	Parents may reach across generational boundaries for comfort and support, often forming unhealthy triangles
	The child who is "triangled" is often the symptom bearer for the family, and responds with mental or physical illnesses, or delinquent behavior
	Stifling and stereotyping of sexual expression; overt or covert incestuous situations may be present
	Communication may be clear at times, but expressed with fear, guilt, or anger
	Communication: not clear, honest, or specific; incongruence between verbal and nonverbal communication; double-bind communications; failure to attend to messages; disqualification through silence, ignoring, evasiveness, or changing the subject
	Anger may be expressed through hitting and other abuse
4. Power	Power and love may be confused as members are controlled through overt or covert coercion, or through "oughts" or "shoulds" that are often stereotyped by gender
	Parents try to get children to "do the right thing" through discipline or coercion
	Children learn power through manipulation rather than learning responsibility
	Roles are defined by gender or beliefs about the person; family behaves as if they are being judged for rightness of actions and beliefs
	Power may be diffuse and does not come from parents
5. Encouragement of autonomy	Not found, or discouraged
	Children are expected to adhere to family norms and power struggles are constant
	Suppression of feelings and creativity
	Children may stay at home well into adulthood or leave early (pseudoautonomy)
	Differences not tolerated, but family identifies a member as "different" and as the cause of the trouble
6. Affective issues	Depression, anxiety, and anger, with resulting conflict expressed openly, or repressed with submission to "oughts" and "shoulds"
	Little empathy shown
	A lot of conflict over rules and family norms
	Caring is controlling rather than growth producing
	Members' self-esteem is low
	Hate, loneliness, and hopelessness are predominant
	With diffuse boundaries: affective tone is exaggerated; members react inappropriately to threats or to one member's difficulties
	With rigid boundaries: affective tone is restricted, depressed, and despairing
	Undue attention (confusing, smothering, and rejecting) is shown to one member

Adapted from Beavers W: *Psychotherapy and growth: a family systems perspective,* New York, 1977, Brunner/Mazel; Kelly A: *Evaluating and improving family health: the holistic health handbook,* Berkeley, Calif, 1978, And/Or Press.

Continued

Table 16-3   Problematic Family Characteristics and Components—cont'd

Characteristic	Component
7. Negotiation and task performance	Accomplished by coercion as parents cannot agree on who does what
	No family meetings, but work is accomplished
	Negotiation is not accomplished
	Tasks vary widely
	With diffuse boundaries: conflict may be overt, constant, and unresolved
	With rigid boundaries: conflict is denied, ignored, and unresolved
8. Transcendent values	Hope and altruism are lacking; change and loss are accepted with enormous pain, anger, and frustration
	Martyrdom may be a stance
	Expect difficulties in the future rather than being hopeful
	Intolerance of loss or differences
	Cynical, hopeless outlook
9. Health measures	Excessive use of alcohol and nonprescription and prescription drugs to relieve the pain of daily living
	Psychophysiological illnesses (headaches, ulcers, obesity, eating disorders)
	Only basic health needs are met
	No health promotion or wellness activities
	Attempts at recreation and exercise, but conflict often occurs when making plans
	Sometimes high anger level leads to hitting, driving at excessive speeds, or running away
	Serious physical illness, usually in one member

Box 16-1   Effects of Mental Illness on the Family

- Denial, anger, fear, worry, sadness, resentment, frustration, grief, sense of betrayal, shame, guilt, perception of being blamed
- Deprivation or loss of dreams, hopes, potential, expectations
- Decline in sense of self-worth and self-esteem
- Threat to security, well-being, safety, control, predictability
- Loss of confidence, integrity, optimism
- Financial strain from costs of treatment, medications
- Decline in income due to absenteeism, unemployment
- Decline in leisure and social activities
- Problems in school
- Increased intergenerational stress
- Decline in social support due to stigmatization
- Threats to physical health due to emotional strain
- Alterations in family interactions, shifts in roles, conflicts
- Need for new or modified decision making, communication, stress management, and coping strategies
- Changes in intimacy and in sexual relationships
- Prolonged parenting or caregiving of an adult child
- Interactions with numerous agency personnel: hospital, aftercare, rehabilitation, insurance, financial, disability, vocational
- Worry about future care of the patient as the caregiver ages

Adapted from Gillis CL: Family nursing research: theory and practice, *Image J Nurs Sch* 23(1):19, 1991; Griffin-Francell C: Psychiatric nurses must be held accountable for their actions, *J Psychosoc Nurs Ment Health Serv* 31(10):5, 1993; Hatfield AB: Incorporating the family's contribution to clinical training. In Letley H, editor: *Clinical training in serious mental illness,* Washington, DC, 1991, National Institute of Mental Health; Koontz E, Cox D, Hasting S: Implementing a short-term family support group, *J Psychosoc Nurs Ment Health Serv* 29(5):5, 1991; Reinhard SC: Perspective on the family's caregiving experience in mental illness, *Image J Nurs Sch* 26(1):71, 1984; Sayles-Cross S: Perceptions of familial caregivers of elder adults, *Image J Nurs Sch* 25(2):88, 1993.

- Noncompliance with medication and treatment
- Bizarre behaviors and communications
- Poor or absent activities of daily living (ADLs)
- Exploitative and provocative behaviors
- Lack of cooperation
- Persistent avoidance behaviors
- Lack of insight; denial; poor judgment
- Social isolation
- Suicidal ideation and attempts
- Hostile, threatening, and abusive behaviors
- Moodiness
- Intrusiveness

Mental illness also causes a disruption in the stages of family development (Doornbos, 1997). Families who experience severe mental illness must come to terms with the loss of an expectation of a productive individual and family life. Saunders (1997) suggests that this loss is actual as well as symbolic.

Reasons for Seeking Family Treatment

Mental illness, relationship problems, and conflict in families can be addressed in several ways (Bowen, 1978; Kerr, 1981). The problems and conflict can (1) be kept between two persons, (2) cause other persons to develop physical illnesses or social acting-out behaviors, (3) cause persons to emotionally distance themselves from each other, or (4) lead to a third person (often a child), pet, or object being "triangled" into the conflict to reduce the tension. The one who is triangled may be labeled as the "person with the problem," rather than the family admitting to the "family problem." The person who is triangled may exhibit disruptive behavior, such as school difficulties, delinquency, and health problems. When families or their individual members can no longer deal with the difficulties, they often seek help for their problems. The person who seeks help provides a valuable family function, as that person becomes the *reason* the family seeks assistance. It is possible that the "identified patient" is not mentally ill and, when the family issues are settled or the illness treated, the person's functioning returns to normal.

The family may have different explanations for or reactions to seeking treatment for family problems. For example, the family may:

- Define the problem as belonging to the "identified patient," but still participate in the treatment
- Have great concern that a family secret of some sort (e.g., incest) may be exposed and avoid treatment
- Identify the existence of a more socially acceptable problem (depression), although a more severe problem exists (spouse abuse) that the family is not willing to discuss
- Be divided in accepting responsibility for the problem and in recognizing the need for treatment
- Not want to be involved with the treatment of the identified patient in any manner

Each problem a patient presents requires a judgment about whether or not it should be approached within the family context. During the family assessment, the nurse must assess for individual problems, such as suicidal, homicidal, or other risky behaviors, in each member. The following situations are common ones for which a family assessment and intervention are desirable:

- A situational crisis causes emotional disruption (e.g., bankruptcy, death, injury).
- A developmental crisis causes emotional disruption (e.g., birth, youngest child leaving home, marriage).
- The family defines a problem as a family issue that needs assistance (e.g., a member diagnosed with mental illness).
- Conflicts exist in family relationships (e.g., partner, elder, or child abuse).
- The patient has difficulty coping with a dysfunctional family or ongoing abuse.
- The family of origin and the present family of a patient are in conflict.
- Mentally ill members of the family of origin and/or the present family create problems for the patient.
- A divorce creates issues to be resolved (e.g., custody, settlements, harassment).
- New members join the family (e.g., adoption, stepparent, stepchildren).
- Treatment goals are undermined by the family.
- The patient is pressured to obtain early discharge to fulfill household responsibilities.
- The patient is pressured to keep family secrets.
- Family members talk with nurses about issues they are not willing to share in family sessions.
- Family members need assistance in talking about sensitive family issues, such as sexuality or alcoholism.

- One spouse attempts to get the other spouse admitted and "labeled" to gain an advantage in a custody battle.
- The family wants the patient to stay sick to continue to get social security/disability/Medicaid on which the family depends financially.
- The patient or family attempts to conspire with staff against other family members.

There are situations that may interfere with or complicate family assessment. A patient may seek independence from the family, and initial involvement of the family may compromise this process. A patient may be too suspicious of family members to participate in a family interview. The family may believe the interview will be damaging to them (for example, fearing an abuse report will be made). Finally, the family may have abandoned the patient completely.

■ Critical Thinking Question

Nursing has always had a family focus, but nurses have not always been encouraged to work with families. What actions can you take to expand the implementation of holistic nursing care?

Family Reactions to Psychiatric Hospitalization

An initial psychiatric admission may be experienced by patients and their families in several ways. They may be devastated or relieved that a family member has been admitted to a psychiatric unit. They may have divergent views: the patient wants help, but the family does not want the patient admitted; the patient wants to be admitted, but not to a psychiatric unit; the patient does not want others to know about the admission; the family wants the patient admitted, but the patient has to be involuntarily committed; or the family and/or others (friends, neighbors, employer) want the patient admitted, and coercion for admission is used.

Infrequent admissions for acute episodes of illness or relationship problems may not be too problematic for some families. If the patient and family have had a long period of constructively addressing problems within the family system, the family may be more eager to engage in family-level problem

solving. If admissions occur chronically, however, the family may experience "burnout." When stress in the family is high, the family may want to admit the identified patient to gain some relief for the family system. Done appropriately (e.g., through a respite day care program), admission for this reason may be helpful to the entire family system. However, a family may inappropriately hospitalize a patient under the guise that the patient is having problems. For example, when the patient begins to confront issues appropriately and tension rises, the family may report that the patient is not taking medication as directed and therefore is having "problem behaviors" again.

Family reactions to psychiatric admissions may be mixed when the admission occurs because of abuse or assault within the family. Some members may experience relief that something has finally been done; others may experience anger, rejection, or humiliation from exposure of the abuse. Some members may be fearful of what the future holds once the abuse is exposed, or that legal action will be taken.

In summary, the nurse must be ready to accept a variety of reasons for and reactions to hospital admission. In each instance, the nurse's responsibility is to respond therapeutically to reactions expressed by patients and family members.

THEORETICAL BASIS FOR FAMILY ASSESSMENT AND INTERACTIONS

Brief Family Nursing Interactions vs. Family Therapy

Interest in the study, treatment, and evaluation of families has increased in all health professions. Both brief family interactions and family therapy are within the scope of professional nursing practice; the nature of the nurse's education and professional licensure/credentials influences the choice. All nurses are generally qualified to conduct brief therapeutic interactions with families and individual patients. Family therapy requires preparation through special certification programs and/or a master's degree.

All nurses need a holistic, contextual view of patients' problems in order to take advantage of opportunities to participate in family-level problem solving and change. The triangle of family health (Figure 16-1) provides a context to understand inter-

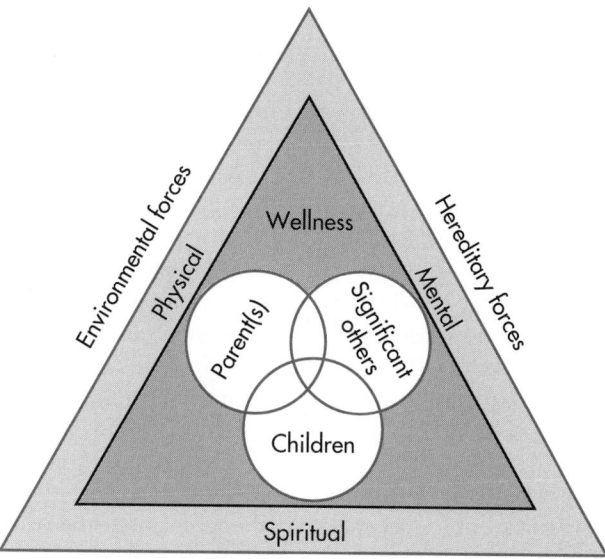

FIGURE 16-1   Triangle of family health

nal and external factors that can affect families and the potential for family change. When working for family change, brief family interventions are more useful now due to the usual short hospitalization of family members.

Using Theories for Family Assessment and Interactions

The nurse who works with patients and their families encounters many different ideas about the components of the problems. Theories help to guide the nurse in family assessments and interactions by providing a framework to contextualize the numerous pieces of information collected about patients and their families (Fawcett, 1989). In working with families, the nurse must choose theories that best explain family situations and that suggest effective nursing goals and interventions (Fawcett, 1989). General systems theory (Bertalanffy, 1968) provides a framework for viewing the relationships between the parts of the family system. Bowen's family systems theory (1978) and the collective language systems approach (Anderson, 1991a; Anderson and Goolishian, 1988) are theoretical bases that can be useful for nursing assessment and intervention.

General systems theory

General systems theory (Bertalanffy, 1968) presents a view in which the organization of the interactive patterns of a system's parts are more important than the component parts of a system. According to Bertalanffy, to understand how something works, we must study the transactional processes occurring between the components of a system, not add up what each part contributes. The following concepts from systems theory may be useful in understanding how an individual fits within his or her family and in understanding the family itself.

- A family system is part of a larger supersystem, composed of many subsystems.
- The family whole is greater than the sum of its parts.
- A change in one family member affects all family members.
- The family is able to create a balance between change and stability.
- Family members' behaviors are best understood as being influenced by many interactions among family members rather than just one direct cause—this is called circular causality (Wright and Leahey, 1994).

Bowen family systems theory

Bowen offers a natural systems theory in which the family is seen as an evolutionary process in nature (Bowen, 1978; Goldenberg and Goldenberg, 1991). Bowen viewed the family as an emotional unit of interlocking relationships that is best understood within its multigenerational context. According to Kerr (1981), Bowen's family systems theory has eight interlocking concepts:

1. Differentiation of self: the extent to which a person can distinguish between experienced intellectual and feeling processes
2. Triangles: at a certain level of intensity, a third person is pulled into a relationship to dilute anxiety
3. Nuclear family emotional system: the fusion of a marital couple's emotional processes that becomes unstable over time
4. Family projection process: parents select the most infantile child as the object of their attention
5. Emotional cutoff: flight from unresolved emotional ties with the family, not true emancipation
6. Multigenerational transmission process: severe dysfunction as the result of the operation of a family emotional system for several generations
7. Sibling position: interactive patterns between marital partners related to their position in the family of origin
8. Societal regression: societal erosion of the forces intent on achieving individuation

When the nurse talks with a family while employing Bowen's family systems theory, the nurse might ask the following questions: "How did each of you in the family deal with Mary's hospitalization?" (differentiation of each family member); "Steve, when you are upset with Gail because she seems more distant and depressed, whom do you talk to in the family?" (triangles); "Gail, what was your reason for leaving home when you were 14 years old?" (emotional cutoff).

Collective language systems approach

This approach views human beings as language-generating, meaning-generating systems engaged in social conversations that are constantly changing, creative, and dynamic (Anderson, 1991a; 1991b).

All words carry unspoken meanings and possible new interpretations that require expression and articulation. In this area of what is "unexpressed," there is the opportunity for evolutionary change in meaning.

Therapeutic interactions with patients and their families is a process of expanding and expressing what has been "the unsaid." Through this dialogue come new ideas, themes, and narratives that create new solutions for problems. Other descriptions and meanings will emerge that are *not* labeled as "problems." In brief, episodic encounters, the nurse can empower families to create new solutions to their present problems (Cox and Davis, 1993).

The collective language systems approach suggests the following questions: "Steve, you have some thoughts about the relationship between Gail, your mother, and your increased anxiety level that you have not shared with us. What would need to happen for you to talk about those ideas here?"; "Gail, what have you been able to do that has been helpful to you in dealing with Mary's depression that you have not talked about with Steve?"

Skills for Working with the Family

To work constructively with patients and their families, the generalist nurse must possess the following skills: self-knowledge skills; assessment skills; therapeutic communication skills; spiritual skills; collaboration skills; and skills regarding referrals, family support, and resources.

Self-knowledge skills

The nurse must be able to identify and own his or her thoughts, beliefs, feelings, actions, and biases. The nurse should become aware of his or her own family dynamics to preclude confusing personal issues with those of patients and their families. The nurse must also attend to personal coping skills, such as exercise, nurturance, and support from colleagues and friends.

Assessment skills

It is important for the nurse to constantly resist the view of one family member as "the problem." Instead, view systematically the interactions *between* all family members as sources for family problem solving. The family is viewed as a collaborative partner with the nurse in problem solving and decision making. As the nurse uses a family assessment guide effectively and efficiently, the most complete information can be available to both the nurse and family as decisions are made based on families' self-discovery of strengths and resources. In this manner, all aspects of information gathering are "'family perceived' as well as 'professional perceived'. The intent of the partnership here is to clarify discrepant views and to discover fresh alternatives for action" (Lapp, Diemert, and Enestvedt, 1993).

Therapeutic communication skills

Therapeutic interactions should be based on family-oriented beliefs, such as the beliefs that families are functioning the best that they can; that families can solve their own problems; that strengths exist in all families; that no one is to blame for the family problems; and that people act in unconstructive ways when protecting and shielding themselves from painful interactions. Family interviewing skills include the ability to interact simultaneously with all family members, with equal amounts of respect and nonjudgment, while focusing on the stated problem (e.g., when one family member has been identified as the perpetrator of violent acts). Attention must be given to observing the interactions *between* members of the system, rather than focusing on the actions of one individual. All information is taken seriously, no matter how astonishing, trivial, or peculiar it seems. Arriving at conclusions about family system problems too quickly may prevent the creation of new meanings and change. Questions are used to bring forth new ideas that connect with other new ideas and form solutions to problems. Facilitation of *multiple* views about the problem maximizes the creation of new meaning. Negotiation and change are possible as new information is exposed within the family dialogue.

The nurse needs knowledge of various teaching strategies and learning principles because all families do not learn information in the same way.

Spiritual skills

Families have identified that facilitative attitudes are one method of coping with a mentally ill member (Doornbos, 1997). Facilitative attitudes included tolerance, patience, acceptance, nonreactiveness, forgiveness, love, encouragement, and hopefulness. These attitudes flow out of the spiritual dimension of individuals (Carson, 1989). The nurse can intervene effectively with family caregivers by providing spiritual care. Skills include entering into a relationship with the caregiver, "becoming a companion in his or her journey," and sharing the caregiver's emotions, such as pain, anger, or sadness (Carson, 1989).

Collaboration skills

The nurse must work effectively as a peer with colleagues in providing care for families and meeting family goals. Nurses collaborate with other disciplines and agencies toward positive family outcomes.

Collaboration skills have been identified by McDaniel and Campbell (1996). The following are the skills that nurses need when working with families and other agencies:

- Maintain attention to collaborative values.
  Focus primarily on capacities as opposed to deficits.
  Promote universal access to health care.
  Empower, educate, and learn from families.
  Value interdependency.
- Become accountable for the use of resources.
  Track statistics and outcomes.
- Discuss, monitor, and deal with issues of shared power among professionals, and between professionals, patients, and families.
  Create space for everyone to have a place in the discourse.
  Examine the relationship between power and helping professions, between competition and collaboration.
  Develop case-specific leadership, dependent on the needs of the patient and the context.
  Learn to be both a leader and a follower.
  Develop the ability to talk about differences.
- Examine issues of culture, race, class, and disabilities in health care.
  Make services culturally responsive.
  Develop ways to accept and support differences.
  Examine cultural countertransference.
- Learn to enhance others' competencies.
- Attend to issues of spirituality.

Skills for referrals, family support, and resources

Referrals are often necessary when working with troubled families whose needs are unmet and whose tasks are not accomplished. The nurse must have the knowledge and skills to support families as they enter the desired system for assistance within the continuum of care.

Application of the Nursing Process to the Family

Assessment

The nurse has several purposes when interviewing and working with families. These purposes begin with the initial assessment of the family and continue through discharge and referral. Assessments include the following:

- Family characteristics: healthy or dysfunctional in the family of origin and the present family
- Developmental stage of the family
- The family's accomplishment of tasks
- The family's and patient's reasons for seeking treatment, and reactions to hospitalization
- The effects of mental illness on the family
- Family coping mechanisms
- The family's understanding of and difficulty with managing the patient's illness and behaviors
- Health problems of family members/significant others

The assessment process begins within the context of the nurse-patient-family relationship. Assessment provides the nurse, patient, and family an opportunity to discuss how they view problems in the system. Questions may be asked when the patient and the whole family are together, when several family members come to visit, or when only the patient is available.

Patients who seek treatment may live with their intact family of origin, a parent who has remarried several times, adoptive parents, foster parents, other relatives, a spouse or significant other, in a residential setting, or they may be visitors to this country or international students. The nurse must consider living arrangements and who will be involved in treatment. Although patients may not live with their family of origin, present problems may be an extension of problems that began there. Alternatively, individual problems may not stem from the family of origin, as in the case of a recent divorce or in the decision to become a parent.

An assessment should also be done concerning other health problems within the family that may be a result of dealing with the mentally ill member or may impinge on care given to that person. Greenberg, et al (1993) found that caregiver subjective burdens related to stigma and worry were significant predictors of negative physical health.

Families cope in different ways when dealing with a family member with a mental illness. Doornbos's research findings (1997) identified the effective coping methods: assuming facilitative attitudes, relying on faith, increasing knowledge of illness, attending support groups, support of family and friends, professional assistance, and distancing from the client. Rose (1996) has suggested that the stage of family development is related to the perception of stressors and identification of coping methods. Assessment of family coping methods will provide valuable data when discussing interventions with the family.

A family assessment guideline can assist in "thinking family systems" (Box 16-2). It uses theory to direct data gathering concerning family interactions, explores family knowledge of health and illness, identifies desired family goals, and indicates family-level interventions. Through guided dialogues, families can be actively engaged in decision making regarding self-health priorities (Lapp, Diemert, and Enestvedt, 1993). "The family perspective serves to expand the scope of practice, to increase insight, to allow for case finding, and to move health intervention to a more holistic dimension" (Lapp, Diemert, and Enestvedt, 1993, p. 281). Theoretical/conceptual perspectives incorporated into this family assessment include general systems theory (Bertalanffy, 1968), family systems theory (Bowen, 1978), family developmental theory (Duvall and Miller, 1985), an integrative approach (Nichols and Everett, 1986), and genograms (McGoldrick and Gerson, 1985).

Below are examples of questions that the nurse may ask when initiating a constructive dialogue during a family assessment. (These questions can be altered depending on which family member[s] the nurse interviews.)

- Composition: "Tell me who is in your family." "Who do you consider to be family members? Do you have any pets that are like family members?"
- Family of origin: "How often do you see your mother and father?" "When you and your

Box 16-2 Family Health and Functioning Assessment

I. Interview the family and obtain the following data:
  A. Demographic and family composition on a genogram
    1. Complete a three-generation genogram with legend and cultural heritage of all family members
    2. Identify the health status of each family member on the genogram
    3. Social networks of first generation members, including neighbor environment
  B. Family interactions
    Identify, discuss, and give examples for each of the following:
    1. Family structure
      a. Subsystems—identify all 5 subsystems
      b. Boundaries—include internal and external
      c. Roles of each family member
      d. Rules of the family—procedural and relational
      e. Triangles—identify all triangles [specify parentification and/or scapegoating]
    2. Family process
      a. Separateness/connectedness—describe this, including sexuality
      b. Enmeshment/disengagement—classify the family by one of these
      c. Communication—who communicates with whom and how
      d. Power—identify who has the power in the family
      e. Secrets/myths—how do they affect family process?
    3. Family spirituality
      a. Method by which family members express their spiritual domain
  C. Family development stage
    1. Identify Duvall's developmental stage[s] and family concerns within the stage[s]
  D. Family knowledge of health and illness
    1. Identify the family's knowledge in the following areas:
      a. Health maintenance and health promotion
      b. Physical and mental illnesses of members
      c. Management of illnesses of members, including medications and side effects
      d. Family coping methods
      e. Resources, such as family support, legal, financial, and community agencies
      f. Treatment options availability
II. Summary
  A. Discuss developmental and health problems in relationship to family (1) structure, (2) process, and (3) spirituality
  B. Discuss family strengths related to structure, process, spirituality, and social networks
  C. Discuss family problems related to structure, process, spirituality, and social networks
  D. Discuss the family's knowledge of health and illness
III. Goals for the family
  As members of the treatment team, ask the family to identify the following:
  A. Changes to be made for a more effective functioning family
  B. Present needs of the family to better care for family members
  C. Family's and/or significant others' role in discharge planning
IV. Interventions
  Indicate interventions and/or referrals related to specific assessment data and family goals

wife have problems, with which family members do you discuss the problems? Do you talk with your mother, father, sister, brother, or wife?"
• Developmental stages: "Tell me about your current family. Are you married? Do you have children? How old are your children who live with you?" "When did your oldest child leave the household?"
• Developmental tasks: "How do you all decide who will do what in your family?" "Who makes the final decisions in your family?"

- Open-system orientation: "When something happens, what type of things do you see as the cause?" "Whom do you see that you need in your life?"
- Boundaries: "Who is concerned about what is happening with John?" "John, whom do you see as involved with your drinking?"
- Contextual clarity: "How much is your mother-in-law involved in decision making in your family?" "How often do you and your wife have time for yourselves?"
- Power: "How do you decide who will do the dishes and who will change a flat tire?" "What type of decisions do you let your children make?"
- Encouragement of autonomy: "When your husband and you have different views, how do you handle it?" "When your child comes to one of you after your partner has said 'no,' how do you handle it?"
- Affective issues: "How do you all deal with feelings in your family?" "Who gets along the best in your family?"
- Negotiation and task performance: "How do you all decide who will feed the dog?" "How do you get along with each other?"
- Transcendent values: "What view do you have about what will happen with this family problem?" "How do you deal with loss in your family? Do you talk with each other about it? Do you believe that loss is a part of life?"
- Health status measures: "Tell me about the physical health of your family members." "How would you deal with family members who use alcohol or drugs?"

Orienting families to inpatient units

Orientation is needed to help families deal with the hospitalization of their family member. The orientation process occurs initially when the patient is admitted and continues as treatment issues arise about which families need information. When orienting families to the hospital unit, the following topics are often included:

1. Unit rules, policies, and schedules; the rationales for these
2. Levels of patients' privileges and precautions; the rationales for these
3. Education and support groups that meet in the hospital for the families

4. Patient confidentiality: patients and family members must be clear how information will be handled. (The nurse must avoid being a *"secret guardian,"* a person who has knowledge from the patient or a family member who has asked that the information not be shared.)
5. The need for the staff to know about patients' destructive behaviors, such as suicidal or homicidal threats and self-mutilation
6. Policies that child or elder abuse must be reported according to law
7. Release forms that families may need to sign if the hospitalized family member is under the age of consent, has been declared legally incompetent, or has a legal guardian
8. Purposes of unit groups, activities, and unit governance
9. Visitation hours and rules: these may depend on the patient's level of precautions and privileges. Unit rules may restrict what items the family may bring to the patient while visiting (e.g., no drugs, alcohol, or food). Items patients are permitted to have should be specified. During family conferences, the family should know under what circumstances the conference can be stopped, such as by the patient's or family's request or when physical violence occurs.
10. Experiencing change: Change is difficult and frightening. Families need to know that they may experience an increased level of discomfort as decisions regarding change approach.
11. Permission for the patient and family to have time to adjust to one another's changes
12. The need to restrict or monitor visitations and phone calls if these are negatively affecting the patient or family
13. Assessing and monitoring visitation by children because of their varying abilities to handle the milieu and other patients
14. Therapeutic passes for home visits—these are now rare due to short hospitalization periods. However, areas to address in preparation may include:
    a. What changes in the patient the family might expect
    b. How the patient and family will manage current behaviors
    c. The rules to be enforced while the patient is at home, such as no alcohol, driving, or over-the-counter medications

d. What the patient wants to accomplish on pass

e. Verbal and/or written evaluations of the home visit by the patient and family

Nurses, patients, and family members must work together constructively to find feasible solutions for these issues. The nurse may talk with families, or family conferences may occur in which these issues can be discussed openly, respectfully, and explicitly with all family members so that more productive solutions can be created.

Nursing diagnosis

Based on the assessments, the nurse develops priority nursing diagnoses, such as those listed in Box 16-3.

Outcome identification

Based on assessments, the nurse works with patients and their families to establish goals to be accomplished during treatment. These goals may be individual goals for a specific family member and/or goals for the family as a whole. Referrals for family therapy may be necessary if supportive interventions do not effect a resolution of family difficulties.

Very troubled families often are encountered on inpatient psychiatric units and need to be referred to family therapy. These families' problems often extend to their environment. Because of this, other agencies may need to be involved or may be involved at the time of initial contact. When establishing goals with these families, the nurse must consider how these agencies will be involved in the treatment process. Agency contact may focus on economic issues, protection for one or more family members, report of abuse to a state agency, contacts with police, or actions of a court order. The nurse can assist these families with finding helpful sources and arranging for these services. These services may include social welfare agencies, churches, emergency food services, voluntary agencies, support groups, hospices, community health services, and psychiatric home-care services. Additional resources for families include the following:

Al-Anon/Alateen
Alcoholics Anonymous
Families Anonymous
Mothers Against Drunk Driving (MADD)
Narcotics Anonymous
National Alliance for the Mentally Ill (NAMI)
Parents Anonymous
Tough Love

Although the family may be involved with these community resources for immediate assistance with an ill family member, families can be encouraged to be advocates for improved mental health care and funding through work with these same agencies.

Box 16-3 Selected Nursing Diagnoses Related to Family Nursing

Impaired verbal communication
Impaired social interaction
Social isolation
Altered role performance
Altered parenting
Potentially altered parenting
Sexual dysfunction
Altered family processes
Parental role conflict
Altered sexuality patterns
Spiritual distress
Impaired adjustment
Defensive coping
Ineffective denial
Ineffective family coping: disabling or compromised

Family coping: potential for growth
Decisional conflict
Health-seeking behaviors
Diversional-activity deficit
Impaired home-maintenance management
Hopelessness
Powerlessness
Knowledge deficit
Dysfunctional grieving
Anticipatory grieving
Potential for violence
Posttrauma response
Anxiety
Fear

From the North American Nursing Diagnosis Association: *NANDA nursing diagnoses: definitions and classifications, 1997-1998,* Philadelphia, 1997, The Association.

Planning/implementation

The skills needed for therapeutic conversations, guided by the collective language systems approach, have been specified earlier. Other interventions the nurse may use when working with patients and their families individually, and in groups on inpatient units, are listed in the box below. Through understanding the family's view of living with a mentally ill member, the nurse can develop interventions that are "relevant, timely, and specific to the needs of the family" (Saunders, 1997, p. 12).

Evaluation

Outcomes of working with patients and their families can be measured by determining whether or not treatment goals have been met, and whether or not patients and families have created new meanings and solutions for present problems. Periodically throughout treatment, the nurse and family system together must evaluate their progress toward the resolutions of their present problems. When appropriate, the nurse can assist patients and families in the reformulation of goals and the creation of posttreatment goals that will be worked toward after discharge from the inpatient unit or outpatient program.

Additionally, recent research (Ascher-Svanum, et al, 1997) indicates interventions should include family education. Findings indicated that families want information concerning their relative's illness and its treatment, and patients want to understand their illness and effective ways to cope with it. The content most preferred by families, with percentages in parentheses, was on the future course of the illness (78%), medications' benefits and side effects (74%), and crisis management (74%). The least preferred content was on substance abuse and comorbidity problems.

Critical Thinking Question

What family-oriented approaches would you use with a woman who is currently choosing to remain with her abusive partner? What referrals might you make as part of discharge planning?

When you strongly suspect that abuse is occurring currently in a family, but they and the patient refuse to discuss it, what approaches might you try?

Key Concepts

1. The nurse who works with families must expect to see many different types of groups who define themselves as a "family."
2. Difficulties in accomplishing family tasks and developmental stages often mean there are problem areas in the family.
3. Individuals must leave their families of origin with healthy communication skills, high self-esteem, few unresolved issues, and a hopeful view of life if relationships in the nuclear family are to be healthy.

Key Nursing Interventions for Working with Families

- Provide empathy, support, acceptance, nonjudgment
- Advocate for and protect patients and families
- Help families build patients' self-esteem, yet have realistic expectations
- Facilitate resolution of normal life-cycle crises
- Prevent additional dysfunction in the family
- Identify troubled families and refer them to a family therapist
- Provide referrals to support groups and family resources
- Teach problem-solving, limit-setting, and conflict-resolution skills
- Help families validate, clarify, negotiate, and communicate feelings appropriately
- Assist families to cope with emotional abuse
- Offer feedback to patients and families

- Negotiate role changes with patients and families
- Provide support for families through brief, problem-focused groups
- Demonstrate candor with patients and families when it is clear that child or elder abuse must be reported
- Teach the principles of "tough love"
- Teach conflict management, communications skills, problem solving, parenting skills, limit setting
- Teach about illnesses, causes, nature, treatments, and prognoses
- Teach about medications, managing side effects, symptoms to be reported, signs of relapse
- Teach and provide a role model for ways to manage the difficult behaviors of patients
- Include the family in discharge planning

4. Individuals who seek help for their "problem" often are assisting the family in receiving help for a family problem.

5. The nurse must ascertain whether a family assessment, family intervention, and/or family therapy is indicated.

6. The nursing process with families requires that the nurse possess self-knowledge skills; assessment skills; therapeutic communication skills; spiritual skills; collaboration skills; and skills regarding referrals, family support, and resources.

7. The nurse must work with families on inpatient units to orient them to the hospital milieu and to provide a constructive environment for change.

Study Questions

(Answer key is in the back of the book.)

Situation: Mary Clark, a single 19-year-old who lives with her parents, has been admitted recently to an inpatient unit. She says that she has not been able to work or take care of her child since her parents announced that they were planning to divorce. Questions 1-3 refer to this situation.

1. During a family meeting with Mary and her parents, what would be the most helpful nursing approach?
   a. Ask each family member his or her ideas about what is occurring in the family.
   b. Make Mary's parents aware of her problems and their part in these problems.
   c. Pay particular attention to Mary and what she needs at this time.
   d. Begin making plans about how the family might solve the problem for Mary.

2. The most appropriate initial nursing intervention is to:
   a. Talk with the parents about how they will take care of Mary's child.
   b. Help Mary's parents to see that she is having a problem with the impending divorce.
   c. Talk with Mary and her parents about what they would like to change in their family.
   d. Encourage the parents to be more supportive of Mary during this difficult time.

3. When defining the Clark family in terms of family composition, the family is:
   a. A nuclear family
   b. An extended family
   c. An alternative family
   d. A blended family

4. An emotional triangle can be described as which of the following?
   a. A phenomenon present only in families with serious problems
   b. A functional method of constructive communication

c. A functional technique found in all healthy relationships
   d. A psychological process for maintaining homeostasis

5. Nursing interventions appropriate to working with families include:
   a. Conveying warmth and acceptance to all family members
   b. Developing an alliance with the patient
   c. Directing each family member in how to help the patient
   d. Assisting the patient with conforming to the family's rules

REFERENCES

Anderson H (speaker): *A collective language systems approach to therapy,* video no. V521, Washington, DC, 1991a, The American Association for Marriage and Family Therapy.

Anderson H (speaker): *Creating a language of change,* video no. V308, Washington, DC, 1991b, The American Association for Marriage and Family Therapy.

Anderson H and Goolishian H: Human systems as linguistic systems: preliminary and evolving ideas about the implications for clinical theory, *Fam Process* 27(4):371, 1988.

Ascher-Svanum H, et al: Educational needs of families of mentally ill adults, *Psychiatr Serv* 48(8):1072, 1997.

Badger T: Living with depression: family members' experiences and treatment needs, *J Psychosoc Nurs Ment Health Serv,* 34(1):21, 1996.

Beavers W: *Psychotherapy and growth: a family systems perspective,* New York, 1977, Brunner/Mazel.

Bertalanffy L: General systems theory: foundation, development, applications, New York, 1968, Braziller.

Bowen M: *Family therapy in clinical practice,* New York, 1978, Jason Aronson.

Carson VB: *Spiritual dimensions of nursing practice,* Philadelphia, 1989, WB Saunders.

Cox RP: The human/animal bond as a correlate of family functioning, *Clin Nurs Res* 2(2):224, 1993.

Cox RP and Davis LL: Social constructivist approaches for brief, episodic, problem-focused family encounters, *Nurse Pract* 18(8):45, 1993.

Dicks H: *Marital tensions,* London, 1967, Routledge & Kegan Paul.

Doornbos MM: The problems and coping methods of caregivers of young adults with mental illness, *J Psychosoc Nurs Ment Health Serv* 35(9):22, 1997.

Duvall E and Miller B: *Marriage and family development,* ed 6, New York, 1985, Harper & Row.

Fawcett J: *Analysis and evaluation of conceptual models of nursing,* ed 2, Philadelphia, 1989, FA Davis.

Gillis CL: Family nursing research, theory and practice, *Image J Nurs Sch* 23(1):19, 1991.

Goldenberg I and Goldenberg H: *Family therapy—an overview,* ed 3, Pacific Grove, Calif, 1991, Brooks/Cole.

Greenberg J, et al: Mothers caring for an adult child with schizophrenia: the effects of subjective burden on maternal health, *Fam Relations* 42:205, 1993.

Griffin-Francell C: Psychiatric nurses must be held accountable for their actions, *J Psychosoc Nurs Ment Health Serv* 31(10):5, 1993.

Grinspoon L: What is new in consumer-operated mental health services, *Harvard Mental Health Letter* 9(2):8, 1992a.

Grinspoon L: Support for recovery, *Harvard Mental Health Letter* 9(5):7, 1992b.

Grinspoon L: Self-help groups–part II, *Harvard Mental Health Letter* 9(10):1, 1993a.

Grinspoon L: Child abuse–part II, *Harvard Mental Health Letter* 9(12):1, 1993b.

Hatfield AB: Incorporating family's contribution to clinical training. In Letley H, editor: *Clinical training in serious mental illness,* Washington, DC, 1990, National Institute of Mental Health.

Hatfield A and Letley H: Surviving mental illness: *Stress, coping and adaptation,* New York, 1993, Guilford Press.

Hellwig K: Psychiatric home care nursing: managing patients in the community setting, *J Psychosoc Nurs Ment Health Serv* 31(12):21, 1993.

Hoffman L: Constructing realities: an art of lenses, *Fam Process* 29(1):1, 1990.

Kelly A: *Evaluating and improving family health: the holistic health handbook,* Berkeley, Calif, 1978, And/Or.

Kerr M: Family systems theory and therapy. In Gurman A and Kniskern D, editors: *Handbook of family therapy,* ed 1, New York, 1981, Brunner/Mazel.

Koontz E, Cox D, and Hasting S: Implementing a short-term family support group, *J Psychosoc Nurs Ment Health Serv* 29(5):5, 1991.

Lapp CA, Diemert CA, and Enestvedt R: Family-based practice: discussion of a tool merging assessment with intervention. In Wegner G and Alexander R, editors: *Readings in family nursing,* Philadelphia, 1993, JB Lippincott.

McDaniel S and Campbell T: Training for collaborative family healthcare, *Families, Systems & Health* 14(2):147, 1996.

McGoldrick M and Gerson R: *Genograms in family assessment,* New York, 1985, WW Norton.

McGoldrick M, Heiman M, and Carter B: The changing family life cycle. In Walsh F, editor: *Normal family processes,* ed 2, New York, 1993, Guilford.

Nichols W and Everett C: *Systemic family therapy: an integrative approach,* New York, 1986, Guilford Press.

North American Nursing Diagnosis Association: *NANDA nursing diagnoses: definitions and classifications, 1997-1998,* Philadelphia, 1997, The Association.

Reinhard SC: Perspectives on the family's caregiving experience in mental illness, *Image J Nurs Sch* 26(1):70, 1994.

Rose LE: Families of psychiatric patients: a critical review and future research directions, *Arch Psychiatr Nurs* 10:67, 1996.

Saunders J: Symbolic interaction issues for families living with severe mental illness, *J Psychosoc Nurs Ment Health Serv* 35(6):8, 1997.

Sayles-Cross S: Perceptions of familial caregivers of elder adults, *Image J Nurs Sch* 25(2):88, 1993.

Scharff D and Scharff J: *Objects relations family therapy,* Northvale, NJ, 1991, Jason Aronson.

Walsh F: Conceptualization of normal family processes. In Walsh F, editor: *Normal family processes,* ed 2, New York, 1993, Guilford.

Walsh SM: Orientation intervention for parents of adolescents after psychiatric hospitalization, *J Psychosoc Nurs Ment Health Serv* 31(7):21, 1993.

Wright L and Leahey M: *Nurses and families: a guide to family assessments and interventions,* ed. 2, Philadelphia, 1994, FA Davis.

CHAPTER 17

Cultural Competence in Psychiatric Nursing: An Interlocking Paradigm Approach

BARBARA JONES WARREN

LEARNING OBJECTIVES

After reading this chapter you should be able to:
- Describe the factors within the interlocking paradigm of cultural competence.
- Explain how incorporation of the paradigm with the psychotherapeutic model can enhance clinical excellence.

CULTURE AND PSYCHIATRIC NURSING

Cultural competence is the process whereby the nurse proficiently develops cultural awareness, knowledge, skill, and encounter for use in education, practice, and research (Campinha-Bacote, 1997b; Warren, 1997). Cultural competence, in conjunction with the psychotherapeutic management model, enhances clinical excellence for psychiatric patients in today's managed care environment.

Because of managed care and other forces, patients and psychiatric nurses have moved from inpatient to community settings and taken their unique individual and hospital cultures with them. They have created a new mental health culture within these community settings (Clement, 1997). Within this new culture the roles of patients have changed and their rights have been more clearly defined. For example, patients have greater knowledge about their illnesses; are active participants in the development and implementation of their treatment process; and know more about themselves, the health care system, and management of their illnesses (Warren, 1997). Patients define this role change as the process of "recovery" (Anthony, 1993; Hogan, 1993, 1996).

Nurses' roles have changed as well. Nurses are now involved with a multitude of patients from diverse cultures and settings. The concept of **cultural diversity** is broader than just race and ethnic diversities but

KEY TERMS

Culture The internal and external manifestation of an individual's, group's, or community's beliefs, values, and norms that are used as premises for everyday life functioning.

The Interlocking Paradigm of Cultural Competence A model that illustrates the use of theoretical, philosophical, process, and assessment factors in the development and incorporation of cultural competence within nursing education, practice, and research.

Ethnonursing The professional culturally competent knowledge used by the nurse in his or her interactions with others and in areas of nursing education, practice, and research to facilitate the well-being and health of persons.

Cultural awareness The process whereby the nurse acknowledges his or her cultural biases and recognizes that other persons, groups, or communities have their unique cultural similarities and differences.

Cultural knowledge The ability of the nurse to learn culturally relevant information about different cultures and apply that knowledge in education, practice, and research areas.

Cultural skill The ability of the nurse to knowledgeably use culturally appropriate information about diverse cultures while conducting cultural assessment and screening procedures.

Cultural encounter The ability of the nurse to actively seek out culturally different experiences to continue the development and expansion of her or his cultural awareness, knowledge, and skill.

Cultural competence The process whereby the nurse has developed cultural awareness, knowledge, skill, and encounter and uses the process in nursing education, practice, and research to promote effective and quality health care delivery for patients.

Cultural diversity The variety of cultural groupings. These groups may include age, gender, socioeconomic status, religion, deafness, race, ethnicity, mental illness, and physically challenged conditions.

Health care actions Those psychological, physical, and spiritual approaches that persons may use in their attempt to maintain their state of wellness or to return themselves to some level of wellness in the event they incur illness.

World view A person's perspective of how they and other individuals function, interact, and behave everyday. This perspective is based upon how an individual's cultural group[s] has developed knowledge, values, and belief systems.

Symbolic imagery A person's use of figurative language, wearing of some article of clothing or jewelry, or a health care action that illustrates a cultural value, belief, or norm.

Symbolic rhythm A person's use of a particular musical, tone, speech, silence, or percussion sound that is based on a cultural value, belief, or norm.

Moxibustion An alternative, cultural, medical treatment approach that utilizes moxi and heat in order to release illness-producing spirits from a person's body, mind, or spirit.

Cupping An alternative, cultural, medical treatment approach that utilizes a small glass or cup in order to conduct the moxibustion treatment.

Skin scraping/coining Another alternative, cultural, medical treatment approach that utilizes a coin in order to reinstate balance and health in a person's body. A healer uses a coin to scrape the skin above meridians in a person's body.

Meridians Lines in a body that are representative of psychological or physical body functions. Cultural healers stimulate meridians and release harmful toxins or illness-producing spirits through the use of alternative treatment approaches such as moxibustion, cupping, coining, or skin scraping.

Hot or cold treatments Those cultural-medical approaches to maintaining or returning a person to a state of wellness. These approaches do not refer to the temperature of a treatment but to the fact that a specific, defined approach is appropriate for each state of wellness or illness.

also encompasses such areas as age, gender, socioeconomic status, religion, deafness, mental illness, and physically challenged conditions (Brink, 1987; Campinha-Bacote, 1994; Comas-Diaz and Green, 1994; Leininger, 1995).

Adding to the challenge for nurses and patients is the fact that programming (i.e., treatment planning)

has become more complicated. The 1990s ushered in developments in technology, increased knowledge about psychobiology (the "Decade of the Brain"), and health care restructuring (American Nurses Association [ANA], 1994). Nurses, other health care professionals, and patients may now think and interact differently with each other because of patient's increased access to health care information through written and electronic media. In addition, resources have been readjusted, reallocated, decreased, and, in some cases, eliminated. Quality, efficiency, and cost savings are key components for the development of successful outcome measures within managed care entities (Charlow, 1996; Clement, 1997). To continue to exist within these entities, psychiatric nurses need to be able to incorporate these components in their patient care (Hughes, 1993).

A growing knowledge and research base indicates patients are more compliant with their health care programs and outcomes are more successful when patients' cultural needs are incorporated into assessment, screening, interventions, and protocols (ANA Expert Panel, 1993; Adebimpe, 1981; ANA, 1986, 1994; Flaskerud, 1992; Meleis, et al, 1995; Pedersen, 1994; Sue and Sue, 1990; Worthington, 1992). Since nurses are often the gatekeepers for health care systems, they need to be knowledgeable in the areas of cultural factors, pharmacology, current community and inpatient milieu strategies, and the biological and psychological correlates of psychiatric wellness and illness. The interlocking paradigm of cultural competence (IPCC) is a model that utilizes specific theoretical, philosophical, process, and assessment strategies to develop and implement cultural competence within the areas of nursing education, practice, and research. The authors have chosen to use this model because of its simplicity, clarity, and applicability to psychiatric nursing. The purpose of this chapter is to explicate the paradigm's applicability to psychiatric nursing.

The Importance of Culture

Culture is a critical component of a person's life and affects one's health care attitudes and actions in relationship to one's ability to understand and utilize the interventions psychiatric nurses develop (Campinha-Bacote, 1994; Warren, 1996a,b). **Culture** is the internal and external manifestation of a person, group, or community's learned and shared values, beliefs, and norms that are used to help individuals function in life and understand and interpret life occurrences (Leininger, 1995; Tylor, 1871; Stewart, 1995; Warren, 1997). In addition to being important to the patient, culture also affects how mental illness may be exhibited. A patient's behaviors may be misinterpreted as pathological if a nurse is not aware of the patient's cultural beliefs and

norms as they relate to health care actions (Warren, 1997). The psychiatric patient who is labeled as being "noncompliant" has frequently not received appropriate or culturally competent nursing care. In reality, it may be the nurse or other health care professionals who are being noncompliant in their ability to develop appropriate health care programming.

Cultural competence is the process whereby the nurse proficiently develops cultural awareness, knowledge, skill, and encounter for use in areas of nursing education, practice, and research in order to promote effective and quality health care delivery for patients (Campinha-Bacote, 1997b; Warren, 1997). A culturally competent psychiatric nurse not only understands the process of cultural competence, but also has incorporated this technique into interactions with peers, students, patients, and other community and professional persons.

INTERLOCKING PARADIGM OF CULTURAL COMPETENCE

The IPCC is a model of how psychiatric nurses can theoretically and philosophically understand, develop, and proficiently use culturally competent strategies and assessment techniques (Figure 17-1). Five factors are involved in the paradigm:

1. The nurse-patient interaction
2. Theory
3. Philosophy
4. Process
5. Assessment

All factors in the IPCC are drawn using an interrelated, overlapping style, which means that the paradigm reflects the interdependence of the factors and the continuous evolving nature of the culturally competent process. The edges of each factor are double sided. This resembles a human cell, which is porous and osmotic. This depiction represents the idea that relationships between the factors are open, fluid, and diffuse. Information is absorbed and assimilated between the factors. In addition, arrows are drawn from the four outer factors into the nurse-patient interaction, which illustrates that information is continuously growing and being supplied to the nurse-patient interaction. The psychotherapeutic management model and the IPCC create a model of clinical excellence when psychiatric nurses use these frameworks to develop health care education, practice, and research strategies and protocols.

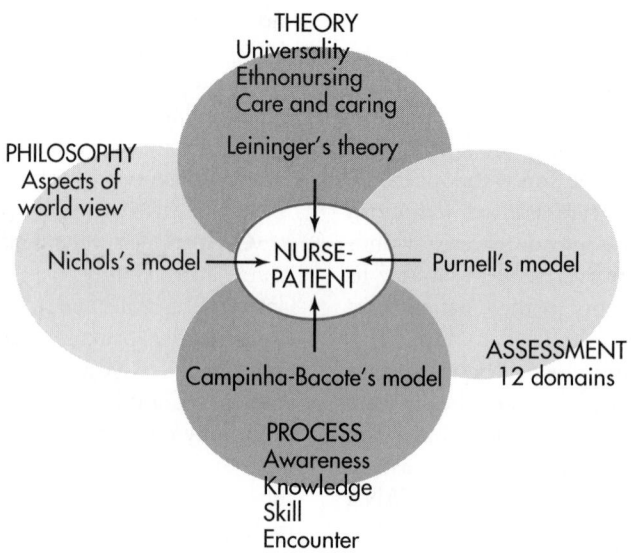

FIGURE 17-1 The Interlocking Paradigm of Cultural Competence.

Nurse-Patient Interaction

The nurse-patient interaction is at the center of the paradigm, illustrating how it serves as the reason, basis, and focal point for development of cultural competence. The interaction may involve an individual, a group, or community. Peplau (1952, 1988) has described the nurse-patient relationship as a psychodynamic relationship in which the nurse not only understands and interprets the patient's behavior but the nurse's as well. Using Peplau's premise, the psychiatric nurse would use the process of cultural competence in conjunction with knowledge regarding therapeutic communication and psychopharmacology to create a therapeutic milieu (Warren, 1996a, 1996b, 1997).

The other four factors in the paradigm are based upon the following four scholars' work:

1. The *theory* factor is grounded in Dr. Madeline Leininger's cultural care diversity and universality theory (1995);
2. Dr. Edwin Nichols's world view model (1987) forms the foundation for the *philosophy* factor;
3. Dr. Josepha Campinha-Bacote's culturally competent model (1994) guides the *process* factor; and
4. Dr. Larry Purnell's twelve domain model for cultural competence (Purnell and Paulanka, 1998) serves as the basis for the *assessment* factor.

The Theory Factor

The theory factor is represented by Leininger's cultural care diversity and universality theory (1995) because her theory provides the grounding for how professional nurses should conduct themselves in their education, practice, and research settings (Table 17-1). This theory has particular use within psychiatric nursing because it examines some of the same components found in the psychotherapeutic management model (e.g., nurse-patient relationship, milieu, role of biology and psychology in illness) and incorporates the importance of culture in relationship to health and wellness.

According to Leininger (1995), nursing knowledge or **ethnonursing knowledge** is that which is learned through formal educational and research processes. This ethnonursing knowledge, for the culturally competent nurse, encompasses information learned regarding the nurse-patient interaction, psychotherapeutic management, nurses' and patients' philosophies, the process of cultural competence, and cultural assessment domains.

Health is defined by a person's cultural perspective in the context of varying states of wellness (Leininger, 1995; Peplau, 1952). An individual's cultural perspective evolves from a world view grounding, environmental influences, relationships with significant others, and available health care systems

Table 17-1 Theory Factor: Leininger's Cultural Care Diversity and Universality Theory

Component	Definition
Ethnonursing knowledge	Knowledge learned through formal nursing education and research processes
Health	Person's state of wellness, defined by one's cultural perspective
Cultural preservation	Nurse's ability to acknowledge, value, and accept a patient's cultural beliefs
Cultural negotiation	Nurse's ability to work within a patient's cultural belief system to develop culturally appropriate and health-focused interventions and protocols
Cultural repatterning	Nurse's ability to incorporate cultural preservation and negotiation to identify patient needs, develop expected outcomes, and evaluate outcome plans
Ethnocentrism	Nurse's perspective that her or his culture is the only one of value and importance
Cultural imposition	Nurse's attempts to impose his or her cultural beliefs, norms, and health care practices upon a patient to replace the patient's cultural belief system with the nurse's because it is of greater value

(Leininger, 1995). The nurse uses empathetic care and caring to provide psychological and physical assistance to patients. The purpose of nursing care is to maintain, restore, or improve patients' level of health (Leininger, 1995). To achieve this purpose, nurses use the techniques of cultural preservation, negotiation, and repatterning (Leininger, 1995). Cultural preservation is the nurse's ability to acknowledge, value, and accept a patient's cultural beliefs. Cultural negotiation is the nurse's ability to work within a patient's cultural belief system to develop culturally appropriate and health-focused interventions and protocols. Cultural repatterning is the nurse's ability to incorporate cultural preservation and negotiation to identify patient needs, develop

expected outcomes, and evaluate outcome plans (Leininger, 1995).

CLINICAL EXAMPLE

All members of the Chen family have been coming to a clinic for their health care. One day Mr. and Mrs. Chen, accompanied by Mr. Chen's father, come to the clinic with their 6-month-old daughter. Mrs. Duong, the clinic nurse who has been following the Chen family's care, notices that the baby has an acute respiratory infection (ARI) and abrasions and surface burns on her back. Mrs. Duong inquires if any treatments have been used on the baby. Mrs. Chen says yes and that Mr. Chen (indicating her father-in-law) has been treating her. Mrs. Duong, realizing that grandfathers are highly respected and are often the treatment providers in Vietnamese culture, asks Mr. Chen if he could describe the treatment he has been using. He states that moxibustion/cupping and coining are the treatments he is using for the baby's cold. Mrs. Duong acknowledges that she understands the purpose of these treatments (i.e., to expel the poisons from the body) (cultural preservation) but also mentions that the baby could develop infections because of the breaks in the skin. She also states that some persons in America might think that the baby is being abused because of the marks on the body. Mrs. Duong makes a suggestion and asks (cultural negotiation) if it is possible for Mr. Chen to use less pressure, cover the coin with a piece of cloth, and slightly cool and cover the moxibustion glass with cloth before he applies it to the skin whenever he uses these treatments (cultural repatterning). Mr. Chen says, "Of course that is possible because I would not want my granddaughter hurt in any way." Mrs. Duong also consults with the clinic physician regarding the baby's ARI, abrasions, and burns. The physician prescribes an antibiotic for the baby's ARI and some ointment for the burns. The Chen family returns to the clinic in 1 week. The baby's ARI is gone, and the bruises and burns are almost completely healed. Mr. Chen states that they have been following all Mrs. Duong's suggestions, including giving the Western medicines.

According to Leininger (1995), ethnocentrism and cultural imposition are the most harmful attitudes a nurse may use with patients. When a nurse acknowledges and values only his or her culture (ethnocentrism), there is no need to develop interventions or strategies based upon the patient's cultural values or beliefs. In fact, the nurse often attempts to impose his or her cultural beliefs and values upon the patient (cultural imposition). Approaches like these may add to the misdiagnosis of patients and produce inaccurate health planning since nurses misinterpret cultural manifestations as symptoms of disease processes (Flaskerud, 1992). For example, a nurse might perceive that a patient is experiencing only physiological problems when the patient states he is "nervous, tired, and having heart problems." However, persons of Hispanic and Latino descent who are depressed may describe themselves using these terms (Homma-True, et al, 1993). Native Americans also may say they are "having heart pain" or are "heartbroken" when they experience depression (Bell, 1994).

The Philosophy Factor

Dr. Edwin Nichols (1987) is a psychologist who has developed a model regarding different world view perspectives (Table 17-2). His model was chosen as the philosophy factor for the IPCC because it provides psychiatric nurses with an understanding of how persons from different cultures have developed their knowledge, values, and belief systems (i.e., **world view**). This factor also adds to ethnonursing knowledge, facilitates nurses' understanding of themselves and their patients' cultural perspectives, and increases the likelihood of productive outcomes for patients (Nichols, 1987).

Nichols (1987) contends there are four components that comprise a world view: (1) *cultural axiology* (value system), (2) *epistemology* (knowledge base), (3) *logic* (reasoning ability), and (4) *process* (development of a relationship with another person, group, or community). In addition, Nichols (1987) delineates four areas of predominant world views: (1) European American, (2) African, African American, Hispanic, and Arabic, (3) Asian, Asian American, and Polynesian, and (4) Native American (Tables 17-3 to 17-6). Nichols determined these world view categories based upon different cultural groups'

Table 17-2 Philosophy Factor: Nichols's World View Model

Component	Definition
Cultural axiology	Person's value system
Epistemology	Person's knowledge base
Logic	Person's reasoning ability
Process	Development of relationship with another person, group, or community

Table 17-3 European American World View

Component	Perspective
Cultural axiology	Value is placed upon the member-object or attainment of the object.
Epistemology	Knowledge is acquired according to the proof of anything's existence being in one's ability to be able to see, hear, touch, taste, or smell it.
Logic	Dichotomous mode of reasoning ability—things are either right or wrong, good or bad. There is no middle or gray shading in life.
Process	Relationships are developed based upon perceived need for them.

Table 17-4 African, African American, Hispanic, and Arabic World View

Component	Perspective
Cultural axiology	Value is placed upon the development and maintenance of interpersonal relationships.
Epistemology	Knowledge bases are developed through use of the affective or feeling senses.
Logic	Reasoning ability is based upon the union of opposites.
Process	Development of interpersonal relationships is based upon the fact that all relationships are interrelated across all continuums.

geographic origination, as well as their commonly shared cultural belief and value system. Nichols (1987) stresses, however, that it is important for nurses to realize that persons within and across cultures may believe or exhibit varying degrees of each one of these views. Or persons may conduct their lives according to a belief based upon one of the views (Nichols, 1987). For example, a European American nurse may conduct his or her education, practice, or research and his or her interactions with other persons based upon a combination of values from each world view area, or she/he may strictly adhere to the European world view. A patient's world view could be exhibited in the same way. Miscommunication between the nurse and the patient might occur if either or both of them did not understand the other person's world view. The outcome of this miscommunication might result in inaccurate patient assessment, development of inadequate interventions, cultural incompetence (i.e., care given without the incorporation of cultural awareness, knowledge, skill, and encounter), and misdiagnosis of a patient's health/illness status.

In addition, Nichols (1987) stresses that a nurse should not place higher value on one world view over another because this is a hierarchical approach that contributes to the development of ethnocentrism and cultural imposition. Psychiatric nurses need to understand their own world view(s), as well as those of their patients, students, and peers, because this approach creates culturally competent interactions that promote understanding, facilitate education, and provide appropriate health care interventions, strategies, and protocols.

European American view

The European American world view's **cultural axiology,** (or value system) is defined by Nichols (1987) as the member-object or attainment of the object by persons. For example, in the United States advertising in newspapers and on television is based upon this premise. Both of these media sources seem to portray and try to convince persons that they will be much happier if they purchase certain name brand items. A nurse would also exhibit this world view when he or she uses psychotherapeutic management and cultural competence while providing patient care. In this case, the attainment of the object (e.g., information about a patient's physical and psychological status) must be accurately and precisely obtained through structured assessment strategies. Interventions and protocols are then developed based upon the attainment of this information. In this case, clinical excellence is enhanced, and the outcome would be the delivery of quality health care to a patient.

Table 17-5	Asian, Asian American, and Polynesian World View
Component	**Perspective**
Cultural axiology	Value is placed on the balance within member-group interactions.
Epistemology	Knowledge bases are developed in striving for transcendence of the mind and body.
Logic	Reasoning ability is based upon the fact that the mind and body can exist independent of the physical world.
Process	Development of relationships is grounded in the thought that everyone and every thing in the physical and spiritual worlds are related.

Table 17-6	Native American World View
Component	**Perspective**
Cultural axiology	Value is placed in the context of a person's relationship to a Greater or Supreme Being.
Epistemology	Knowledge bases are developed based upon a person's understanding of one's relationship with the Greater or Supreme Being.
Logic	Reasoning ability is grounded in the belief that every person is innately good and has no evil within.
Process	Development of relationships with another person, group, or community is grounded in the idea that the Greater or Supreme Being is in every person, hence all persons should be valued.

The **epistemology** or knowledge base for a person exhibiting the European American world view is grounded in the cognitive, or "seeing is believing" (Nichols, 1987). A nurse who exhibits this perspective would think she or he has to be able to see, touch, smell, or hear patients symptoms and that patients believe the same premise. This nurse might say, "I can't get Mrs. Alvarez to take her insulin this morning. She keeps telling me someone put an 'evil eye' on her and only her 'healer' can make the spell go away and cure her disease. I'm not sure where she got that idea from. I was taught in my nursing education that the cause of illness is due to the body not functioning correctly, deterioration of the body or its system, or the invasion of viruses and germs. I've never heard about any spells. Perhaps there's a chance that Mrs. Alvarez may need a psychiatric consult since it seems she is delusional and perhaps psychotic." Of course, there are many situations in which a nurse must be able to see, touch, smell, or hear the symptom of a patient to adequately and safely assess patient status, develop grades for students, or document achievements and goals for expected outcomes related to a patient's or the nurse's performance standards.

Logic or reasoning ability for the European American view is grounded in the dichotomous, clearly defined mode: things are either/or, right/wrong, good/bad (Nichols, 1987). For example, managed care and insurance companies give priority to payment for certain conditions over others. Determination of the payment status of all conditions is done according to clearly defined criteria. In other words, a condition is viewed as either being within a payment category or not, and there are very few instances in which payment decisions are changed or altered from categories. In fact, companies use this approach based upon the reasoning that payment criteria must be adhered to in order to provide good or right (i.e., quality) care to patients and prevent nurses, physicians, and patients from abusing the health care payment system. Another example of the European American logic would be the determination of antipsychotic medication use for psychiatric patients. The older antipsychotics, such as chlorpromazine or haloperidol, are cheaper but are generally less effective and create more side effects than the newer atypical antipsychotics, such as clozapine or olanzapine. However, determination of who gets what medication may be based upon what the patient can pay, not the appropriateness of the medication for the patient's symptoms.

The **process** or development of a relationship with another person, group, or community is formed and based upon perceived need. A person exhibiting the European American process may state, "I really must spend my time trying to develop my career. Everything else is on hold for now." Another example entails a patient who comes to a health care facility because he or she may need a physical prior to starting employment at a company. This patient comes with the intent or purpose to receive information and/or treatment about health. Nurses are at the facility for the purpose of providing health care for patients and being employed for monetary gain. In addition, a nurse educator or researcher may have the intent of educating students and finding and then following research participants for clinical studies. Students are there for the purpose of knowledge development and to satisfy requirements for their educational process.

African, African American, Hispanic, and Arabic view

Cultural axiology, or the value system for persons exhibiting the African, African American, Hispanic, and Arabic view, is grounded in the development and maintenance of interpersonal relationships (Nichols, 1987). This development is based upon the fact that the participants in the interpersonal relationship are joined because of mutual liking and respect for one another. An example of this view would be the patient who says, "You can always count on your family and friends. They're the key to life." Devotion to another person, group, or community may have positive or negative outcomes for the participants in the relationship(s). Examples of positive outcomes include participation in social or self-help groups such as religious communities, Girl or Boy Scouts, parenting support groups, and health care professions. Negative outcomes may occur, however, for children and adolescents involved in community gangs.

The **epistemology** or knowledge base for this view is grounded in the affective or feeling senses. Such things as symbolic imagery and rhythm are important to a nurse or patient who believes in this world view (Nichols, 1987). Symbolic imagery can be illustrated by a person wearing a certain metal representation of a religious saint as a safeguard against injury. A patient may also utilize specific herb(s) on a daily basis to maintain his or her health or use them during an illness to restore health based upon family teaching. Rhythm can be represented by the different musical or rhythmic sounds that a person may enjoy or use as meditation and relaxation techniques. The nurse who states she can just "tell" when something is going to happen with a patient even if all physical signs are within normal limits is illustrative of the "feeling senses" grounding within the African, African American, Hispanic, or Arabic epistemology. Patients exhibiting this perspective may tell family, nurses, and physicians if and when they are going to die. Nurses or patients exhibiting this epistemology may describe themselves as being "spiritual, believing in fate, and being part of a greater plan in the universe."

The **logic** or reasoning ability for the African, African American, Hispanic and Arabic world view is described by Nichols (1987) as the union of opposites. Today's blending of gender roles and traits is an example of this view. The "traditionally" described gender role derivations divide the behaviors, attitudes, beliefs, and norms for men and women into clearly distinct classifications (Comas-Diaz and Green, 1994). However, women and men exhibiting African, African American, Hispanic, and Arabic logic or reasoning ability do not describe their roles within these clearly defined divisions. A nurse who manifests this view may say, "I think being a good pediatric nurse has nothing to do with gender. Look at Mr. Jay and Ms. Jones. Both of them are great! They're sensitive and very knowledgeable. They also do great teaching with the kids and their families. Each one seems to combine just the right amount of sensitivity, caring, precision, and logic in their nursing practices."

The **process** or view of how relationships are developed is grounded in what Nichols (1987) terms *ntuology,* or the fact that relationships are interrelated across all continuums through networks and spiritual connections. A patient with this view might seek health advice from multiple sources, including his or her family, friends, community healers, and ministers in conjunction with traditional medical treatment sources. This patient may also feel a spiritual connection to family members or friends who have died and may seek the advice of these individuals or their intercession when the patient is experiencing difficulties in life. And the patient's community would offer up "prayers" and "thoughts" for him or her.

Asian, Asian American, or Polynesian view

Persons exhibiting the Asian, Asian American, or Polynesian world view have their **cultural axiology** or value system in the member-group interaction and balance in life (Nichols, 1987). For example, a person with this axiology is careful to make certain that his or her wants or actions never supersede or conflict with those of his or her family or community. Health is defined according to the balancing of natural forces within and outside of the body, and illness occurs when these forces become imbalanced (Nichols, 1987). The effect of the peer group in Asian American society is another example of this axiology. Persons often defer to group wants over their own in an attempt to keep balance and cohesion between themselves and the other group members (Purnell and Paulanka, 1998). A person may take vitamins, minerals, and herbal medications as another way of balancing the body and promoting health (Giger and Davidhizar, 1995). Exercising, meditation, and relaxation techniques may also be used for this purpose.

The **epistemology** or knowledge base for the Asian, Asian American, and Polynesian world view is in the connative or striving for transcendence (i.e., elevation or improvement of the mind from the body). An example of this would be a nurse or patient who uses meditation techniques to clear the mind and release tensions in the body. Another example would be the patient with intractable pain who images the pain as decreasing or leaving the body as a means of control over the level of discomfort (Andrews and Boyle, 1995; Giger and Davidhizar, 1995; Spector, 1996).

The **logic** or the reasoning ability for this world view is represented by *nyaya,* or seeing the objective world as being independent of thought and mind (Nichols, 1987). An example of this would be the nurse or patient who uses tai chi, a body movement and relaxation technique for the purpose of harmonizing energy processes in the body, integrating (i.e., balancing) the mind and body, and placing themselves in the natural order of the universe (e.g., returning themselves to health) (Dunn, 1996). Yoga is another illustration of *nyaya* as persons practice it to reenergize the mind and body and, thus, elevate and release the mind from the body through the use of meditation, concentration, and structured body positions (Villarosa, 1994).

Process, or the development of relationships with another person, group, or community, is grounded in the thought that everyone and everything are interrelated. The breaking up of relationships not only creates a disharmony between the persons involved but also affects others in society. For example, a person believing in this process might see societal problems (e.g., interaction problems between people and truancy in schools) as being related to the increasing divorce rate in the United States (Nichols, 1987). Or the increased use of drugs might be seen as being an outcome of persons not feeling a part of society and, in their attempt to feel better, they use some chemical substance. Persons' participation in social groups is based upon the fact that these groups provide a support system for the involved persons and give greater harmony to society as the group members often do "charitable" or helpful works for others. Examples of this include volunteer participation at homeless shelters, food banks, support groups, and help/hot lines.

Native American view

Persons exhibiting the Native American world view have their **cultural axiology,** or value system, in the

Table 17-7   Process Factor: Campinha-Bacote's Model of Cultural Competence

Component	Definition
Cultural awareness	Nurse's ability to acknowledge the fact that cultural similarities and differences exist and to acknowledge specific biases
Cultural knowledge	Nurse's ability to formally learn accurate facts about diverse cultures and apply that knowledge in a effective way to appropriately program with persons from diverse groups
Cultural skill	Nurse's ability to knowledgeably and proficiently use information regarding cultural issues in assessment and screening processes
Cultural encounter	Nurse's ability to actively and purposively seek out culturally different experiences to expand and develop cultural awareness, knowledge, and skill

context of their relationship to a Greater or Supreme Being (Nichols, 1987). Nurses and patients who exhibit this cultural axiology may say that they "feel a connection to a Supreme Being" and "must conduct" themselves in life and in their interactions with others according to that relationship belief. Many religious or secular groups' norms and actions are grounded in this cultural axiology.

In conjunction with the axiology is the idea that the epistemology, or the knowledge base, is grounded in understanding one's relationship with the Greater or Supreme Being. An example of this is the work of religious health care orders who make decisions regarding health care based upon the fact that the Greater or Supreme Being would direct them to whom to care for and how to care. In addition, a nurse exhibiting this epistemology would see this approach as maintaining harmony and balance in health and life.

Logic, or the reasoning ability for persons with the Native American world view states that persons are intrinsically all good. A patient exhibiting this view would not question any health care professional's advice regarding his or her treatment and would leave any decisions about care up to the professional since he or she would believe that person would have one's best interests in mind.

Process, or the development of relationships with another person, group, or community, is grounded in the idea that a Spirit or the Supreme Being exists in everything. "I know we are all part of a greater plan and direction and must do everything in our power to preserve and protect the Earth" represents this view. For some persons, the current thrust and support toward ecology and protection of the earth is founded in this thought. The earth, viewed as part of the greater continuum that contains the Greater or Supreme Being, should be guarded because of this connection.

The Cultural Competence Process Factor

Campinha-Bacote's model of cultural competence serves as the basis for this factor since it provides specific guidelines for developing basic cultural competence (Table 17-7). According to Campinha-Bacote (1994), the process of cultural competence involves development of four components: (1) cultural awareness, (2) cultural knowledge, (3) cultural skill, and (4) cultural encounter.

Cultural awareness

Cultural awareness is the initial component for development of basic cultural competence. It represents one's ability to acknowledge the fact that cultural similarities and differences exist. In addition, one's biases must be acknowledged. For example, a nurse who acknowledges his or her biases might say, "I know that there are different reasons for persons to develop HIV-AIDS and I should be understanding and caring toward anyone with the disease. But I have so many negative feelings about taking care of some persons who contract the disease."

Cultural knowledge

Cultural knowledge is the ability of a nurse to formally learn accurate facts about diverse cultures and apply that knowledge in an effective way so as to appropriately program (e.g., assess, develop appropriate intervention plans, and evaluate plans) with persons from the diverse groups. Cultural knowledge is another component within Leininger's ethnonursing knowledge and it influences psychiatric nurses' use of psychotherapeutic techniques with their patients.

One of the major areas of knowledge that psychiatric nurses should develop and use concerns persons' beliefs regarding health and illness. Persons generally believe in either folk medicine or Western medicine (Campinha-Bacote, 1997a). The folk medicine belief states that illnesses have natural or unnatural causes (Giger and Davidhizar, 1995). Cultural groups who may subscribe to these beliefs include Appalachian, Asian, African American, Mexican American, Haitian, West Indian, Native American, or Trinidadian groups (American Psychiatric Association [APA], 1994; Giger and Davidhizar, 1995; Hinton and Chen, 1993; Purnell and Counts, 1998). Nurses need to be aware of and knowledgeable about the fact that each one of these cultural groups may subscribe to one world view or have a combination of world views. For example, persons from the Appalachian culture exhibit a combination of world views since they incorporate a variety of ethnic racial group influences. While the original Appalachian culture stemmed from Europeans such as the English and Scots, current Appalachian culture has incorporated other ethnic racial groups, including African American and Native American (Purnell and Counts, 1998). Consequently, the Appalachian culture incorporates not only the European American world views but also those of the African, African American, Hispanic, Arabic, and Native American cultures. Persons from the Mexican American culture may incorporate the world views of African, African American, Hispanic, Arabic, and Native American groups. Persons from Haitian, West Indian, and Trinidadian cultural groups may also incorporate the world views of African, African American, Hispanic, and Arabic and Native American. It is also important for nurses to remember that every person is a unique human being and may have individual world views that are different from the predominant ethnic, racial, or cultural group with which the person identifies himself or herself.

A person who believes in the natural cause of illness or disease feels that everyone and everything in the world is interconnected (Giger and Davidhizar, 1995; Spector, 1996). In addition, an alteration in any person or thing changes the environment, and these changes may produce illness or disease. Natural causes of illness are those normal alterations in a person's air, food, or water environment that produce disharmony and imbalance within the person's equilibrium (Campinha-Bacote, 1994). These changes occur "naturally" in nature (i.e., they are not caused by outside forces). Persons who believe in the importance of maintaining the ecology subscribe to the natural causes belief of illness and disease. For example, individuals from Asian and Greek cultures may utilize specific treatments that restore the body's equilibrium (Andrews and Boyle, 1995; Tripp-Reimer and Sorofman, 1998). Such treatments might include the use of acupuncture, acupressure, nutritional therapies, skin scraping/coining, moxibustion, and cupping. Linear and circular lines throughout the body, known as *meridians,* are stimulated to restore balance through the use of needles *(acupuncture)* inserted into meridian areas or when pressure *(acupressure)* is exerted upon them (Giger and Davidhizar, 1995). Nutritional therapies may include the use of certain foods or herbs. Skin scraping/coining, moxibustion, and cupping are used to restore balance by bringing heat to the skin surface, which allows the release of the toxin or evil spirit from the affected body area (Giger and Davidhizar, 1995). In the case of **skin scraping/ coining,** a person, generally a healer in the community, uses a coin and briskly rubs or scrapes the skin surface. In **moxibustion,** a cotton ball containing the substance moxa, is ignited with a match in a small glass or cup. This glass or cup is then placed on the skin above a meridian. The idea is that the illness or evil is released from a person's body when heat is generated above the meridians. As noted in the clinical example, skin abrasions and contusions, often occurring on the skin as a result of skin scraping/coining, moxibustion, and cupping, may provide a climate for infection. Consequently, nurses needs to be knowledgeable regarding Leininger's concepts of cultural preservation, cultural negotiation, and repatterning to assist healers to use less heat and pressure when using these treatments (see clinical example). A nurse might suggest that a person place a small piece of cloth over the coin in addition to using less pressure. These negotiation strategies reduce the possibility of infection yet permit individuals to practice their beliefs.

When outside forces are involved in the cause of an illness or disease, it is termed unnatural. An example of an outside force is a magician, witch, ghost, or supernatural being that a person believes may use a spell or hex to cause an imbalance and produce illness or disease within the person (Giger and Davidhizar, 1995). A person of Hispanic descent may say that one's soul was lost *(susto)* because of another person's ability to cause a frightening experience or to place an evil eye *(mal ojo)* upon him or her (Campinha-Bacote, 1994; Purnell and Paulanka, 1998). Since good health is contingent upon the restoration of a person's equilibrium, an ill person may consult a healer or root doctor to help break the spell of the evil eye and return the lost soul (Giger and Davidhizar, 1995). Nurses need to be knowledgeable about these beliefs. In addition, the nurse may need to have the healer or root doctor included in the assessment and planning process of a patient for the plan and outcome to be successful. This consultation with the healer or root doctor is another example of the nurse using cultural preservation, cultural negotia-

tion, and repatterning to produce culturally competent care for patients. Another cultural example is illustrated by some groups' belief that certain liquids, foods, or medicines must be taken in balance with one another to restore health (Kuhn, 1998). A medicine might be labeled as hot and need to be taken in conjunction with a cold liquid or food to be effective. The terms *hot* and *cold* have nothing to do with temperature but are indicative of how the substance reacts within the body to restore equilibrium.

In addition, a person who believes in the unnatural cause of illness may see his or her illness as a divine punishment for bad or sinful behavior (Carson, 1989; Plummer, 1996; Zumbro Valley Medical Society, 1978). In this case, the person may not want to use medical intervention to treat his or her illness since the illness would be viewed as "part of life experience, punishment for what they did, or a way of atonement for sins." However, the person's minister or religious healer might be able to intercede by asking God for a "cure" through the use of prayer and meditation (Purnell and Paulanka, 1998). The psychiatric nurse would again need to use cultural preservation, cultural negotiation, and repatterning and include the patient, his identified family and friends, the healer, root doctor, and minister in the health assessment and planning process.

Persons who believe in Western medicine think there are specific scientific explanations for every illness and disease (Campinha-Bacote, 1994; Warren, 1996a, 1996b, 1997). The causes of illness and disease are viruses, bacteria, germs, biological change, and degenerative processes that can be seen or located through the use of blood tests, x-ray examination, scanning procedures, or other tests. This belief is grounded in the European world view in which the sources of illness can be seen, counted, and measured. Cures are based upon eradication of the causative agent. This belief regarding the cause of illness and disease provides an important basis for how many illnesses and diseases can be stabilized or cured since the causative agent can be located and targeted for treatment.

Ethnopharmacology

Ethnopharmacology is the study of the biological and psychological genetic influences *(pharmacoge-*

netics), effect *(pharmacodynamics)*, and metabolism *(pharmacokinetics)* of medications on different ethnic, racial, and cultural groups (Levy, 1993; Lin, Poland, and Anderson, 1995; Warren, 1996a, 1996b, 1997). This is another area in which psychiatric nurses need to develop their ethnonursing knowledge. Persons react to pharmacologic interventions based upon their normal biological makeup, environmental influences, and nonbiological factors (e.g., cultural influences) (Kudzma, 1992; Levy, 1993; Lin, Poland, and Anderson, 1995). Keltner (1995) has indicated that nurses need to examine three major components in their administration of psychotropic medications:

1. Five rights of administration (right patient, drug, dose, time, and route)
2. Knowledge regarding drug characteristics
3. Application of the nursing process

These components are part of the ethnonursing knowledge and cultural knowledge in the interlocking paradigm.

Specific ethnic, racial, and cultural differences affect a patient's medication options and dosage requirements. In general, children, women, and older patients require lower doses to achieve therapeutic effects and avoid toxic levels of medications (Kuhn, 1998). The use of medications by pregnant women should be carefully evaluated and monitored by physicians and nurses since very little conclusive research has been conducted on pregnant women, and there may be the risk of fetal malformations (Keltner, 1995; Kuhn, 1998). Nurses should also evaluate patients' use of alcohol and caffeine since use of these may potentiate the action of antidepressants and psychotropics and lead to toxicity (Kuhn, 1998).

Levy's (1993) findings have indicated that certain ethnic racial groups have a pharmacokinetic variation that causes them to be fast or slow metabolizers. Asian Americans may need smaller doses of psychotropic drugs since they reach higher plasma levels more quickly than do other ethnic racial groups (Kuhn, 1998). Free circulating drugs may accumulate in a patient's body when medications are metabolized too slowly. However, increased dosages may be required for persons who are fast metabolizers to produce the desired therapeutic effect since medications are too quickly metabolized and excreted (Levy, 1993).

Drug tolerance and effect may also be related to structural defects in drug receptor sites, which leads to improper binding of the drug at the receptor site and ineffective action of a medication even though the serum levels appear to be within the therapeutic range (Kudzma, 1992; Kuhn, 1998). For example, European Americans have a sensitivity to isoniazid (INH) toxicity and resultant peripheral neuritis. Asian American individuals have a very slow metabolism rate with tricyclic antidepressants, lithium, and haloperidol. Clozapine-induced agranulocytosis is higher in Ashkenazi Jewish and Native American populations than others.

Nurses need to be knowledgeable regarding the specific pharmacogenetic, pharmacodynamic, and pharmacokinetic alterations for African Americans regarding antihypertensives, antidepressants, and psychotropics. The angiotensin-renin and sodium-lithium countertransport systems may function differently in many African Americans than in European Americans. It has also been hypothesized that many African Americans have excessive renin production and a sensitivity to sodium that creates increased sodium and water reabsorption and resultant hypertension (Kudzma, 1992; Kuhn, 1998). In addition, African Americans who take diuretics to control their hypertension may have an intensified response to the action of psychotropics and antidepressants because of the altered sodium and water levels (Warren, 1996a, 1996b, 1997). All of these variations in pharmacogenetics, pharmacodynamics, and pharmacokinetics may contribute to higher rates of hypertension, higher red blood cell/serum lithium ratios, and higher rates of central nervous system-related side effects and toxicity in African Americans.

Since little research has been conducted on persons of Hispanic descent, less is known regarding pharmacogenetics, pharmacodynamics, and pharmacokinetics in this population (Kuhn, 1998). It has been reported, however, that Hispanics taking tricyclic antidepressants have required lower doses of the drugs and incur greater side effects than European Americans (Kuhn, 1998).

In addition, many persons of Hispanic and Asian descent may define certain medications, herbs, and illnesses according to "hot" and "cold" terms (Campinha-Bacote, 1994; Kuhn, 1998; Warren, 1996a, 1996b, 1997). Decisions regarding taking medications and herbs are made to maintain or restore physiological and psychological balance within a person (Kuhn, 1998). Hence, it is prudent that a nurse ask, "What is the accepted practice or the current treatment for my patient?"

Herbal therapies

Psychiatric nurses also need to assess patients' use of herbal therapies because patients often use herbs to maintain their health and to treat illness (Table 17-8). Korean ginseng is thought to be a "panacea" for treatment of a variety of psychological ailments, including insomnia, eating disorders, memory and concentration problems, nervousness and anxiety, alcoholism, and agoraphobia (Heineman, 1997). The Nigerian root extract is used to treat psychosis in some African populations (Lin, Poland, and Anderson, 1995). Some herbal therapies, however, may interfere with traditional Western medications' actions and metabolism. The Japanese herbs swertia japonica and kamikiki-to and the Cuban herb datura candida potentiate the actions of tricyclic antidepressants and low-potency antipsychotics (Lin, Poland, and Anderson, 1995). South American holly is analogous to caffeine and counteracts the sedative and anxiolytic effects of the benzodiazepines (Lin, Poland, and Anderson, 1995).

Summary

Nonbiological factors that influence pharmacologic metabolism and action include the person's personality, cultural beliefs and practices, stress, social support levels, and the attitudes of physicians and nurses regarding persons from diverse cultures. And finally, nurses' lack of knowledge regarding ethnopharmacology and patients' beliefs about the cause of illness may lead to the underdiagnosis, overdiagnosis, or misdiagnosis of patients from diverse cultural groups. Normal cultural variations and patterns may be misinterpreted as a sign of some illness when none is present. Or nurses may not adequately assess a cultural belief or practice and then fail to accurately observe changes or alterations within a patient.

Cultural skill

Cultural skill is the ability of a nurse to knowledgeably and proficiently use information regarding cultural issues in the assessment and screening procedures process. A variety of cultural assessment tools are available, including: Berlin and Fowkes's LEARN model (1982), Bloch's ethnic/cultural assessment guide (1983), Giger and Davidhizar's cultural assessment (1995), Leininger's sunrise model (1995), and Purnell's twelve domain model for cultural competence (Purnell and Counts, 1998) (Table 17-9).

Nurses should choose a cultural assessment tool based upon their cultural expertise, comfort level with the tool, the patient, and the amount of information needed. There are, however, some basic content areas a nurse should look for when deciding which assessment tool to use. These include communication, orientation, nutrition, family relationships, health beliefs, education, spiritual/religious, and biological/physiological elements. Table 17-10 contains an example of a cultural assessment worksheet with specific questions. Warren, Campinha-Bacote, and Munoz (1994) adapted this worksheet from Fong's assessment model (1985) and redeveloped it for use within the public mental health system of Ohio. The sheet has been modified by Warren (1997) and can now be used as an assessment guide for any patient and/or cultural group.

The cultural assessment

Cultural assessments should be a part of every psychological and physical assessment process that nurses conduct since every person has a unique culture that influences his or her health care be-

Table 17-8   Herbal Therapies

Herb	Property
Korean ginseng	Treatment for insomnia, eating disorders, memory and concentration problems, nervousness and anxiety, alcoholism, and agoraphobia
Nigerian root extract	Treatment of psychosis
Japanese swertia japonica and kamikiki-to	Potentiate the action of tricyclic antidepressants and low-potency antipsychotics
Cuban datura candida	Same as swertia and kamikiki-to
South American holly	Caffeine basis, counteracts the sedative anxiolytic effects of benzodiazepines

liefs and actions (Warren, 1996b, 1997). In addition, questions and observations should be smoothly and sensitively incorporated into any assessment process so it does not appear to the patient that the nurse is being rude or intrusive. For example, a nurse should *not* ask, "Do you believe that people are good or bad or a combination of both?" Instead, the nurse should observe the patient's attitudes and reactions in order to obtain this information. However, the nurse could directly ask a patient, "Is there anyone I could notify for you, or is there someone you would like to have here with you?" This would let the patient know that the nurse is concerned about his or her practices and would provide the nurse with the opportunity to include significant persons in the assessment and planning process. This nursing approach also increases ethnonursing knowledge and promotes cultural preservation, cultural negotiation, and repatterning as recommended by Leininger (1995) for effective and quality health care.

Cultural encounter

Cultural encounter is the ability of the nurse to actively and purposively seek out culturally different experiences to develop and expand cultural awareness, knowledge, and skill abilities (Campinha-Bacote, 1994). This is the nurse's use of Leininger's (1995) repatterning technique to identify areas in which the nurse would need further experience and knowledge to improve patients' health status. By definition, the nurse who exhibits cultural skill exhibits

cultural proficiency in areas of education, practice, and research.

The Assessment Factor

The assessment factor is represented by Purnell's (Purnell and Paulanka, 1998) twelve domain model for cultural competence (see Table 17-11 on p. 215). His model was chosen for the assessment factor because it provides a systematic psychological, physiological, and cultural guideline for the assessment of patients. In addition, it expands the theoretical, philosophical, and process knowledge bases for nurses, which supports the theoretical work of Leininger's concept (1995) of ethnonursing knowledge, Nichols's philosophy (1987) of world views, and Campinha-Bacote's process (1994) of cultural competence. And finally, the systematic style of Purnell's model (Purnell and Paulanka, 1998) makes it ideal for use in nursing education, practice, and research when precise assessment and data collection are required.

Purnell (1998) advises health care professionals to elicit cultural information based upon identification and exploration of the following assessment domains: (1) overview and heritage, (2) communication, (3) family roles and organization, (4) workforce issues, (5) biocultural ecology, (6) high-risk behaviors, (7) nutrition, (8) pregnancy and childbearing practices, (9) death rituals, (10) spirituality, (11) health care practices, and (12) health care practitioners. Purnell's model (1998) incorporates the European American world view concept in

---

Table 17-9   Cultural Assessments

Assessment Name	Assessment Domains
Berlin and Fowkes's LEARN model	Listen, explain, acknowledge, recommend, and negotiate when conducting a cultural assessment
Bloch's ethnic/cultural assessment guide	Collection of data in cultural, sociological, physiological, and psychological areas
Giger and Davidhizar's cultural assessment	Communication, space, social organization, time, environmental control, and biological variations
Leininger's sunrise model	Systematic examination of cultural beliefs, values, and practices
Purnell's twelve domain model for cultural competence	Overview and heritage, communication, family roles and organization, workforce issues, biocultural ecology, high-risk behaviors, nutrition, pregnancy and childbearing practices, death rituals, spirituality, health care practices, and health care practitioners

Table 17-10   Warren, Campinha-Bacote, and Munoz's Cultural Assessment Worksheet

Assessment Area	Questions or Areas of Inquiry
Communication	1. Do you speak any languages? 2. Is English your first language? 3. Does the patient speak English fluently? 4. Does the patient prefer an interpreter? 5. Does the patient feel appropriate touching is acceptable? 6. Are there ethnic behaviors that the patient uses?
Orientation	1. How long have you lived where you now live? 2. Where were you born? 3. What ethnic, racial, or cultural group do you identify yourself with? 4. How closely do you follow the traditional values, beliefs, and practices of your self-identified group? 5. What are the patient's thoughts on the following: human nature, development of knowledge, work ethic, relationship with nature.
Nutrition	1. Do you have certain foods you prefer? 2. What kind of foods do you eat when you are ill? 3. Do you avoid certain foods because of your beliefs?
Significant others and/or family	1. Who do you consider as important to you? 2. Is there anyone you would like for me to contact or not contact while you are here for treatment? 3. How are decisions made in your home environment? 4. In your home, what are the roles for children, women, and men? 5. What are some of the social customs or practices that you do at home? 6. Share with me three of your most important values.
Health	1. What brought you here for treatment today? 2. What do you think will help you feel better or get well? 3. Have you used treatments in the past that were helpful for you? 4. What type of treatments don't you like or feel comfortable receiving? 5. Is there something you think I can assist you with to help you improve? 6. Who do you usually go to for help or treatment when you're ill? 7. What do you think causes physical and mental problems?
Education	1. How do you prefer to learn new things, tasks (e.g., reading, watching television or videos, talking with someone)? 2. How have you gotten your education (e.g., in school, by self-instruction)? 3. How would you prefer to pay for your treatment?
Spirituality/religion	1. Do you consider yourself spiritual or religious? If so, what does that mean to you? 2. Do you have a religious preference? 3. Are there certain persons you like to talk to regarding your spiritual, religious beliefs, or health care, or are there practices that you like to participate in?
Biology/physiology	1. Do you have any specific health problems or disease conditions in your family of origin? 2. Are there certain medications, herbs, or any therapies that you avoid because they make you ill? 3. Are there specific skin, hair, grooming, or health care needs that you prefer? 4. Are you taking any medications now? (Include an examination of vitamin, nutritional, and herbal approaches.) 5. How many cigarettes do you smoke every day? 6. How many glasses of wine do you drink per week? 7. How many cans or bottles of coke, root beer, or beer do you drink per week? 8. How many cups of tea or/and coffee do you drink per day? 9. Are there any other beverages you drink every day? 10. How many bars or pieces of chocolate do you eat every day?

Table 17-11   **Assessment Factor: Purnell's Twelve Domain Model for Cultural Competence**

Component	Definition
Overview and heritage	Origins, residence, topography, economics, politics, education, and occupation for the patient
Communication	Dominant language, dialects, contextual use, volume and tone, spatial distancing, eye contact, facial expressions, greetings, temporality, time, preferred name and title, use of touch
Family roles and organization	Head of household, gender roles, goals and priorities, roles of aged, developmental tasks, extended family, social status, alternative life-styles
Workforce issues	Acculturation, autonomy, language barriers
Biocultural ecology	Biological variations, skin color, heredity, genetics, economics, drug metabolism
High-risk behaviors	Use of tobacco, alcohol, recreational drugs, level of physical activity, issues of safety
Nutrition	Meaning of food, common food preferences, food rituals, deficiencies, limitations, health promotion
Pregnancy	Fertility practices, views regarding pregnancy, birthing practices, postpartum
Death rituals	Rituals and bereavement practices
Spirituality	Religious or spiritual practices, use of prayer, meaning of life, individual areas of strength, relationship to health
Health care practices	Focus of health care, traditional practices, major beliefs, responsibility for health, self-medication, role of pain, illness, mental health beliefs
Health care practitioners	Perceptions of health care practitioners, role of folk practitioners or healers, gender and health care status

its systematic approach to collection of data on a person. However, he also has included a number of areas that specifically direct the nurse to examine the patient's perception and beliefs regarding the other three predominant world views. Among these areas are overview and heritage, communication, family roles and organization, death rituals, and spirituality.

Purnell's visual depiction of his model is circular with a solid circle in the middle representative of unknown phenomena. The global society is on the outside of three concentric circles representing community, family, and person. The twelve assessment domains are spokes connected to the unknown phenomena circle. Purnell's model also provides suggestions for the health care provider to identify, observe, and explore within each domain. Examples of these in the overview and heritage domain are to identify the part of the world from which this group may originate and assess what is considered education, as well as the person's level of education within that cultural framework.

SUMMARY

Cultural competence adds to the clinical excellence of psychiatric nursing practice when it is incorporated into psychotherapeutic management techniques. This combination is even more critical because of today's increasing numbers of culturally diverse groups and the rapidly evolving managed care environment. The interlocking paradigm of cultural competence incorporates five factors in the development of the process of cultural competence: nurse-patient interaction, theory, philosophy, process, and assessment. Each of the factors involves the development and use of specific cultural knowledge regarding persons' physiological, psychological, and spiritual beliefs and practices as they relate to various levels of health.

Key Concepts

1. Cultural competency is an important process for nursing because it can promote understanding between patients, nurses, and other health care professionals as

well as enhance clinical excellence in the areas of education, practice, and research.

2. Culture is important for nurses to understand because it is a critical component of peoples' lives. Culture affects their health care attitudes and actions in relationship to their ability to understand and utilize the interventions that psychiatric nurses develop.

3. The Interlocking Paradigm of Cultural Competence serves as a model of how nurses can theoretically and philosophically understand, develop, and proficiently use culturally competent strategies and assessment techniques.

4. Cultural incompetence can create patient noncompliance and inadequate interventions because it negates the importance of culture.

5. Ethnonursing, a combination of nursing practice and cultural knowledge, promotes culturally competent nursing care.

6. Ethnopharmacology is a key concept for nurses to understand and use as it helps them to incorporate knowledge regarding the biological and psychological influences of medications on different ethnic, racial, and cultural groups.

7. Herbal therapies are alternative medicinal approaches to treating patients' psychological and physiological illnesses.

8. A cultural assessment is an examination of a patient's cultural perspective that needs to be part of any nursing assessment process.

▌ Study Questions

(Answer key is in the back of the book.)

1. Which of the following factors in the Interlocking Paradigm of Cultural Competence support the psychotherapeutic management model of care by providing effective nursing care for patients?
   a. Leininger's cultural care diversity and universality theory.
   b. Nichols's philosophy of world views.
   c. Campinha-Bacote's model of cultural competence.
   d. Purnell's cultural assessment domains.
   e. All of the above.

2. A mother of Asian descent brings her 18-month-old daughter to the pediatrician's office for a well-baby visit. The pediatric nurse practitioner (PNP) discovers that the little girl has multiple long lines of contusions and abrasions on her back. When the PNP asks the mother what happened, she responds with, "She was feverish, and I helped her get better." After further assessment of the child and talking with the mother, the nurse comes to the following conclusion(s) regarding the situation:
   a. The child is a victim of abuse by the mother.
   b. The child fell when she was ill.

   c. The mother used "coining," a healing technique recommended by the child's grandmother, to reduce her temperature.
   d. The child may be presenting early symptoms of a blood dyscrasia and should be seen by a hematologist.
   e. b and c

3. What is (are) the next step(s) that the PNP would use in developing a plan of care for the mother and child?
   a. Notify the child authorities that she suspects the child is being abused by the mother.
   b. Examine the child for further injuries.
   c. Ask the mother to explain what she meant when she said she "helped her get better."
   d. Use cultural negotiation and assist the mother in being able to "help" her daughter in the future when or if she becomes ill.
   e. b, c, and d

REFERENCES

ANA Expert Panel Report: ANA expert panel report: culturally competent health care, *Nurs Outlook* 40(6): 277, 1993.

Adebimpe V: Overview: white norms in psychiatric diagnosis of Black American patients, *J Psychiatry* 138(3): 279, 1981.

American Nurses Association: *A statement on psychiatric mental-health nursing practice*, Washington, DC, 1994, The Association.

American Nurses Association: *Cultural diversity in the nursing curriculum: a guide for implementation*, Kansas City, Mo, 1986, The Association.

American Psychiatric Association: *Diagnostic and statistical manual of mental disorders-IV (DSM-IV)*, ed 4, Washington, DC, 1994, The Association.

Andrews MM and Boyle JS: *Transcultural concepts in nursing care*, ed 2, Philadelphia, 1995, JB Lippincott.

Anthony WA: Recovery from mental illness: the guiding vision of the mental health services in the 1990's, *Psychiatr Rehabil J* 2(3): 17, 1993.

Bell R: Prominence of women in Navajo healing beliefs and values, *Nurs Health Care* 15(1): 232, 1994.

Berlin J and Fowkes W: A teaching framework for cross-cultural health, *West J Med* 139(6), 934, 1982.

Bloch B: Bloch's assessment guide for ethnic/cultural variations. In Orque M and Monry L, editors: *A multicultural approach*, St. Louis, 1983, Mosby.

Brink P: Cultural aspects of homosexuality, *Holistic Nurs Pract* 1(4): 12, 1987.

Campinha-Bacote J: *The process of cultural competence in health care: a culturally competent model of care*, ed 2,

Wyoming, Ohio, 1994, Transcultural C.A.R.E. Associates, Perfect Printing Press.

Campinha-Bacote J: Readings and resources in transcultural health care and mental health, *Monographs from Transcultural C.A.R.E.,* ed 9, Wyoming, Ohio, 1997a, Perfect Printing Press.

Campinha-Bacote J: Understanding the influence of culture. In Haber J, et al: *Comprehensive psychiatric nursing,* ed 5, St. Louis, 1997b, Mosby.

Carson V: *Spiritual dimensions of nursing practice,* Philadelphia, 1989, WB Saunders.

Charlow BA: Rational care or rationed care? The choice could be up to you, *The Journal* 7(1): 14, 1996.

Clement J: Managed care and recovery: opportunities for psychiatric nursing, *Arch Psychiatr Nurs* 11(5): 231, 1997.

Comas-Diaz L and Green B: Women of color: integrating ethnic and gender identities in psychotherapy, New York, 1994, Guilford.

Dunn T, director and producer: *Tai chi for health*, Venice, Ca, 1996, Healing Arts Publishing, Inc. (videotape).

Flaskerud J: Racial/ethnic identity and amount and type of psychiatric treatment, *Am J Psychiatry* 149: 379, 1992.

Fong CM: Ethnicity and nursing practice, *Top Clin Nurs* 7(3): 1, 1985.

Giger JN and Davidhizar RE: *Transcultural nursing: assessment and intervention,* ed 2, St. Louis, 1995, Mosby.

Heineman J: *Healing power herbs,* Boca Raton, Fla, 1997, Globe Digests.

Hinton W and Chen Y: DSM-III disorders in Vietnamese refugees, *JAMA* 181(2): 113, 1993.

Hogan MF: *Recovery: the new force in mental health.* Paper presented at the meeting of the Lake County Mental Health Board, Cleveland, 1993.

Hogan MF: *Living in community,* Columbus, Ohio, 1996, Ohio Department of Mental Health.

Homma-True R, et al: Ethnocultural diversity in clinical psychology, *Clin Psychol* 46: 50, 1993.

Hughes C: Culture in clinical psychiatry. In Gaw A, editor: *Culture, ethnicity, and mental illness,* Washington, DC, 1993, American Psychiatric Press.

Keltner NL: Introduction to psychotropic drugs. In Keltner NL, Schwecke LH, and Bostrom CE, editors: *Psychiatric Nursing,* ed 2, St. Louis, 1995, Mosby.

Kudzma E: All bodies are not created equal, *Am J Nurs* 12: 48, December 1992.

Kuhn M: *Pharmaco-therapeutics: a nursing process approach,* ed 4, Philadelphia, 1998, FA Davis.

Lawson W: Racial and ethnic differences in psychiatric research, *Hosp Community Psychiatry* 37: 50, 1986.

Leininger M: Transcultural nursing: concepts, theories and practices, New York, 1995, McGraw-Hill.

Levy R: *Ethnic and racial differences in responses to medications,* Reston, Va, 1993, National Pharmaceutical Council.

Lin K, Poland RE, and Anderson D: Psychopharmacology, ethnicity and culture, *Transcultural Psychiatr Res Rev* 32: 1, 1995.

Lipson JG, Dibble SL, and Minarik PA: *Culture and nursing care: a pocket guide,* San Francisco, 1996, UCSF Nursing Press.

Meleis AI, et al: *Diversity, marginalization, and culturally competent health care: issues in knowledge development,* Washington, DC, 1995, American Academy of Nursing.

Nichols E: *Nichols' model of the philosophical aspects of cultural difference.* Paper presented at meeting of faculty, The Ohio State University, Columbus, Ohio, June 1987.

Pedersen P: *A handbook for developing multicultural awareness,* ed 2, Alexandria, Va, 1994, American Counseling Association.

Peplau H: *Interpersonal relations in nursing,* New York, 1952, Putnam.

Peplau H: The art and science of nursing, *Nurs Sci Q* 1: 8, 1988.

Plummer P: Developing culturally responsive psychosocial rehabilitative programs for African Americans, *Psychiatr Rehabil J* 19(4): 38, 1996.

Purnell L and Counts M: Appalachians. In Purnell L and Paulanka P, editors: *Transcultural health care: a culturally competent approach,* Philadelphia, 1998, FA Davis.

Purnell L and Paulanka P: Purnell's model for cultural competence. In Purnell L and Paulanka P, editors: *Transcultural health care: a culturally competent approach,* Philadelphia, 1998, FA Davis.

Spector R: *Cultural diversity in health and illness,* ed 4, Stamford, Conn, 1996, Appleton & Lange.

Stewart B: Overview of culture and behavior. In Antai-Ontong D, editor: *Psychiatric nursing: biological and behavioral concepts,* Philadelphia, 1995, WB Saunders.

Sue DW and Sue D: *Counseling for the culturally different: theory and practice,* ed 2, New York, 1990, John Wiley.

Tripp-Reimer T and Sorofman B: Greek-Americans. In Purnell L and Paulanka P, editors: *Transcultural health care: a culturally competent approach,* Philadelphia, 1998, FA Davis.

Tylor E: *Primitive culture,* vol I, London, 1871, Bradbury, Evans, & Co.

Villarosa L, editor: *Body and soul: the black woman's guide to physical health and emotional well-being,* New York, 1994, Harper Perennial.

Warren BJ: *Cultural competency: implications for nursing education, practice, and research. Integrating psychiatric mental health nursing into education, research, and practice.* Symposium conducted at the 1996 Annual Conference of the Society for Education and Research in Psychiatric Mental Health Nursing (SERPN), Nashville, Tenn, November 1996a.

Warren BJ: Cultural competency: implications for nursing, *SERPN News Series* 1(3): 1, 1996b.

Warren BJ: *Cultural competence: the critical connection.* Workshop symposium presented for the meeting of the ADAMHS Board, CompDrug, Columbus, Ohio, 1997.

Warren BJ, Campinha-Bacote J, and Munoz C: *Cultural assessment worksheet,* Columbus, Ohio, 1994, Unpublished.

Worthington C: An examination of factors influencing the diagnosis and treatment of black patients in the mental health system, *Arch Psychiatr Nurs* 6(33): 195, 1992.

Zumbro Valley Medical Society, Medicine and Religion Committee: *Religious aspects of medical care: a handbook of religious practices of all faiths,* ed 2, St. Louis, 1978, Catholic Hospital Association.

Psychopharmacology

CHAPTER 18

Introduction to Psychotropic Drugs

NORMAN L. KELTNER

LEARNING OBJECTIVES

After reading this chapter you should be able to:
- Define the role of psychopharmacology in psychotherapeutic management.
- Identify the nurse's responsibilities in administering psychotropic drugs.
- Describe the function and inactivation of neurotransmitters.
- Discuss the function of the blood-brain barrier and the significance of lipid solubility.
- State the benefits of teaching patients about psychotropic drugs.

"Telling me that I have a brain disease and that I should take medications does not solve my problems." (Riffer NW: It's a brain disease, *Psychiatric Services,* 48(6):773, 1997)

We are a drug-taking society. People take all kinds of drugs: drugs to sleep, drugs to wake up, drugs to fight infections, drugs to lower blood pressure, drugs to lower cholesterol, drugs to lose weight. We take drugs for all kinds of reasons. We take prescription drugs, over-the-counter drugs, legal drugs, and illegal drugs. Drugs, drugs, drugs! We take drugs to fix things. And, of course, we take drugs for mental and emotional problems.

Among these drugs are those that will reduce "crazy" thinking (antipsychotics), slow down the manic mind (mood stabilizers or antimanic agents), improve mood (antidepressants), calm the nerves (antianxiety drugs), improve thinking (drugs for Alzheimer's disease), and even drugs to correct problems caused by the drugs just listed (e.g., antiparkinson drugs).

The introductory quote from Dr. Riffer, when coupled with the pejorative tone of the opening paragraph, would suggest a negative view of psychotropic drugs by the authors. Nothing could be further from the truth. In fact, no other psychiatric nursing textbook has historically emphasized the

KEY TERMS

Axon   The part of a neuron that transmits impulses away from the cell body

Blood-brain barrier   A barrier that guards the brain from fluctuations in body chemistry. It regulates the amount and speed with which substances in the blood enter the brain.

Dendrites   The part of the neuron that transmits impulses toward the cell body

Lipid solubility   The ability of a substance to dissolve in fat

Neurotransmitters   Chemical substances in the nervous system that facilitate the transmission of nerve impulses across synapses between neurons

Noncompliance   Failure to take medication as prescribed

Precursor   Something that precedes. Tyrosine is a precursor to dopamine in the synthesis of dopamine in the body.

Synapse   The microscopic space between two neurons

Vesicle   Storage sac at the synaptic terminal

---

importance of these agents more than this text has. Nevertheless, this somewhat negative observation suggests several important points:

1. Psychotropic drugs alone are seldom the answer.
2. Americans are looking for answers in the form of a pill.
3. The use of psychotropic medications must be more than an unhealthy extension of #2.

Ideally, psychotropic drugs should be prescribed based on an accurate diagnosis and then taken until an acceptable mental/emotional state can be obtained. At that point, the patient could hopefully be withdrawn from the medication and then proceed with his or her life. Unfortunately, this does not always occur. Some individuals recover never to need these medications again, others become dependent on these agents as proposed in (2) above, and still others need the chemistry-correcting properties of these drugs for the foreseeable future.

In Chapter 1, a brief historical review of the development of psychotropic drugs is presented. Box 18-1 outlines a summary of significant points in the evolution of psychopharmacology. A careful reading of this summary reveals that antipsychotics, antidepressants, and antimanic agents were all developed before 1960. Though many related drugs were eventually synthesized from the prototypes of each class, the "clones" were remarkably similar to the original. In the past decade, however, several substantially different kinds of drugs have emerged. Clozapine (Clozaril) and other atypical antipsychotic medications are very different from the traditional antipsychotics. Fluoxetine (Prozac) and other

selective serotonin reuptake inhibitors (SSRIs) are quite different from the earlier antidepressants. Finally, new drugs in the treatment of Alzheimer's disease (tacrine [Cognex], donepezil [Aricept]) are providing hope and encouragement to many patients and families plagued by this illness. These examples point to the continuous effort by clinicians and researchers to effectively address the mental, emotional, and addictive disorders afflicting approximately 25% of Americans. These exciting new developments in psychopharmacology are creating a climate at the end of the "decade of the brain" that should challenge every nurse to understand and apply psychopharmacological concepts to practice.

NURSING RESPONSIBILITIES

Psychopharmacology is the second component of the psychotherapeutic management model. The effectiveness of treatment with antipsychotic, antidepressant, and antimanic drugs is not questioned. These drugs have enabled millions of persons to live more satisfying and productive lives. The least restrictive alternative or environment, a concept that captures the community mental health effort to allow individuals to live their lives in an unrestrictive atmosphere, has evolved primarily as a result of the impact of these drugs.

Because nursing provides 24-hour care, the nurse is in an advantageous position to assess drug side effects, evaluate desired effects, and apply preventative care to reduce potential problems. In addition, the nurse most often makes decisions concerning prn

Box 18-1   Significant Points in the Evolution of Psychotropic Drugs

1930s Benzodiazepines are first synthesized by Sternbach.

1948 Rapport, Green, and Page isolate "serotonin" from beef serum.

1949 John Cade, an Australian psychiatrist, reports on the efficacy of lithium in mania.

1949 The U.S. Food and Drug Administration bans lithium because of deaths in patients with cardiac disease.

1951 Chlorpromazine is developed as a nonsedating antihistamine. Laborit and others report diminished surgical anxiety in conscious patients.

1952 Delay and Deniker, two psychiatrists working with Laborit, administer chlorpromazine to a manic patient with successful results.

1952 Iproniazid, a derivative of the antituberculosis agent isoniazid, is identified as a monoamine oxidase inhibitor (MAOI).

1953 Bein isolates reserpine from rauwolfia. Reserpine, effective in treating psychosis, causes severe depression related to depletion of norepinephrine.

1954 Lehman publishes the first American article on chlorpromazine in the *Archives of Neurology and Psychiatry*.

1955 Researchers alter the molecular structure of chlorpromazine, developing new antipsychotic agents, e.g., haloperidol and fluphenazine.

1957 The first papers appear on MAOIs as antidepressants.

1957 Haloperidol (Haldol) is developed.

1958 Kuhn publishes the first article on tricyclic antidepressants in the *American Journal of Psychiatry*.

1960 Harris presents the first paper on the effectiveness of benzodiazepines in *The Journal of the American Medical Association*.

1970 The ban on lithium is lifted in the United States.

1980s A new class of antidepressants is developed, the selective serotonin reuptake inhibitors (SSRIs).

1980s The antiepileptic drugs carbamazepine and valproate are reported to have mood-stabilizing properties.

1990s Clozapine (Clozaril) and risperidone (Risperdal), the first truly new antipsychotic agents in 40 years, are released in the United States.

1990s Tacrine (Cognex), a drug used to treat patients with Alzheimer's disease, is made available. Studies indicate that about 20% to 30% of cases improve.

From Ayd FJ: The early history of modern psychopharmacology, *Neuropsychopharmacology* 5(2):71, 1991; Kuhn R: The treatment of depressive states with G 22355 (imipramine hydrochloride), *Am Psychiatry*, 115(5):459, 1958; Rifkin A: Extrapyramidal side effects: a historical perspective, *J Clin Psychiatry*, 48(9):3, 1987.

medications. Nearly one half of all orders for antipsychotic drugs are written prn (Blair, 1990). The nurse, therefore, needs to understand key dimensions of psychotropic drug use. Box 18-2 outlines nursing responsibilities for psychotropic drug administration based on the American Nurses Association's (ANA's) guidelines on psychopharmacology.

Each chapter in Unit Four provides a discussion of pharmacological effects (desired effects); absorption, distribution, and administration; side effects (undesired effects); and drug interactions. Equally important, a discussion of nursing implications emphasizes nursing interventions related to therapeutic vs. toxic drug levels, use during pregnancy, use in the elderly, side effects, interactions, and teaching patients.

Understanding psychopharmacology involves more than memorizing facts. The nurse must understand two concepts: *neurotransmitters* and the *blood-brain barrier*. These two concepts are central to understanding the categories of drugs discussed in this book. An overview of these two important concepts is given in this chapter and should be studied before reading about specific psychotropic drugs. A third concept, the science and art of teaching patients about psychotropic agents, crosses all drug categories and should be included in discussions with patients and their families. A brief overview of patient teaching strategies concludes the chapter. Drug-specific issues concerning teaching are found in each chapter.

■ Critical Thinking Question

Some nurses may have little knowledge about some drugs they administer. Do you consider this unethical, unprofessional, unsafe, or simply a reality of the nursing profession? Since no one can know every drug, what basic information should a nurse know before giving medication?

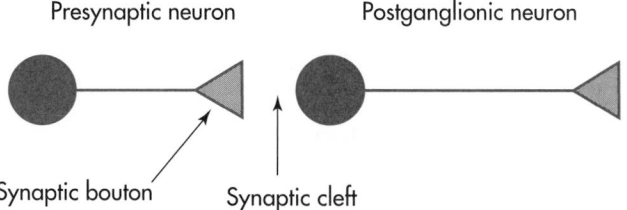

Presynaptic neuron   Postganglionic neuron

Synaptic bouton   Synaptic cleft

FIGURE 18-1 Two-neuron chain showing the presynaptic and postsynaptic neurons interconnected by a synapse. The synapse is composed of a synaptic bouton *(triangle)* that is on the presynaptic membrane, the synaptic cleft, and the postsynaptic membrane, which in this instance is the dendrite or cell body *(circle)* of the postsynaptic neuron. (From Keltner N and Folks D: *Psychotropic Drugs,* St. Louis, 1997, Mosby.)

Box 18-2 Objectives from the ANA Guidelines on Psychopharmacology

The psychiatric mental health nurse can:

1. Describe psychopharmacological agents based on similarities and differences
2. Discuss actions of psychopharmacological agents from global responses to cellular responses
3. Differentiate psychiatric symptoms from medication side effects
4. Apply basic principles of pharmacokinetics and pharmacodynamics
5. Identify appropriate use of psychopharmacological agents in special populations
6. Involve clients and their families
7. Identify factors that may prevent the active involvement of clients in their care
8. Describe appropriate nonpsychopharmacological interventions
9. Discuss the use of standardized rating scales
10. Demonstrate the knowledge necessary to develop psychopharmacological education and treatment plans

Adapted from Laraia MT, et al: *Psychiatric Mental Health Nursing Psychopharmacology Project,* Washington, DC, 1994, American Nurses Association.

NEUROTRANSMITTERS

Nerve cells, or neurons, comprise the basic unit of the nervous system. Nerve cells are designed to receive and give information. Dendrites are the projections from the neuron that receive information and transmit it to the cell body. Axons send information from the nerve cell to the dendrites, axons, or cell bodies of other neurons. Axons of one cell are separated from the dendrites, axons, or cell body of another by a microscopic space known as a synapse (Figure 18-1). Figure 18-2 depicts the relationship between neurotransmitters, neurons, and psychotropic drugs.

Information, in the form of an electrochemical excitation, is communicated between cells in a specific manner. An electrochemical impulse runs from the cell body through the axon to the presynaptic terminal. Neurotransmitters are stimulated and released from the presynaptic terminal into the synaptic cleft and combine with the postsynaptic receptors on the dendrites of the neuron, evoking a neuronal response. Lest the student be misled, it should be explained that neurons are not strung throughout the brain end on end. The neuronal system is very complex, with some neurons receiving input from thousands of other neurons. Furthermore, the arborization or branching of dendrites continues into late adolescence and may partially account for the emergence of schizophrenia at this time of life.

Neurotransmitters are synthesized from natural precursors (e.g., amino acids) in the body (Box 18-3). These precursors are extracted from the bloodstream and are synthesized in the cell into neurotransmitters. Neurotransmitters are stored in storage vesicles in the presynaptic terminals of the cell. There are many kinds of neurotransmitters, and they combine with specific receptors. For instance, the neurotransmitter norepinephrine combines only with a norepinephrine receptor. Once norepinephrine electrochemically stimulates the norepinephrine receptor, information is transmitted from the dendritic outgrowth to the cell body, which in turn communicates to the next neuron, and so on. Once

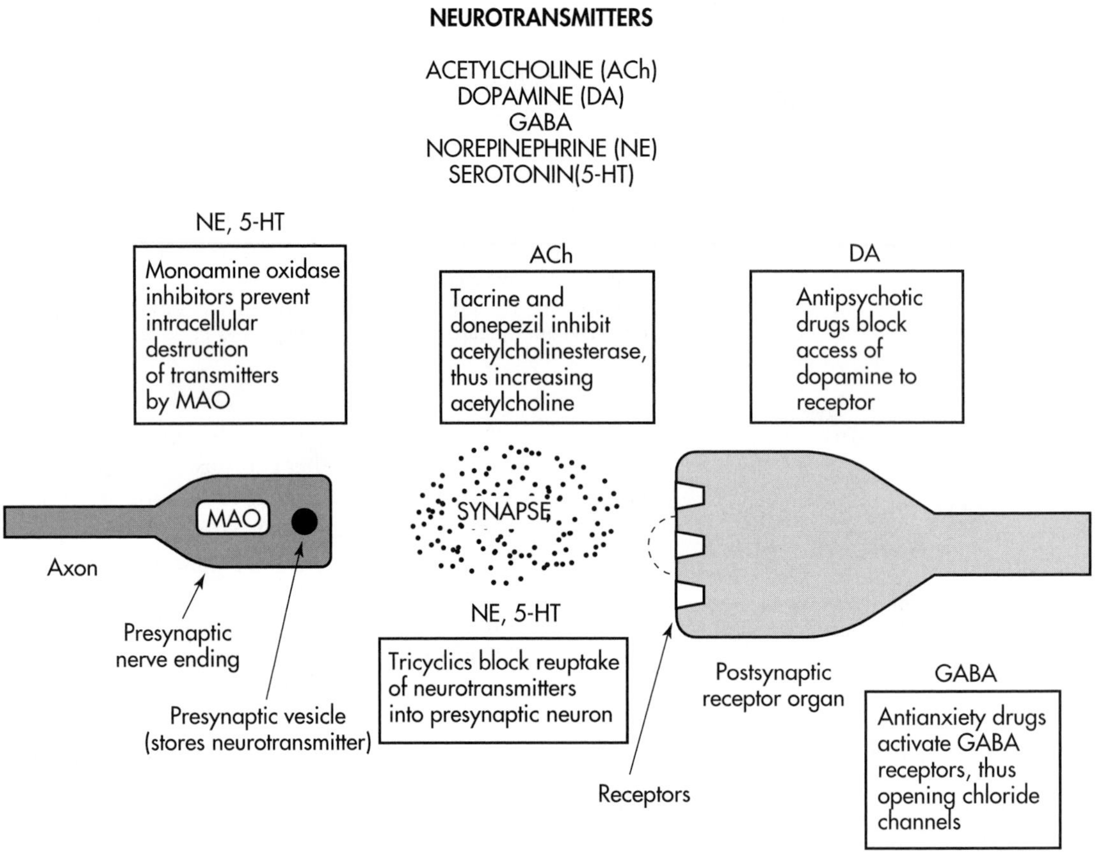

FIGURE 18-2 Explanation of how the five major neurotransmitters are affected by psychotropic drugs. (Adapted from Stuart G and Sundeen S: *Principles and practice of psychiatric nursing,* ed 5, St. Louis, 1995, Mosby.)

Box 18-3   Four Neurotransmitter Systems*

Monoamines
Dopamine (a catecholamine)
Norepinephrine (a catecholamine)
Serotonin (an indolamine)

Cholinergic
Acetylcholine

Amino acids
Gamma-aminobutyric acid (GABA)

Peptides
Enkephalins

*See Table 5-1 for greater detail.

---

in the synaptic cleft, the neurotransmitter can, until it is inactivated, continue to stimulate the postsynaptic receptor. Neurotransmitters are inactivated in two ways: they are metabolized by enzymes, or, more often, they are taken back into the presynaptic storage vesicles (referred to as reuptake). Knowledge of this inactivation process has facilitated the evolution of psychopharmacology. The most important neurotransmitters for psychiatric nursing students to understand are presented in Box 18-4 and 18-5.

Psychotropic drugs can affect neurotransmitters in several ways (Figure 18-2):

1. The release of a neurotransmitter can be affected. Some drugs cause the release of stored neurotransmitters. For example, amantadine (Symmetrel), an antiparkinson drug, causes the release of the neurotransmitter dopamine.

2. Psychotropic drugs can combine with a receptor and prevent the "natural" neurotransmitter from combining with it. Antipsychotic drugs such as chlorpromazine (Thorazine) block dopamine receptors.
3. Psychotropic drugs can affect the response of a receptor to a neurotransmitter. For example, tricyclic antidepressants (TCAs) are thought to "down-regulate" postsynaptic receptors thus changing these receptors' sensitivity to neurotransmitters.
4. Psychotropic drugs can terminate the inactivation of neurotransmitters. Tricyclic antidepressants block the reuptake of neurotransmitters; antidepressants of another class, the monoamine oxidase inhibitors, block the enzymatic reduction of neurotransmitters (Brown and Mann, 1987).

Box 18-4 Most Important Neurotransmitters for Psychiatric Nursing Students to Know

Psychotropic drugs work by affecting neurotransmitter systems. The authors believe the foundation for understanding psychotropic drugs rests on knowledge of just five neurotransmitters. Though there is much to be learned, we are satisfied that understanding how psychotropic drugs affect acetylcholine, dopamine, gamma-aminobutyric acid (GABA), norepinephrine, and serotonin is the starting point. As the following chapters will discuss:

Acetylcholine is important in conceptualizing the pathology and treatment of Alzheimer's disease and parkinsonism.

Dopamine is important in conceptualizing the pathology and treatment of schizophrenia and parkinsonism.

GABA is important in conceptualizing the pathology and treatment of anxiety.

Norepinephrine is important in conceptualizing the pathology and treatment of mania and depression.

Serotonin is important in conceptualizing the pathology and treatment of mania and depression.

Box 18-5 illustrates the relationship between these neurotransmitters and specific mental disorders.

BLOOD-BRAIN BARRIER

The second concept, the blood-brain barrier, is also important for understanding psychotropic drug activity (Goldstein and Betz, 1986). Life depends on homeostasis, or balance. The brain, more than other organs of the body, requires a constant internal milieu. Whereas other parts of the body experience fluctuations in body chemistry, even small changes in the brain produce serious problems. The brain is protected from fluctuations by the blood-brain barrier. This barrier regulates the amount and speed of substances in the blood entering the brain. Water, carbon dioxide, and oxygen readily cross the barrier; other substances are excluded from the brain.

The blood-brain barrier has three dimensions: an anatomical dimension, a physiological dimension, and a metabolic dimension. The anatomical dimension is the structure of the capillaries that supply blood to the brain and prevent many molecules from "slipping" through.

The physiological dimension is a chemical and transport system that recognizes and then allows certain molecules into the brain. Lipid solubility is the most important of the chemical properties that determine whether a molecule will pass through the blood-brain barrier. Highly lipid-soluble substances pass the blood-brain barrier with relative ease.

Box 18-5 Neurotransmitters and Related Mental Disorders*

Neurotransmitter Action	Related Mental Disorder
Increase in dopamine	Schizophrenia
Decrease in norepinephrine	Depression
Decrease in serotonin	Depression
Decrease in acetylcholine	Alzheimer's disease
Decrease in gamma-aminobutyric acid (GABA)	Anxiety

*The authors realize this is an overly simplistic explanation but the box does serve to convey the basic neurotransmitter theories for the related mental disorder.

Highly water-soluble substances penetrate this barrier slowly and in insignificant amounts. Nicotine, ethanol, heroin, caffeine, and diazepam (Valium) are examples of highly lipid-soluble substances. Penicillin, dopamine, epinephrine, and potassium are not highly lipid-soluble and do not penetrate the blood-brain barrier well. This is clinically significant because only drugs that can pass through this barrier in significant amounts are effective in treating a psychiatric or medical disorder of the brain. Certain non–lipid-soluble substances such as glucose, the brain's primary energy source, and essential amino acids, which are needed for the synthesis of neurotransmitters, are required for normal brain function. Special transport systems carry these essential substances across the blood-brain barrier. A discussion of transport systems is beyond the scope of this book; however, a detailed review can be found in an article by Goldstein and Betz (1986).

The metabolic barrier prevents molecules from entering the brain by enzymatic action within the endothelial lining of the brain capillaries. For example, levodopa can pass the blood-brain barrier, but much of it is reduced to dopamine before it can pass completely through the capillary wall into the brain. The metabolic product, dopamine, does not readily pass this barrier, thus illustrating the third way our brains protect us from substances in peripheral circulation.

The importance of understanding the blood-brain barrier for the psychiatric nurse can be illustrated by several examples. If, for instance, penicillin were the only antibiotic available (which was true at one time), large doses would be needed for a central nervous system (CNS) infection because this water-soluble drug does not pass the blood-brain barrier easily. When a large dose of penicillin is given only a fraction of that dose enters the brain. Most of the penicillin stays in the peripheral system. This does not cause alarm because penicillin has relatively few adverse effects. On the other hand, dopamine (and many other drugs), which is used to treat parkinsonism (a dopamine-deficiency disease), has many adverse affects on the body. The dosage needed to adequately affect the brain (a central effect) is so large that it would have serious adverse effects on the rest of the body (e.g., cardiac stimulation, a peripheral effect). Understanding the blood-brain barrier helps the nurse accurately conceptualize drug therapy. It

also provides a base for understanding how highly lipid-soluble substances such as alcohol and heroin can be so addicting.

■ Critical Thinking Question

Many patients with parkinsonism are also often depressed. The major neurotransmitter deficit associated with parkinsonism is dopamine, yet dopamine deficiency often is not mentioned in the depression literature. Can you explain this from a physiological perspective? (Hint: look at the figures in the next chapter.)

TEACHING PATIENTS

The importance of teaching patients cannot be overemphasized. Macpherson, et al (1993) found that 72% of psychiatric patients demonstrated no understanding of their medications. Geller (1982), in an oft-quoted report a few years earlier, found that only 8% of psychiatric inpatients knew the name, dosage schedule, and desired effect of the drugs they were receiving. Clinical experience indicates that this percentage has improved somewhat; still, there is much ignorance about these drugs to overcome. Added to this ignorance of drugs is the sobering statistic that up to 92% of rehospitalizations are related to patients' nonadherence to medication schedules (Coudreaut-Quinn, Emmons, and McMorrow, 1992). As knowledge deficits are removed, better compliance can be anticipated.

Despite a certain risk associated with discussing medications and side effects with patients, nurses have a professional duty to do so with knowledge and sensitivity, that is, with balance. The nurse may frighten patients with too much or inappropriate information. Good professional judgment is important, including teaching patients about what effects are visible, what can be felt, and what the possibilities are of becoming drug-dependent (e.g., benzodiazepines). The nurse should also emphasize regular checkups and tests.

Teaching patients about their medications enables them to be mature participants in their own care and can decrease undesirable side effects (Brown and Mann, 1987). Furthermore, noncompliance or the failure to take medications as prescribed, can be reduced by effective teaching. Each chapter in this unit outlines patient education issues specific to each class of drugs discussed.

■ Critical Thinking Question

In this chapter the authors state that the nurse should use balance when giving information to a patient about a drug. What is the balance between arousing unneeded apprehension in a patient vulnerable to suggestion and treating that adult patient like a child? Obviously, in your role as student and later as nurse, you would not want to do either.

◆ Key Concepts

1. Psychopharmacology is the second component of psychotherapeutic management. Psychotropic drugs have enabled millions of persons to live more productive lives in the "least restrictive alternative/environment."
2. Nurses assess for drug side effects, evaluate desired effects, and make decisions about prn medications, so it is important for nurses to understand general principles of psychopharmacology and to have specific knowledge concerning frequently used psychotropic drugs.
3. Neurotransmitters, which are neurochemical substances in the brain, evoke a neuronal response, are synthesized by cytoplasmic enzymes, and are typically stored in storage vesicles in the presynaptic terminals of the neuron.
4. Since both neurotransmitter deficiency (e.g., norepinephrine and serotonin in depression) and excess (e.g., dopamine in schizophrenia) are related to mental disorders, psychotropic drugs are effective because they cause an increase or decrease in the brain's ability to use a specific neurotransmitter.
5. The blood-brain barrier protects the brain from the physiological fluctuations experienced by the rest of the body and regulates the amount of substances entering the brain and the speed with which they enter.
6. Highly lipid-soluble drugs such as ethanol, heroin, and diazepam (Valium) pass the blood-brain barrier with ease. This partially accounts for the high abuse of these drugs.
7. Only drugs that pass the blood-brain barrier can affect the central nervous system. Consequently, these agents are useful in the treatment of mental disorders but also can cause drug dependence.

9. Teaching patients can decrease the incidence of side effects while increasing compliance with the drug regimen. The nurse should use good clinical judgment when deciding what to share with patients and their families.

◆ Study Questions

(Answer key is in the back of the book.)

1. Psychotropic drugs were partially responsible for the development of which of the following concepts?
   a. Least restrictive alternative/environment
   b. Psychotherapeutic management
   c. Psychotherapy
   d. Behavior therapy
2. Which of the following has been proclaimed the first legitimately new antipsychotic since Thorazine?
   a. Prozac
   b. Clozapine
   c. Zoloft
   d. Mellaril
3. A substance that changes the resting potential of a postsynaptic membrane is a(n):
   a. Psychoactive agent.
   b. Cerebrospinal antagonist.
   c. Amino acid.
   d. Neurotransmitter.
4. Neurotransmitters
   a. Are synthesized from natural precursors.
   b. Are stored in storage vesicles in the presynaptic terminals.
   c. Combine with specific receptors.
   d. All of the above
5. Psychotropic drugs affect neurotransmitters in several ways. They can:
   1. Release stored neurotransmitters.
   2. Block receptors.
   3. Affect the response of neurotransmitters.
   4. Stop the inactivation of a neurotransmitter.
   5. Increase the number of neurons releasing neurotransmitters.
      a. 1, 2, 3, 4
      b. 1, 2, 3, 5
      c. 2, 4, 5
      d. All of the above
6. The brain is protected from fluctuations in the body by the:
   a. Spinal cord.
   b. CNS.
   c. Blood-brain barrier.
   d. All of the above

7. The most important chemical property influencing a drug's ability to pass easily through the blood-brain barrier is:
   a. Water solubility.
   b. Lipid solubility.
8. Which of the following drugs can most easily pass the blood-brain barrier?
   a. Penicillin
   b. Ethanol
   c. Dopamine
9. Macpherson, et al found what percentage of psychiatric patients ignorant of basic information about the drugs they were taking?
   a. 10%
   b. 30%
   c. 50%
   d. More than 70%

REFERENCES

Ayd FJ: The early history of modern psychopharmacology, *Neuropsychopharmacology* 5(2):71, 1991.

Berman I, Sapers BL, and Salzman C: Psychopharmacology: sertraline: a new serotonergic antidepressant, *Hosp Community Psychiatry* 43(7):671, 1992.

Blair DT: Risk management for extrapyramidal symptoms, *Qual Assur Rev Bull* 17:116, 1990.

Brown RP and Mann JJ: A clinical perspective in the role of neurotransmitters in mental disorders, *Hosp Community Psychiatry* 36:141, 1987.

Coudreaut-Quinn EA, Emmons MA, and McMorrow MJ: Self-medication during inpatient psychiatric treatment, *J Psychosoc Nurs Ment Health Serv* 30(12):32, 1992.

Geller JL: State hospital patients and their medications: do they know what they take? *Am J Psychiatry* 139:611, 1982.

Goldstein GW and Betz AL: The blood-brain barrier, *Sci Am* 255:74, 1986.

Macpherson R, et al: Long-term psychiatric patients' understanding of neuroleptic medication, *Hosp Community Psychiatry* 44(1):71, 1993.

O'Connor FW, Sprunger JE, and Petry SD: A clozapine treatment program for patients living in the community, *Hosp Community Psychiatry* 43(9):909, 1992.

Wilson WH: Clinical review of clozapine treatment in a state hospital, *Hosp Community Psychiatry* 43(7):700, 1992.

CHAPTER 19

Antiparkinson Drugs

NORMAN L. KELTNER
BETTE R. KELTNER

LEARNING OBJECTIVES

After reading this chapter you should be able to:
- Differentiate Parkinson's disease and parkinsonism
- Discuss the causes and symptoms of parkinsonism.
- Identify the two neurotransmitters primarily associated with Parkinson's disease.

- Explain the difference between the extrapyramidal system and the pyramidal system.
- Describe the biochemical relationship between Parkinson's disease and extrapyramidal side effects.
- Discuss side effects of antiparkinson drugs.

Note to the Student: You might find it odd that a chapter is dedicated to antiparkinson drugs in a psychiatric nursing textbook. Actually this chapter has a lot to do with psychiatric nursing. Here are some good reasons for including this chapter:

1. Understanding Parkinson's disease sets the stage for a better biochemical understanding of schizophrenia.
2. Parkinson's disease and some serious side effects of antipsychotic drugs are related.
3. Parkinson's disease, as a neurodegenerative disorder, is associated with specific mental disorders.
4. This chapter reinforces that many, but not all, mental disorders are brain disorders.

PARKINSON'S DISEASE AND PARKINSONISM

Idiopathic parkinsonism or Parkinson's disease is a progressive, chronic, degenerative disease of unknown cause that involves the area of the brain called the extrapyramidal system. It is the only neurodegenerative disease that can be successfully treated on a long-term basis (Agid, 1991). While Parkinson's disease and parkinsonism are not synonymous (see Key Terms) they present basically the same clinical picture related to extrapyramidal system disorder. The extrapyramidal system is associated with involuntary movements and when compromised causes tremors, bradykinesia, rigidity, and a host of other associated symptoms. The extrapyramidal system is distinguished from the pyramidal system in several ways. Functionally, the extrapyramidal system serves to coordinate and support involuntary movement, whereas the pyramidal system is responsible for voluntary movement. Weakness and paralysis are the result of damage to the pyramidal system whereas alterations in tone and posture reflect extrapyramidal system involvement.

Anatomically, the extrapyramidal system lies in front of the pyramidal system in the premotor area

KEY TERMS

Akathisia   Motor restlessness generally expressed as the inability to sit still. Akathisia is an extrapyramidal side effect (EPSE).

Anticholinergic effect   An effect caused by drugs that block acetylcholine receptors. Common anticholinergic effects include dry mouth and blurred vision. See the anticholinergics side effects table on p. 239 for more symptoms.

Basal ganglia   Subcortical structures that fine-tune involuntary movement, including the caudate nucleus, putamen, and globus pallidus

Bradykinesia   Slow or retarded movement

Dyskinesia   Abnormal voluntary skeletal muscle movement usually producing a jerky motion. Dyskinesia is an EPSE.

Dysphagia   Difficulty in swallowing

Dystonia   Rigidity in muscles that control posture, gait, or ocular movement. Dystonia is an EPSE.

Extrapyramidal system   Outside the pyramidal (voluntary) tract; coordinates involuntary movements

Extrapyramidal side effects (EPSEs)   Side effects caused by drugs that block dopamine, thus creating a dopamine-acetylcholine (ACh) imbalance. EPSEs include akathisia, akinesia, dyskinesia, dystonia, drug-induced parkinsonism, and neuroleptic malignant syndrome.

Monoamine oxidase   An enzyme that metabolizes monoamines such as dopamine, norepinephrine, and serotonin

Neuroleptic drug   Another term for antipsychotic drug

Oculogyric crisis   Involuntary tonic muscle spasms of the eye in which the eye usually rolls upward in a fixed stare. This is a very frightening dystonic reaction caused by antipsychotic drugs.

Parkinson's disease   Or idiopathic parkinsonism, where the cause is unknown. It presents pathologically by a loss of dopaminergic neurons in the substantia nigra and clinically by a variety of motor and nonmotor signs and symptoms.

Parkinsonism   Causes of the disease are known, such as brain injury, antipsychotic drugs, carbon monoxide

Substantia nigra   Literally, black substance; a pigmented area of the midbrain where dopamine is synthesized

Tardive dyskinesia   Literally, a late-appearing dyskinesia; usually affects the muscles of the mouth and face and rarely the trunk. Signs include lip smacking, grinding of teeth, and a rolling or protruding tongue. The side effects can be irreversible.

---

of the frontal lobe and extends to the basal ganglia and midbrain. The pyramidal system begins in the motor strip, extends down through the brain to the brainstem, crosses over, and continues to various points in the spinal cord (this is the corticospinal tract). The crossing over (decussation) accounts for the fact that a stroke on the right side of the brain manifests on the left side of the body.

The major cause of extrapyramidal system malfunction is a deficiency in the neurotransmitter dopamine and a subsequent decrease in dopamine transmission to the basal ganglia (Figure 19-1). Dopamine is primarily produced in a pigmented area (melanin-containing cells) of the midbrain called the substantia nigra (Figure 19-2). In Parkinson's disease the substantia nigra loses its pigmented cells and consequently its ability to produce dopamine. The rate of loss for a normal individual is about 0.5% per year. In persons with Parkinson's disease that rate is doubled to 1% per year, or about 10 neurons per day (Scherman, et al, 1989). Total loss of pigmented cells in the substantia nigra can approach 90% in some cases (Agid, 1991). A certain number of cells (a threshold) must be lost before symptoms are noticeable: 50% to 60% of the dopaminergic neurons in the substantia nigra and perhaps 70% to 80% of the neuronal terminals that project to the basal ganglia (Agid, 1991). This concept of threshold is consistent with other body pathologies with which the student might be familiar wherein much of an organ deteriorates before symptoms are apparent. The fact that individuals with significant neuronal loss (presumably up to nearly 50% in the substania nigra) can continue to function normally is due to increased activity in dopamine production by the remaining cells.

The motor problems associated with Parkinson's disease and parkinsonism are caused by the imbal-

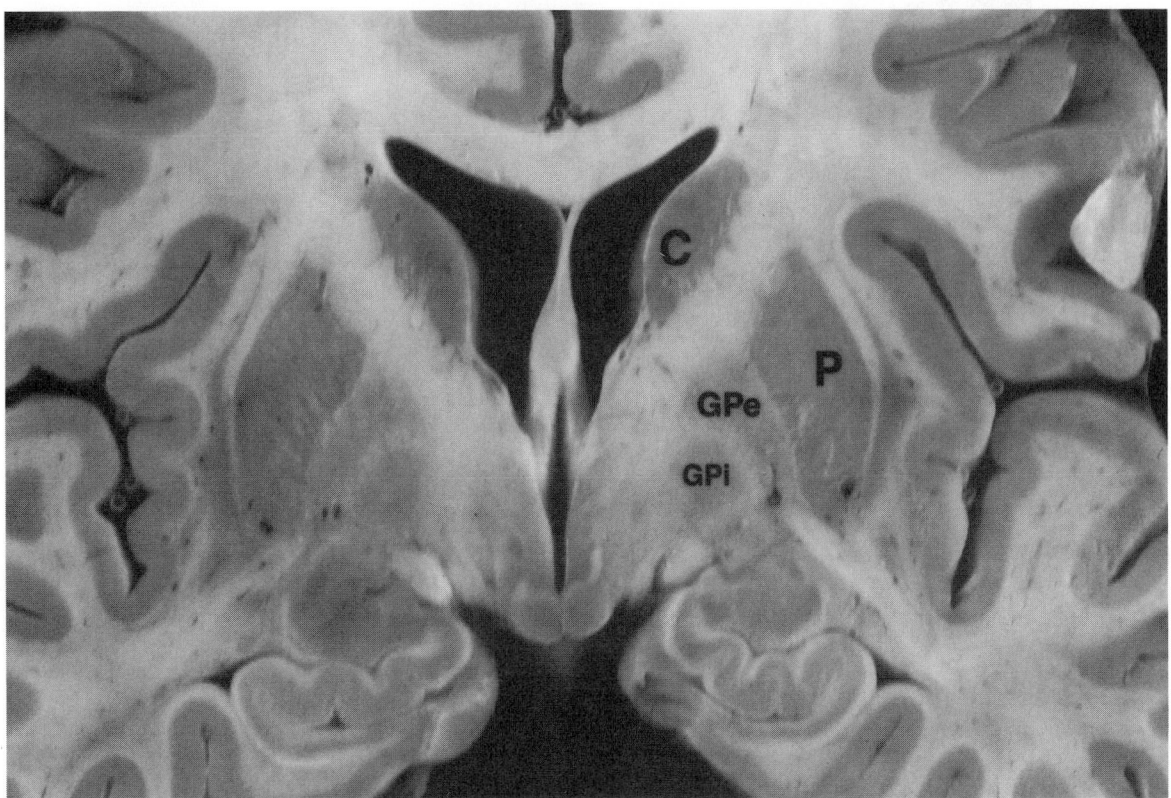

FIGURE 19-1   Basal ganglia. The basal ganglia are composed of several subcortical (below the surface of the brain gray matter) nuclei, including the caudate nucleus *(C)*, the putamen *(P)*, and the globus pallidus. The globus pallidus can be further divided into the globus pallidus externa *(GPe)* and the globus pallidus interna *(GPi)*. (Courtesy Dr. Richard E. Powers, Director, University of Alabama at Birmingham Brain Resource Program.)

ance of dopamine with another neurotransmitter, acetylcholine (ACh). The balance of these two neurotransmitters enables the extrapyramidal system to control posture, balance, walking, and other movements. The three primary symptoms of Parkinson's disease mentioned above (tremor, bradykinesia, and rigidity) cause a host of secondary symptoms (Keltner, et al, 1998).

Tremors occur in approximately 75% of cases. Historically, the terms *paralysis agitans* and *shaking palsy* were also used to identify Parkinson's disease. These diagnostic labels emerged because tremors were the most noticeable symptom. Tremors can usually be detected in one arm or hand when the person is at rest. Stress and emotional upset increase the severity of tremors (Lang and Fahn, 1989). Note that these resting tremors (involuntary movements) are in contrast with the tremors associated with alcoholism, which are evoked during voluntary

movement. The lesion responsible for the alcoholic tremor is located in the cerebellum, the "fine-tuner" of voluntary movement. Parkinsonian tremors are more amenable to treatment than some other symptoms of Parkinson's disease.

Bradykinesia, a generalized motor slowing, also manifests as masked facies (face movements slow down) and decreased associated movements; for example, arm swings. Movements are difficult to initiate, are slow, and are difficult to stop.

Rigidity, commonly referred to as cogwheel or lead-pipe rigidity, makes movement and normal responses difficult (Lannon, et al, 1986). Other symptoms include postural difficulties; a gait disorder characterized by slow, shuffling steps; and orthostatic hypotension. Falls can be a serious consequence. Finally, changes in mental status, such as dementia and depression, are not uncommon. Cerebral cortex damage occurs as the disease progresses including a

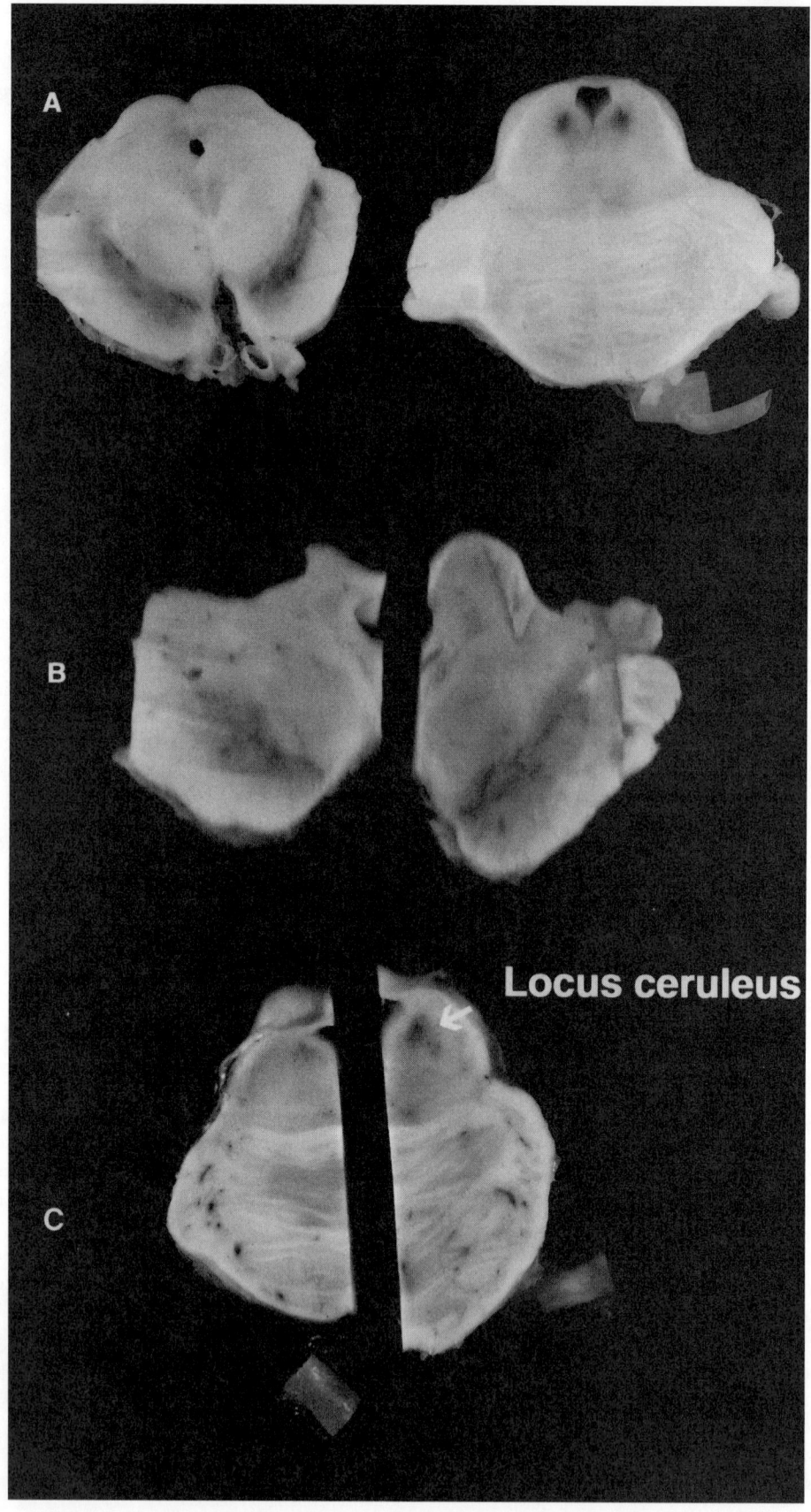

Locus ceruleus

FIGURE 19-2 For legend see opposite page.

major site of acetylcholine synthesis, the nucleus basalis of Meynert (Agid, 1991). This may contribute to the dementia that is observed in 15% to 30% of these patients (Cummings, 1992; Clough, 1991). Depression is the most common psychiatric disorder among patients with Parkinson's disease, perhaps occurring in about 40% of this population (Cummings, 1992). A substantial portion of these patients have what is categorized as less severe depressive symptoms (Tandberg, et al, 1996).

Secondary symptoms are caused by primary symptoms. Dysphagia, or difficulty in swallowing, creates problems with eating and can cause excessive accumulation of saliva that, in turn, leads to drooling (sialorrhea). Weight loss and choking are more important considerations of dysphagia. Bradykinesia and rigidity combine to impair respiratory, bladder, and bowel function; compromise breathing; and cause urinary retention and constipation.

The prevalence rate for Parkinson's disease in the United States is reported to be from 94 per 100,000 to 347 per 100,000 (Tanner and Goldman, 1996). When these same symptoms appear and the cause is identifiable it is referred to as parkinsonism. Known causes include reserpine, brain injury, and environmental toxins such as carbon monoxide and manganese. 1-Methyl-4-phenyl-1,2,3,6-tetrahydropyridine (MPTP), a contaminant of some street drugs and potent neurotoxin, causes selective destruction of dopaminergic neurons in the substantia nigra (Jenner, 1992) and is responsible for causing parkinsonism in some young people who take street drugs. Another important cause of parkinsonism is the antipsychotic drugs frequently prescribed for patients with schizophrenia and other psychotic disorders.

NEUROTRANSMITTERS

A balance between ACh and dopamine is required for normal movement. Dopamine serves as an inhibitory neurotransmitter and ACh as an excitatory neurotransmitter. A parkinsonian imbalance (too little dopamine) can occur in these three ways:

1. The brain may produce less dopamine, as in degeneration of the substantia nigra in Parkinson's disease.
2. Neuronal dopamine can be depleted chemically; for example, with reserpine.
3. Dopamine can be blocked at the postsynaptic receptor, as occurs with antipsychotic drugs.

When this imbalance occurs, motor neurons experience a continual "switched on" effect without the switching off needed for normal movement. Figure 19-3 illustrates a normal and an imbalanced state of these two neurotransmitters. Drug treatment of Parkinson's disease is aimed at rebalancing the

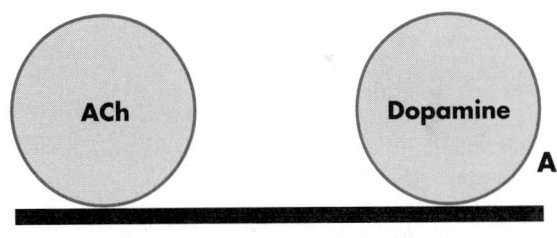

Normal balance with normal movement

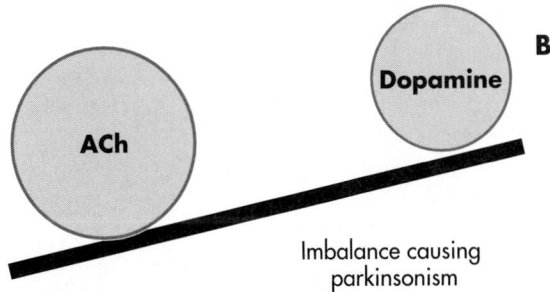

Imbalance causing parkinsonism

FIGURE 19-3 A, Balance between acetylcholine (ACh) and dopamine resulting in normal movement. **B,** Imbalance (too little dopamine) resulting in movement disorder.

FIGURE 19-2 The effects of aging and disease on catecholamine centers in the brainstem. **A,** Normal pigment in the substantia nigra *(left)* and locus ceruleus *(right)* of a young individual. **B,** Mild age-related loss of pigment in the brainstem of a normal individual *(right)* and loss of pigmented neurons in the brainstem of an individual with parkinsonism *(left)*. **C,** Mild depigmentation of the locus ceruleus in an aged individual *(right)* and severe depigmentation in parkinsonism *(left)*. (Courtesy Dr. Richard E. Powers, Director, University of Alabama at Birmingham Brain Resource Program.)

neurotransmitters ACh and dopamine. Balance is accomplished in three ways:

1. Drugs are used to increase the level of dopamine (dopaminergic agents).
2. Drugs are used to decrease the level of ACh (anticholinergic agents).
3. A combination of these two drugs is used to increase dopamine and decrease ACh simultaneously (dopamine agents plus anticholinergic agents). Box 19-1 lists selected antiparkinson drugs.

Parkinson's Disease and Depression

As noted above, depression is commonly associated with Parkinson's disease (Santamaria and Tolosa, 1992). The biochemical explanation of depression implicates a reduced bioavailability of norepinephrine as a primary cause of depression. Norepinephrine is a metabolite of dopamine. If there is not adequate dopamine in the brain, as in Parkinson's disease, then it follows that there may not be adequate levels of norepinephrine. And, this does occur. Norepinephrine is synthesized in the substantia

nigra and a 50% reduction has been observed there in Parkinson's disease (Cummings, 1992).

Also, as the substantia nigra in the brainstem suffers excessive neuronal loss, it is not surprising to find that another pigmented brainstem nuclei, the locus ceruleus, also experiences depigmentation. The locus ceruleus is a major site of norepinephrine synthesis in the brain (see Chapter 5). Figure 19-2 illustrates the depigmentation of these two melanin-containing nuclei.

Finally, a 60% reduction (Cummings, 1992) in dopamine has been reported in the nucleus accumbens, a major site in the so-called reward pathway. Accumulating information reinforces the role of dopamine in our ability to experience pleasure. This level of loss would explain any anhedonia associated with Parkinson's disease.

DOPAMINERGIC AGENTS

If this were a book on Parkinson's disease the authors would devote considerable space to describing the pharmacological characteristics of dopaminergic

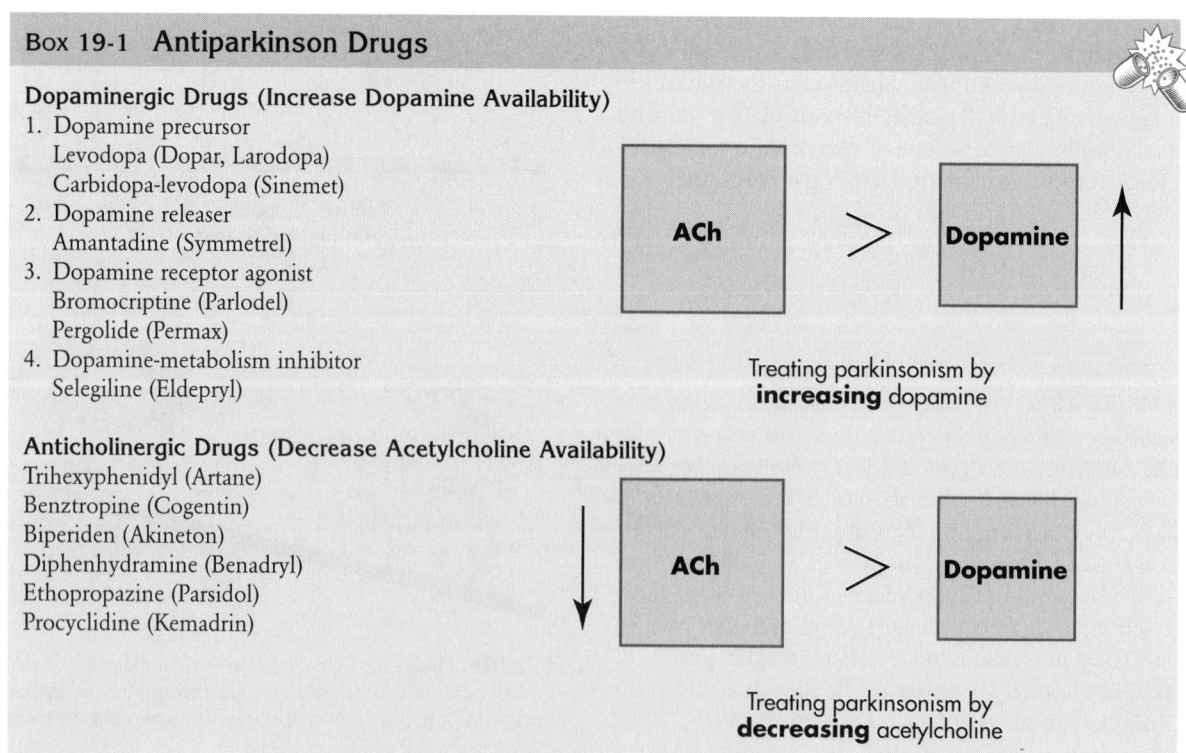

Box 19-1 Antiparkinson Drugs

Dopaminergic Drugs (Increase Dopamine Availability)
1. Dopamine precursor
   Levodopa (Dopar, Larodopa)
   Carbidopa-levodopa (Sinemet)
2. Dopamine releaser
   Amantadine (Symmetrel)
3. Dopamine receptor agonist
   Bromocriptine (Parlodel)
   Pergolide (Permax)
4. Dopamine-metabolism inhibitor
   Selegiline (Eldepryl)

ACh > **Dopamine**

Treating parkinsonism by
increasing dopamine

Anticholinergic Drugs (Decrease Acetylcholine Availability)
Trihexyphenidyl (Artane)
Benztropine (Cogentin)
Biperiden (Akineton)
Diphenhydramine (Benadryl)
Ethopropazine (Parsidol)
Procyclidine (Kemadrin)

ACh > **Dopamine**

Treating parkinsonism by
decreasing acetylcholine

agents. Such an effort would be beneficial because these drugs help us understand a great deal about the blood-brain barrier and neurotransmitter precursors, metabolism, and receptors. For example, as noted in Box 19-1, dopaminergic agents (agents that increase dopamine) can be divided into four categories. A description of those four categories has heuristic value and will be presented briefly. A broader discussion of dopaminergics will be deferred to a neurology nursing text.

Figure 19-3 and Box 19-1 illustrate the deficiency of dopamine in Parkinson's disease (PD). Further, the imbalance with acetylcholine is causative of the motor symptoms associated with PD. Dopaminergic drugs are used to restore the balance one dimensionally (that is, working only on the dopamine aspect of the imbalance). There are four approaches to doing this.

First, however, it is important to recall the metabolic steps in the synthesis of catecholamines (e.g., dopamine, norepinephrine):

Phenylalanine>>tyrosine>>levodopa>>dopamine>>norepinephrine

1. Dopamine precursor (levodopa, "levodopa and carbidopa" [Sinemet]): these drugs increase dopamine by increasing the bioavailability of its immediate precursor, levodopa. That is, if there is more levodopa, then there should be more dopamine.
2. Dopamine releaser (amantadine [Symmetrel]): this drug use is based on the knowledge that some dopamine remains in the system, and amantadine causes the remaining dopamine to be better utilized.
3. Dopamine agonist (bromocriptine [Parlodel] and pergolide [Permax]): agonists are drugs that mimic a neurotransmitter; in this case, dopamine. The dopamine receptor "thinks" that these agonists are dopamine. Both directly stimulate the dopamine postsynaptic receptor.
4. Dopamine-metabolism inhibitor (selegiline [Eldepryl]): this drug blocks the metabolism of dopamine by inhibiting monoamine oxidase B.

So, there are four ways pharmacologists have developed to restore the balance between acetylcholine and dopamine. Scientists have developed drugs to increase dopamine by:

1. Adding a dopamine precursor to the system
2. Better utilizing existing dopamine

3. "Tricking" the brain with agonists
4. Inhibiting a metabolizer of dopamine

It should be reiterated that these four approaches only address one side of the equation—the dopamine side.

For the purposes of this book, the other side of the equation—the acetylcholine side—is more germane. These are the drugs used to restore the imbalance caused by antipsychotic drugs. As will be noted in the following chapter, antipsychotic agents block (or antagonize) dopamine receptors. This dopamine receptor antagonism causes a man-made or iatrogenic parkinsonian-like syndrome—the aforementioned extrapyramidal side effects (EPSEs). But restoring the balance with a dopaminergic is not appropriate because, as will be emphasized in the chapter on schizophrenia, the most compelling hypothesis for schizophrenia is the presence of too much dopamine. Hence, anticholinergics (drugs that block acetylcholine receptors) are used to restore the balance (Box 19-2).

The following outline is repetitive but may be helpful:

1. Individuals with schizophrenia have too much dopamine.
2. Antipsychotic agents block dopamine.
3. When dopamine is blocked, an iatrogenic parkinsonism can develop.
4. An antiparkinson drug is needed to "fix" the problem created by the antipsychotic.
5. If dopaminergic antiparkinson drugs are given, schizophrenia may worsen. (See Table 19-1 for psychiatric side effects of dopaminergics).
6. So, anticholinergic drugs are given to restore acetylcholine/dopamine balance.

Table 19-1	Psychiatric Side Effects of Dopaminergics*	
Drugs	**Psychiatric Side Effects***
Amantadine	Confusion
Bromocriptine	Hallucinations
Levodopa	Delusions
Pergolide	Paranoid ideation
Selegiline	Depression
Sinemet	Agitation
	Anxiety
	Euphoria

*Common to most of these drugs.

Box 19-2   Model for Drug-Induced Parkinsonism

Clinical Manifestation	Theoretical Understanding	Intervention	Possible Effect of Intervention
1. Positive symptoms of schizophrenia	2. Increased bioavailability of dopamine	3. Antipsychotic drug(s) (dopamine antagonists)	4. Improvement of psychotic symptoms and possible development of EPSEs

[Diagram: Theoretical Understanding column shows two bars — a tall bar labeled "Dopamine" and a shorter bar labeled "Acetylcholine." Possible Effect of Intervention column shows a short bar labeled "Dopamine" and a tall bar labeled "Acetylcholine."]

Clinical Manifestation	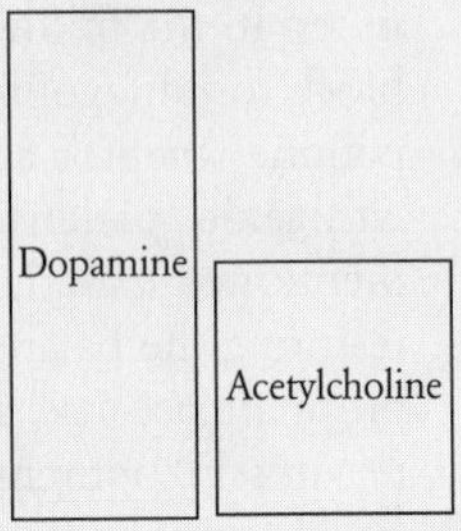 Theoretical Understanding	Intervention	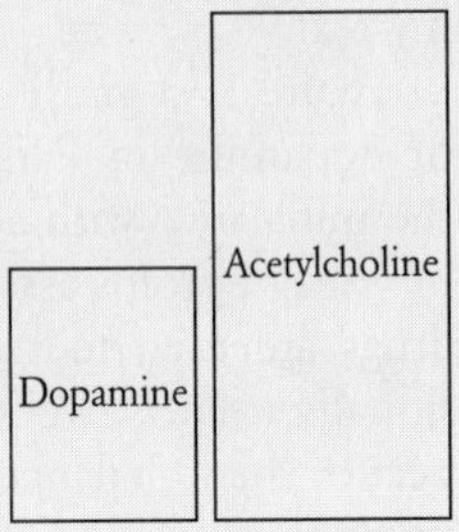 Possible Effect of Intervention
5. EPSEs (e.g., parkinsonism, akathisia)	6. An iatrogenic imbalance between ACh and dopamine has occurred	7. Add anticholinergic drug to treatment regimen	8. Continued improvement in psychotic symptoms and amelioration of EPSEs (restored balance between dopamine and acetylcholine)

[Diagram: Possible Effect of Intervention column shows two equal bars labeled "Dopamine" and "Acetylcholine."]

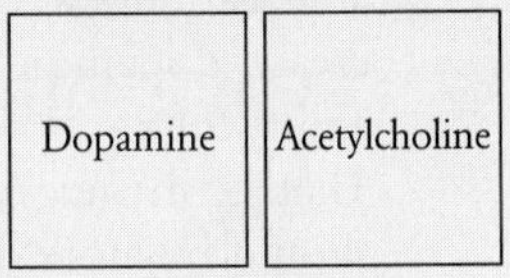

Source: From Keltner NL, Folks DG, Palmer CA, Powers RE: *Psychobiological foundations of psychiatric care,* St. Louis, 1998, Mosby.

■ Critical Thinking Question

What is the connection between Parkinson's disease and schizophrenia from a neurotransmitter perspective?

ANTICHOLINERGIC AGENTS

As previously noted, another way to restore the dopamine-ACh balance is to decrease the availability of ACh. Anticholinergic antiparkinson drugs are useful in the early stages of Parkinson's disease. These drugs are used to treat drug-induced parkinsonism as well as parkinsonism from other causes. All anticholinergic drugs that act on the central nervous system (CNS) and that are discussed in this chapter are similar to trihexyphenidyl (Artane). Trihexyphenidyl was the first of this class to be used extensively; however, benztropine (Cogentin) is more likely to be prescribed today. In the context of this text, when a dosage is appropriate for clarification of a point, trihexyphenidyl will most often be used for the example. Brief comments about the other anticholinergics are found at the end of the chapter. The relative anticholinergic potency of selected psychotropic drugs is found in Table 19-2. Atropine, the prototypical anticholinergic drug used before surgery, is twice as potent as benztropine and five times as potent as trihexyphenidyl on a milligram-per-milligram basis. See Box 19-3 for the adult dosages of these drugs.

Table 19-2   Anticholinergic Effect of Frequently Prescribed Psychotropic Drugs Compared to Trihexyphenidyl

Drug	Equivalent in Milligrams	Typical Use
Atropine	0.5	Given before surgery
Benztropine (Cogentin)	1.0	Antiparkinson
TRIHEXYPHENIDYL (ARTANE)	2.5	Antiparkinson
Biperiden (Akineton)	1.0	Antiparkinson
Amitriptyline (Elavil)	10	Antidepressant
Doxepin (Sinequan)	30	Antidepressant
Nortriptyline (Pamelor)	60	Antidepressant
Imipramine (Tofranil)	75	Antidepressant
Desipramine (Norpramin)	150	Antidepressant
Amoxapine (Asendin)	600	Antidepressant
Clozapine (Clozaril)	15	Antipsychotic
Thioridazine (Mellaril)	50	Antipsychotic
Chlorpromazine (Thorazine)	370	Antipsychotic
Diphenhydramine (Benadryl)	50	Antihistamine

According to this table, 50 mg of thioridazine has the same anticholinergic effect as 1 mg of benztropine.
Adapted from de Leon J, et al: A pilot effort to determine benztropine equivalents of anticholinergic medications, *Hosp Community Psychiatry* 45(6):606, 1994.

Pharmacologic Effects (Desired Effects)

Anticholinergic drugs act primarily by inhibiting ACh, thus preventing its stimulation of the cholinergic excitatory pathways. These drugs may also inhibit reuptake of dopamine. Of course, both of these effects contribute to the restoration of the ACh-dopamine balance. Anticholinergics are effective alone or in combination with dopaminergic agents in the treatment of Parkinson's disease, but are used alone in the treatment of parkinsonism induced by antipsychotic drugs.

Treating Parkinson's disease

The initial dose of trihexyphenidyl is 1 to 2 mg; this is increased by 2 mg every 3 to 5 days to a total daily dose of 6 to 10 mg.

Treating drug-induced extrapyramidal side effects

Antipsychotic drugs block dopamine receptors, frequently causing EPSEs. Many of the symptoms associated with "naturally" occurring Parkinson's disease—tremors, rigidity, and bradykinesia—are present in drug-induced parkinsonism along with related

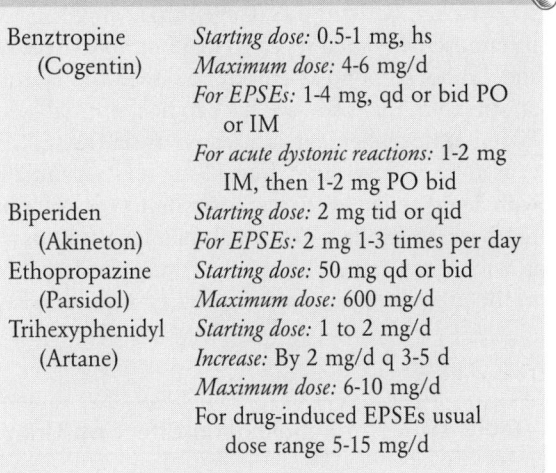

Box 19-3   Anticholinergic Drug Dosages*

Benztropine (Cogentin)	*Starting dose:* 0.5-1 mg, hs *Maximum dose:* 4-6 mg/d *For EPSEs:* 1-4 mg, qd or bid PO or IM *For acute dystonic reactions:* 1-2 mg IM, then 1-2 mg PO bid
Biperiden (Akineton)	*Starting dose:* 2 mg tid or qid *For EPSEs:* 2 mg 1-3 times per day
Ethopropazine (Parsidol)	*Starting dose:* 50 mg qd or bid *Maximum dose:* 600 mg/d
Trihexyphenidyl (Artane)	*Starting dose:* 1 to 2 mg/d *Increase:* By 2 mg/d q 3-5 d *Maximum dose:* 6-10 mg/d For drug-induced EPSEs usual dose range 5-15 mg/d

*Dosages for adults.

symptoms such as akathisia, dystonic reactions, and dyskinesias. Blockade or depletion of dopamine in the basal ganglia or the nigrostriatal tract produces EPSEs. High-potency antipsychotic agents such as haloperidol cause EPSEs more often than do low-potency agents (McEvoy, 1991). In addition, several nonneuroleptic drugs cause EPSEs including certain antidepressants, antiemetics, and lithium (Blair and Dauner, 1993). These symptoms contribute to the discomfort, anxiety, and frustration of this already troubled population and are major contributors to noncompliance (Forman, 1993). Patients taking antipsychotic drugs can experience a gradual or sudden onset of symptoms. As an illustration of how suddenly these side effects can occur, the following clinical example is provided.

CLINICAL EXAMPLE

A 25-year-old Hispanic woman who is taking an antipsychotic drug (haloperidol) starts to experience psychomotor slowing as she walks down the hallway of the hospital. Before she reaches the end of the hall, she requires assistance. Within 2 minutes of sitting down she experiences a severe dystonic reaction. Her neck becomes rigidly hyperextended, and the eyes roll upward in a fixed stare (oculogyric crisis). Her breathing becomes labored because of the position of her neck and she is frightened. Because she is also delusional, it is difficult to imagine what this frightening side effect of her medication represents to her. Benztropine (Cogentin), 2 mg, is given intramuscularly then repeated in 15 minutes because she did not respond as quickly as hoped for. Within another 5 minutes she was back to her "normal" self. When trihexyphenidyl is used to treat the EPSEs caused by antipsychotic drugs, 1 mg is given initially with 1 mg added every few hours until the reaction has been controlled. The usual maintenance dosage is 5 to 15 mg per day. The crisis situation described in the preceding paragraph obviously required a less conservative approach. Trihexyphenidyl is not available in parenteral form, and the oral form does not act rapidly enough to control oculogyric crises or other severe dystonic reactions. In a situation similar to the clinical example, benztropine (Cogentin) is more appropriate because it is available in parenteral form.

Side Effects

Anticholinergic drugs produce both CNS and peripheral nervous system (PNS) side effects, which are listed in the anticholinergics side effects box on the next page. These effects are similar to those of atropine. CNS effects include confusion, agitation, dizziness, drowsiness, and disturbances in behavior. The cholinergic system is implicated in memory and learning, and anticholinergic drugs affect this system also. PNS anticholinergic effects such as dry mouth, blurred vision, nausea, and nervousness occur in 30% to 50% of these patients.

Peripheral anticholinergic side effects basically result from blocking the parasympathetic system (a cholinergic [ACh] system) (Table 19-3). For instance, blurred vision results from pupils that dilate because of the blocking of ACh receptors of the third cranial nerve (oculomotor nerve). The third cranial nerve constricts the pupil; when it is blocked, the pupil dilates. Dry mouth results when cranial nerves VII and IX (facial and glossopharyngeal) are blocked from causing salivation. Decreased tearing is related to cranial nerve VII. Although these problems are annoying, they are not typically major health hazards. On the other hand, when cranial nerve X (vagus nerve) is blocked, tachycardia can occur and cause serious

Table 19-3   Anticholingeric Effect on Cranial Nerves with Parasympathetic Functions

Cranial Nerve	Parasympathetic Function	Anticholingeric Effect
III	Constricts pupils	Mydriasis (dilates pupils), blurred vision
	Alters shape of lens	Impairs accommodation
VII	Salivation	Dry mouth
	Lacrimation	Decreased tearing
	Nasal mucous secretion	Dry nasal passage
IX	Salivation	Dry mouth
	Nasal mucous secretion	Dry nasal passage
X	Slows heart rate	Tachycardia
	Promotes peristalsis	Slows peristalsis—constipation
	Constricts bronchi	Dilates bronchi

problems. The sinoatrial (SA) node has a beat of 100 to 120 impulses per minute. The reason our hearts do not beat that fast is because the parasympathetic system provides a braking action. When anticholinergic drugs are given, part of the brake is re-

moved. This can result in major problems, particularly for older individuals.

Constipation, a problem with parkinsonism patients because of rigidity, can be worsened by anticholinergics. Urinary hesitance and retention and

Side Effects and Nursing Interventions for Anticholinergics

Side Effects	Interventions
Peripheral Nervous System Effects	
Dry mouth	Sugarless hard candy and chewing gum; frequent rinses; take before meals
Nasal congestion	Over-the-counter nasal decongestant if approved by physician
Urinary hesitation	Running water, privacy, warm water over perineum
Urinary retention	Catheterize for residual fluids, encourage frequent voiding
Blurred vision, photophobia	Reassurance (normal vision typically returns in a few weeks), sunglasses, caution when driving, tolerance develops
Constipation	Laxatives as ordered, diet with roughage, 2500 to 3000 ml of water per day
Mydriasis	If eye pain develops could indicate undiagnosed narrow angle glaucoma—immediate attention is warranted
Orthostatic hypotension	Request patient to get out of bed slowly, to sit on the edge of the bed a short while, and rise slowly
Sedation	Help the patient get up early and get the day started
Decreased sweating	This can lead to fever; take temperature; if fever occurs, reduce body temperature (e.g., sponge baths)
Temperature	Limit strenuous activity, wear appropriate clothing
Central Nervous System Effects	
Akathisia	Be patient and reassure patient who is "jittery" that you understand the need to move and that appropriate drug interventions can help differentiate akathisia and agitation. Since akathisia is the chief cause of noncompliance with antipsychotic regimens, switching to a different class of antipsychotic drug may be necessary to achieve compliance.
Dystonias	If a severe reaction such as oculogyric crisis or torticollis occurs, give antiparkinson drug (e.g., benztropine [Cogentin]) or antihistamine (e.g., diphenhydramine [Benadryl]) immediately, as needed, and offer reassurance. More than likely an order for intramuscular administration will not have been written, so call the physician at once to obtain the order. For less severe dystonias, notify the physician when an order for an antiparkinson drug is warranted.
Drug-induced parkinsonism	Assess for the three major parkinsonism symptoms, tremors, rigidity, and bradykinesia, and report to physician. Antiparkinson drugs will probably be indicated.
Tardive dyskinesia	Assess for signs by using the abnormal inventory movement scale. Drug holidays may help prevent tardive dyskinesia. Anticholinergic agents will worsen tardive dyskinesia, so question their indiscriminate prophylactic use.
Neuroleptic malignant syndrome	Be alert for this potentially fatal side effect. *Routinely* take temperatures and encourage adequate water intake among all patients on a regimen of antipsychotic drugs, and *routinely* assess for rigidity, tremor, and similar symptoms.
Seizures	Seizures occur in approximately 1% of patients receiving antipsychotic drug treatment. *Clozapine* causes an even higher rate, up to 5% of patients taking 600 to 900 mg/day. For dosages of clozapine greater than 600 mg/day a normal EEG should be performed. If a seizure occurs, it may be necessary to discontinue clozapine.*

*From Jaretz N, Flowers E, and Millsap L: Clozapine: nursing care considerations, *Perspect Psychiatr Care* 28:19, 1992.

decreased sweating are other PNS effects. Interestingly, dry mouth and decreased sweating may be welcomed by parkinsonism patients who drool or perspire excessively.

Interactions with Other Anticholinergics

The anticholinergic response is intensified when anticholinergics are administered with drugs that have similar effects. Important drugs in this group include:

- Amantadine: a dopaminergic antiparkinson drug that has anticholinergic properties as well
- Chlorpromazine: additive anticholinergic effect
- Monoamine oxidase inhibitors: additive anticholinergic effect
- Antihistamines: additive anticholinergic effect
- Antiarrhythmic drugs: additive anticholinergic effect

Other interactions include an intensification of sedative effects when combined with CNS depressants and a decrease in absorption when combined with antacids and antidiarrheal drugs.

Nursing Implication for Anticholinergic Drugs

Therapeutic vs. toxic dosage levels

Therapeutic ranges

The therapeutic range for trihexyphenidyl is 6 to 10 mg a day for Parkinson's disease and 5 to 15 mg a day for drug-induced EPSEs (see Box 19-3). Overdose may result in CNS hyperstimulation (confusion, excitement, hyperpyrexia, agitation, disorientation, delirium, or hallucinations) or CNS depression (drowsiness, sedation, or coma). The atropine-like effects previously mentioned intensify. The cardiovascular, urinary, and gastrointestinal systems are particularly involved. The eyes are also affected. High fevers are due to the CNS effects of trihexyphenidyl and its ability to decrease sweating.

Intervention for toxic levels

Gastric lavage is the preferred treatment if the patient is conscious. A short-acting barbiturate (e.g., thiopental) may be ordered by the physician if CNS stimulation occurs, but the nurse and the physician must be aware that stimulation may precede CNS depression. Supportive care is important and may require maintenance of an airway and mechanical assistance with breathing. Hyperthermia should be monitored, and assessment should be made for signs of convulsions, which may follow high fevers. Hyperthermia can be controlled with tepid baths or other nursing measures.

Use in pregnancy

Anticholinergics should be used cautiously during pregnancy. Theoretically, these drugs will decrease milk flow during lactation.

Use in the elderly

As has been emphasized above and in a number of chapters in this text, elderly individuals are particularly sensitive to anticholinergic agents. Cognitive, cardiovascular, and gastrointestinal side effects are more pronounced in this age group. Older men with prostatic enlargement can have those difficulties exacerbated with these agents.

Side effects

Numerous annoying side effects are associated with anticholinergic drugs (see the anticholinergics side effects box). Several nondrug alternatives to help the patient are listed in this table.

Interactions with anticholinergic drugs

The nurse should alert the patient to the danger of over-the-counter drugs and other prescription drugs that intensify the atropine-like effects of centrally acting anticholinergics. Antihistamines, commonly a component of cold remedies, add to the anticholinergic effects. Alcohol and other depressants can increase drowsiness and should be avoided if possible. Over-the-counter antacids should not be taken unless ordered by the physician. Complications can be modified by giving antacids or antidiarrheals 1 to 2 hours before anticholinergics are taken.

Teaching patients

In addition to teaching appropriate information about side effects, the nurse should also emphasize certain points. The patient and family should be advised of the following:

- Not to discontinue these drugs abruptly. Tapering off over a 1-week period is advised.
- To avoid driving or other hazardous activities until tolerance occurs and drowsiness and blurred vision diminish.
- To avoid over-the-counter medications (e.g., cough and cold preparations) that have anticholinergic or antihistamine properties; alcohol, which will add to CNS depression; and antacids, which will interfere with absorption of anticholinergics.

Selected Centrally Acting Anticholinergic Drugs

Benztropine (Cogentin)

Benztropine is used to treat all parkinson-like disorders, including drug-induced EPSEs. It is probably the most frequently prescribed anticholinergic antiparkinson drug. Because benztropine is from a different chemical class than trihexyphenidyl, it may be more effective in some patients. It is usually given orally at a dose of 1 to 4 mg a day. It can be given intramuscularly (1 to 2 mg) for noncompliant psychotic patients and intramuscularly or intravenously (1 to 2 mg) for acute dystonic reactions. Benztropine causes greater and longer-lasting sedation than trihexyphenidyl; when given at bedtime, this may be a desirable effect.

Biperiden (Akineton)

Biperiden is used adjunctively in all parkinson-like disorders, including drug-induced EPSEs. It is similar to trihexyphenidyl and should be effective if trihexyphenidyl is effective. Typically, 2 mg three to four times daily is used for all forms of parkinson-like disorders except drug-induced EPSEs, for which 2 mg one to three times daily is given. For acute symptoms, 2 mg is given intramuscularly or intravenously every half hour prn (up to 8 mg in 24 hours).

Diphenhydramine (Benadryl)

Diphenhydramine, the prototype antihistamine, is effective for most parkinson-like disorders. The usual dose is 25 to 50 mg three to four times daily. It can cause considerable sedation in some persons and little in others. It is 50 times less potent than benztropine (Table 19-2).

Ethopropazine (Parsidol)

Ethopropazine is a phenothiazine derivative. This is interesting because phenothiazines are generally used as antipsychotics, which tend to make Parkinson's disease worse. The initial dosage is 50 mg orally once or twice a day. Maintenance dose ranges from 100 to 600 mg per day.

Procyclidine (Kemadrin)

Procyclidine is used for all parkinson-like disorders, including drug-induced EPSEs. It is found to be most effective for the symptomatic treatment of rigidity and sialorrhea (excessive salivation). It may increase tremors. The usual starting dose is 2.5 mg orally three times daily, and it can be increased to 5 mg three or four times a day (after meals and at bedtime). If procyclidine is replacing another anticholinergic drug, it should be started at a lower dose and the other drug gradually decreased.

Trihexyphenidyl (Artane)

Trihexyphenidyl was the first anticholinergic used extensively for EPSEs. Dosage for both Parkinson's disease and EPSEs have been noted above.

Critical Thinking Question

The rate-limiting step in the "natural" synthesis of dopamine is the availability of the enzyme tyrosine hydroxylase that converts tyrosine to levodopa (or L-dopa or dopa). How does this fact determine what is given to increase dopamine in the Parkinson's disease patient?

Key Concepts

1. Parkinson's disease is related to degeneration of the substantia nigra, the dopamine-generating portion of the brain; however the cause is unknown. Parkinsonism includes those disorders in which the cause is known, e.g., antipsychotic drug-induced, carbon monoxide brain damage, etc.

2. Normal muscle activity requires a balance between dopamine and ACh; consequently, a dopamine deficiency is responsible for symptoms of Parkinson's disease.

3. There are three primary symptoms associated with Parkinson's disease: tremors, bradykinesia, and rigidity.

4. Secondary symptoms of Parkinson's disease (i.e., difficult swallowing, respiratory problems, and constipation) are caused by primary symptoms.

5. Drug treatment of Parkinson's disease is based on reestablishing a balance between dopamine and ACh.

6. There are three basic approaches to reestablishing this balance: using dopaminergic drugs to increase dopamine levels, using anticholinergic drugs to decrease ACh levels, or a combination of these approaches.

7. There are four types of dopaminergic drugs: dopamine precursors, dopamine releasers, dopamine agonists, and dopamine metabolism inhibitors.

8. Dopamine precursors, such as levodopa and carbidopa-levodopa (Sinemet), work by adding new dopamine to the system.

9. The dopamine releaser amantadine (Symmetrel) works by enhancing the release of existing dopamine and also, perhaps, by inhibiting the reuptake of dopamine.

10. Bromocriptine (Parlodel), a dopamine agonist, mimics dopamine and directly stimulates dopaminergic postsynaptic receptors.

11. The dopamine-metabolism inhibitor selegiline (Eldepryl) blocks the metabolism of dopamine.

12. Major anticholinergic antiparkinson drugs include trihexyphenidyl (Artane) and benztropine (Cogentin).

13. Anticholinergic drugs are used to treat antipsychotic drug-induced parkinsonism and other EPSEs.

14. EPSEs are a drug-induced imbalance of acetylcholine and dopamine.

15. Anticholinergic agents help restore the balance.

16. Dopaminergic drugs are inappropriate to use because these drugs could theoretically worsen the psychosis by adding more dopamine (see Chapters 20 and 27).

17. Anticholinergic drugs have many side effects. Elderly individuals are particularly sensitive to these side effects.

2. A decreased availability of dopamine in the brain is responsible for:
   a. Parkinsonism.
   b. Schizophrenia.
   c. Tardive dyskinesia.

3. Which of the following drugs taken PO (assuming dosage is the same) has the greatest potential for aggravating schizophrenia? Why?
   a. Dopamine
   b. Levodopa
   c. Carbidopa-levodopa (Sinemet)   *Passes blood-brain barrier*
   d. Chlorpromazine

4. The pharmacological goal in treating parkinsonism is to:
   1. Increase acetylcholine to balance dopamine.
   2. Increase dopamine to balance acetylcholine.
   3. Decrease acetylcholine to balance dopamine.
   4. Decrease dopamine to balance acetylcholine.
      a. 1, 2
      b. 1, 3
      c. 2, 3
      d. 2, 4

5. EPSEs are related to Parkinson's disease because:
   a. Both are related to decreased availability of dopamine.
   b. Both are related to increased availability of dopamine.
   c. They are not related.

6. A patient in oculogyric crisis (a severe dystonic reaction) needs immediate intervention. Which of the following drugs is appropriate? Why?
   a. Artane
   b. Cogentin   *can be given IM*
   c. Kemadrin
   d. Parsidol

7. A patient taking benztropine (Cogentin) complains of blurred vision. Which cranial nerve is being affected by the benztropine?
   a. CN II
   b. CN IV
   c. CN VII
   d. CN III

Study Questions

(Answer key is in the back of the book.)

1. Parkinsonian symptoms can be caused by:
   a. An imbalance between dopamine and acetylcholine.
   b. Age-related degeneration of the extrapyramidal system.
   c. Dopamine-depleting drugs such as antipsychotics.
   d. All of the above.

REFERENCES

Agid Y: Parkinson's disease: pathophysiology, *Lancet* 337:1321, 1991.

Blair DT and Dauner A: Nonneuroleptic etiologies of extrapyramidal symptoms, *Clin Nurs Specialist* 7(4):225, 1993.

Calesnick B: Selegiline for Parkinson's disease, *Am Fam Physician* 41:589, 1990.

Caligiuri MP, Lohr JB, and Jeste DV: Parkinsonism in neuroleptic-naive schizophrenia patients, *Am J Psychiatry* 150(9):1343, 1993.

Clough DG: Parkinson's disease: management, *Lancet* 337:1324, 1991.

Cummings JL: Depression and Parkinson's disease, *Am J Psychiatry* 149:4:443, 1992.

Forman L: Medication: reasons and interventions for noncompliance, *J Psychosoc Nurs Ment Health Serv* 31(10):23, 1993.

Garrett E: Parkinsonism: forgotten considerations in medical treatment and nursing care, *J Neurosurg Nurs* 14:1318, 1982.

Jenner P: What process causes nigral cell death in Parkinson's disease? *Neurol Clin* 10(2):387, 1992.

Keltner NL, et al: *Psychobiological foundations of psychiatric care,* St. Louis, 1998, Mosby.

Lang ET and Fahn S: Assessment of Parkinson's disease. In Munsat TL, editor: *Quantification of neurologic deficit,* London: 1989, Butterworth.

Lannon MC, et al: Comprehensive care of the patient with Parkinson's disease, *J Neurosci Nurs* 18:121, 1986.

McEvoy GK: Central nervous system agents. In *American Hospital formulary service drug information,* Bethesda, Md, 1991, American Society of Hospital Pharmacists.

Olin BR: *Facts and comparisons,* Philadelphia, 1990, JB Lippincott.

Santamaria J and Tolosa E: Clinical subtypes of Parkinson's disease and depression. In Huber SJ and Cummings JL, editors: *Parkinson's disease: neurobehavioral aspects,* New York, 1992, Oxford University Press.

Scherman D, et al: Striatal dopamine deficiency in Parkinson's disease: role of aging, *Am Neurol* 26:551, 1989.

Tandberg E, et al: The occurrence of depression in Parkinson's disease: a community-based study, *Arch Neurol* 53:175, 1996.

Tanner CM and Goldman SM: Epidemiology of Parkinson's disease, *Neurol Clin North Am,* 12:317, 1996.

Tetrud JW and Langston JW: The effect of deprenyl (selegiline) on the natural history of Parkinson's disease, *Science* 245:519, 1989.

Watsky ES and Salzman C: Psychotropic drug interactions, *Hosp Community Psychiatry* 42:247, 1991.

CHAPTER 20

Antipsychotic Drugs

NORMAN L. KELTNER

LEARNING OBJECTIVES

After reading this chapter you should be able to:
- Explain the concept of *neurotransmitters*, specifically dopamine, in relation to psychosis.
- Identify the clinical uses of antipsychotic drugs.
- Recognize differences between high-potency and low-potency antipsychotic drugs.
- Identify a representative high-potency, low-potency, and atypical antipsychotic drug, including the specific side effects and drug interactions of that drug.
- Describe signs and symptoms associated with extrapyramidal side effects (EPSEs).
- Recognize therapeutic vs. toxic levels of antipsychotic drugs.
- Describe potential interactions of antipsychotic drugs.
- Discuss implications for teaching patients about antipsychotic drugs.

Antipsychotic or neuroleptic drugs are used to treat schizophrenia and other psychoses. Additionally, various other manifestations of mental illness are amenable to these agents. Traditional antipsychotic drugs are most effective for treating acute psychoses and the agitation associated with mania and other mental disturbances. Newer atypical agents such as clozapine (Clozaril), risperidone (Risperdal), olanzapine (Zyprexa), quetiapine (Seroquel), ziprasidone (Zeldox) and perhaps sertindole (Serlect)* appear to be effective in the treatment of more chronic forms of psychoses as well. Other uses of antipsychotics, such as in the treatment of hiccoughs and as antiemetics, will not be addressed in this book.

---

*At this writing (5/98) Abbott Laboratories has withdrawn its new drug application for Serlect.

HISTORICAL PERSPECTIVE

Chlorpromazine (Thorazine), from the phenothiazine family of drugs, is considered the first antipsychotic drug. It was synthesized from another phenothiazine (promethazine [Phenergan]) that had been developed earlier in the century. Promethazine, although sharing the antiemetic properties of chlorpromazine, did not produce an antipsychotic response. The "discovery" of the first antipsychotic was somewhat serendipitous. In 1950 a French scientist, while hoping to develop a new antihistamine, synthesized chlorpromazine. Although not classically antihistaminic, this new drug did prove quite sedating. Labroit, a physician, utilized this property to calm jittery patients prior to surgery. He noted, "There is not any loss of consciousness, not any

KEY TERMS

Akathisia   Motor restlessness generally expressed as the inability to sit still. Akathisia is an EPSE.

Anticholinergic effect   An effect caused by drugs that block acetylcholine receptors. Common anticholinergic effects include dry mouth and blurred vision.

Basal ganglia   Subcortical structures that fine-tune involuntary movement

Bradykinesia   Slow or retarded movement

Dyskinesia   Abnormal voluntary skeletal muscle movement usually producing a jerky motion. Dyskinesia is an EPSE but is probably related to dopamine receptor sensitivity rather than dopamine receptor blockade.

Dysphagia   Difficulty in swallowing

Dystonia   Rigidity in muscles that control posture, gait, or ocular movement. Dystonia is an EPSE.

Extrapyramidal system   Outside the pyramidal (voluntary) tract. Coordinates involuntary movements

Extrapyramidal side effects (EPSEs)   Side effects caused by drugs that block dopamine, thus creating a dopamine-acetylcholine (ACh) imbalance. EPSEs include akathisia, akinesia, dyskinesia, dystonia, drug-induced parkinsonism, and neuroleptic malignant syndrome (NMS). See dyskinesia definition for a distinction in pathophysiology.

Monoamine oxidase   An enzyme that metabolizes monoamines such as dopamine, norepinephrine, or serotonin

Neuroleptic drug   Another term for antipsychotic drug

Oculogyric crisis   Involuntary tonic muscle spasms of the eye in which the eye usually rolls upward in a fixed stare. This is a very frightening dystonic reaction caused by antipsychotic drugs.

Substantia nigra   Literally, black substance; a pigmented area of the midbrain where dopamine is synthesized

Tardive dyskinesia   Literally, a late-appearing dyskinesia; usually affects the muscles of the mouth and face. Signs include lip smacking, grinding of teeth, and a rolling or protruding tongue. The side effects can be irreversible.

Ventral tegmental area (VTA)   Another site of dopamine synthesis. Also located in midbrain near the substantia nigra. The VTA is not pigmented.

---

change in the patient's mentality, but a slight tendency to sleep and above all a disinterest for what goes on around him" (Ayd, 1991). At Labroit's suggestion, two French psychiatrists administered this drug to 38 acutely psychotic patients with encouraging results (Ayd, 1991). These two men, J. Delay and P. Deniker, are credited with discovering the first in a long series of antipsychotic medications.

Before the introduction and acceptance of chlorpromazine and the many related drugs, hundreds of thousands of patients with severe psychiatric disturbances were hospitalized under sometimes poor conditions. These patients were isolated, physically restrained, and occasionally subjected to psychosurgery (lobotomy). The treatments rarely restored patients to a state that enabled them to function productively or to interact in a reasonably normal way with others.

Although all the hopes for antipsychotic drugs have not been realized, these drugs have had a dramatic impact on psychiatric care. Their use by the psychiatric community resulted in the abandonment of most early and ineffective treatments, and long-term hospitalizations fell from more than 500,000 in 1955 (before the widespread use of antipsychotic drugs) to about 70,000 in 1997 (Figure 20-1). Antipsychotic drug use in public hospitals began in about 1954. Most patients who once would have been hospitalized now live and function well in their homes and jobs because of antipsychotic drug treatment. On the other hand, many previously hospitalized patients are not doing well outside the hospital setting, indicating that psychopharmacological treatment alone is not enough for many patients.

The drugs discussed in this chapter are generally called antipsychotic agents, but historically they have also been referred to as major tranquilizers, ataractics (drugs that produce calmness or serenity), and neuroleptics (because they can produce neurological symptoms).

CLASSIFICATION SYSTEMS

Antipsychotic drugs are generally conceptualized in three overlapping ways. The first and most accurate

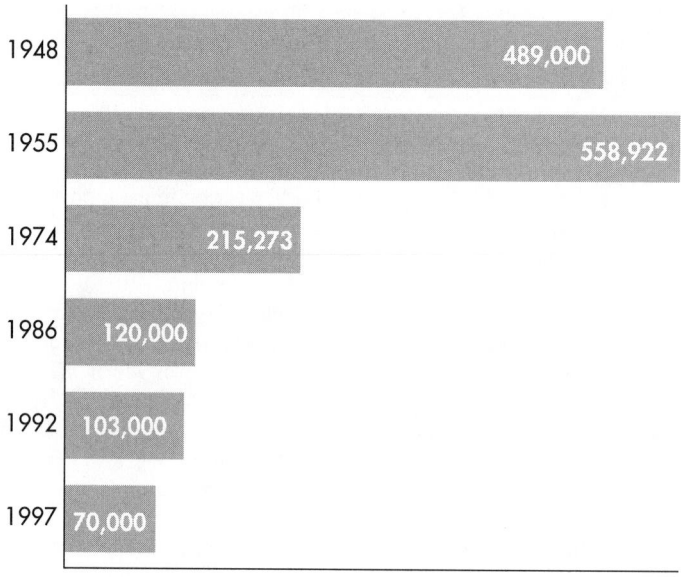

FIGURE 20-1   Mental patients hospitalized in public hospitals in the years surrounding and since the discovery of antipsychotic drugs.

classification system is based on chemical class, as listed in Table 20-1. These drugs have diverse chemical properties, but they all effectively reduce various psychiatric symptoms. Because of the differences in chemical class, the type, intensity, and frequency of side effects vary among these drugs. Therefore, when a drug is "not working," it should be substituted with a drug of a *different* class.

The second classification of antipsychotic drugs is based on potency (Box 20-1). This is a less "scientific" approach than classification by chemical class but has gathered support because of its clinical utility. Essentially, some drugs require much higher dosages than others to achieve similar clinical results (i.e., specific dopamine receptor blockade) (see Table 20-1). For instance, about 100 mg of chlorpromazine (Thorazine) is required to achieve the same clinical effect as 2 mg of haloperidol (Haldol). Drugs that are one to four times as potent as chlorpromazine are designated as *low potency;* those 20 or more times as potent are considered *high potency* (Gomez and Gomez, 1990).

This classification system in not as "clean" as the chemical classification system. A few drugs such as loxapine, molindone, and perphenazine do not fall comfortably into either high- or low-potency groups.

Nonetheless, clinically this dichotomy is significant because low-potency drugs tend to cause more

Box 20-1   Classification of Traditional (i.e., Typical) Antipsychotic Drugs Based on Potency

High-Potency Antipsychotic Drugs
Fluphenazine (Prolixin)
Haloperidol (Haldol)
Thiothixene (Navane)
Trifluoperazine (Stelazine)

Moderate-Potency Antipsychotic Drugs
Loxapine (Loxitane)
Molindone (Moban)
Perphenazine (Trilafon)

Low-Potency Antipsychotic Drugs
Chlorpromazine (Thorazine)
Chlorprothixene (Taractan)
Mesoridazine (Serentil)
Thioridazine (Mellaril)

intense anticholinergic effects (e.g., dry mouth, blurred vision), whereas high-potency drugs cause more extrapyramidal side effects (EPSEs) (e.g., dystonias, parkinsonism). Knowing this prepares the nurse for the most obvious set of side effects.

TABLE 20-1   Major Traditional and Atypical Antipsychotic Drugs

	Dosage* Range (mg/Day)	EPSEs†	Anticholinergic	Orthostasis	Sedation	Effect on Negative Symptoms
Traditional Antipsychotic Drugs						
High-Potency Antipsychotic Drugs						
Fluphenazine (Prolixin)	0.5-20	Severe	Mild	Mild	Mild	
Haloperidol (Haldol)	1-15	Severe	Mild	Mild	Mild	
Thiothixene (Navane)	8-30	Severe	Mild	Mild	Mild	
Trifluoperazine (Stelazine)	2-80	Severe	Mild	Mild	Mild	
Moderate-Potency Antipsychotic Drugs						
Loxapine (Loxitane)	20-250	Severe	Mild	Moderate	Moderate	
Molindone (Moban)	50-255	Severe	Mild	Mild	Mild	
Perphenazine (Trilafon)	12-64	Severe	Mild	Mild	Mild	
Low-Potency Antipsychotic Drugs						
Chlorpromazine (Thorazine)	30-800	Moderate	Moderate	Severe	Significant	
Thioridazine (Mellaril)	150-800	Mild	Severe	Severe	Significant	
Chlorprothixene (Taractan)	75-600	Moderate	Moderate	Moderate	Significant	
Atypical Antipsychotic Drugs						
Clozapine (Clozaril)	300-900	Mild	Severe	Severe	Significant	Significant
Risperidone (Risperdal)	4-16	Mild‡ to very low	Mild	Mild	Mild	Significant
Olanzapine (Zyprexa)	5-20	Mild§	Mild	Mild	Moderate to significant	Significant
Quetiapine (Seroquel)	300-400	Mild to low	Mild	Mild	Mild	Significant
Sertindole (Serlect)	12-24	Mild to low	Mild to moderate	Mild	Mild	Significant
Ziprasidone (Zeldox)	80-160	Mild	Mild	Mild	Mild	Significant

*Adult daily dosage in milligrams.
†Extrapyramidal side effects.
‡Risperidone does cause significant levels of EPSEs at higher dosages.
§Akathisia occurs more than other EPSEs.

Anticholinergic side effects and EPSEs will be discussed in the section on side effects. It is interesting to note that anticholinergic antiparkinson drugs are used to treat EPSEs, and the fact that low-potency antipsychotic drugs have fewer EPSEs is related to this property. Table 20-1 illustrates that, as a general rule, those drugs with greater anticholinergic effects have less intense EPSEs.

The third means of categorizing these drugs is based on "typicality." That is, drugs developed between 1950 (i.e., chlorpromazine) and 1990 are considered traditional or typical antipsychotics. The newer agents, which will be discussed later in the chapter, are referred to as atypical because of these characteristics:

1. Fewer EPSEs
2. Effective for negative symptoms
3. Do not elevate prolactin
4. Potent antagonists of $5HT_2$

These agents are much more effective than typical agents in modifying negative symptoms of schizophrenia. See Table 20-2 for a brief synopsis of positive and negative symptoms.

Table 20-2   Positive and Negative Symptoms of Schizophrenia

Symptom Category	Symptoms
Positive (Type I) Prognosis: good Precipitating factors: yes Onset: acute Sensorium: dreamlike quality Intellectual impairment: none Pathophysiology: D_2 hyperactivity Pathoanatomy: VBRs* normal Response to typical neuroleptics: good Effect of levodopa: increases symptoms	Abnormal thought form Agitation, tension Associational disturbances Bizarre behavior Conceptual disorganization Delusions Excitement Feelings of persecution Grandiosity Hallucinations Hostility Ideas of reference Illusions Insomnia Suspiciousness
Negative (Type II) Prognosis: poor Onset: chronic Family history: more than type I Sensorium: clear Intellectual impairment: yes Pathophysiology: possibly hypodopaminergic, decreased CBFs* Pathoanatomy: increased VBRs,* other changes (see text) Response to typical neuroleptics: varies Response to atypical neuroleptics: good Effect of levodopa: minimal	Alogia Anergia Anhedonia Asocial behavior Attention deficits Avolition Blunted affect Communication difficulties Difficulty with abstractions Passive social withdrawal Poor grooming and hygiene Poor rapport Poverty of speech

From Harris D and Keltner NL: Medication management. In Worley NK, editor: *Mental health in the community*, St. Louis, 1997, Mosby.
*CBF = cerebral blood flow; VBRs = ventricular brain ratios.

NEUROCHEMICAL THEORY OF SCHIZOPHRENIA

Although various theories of schizophrenia exist and are vigorously debated, the neurochemical theory affords the best explanation for the effectiveness of antipsychotic agents. The neurochemical theory states that schizophrenia and psychotic symptoms (e.g., hallucinations and delusions) are caused by increased levels of dopamine in the limbic system of the brain. Because antipsychotic drugs are dopamine blockers, it follows that their effectiveness can be attributed to this dopamine-blocking activity. Further-

more, this theory of schizophrenia is supported by clinical observations and clinical research, both of which demonstrate that high doses of levodopa and amphetamines can produce schizophrenic symptoms. These drugs increase dopamine levels.

This explanation, however, does not answer all the questions surrounding the issue, most specifically questions regarding negative symptoms. Figure 20-2 provides more useful information. As shown in this figure, there are several dopaminergic tracts in the brain. Dopamine is synthesized primarily in the substantia nigra and ventral tegmental area

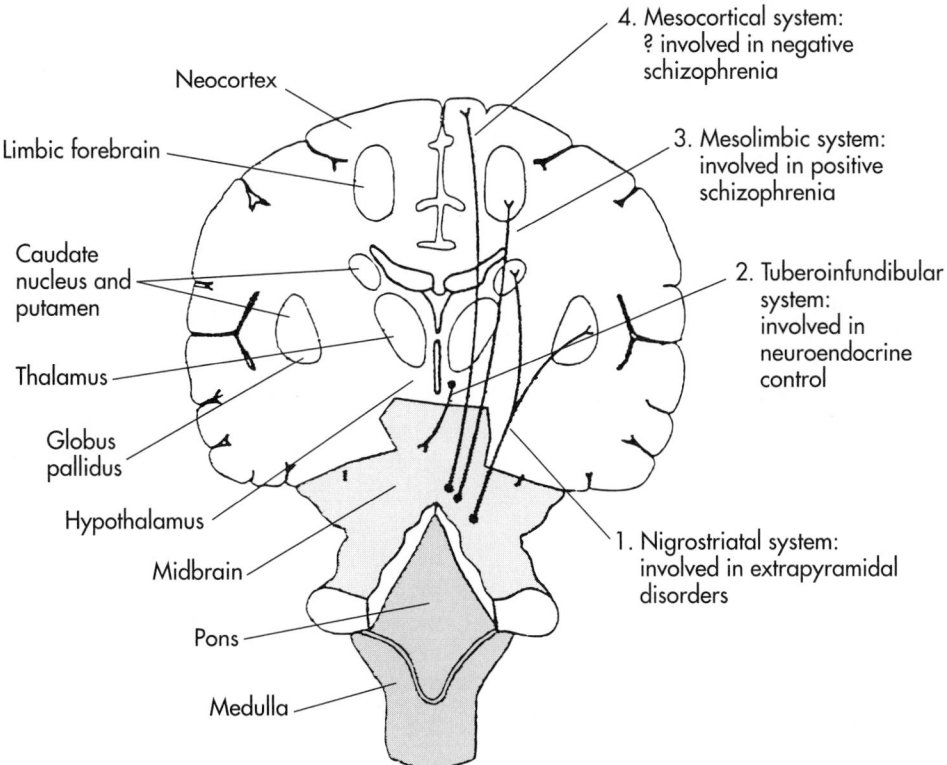

FIGURE 20-2   Four dopaminergic tracts important for understanding the actions of antipsychotic drugs. *1,* Nigrostriatal system: when antipsychotic drugs antagonize this system, a pseudoparkinsonism or extrapyramidal effect occurs. *2,* Tuberoinfundibular system: when antipsychotic drugs antagonize this system, the dopamine inhibition of the hypothalamic hormone prolactin is lifted and can lead to gynecomastia and galactorrhea. *3,* Mesolimbic system: when antipsychotic drugs antagonize this system, a decrease in the symptoms of schizophrenia occurs (primarily positive symptoms). This is the effect that makes these drugs antipsychotic. *4,* Mesocortical system: when antipsychotic drugs antagonize this system, it is thought the disorder can be worsened in some patients. Risperidone is thought to antagonize serotonin receptors in the cortex that, in turn, liberate dopamine there. That is, it is suspected that a mesocortical hypodopaminergic state may contribute to negative symptoms. Much remains to be understood about the role, if any, of the mesocortical dopaminergic tract in schizophrenia. (From Roberts GW, Leigh PN, and Weinberger DR: *Neuropsychiatric disorders,* London, 1993, Wolfe Publishing.)

(Perry et al, 1991) and is delivered to "distant" sites via dopaminergic tracts. The dopaminergic projections to the limbic site (3), the site that is thought to be dysfunctional in positive schizophrenia, may be hyperactive (accounting for positive symptoms of schizophrenia), whereas the nigrostriatal tract (1), the dopaminergic tract to the basal ganglia, may be hypoactive (accounting for parkinson symptoms). Furthermore, according to some theorists, hypoactivity in the mesocortical tract (4) may cause a decline in the function of that area (e.g., decreased cognition), accounting for negative symptoms. To fully appreciate the complexity of psychopharmacological treatment of psychoses, the student must recognize that there are dopamine-dependent areas of the brain that communicate with dopamine-synthesizing areas (substantia nigra and ventral tegmental areas in the midbrain) via different neuronal tracts.

The ultimate antipsychotic agent may be one that blocks dopamine receptors in the mesolimbic area (treating positive symptoms); blocks serotonin receptors (i.e., $5HT_2$) and liberates dopamine in the mesocortical area (treating negative schizophrenia); while not obstructing the function of the nigrostriatal tract (that is, not causing a drug-induced parkinsonism or other EPSEs) or blocking receptors in the tuberoinfundibular tract (i.e., not elevating prolactin levels).

PHARMACOLOGICAL EFFECTS (DESIRED EFFECTS)

Chlorpromazine and the other antipsychotic drugs are used primarily to treat psychotic disorders, specifically, schizophrenia and other chronic mental illness. Psychosis is a phenomenon of brain activity; therefore, the sought-after effects of these drugs occur in the central nervous system (CNS). Tolerance to an antipsychotic effect is uncommon. Peripheral nervous system (PNS) effects will be discussed under the section on side effects (undesired effects). It should be noted, however, that some peripheral effects are not totally unappreciated. For instance, the antiemetic effect of antipsychotic drugs may be welcomed by some patients.

CNS Effects

CNS effects include the sedation, emotional quieting, and psychomotor slowing originally described by Labroit and others. This explains why these drugs were once generally referred to as "major tranquilizers." Emotional quieting enables the patient to take advantage of other forms of therapeutic intervention; for example, the therapeutic nurse-patient relationship and the well-managed milieu.

Sedation decreases insomnia, a frequent complaint of psychotic patients. It is not fully understood whether this is due to the sedating effect itself or to being "freed" from disturbing thoughts (or a combination of the two). Not all antipsychotic drugs are significantly sedating. High-potency drugs are less sedating than low-potency drugs. For example, haloperidol (Haldol) and fluphenazine (Prolixin) are not particularly sedating but are quite effective. It is reasonable to conclude that the effectiveness of antipsychotic agents results from more than their tranquilizing qualities alone.

Psychiatric Symptoms Modified by Antipsychotic Drugs

Antipsychotic drugs are most effective in treating what have been called the "positive" symptoms of schizophrenia (see Table 20-2). Positive symptoms include hallucinations and delusions. Symptoms less responsive to antipsychotic drugs, or "negative" symptoms, include those developed over an extended period of time, such as a flattened affect, verbal paucity, and a lack of drive or goal-directed activity. Referring once again to Figure 20-2, the student can infer that positive symptoms arise from too much dopamine in the limbic area (hyperactive mesolimbic tract) and that negative symptoms arise from too little dopamine in the cortex (hypoactive mesocortical tract). It stands to reason, then, that antipsychotic drugs that are dopamine antagonists are better at decreasing the effect of dopamine in the limbic area than they are at increasing the effect of dopamine to the cerebral cortex. Ultimately, improvement in objective and subjective or positive and negative symptoms is the measurement of progress. Psychotic symptoms associated with other mental disorders, such as mania and cognitive disorders, also improve with these drugs.

Alterations of perception

As a rule, the more bizarre the behavior of a person experiencing psychotic symptoms (the more positive symptoms), the more likely that an antipsychotic drug will be beneficial. Hallucinations and illusions are reduced with these drugs. Even when the symptoms are not fully eradicated, antipsychotic drugs may enable the person to understand that hallucinations and illusions are not real. This is an improvement.

Alterations of thought

Antipsychotic drugs improve reasoning, decrease ambivalence, and decrease delusions. Because clouded reasoning, ambivalence, and delusional thoughts are frustrating and, at times, frightening, antipsychotic agents can free the patient to think more clearly and better communicate with others.

Alterations of activity

Often persons with schizophrenia are hyperactive because of their internal turmoil and, perhaps, their neurochemical state. Antipsychotic drugs slow psychomotor activity. Low-potency drugs, such as chlorpromazine (Thorazine), are sedating and may be used for agitated and combative persons.

Alterations in consciousness

Mental clouding and confusion are anxiety-producing symptoms associated with psychosis. Some mental health professionals believe these disorders are the most disabling. Antipsychotic drugs are effective in decreasing confusion and clouding.

Alterations in personal relationships

Patients with schizophrenia often have histories of social withdrawal and may have few, if any, close personal relationships. If there are relationships with family members, they are often strained. Persons with schizophrenia may invest little effort in their appearance and may not be particularly careful about their behaviors. The combination of introspection, rumination, and self-focused speech produces ineffective communication patterns that reinforce isolation and alienation. In the give-and-take of society, persons with schizophrenia often have little to give and, as a result, are basically socially unattractive to most people. Antipsychotic drugs enable patients to become less focused on themselves and

more focused on others. The socially damaging, self-absorptive thinking experienced by patients with schizophrenia may be due to the considerable energy they must expend to maintain some degree of equilibrium in the face of psychological turmoil. This is similar to the way many people give less attention to their appearance or behavior during an illness. Antipsychotic drugs reduce the inner turmoil, freeing psychic energy for normal interpersonal relationships and for the therapeutic nurse-patient relationship.

Alterations of affect

Affective disorders alone are not treated with antipsychotic drugs, but affective flattening, inappropriateness, and lability are affective symptoms sometimes associated with schizophrenia, and they often respond to antipsychotic drugs. However, a flat affect is a cardinal symptom of negative schizophrenia and may only respond to an atypical antipsychotic drug.

> ### ■ Critical Thinking Question
>
> *If* the positive symptoms of schizophrenia are caused by excessive bioavailability of dopamine, and *if* antipsychotic drugs are effective because they are dopamine antagonists, and *if* decreased dopamine levels contribute to EPSEs, *then* why don't all patients receiving antipsychotic drugs develop EPSEs, even when taking sufficient antipsychotic medication to manage their psychotic symptoms? (Hint: Review the four major dopaminergic tracts in the brain.)

PHARMACOKINETICS

A pharmacokinetic discussion of each antipsychotic agent would be prohibitive. Instead, the first antipsychotic, chlorpromazine, will serve as a prototype in the discussion of pharmacokinetic parameters. Atypical drugs will be discussed separately, and an overview of their pharmacokinetic properties will be addressed at that point.

Chlorpromazine enters the CNS rapidly. A tranquilizing effect occurs within 60 minutes of an oral dose and within 10 minutes of an intramuscular dose. In some persons, however, the actual antipsychotic effect may not be realized for several weeks to several months. Chlorpromazine accumulates in fatty tissue and is released slowly. Traces of metabolites of this drug are found in the urine months after therapy has stopped. This may explain why patients who abruptly stop taking this medication continue to experience an antipsychotic effect for a while; that is, the chlorpromazine continues to be released from fatty storage sites after being discontinued. This slow release from fatty stores may also account for noncompliance, because the patient who stops taking this medication does not experience an immediate return of symptoms. The following clinical example probably represents this phenomenon.

CLINICAL EXAMPLE

Bob, a 48-year-old military veteran with a long history of mental illness, has been taking chlorpromazine for 20 years. Over that time, the nursing staff at the Veterans Administration (VA) hospital has gotten to know Bob well because he periodically requires hospital-based intervention. One day Bob calls the nursing office on the psychiatric floor and tells the nurse that he feels he can conquer his problems by "mind over matter." He is going to stop all psychotropic medications. Bob seems to do quite well for several weeks, causing some of the nursing staff to wonder about the new approach. At the end of 3 weeks Bob is brought to the hospital in a very disturbed psychotic state. Chlorpromazine is reinstituted, and Bob's delusional thoughts subside.

Because 95% to 98% of chlorpromazine is bound to plasma proteins (protein-bound drugs cannot cross the blood-brain barrier), only a fraction of the drug affects the CNS. Physiological changes that even slightly disrupt this level of protein-binding action may increase the percentage of free drug and potentially have a greater effect. Theoretically, chlorpromazine may have a more potent effect on older persons because of their decreased protein-binding capabilities, but it is not clear if the effect is substantial. Chlorpromazine is metabolized in the liver and has a half-life of 10 to 30 hours. Impaired hepatic function extends its half-life and therefore its effect.

Although many traditional antipsychotic drugs are available, there is little documentation that one drug is more effective than another. Some patients, for example, respond to chlorpromazine and some respond to haloperidol. Therefore, the choice of which antipsychotic drug to prescribe is usually based on the prescriber's preference and experience, the likelihood that a certain drug will be helpful (e.g., on the basis of the patient's previous response to a certain drug), and an educated guess about the chance of drug-induced side effects. The last factor can be used therapeutically. For instance, a patient might benefit from a drug that has a sedating effect.

Because of nurses' prolonged contact with inpatients and periodic contact with outpatients, few psychiatric professionals have a better opportunity to assess both desired and undesired responses that help identify the best drug for a particular patient. Additionally, because nearly half of all orders for antipsychotic medications are written as prn orders, and because nurses typically make decisions about prn medications, nurses have an added reason to evaluate the responses to these drugs (Blair, 1990).

Most antipsychotic drugs are available in oral and parenteral forms. Oral administration is the preferred route for a variety of reasons, including the fact that patients generally prefer this route. Tablets, however, have consistently created a problem because they are so easy to "cheek." "Cheeking" occurs when patients place the tablet to one side of the mouth and pretend to have swallowed it. An estimated 46% of patients—both inpatient and outpatient—take less medication than is ordered (Blair, 1990). Noncompliance is thought to be the single most important cause of symptom exacerbation and rehospitalization (Forman, 1993). Psychiatric patients may not want to take their medication for several reasons, including the admission of illness that taking medication may imply, paranoid fears of poisoning, or unpleasant reactions or side effects. Many inpatient units use liquid forms of antipsychotic drugs to counteract noncompliant tendencies. Liquids or concentrates usually have an unpleasant taste and should be diluted.

Another form of administration is the parenteral route. Parenteral drugs are usually used to treat acutely disturbed persons or patients who represent significant compliance risks.

Both haloperidol decanoate and fluphenazine decanoate are long-acting injectable forms that require injection as seldom as once per month or at longer intervals. These long-acting injections are particularly beneficial for outpatients or patients who are noncompliant. Commonly prescribed antipsychotics available in parenteral form are found in Box 20-2.

Box 20-2 Major Parenteral Antipsychotics

Chlorpromazine (Thorazine)
Chlorprothixene (Taractan)
Fluphenazine (Prolixin)
Fluphenazine decanoate (Prolixin Decanoate)
Haloperidol (Haldol)
Haloperidol decanoate (Haldol Decanoate)
Loxapine (Loxitane)
Thiothixene (Navane)
Trifluoperazine (Stelazine)

When a patient does not respond to antipsychotic drug therapy, the nurse's assessment of the patient may be quite helpful to the prescriber. Three principles should be kept in mind when assessing a patient's response and the possibility of changing drugs:

1. If the patient is not taking the original drug as ordered, it is impossible to evaluate its potential therapeutic value. If at all possible, the nurse should establish whether or not the patient is compliant.

2. The drug currently being used should be given a fair trial. Daily therapy for 3 to 6 weeks or more may be needed before a drug's effectiveness (or ineffectiveness) can be ascertained. The emphasis on short hospital stays may make evaluation more difficult.

3. If a change of medication is indicated, the new agent should be taken from a different chemical class or subclass (of the phenothiazines) for the patient to profit from inherent differences between classes. Drugs within a class or subclass act similarly and offer no therapeutic advantage.

SIDE EFFECTS

Antipsychotic drugs produce numerous side effects because of PNS and CNS actions (see Table 20-1 and Box 20-3). Side effects due to PNS autonomic blocking (i.e., anticholinergic, antiadrenergic) actions are more likely to be caused by low-potency forms, such as chlorpromazine. CNS EPSEs are more likely to be caused by high-potency drugs, such as haloperidol. As a general rule, EPSEs are more dev-

astating and contribute to patients' refusals to continue taking the medications.

PNS Effects

PNS anticholinergic effects—dry mouth, blurred vision, and constipation—are common and can often be managed with nondrug interventions. Mydriasis can cause an increase in intraocular pressure that can aggravate narrow-angle glaucoma. Other relatively common anticholinergic effects are constipation and urinary hesitancy. Patients with a history of glaucoma or prostatic hypertrophy are not ordinarily placed on these drugs. Tachycardia is another PNS effect, and persons with cardiovascular disease should be carefully evaluated before being given these drugs. Antipsychotic drugs have caused sudden death related to arrhythmias and decreased cardiac output.

Hypotension is the major antiadrenergic effect of antipsychotic drugs. Hypotension is caused by blocking alpha-1 receptors. Blocking these sympathetic receptors on peripheral blood vessels prevents these vessels from responding (constricting) automatically to changes in position. Hypotension occurs most often in the elderly. Hypotension often occurs when the individual stands or changes positions suddenly (orthostatic hypotension); thus, precautions against falls must be instituted. In a normal, younger person, accommodation usually occurs within 2 weeks; however, many patients cannot tolerate orthostatic hypotension for that long.

Hypotension also causes a reflex tachycardia that can, in turn, causes general cardiovascular inefficiency. A reflex tachycardia is, by definition, tachycardia that automatically occurs as an adaptive function to compensate for lower extremity vasodilation. Antipsychotic drugs are prescribed cautiously for persons with severe hypotension, heart failure, or a history of arrhythmias.

CNS EPSEs

EPSEs → noncompliance → relapse → rehospitalization

It is estimated that up to 75% of all patients receiving antipsychotic medications have EPSEs (Blair, 1990) and, in turn, EPSEs may account for up to 50% of readmissions (cited in Blair and Dauner, 1993a). Abnormal involuntary movement disorders develop because of drug-induced imbalances

Box 20-3   Major Adverse Responses to Antipsychotic Drugs in Summary

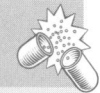

Neuroleptic Malignant Syndrome (NMS)
Caused by: a hypodopaminergic state
Offending agents: high-potency antipsychotics primarily
Signs and symptoms:
 Agitation
 Altered levels of consciousness
 Autonomic hyperactivity
 Electrolyte imbalance
  Hyperkalemia
  Hyponatremia
  Metabolic acidosis
 Hyperreflexia
 Hyperthermia
  Diaphoresis
  Tachypnea
 Impaired breathing
 Muscular rigidity
 Muteness
 Pallor
 Rhabdomyolysis-acute myoglobinuric renal failure

Anticholinergic Side Effects
Caused by: blockade of cholinergic receptors (muscarinic receptors)
Offending agents: anticholinergic drugs such as the low-potency antipsychotics and anticholinergic antiparkinson drugs.
Signs and symptoms:
 Anhidrosis
 Blurred vision

Signs and symptoms—cont'd:
 Constipation
 Diminished lacrimation
 Dry mouth
 Mydriasis
 Tachycardia
 Urinary hesitancy
Mechanism: blocks the cholinergic receptors on the four cranial nerves that have parasympathetic components:

Cranial nerve	When blocked causes these symptoms
III (oculomotor)	Blurred vision and impairs accommodation
VII (facial)	Dry mouth, decreased tearing, dry nasal passage
IX (glossopharyngeal)	Dry mouth, dry nasal passage
X (vagus)	Tachycardia, constipation, dilates bronchi

Extrapyramidal Side Effects (EPSEs)
Caused by: hypodopaminergic state
Offending agents: typically high-potency antipsychotics
Signs and symptoms:
 Akathisia
 Akinesia
 Dystonia
 Dyskinesia*
 Drug-induced parkinsonism

*Tardive dyskinesia is thought to be related to dopamine hypersensitivity rather than the actual hypodopaminergic state.

between two major neurotransmitters, dopamine and ACh, in specific parts of the brain. This imbalance seems to be caused more often by high-potency antipsychotic drugs such as haloperidol. EPSEs can be grouped as follows: akathisia; dystonias; tardive dyskinesia (TD); drug-induced parkinsonism; and neuroleptic malignant syndrome (NMS). TD, a late-appearing dyskinesia, is one of the most serious and least treatable of all the EPSEs. Guidelines for minimizing EPSEs are found in Box 20-4.

Akathisia

Akathisia, literally the "inability to sit," is an almost unbearable need to move and is an unpleasant

subjective and objective response to antipsychotic drugs. It is the most common EPSE (20% to 50% of all patients taking neuroleptics experience akathisia, and this EPSE represents about 50% of all reported EPSE cases) and probably accounts for more noncompliant behavior than other side effects. Akathisia has been linked to suicide attempts in this population (cited in Blair and Dauner, 1993a). It was first described in 1911, long before antipsychotic drugs were available, which suggests that other variables must contribute to this distressing side effect.

Subjectively, patients with akathisia feel jittery or uneasy and may report a lot of "nervous energy." *Objectively,* patients are restless and cannot sit still, even during group activities. Unfortunately, restlessness and verbal reflections of subjective anguish can be misinterpreted as psychiatric deterioration. *If an additional antipsychotic drug is given because of this misinterpretation, these patients will suffer much more.* Akathisia usually responds to anticholinergic drugs, such as trihexyphenidyl (Artane) or benztropine (Cogentin) (see Chapter 19). The following clinical example represents a misinterpretation of patient behavior with an unfortunate outcome.

▪ Critical Thinking Question

The chapter states that low-level antipsychotic drugs have fewer EPSEs than high-potency drugs. Why might that be so? (Hint: The answer may be related to the kind of effects that are more prominent with low-potency drugs and the kind of drugs that are used to treat EPSEs.)

CLINICAL EXAMPLE

During a group therapy session in a state public hospital, Bill continuously stands up and cannot sit down. The moment the group leader instructs Bill to sit down, he stands up again. The group leader misinterprets Bill's behavior as defiance. This misinterpretation escalates into a confrontation that culminates when Bill is forceably restrained and given a prn injection of an antipsychotic agent.

Had the group leader been more aware of EPSEs, she would have suspected akathisia and realized that an antipsychotic would only make the patient worse.

Dystonias

Dystonic reactions may cause rigidity in muscles that control posture, gait, or ocular movement. In oculogyric crisis the eyes roll back, which is very frightening. Torticollis, another dystonic reaction, is a contracted state of the cervical muscles that produces torsion on the neck. Laryngeal-pharyngeal dystonia, associated with gagging, cyanosis, respiratory distress, and asphyxia, is life-threatening. Up to 46% of patients who do not receive prophylactic anticholinergic drugs develop dystonic reactions (Tesar, 1993). Although these reactions are frightening to the patient and observers, most are usually benign and respond to intramuscular anticholinergic antiparkinson drugs, such as benztropine.

Box 20-4 Guidelines for Minimizing EPSEs

1. Antipsychotic drugs should not be used for nonapproved indications; for example, they should not be used to treat simple anxiety.
2. The dose for certain groups should be limited. Older persons, for instance, are especially susceptible to hypotension and TD.
3. As with all drugs, but especially because there seems to be a dose-EPSE relationship, the lowest effective dose of an antipsychotic drug should be given. Since these drugs are metabolized primarily in the liver, persons with reduced liver function due to old age or liver disease should be given comparatively lower doses.
4. Drug holidays (brief periods when the patient is taken off drugs) can decrease side effects without jeopardizing the therapeutic value of the drug for many patients.

Drug-induced parkinsonism

Antipsychotic drugs can produce symptoms peculiar to parkinsonism. Tremors, rigidity, and akinesia are possible consequences of antipsychotic drug therapy. Antipsychotic drugs can intensify existing "naturally occurring" parkinsonism, so they are seldom prescribed for persons with this condition. The preceding chapter provides a comprehensive description of parkinsonism.

Akinesia refers to an absence of movement and a diminished mental state. It is experienced by about 33% of patients taking antipsychotic drugs (VanPutten and Marder, 1987). Physical manifestations are more often a state of bradykinesia, or a slowing of movement. Movement is difficult to initiate and difficult to maintain. The patient lacks spontaneity in movement and speech, and experiences a slowing of the mental process. Subjectively the patient feels sedated and sleepy, and presents with a fixed, flat expression and dulled speech (Blair and Dauner, 1993a).

Paradoxically, these same symptoms (for different reasons) are common in schizophrenia and are, therefore, the focus of treatment. Historically, it has been common for nurses to mistake bizarre postures caused by EPSEs for exacerbation of schizophrenic symptoms. The dilemma is real. If a manifestation of schizophrenia occurs, then more medication may be indicated. If it is an EPSE, more medication will worsen the symptoms.

Tardive Dyskinesia

Dyskinesia refers to abnormal voluntary skeletal muscle movements, which usually produce a jerky motion. Treatment with any antipsychotic drug involves the risk of TD, one of the most serious EPSEs. The term *tardive* means late-appearing. Typically, TD appears after months or years of drug use, but it can appear sooner. Although the other EPSEs are caused by a dopamine deficiency much like that in parkinsonism, TD is thought to be caused by a hypersensitivity to dopamine and a cholinergic deficit. Anticholinergic drugs such as trihexyphenidyl and benztropine may aggravate TD. TD probably affects 15% to 20% of all patients taking antipsychotic drugs.

TD usually affects the muscles of the mouth and face. Signs of TD include lip smacking, grinding of the teeth, rolling or protrusion of the tongue, tics, and diaphragmatic movements that may impair breathing (American Psychiatric Association [APA], 1980). These involuntary movements are generally coordinated, fluctuate in severity, and disappear during sleep. Patients with TD are three times as likely to have an impaired gag reflex.

Because TD is considered to be irreversible (except in the early stages), the physician who prescribes the antipsychotic drug should be notified if TD is suspected. The abnormal involuntary movement scale (AIMS) (see Appendix F) provides a valuable assessment tool for TD. The dopamine agonist bromocriptine (Parlodel) has been found to be effective in treating this side effect.

Neuroleptic malignant syndrome

NMS is a potentially fatal reaction to antipsychotic drugs (Keltner and McIntyre, 1985; Persing, 1994). It was once thought to occur in about 1% of patients taking antipsychotics with an accompanying mortality rate of up to 30% (Keltner, 1997a). Increased vigilance by nurses and others has significantly reduced both morbidity and mortality rates (Keck, Pope, and McElroy, 1991; Shalev, Hermesh, and Munitz, 1989). Still, NMS remains a major concern for patients receiving antipsychotics.

NMS occurs most often when high-potency antipsychotic drugs are prescribed. Haloperidol (Haldol) is frequently cited as the causative neuroleptic. NMS is not related to toxic drug levels and may occur after only a few doses. Typically, onset is from 3 to 9 days after initiation of an antipsychotic (Kline, et al, 1989). NMS shares some symptoms with other EPSEs. It is manifested by muscular rigidity, tremors, impaired ventilations, muteness, altered consciousness, and autonomic hyperactivity. Perhaps the cardinal symptom is high body temperature. Temperatures as high as 108°F (42.2°C) have been reported, although temperatures are more likely to be 101° to 103°F. Because an increased temperature is the chief sign of NMS, the nurse should monitor temperatures closely.

Dantrolene (Dantrium) and bromocriptine (Parlodel) are the drugs of choice for treating NMS and should be continued for 8 to 12 days after improvement. Antipsychotics should not be reinstituted for at least 2 weeks after complete resolution of NMS symptoms.

Other side effects

Other side effects that may occur in patients taking antipsychotic drugs include hyperglycemia, jaundice, blood dyscrasias, susceptibility to hyperthermia, sun-sensitive skin (sunburn), nasal congestion, wheezing, galactorrhea (seepage from breast), gynecomastia (enlarged breast in either sex), impaired ejaculation, and amenorrhea.

A non-EPSE CNS effect is memory loss. Because the cholinergic system is implicated in memory and learning, anticholinergic antiparkinson drugs and low-potency antipsychotic drugs could play a role in this cognitive symptom. Clozapine (Clozaril) causes agranulocytosis in 1% of patients and is potentially fatal.

Prophylactic treatment of EPSEs

Prophylactic use of anticholinergic agents has been questioned, but newer evidence suggests they are safe and effective for preventing dystonic reactions. Before considering prophylactic use of anticholinergic agents, a simple risk assessment can be done. (See Box 20-5 for the EPSE risk-assessment tool.) Dystonic reactions occur in up to 13% of patients taking prophylactic anticholinergics, as opposed to up to

46% in patients not receiving this prophylaxis (Tesar, 1993). Because 90% of dystonic reactions occur within the first 5 days of treatment, the anticholinergic can probably be discontinued after 2 weeks (Tesar, 1993). Of course, the risk for other EPSEs can continue for several months. Benztropine (Cogentin) 2 mg or trihexyphenidyl (Artane) 2 to 5 mg orally (PO) or intramuscularly (IM) for patients beginning high-potency antipsychotic treatment is appropriate.

NURSING IMPLICATIONS

Therapeutic vs. Toxic Levels

Overdoses of antipsychotic drugs are seldom fatal, and treatment is supportive (e.g., gastric lavage to empty the stomach). Overdose can cause severe CNS depression (somnolence to coma), hypotension, and EPSEs. Restlessness or agitation, convulsions (antipsychotic drugs lower the seizure threshold), hyperthermia, increased anticholinergic

---

Box 20-5   Extrapyramidal Symptoms: Patient Risk Factor Assessment Tool

Patient-Specific Risks:

Age:	Above 55	3 points
	40-55	2 points
	Below 40	1 point
Sex:	Female	2 points
	Male	1 point
	Male under 30 years	2 points
History:	Exposure to ECT (electroconvulsive therapy)	1 point
	Previous EPSE (extrapyramidal side effect)	2 points
Diagnosis:	Organic brain syndrome	3 points
	Schizoaffective and/or affective disorder	1 point
TOTAL		_____

Score of 2-5 points—low predisposition for EPSE
Score of 6-8 points—high predisposition
Score of 9-12 points—extreme predisposition

Agent-Specific Risks:

High-potency medication	4 points
Moderate potency	3 points
Low potency	2 points
Exposure over 60 days	2 points
Exposure over 2 years	3 points
Depot injections	2 points
Concurrent lithium therapy	2 points
Two or more antipsychotics	2 points
TOTAL	_____

Scores of 2-5 points—low risk
Scores of 6-8 points—moderate risk
Score above 8 points—extreme risk

Treatment-Specific Risks:

No prophylaxis and no prn for anti-EPSE medication	5 points
No prophylaxis, but prn order for EPSE medication is written	3 points
Prophylactic medication for EPSE but no prn order	2 points
Prophylaxis and prn coverage	1 point
prn of antipsychotics more than 5 times a week	4 points
prn of antipsychotics 3-5 times a week	3 points
prn of antipsychotics 2-3 times a week	2 points
Ratio of antipsychotic prns to anti-EPSE prns is greater than 3 to 1	4 points
TOTAL	_____

Score of 1-4 points—low treatment risk
Score of 5-8 points—high treatment risk
Score of 9-13 points—severe risk

Total Risk Management Designations: Grand Total _____

4-15 points	low risk
16-21 points	high risk
Greater than 21 points	extreme risk

symptoms, and arrhythmias are other indicators of an overdose.

Use in Pregnancy

FDA Pregnancy Categories range from category B to category D (definite fetal risks). These drugs readily pass the placental barrier, reach significant levels in the fetus, and have been documented to cause EPSEs in some newborns (Arana and Hyman, 1991).

Although the risks to the fetus are statistically low, exposure to antipsychotic drugs during the first trimester should nonetheless be avoided. During the remainder of the pregnancy, tapering to the lowest possible dose is desirable. If possible, antipsychotic drugs should be discontinued to reduce the risk of transient neonatal toxicity (Cohen, 1989).

Use in Elderly

Since elderly individuals have decreased hepatic metabolism capability, it is prudent to reduce dosage in this age group. Further, age-related nigrostriatal and cholinergic degeneration cause pharmacodynamic responses that are more intense than those experienced by younger individuals. For example, el-derly patients have a more robust response to the dopaminergic and cholinergic antagonism of these agents. Hence, both extrapyramidal and anticholinergic effects can be heightened. Dosages equivalent to 0.5 to 2 mg of haloperidol (Haldol) daily are typically adequate.

Side Effects

PNS anticholinergic and antiadrenergic effects of antipsychotic drugs are troublesome but are not always as serious or as disturbing to the patient as CNS EPSEs. Nurses are often the first psychiatric professionals to observe these side effects. There are several specific interventions the nurse can provide to ameliorate side effects or to prevent serious consequences (see the antipsychotic drugs side effects box).

Interactions

Antipsychotic drugs interact with many other drugs. Because these interactions can be serious, it is important for the nurse to know potential offending agents and then advise the family and patient accordingly. CNS depressants such as alcohol, anti-

Side Effects and Nursing Interventions of Antipsychotic Drugs

Side Effects	Interventions
Peripheral Nervous System Effects	
Constipation	Encourage high dietary fiber and increased water intake; give laxatives as ordered.
Dry mouth	Advise patient to take sips of water frequently; provide sugarless hard candies, sugarless gum, and mouth rinses.
Nasal congestion	Give over-the-counter nasal decongestant if approved by physician.
Blurred vision	Advise patient to avoid potentially dangerous tasks. Reassure patient that normal vision typically returns in a few weeks, when tolerance to this side effect develops. Pilocarpine eyedrops can be used on a short-term basis.
Mydriasis	Advise patient to report eye pain immediately.
Photophobia	Advise patient to wear sunglasses outdoors.
Hypotension or orthostatic hypotension	Ask patient to get out of bed or chair slowly. Patient should sit on the side of the bed for 1 full minute while dangling feet, then slowly rise. If hypotension is a problem, measure blood pressure before each dose is given. Observe to see whether a change to another antipsychotic agent is indicated.

Side Effects and Nursing Interventions of Antipsychotic Drugs—cont'd

Side Effects	Interventions

Peripheral Nervous System Effects—cont'd

Tachycardia — Tachycardia is usually a reflex response to hypotension. When intervention for hypotension (previously described) is effective, reflex tachycardia usually decreases. With *clozapine,* hold the dose if pulse rate is greater than 140 pulsations per minute.*

Urinary retention — Encourage frequent voiding and voiding whenever the urge is present. Catheterize for residual fluids. Ask patient to monitor urine output and report output to nurse. Older men with benign prostatic hypertrophy are particularly susceptible to urinary retention.

Urinary hesitation — Provide privacy, run water in the sink, or run warm water over the perineum.

Sedation — Help patient get up early and get the day started.

Weight gain — Help patient order an appropriate diet; diet pills should not be taken.

Agranulocytosis — A high incidence of agranulocytosis (<1%) is associated with *clozapine.* White blood cell count (WBC) should be performed weekly. When baseline WBC is less than 3500 cells/mm³, treatment should not be initiated. After treatment begins, a WBC of less than 3000 cells/mm³ and a granulocyte count of less than 1500 cells/mm³ indicate treatment interruption to monitor for infection. If no signs of infection are present, treatment can resume. If WBC is less than 2000 cells/mm³ and granulocyte count is less than 1000 cells/mm³, stop therapy and do not rechallenge the patient. If infection develops, antibiotics should be prescribed.

Central Nervous System Effects

Akathisia — Be patient and reassure patient who is "jittery" that you understand the need to move and that appropriate drug interventions can help differentiate akathisia and agitation. Since akathisia is the chief cause of noncompliance with antipsychotic regimens, switching to a different class of antipsychotic drug may be necessary to achieve compliance.

Dystonias — If a severe reaction such as oculogyric crisis or torticollis occurs, give antiparkinson drug (e.g., benztropine [Cogentin]) or antihistamine (e.g., diphenhydramine [Benadryl]) immediately, as needed, and offer reassurance. More than likely an order for intramuscular administration will not have been written, so call the physician at once to obtain the order. For less severe dystonias, notify the physician when an order for an antiparkinson drug is warranted.

Drug-induced parkinsonism — Assess for the three major parkinsonism symptoms, tremors, rigidity, and bradykinesia, and report to physician. Antiparkinson drugs will probably be indicated.

Tardive dyskinesia — Assess for signs by using the abnormal inventory movement scale. Drug holidays may help prevent tardive dyskinesia. Anticholinergic agents will worsen tardive dyskinesia, so question their indiscriminate prophylactic use.

Neuroleptic malignant syndrome — Be alert for this potentially fatal side effect. *Routinely* take temperatures and encourage adequate water intake among all patients on a regimen of antipsychotic drugs, and *routinely* assess for rigidity, tremor, and similar symptoms.

Seizures — Seizures occur in approximately 1% of patients receiving antipsychotic drug treatment. *Clozapine* causes an even higher rate, up to 5% of patients taking 600 to 900 mg/day. For dosages of clozapine greater than 600 mg/day a normal EEG should be performed. If a seizure occurs, it may be necessary to discontinue clozapine.

*Jaretz, Flowers, and Millsap, 1992.

histamines, antianxiety drugs, antidepressants, barbiturates, meperidine, and morphine have additive effects that can cause profound CNS depression.

Prescription drugs

The nurse should review prescriptions to serve as a safety net for the prescriber who might make an inadvertent error. This is also important because nurses find themselves acting as case managers/advocates for the patients who are seeing and receiving prescriptions from multiple providers. The latter scenario happens often and is relevant for all medications.

Nonprescription drugs

Many nonprescription drugs have potentially harmful interactive effects with antipsychotic drugs. CNS depressants such as alcohol, cold and flu agents, and sleep aids can have additive effects. Other drugs decrease the effect of antipsychotics. For instance, antacids decrease absorption of antipsychotic drugs. Table 20-3 provides a list of some of the important interactions between antipsychotic and other drugs.

Teaching Patients

Teaching patients is an important dimension of nursing care for patients who are taking antipsychotic drugs. The nurse should use discretion in selecting the content of educational sessions because some patients have a tendency to become anxious about potential side effects. The nurse should focus on symptoms that can be seen or felt. The patient should be given a simply written description of drug benefits and side effects with instructions on how to cope with the side effects. Having this information in a

TABLE 20-3   **Adverse Interactions of Antipsychotics with Other Drugs**

Drug	Effect of Interaction
Amoxapine, fluoxetine	Increased EPSEs
Amphetamines	Decreased antipsychotic effect
Anticholinergic/antiparkinson drugs	Increased anticholinergic effect; delayed onset of the effects of oral doses of antipsychotics; potentially increased risk of hyperthermia
Barbiturates, nonbarbiturate hypnotics	All cause respiratory depression and increase sedation; all decrease antipsychotic serum levels; hypotension
Benzodiazepines	Increased sedation; respiratory depression with lorazepam and loxapine
Beta-adrenergic blocking agents (propranolol)	Effects of either or both drugs increased
Cimetidine	Chlorpromazine absorption decreased; increased sedation with chlorpromazine
Diazoxide	Can cause severe hyperglycemia
Dopaminergic antiparkinson drugs (e.g., bromocriptine)	Antagonizes the antipsychotic effect
Guanethidine	Control of hypertension is decreased
Insulin, oral hypoglycemics	Control of diabetes is weakened
L-dopa	Decreased antiparkinson effect of L-dopa; may exacerbate psychosis
Lithium	Decreases antipsychotic effect; may cause neurotoxicity when combined with haloperidol; lithium toxicity may be masked by antiemetic effect of antipsychotic drugs; increases EPSEs
Narcotics	Hypotension with chlorpromazine and meperidine; increased sedation; hypotension augmented; respiratory depression augmented
Phenytoin	May increase phenytoin toxicity; decreased antipsychotic blood serum levels
Trazodone	Additive hypotension with phenothiazines
Tricyclics	Possible ventricular arrhythmias with thioridazine; possible increased blood serum levels of both; hypotension; sedation; anticholinergic effect; increased risk of seizures

From Keltner NL and Folks DG: *Psychotropic drugs,* ed 2, St. Louis, 1997, Mosby.

written format helps the patient and family feel more in control and, therefore, act as collaborators in treatment.

In addition to the education issues already mentioned, the patient and family should be taught the following:

- Avoid immersion in hot water because hypotension may occur, causing falls.
- Avoid abrupt withdrawal of medication because EPSEs can occur.
- Utilize a sunscreen to prevent sunburn and use a maximum-strength variety if sunbathing.
- Take the drug as prescribed. Noncompliance is the leading cause of the return of symptoms and a leading cause of readmission (Forman, 1993).
- Immediately report signs of a sore throat, malaise, fever, or bleeding. Such signs may indicate a blood dyscrasia.
- Dress appropriately in hot weather and drink plenty of water to avoid heatstroke.

Critical Thinking Questions

Some clinicians believe that unless a patient has some level of EPSEs, the patient is not receiving enough medication. What might the rationale be for this view?

TRADITIONAL DRUGS BY CHEMICAL CLASS

This section of the chapter provides a little more detail about the traditional antipsychotics. These drugs are arranged by chemical class; however, as has been mentioned earlier, thinking of them in terms of high vs. low potency has more clinical utility. Though a great deal of attention is directed towards the newer atypical antipsychotics, it should not be assumed that the older, more traditional medications are no longer useful. Haloperidol, for instance, is a frequently prescribed drug and is very effective. Further, economic considerations alone dictate that older, less expensive drugs continue to be prescribed.

As mentioned in the historical section, antipsychotics were first synthesized around 1950. All drugs developed until 1990 were molecular variations that

essentially targeted the same receptors. Of the many drugs developed, only a relative few withstood the demands of clinical use. Below is a discussion of those few. Usage of these drugs is not equal as some are prescribed much more often than others.

Other Phenothiazines

Phenothiazines are divided into three chemical subclasses: the **aliphatics** (chlorpromazine comes from this subclass), the **piperidines** (Mellaril comes from this subclass), and the **piperazines** (Prolixin and Stelazine come from this subclass). Within each subclass some are seldom prescribed. Only those agents that are somewhat commonly used are discussed below.

Thioridazine (Mellaril)

Thioridazine (Mellaril) is almost as old as chlorpromazine and was the best-selling antipsychotic in the United States at one time (Wysowski and Baum, 1989). Some patients tend to respond to it better than to other drugs. Thioridazine is also used for the short-term treatment of marked depression accompanied by anxiety in adult patients, and for agitation, anxiety, depressed mood, tension, sleep disturbances, fears, and other symptoms in geriatric patients. Thioridazine has been therapeutic in children with severe behavioral problems marked by combativeness. This drug has a maximum upper limit of 800 mg per day because of the possibility of pigmentary retinopathy, which decreases visual acuity, impairs night vision, and is characterized by pigment deposits on the fundus.

Fluphenazine (Prolixin)

Fluphenazine (Prolixin), a high-potency antipsychotic, is commonly prescribed and considered to be an effective medication. Fluphenazine decanoate (Prolixin Decanoate), the long-acting form, is beneficial for patients who do not comply with a daily oral medication regimen. This injection can be given every 2 to 4 weeks.

Trifluoperazine (Stelazine)

Trifluoperazine (Stelazine) is prescribed relatively often. This drug is indicated for excessive anxiety, tension, and agitation, as well as for psychotic manifestations.

Perphenazine (Trilafon)

Perphenazine (Trilafon) is often used with antidepressants for patients who are both psychotic and depressed. It can be given separately or is available in a fixed-dose combination with amitriptyline (Elavil). The fixed-dose combination of perphenazine-amitriptyline is called Triavil. This combination drug is seldom prescribed.

Butyrophenone: Haloperidol

Haloperidol (Haldol) is from the butyrophenone chemical class of antipsychotic drugs. It is a high-potency drug (2 mg of haloperidol is equivalent to 100 mg of chlorpromazine) that tends to cause more EPSEs and fewer anticholinergic side effects than do the low-potency drugs. Haloperidol is a frequently prescribed antipsychotic that is used extensively in the elderly (because of fewer anticholinergic effects) and in pediatric psychiatry. New evidence suggests a clear correlation between plasma levels of haloperidol and therapeutic response. Bernardo, et al (1993) found that both very high and very low plasma concentrations of haloperidol are not therapeutic and that a therapeutic window exists for an optimal effect.

A problem of ongoing concern to psychiatric nurses is the threat of aggressive behavior of psychiatric patients. Chemical restraint, an unfortunate choice of words for describing psychopharmacological intervention of this kind, is a means of relieving a patient of distressing symptoms that lead to aggressive behavior. Parenteral haloperidol alone or in combination with the benzodiazepine, lorazepam (Ativan), is an excellent approach to helping patients stay in control. These two agents can be drawn up in the same syringe and administered as a single injection.

Haloperidol is also used for Gilles de la Tourette's disease, which is characterized by facial grimaces; tics; purposeless movements of the upper body, shoulder, and arms; coprolalia (frequent, extreme profanity); and echolalia (repetition of another person's words).

Haloperidol decanoate is a long-acting form and can be given at 2- to 4-week (or longer) intervals. It is particularly beneficial for persons who struggle with compliance.

Thioxanthenes: Chlorprothixene and Thiothixene

Chlorprothixene (Taractan) and thiothixene (Navane) have different potencies. Chlorprothixene is similar in potency to chlorpromazine. Thiothixene is 20 times as potent as chlorpromazine (see Table 20-1), similar to haloperidol in potency. Thiothixene is prescribed relatively often. Thiothixene exhibits rather weak anticholinergic properties but relatively powerful EPSEs (see Table 20-1).

Dibenzoxazepine: Loxapine

Loxapine (Loxitane) is a moderately potent antipsychotic (about 10 times as potent as chlorpromazine), so the generalizations associated with the high- vs. low-potency categorizations are not as helpful. Table 20-1 reveals severe EPSEs, moderate orthostasis and sedation, and low anticholinergic side effects.

Specific EPSEs have been reported frequently (in approximately 20% of patients), particularly during the first few days of treatment. Specific EPSEs include akathisia and parkinsonism symptoms (tremors, rigidity, sialorrhea, and masked facies).

Dihydroindolone: Molindone

Molindone (Moban) is also a moderate-potency drug and about 10 times as potent as chlorpromazine (see Table 20-1). It is used exclusively for the treatment of psychosis. Some studies indicate that molindone may be the ideal antipsychotic because it produces fewer overall side effects (Richelson, 1984). Molindone provokes heavy menstruation in previously amenorrheal women.

ATYPICAL DRUGS BY CHEMICAL CLASS

Atypical antipsychotics are atypical because they work differently than do the traditional drugs and have a greater effect on negative symptoms. One of the differences is their blockade of serotonin receptors that, in turn, is thought to liberate dopamine in the cortex. *This theoretical understanding explains the reduction in negative symptoms, that is, if negative schizo-phrenia is related to reductions in dopamine in the cortex and if atypical antipsychotics increase dopamine levels in the cortex, then this serotonin-antagonizing property is potentially therapeutic.* Because of laboratory findings and clinical improvements, these drugs are also being described in the literature as *serotonin/dopamine antagonists* or SDAs.

Dibenzodiazepine: Clozapine

Clozapine (Clozaril) was the first new antipsychotic agent to be introduced in the United States in 40 years when it was released to the retail market in 1990. Although clozapine had been used in Europe and China for some time, it was not approved in America because of the seriousness of a major side effect, agranulocytosis.

In Finland during the months of June and July of 1975, 9 out of 18 patients who developed clozapine-induced agranulocytosis died (Idanpaan-Heikkila, et al, 1975). This alarming event sent shudders through the psychiatric community, thus clozapine was not approved in the United States for another 15 years. By the mid-1980s, studies revealed a more optimistic picture of this drug tempered by a still too high morbidity rate of 1% to 2% for agranulocytosis and a mortality rate of about one third of those developing this blood dyscrasia (Keltner, 1997b).

The 1990 Food and Drug Administration (FDA) approval of clozapine was achieved partly because of rigid treatment protocols that the manufacturer, Sandoz, Inc, required of those prescribing the drug. From its introduction into the U.S. market in 1990 until June of 1996, 728 cases of leukopenia (defined as a white blood cell count [WBC] between 2000 and 3000 cells/mm^3 or a granulocyte count of 1000 to 1500 cells/mm^3) and 464 cases of agranulocytosis were reported as a result of clozapine therapy (Feldman, 1996). During that same period of time, 13 deaths were reported (Sandoz, Inc, 1995). Currently investigations infer a slightly lower morbidity rate of less than 1%. The mortality rate has significantly declined as well (Alvin and Lieberman, 1994). When deaths do occur related to agranulocytosis, they occur early in treatment (Alvin and Lieberman, 1994).

In the previous discussion of how antipsychotic agents work, it was noted that traditional antipsychotic drugs antagonize or block dopamine receptors. A more accurate statement is that traditional antipsychotic drugs block dopamine-D$_2$ receptors. Clozapine has greater affinity for dopamine-D$_1$, dopamine-D$_4$, and serotonin (5HT$_2$) receptors. See Boxes 20-6 and 20-7. Although differentiating

---

Box 20-7 Areas of Concentration for Dopamine Receptor Subtypes

D$_1$: Motor neurons in the basal ganglia and may be the principal dopamine-stimulating receptor for motor function.
- It has no direct role in controlling psychotic symptoms
- It does influence D$_2$ receptor function.

D$_2$: Located in neurons of both the limbic and motor centers. Dopamine stimulation of D$_2$ receptors activates psychomotor pathways.
- Overactivation thought to be cause of positive symptoms.
- D$_2$ receptors are modulated when the D$_1$ receptor is blocked but this does not occur in schizophrenia.

D$_3$ and D$_4$: Found primarily in limbic centers. Dopamine stimulation of D$_3$ may suppress behavior; overstimulation of D$_3$ may be associated with negative symptoms. D$_4$ receptors are located on neurons that influence thought processes and may be related to positive symptoms.

D$_5$: Found only in the limbic regions including hippocampal gyrus and nucleus accumbens. May be an important dopamine-stimulating receptor for behavior.

Seeman P. Dopamine receptors as new targets for novel drugs. *Current Approaches to Psychoses*, 4:8-9, 1995.

Box 20-6 Percentage of Dopamine D$_2$ Receptors Blocked by Certain Drugs

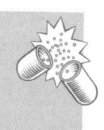

Haloperidol (Haldol): 80%
Clozapine (Clozaril): 10%
Risperidone (Risperdal): 25%
Olanzapine (Zyprexa): 20%

subtypes of receptors is somewhat beyond the scope of a basic psychiatric nursing textbook, such a differentiation does serve as a vehicle for the understanding of two important points. First, this difference in receptor affinity helps to explain why clozapine was called the first truly new antipsychotic in 40 years. Second, it confirms the fact that there is much to learn in psychiatric nursing, and that there is still much that is unknown about the brain, how it works, and how drugs affect it. For example, Seeman and Van Tol (1994) have identified a total of 26 dopamine receptor subtypes (D_1-D_5) and their variants.

Clozapine has proven successful in helping patients who have not been helped by chlorpromazine (Thorazine) and haloperidol (Haldol), probably because of the difference in receptor affinity. Remarkable case studies of patients who have not responded to other treatment strategies, but who have responded to clozapine, have encouraged mental health professionals to learn more about this drug. Research indicates that 10% to 20% of schizophrenic patients never respond adequately to traditional antipsychotic drugs and another 20% to 30% who are initially responsive stop responding within a year. Some studies suggest that as many as 64% of these treatment-resistant patients respond to clozapine (Perry, et al, 1991).

This relative lack of EPSEs, particularly TD, coupled with its remarkable therapeutic results in patients with schizophrenia, would seemingly make clozapine the drug of choice. However, as with many "wonder drugs," there are problems. Clozapine produces a life-threatening side effect, the previously mentioned agranulocytosis, and it is a very expensive drug.

■ Critical Thinking Questions

Clozapine remains an expensive drug and can cause fatal agranulocytosis. It is easy to say that everyone who needs clozapine should have it. Focus on the population who is most resistant to traditional drugs as well as the compliance problems among this population. Consider a delivery system for getting this drug to the people who need it. How can this be done? What role can nursing play in the solution to this problem?

CLINICAL EXAMPLE

Fred White is a 37-year-old man who has struggled with schizophrenia since late adolescence. Because his illness was not manageable at times, he experienced several short hospitalizations. He eventually was placed involuntarily in the state hospital and was living there in 1990 when clozapine became available. After 4 months of taking clozapine, Fred was discharged from the state hospital. A nurse clinician who has known Fred over this time period states that "he was doing well on clozapine and stayed on the drug for almost three years." In late 1992 Fred's WBC count began to drop, and he was withdrawn from clozapine and placed on large dosages of haloperidol. He was hospitalized "locally" on several occasions and then as a "last-ditch effort" the psychiatrist rechallenged Fred with clozapine after gaining approval from the manufacturer. He improved again but several months later was hospitalized for a decreased WBC count. Fred's presenting symptoms were sore throat (so sore that he gave up eating and had trouble speaking), malaise, and a high temperature (103°F). He was withdrawn from clozapine again never to be rechallenged. Today he is back in the state hospital.

Agranulocytosis is clinically defined as a granulocyte count below 500/mm³ (Box 20-8). Because of its life-threatening potential, the manufacturer of Clozaril requires that patients be closely monitored by the manufacturer or its representative. As of March 1998 patients are to be monitored weekly for the first 6 months and then bi-weekly thereafter for patients with acceptable white blood counts.

Clozapine is associated with several important side effects, including dose-related seizures (the higher the dosage of clozapine, the greater the likelihood of seizures) and sialorrhea (excessive salivation). In clinical testing, up to 5% of patients who took 600 to 900 mg of clozapine per day experienced seizures. Sialorrhea occurred in 31% of the patients. Some patients carry paper cups to spit in due to excessive salivation.

Benzisoxazole: Risperidone

The second atypical antipsychotic to be developed was risperidone (Risperdal). It was approved in 1994 and at this time is the most often prescribed antipsychotic agent (Marder, 1997). It is atypical yet different than clozapine. Risperidone has a greater affinity for

Box 20-8   **Possible Mechanisms of Agranulocytosis**

1. The clozapine metabolite, desmethylclozapine, may have direct cytotoxic effect on marrow cells.
2. Release of granulocyte-stimulating factor may be suppressed by clozapine, resulting in hematologic imbalance.
3. Clozapine may induce antibody formations that are toxic to peripheral blood neutrophils and their committed precursors.

Adapted from Feldman J: Clozapine and agranulocytosis, *Psychiatr Serv* 47(11):1177, 1996.

dopamine D_2 receptors and a similar antagonism of serotonin $5HT_2$ receptors, so theoretically it has a good receptor profile for both positive and negative schizophrenia (Keltner, 1995). Risperidone's lack of serious side effects make it a well-tolerated drug as well. Risperidone has little affinity for muscarinic (i.e., cholinergic receptors), so anticholinergic side effects are minimized (see Table 20-1). Neither does it appear to cause agranulocytosis, EPSEs, tardive dyskinesias, or NMS. Further, it appears to be a safe drug, with patients surviving amounts many times higher than therapeutic doses (Brown, 1993).

Though risperidone is considered to have a good side effect profile, an important side effect is its blockade of alpha-1 receptors, resulting in significant orthostatic hypotension. Other side effects include insomnia, agitation, headache, anxiety, and rhinitis. Risperidone is readily absorbed from the gastrointestinal tract, and its metabolite, 9-hydroxyrisperidone, is active. The half-life of these active molecules is about 24 hours (Land and Salzman, 1994). The expense of Risperdal has caused some governments and health maintenance organizations (HMOs) to deny its use. For example, a 30-day supply of Risperdal costs $240, whereas the same amount of Haldol costs only $2.50 (News, 1997).

NEW ATYPICAL ANTIPSYCHOTICS

Olanzapine

Olanzapine (Zyprexa) was released to the market in September 1996 and is comparable to risperidone in efficacy and side effect profile, and does not cause agranulocytosis. It has a broad affinity for several neurotransmitters now thought to be implicated in schizophrenia (Tollefson, 1997). In addition, olanzapine seems to demonstrate regionally specific activity in the brain. Olanzapine modulates mesolimbic function without a significant effect on the extrapyramidal system (Tollefson, 1997). Further, olanzapine normalizes N-methyl-D-aspartate (NMDA) receptor function, thus blocking some signs and symptoms associated with schizophrenia. The typical dose of olanzapine is between 5 mg and 20 mg per day. Olanzapine has a good side effect profile with few incidents of EPSEs. Early clinical studies indicate its efficacy in the treatment of both positive and negative symptoms. The following clinical example illustrates how olanzapine has made a significant difference in one man's life.

CLINICAL EXAMPLE

Bill, a male in his early 30s, was first diagnosed with schizophrenia when he was 19 years of age. He experienced a sudden onset and was hospitalized locally five times in 6 months. In 1992 he was admitted to the state hospital; clozapine was prescribed within a few weeks, and he responded favorably. Bill was discharged from the hospital after 5 months to a day treatment program in rural Alabama and did well in that program and on a regimen of clozapine for several years. As protocols required, he was monitored for blood work on a weekly basis and eventually experienced a drop in his WBC count. Clozapine therapy was discontinued, and olanzapine therapy was started. Bill is doing very well with olanzapine. His thought content improved (at least his ability to express his thoughts improved), his affect was brighter and more appropriate, and his parents described him as being as well or better than before he became ill. After years in the day treatment program and only a few months taking olanzapine, he was discharged and now lives on his own. He works 4 days a week at a large store and attends supportive treatment 1 day per week.

Quetiapine

Quetiapine (Seroquel) is a new atypical antipsychotic made available in September 1997 (Arvanitis,

1997). Quetiapine, like other atypical agents, has a lower affinity for dopamine D_2 receptors than it does for serotonin $5HT_2$ receptors. It has little affinity for muscarinic cholinergic receptors, so few anticholinergic side effects are expected. Clinically, it is expected that quetiapine will be effective in the treatment of both positive and negative symptoms, provoke few EPSEs, and will not increase serum prolactin levels significantly. Quetiapine can be given with or without food with the initial dose range between 300 and 400 mg/day, given in two doses. Quetiapine has a low potential for interactions with other drugs.

Sertindole

Sertindole (Serlect) is a new atypical antipsychotic drug with potent dopamine D_2 and serotonin $5HT_2$ antagonism (Silber, 1997). Further, sertindole does not significantly affect histamine and muscarinic receptors. Hence sertindole is expected to be efficacious for both positive and negative schizophrenia without important sedative, anticholinergic, or extrapyramidal side effects. A prolonged QT interval has been observed with this drug, and it is recommended that a baseline electrocardiogram and other cardiovascular parameters be assessed before therapy is initiated. Dosage ranges from 12 to 24 mg/day, given in one dose. Serlect has recently been withdrawn from the drug approval process.

Ziprasidone

Ziprasidone (Zeldox) is a very new atypical antipsychotic that has not been released for marketing at this writing. It acts on several neurotransmitter systems (Tandon, 1997). It potently blocks dopamine D_2 and serotonin $5HT_2$ receptors, behaves as an agonist at the serotonin $5HT_{1A}$ receptor, and blocks the reuptake of serotonin and norepinephrine. These pharmacological properties suggest a drug that will be effective for both positive and negative schizophrenia with the potential to provide effective treatment for depression and anxiety, which are so commonly associated with schizophrenia. Ziprasidone should cause few EPSEs, few anticholinergic side effects, and mild antihistaminic effects. Ziprasidone is given at a dosage of 40 to 80 mg twice daily. A rapid-acting intramuscular form of ziprasidone is in development.

Critical Thinking Question

Perhaps you are caring for a person who needs medication but will not take it; for example, a patient with paranoid delusions might truly believe that you are poisoning her with the antipsychotic drug. What are your legal and ethical grounds for nursing care in this situation?

Key Concepts

1. The dopamine hypothesis of schizophrenia states that schizophrenia is caused by an excessive level of dopamine in the brain.
2. Antipsychotic drugs block dopamine receptors, reducing the effect of excessive availability of dopamine in the brain.
3. Antipsychotic drugs are classified in three ways: on the basis of chemical class, on the basis of potency, and on "typicality."
4. Desired effects of antipsychotic drugs include sedation, emotional quieting, psychomotor slowing, and the alleviation of major symptoms of schizophrenia (i.e., alterations in perceptions, thoughts, consciousness, interpersonal relationships, and affect).
5. Anticholinergic side effects (e.g., dry mouth, blurred vision, and constipation) and EPSEs, including akathisia, dystonic reactions, akinesia, drug-induced parkinsonism, and TD, are the major categories of side effects associated with antipsychotic drugs.
6. High-potency antipsychotic drugs, such as haloperidol (Haldol) and fluphenazine (Prolixin), tend to cause more EPSEs. Low-potency antipsychotic drugs, such as chlorpromazine (Thorazine) and thioridazine (Mellaril), tend to cause more anticholinergic side effects.
7. NMS is a serious adverse effect of antipsychotic drugs (primarily high-potency drugs).
8. Overdosages with antipsychotic drugs are seldom fatal.
9. Antipsychotic drugs interact with other CNS depressants such as alcohol, meperidine (Demerol), and morphine, thereby increasing CNS depression.
10. Teaching patients should focus on the recognition of side effects and the avoidance of CNS depressants.
11. The nurse should routinely assess for NMS by taking the patient's temperature and evaluating for rigidity and/or tremors.
12. Clozapine (Clozaril) is the first truly new antipsychotic drug in 40 years.
13. Clozapine has a greater affinity for dopamine D_1, D_4 and serotonin $5HT_2$ receptors, produces few EPSEs, and has had remarkable success in treatment-resistant patients.

14. Clozapine causes agranulocytosis, a potentially fatal illness, and is relatively expensive.
15. Risperidone (Risperdal), olanzapine (Zyprexa), and other new atypical antipsychotics are promising drugs in the treatment of schizophrenia and do not cause the life-threatening illness, agranulocytosis.

Study Questions

(Answer key is in the back of the book.)

Bill Nunes is a 41-year-old man with a long history of schizophrenia. Bill has been divorced for 15 years, has not seen his children for 6 years, and lives in a cheap, downtown hotel. He was admitted to your unit 3 days ago after he caused problems in a 24-hour food mart. He entered the store about 5 AM and began shouting, waving his fists in the air, and talking loudly to himself. The police were called, and Mr. Nunes was admitted to the psychiatric evaluation unit. Several of the questions below are based upon this clinical example.

1. Mr. Nunes enters the nursing station at about 4 PM with his eyes fixed upward. He is screaming that he cannot move his eyes, and he is obviously afraid. A brief review of his chart indicates he is on haloperidol 5 mg tid, is attending a low-stimulation group activity, and is involved in occupational therapy. Your assessment would be that he is:
   a. Experiencing an oculogyric crisis.
   b. Seeking attention in a counterproductive manner.
   c. Experiencing an exacerbation of psychotic symptoms.
   d. Any of the above might be true.
2. Your first nursing intervention should be to:
   a. Ignore Mr. Nunes; to attend to this behavior will only reinforce it.
   b. Call the physician. This could be a life-threatening side effect of haloperidol.
   c. Give a prn anticholinergic drug to counteract the effects of haloperidol.
   d. Give a prn antipsychotic drug to treat this bizarre behavior.
3. The first antipsychotic drug introduced in the United States was:
   a. Chlorpromazine.
   b. Lithium.
   c. Haloperidol.
   d. Clozapine.
4. Antipsychotic drugs were first generally available to state hospitals in about:
   a. 1948.
   b. 1954.

   c. 1959.
   d. 1963.
5. High-potency drugs are more likely to have severe ____ side effects than low-potency antipsychotics.
   a. Sedative
   b. Extrapyramidal (EPSEs)
   c. Anticholinergic
   d. Orthostatic hypotension
6. Which of the following side effects should the nurse anticipate being particularly bothersome to a 65-year-old man with benign prostatic hypertrophy (BPH)? Why?
   a. Sedative
   b. EPSEs
   c. Anticholinergic
   d. Orthostatic hypotension
7. Your intervention for Mr. Nunes was successful. A week later, however, you notice that he cannot sit still in his group activity. He continuously gets up and has to be reminded to sit down. He complains, "My legs are on fire. I just can't sit here anymore." You realize:
   a. That he is experiencing akathisia.
   b. That he is having a kinesthetic hallucination.
   c. That he is experiencing a parkinsonian effect.
   d. That he is trying to avoid confrontation of his own feelings in group.
8. Another patient has been taking antipsychotic drugs for years. You notice that he begins to grind his teeth and moves and smacks his lips frequently. Your assessment would include:
   a. Oculogyric crisis.
   b. Gustatory hallucinations.
   c. Tardive dyskinesia.
   d. Neuroleptic malignant syndrome.
9. Which of the side effects of antipsychotic drugs is most lethal? What are the major signs and symptoms of this side effect?
   a. Oculogyric crisis
   b. Gustatory hallucinations
   c. Tardive dyskinesia
   d. Neuroleptic malignant syndrome
10. Mr. Nunes was discharged about a month ago. Unfortunately, there were no realistic options for him but to return to his downtown hotel. He does have appointments to see a community mental health nurse on a weekly basis. He complains of hearing voices and admits during one of his appointments that he is not taking his medication. Which of the following medication strategies would best suit a patient in Mr. Nunes's situation?
    a. Chlorpromazine once per day at the clinic
    b. Haloperidol decanoate once every 2 weeks
    c. Fluphenazine 5 mg tid given to the hotel manager to administer
    d. Electroconvulsive therapy

11. When drugs are provided without the benefit of a well-managed milieu or strong nurse-patient relationships, patients will:
    a. Decompensate.
    b. Be receiving custodial care.
    c. Be free to grow in their own ways.
12. The side effects of rigidity, tremor, and bradykinesia are related to: *triad of symptoms assoc. c parkonsonism.*

REFERENCES

Alvin JM and Lieberman JA: Agranulocytosis: incidence and risk factors, *J Clin Psychiatry* 55(Suppl B):137, 1994.

American Psychiatric Association: *Tardive dyskinesia: a task force report*, Washington, DC, 1992, The Association.

American Psychiatric Association Task Force on Tardive Dyskinesia: The task force on late neurological effects of antipsychotic drugs: tardive dyskinesia: summary of a task force report of the American Psychiatric Society, *Am J Psychiatry* 137:1163, 1980.

Arana GW and Hyman SE: *Handbook of psychiatric drug therapy*, ed 2, Boston, 1991, Little Brown.

Arvanitis L: Quetiapine (Seroquel), *The Decade of the Brain* 8(3):9, 1997.

Ayd FJ: The early history of modern psychopharmacology, *Neuropsychopharmacology* 5(2):71, 1991.

Bernardo M, et al: Monitoring plasma level of haloperidol in schizophrenia, *Hosp Community Psychiatry* 44(2):115, 1993.

Blair DT: Risk management for extrapyramidal symptoms, *Qual Assur Rev Bull* 17:116, 1990.

Blair DT and Dauner A: Nonneuroleptic etiologies of extrapyramidal symptoms, *Clin Nurse Specialist* 7(4):225, 1993a.

Blair DT and Dauner A: Neuroleptic malignant syndrome: liability in nursing practice, *J Psychosoc Nurs Ment Health Serv* 31(2):5, 1993b.

Brown K, et al: Overdose of risperidone, *Ann Emerg Med* 22(12):140, 1993.

Cohen LS: Psychopharmacology: psychotropic drug use in pregnancy, *Hosp Community Psychiatry* 40:566, 1989.

Czobor P and Volavka J: Quantitative electroencephalogram examination of effects of risperidone in schizophrenic patients, *J Clin Psychopharmacol* 13(5):332, 1993.

Ereshefsky L and Lacombe S: Pharmacological profile of risperidone, *Can J Psychiatry* 38(Suppl 3):S80, 1993.

Feldman J: Clozapine and agranulocytosis, *Psychiatr Serv* 47(11):1177, 1996.

Forman L: Medication: reasons and interventions for noncompliance, *J Psychosoc Nurs Ment Health Serv* 31(10):23, 1993.

Geller JL, Gaulin BD, and Barreira PJ: A practitioner's guide to use of psychotropic medication in liquid form, *Hosp Community Psychiatry* 43(10):969, 1992.

Gomez GE and Gomez EA: The special concerns of neuroleptic use in the elderly, *J Psychosoc Nurse Ment Health Serv* 28:7, 1990.

Hooper JF, Herren CK, and Goldwasser H: Neuroleptic malignant syndrome, *J Psychosoc Nurs Ment Health Serv* 27:13, 1989.

Idanpaan-Heikkila J, et al: Clozapine and agranulocytosis *Lancet* 2:611, 1975, (letter).

Jaretz N, Flowers E, and Millsap L: Clozapine: nursing care considerations, *Perspect Psychiatr Care* 28:19, 1992.

Keck PE, Pope HG, and McElroy SL: Declining frequency of neuroleptic malignant syndrome in a hospital population, *Am J Psychiatry* 148:880, 1991.

Keltner NL: Catastrophic consequences secondary to psychotropic drugs. Part I. *J Psychosoc Nurs Ment Health Serv* 35(4):41, 1997a.

Keltner NL: Catastrophic consequences secondary to psychotropic drugs. Part II. *J Psychosoc Nurs Ment Health Serv* 35(5):48, 1997b.

Keltner NL: Risperidone: the search for a better antipsychotic, *Perspect Psychiatr Care* 31(1):30, 1995.

Keltner NL and Folks DG: *Psychotropic drugs*, St. Louis, 1993, Mosby.

Keltner NL and McIntyre CW: Neuroleptic malignant syndrome, *J Neurosurg Nurs* 17:362, 1985.

Kline S, et al: Serotonin syndrome versus neuroleptic malignant syndrome as a cause of death, *Clin Pharmacol* 8:510, 1989.

Land W and Salzman C: Risperidone: a novel antipsychotic medication, *Hosp Community Psychiatry* 45(5): 434, 1994.

Littrell K and Magill AM: The effect of clozapine on preexisting tardive dyskinesia, *J Psychosoc Nurs Ment Health Serv* 31(9):14, 1993.

Marder SR: Risperidone (Risperdal), *The Decade of the Brain* 8(3):5, 1997.

Mehtonen OP, et al: A survey of sudden death associated with the use of antipsychotic or antidepressant drugs: 49 cases in Finland, *Acta Psychiatr Scand* 84:58, 1991.

Middlemiss MA and Beeber ZS: Depot antipsychotics, *J Psychosoc Nurs Ment Health Serv* 27:36, 1989.

News: Schizophrenia drug cut off by California HMO, *J Psychosoc Nurs Ment Health Serv* 35(3):8, 1997.

Overall JE, et al: Justifying neuroleptic drug treatment, *Hosp Community Psychiatry* 40:749, 1989.

Perry PJ, et al: Clozapine and norclozapine plasma concentrations and clinical response of treatment of refractory schizophrenic patients, *Am J Psychiatry* 148(2): 231, 1991.

Persing JS: Neuroleptic malignant syndrome: an overview, *S D J Med* 47(2):51, 1994.

Richelson E: Neuroleptic affinities for human brain receptors and their use in predicting adverse effects, *J Clin Psychiatry* 45:331, 1984.

Sandoz, Inc: Clozaril systems data, *Treatment Trends* 1:2, 1992.

Sandoz, Inc: Personal communication, 1995.

Seeman P and Van Tol HH: Dopamine receptor pharmacology, *Trends Pharmacol Sci* 57(7):264, 1994.

Shalev A, Hermesh H, and Munitz H: Mortality from neuroleptic malignant syndrome, *J Clin Psychiatry* 50(1):18, 1989.

Silber C: Sertindole (Serlect), *The Decade of the Brain* 8(3):11, 1997.

Tandon R: Ziprasidone (Zeldox), *The Decade of the Brain* 8(3):13, 1997.

Tesar GE: The agitated patient. Part II. Pharmacologic treatment, *Hosp Community Psychiatry* 44(7):627, 1993.

Tollefson GD: Olanzapine (Zyprexa), *The Decade of the Brain* 8(3):7, 1997.

VanPutten T and Marder SR: Behavioral toxicity of antipsychotic drugs, *J Clin Psychopharmacol* 7:243, 1987.

Wysowski DK and Baum C: Antipsychotic drug use in the United States, 1976-1985, *Arch Gen Psychiatry* 46:929, 1989.

Yassa R, et al: Factors in the development of severe forms of tardive dyskinesia, *Am J Psychiatry* 147:1156, 1990.

CHAPTER 21

Antidepressant and Antimanic Drugs

NORMAN L. KELTNER

LEARNING OBJECTIVES

After reading this chapter you should be able to:
- Understand neurobiological concepts of depression.
- Describe the differences among the three major classes of antidepressant drugs (TCAs, SSRIs, and MAOIs).
- Explain the mechanism of action of antidepressant and antimanic drugs.
- Discuss side effects of antidepressant and antimanic drugs.
- Identify therapeutic vs. toxic serum levels of lithium.
- Describe potential interactions of antidepressant and antimanic drugs.
- Discuss implications of teaching patients about antidepressant and antimanic drugs.

Antidepressant and antimanic drugs are used in the treatment of mood disorders. In conceptualizing a "mood continuum," depression (or dysphoria) is placed on one end and elation (euphoria/mania) on the other. Although these extremes in emotions are seemingly opposite, they are related. This chapter will focus on the psychopharmacological classes of drugs used to treat mood disorders, the *antide-* *pressant* and the *antimanic* drugs (Box 21-1). A complete discussion of mood disorders is found in Chapter 28.

ANTIDEPRESSANTS

HISTORICAL PERSPECTIVE

In the early 1950s, Bein (Ayd, 1991) isolated reserpine from rauwolfia serpentina, a naturally occurring medicinal agent that had been used to treat hypertension. Reserpine was found to have additional value in the treatment of psychosis, but with profound side effects, primarily severe depression and suicidal ideation. The researchers related this action of reserpine to norepinephrine depletion. From this early linking of neurotransmitter depletion to depression, scientists began conceptualizing pharmacological interventions for depression.

The crucial step in the development of antidepressant drugs was the synthesizing of agents that would increase the intrasynaptic availability of certain neurotransmitters. The treatment of depression was revolutionized in the late 1950s when tricyclic antidepressants (TCAs) were first introduced. In the first research report, Kuhn (1958), referring to

KEY TERMS

Anticholinergic effect   An effect caused by drugs that block acetylcholine receptors. Common anticholinergic effects include dry mouth, blurred vision, constipation, and urinary hesistancy.

Bipolar disorder   A mood disorder that is characterized by one episode of manic behavior, with or without a history of episodes of depression

Depression   Mood disturbance characterized by feelings of sadness, despair, apathy, and discouragement caused by loss in the person's life or by neurobiological imbalance of neurotransmitters

Dysthymia   A chronic mood disturbance characterized by a depressed mood that lasts for at least 2 years

Mania   A condition characterized by a mood that is elevated, expansive, or irritable

Monoamines   Neurotransmitters such as dopamine, norepinephrine, and serotonin

Monoamine oxidase   An enzyme that metabolizes monoamines such as dopamine, norepinephrine, and serotonin

Monoamine oxidase inhibitors (MAOIs)   Antidepressant drugs that increase certain neurotransmitters by interfering with their metabolism

Suicide   Self-inflicted death

Tyramine   A substance derived from the amino acid, tyrosine, and found in many common foods such as aged cheeses, yogurt, and avocados (see Box 21-4). Tyramine-rich foods can cause a hypertensive crisis in a person being treated with MAOIs.

Tyrosine   An amino acid that is the precursor to levodopa, dopamine, norepinephrine, and epinephrine

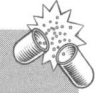

Box 21-1   Antidepressant and Antimanic Drugs Based on Traditional Classification

Tricyclic and Related Nonselective Cyclic Antidepressant Drugs
Amitriptyline (Elavil)
Amoxapine (Asendin)
Bupropion (Wellbutrin)
Desipramine (Norpramin)
Doxepin (Sinequan)
Imipramine (Tofranil)*
Maprotiline (Ludiomil)
Nefazodone (Serzone)
Nortriptyline (Aventyl, Pamelor)
Protriptyline (Vivactil)
Trazodone (Desyrel)
Trimipramine (Surmontil)
Venlafaxine (Effexor)

Selective Serotonin Reuptake Inhibitors
Fluoxetine (Prozac)
Fluvoxamine (Luvox)
Paroxetine (Paxil)
Sertraline (Zoloft)

Monoamine Oxidase Inhibitors
Moclobemide (Manerix)
Phenelzine (Nardil)
Tranylcypromine (Parnate)

Antimanic Drugs
Carbamazepine (Tegretol)
Lithium carbonate (Eskalith)
Valproic acid (Depakene)

*First antidepressant discovered and prototype of class.

imipramine (Tofranil), stated that patients "again became interested in things, are able to enjoy themselves, despondency gives way to a desire to undertake something, despair gives place to renewed hope in the future." Subsequent vigorous clinical research over the years has consistently underscored the efficacy of these drugs in the treatment of depression.

There are a number of theories concerning the cause of depression, but the efficacy of antidepressants is best understood from a neurochemical perspective. According to one neurochemical theory, depression is caused by an imbalance or decreased availability of certain neurotransmitters; specifically, deficiencies of norepinephrine, serotonin, and possibly dopamine. Psychopharmacological treatment is

Goals for Treatment with Antidepressants

1. Reduce and ultimately remove all signs and symptoms of the depression
2. Restore occupational and psychosocial function to that of the asymptomatic state
3. Reduce the likelihood of relapse and recurrence

Course of Treatment Once Diagnosis Is Made

1. Start treatment and assess every 1-2 weeks. Clinical improvement usually takes 2-4 weeks.

Patient outcomes:

Improvement: At 6 weeks *if better* continue same treatment for 6 more weeks. If improvement continues and complete remission occurs continue antidepressant for 4-9 months.

No Improvement: At 6 weeks *if not improved* augment treatment approach or change antidepressant. If after the 12th week patient is still not better, change treatment strategies.

From US Department of Health and Human Services: *Depression in primary care, vol 2, Treatment of major depression*, Washington, DC, 1993, The Department.

based on restoration of normal levels of these neurotransmitters through drugs in one of three ways (Brown and Mann, 1985):

1. By blocking neurotransmitter reuptake into nerve endings
2. By inhibiting neurotransmitter breakdown
3. By reducing stimulation of beta-adrenergic receptors

Much more is known about the first two views of drug efficacy. However, the third hypothesis is supported by the fact that some antidepressants (e.g., trazodone, bupropion, and nefazodone) do not significantly inhibit neurotransmitter reuptake but effectively treat depression.

The three major classes of antidepressants are TCAs and several nonselective cyclic antidepressants, selective serotonin reuptake inhibitors (SSRIs), and MAOIs. The term *tricyclic* refers to molecular configuration and several new agents are more accurately referred to as *bicyclic, tetracyclic,* or corporately as *heterocyclic*. However this chapter uses the generic terms *antidepressant* and *tricyclic* somewhat interchangeably to represent all of these agents. A more accurate term would be to simply designate these

Antidepressant Classifications with Greater Specificity

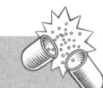

I. Classification Based on Specificity for Reuptake Inhibition of Brain Neurotransmitters

Selective serotonin reuptake inhibitors (SSRI)
Fluoxetine (Prozac)
Fluvoxamine (Luvox)
Paroxetine (Paxil)
Sertraline (Zoloft)

Selective dopamine reuptake inhibitor (SDRI)
Bupropion (Wellbutrin)

Selective serotonin/norepinephrine reuptake inhibitor* (SNRI)
Venlafaxine (Effexor)

Nonselective cyclic antidepressants
Mixed serotonin/norepinephrine reuptake inhibitors*
  Amitriptyline (Elavil)
  Amoxapine (Asendin)
  Doxepin (Sinequan)
  Imipramine (Tofranil)

Nortriptyline (Aventyl, Pamelor)
Protriptyline (Vivactil)
Norepinephrine Reuptake Inhibitors*
  Desipramine (Norpramin)
  Maprotiline (Ludiomil)
Serotonin Reuptake Inhibitor
  Clomipramine (Anafranil)
Serotonin Reuptake Inhibitor/Receptor Blockers*
  Nefazodone (Serzone)
  Trazodone (Desyrel)

II. Classification Based on Specificity of Enzyme Inhibition

Nonselective irreversible inhibitors of MAO
Phenelzine (Nardil)
Tranylcypromine (Parnate)

Reversible inhibitor of MAO-A (RIMA)
Moclobemide (Manerix)

Selective MAO-B inhibitor
Selegiline (Eldepryl)

*Terms first noted in Bezchlibryk-Butler KZ and Jefferies JJ; *Clinical handbook of Psychotropic drugs*, Seattle, 1997, Hogrefe and Huber Publishers.

drugs as cyclic antidepressants. Yet for the sake of consistency the authors will continue to use the term tricyclic.

Monoamine oxidase inhibitors are always referred to as MAOIs and selective serotonin reuptake inhibitors are always referred to as SSRIs. Figure 21-1 illustrates the mechanisms of action for these antidepressants.

TRICYCLIC ANTIDEPRESSANTS

As previously noted, the term *tricyclic* is derived from the chemical structure of these drugs (i.e., tricyclic antidepressants contain three hydrocarbon rings). The related drugs inhibit neurotransmitter uptake but have different chemical structures; for example, maprotiline (Ludiomil) has four hydrocarbon rings (a tetracyclic). Most of these drugs share important properties with imipramine, the first TCA (introduced by Kuhn in 1958).

Antidepressants are not used for all types of depression (e.g., they are not typically prescribed for depressions related to loss). When they are indicated, however, approximately 67% of patients treated experience a remission of symptoms (Glod, 1997). These drugs do not cure depression, but long-term use has been successful. Most relapses are associated with patient-initiated tapering off or discontinuance.

TCAs have been around for some time and are still the first choice of some clinicians. However SSRIs are the first-line agent selected by many clinicians for several reasons that will be discussed.

MAOIs are usually the last choice because of their serious side effects; however, certain types of depressive symptoms may respond more rapidly to MAOIs. Newer MAOIs, such as moclobemide (Manerix), will have fewer serious side effects. Another effective treatment approach, electroconvulsive therapy (ECT), is discussed in Chapter 37. Obviously, consideration of various forms of psychotherapy

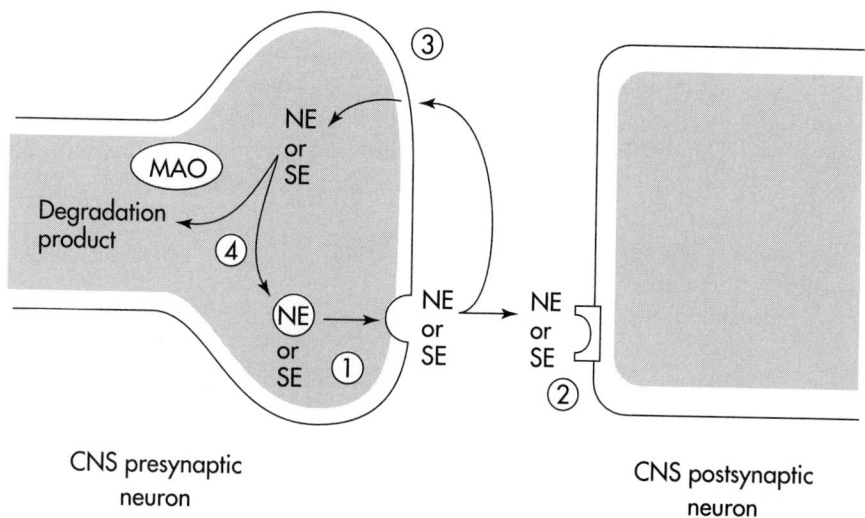

CNS presynaptic neuron   CNS postsynaptic neuron

FIGURE 21-1 Depression results from an amine (norepinephrine, serotonin) concentration too low to activate sufficient receptors; mania results from overabundance of amines acting at receptors. Biogenic amine theory of depression is applied to actions of antidepressant drugs, tricyclic antidepressants, selective serotonin reuptake inhibitors, and MAO inhibitors, and to the action of lithium, used to treat mania. *1,* Lithium inhibits release of norepinephrine and serotonin. *2,* TCAs and MAOIs increase receptor sensitivity to norepinephrine. *3,* TCAs block reuptake of norepinephrine and serotonin; SSRIs block reuptake of serotonin. Lithium enhances reuptake of norepinephrine and serotonin. *4,* MAOIs prevent degradation of norepinephrine and serotonin. NE = norepinephrine; SE = serotonin (From Clark J, Queener S, and Karb V: *Pharmacologic basis of nursing practice,* ed 4, St. Louis, 1993, Mosby.)

and psychotherapeutic interaction is always indicated. TCAs produce both central nervous system (CNS) effects (increasing neurotransmitter availability) and undesired peripheral nervous system (PNS) effects (anticholinergic responses).

Pharmacological Effects (Desired Effects)

Theoretically, the serum level of biogenic amines in the depressed person is so low it makes it impossible to achieve a normal mood. TCAs alleviate the symptoms of depression by blocking the reuptake of these released neurotransmitters (i.e., amines).

Because neurotransmitter activity is terminated by reuptake, this blocking causes greater neurotransmitter availability and thus prolongs their stimulating action. Paradoxically, clinical studies have shown that this specific effect occurs quickly; yet there is a lag period of 2 to 4 weeks before an antidepressant effect is experienced. Exactly what this means is not clear; however, it seems to indicate that more than neurotransmitter availability is involved in depression.

TCAs can be categorized further as secondary amines or tertiary amines (Table 21-1). Drugs that tend to increase the availability of norepinephrine more than serotonin are termed *secondary amines* and drugs that tend to increase serotonin availability more than norepinephrine are called *tertiary amines*. Secondary amines have fewer side effects in elderly patients (Smith and Buckwalter, 1992). Clomipramine (Anafranil), although it is a strong potentiator of serotonin, is typically not prescribed for depression but is the drug of choice for obsessive-compulsive disorder.

Other therapeutic effects of TCAs

Sedation is a therapeutic effect of these drugs. Insomnia and agitation are experienced by some depressed persons, so sedation is often welcomed by those individuals. Tolerance to this sedation usually develops.

On the other hand, some individuals who are depressed are lethargic. A few TCAs are referred to as "activating antidepressants" because they increase psychomotor activity.

Another positive side effect is improved appetite. Anorexia is sometimes a symptom of depression, so appetite stimulation is significant. Whether this is due to a central antihistaminic effect (which some researchers suspect) or to improved mood is not clear. It should be noted that weight gain can be significant and may contribute to a new set of problems.

TCAs have other therapeutic uses as well. Recommended uses include treatment of anxiety associated with depression, alcoholism, and neurotic disorders; treatment of panic attacks; and treatment of phobic anxieties. A typically undesired peripheral effect of imipramine, urinary hesitancy, can be capitalized on to treat childhood enuresis (bedwetting).

In summary, TCAs are thought to treat depression by increasing the availability of specific neurotransmitters. In addition to this desired effect, TCAs often produce the welcomed side effects of sedation and improved appetite.

TABLE 21-1   Secondary and Tertiary Amines

Secondary Amines	Tertiary Amines
Amoxapine (Asendin)	Amitriptyline (Elavil)
Desipramine (Norpramin)	Doxepin (Sinequan)
Nortriptyline (Aventyl, Pamelor)	Imipramine (Tofranil)
Protriptyline (Vivactil)	

FDA Approved Indications

Antidepressants
Major depression
Prophylaxis of recurrent major depression
Depression secondary to other mental illnesses
Depressive phase of bipolar disorder
Obsessive-compulsive disorder (SSRIs and clomipramine)
Enuresis in children (imipramine)
Panic disorders (paroxetine)

Antimanic
Long-term control or prophylaxis of bipolar disorder
Treatment of acute mania

Pharmacokinetics and Dosing

TCAs are absorbed well from the gastrointestinal tract and are usually given orally (PO).

TCAs are metabolized in the liver, and some metabolites have antidepressant effects (desipramine is a metabolite of imipramine; nortriptyline is a metabolite of amitriptyline).

Peak plasma concentrations are reached in 2 to 4 hours on average; however, due to a significant first pass through the liver, only about 30% to 70% of the oral dosage is available in the bloodstream (DeVane, 1986). TCAs are highly bound to plasma proteins (e.g., amitriptyline, 97%). Their effects are due to a small fraction of free drug, so even a small increase in free drug is potentially serious. Persons with diminished liver function (e.g., the elderly, the young, alcoholics, and those with a history of hepatitis) or those with decreased plasma protein levels (e.g., the elderly) may be at special risk of elevated serum levels. People over the age of 55 are usually started at half the regular adult dosage.

The relatively long half-lives of these drugs usually allow once-per-day dosing schedules. A steady state is typically reached in about 5 days. These drugs are initiated at low doses and increased every 3 to 5 days until the patient becomes intolerant of side effects.

All TCAs seem to be equally effective. Table 21-2 captures several important treatment parameters of antidepressants.

Side Effects

Patients taking TCAs experience undesirable side effects of both the PNS and the CNS. Tertiary amines have more frequent and more severe side effects than do the secondary amines or the other non-MAOI antidepressants (Gomez and Gomez, 1992).

PNS side effects

The major side effects are the anticholinergic effects on the peripheral autonomic nervous system. Dry mouth is common but not dangerous. Visual disturbances include blurred vision, dry eyes, and photosensitivity due to mydriasis (pupil dilation). These symptoms, too, are more annoying than dangerous. (However, mydriatic action can precipitate an acute attack of glaucoma, particularly in persons with undiagnosed narrow-angle glaucoma.)

Other anticholinergic side effects include slowing of the gastrointestinal tract that leads to constipation, and slowing of bladder function that leads to urinary hesitancy or retention. The elderly are most susceptible to these side effects, and elderly men with benign prostatic hypertrophy are at a special risk for bladder problems. Anhidrosis (decreased sweating) impairs body cooling. Anticholinergic effects on the cardiovascular system are common enough to warrant serious consideration. Essentially, the parasympathetic system serves as a "brake" for the heart and, when this system is blocked by anticholinergics, the brake is released and the heart speeds up. Tachycardias and arrhythmias can lead to myocardial infarction. TCAs can also have a quinidine-like effect that delays conduction. In susceptible patients this can lead to heart block.

Patients with a history of heart problems must be carefully evaluated.

Children have shown troublesome cardiovascular responses to TCAs (notably desipramine) that warrant serious consideration. Since these concerns were first noted, several deaths have occurred in children taking these drugs. In each case, sudden death, usually associated with physical activity, was the cause.

The serum level may be 42% higher in children than adults at the same dose (Bezchlibnyk-Butler and Jeffries, 1997). Children receiving these drugs need to be carefully monitored (Biederman, et al, 1989; Fletcher, et al, 1993).

These drugs also block alpha-1 adrenergic receptors on peripheral blood vessels and inhibit the body's natural vasoconstricting reaction when a person stands. A pooling of blood occurs in the lower extremities, leading to inadequate cerebral perfusion. The heart responds with a reflex tachycardia in order to help the body adapt (McCarthy and Synder, 1992). Dimming of vision, dizziness, and fainting cause a sense of loss of control and can lead to falls and serious injury. Box 21-2 provides a reference for orthostatic hypotension, a significant and disabling side effect of both antidepressant and antipsychotic drugs. Healthy persons, however, frequently accommodate cardiovascularly, and this side effect diminishes within a few weeks. Patients with a history of heart problems must be carefully evaluated and closely monitored.

Amitriptyline (Elavil) is considered the most cardiotoxic antidepressant and, with its high levels of

TABLE 21-2 Comprehensive Table of Antidepressants: Dosage and Pharmacokinetics;
Specificity for NT Reuptake; Receptor Antagonism; and Side-Effect Profile

	Dosage\Pharmacokinetics			Specificity for NT† Reuptake		
	Daily Dosage/ Range (mg)	Half-Life* (hrs)	Protein Binding (%)	NE†	5-HT†	DA†
I. Cyclic Antidepressants						
Tricyclic Antidepressants (TCAs)						
Amitriptyline (Elavil)	75-300	31-46	97	1	3	1
Amoxapine (Asendin)	100-300	8-30	92	3	1	1
Clomipramine (Anafranil)	75-200	19-37	97	1	4	1
Desipramine (Norpramin)	75-300	12-24	90-95	5	1	1
Doxepin (Sinequan)	75-300	8-24	>90	1	2	1
Imipramine (Tofranil)	75-300	11-25	89-95	2	3	1
Maprotiline (Ludiomil)	75-300	21-25	88	2	1	1
Nortriptyline (Pamelor, Aventyl)	50-200	18-44	92	3	2	1
Protriptyline (Vivactil)	40-60	67-89	92	5	2	1
Trimipramine (Surmontil)	75-300	7-30	95	1	1	1
Selective Serotonin Reuptake Inhibitors (SSRIs)						
Fluoxetine (Prozac)	10-60	48-216	95	0	3	1
Fluvoxamine (Luvox)	100-300	15-19	80	0	4	1
Paroxetine (Paxil)	20-60	3-20	95	1	5	1
Sertraline (Zoloft)	25-200	26-98	98	0	4	2
Novel Cyclic Antidepressants						
Bupropion (Wellbutrin)	150-450	8-15	80	0/1	0	2
Mirtazapine (Remeron)	20-35	20-40	85	0	0	0
Nefazodone (Serzone)	100-600	2-4	99	0	3	1
Trazodone (Desyrel)	150-450	4-9	89-95	0	2	1
Venlafaxine (Effexor)	150-450	5-11	23	2	3	1
II. Monoamine Oxidase Inhibitors (MAOIs)						
Irreversible MAOIs						
Phenelzine (Nardil)	30-90	–	–	–	–	–
Tranylcypromine (Parnate)	20-60	–	–	–	–	–
Reversible Inhibitor of MAO-A (RIMA)						
Moclobemide (Manerix)	300-600	1-3	50	–	–	–

*With active metabolite.
†*NT,* neurotransmitter; *NE,* norepinephrine; *5-HT,* serotonin; *DA,* dopamine; *ACh,* acetylcholine; *H₁,* histamine; *Alpha-1,* alpha adrenergic; *OH,* orthostatic hypotension.
‡Scale for receptor antagonism specificity: *1,* low; *5,* high; *S,* <2%; *X,* >2%; *XX,* >10%; *XXX,* >30%.
§Percentage of patients experiencing side effects (Bezchlibnyk-Butler and Jeffries, 1997).

Receptor Antagonism‡				Side-Effect Profile (%)§					
ACh†	H₁†	Alpha-1†	OH†	Dry Mouth	Insomnia	Sedation	Seizures	Sexual Dysfunction
3	4	3	XX	XXX	X	XXX	S	X
2	3	3	XX	XXX	XX	XX	S	–
3	3	3	XX	XXX	XX	X	S	XXX
2	2	2	X	XX	XX	XX	S	X
3	5	3	XX	XXX	XX	XXX	S	X
3	3	3	XXX	XXX	XX	XX	S	XXX
2	4	3	X	XXX	S	XX	X	S
2	3	3	X	XX	S	X	S	X
3	3	2	XX	XX	XX	S	S	S
1	5	3	XX	XX	X	XXX	S	–
1	1	1	XX	XX	XX	XX	S	XXX
1	–	1	XX	XX	XX	XX	S	XXX
2	1	2	XX	XX	XX	XX	S	XXX
2	1	1	XX	XX	XX	XX	S	XX
1	1	1	X	XX	XX	X	X	S
1	5	2	X	XX	XX	XXX	S	X
1	1	3	XX	XX	XX	XX	S	S
–	2	3	XX	XX	XX	XXX	S	S
–	–	–	XX	XX	XX	XX	S	X
2	2	2	XX	XXX	XX	XX	S	XXX
2	2	2	XX	XX	XX	XX	–	X
2	1	2	XX	XX	XX	XX	S	S

sedation, anticholinergic activity, and orthostatic hypotension, it is a less desirable drug, particularly in the elderly (Gomez and Gomez, 1992).

■ Critical Thinking Question

Examine Table 21-2 and identify the factors that make the SSRIs so appealing.

CNS side effects

A number of CNS effects have been reported. These effects are related to blocking of histamine H₁, adrenergic alpha-1, and anticholinergic receptors. Sedation is a common side effect and can be helpful because insomnia is a frequent symptom of depression. Problematic CNS effects include confusion, disorientation, delusions, agitation, hallucinations, and lowering of the seizure threshold. These psychiatric side

Box 21-2   Orthostatic Hypotension (OH) Caused by Antidepressant and Antipsychotic Drugs

Definition:	Upon standing the patient will experience:
	Systolic blood pressure: a drop of 10-25 mm Hg
	Diastolic blood pressure: a drop of 5-10 mm Hg
	Heart rate: an increase of 5-20 beats/minute
OH in the elderly:	20% of patients >65
	50% of patients >75
	20% of falls attributed to OH
Risk factors:	Age 65 or older
	Dehydration
	Recent immobility
	Fluid loss (i.e., diarrhea)
	Diuretics
	Cardiac medications
Interventions:	Regularly monitor OH vital signs
	Caffeine
	Sodium chloride tablets
	Teach the patient to rise slowly, dangle feet before standing
	Teach the patient that OH is worse in the morning
	Teach the importance of adequate fluids
	Teach the patient to avoid hot showers and baths
	Teach the patient that symptoms decrease with time
	Support stockings

Adapted from McCarthy P and Snyder JC: Orthostatic hypotension: a potential side effect of psychiatric medications, *J Psychosoc Nurs Ment Health Serv* 30(8):3, 1992.

effects may be found in as many as 5% to 15% of patients treated with TCAs (Meador-Woodruff, 1990). The effects usually occur when serum TCA levels are elevated and most often affect elderly patients. TCAs may aggravate an existing dementia or may mimic dementia (Gomez and Gomez, 1992). Other potential CNS effects include anxiety, insomnia, nightmares, ataxia, and tremors. Some patients report nightmares so terrifying that they avoid sleep, even though they are sleep-deprived.

Suicide

There is a clear association between suicide and depression. In fact, 50% to 70% of those who commit suicide are found to have demonstrated characteristics of depression (Keltner and Folks, 1993). Consequently, there is considerable evidence to support treating suicidally depressed individuals with antidepressants. Paradoxically, however, antidepressants can energize patients who have been too depressed to act on their suicidal thoughts. As the antidepressants suc-

ceed and the depression lifts, patients may then have the energy to act. Therefore, suicidally depressed persons warrant special nursing consideration after antidepressant therapy is initiated. Activating antidepressants such as desipramine and fluoxetine may be more likely to energize a patient in this manner. Furthermore, as will be discussed later, TCAs, for the most part, are very toxic. This means that the very drugs a patient is taking to treat depression can be used to overdose and die. TCAs account for nearly 7% of all deaths from intentional drug overdose (Zimmermann, 1997).

■ Critical Thinking Question

Many people who are depressed are also suicidal. Antidepressants are effective in the treatment of depression but can also contribute to suicidal risk. Discuss how each of these variables can contribute to suicide:

a. Lag time
b. Narrow therapeutic index
c. Energizing effect of some antidepressants
d. Serious interactions, particularly with MAOIs

Trazodone (Desyrel) and bupropion (Wellbutrin) do not have lethal overdose potential, so these drugs may be better suited for actively suicidal patients (Martin, 1990).

Interactions

Several serious drug interactions occur with TCAs, including CNS depression, cardiovascular and hypertensive effects, and additive anticholinergic effects. Other problematic interactions may also occur. See Table 21-3 for a reference to these interactions.

CNS depression

Increased CNS depression may occur when TCAs are taken with CNS depressants such as alcohol, anticonvulsants, antipsychotics, benzodiazepines, sedatives, and some antihypertensives (e.g., beta-blockers, reserpine).

Cardiovascular and hypertensive effects

Cardiovascular arrhythmias or hypertension can occur when sympathomimetic drugs are given with TCAs. Because TCAs block the reuptake of norepinephrine, drugs with sympathomimetic agents cause an increase in norepinephrine in the synaptic cleft. Interactants to avoid include norepinephrine, dopamine, ephedrine, and phenylpropanolamine (found in many over-the-counter stimulants). MAOIs, another class of antidepressants, must be completely avoided. Severe reactions, including high fever, seizures, and a fatal hypertensive crisis, can occur. MAOIs are not usually prescribed unless TCAs have failed. When changing to MAOIs, the patient must discontinue TCAs for 14 days before the new drug is given.

In addition, TCAs block alpha-adrenergic receptors, thus compromising the effectiveness of many antihypertensives to control hypertension.

Additive anticholinergic effects

Additive anticholinergic effects can occur when TCAs are given with other anticholinergic drugs, including antipsychotic drugs, atropine, scopolamine, anticholinergic antiparkinson drugs, and antihistamines. This is particularly true in elderly patients. All the PNS and CNS anticholinergic effects mentioned earlier can be worsened.

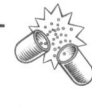

TABLE 21-3	Drug Interactions with Tricyclic Antidepressants	
Drug	**Effect of Interaction**
Cimetidine	Increased TCA serum levels
MAOIs	Hyperpyrexia, excitability, muscular rigidity, convulsions, fatal hypertensive crisis, mania
Sympathomimetics	Cardiac arrhythmias, hypertension
Clonidine, guanethidine	Decreased antihypertensive effect, decreased antidepressant effect
Warfarin	Increased bleeding
Barbiturates, carbamazepine, phenytoin	Decreased TCA effect
Antipsychotics	Increased extrapyramidal side effects (EPSEs), sedation, hypotension; risk of seizures; anticholinergic effect
Procainamide, quinidine	Prolongation of cardiac conduction
Anticholinergics	Increased anticholinergic effect
L-dopa	Increased agitation, tremor, and rigidity
Alcohol, anticonvulsants, benzodiazepines	Increased sedation

Adapted from Watsky EJ and Salzman C: Psychotropic drug interactions, *Hosp Community Psychiatry* 42(3):247, 1991.

Nursing Implications

Therapeutic vs. toxic blood levels

TCAs do not produce euphoria and are not addicting, so the potential for abuse is not great. Overdose, however, is a real issue.

TCA overdose accounts for about 7% or so of all deaths from intentional overdose (Zimmermann, 1997). The difference between a therapeutic dose and a lethal dose is small. Just three times the maximum therapeutic dose (see Table 21-2) can be lethal (Bezchlibnyk-Butler and Jeffries, 1997). For this reason, it is not uncommon for outpatients to be restricted to a 7-day supply if suicide is a risk.

Toxic blood levels may result in sedation, ataxia, agitation, stupor, coma, respiratory depression, and convulsions. Exaggeration of side effects previously mentioned can also occur. Cardiovascular reactions can occur suddenly and cause acute heart failure, even several days after the overdose. Lengthening of the QRS complex (normal is 0.08 to 0.11) to greater than 0.12 is a danger sign (Bezchlibnyk-Butler and Jeffries, 1997). On the other hand, cardiovascular reactions can be "delayed"; that is, they can occur after "recovery" from depression. For these reasons, all antidepressant overdoses should be considered serious, and the patient should be admitted to a hospital for monitoring.

The nurse should be aware of several assessment and intervention strategies when a toxic level of TCAs is suspected (see the TCA nursing interventions box below).

Use in pregnancy

These drugs have not been clearly found to cause teratogenic effects but should be avoided in the first trimester. Since depressive symptoms, such as loss of appetite, can interfere with fetal development by preventing adequate fetal weight gain, antidepressants may be prescribed to pregnant women. Antidepressants are typically placed in FDA pregnancy categories B or C. During pregnancy, TCAs with low anticholinergic effects (e.g., nortriptyline and desipramine) are preferred to those with high anticholinergic effects. TCAs need to be tapered off before delivery to avoid transient perinatal toxicity (Cohen, 1989). About 1% of a mother's dose is excreted in breast milk (Bezchlibnyk-Butler and Jeffries, 1997).

Use in the elderly

TCAs should be given in lower doses to elderly patients. The maxim "start low and go slow" is particularly true for this population. The secondary amines (i.e., amoxapine, desipramine, nortriptyline, protriptyline) are preferred. Side effects previously mentioned such as cardiovascular effects, orthostatic hypotension, cognitive impairment, and all peripheral anticholinergic effects are more pronounced in this age group.

Side effects

Selected side effects and appropriate nursing interventions are listed in the side effects box on p. 281.

Interactions

The nurse should be aware of the interactants mentioned in Table 21-3. As a general rule, persons taking TCAs should avoid certain categories of drugs, including over-the-counter drugs:

Drugs that have anticholinergic properties
Drugs that depress the CNS
Drugs that stimulate the CNS
MAOIs (deaths have been reported from this combination)

A history of hypersensitivity to TCAs precludes their use. Because TCAs lower the seizure threshold, concomitant use of ECT should be considered only after careful evaluation.

Teaching patients

The nurse should discuss side effects and several important principles with patients and their families:

Key Nursing Interventions for TCA Overdose

- Monitor blood pressure, heart rate and rhythm, and respirations.
- Maintain patent airway.
- ECG is recommended.
- Cathartics or gastric lavage with activated charcoal *to prevent further drug absorption* (for up to 24 hours).

- The antidote for severe TCA poisoning (anticholinergic toxicity) is physostigmine (Antilirium), an acetylcholinesterase inhibitor *(inhibits the breakdown of acetylcholine)*. Should be given only in patients with life-threatening symptoms (e.g., coma, convulsions) because of risk associated with physostigmine use.

- A "lag period" of 2 to 4 weeks occurs before full therapeutic effects are experienced.
- Certain drugs must be avoided, including over-the-counter preparations.
- Abrupt discontinuation can cause nausea, headache, and malaise.
- Eye pain must be reported immediately, particularly in the elderly, where undiagnosed narrow-angle glaucoma can lead to an emergency situation.
- Some side effects will lessen after patients adjust to the medication.

Individual TCAs

Following are brief descriptive statements about tricyclic antidepressants. Only unique features of usage, side effects, etc., are mentioned here. Uses and side effects that are common to all of the drugs are not discussed nor is information that can be gleaned from tables in this chapter.

Amitriptyline

Amitriptyline (Elavil) is prescribed often but because of its side-effect profile is not a first-choice agent for the elderly (Nakra and Grossberg, 1990). Amitriptyline is highly anticholinergic and one of the most sedating and cardiotoxic antidepressants (Nakra). It is available in parenteral form and in a fixed-dose combination with the antipsychotic perphenazine (this combination is named Triavil).

Amoxapine

Amoxapine (Asendin) is a secondary amine. It is a *metabolite of the antipsychotic drug loxapine* and blocks

Side Effects and Nursing Interventions for Antidepressants

Side Effects	Interventions
Peripheral Nervous System	
Dry mouth	Advise frequent sips of water, hard candies, sugarless gum.
Mydriasis	Advise wearing of sunglasses outdoors.
Diminished lacrimation	Suggest artificial tears.
Blurred vision	Caution about driving and potential for falls. Usually subsides in 1 to 2 weeks. The patient should remove objects in the house that might be tripped over (e.g., throw rugs, small tables).
Eye pain	Advise patient to report eye pain immediately, as it may indicate an acute glaucoma attack. All elderly persons should be screened for glaucoma before treatment with TCAs is initiated.
Urinary hesitancy/retention	Monitor fluid intake. Patient should be told to avoid putting off urinating. Catheterization may be needed.
Constipation	Monitor fluid and food intake. Urge patient to heed the urge to defecate. A high-fiber diet and large amounts of water (2500 to 3000 ml per day) are helpful.
Anhidrosis	Decreased sweating can lead to increased body temperature. Adequate fluids, appropriate clothing, and sensible exercise should be stressed.
Cardiovascular effects	TCAs are contraindicated during the recovery phase of myocardial infarction.
Orthostatic hypotension	See Box 21-2.
Central Nervous System	
Sedation	Caution patient about driving.
Delirium or mania	Discontinue the drug and call the physician.
Suicidal patients	Observe patients closely since antidepressants may increase energy for suicide.

dopamine receptors. As one might expect, amoxapine can cause side effects typically associated with neuroleptics (e.g., extrapyramidal side effects [EPSEs] and tardive dyskinesia). Because of its potential to cause tardive dyskinesia, amoxapine should be avoided in the elderly if possible (Gomez and Gomez, 1992). Amoxapine may be beneficial for patients who are both psychotic and depressed.

Desipramine

Desipramine (Norpramin) is a secondary amine and a *metabolite of imipramine*. Some clinicians believe it to be a good choice for depressed elderly patients who are known to be sensitive to anticholinergic side effects (the elderly with narrow-angle glaucoma or prostatic hypertrophy) because it has relatively minor anticholinergic effects. Desipramine is also less sedating. It is an *activating antidepressant* and thus may be advantageous for apathetic, lethargic, and hypersomnic patients. Due to its aforementioned effects on cardiovascular systems of children, it should be used with care in this age group. Desipramine is particularly therapeutic in the treatment of panic attacks and dysthymia (Bezchlibnyk-Butler and Jeffries, 1997).

Doxepin

Doxepin (Sinequan) potentiates serotonin. It is sedating, has anticholinergic activity, and relatively high antianxiety effects. Doxepin has few cardiovascular effects, but orthostatic hypotension and weight gain occur in over 10% of patients taking this drug. Doxepin may have antiulcer properties.

Imipramine

Imipramine (Tofranil) is the oldest TCA. None of the newer antidepressants have proven to be more effective. Imipramine pamoate (Tofranil-PM) is available in a single bedtime dose for adults. Imipramine, due to its anticholinergic properties, has proven effective in the treatment of childhood enuresis. Imipramine is a first-line drug in the treatment of panic disorder and is the standard by which newer drugs are measured (Shelton, 1993). It should be used with care in children due to its cardiovascular effects.

Maprotiline

Maprotiline (Ludiomil) potentiates norepinephrine, has anticholinergic effects, and is sedating. It produces a strong antianxiety effect and may be indicated in patients who present with anxiety. Maprotiline is well tolerated and poses no cardiovascular risk (Gomez and Gomez, 1992).

Nortriptyline

Nortriptyline (Aventyl, Pamelor), a secondary amine TCA, is preferred for persons with a history of unfavorable responses to antidepressants because it has a good side-effect profile. It has less tendency to cause orthostatic hypotension, so it is a good choice for elderly patients, or for patients who are beset by dizziness or who have a tendency to fall. Because nortriptyline is somewhat sedating and has a good side-effect profile, it is often prescribed for elderly depressed patients who are agitated and suffering from insomnia. It is a metabolite of the tertiary amine, amitriptyline.

Protriptyline

Protriptyline (Vivactil) is a secondary amine that potentiates norepinephrine much more than serotonin. It produces a greater incidence of tachycardia, cardiovascular problems, and orthostatic hypotension because of its stimulating effects. Because some depressed patients experience hypersomnia instead of insomnia, protriptyline may enable those persons to reduce their amount of sleep. It has significant anticholinergic effects.

Novel Cyclic Antidepressants
Bupropion

Bupropion (Wellbutrin) is unique. Whereas traditional antidepressants increase the bioavailability of norepinephrine or serotonin, bupropion *inhibits dopamine reuptake*. Bupropion has a good side-effect profile. Clinical tests indicate that orthostatic hypotension, cardiovascular conduction problems, anticholinergic effects, and daytime sedation are minimal with bupropion compared to other antidepressants. On the other hand, agitation is not uncommon because, like fluoxetine and desipramine, bupropion is an *activating antidepressant*. Unlike those two drugs and most other antidepressants, bupropion does not have a lethal overdose potential (Martin, 1990). Bupropion is contraindicated for patients with seizure disorders, and it lowers the seizure threshold for all patients (particularly at doses above 450 mg/day). It is thought to be four times more likely than other antidepressants to cause seizures (Olin, 1990). Patients who are suffering from bulimia or anorexia should not be given bupropion because of its tendency to cause weight loss. It should not be given in combination with MAOIs, fluoxetine, or dopaminergic drugs (e.g., levodopa). Finally, bupropion has proven to be an effective replacement for SSRIs when those drugs cause sex-related problems (e.g., decreased libido), and it also reduces the craving for cigarettes in smokers who have quit or who want to quit (under the trade name Zyban).

Nefazodone

Nefazodone (Serzone) is a relatively new antidepressant and is a first-line agent for depression. It is chemically related to trazodone but is not associated with the same level of orthostatic hypotension and certain other cardiovascular effects as trazodone. It also does not have the same potential for priapism as trazodone. Nefazodone blocks serotonin receptors and inhibits the reuptake of both norepinephrine and serotonin. It has a good side-effect profile and does not cause insomnia, sexual dysfunction, or nervousness. It is a potent inhibitor of the cytochrome P-450 enzyme system, thus those drugs reduced by this system will have their plasma levels increased if given with nefazodone. This is particularly important for drugs that have a potential for cardiotoxicity, such as terfenadine (Seldane) and astemizole (Hismanal).

Mirtazapine

Mirtazapine (Remeron) is the newest antidepressant and is approved for major depression only. Its pharmacological effect is different from other antidepressants. It selectively blocks alpha-2 autoreceptors, which increases norepinephrine and serotonin by utilizing the presynaptic feedback system; that is, blockade of alpha-2 autoreceptors signals the need for more of these neurotransmitters. Mirtazapine has a moderately high protein binding (85%) and a relatively long half-life (20 to 40 hours).

Mirtazapine is not accompanied by the anticholinergic and alpha-1 antagonism associated with TCAs. Sedation is reported in over 20% of patients taking mirtazapine, weight gain in about 10%, and an increase in serum cholesterol in 15% of patients. Other side effects can be found in Table 21-2.

Trazodone

Trazodone (Desyrel) potentiates serotonin but not norepinephrine. It is prescribed often because it has almost no anticholinergic effects and few cardiac effects. It is a sedating drug and is prescribed for patients who are insomnic. Trazodone is often prescribed for sleep in nondepressed individuals. Though often prescribed for elderly depressed patients, it has a specific interaction with digoxin and should be used purposefully in such situations (Jenike, 1985). *Trazodone's absorption is increased by 20% if it is taken right after a light meal.* One unusual adverse reaction to this drug is *priapism* (prolonged penile erection). Surgical intervention has been required in a significant percentage of affected men. If priapism occurs, the nurse should stop the medication and notify the prescriber.

Venlafaxine

Venlafaxine (Effexor) is a relatively new antidepressant released in 1994. It is structurally unrelated to any currently marketed antidepressant. It is classified as a selective serotonin norepinephrine reuptake inhibitor (Bezchlibnyk-Butler and Jeffries, 1997). Venlafaxine appears to combine the best qualities of TCAs and SSRIs in that it inhibits the reuptake of both norepinephrine and serotonin as do the TCAs and, like the SSRIs, does not bind significantly to muscarinic, histaminergic, or adrenergic receptors. Theoretically, few anticholinergic, antihistaminic, or antiadrenergic side effects should occur. However, elevation in blood pressure has occurred in some patients (less than 13%) especially at higher dosages (e.g., 300 mg/day or more). Venlafaxine has a lower potential for drug interaction than other antidepressants and does not exaggerate the effects of alcohol. Venlafaxine has a much lower protein-binding ratio (23%) when compared to the SSRIs (which average about 96%) but the clinical significance of this characteristic is not yet known. Venlafaxine may be effective in treating SSRI-induced sexual dysfunction, obsessive-compulsive disorder, and panic disorders.

SELECTIVE SEROTONIN REUPTAKE INHIBITORS

SSRIs are effective antidepressants that have fewer side effects than TCAs and are first-choice drugs for treatment of depression. These newer agents have fewer anticholinergic, cardiovascular, and sedating side effects (Berman, Sapers, and Salzman, 1992). Fluoxetine (Prozac) was the first SSRI marketed in the United States. Stories of near-miraculous recoveries were followed by reports of major problems associated with this drug. Early anecdotal information, coupled with some research findings, associated fluoxetine with suicidal and homicidal behaviors. Subsequent efforts indicate that fluoxetine is an effective antidepressant and that suicidal patients taking this drug (as well as other antidepressants) should be closely monitored as they become energized by fluoxetine's activating properties.

Pharmacological Effect (Desired Effect)

The antidepressant effect of SSRIs is thought to be linked to their inhibition of serotonin reuptake in neurons. These drugs do not bind significantly to histaminic, cholinergic, dopaminergic, or adrenergic receptors, thus reducing many of the side effects that plague people taking TCAs.

Absorption, Distribution, Administration

SSRIs are absorbed in the gastrointestinal tract. Peak plasma levels are achieved for most of these drugs between 4 and 6 hours. They are metabolized in the liver and have relatively long serum half-lives. The long half-lives allow once-a-day dosing schedules.

Both fluoxetine and sertraline have active metabolites that significantly extend their half-lives.

Side Effects

As noted above, the SSRIs have relatively few anticholinergic, antihistaminic, or antiadrenergic effects; thus they do not cause the same intensity of side effects associated with TCAs. Dry mouth, blurred vi-

sion, sedation, and cardiovascular symptoms are not nearly as common with these agents. However, gastrointestinal symptoms such as nausea, diarrhea, loose stools, and weight loss are relatively common (Berman, Sapers, and Salzman, 1992).

CNS effects include headache, dizziness, tremors, nervousness, decreased libido, and decreased orgasm. Some research indicates some level of sexual dysfunction in 27% of women and 45% of men taking antidepressants (News, 1998). Due to the overall less severe side-effect profile, SSRIs are well tolerated by elderly patients.

Interactions

SSRIs interact with several drugs (Table 21-4), and some of these interactions are related to SSRI-inhibition of the cytochrome P-450 enzyme system. SSRIs and MAOIs have proven to be a fatal combination. Beasly, et al (1993) document the case histories of seven individuals who died because of this interaction. This phenomenon is called the serotonin syndrome, which is discussed in Box 21-3. Watsky and Salzman (1991) recommend a 5-week interval between discontinuing fluoxetine and beginning an MAOI.

Toxicity

SSRIs have a low potential for overdose. Even high doses have not resulted in fatalities. Toxic symptoms

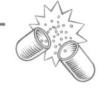

TABLE 21-4	Significant Drug Interactions with SSRIs
Drug	**Effect of Interaction**
Irreversible MAOIs	AVOID; this combination can be fatal, i.e., serotonin syndrome
Lithium	Increased lithium levels, increased serotonergic effect
Antipsychotics	Increased EPSEs
Benzodiazepines	Increased benzodiazepine half-life
TCAs	Increased TCA serum levels → toxicity
	Displacement of TCAs from serum proteins → toxicity
Carbamazepine, phenytoin	Increased anticonvulsant serum levels

include nausea, vomiting, tremor, myoclonus, and irritability. Treatment is symptomatic and supportive.

Use During Pregnancy

SSRIs are pregnancy category B drugs (meaning that risks to the fetus have not been established). However, these drugs should be avoided during the first trimester as a prudent precaution. The long half-lives of fluoxetine and sertraline could also be significant factors in treating the pregnant patient.

Use in the Elderly

SSRIs are safe for use in the elderly because of their side-effect profile. As with most medications, SSRI dosage should be reduced in the elderly. Their potential for weight loss must be monitored in elderly patients, however. The half-life of paroxetine (Paxil) increases 2 or 3 times in the elderly, thus extra precautions are warranted.

Individual SSRIs

Fluoxetine

Fluoxetine (Prozac) was the first SSRI and is the most frequently prescribed antidepressant in the United States. It is an effective antidepressant and has found some clinical utility, albeit unapproved by the Food and Drug Administration (FDA), as a weight loss treatment and as a treatment to control explosive outbursts. Beyond the more typical uses of fluoxetine, it is approved for the treatment of

---

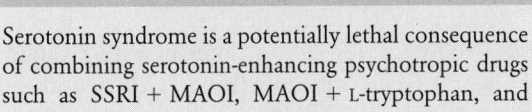

Box 21-3 Serotonin Syndrome

Serotonin syndrome is a potentially lethal consequence of combining serotonin-enhancing psychotropic drugs such as SSRI + MAOI, MAOI + L-tryptophan, and clomipramine (Anafranil) + MAOI.

Patients suffering from the serotonin syndrome experience hyperreflexia, hyperthermia, myoclonus, and other symptoms suggestive of the better-known neuroleptic malignant syndrome (NMS).

Clinical Example

A woman after taking one dose of sertraline (100 mg), became unconscious, hyperthermic (108°F), and myoclonic, and died within a few days. The patient, who had been taking an MAOI, was prescribed an SSRI by another clinician and did not wait the required 14 days before initiating therapy.

Nurses should be aware that:

1. MAOIs and SSRIs should not be given concomitantly.
2. A period of 14 days is required between stopping an MAOI and starting an SSRI.
3. A period of 5 weeks is required between stopping the SSRI fluoxetine (Prozac) and starting an MAOI.
4. MAOIs and clomipramine (Anafranil) should not be given concomitantly.

From Keltner NL and Harris C: Serotonin syndrome: a case of fatal SSRI/MAOI interaction, *Perspect Psychiatr Care*, 1994.

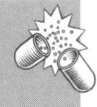

Sources of Drug Interactions in SSRIs and Novel Antidepressants

Pharmacokinetics

What the body does to a drug includes key factors for nurses to understand: absorption, distribution, metabolism, and elimination of drugs. Two of these processes are considered here to explain two important dimensions of drug interactions for SSRIs and some novel antidepressants.

Competition for Protein Binding

SSRIs are highly bound to proteins, and when given with other highly bound drugs (e.g., TCAs) they compete for binding sites. This results in displacement from protein binding sites and a consequent increase in free (i.e., unbound) molecules.

Inhibition of Cytochrome P-450 Enzymes

SSRIs and some novel antidepressants inhibit cytochrome P-450 hepatic enzymes. There are several variants or isoenzymes within the P-450 system (e.g., IA2, II9, IID6, IIC, IIIA4), but that discussion is beyond the scope of this text. Drugs metabolized by P-450 enzymes can have their metabolic process slowed if given with SSRIs or nefazodone, thus leading to increased serum levels.

bulimia, and unapproved uses include pain management and smoking cessation (Bezchlibnyk-Butler and Jeffries, 1997).

Sertraline

Sertraline (Zoloft) is a widely marketed SSRI and is the second drug of this class to be used in the United States. It is a more potent inhibitor of serotonin reuptake than fluoxetine. Sertraline, too, can be given once a day, morning or evening, with or without food. Sertraline may delay or totally inhibit ejaculation in men and orgasm in women, but patients often do not disclose this side effect. Orgasmic ability returns 2 to 3 days after drug cessation.

Paroxetine

Paroxetine (Paxil) is the most potent serotonin reuptake blocker and is approved for the treatment of panic attacks.

Because its metabolites are not active, paroxetine has a shorter half-life and fewer problems should the need arise to discontinue it. The most common side effect is nausea, but this effect rarely leads to dose reduction or drug discontinuation. It has also been shown to be effective for the prevention of depressive relapse (Nemeroff, 1993). Like the other SSRIs, paroxetine can be given on a once-a-day basis. Like sertraline, paroxetine delays or inhibits orgasm.

Fluvoxamine

Fluvoxamine (Luvox) is the newest SSRI and is specifically approved for the treatment of obsessive-compulsive disorder. It does not have an active metabolite and has a side-effect profile similar to other SSRIs.

MONOAMINE OXIDASE INHIBITORS (MAOIs)

MAOIs, the third class of antidepressants, are usually administered to hospitalized patients or to persons who can be closely supervised. In the early 1950s, a derivative of the tuberculosis drug isoniazid was developed (Ayd, 1991). A derivative, iproniazid, an MAOI, was found to have mood-elevating properties. After several clinical trials, iproniazid was found to cause fatal hepatitis and was banned by the FDA. Soon, other MAOIs were synthesized to replace the banned drug. Two of these drugs (phenelzine [Nardil] and tranylcypromine [Parnate]) have survived the test of time and are still used. They are referred to as irreversible nonselective inhibitors of both monoamine oxidase-A (MAO-A) and monoamine oxidase-B (MAO-B). Moclobemide (Manerix), a new MAOI, is a reversible selective inhibitor of MAO-A (RIMA). Selegiline (Eldepryl), most well known as an antiparkinson drug, is a selective MAO-B inhibitor at low dosages (i.e., 10 to 15 mg) but becomes nonselective at higher doses. It has some antidepressant value.

The older, irreversible drugs are almost always prescribed after several TCAs have failed, although an argument can be made that MAOIs are particularly effective in treating atypical depression (e.g., hypersomnia and excessive eating). This second-class status reflects the seriousness of the adverse reactions to these drugs, especially life-threatening hypertension. Although many expert clinicians believe this fear of MAOIs is unwarranted, there is a widespread reluctance to use them.

Moclobemide and selegiline (in its selective state) at low doses do not interact with tyramine-containing foods, therefore they lack the serious side effects of the older MAOIs.

Pharmacological Effects (Desired Effects)

MAOIs block monoamine oxidase, a major enzyme involved in the metabolic decomposition and inactivation of norepinephrine, serotonin, and dopamine. This enzyme inhibition lasts for 10 days in the irreversible MAOIs and 24 hours in moclobemide. The enzyme inhibition increases the levels of these neurotransmitters in the PNS and the CNS. According to the neurochemical theory of depression, depressed persons have lower than normal amounts of these neurotransmitters available. MAOIs help to achieve the normal amounts by slowing the deactivation of these amines. This is in contrast to the TCAs, which help achieve normal amounts by preventing the reuptake of amines by the neurons. It takes 10 days to 4 weeks for the antidepressant effect of MAOIs to occur; however, as with the TCAs, the physiological action (the inhibition of monoamine oxidase) occurs right away. This suggests that factors other than low levels of specific neurotransmitters are involved in depression.

In the PNS, the slowed release of norepinephrine causes decreased heart rate, decreased vasoconstriction, and hypotension. MAOIs also inhibit monoamine oxidase in the liver, which leads to elevated levels of other drugs that are normally metabolized in the liver by monoamine oxidase.

Absorption, Distribution, Administration

MAOIs are well absorbed from the gastrointestinal tract and are given PO. They are metabolized in the liver. Moclobemide has a high first-pass metabolism. Age does not affect moclobemide's pharmacokinetic activities.

Side Effects

MAOIs cause CNS, cardiovascular, and anticholinergic side effects. Serious, life-threatening reactions can occur when irreversible MAOIs interact with certain drugs or foods (see the following discussion on interactions).

Because MAOIs increase the availability of biogenic amines in the brain, CNS hyperstimulation may occur, causing agitation, acute anxiety attacks, restlessness, insomnia, and euphoria. In persons thought to have quiescent schizophrenia (an unrecognized, latent form), full schizophrenic episodes have erupted. Hypomania (less severe than full mania) is a more common effect.

Hypotension is a common cardiovascular effect. This is due to the slowdown in the release of norepinephrine. Unlike the effect of TCAs, a reflex tachycardia does not occur, because the slowed release of norepinephrine is also experienced by other adrenergic nerves, and the heart does not reflexively speed up. Hypotension, combined with failure of a compensatory increased heart rate, can lead to heart failure.

MAOIs can cause anticholinergic effects, such as dry mouth, blurred vision, urinary hesitancy, and constipation. Hepatic and hematological dysfunctions can occur and, although rare, are potentially serious. Blood counts and liver function tests should be obtained before therapy begins.

Interactions

MAOIs have a number of serious interactions. Potentially lethal interactants include both drugs and foods.

Drug-drug interactions

The nurse should be aware of several types of drug interactions (Table 21-5):
- Those that cause *hypertension* (including hypertensive crisis)
- Those that cause severe *anticholinergic responses*
- Those that can cause profound *CNS depression*

Sympathomimetic drugs are classified as direct-acting, indirect-acting, and mixed-acting (having both

TABLE 21-5 **Significant Drug Interactions with Irreversible Nonselective MAOIs***

Drugs	Effect of Interaction
Anticholinergic drugs	Compound anticholinergic response
Anesthetics (general)	Deepen CNS depression
Antihypertensive (diuretics, beta-blockers, hydralazine)	Cause hypotension
CNS depressants	Intensify CNS depression
Guanethidine, methyldopa, reserpine	Produce severe hypertension
Sympathomimetics (mixed and indirect acting): amphetamines, methylphenidate, dopamine, phenylpropanolamine (in many over-the-counter hay fever, cold, and diet medications)	Precipitate hypertensive crisis, cardiac stimulation, arrhythmias, cerebrovascular hemorrhage
Sympathomimetics (direct-acting): epinephrine, norepinephrine, isoproterenol; less likely to cause problems	Same as above but *theoretically* should not produce as severe a reaction
Tricyclic antidepressants	Same as above
Serotonergic drugs (e.g., SSRIs)	Avoid. This combination can be fatal.

*Less severe interaction with these drugs also occur with the RIMA, moclobemide.

direct and indirect properties). Indirect-acting and mixed-acting sympathomimetics cause serious and sometimes fatal hypertension. Direct-acting sympathomimetics act by adding new norepinephrine to the body, whereas indirect-acting sympathomimetics release existing norepinephrine from the neurons. Because MAOIs increase the amount of stored norepinephrine in the PNS, there is a potential for indirect-acting and mixed-acting sympathomimetics to release relatively large amounts of norepinephrine. This makes it crucial to avoid these interacting drugs. Even small amounts can trigger a hypertensive crisis. Typical indirect-acting and mixed-acting sympathomimetics include amphetamines, cocaine, methylphenidate (Ritalin), dopamine, mephentermine, and ephedrine. Over-the-counter weight-loss and stimulant products contain phenylephrine, phenylpropanolamine, and pseudoephedrine, which are mixed- or indirect-acting sympathomimetics. Direct-acting sympathomimetics such as norepinephrine, epinephrine, and isoproterenol theoretically should not trigger the release of existing norepinephrine. Moclobemide should not be combined with the irreversible MAOIs or with narcotics. Finally, MAOIs should not be given in combination with TCAs except in unusually refractory cases and never in combination with SSRIs.

The initial symptoms of hypertensive crisis are palpitation; tightness in the chest; stiff neck; and a throbbing, radiating headache. Very high blood pressure with elevation of the heart rate is common. Cardiovascular consequences have included myocardial infarction, cerebral hemorrhage, myocardial ischemia, and arrhythmias. Diaphoresis and pupillary dilation are also prominent signs.

Anticholinergic effects can be severe if other anticholinergic drugs are given with MAOIs. Typical anticholinergic side effects can be reviewed in the discussion of TCA side effects.

Finally, because MAOIs "inhibit" monoamine oxidase in the liver, some drugs, particularly CNS depressants, are not as rapidly metabolized there and create serum levels high enough to seriously depress the CNS.

Meperidine (Demerol) is specifically contraindicated. A marked potentiation of these drugs can occur, and deaths are documented. Hypotensive drugs are also potentiated by MAOIs. The nurse should be aware that MAOI inhibition continues for up to 10 days after tranylcypromine and phenelzine are discontinued. In other words, the potential for serious interactions continues for some time after MAOIs are discontinued.

Food-drug interactions

Food-drug interactions center on the amino acid tyramine, a precursor to dopamine, norepinephrine, and epinephrine. Tyramine is found in many foods commonly consumed in the North American diet (Box 21-4). Aged cheese, bananas, salami, and coffee are a few foods containing tyramine that must be

---

Signs and Symptoms of Hypertensive Crisis

Occipital headache
Stiff neck
Sore neck
Nausea and vomiting
Sweating
Dilated pupils and photophobia
Sudden, unexplained nosebleed
Tachycardia, bradycardia
Constricting chest pain

Box 21-4 Tyramine-Rich Foods to Avoid with MAOIs

Alcoholic beverages	Meats
Beer and ale	Bologna
Chianti and sherry	Chicken liver
wine	Fish, dried
Alcohol-free beer	Liver
Dairy products	Meat tenderizer
All mature cheese:	Pickled herring
cheddar, blue, brie,	Salami
mozzarella	Sausage
Sour cream	Other foods
Yogurt	Caffeinated coffee,
Fruits and vegetables	colas, tea (large
Avocados	amounts)
Bananas	Chocolate
Fava beans	Licorice
Canned figs	Sauerkraut
	Soy sauce
	Yeast

avoided by the patient (Gelenberg, 1998). In fact, all high-protein foods that have undergone protein breakdown by aging, fermentation, pickling, or smoking should be avoided. Hypertension and hypertensive crisis can develop from this food-drug combination.

Nursing Implications

Therapeutic vs. toxic drug levels

An intensification of the effects already discussed occurs with overdose. A lethal dose of MAOIs is only 6 to 10 times the daily dose (see Table 21-2 for dosages). Careful monitoring when these medications are given is important. "Cheeking" and hoarding of these drugs could be disastrous. If MAOI overdose is suspected, the nurse should know the following:

- Emesis and gastric lavage may be helpful if performed early.
- Monitoring of vital signs is important.
- External cooling is warranted if high fevers occur.
- Hypotension should be treated in the standard manner.

Use in pregnancy

MAOIs should be avoided during the first trimester. Later in the pregnancy use them only if the anticipated benefit justifies the potential risks to the fetus.

Use in the elderly

MAOIs may be effective in older patients because monoamine oxidase activity increases with age (Bezchlibnyk-Butler and Jeffries, 1997). Precautions for orthostatic hypotension should be observed in this age group however.

Side effects

The nurse should be familiar with the common side effects of MAOIs and the appropriate nursing interventions (see the MAOIs side effects box).

Interactions and contraindications

It is important for the nurse to understand that drug-drug and food-drug interactions are serious and potentially fatal. The nurse should know the following:

- Sympathomimetic drugs should not be combined with MAOIs.
- Foods containing tyramine must not be ingested by the patient who is taking MAOIs.

MAOIs are contraindicated in patients:

- With a history of stroke or cardiovascular disease
- With a pheochromocytoma, a tumor that secretes pressor substances
- Undergoing elective surgery (because of the hypotensive potential of combining MAOIs and anesthesia)

MAOIs should not be given in combination with:

- Other MAOIs
- TCAs or SSRIs
- Meperidine (Demerol)

Side Effects and Nursing Interventions for MAOIs

Side Effects	Interventions
CNS hyperstimulation	Reassure the patient. Assess for developing psychosis, hypomania, or seizures. If symptoms warrant, withhold the drug and notify the physician.
Hypotension	Monitor blood pressure frequently and intervene to prevent falls and injuries; having patient lie down may help return blood pressure to normal.
Anticholinergic effects	See antidepressant side effects for appropriate nursing interventions.
Hepatic and hematological dysfunction	Blood counts and liver function tests should be performed. If dysfunction is apparent, MAOI should be discontinued.

Hypertensive crisis is a major concern. If it occurs the nurse should:

- Discontinue MAOIs and contact the physician.
- Know that therapy to reduce the blood pressure is warranted and that phentolamine (Regitine) is the appropriate drug or nifedipine (Procardia) 10 mg bitten and swallowed (Bezchlibnyk-Butler and Jeffries, 1997).
- Monitor vital signs.
- Have patient walk (will lower blood pressure somewhat).
- Manage fever by external cooling.
- Institute supportive nursing care as indicated.

■ Critical Thinking Question

Bill took some amphetamines while on an MAOI. Will these drugs interact? If so, what will happen? If not, why not?

Teaching patients

The nurse must be persistent in teaching patients and their families about MAOIs and their side effects. Although most of these drugs are administered in a closely supervised setting, the nurse is nonetheless responsible for educating patients. Because patients taking MAOIs can experience serious reactions to certain other drugs and foods, the nurse must clearly convey this information.

- Therapeutic effects are achieved within 10 days to 4 weeks.
- Driving must be avoided if the patient is drowsy.
- Certain over-the-counter drugs should be avoided, and *all* of the patient's health-care providers should be aware that the patient is taking an MAOI.
- High-tyramine foods should be avoided.
- Headaches, palpitations, and stiff neck should be reported immediately.

Irreversible MAOIs

Two irreversible MAOIs are used in the treatment of depression.

Phenelzine

Phenelzine (Nardil) has been found to be most effective in depressed persons who are clinically char-

acterized as "atypical." It is considered the most effective MAOI and is the most sedative. A clinical response is experienced in about 4 weeks. It has also been used as a deterrent to cocaine abuse and for panic attacks.

Tranylcypromine

Tranylcypromine (Parnate) seems most effective for severe reactive or endogenous depression. A clinical effect is experienced in about 10 days, sooner than with the other MAOIs. It is the most stimulating. Tranylcypromine is contraindicated in patients over 60 years of age. Due to severe hypertension leading to death in some patients, tranylcypromine was banned by the FDA in 1961. Sharp protests by influential psychiatrists eventually led to a reversal of the FDA position (Ayd, 1991).

Reversible Inhibitor of MAO-A

Moclobemide

Moclobemide (Manerix) is a new class of MAOI. It is selective in that it inhibits only the A type of monoamine oxidase. Its inhibition lasts just 24 hours versus 10 days for the older MAOIs; thus it is considered reversible. Its dosing is not affected by age or renal function. Though moclobemide does not have the classic and significant reactions to tyramine-containing foods that phenelzine and tranylcypromine have, it is still recommended that it be taken after meals to reduce tyramine-related responses (Bernstein, 1995; Bezchlibnyk-Butler and Jeffries, 1997).

ANTIMANIC DRUGS

LITHIUM

Lithium, a naturally occurring element, is not much different from sodium. The differences, however, are significant enough to make lithium useful in the treatment of manic depression. Lithium was discovered in 1817 by Arfwedson, who named it after the Greek word for stone. Lithium was touted as a cure for epilepsy, gout, and other problems. In the 1940s, lithium was used as a salt substitute for cardiac patients in the United States. In 1949, an Australian,

John Cade, reported his research in the *Medical Journal of Australia,* showing lithium to be effective in the treatment of manic depression. In that same year, the March 12 issue of *JAMA* reported two accounts of fatal lithium poisoning. This sounded the death knell for lithium in this country (Ayd, 1991). Fears of lithium were compounded by a lack of interest on the part of drug companies. As a natural element, lithium is not patentable, and consequently a drug company could invest research funds only to have another pharmaceutical company legally use the findings (Ayd, 1991). Lithium was not made available in the United States until 1970.

Lithium is now used for the treatment and prophylaxis of the manic phase of manic-depressive illness. There is also a growing body of clinical research that supports its use as an antidepressant and for augmentation with antidepressants in refractory depression.

Pharmacological Effects (Desired Effects)

Although precisely how lithium achieves its normalizing effect on mania is not known, it is thought that the lithium ion substitutes for the sodium ion in neurons. This compromises the ability of the neurons to release, inactivate, and respond to neurotransmitters. See Figure 21-1, which illustrates the mechanisms of action for lithium.

Absorption, Distribution, Administration

Lithium is well absorbed from the gastrointestinal tract. It is given PO in tablets, capsules, or concentrate. Peak blood levels are reached in 1 to 3 hours. More than 95% of the amount ingested is excreted by the kidneys unchanged. Lithium is not metabolized. Hence, renal disease lengthens the half-life, necessitating a reduction in dosage. Its typical plasma half-life is about 24 hours. The absorption and excretion of lithium and sodium are closely linked. Lithium is reabsorbed with sodium in the proximal tubule. Diuretics, particularly those affecting the loop of Henle and the distal tubule, lead to increased retention of lithium (Horne, Heitz, and Swearingen, 1991; Trimble, 1996). If dietary sodium intake increases, it is likely that plasma lithium levels will drop as lithium is excreted more rapidly. Con-versely, if sodium in the diet decreases, or if sodium is lost in ways other than through the kidneys (e.g., sweating or diarrhea), lithium levels increase. These are important considerations because a therapeutic serum level of lithium is not much lower than a toxic serum level. Diet and activity levels should not change abruptly.

Lithium is effective in 60% to 80% of cases (Calabrese, et al, 1993); however, it takes 7 to 10 days to achieve a clinical response. Lithium dosage is based on both clinical response and serum lithium levels. The typical dose for acute mania is 600 mg three times per day, which usually produces a serum level of 1 to 1.5 mEq/L. Desirable maintenance blood levels are 0.6 to 1.2 mEq/L and can be maintained on 900 to 1200 mg per day. Blood levels over 1.5 mEq/L can be toxic.

Side Effects

Lithium's side effects are linked to serum blood levels. Blood levels over 1.5 mEq/L can be considered toxic. Common side effects are nausea, dry mouth, diarrhea, and thirst. Drowsiness, mild hand tremor, polyuria, weight gain, a bloated feeling, sleeplessness, and light-headedness are other relatively common side effects. Polyuria and polydipsia occur in about 70% of patients taking lithium (Martin, 1993). These effects occur at therapeutic levels but usually cease after the sixth week. However, these same side effects increase in severity at toxic serum levels.

Side effects unrelated to serum levels include weight gain, a metallic taste, headache, edema of the hands and ankles, and pruritus. Even at therapeutic levels, lithium can affect thyroid gland function. Some patients may require thyroid hormone. Lithium may also impair the mental or physical abilities required for driving.

Lithium is generally contraindicated in persons with cardiovascular disease. Lithium may also harm the fetus and is an FDA category D drug (evidence of fetal risk has been established). Adverse reactions to toxic blood levels are discussed below. Lithium therapy is contraindicated for persons with renal disease; if lithium is necessary, there should be close supervision of these patients. Lithium-induced renal insufficiency (creatinine level consistently over 2 mg/100 ml) is apparently uncommon (Gitlin, 1993). However, polyuria and diabetes insipidus are seen in 12% to 20% of patients taking lithium

(Martin, 1993). Nephrogenic diabetes insipidus is caused by inhibition of the cAMP-dependent action of antidiuretic hormone (ADH) on the distal tubule and collecting duct cells. When ADH is blocked, the patient suffers from polyuria (defined as urinating in excess of 3 L per day). The following clinical example highlights nephrogenic diabetes insipidus and the attempts to treat it.

■ Critical Thinking Question

If a person taking lithium suffers from serious diarrhea, what will happen to the person's serum level?

CLINICAL EXAMPLE

Mr. Jones, a 67-year-old male on the geropsychiatric unit, drinks approximately 4 L of water per day. He urinates more than 3 L per day. His creatinine level is 2 mg/dL. Mr. Jones is diagnosed with nephrogenic diabetes insipidus related to long-term lithium treatment. His potassium level is 3 mEq/L. He complains of shakiness, tremors, weakness, and general malaise. He is on daily fluid balance profiles. Treatment follows a stepwise approach:
1. Lithium is discontinued.
2. Potassium supplement is started.
3. Amiloride is begun to enhance ADH activity.

Interactions

Familiarity with the drugs that can elevate lithium serum levels is essential. Diuretics (except acetazolamide) decrease lithium excretion and thereby elevate serum lithium levels. Indomethacin and other nonsteroidal antiinflammatory drugs increase serum lithium levels by reducing renal elimination of lithium. Switching to a low-salt diet also elevates serum lithium levels.

Some drugs decrease serum lithium levels and pose the problem of inadequate treatment and symptom exacerbation. Drugs decrease serum levels in one of two ways: by increasing lithium excretion or by decreasing lithium absorption. Drugs that increase lithium excretion include acetazolamide (Diamox), caffeine, and alcohol.

It is not uncommon for lithium to be combined with antipsychotic drugs or benzodiazepines. These drugs are ordered with lithium because of lithium's clinical-response lag time of 1 to 2 weeks. Antipsychotic agents are prescribed to produce a neuroleptic effect until the lithium produces a clinical response. A potential problem with this combination is that the antiemetic properties of the antipsychotic mask early signs of lithium toxicity—nausea and vomiting. A second concern centers on the specific combination of lithium and haloperidol. Some studies report a significantly higher percentage of neurotoxicity with this combination.

Lithium also prolongs the paralyzing effect of neuromuscular blocking agents given before surgery and ECT. Apnea and oxygen deprivation can be avoided if appropriate steps are taken (e.g., extra oxygenation).

■ Critical Thinking Question

Johnny is a good basketball player. He is 23 years old and is taking lithium. Since Johnny perspires a great deal on the days he plays (about 4 times per week), his nurse is concerned about his serum levels being consistent. What is this nurse considering?

Nursing Implications

Therapeutic vs. toxic drug levels

Therapeutic serum lithium levels are 0.6 to 1.2 mEq/L. At serum levels above 1.5 mEq/L, adverse reactions can occur. Typically, the higher the serum levels, the more severe the reaction. Mild to moderate toxic reactions occur at levels from 1.5 to 2.5 mEq/L, and moderate to severe reactions occur at 2 to 2.5 mEq/L. Diarrhea, vomiting, drowsiness, muscular weakness, and lack of coordination can be early signs of lithium toxicity. At higher levels, ataxia, giddiness, tinnitus, blurred vision, and large output of dilute urine may be seen. At serum levels above 3 mEq/L, multiple organs and organ systems may be involved, leading to coma and death (Sugarman, 1984). Levels above 4 mEq/L are associated with poor outcomes. Interestingly, persons with serum levels as high as 10 mEq/L have survived. Serum levels should be monitored and not allowed to exceed 2 mEq/L.

There is no antidote for lithium poisoning. Discontinuing the drug may be enough when supportive nursing care is available. Gastric lavage has been used successfully. Parenteral normal saline may provide enough volume and sodium to prevent major problems for serum levels below 2.5 mEq/L. For severe lithium poisoning, forced diuresis or hemodialysis may be needed.

Use in pregnancy

Cessation of lithium during pregnancy is suggested because of cardiovascular malformation when used in the first trimester. If antimania treatment is essential in the first trimester, carbamazepine may be beneficial. When lithium is prescribed in the second and third trimesters, dosages should be reduced by as much as 50% before delivery because of possible neonatal toxicity from high maternal serum levels of lithium (Cohen, 1989). Major congenital abnormalities for lithium-taking mothers is 4% to 12% as opposed to 2% to 4% in non–lithium-taking mothers. For anticonvulsants the risk is 4% to 6% (Fact Sheet, 1998). Lithium is present in breast milk at 30% to 100% of mother's serum level (Bezchlibnyk-Butler and Jeffries, 1997).

Use in the elderly

Elderly patients can benefit from lithium but, due to the severity of side effects and adverse reactions, these patients must be assessed for renal function and dietary history. Most lithium-induced reactions are more likely in this age group. Serum levels of 0.4 to 0.8 mEq/L are appropriate for elderly patients.

Side effects

Because lithium has a narrow therapeutic index, serum lithium levels should be determined frequently. Daily levels are not uncommon in some acute treatment units. Once the patient is stabilized, monthly or even less frequent serum level determinations are usually adequate. Blood levels are usually drawn before the first dose in the morning (usually 8 to 12 hours after the last dose). However, the nurse should not rely on laboratory tests alone and should continue clinical evaluation of the patient (see the lithium nursing interventions box).

Interactions

The nurse should help patients to understand the basic mechanisms affecting serum lithium levels. Drug interactions that increase or decrease serum levels should be reviewed. The nurse must impress upon all patients the necessity for alerting all other health-care providers to the lithium treatment, even though some patients may be reluctant to do so.

Teaching patients

The nurse should teach patients and their families the following:

- The symptoms of minor toxicity, which include vomiting, diarrhea, drowsiness, muscular weakness, and lack of coordination
- The symptoms of major toxicity, which include giddiness, tinnitus, blurred vision, and dilute urine
- The side effects associated with lithium and when to notify the physician
- To avoid conception, since lithium may harm the fetus
- To avoid driving until stabilized on the lithium

See Box 21-5 for patient guidelines for taking lithium.

Key Nursing Interventions for Patients Taking Lithium

- Prepare the patient for expected side effects without instilling anxiety.
- Discuss which side effects should subside (nausea, dry mouth, diarrhea, thirst, mild hand tremor, weight gain, bloatedness, insomnia, light-headedness).
- Identify the side effects that require immediate notification of the physician (e.g., vomiting, severe tremor, sedation, muscle weakness, vertigo).

- Suggest taking lithium with meals *to reduce nausea.*
- Suggest drinking 10 to 12 8-oz (240 ml) glasses of water per day *to reduce thirst and maintain normal fluid balance.*
- Advise patient to elevate feet *to relieve ankle edema.*
- Advise patient to maintain a consistent dietary sodium intake, but to increase sodium if there is a major increase in perspiration.

Box 21-5 Patient Guidelines for Taking Lithium

To achieve a therapeutic effect and prevent lithium toxicity, patients taking lithium should be advised of the following:

1. Lithium must be taken on a regular basis, preferably at the same time daily. For example, a patient taking lithium on a three-times-daily schedule, and who forgets a dose, should wait until the next scheduled time to take the lithium, but should not take twice the amount at that time, because lithium toxicity could occur.
2. When lithium treatment is initiated, mild side effects, such as a fine hand tremor, increased thirst and urination, nausea, anorexia, and diarrhea or constipation, may develop. Most of the mild side effects are transient and do not represent lithium toxicity. Also, in some patients taking lithium, some foods such as celery and butter fat will have an unappealing taste.
3. Serious side effects of lithium that necessitate its discontinuance include vomiting, extreme hand tremor, sedation, muscle weakness, and vertigo. The prescribing physician should be notified immediately if any of these occur.
4. Lithium and sodium are eliminated from the body through the kidneys. An increase in salt intake increases lithium elimination, and a decrease in salt intake decreases lithium elimination. Thus, it is important that the patient maintain a balanced diet and salt intake. The patient should consult with the prescribing physician before making any dietary alterations.
5. Various situations can require an adjustment in the amount of lithium administered to a patient; for example, the addition of a new medication to the patient's drug regimen, a new diet, or an illness with fever or excessive sweating.
6. For determination of lithium levels, blood should be drawn in the morning approximately 8 to 12 hours after the last dose was taken.

ALTERNATIVES TO LITHIUM: CARBAMAZEPINE AND VALPROIC ACID

Though lithium is often the first drug prescribed for bipolar disorder, only about 60% to 80% of patients respond (Calabrese, et al, 1993). Due to the seriousness of bipolar disorder, researchers have diligently sought alternatives for patients who do not respond to lithium. The two most promising alternatives are the anticonvulsants carbamazepine (Tegretol) and valproic acid (Depakene).

Carbamazepine

Carbamazepine is effective for most patients who do not respond to lithium or for whom lithium is contraindicated (e.g., in pregnancy or in allergic reactions). Although it is an effective anticonvulsant, it is chemically related to tricyclic antidepressants. Patients who seem more apt to be unresponsive to lithium and who, in turn, do respond to carbamazepine, are patients with a rapidly cycling bipolar episode. Carbamazepine may, at times, be given in combination with lithium. It is thought that the effectiveness of carbamazepine may be related to its inhibition of "kindling" activity in the brain. In other words, just as kindling in the fireplace is the first step in building a fire, so it is thought that some abnormal brain activities begin as "kindling" and spread. A cup of water can dowse the fire from kindling but is ineffective in the control of a raging fire. The concept of kindling is used to explain seizure activity in the brain. Carbamazepine's antimanic serum levels are related to its therapeutic anticonvulsant serum levels.

Nausea, anorexia, and occasional vomiting are side effects of carbamazepine. Sedation and drowsiness are other relatively common side effects. The most serious potential side effect of carbamazepine is agranulocytosis. Complete blood counts should be performed weekly when this drug treatment is initiated. Therapeutic serum levels for carbamazepine are from 4 to 12 μg/ml.

Significant drug interactions with carbamazepine include antibiotics, other anticonvulsants, lithium, calcium channel blockers, or angiotensin-converting enzyme (ACE) inhibitors.

Valproic Acid

Valproic acid (Depakene) is another anticonvulsant with antimanic properties. Approximately 70% to 80% of patients who do not respond to lithium suffer from the rapid-cycling variant of bipolar disorder (Dunner and Fieve, 1974). Valproic acid seems to be particularly effective for this group of patients. Therapeutic serum levels are from 50 to 100 μg/ml.

Advantages of valproic acid include its rapid onset, the fact that it can be used initially without attempting lithium, and it is well tolerated with little effect on cognition. Disadvantages of valproic acid include transient hair loss, weight gain, tremors, gastrointestinal upset, and dose-related thrombocytopenia.

🔖 Key Concepts

1. According to the neurochemical theory, depression is the result of a decreased availability of the neurotransmitters norepinephrine, serotonin, and possibly dopamine in the brain.
2. There are three major classes of antidepressants: tricyclic antidepressants (TCAs), selective serotonin reuptake inhibitors (SSRIs), and monoamine oxidase inhibitors (MAOIs).
3. TCAs and SSRIs block the reuptake of neurotransmitters back into the nerve ending, thereby increasing their availability.
4. MAOIs slow the breakdown of these neurotransmitters by inhibiting the enzyme, monoamine oxidase, thereby increasing the availability of these neurotransmitters.
5. Common side effects of TCAs (dry mouth, blurred vision, constipation, and tachycardia) are associated with their anticholinergic properties.
6. Because TCAs have a narrow therapeutic index, amounts even slightly greater than therapeutic dosages can be fatal. TCAs account for about 7% of all deaths from intentional overdose.
7. Patients should be taught about the "lag time" of 2 to 4 weeks that it takes for a full therapeutic effect to be experienced with TCAs.
8. SSRIs have fewer anticholinergic, antihistaminic, antidopaminergic, and antiadrenergic side effects than do TCAs.
9. SSRIs are first-choice drugs for the treatment of depression.
10. SSRIs are highly bound to serum proteins and can displace other protein-bound drugs.
11. All SSRIs affect cytochrome P-450 metabolizing enzymes and affect the metabolism of other drugs metabolized by this system.
12. MAOIs can cause central (stimulation), cardiovascular (hypotension), and anticholinergic side effects.
13. Traditional irreversible nonselective MAOIs interact with several foods that contain tyramine (e.g., aged cheese, bananas, salami) and with indirect- and mixed-acting sympathomimetic drugs (e.g., amphetamines and methylphenidate [Ritalin]) to cause hypertensive crisis. Reversible inhibitors of MAO-A (RIMA) seem to have minimal interactions with foods containing tyramine.
14. MAOIs have a lag time of 10 days to 4 weeks.
15. Lithium is the drug of choice for the manic phase of bipolar disorder.
16. Clinically therapeutic serum levels are 0.6 to 1.2 mEq/L, but at higher serum levels, serious or even fatal reactions occur.
17. Common side effects of lithium include nausea, dry mouth, diarrhea, thirst, and mild hand tremor.
18. Lithium has a narrow therapeutic index and a lag time of 7 to 10 days.

🔖 Study Questions

(Answer key is in the back of the book.)

1. During the first day of treatment with a TCA you expect:
   a. An improvement in appetite
   b. An improvement in mood
   c. Anticholinergic side effects (e.g., dry mouth)
   d. Signs of toxicity

John Johnson, a 69-year-old retired truck driver, has been very despondent for some time. After careful assessment, it is determined that Mr. Johnson is depressed. The next two questions are based on this example.

2. Which of the following TCA side effects would be a special concern for Mr. Johnson?
   a. Mania
   b. Sialorrhea
   c. Dry mouth
   d. Urinary retention

3. Other side effects that might concern Mr. Johnson's nurse are:
   1. Undiagnosed narrow-angle glaucoma
   2. A history of herpes
   3. Constipation
   4. Cataracts
      a. All of the above
      b. 1, 3
      c. 2, 3, 4
      d. 3 only

4. Which one of the following statements is *not* true of TCAs?
   a. They can be given PO.
   b. They have a narrow therapeutic index.
   c. Beneficial, therapeutic effects occur within hours.
   d. Many side effects disappear after a few weeks.

5. Which TCA is the most sedating? (Use Table 21-2.)
   a. Amitriptyline
   b. Desipramine
   c. Protriptyline
   d. Nortriptyline
6. Which antidepressant class has the fewest anticholinergic side effects?
   a. TCAs
   b. MAOIs
   c. SSRIs
7. Which antidepressant class is the least sedating?
   a. TCAs
   b. MAOIs
   c. SSRIs
8. Which antidepressant potentiates norepinephrine most effectively?
   a. Amitriptyline
   b. Desipramine
   c. Fluoxetine
   d. Paroxetine
9. Depression treated with TCAs should be relieved within:
   a. 24 hours
   b. 1 week
   c. 2 to 4 weeks
   d. 6 to 8 weeks
10. Bill Smith is placed on an MAOI after TCAs proved to be ineffective. Which of the following are definitely contraindicated for Bill?
    1. Aged cheese, figs, certain wines
    2. Indirect-acting stimulants
    3. Mixed-acting stimulants
    4. Direct-acting stimulants
    a. All the above
    b. 1, 4
    c. 1, 2, 3
    d. 3, 4
11. According to the chapter discussion, TCAs achieve their effect by:
    a. Blocking the reuptake of serotonin and norepinephrine at presynaptic neurons
    b. Blocking neurotransmitter metabolism
    c. Inhibiting monoamine oxidase
    d. Decreasing acetylcholine levels
12. According to the text, MAOIs achieve their effect by:
    a. Blocking the reuptake of serotonin and norepinephrine at the presynaptic neuron
    b. Blocking neurotransmitter metabolism
    c. Increasing dopamine bioavailability
13. Which of the following statements about lithium are true?
    1. Lithium is a naturally occurring element.
    2. Lithium has always been used for treatment of elevated mood.

    3. Lithium levels should be taken once per month after a patient is stabilized.
    4. A mild hand tremor is an early side effect.
    a. 1, 2
    b. 1, 4
    c. 1, 3, 4
    d. All of the above
14. The serum parameters for a therapeutic response to lithium are:
    a. 0.2 to 0.6 mEq/L
    b. 0.6 to 1.2 mEq/L
    c. 1 to 1.6 mEq/L
    d. 2 to 3 mEq/L

REFERENCES

Ayd FJ: The early history of modern psychopharmacology, *Neuropsychopharmacology* 5(2):71, 1991.

Beasley CL, et al: Possible monoamine oxidase inhibitor-serotonin uptake inhibitor interaction: fluoxetine clinical data and preclinical findings, *J Clin Psychopharmacol* 13(5):312, 1993.

Berman I, Sapers BL, and Salzman C: Sertraline: a new serotonergic antidepressant, *Hosp Community Psychiatry* 43(7):671, 1992.

Bernstein JG: *Handbook of drug therapy in psychiatry,* ed 3, St. Louis, 1995, Mosby.

Bezchlibnyk-Butler KZ and Jeffries JJ: *Clinical handbook of psychotropic drugs.* Seattle, 1997, Hogrefe and Huber Publishers.

Biederman J, et al: A double-blind placebo-controlled study of desipramine in the treatment of ADD. II. Serum drug levels and cardiovascular findings, *J Am Acad Child Adolesc Psychiatry* 28(6):903, 1989.

Brown RP and Mann JJ: A clinical perspective of the role of neurotransmitters in mental disorders, *Hosp Community Psychiatry* 36:141, 1985.

Calabrese JR, et al: Brief report: predictors of valproate response in bipolar rapid cycling, *J Clin Psychopharmacol* 13(4):280, 1993.

Cohen LS: Psychotropic drug use in pregnancy, *Hosp Community Psychiatry* 40:566, 1989.

DeVane CL: Cyclic antidepressants. In Evans WE, Schentag JJ, and Jusko WJ, editors: *Applied pharmacokinetics: principles of therapeutic drug monitoring,* Spokane, Wash, 1986, Applied Therapeutics.

Dunner DL and Fieve RR: Clinical factors in lithium carbonate prophylaxis failure, *Arch Gen Psychiatry* 30:229, 1974.

Fact Sheet: Taking mood stabilizers during childbearing years. *NAMI Advocate* 19(4):16, 1998.

Fletcher SE, et al: Prospective study of ECG effects of imipramine in children, *J Pediatr* 12(4):652, 1993.

Gelenberg AJ: The MAOI diet. *Biological Therapies in Psychiatry Newsletter* 21(2):1, 1998.

Gitlin MJ: Lithium-induced renal insufficiency, *J Clin Psychopharmacol* 13(4):276, 1993.

Glod CA: Factors in antidepressant selection: sorting out the issues, *APNA News* 9(3):3, 1997.

Gomez GE and Gomez EA: The use of antidepressants with elderly patients, *J Psychosoc Nurs Ment Health Serv* 30(11):21, 1992.

Gomez GE and Gomez EA: Depression in the elderly, *J Psychosoc Nurs Ment Health Serv* 31(5):28, 1993.

Harsch HH and Holt RE: Use of antidepressants in attempted suicide, *Hosp Community Psychiatry* 39:990, 1988.

Horne MM, Heitz UE, and Swearingen PL: *Fluid and electrolyte balance,* St. Louis, 1991, Mosby.

Jenike MA: *Handbook of geriatric psychopharmacology,* Littleton, Mass, 1985, John Wright-PSG.

Keltner NL and Folks DG: Alternatives to lithium in the treatment of bipolar disorder, *Perspect Psychiatr Care* 27(2):36, 1991.

Keltner NL and Folks DG: *Psychotropic drugs,* St. Louis, 1993, Mosby.

Kuhn R: Treatment of depressive states with G22355 (imipramine hydrochloride), *Am J Psychiatry* 115:459, 1958.

Martin A: Clinical management of lithium-induced polyuria, *Hosp Community Psychiatry* 44(5):427, 1993.

Martin RL: Geriatric psychopharmacology: present and future, *Psychiatr Annals* 20:682, 1990.

McCarthy P and Snyder JC: Orthostatic hypotension: a potential side effect of psychiatric medications, *J Psychosoc Nurs Ment Health Serv* 30(8):3, 1992.

Meador-Woodruff JH: Psychiatric side effects of tricyclic antidepressants, *Hosp Community Psychiatry* 41:84, 1990.

Monroe LR: New weapons in the assault on depression, *Los Angeles Times,* p E1, 4, January 2, 1990.

Nakra BRS and Grossberg GT: Mood disorders. In Bienenfeld D, editor: *Verwoerdt's clinical geropsychiatry,* Baltimore, 1990, Williams & Wilkins.

Nemeroff CB: Paroxetine: an overview of the efficacy and safety of a new selective serotonin reuptake inhibitor in the treatment of depression, *J Clin Psychopharmacol* 13(6)(suppl 2):10, 1993.

News: A steep price to pay. *J Psychosoc Nurs Ment Health Serv* 36(5):10, 1998.

Olin DR: *Drug facts and comparisons,* St. Louis, 1990, JB Lippincott.

Shelton RC: Psychopharmacology: pharmacotherapy of panic disorder, *Hosp Community Psychiatry* 44(8):725, 1993.

Smith M and Buckwalter KC: Medication management, antidepressant drugs, and the elderly: an overview, *J Psychosoc Nurs Ment Health Serv* 30(10):30, 1992.

Sugarman JR: Management of lithium intoxication, *Fam Pract* 18:237, 1984.

Trimble MR: *Biological psychiatry.* New York, 1996, John Wiley and Sons.

Watsky EJ and Salzman C: Psychotropic drug interactions, *Hosp Community Psychiatry* 42(3):247, 1991.

Zimmermann PG: Tricyclic antidepressant overdose, *Am J Nurs* 97(10):39, 1997.

CHAPTER 22

Antianxiety Drugs

NORMAN L. KELTNER

LEARNING OBJECTIVES

After reading this chapter you should be able to:
- Describe the differences between benzodiazepines and buspirone.
- Identify when benzodiazepines are indicated.
- Discuss the side effects of benzodiazepines.
- Identify benzodiazepines appropriate for the elderly.
- Identify the specific antidote for benzodiazepine overdose.
- Describe potential drug interactions with benzodiazepines, particularly with CNS depressants such as alcohol.
- Discuss the implications for teaching patients about antianxiety drugs.

People have been seeking relief from anxiety since the beginning of recorded history. Alcohol is the oldest drug to be used to reduce anxiety and has been used by countless millions to self-medicate fears, phobias, and "nerves." From biblical times through the present, men and women have taken alcohol to calm down, to forget, and/or to escape reality. It is still the most often self-prescribed anxiolytic. However, individuals who drink alcohol for these reasons have found alcohol to be a two-edged sword—with relief has come abuse, dependence, and assorted other problems.

In recent times other drugs have been developed to alleviate anxiety. In the early 1990s, bromo seltzers were advertised to have anxiolytic properties, but problems surfaced with bromide dependency, and bromo seltzers had to be withdrawn from the market (Harvey, 1985). In the 1930s and 1940s, barbiturates were heralded as having potential to treat anxiety, but they too were found to have many adverse effects, including seizures, dependence, addiction, and withdrawal.

The first drug specifically for the treatment of anxiety was meprobamate (Miltown, Equanil), developed in 1955 (Ayd, 1991). This drug, with its ability to calm nerves, blur the reality of stressors, and, in general, make persons feel better, was a national sensation. Ayd (1991) describes the impact of meprobamate as follows:

"In the months thereafter the demand for Miltown, a name derived from the New Jersey town in which Wallace Laboratories manufactured meprobamate, far exceeded that for any drug previously marketed in the United States. For a time Milton Berle was renamed Miltown Berle, magicians pulled Miltown instead of rabbits from their magical hats, and newspaper and national coverage of this drug was unprecedented."

KEY TERMS

Abuse Excessive use of a substance that differs from societal norms

Anxiety A feeling of apprehension, uncertainty, or tension

Anxiolytic An antianxiety drug

Dependence A state in which a drug user must take a usual or increasing dose of a drug in order to prevent the onset of abstinence symptoms/withdrawal. The drug user must take the drug to feel "normal."

Disinhibition A state in which a person is not able to suppress urges or statements that may be socially unacceptable (e.g., telling a dirty joke in an inappropriate situation or making sexual comments to the boss's wife)

Tolerance The need for increasing amounts of a substance to achieve the same effects. Pharmacokinetic tolerance results when the drug is metabolized more rapidly. Pharmacodynamic tolerance occurs when more drug is required at the receptor sites in order to achieve the same effect.

Withdrawal Physical signs and symptoms that occur when the addictive substance is reduced or withheld; also referred to as *abstinence syndromes*

This reception probably says far more about the American psyche than it does about the efficacy of meprobamate. Obviously, the nation was ready for a drug to buffer the stressors of a busy society. For several years, meprobamate was a widely prescribed medication, but as with alcohol, bromo seltzer, and barbiturates, problems surfaced. Individuals using meprobamate were subject to abuse, tolerance, and lethal overdose. Its appeal as an antianxiety agent began to diminish. Fortunately, waiting in the wings were new agents to calm the trembling hands of a nation beseiged with anxiety.

Before the 1950s were over, another class of antianxiety drugs was developed, the benzodiazepines. These drugs had advantages over barbiturates: they were less likely to be abused and were safer when overdoses occurred (Hollister, 1994). Though first synthesized in the 1930s, benzodiazepines were not discovered to have a psychiatric effect until the late 1950s. Ayd (1991) outlines the nearly serendipitous nature of the development of chlordiazepoxide (Librium), the first benzodiazepine. After nearly 40 benzodiazepine derivatives had been synthesized and found lacking in therapeutic qualities, the last one was laid to the side only to be tested 20 years later. During that testing, psychotropic properties were noted. The first written report of those properties was published by Harris in the *Journal of the American Medical Association* in 1960. Eventually, several thousand benzodiazepine derivatives would be synthesized, including familiar drugs such as diazepam (Valium), lorazepam (Ativan), alprazolam (Xanax), oxazepam (Serax), and clonazepam (Klonopin).

However, as with all the drugs mentioned above, these drugs too are linked to significant problems. Benzodiazepines were (and continue to be) abused, they induced tolerance, and they were implicated in lethal overdoses (though always when combined with other drugs).

Clinical researchers and drug manufacturers continue to search for the perfect antianxiety drug, the drug that will ameliorate anxiety without significant adverse effects. A nonbenzodiazepine antianxiety agent that is widely marketed is buspirone (BuSpar). Buspirone apparently does not have the potential for abuse, dependency, and withdrawal that is associated with other antianxiety agents. A large group of unrelated drugs seem to have antianxiety properties, or at least have been found useful in the treatment of specific anxiety-like syndromes. Examples of drugs with antianxiety properties include some beta-blockers (e.g., propranolol), antihistamines, monoamine oxidase inhibitors, tricyclic antidepressants (TCAs), phenothiazines, hydroxyzine (Vistaril), and opioids. Beta-blockers and TCAs are briefly mentioned at the end of the chapter. Finally, a host of potentially new antianxiety drugs are currently being tested.

■ Critical Thinking Question

In the introductory paragraphs to this chapter, a review of historical data reflects our nation's passion for solutions to our anxieties and fears. What is happening in our society to contribute to this? Do you think this is unique to America?

BENZODIAZEPINES

Historically, antianxiety agents have been referred to as *anxiolytics* or *minor tranquilizers.* The major class of antianxiety drugs is benzodiazepines; these drugs are used most often to treat anxiety. Benzodiazepines are widely used by both psychiatric and general-medicine patients. They are used regularly by some persons with chronic anxiety and for time-limited periods by persons going through crises. Benzodiazepines are also commonly used to decrease presurgery "jitters." Evidence also suggests their effectiveness as antipanic agents (Lydiard, Roy-Byrne, and Ballinger, 1988).

Anxiety is a subjective experience that can be observed by others. The anxious person feels excessively alert, is easily startled, is restless, talks too much, visually scans the environment, has tremors, and may have dilated pupils. While many people use these drugs prn, benzodiazepines should not usually be taken for the stresses of everyday living. Benzodiazepines have no therapeutic value in the treatment of psychosis, but may be effective in treating the anxiety that is often associated with neuroleptic dose reduction (Garcia, et al, 1990).

Pharmacological Effect (Desired Effect)

Benzodiazepines have a generally depressing effect on the central nervous system (CNS) including the limbic system, the thalamus, the hypothalamus, and the reticular activating system (which projects to the thalamus and hypothalamus). Because the reticular activating system is depressed, incoming stimuli are muted and evoke less reaction. This effect is probably achieved by the potentiation of gamma-aminobutyric acid (GABA), an inhibitory neurotransmitter, binding to a benzodiazepine recognition site.

To illustrate the concept of *muting,* two of the symptoms listed above will be highlighted. Hyperalertness and environmental scanning are defensive reactions utilized by the anxious person to guard against an environment perceived to be threatening. The "stressed out" person might overreact to being startled because the body's system is on alert. As the antianxiety agent "decreases" environmental input, there is a general relaxing of the anxious posture.

These drugs can cause several levels of CNS depression, from sedation to anesthesia. Benzodiazepines do this by sedating the patient and depressing the inhibitory neurons affecting arousal. The latter effect causes a state of disinhibition, or loosening of inner impediments to conduct. Disinhibition results in feelings of euphoria and excitement that, in turn, can lead to poor judgment. The natural restraint that minimizes social blunders is depressed.

In order to visualize the potential allure of benzodiazepines, visualize a tension continuum with anxiety on one end and a carefree sense of being on the other. Benzodiazepines have the potential to move the anxious person from the agony of the anxiety end to the relaxed-feeling of the carefree end. In therapeutic doses, this degree of shift from anxiety to disinhibition is not gained or sought, but because of the possibility of reaching a carefree zone, benzodiazepines have become drugs of abuse (Schedule IV; see Appendix I).

Pharmacokinetics

Benzodiazepines are readily absorbed after oral ingestion; however, intramuscular (IM) administration produces slow and inconsistent absorption for most of these drugs (lorazepam [Ativan] is an exception). The benzodiazepines are very lipid-soluble and therefore readily cross the blood-brain barrier. The benzodiazepines are metabolized by the liver but do not significantly induce their own hepatic metabolism compared to barbiturates. They are excreted in the urine. The active metabolites can exert an effect for up to 10 days. In fact, a convenient way of categorizing benzodiazepines is to divide them into those with short half-lives (less than 20 hours) and those with longer half-lives (more than 20 hours). Of the selected benzodiazepines with shorter half-lives listed in Table 22-1, lorazepam (Ativan), oxazepam (Serax), and temazepam (Restoril) are preferable for use in the elderly. Clorazepate (Tranxene), chlordiazepoxide (Librium), and diazepam (Valium) have longer half-lives and hence have longer duration of action. Accordingly, they are less suited for use in older patients.

However, looking at half-lives alone is misleading. An important factor in half-life determination over time is the metabolic process that each benzodiazepine undergoes. Most benzodiazepines are oxidized in the liver, but since hepatic function and vol-

TABLE 22-1   **Antianxiety Agents: Adult Dosage, Speed of Onset, Half-Life, Elderly Dosage, and Metabolic Process**

Drug	Adult Dosage Range (mg/day)	Speed of Onset (PO)	Elimination Half-Life (hr)*	Elderly Dosage (mg)**	Metabolic Process
Alprazolam (Xanax)	0.75-4	Intermediate	12-15		Oxidation
Chlordiazepoxide (Librium)	15-60	Intermediate	5-30		Oxidation
Clonazepam (Klonopin)	1.5-10	Intermediate	18-60	0.25-3 in divided doses	Oxidation
Clorazepate (Tranxene)	15-60	Fast	30-100		Oxidation
Diazepam (Valium)	4-40	Very fast	20-80		Oxidation
Lorazepam (Ativan)	2-4	Intermediate	10-20	1-2 in divided doses	Conjugation
Oxazepam (Serax)	30-60	Intermediate to slow	5-20	10 tid	Conjugation
Buspirone (BuSpar)	15-40	Intermediate	2-11	Up to 15 in divided doses	Oxidation

Adapted from Olin BR: *Drug facts and comparisons*, St. Louis, 1996, JB Lippincott.
*Range of half-life over the life span.
**Only for those drugs recommended for use in the elderly.

ume change with age the liver becomes less efficient at metabolizing these drugs over a lifetime. For instance, the half-life of diazepam is about 20 hours in a young man but stretches to 80 hours in a man 80 years of age. On the other hand, a few benzodiazepines are metabolized by a different process (i.e., conjugation), a process not significantly affected by the aging process. These benzodiazepines are lorazepam, oxazepam, and temazepam. Because their half-lives remain fairly stable over the life span and because they do not have active metabolites, they are better suited for use in the elderly (see Table 22-1). Since temazepam is primarily used as a sedative there will be no further discussion of this drug.

Because hepatic metabolism is the primary mechanism for drug disposition, drugs that interfere with liver metabolism (e.g., alcohol) dangerously compound the effect of benzodiazepines.

Table 22-1 presents information on these drugs, including the usual adult dosages, speed of onset after oral administration, elimination half-life over the life span, typical dosages for those drugs recommended for use in the elderly, and metabolic process.

Side Effects

Commonly, CNS side effects are manifested, including drowsiness, fatigue, and decreased coordina-

tion. A certain mental impairment and slowing of reflexes also occur. Less frequently, confusion, depression, and headache may be present. Peripheral nervous system (PNS) effects include occasional constipation, double vision, hypotension, incontinence, and urinary retention. Benzodiazepines can exacerbate narrow-angle glaucoma.

Beyond these undesired effects are the triple problems of dependence, withdrawal, and tolerance (Beeber, 1989). Dependence can be defined as a state in which the body functions "normally" when the drug is present. The body, in turn, functions "abnormally" when the drug is not present. When benzodiazepine is withdrawn from the dependent person, such symptoms as agitation, tremor, irritability, insomnia, vomiting, sweating, and even convulsions may be experienced. Abrupt withdrawal from benzodiazepines can have serious effects (e.g., convulsions); thus, gradual tapering in dosage is important. Withdrawal probably creates a situation in which the function of the GABA-binding sites is compromised, reducing GABA-induced inhibition (Rapport and Covington, 1989).

Since GABA is an inhibitory neurotransmitter, releasing the "inhibition" results in a "taking off the brake" phenomenon. Hence, the effects just mentioned occur. This inhibiting effect of benzodiazepines accounts for their anticonvulsive activity. Intravenous diazepam (Valium) and lorazepam

Side Effects and Nursing Interventions for Benzodiazepines

Side Effects	Interventions
Dry mouth	Advise rinsing mouth with water often, eating sugarless hard candies, and chewing sugarless gum.
Ataxia	Provide assistance with ambulation.
Dizziness, drowsiness	Assist with ambulation and with getting in and out of bed. Caution about driving.
Nausea	Take with food.
Withdrawal symptoms (increased anxiety, flulike symptoms, tremors)	Contact prescriber.

(Ativan) are first-line agents for status epilepticus, and clonazepam (Klonopin) is regularly prescribed as an anticonvulsant. Tolerance to sedation occurs, however; dose escalation is not pronounced for antianxiety effects in those patients adhering to the prescriptive regimen. Older persons with impaired liver or renal function and debilitated persons experience more side effects, and consequently should receive less of these drugs (see nursing interventions box and discussion of pharmacokinetics).

Interactions

Benzodiazepines are CNS depressants and interact *additively* with other CNS depressants. Alcohol, TCAs, monoamine oxidase inhibitors (MAOIs), nefazodone (Serzone), opioids, antipsychotics, and antihistamines increase the sedative effects of benzodiazepines (Watsky and Salzman, 1991). Table 22-2 lists major interactants for the benzodiazepines.

Nursing Implications

Therapeutic vs. toxic drug levels

Benzodiazepines taken alone are relatively safe drugs. Overdoses hundreds of times higher than a therapeutic dose have been reported without resulting in death. However, if benzodiazepines are combined with other drugs, such as alcohol, effects can be fatal. Signs and symptoms of overdose include somnolence, confusion, coma, diminished reflexes, and hypotension. Effective treatment begins with emptying the stomach by induced vomiting and gastric lavage, followed by activated charcoal. The nurse should

Table 22-2   Major Interactions with Benzodiazepines

Alcohol and other CNS depressants	Increased sedation, CNS depression
Antacids	Impaired absorption rate of benzodiazepine
Disulfiram (Antabuse) and Cimetidine (Tagamet)	Increase the plasma level of benzodiazepines that are oxidized
Nefazodone (Serzone)	Inhibits metabolism of alprazolam and triazolam
Phenytoin	Increased anticonvulsant serum level
TCAs	Increased sedation, confusion, impaired motor function
MAOIs	CNS depression
Succinylcholine	Decreased neuromuscular blockade

monitor blood pressure, pulse, and respirations and provide supportive care as indicated. Hypotension can be treated with levarterenol (Levophed). Physostigmine is a very potent antidote for acute diazepam poisoning and can be effective for respiratory depression associated with diazepam overdose (Ciraulo, et al, 1989). Dialysis has limited value.

Flumazenil (Mazicon), is a benzodiazepine receptor blocker. It selectively blocks benzodiazepine receptors but does not block adrenergic or cholinergic receptors. Because it does not stimulate the CNS and does not block other receptors, it can be given when benzodiazepine overdose is suspected without fear of unexpected interactions. A response to flumazenil typically occurs within 30 to 60 seconds. Two important considerations when giving flumazenil are that it does not speed the metabolism or excretion of benzodiazepines and that it has a short duration of action. This presents a clinical management problem. If the patient responds to flumazenil, then benzodiazepines are present, but because flumazenil does not speed metabolism and has a short duration of action, the patient may "recover" only to return to a "preflumazenil" state. This requires constant vigilance by the nurse and repeated doses of flumazenil as the body eliminates the benzodiazepine from the system.

Use in pregnancy

The association of benzodiazepine use and fetal abnormalities is not supported (Cohen, 1989). There is some concern that benzodiazepines may be associated with cleft lip and cleft palate in the first trimester, but the evidence is not conclusive. Even such inconclusive findings might warrant discontinuance during pregnancy. Benzodiazepines are also known to enter breast milk so nursing mothers should not use these drugs. However, if the drug cannot be discontinued without exacerbation of symptoms, tapering to the lowest possible dosage is desirable.

Use in the elderly

As has been mentioned in the pharmacokinetic discussion, specific benzodiazepines are acceptable for use in the elderly, but most are not recommended. This dichotomy is based on metabolic processes. Lorazepam (Ativan) and oxazepam (Serax) are considered to be the best benzodiazepines for older individuals. Temazepam (Restoril) and, occasionally, alprazolam (Xanax) are also used in this age group. The other benzodiazepines, including diazepam (Valium) and chlordiazepoxide (Librium), have extended half-lives and active metabolites and should not be routinely prescribed for older patients.

Side effects

The most common side effects are related to mental alertness. The patient should be cautioned about driving or operating hazardous machinery. Tolerance to most side effects quickly develops. Blood pressure

Use of Benzodiazepines (BZs) for Anxiety in the Elderly

Good BZs	BZs to avoid
Lorazepam (Ativan)	Diazepam (Valium)
Oxazepam (Serax)	Chlordiazepoxide (Librium)

of inpatients should be monitored routinely, and a drop of 20 mm Hg (systolic) on standing warrants withholding the drug and notifying the physician. Other side effects and nursing interventions are listed in the box on page 302.

Interactions

Benzodiazepines interact with a number of CNS depressants. The nurse should explain this carefully to patients who are taking benzodiazepines. A high percentage of psychiatric patients abuse drugs (Carey, 1989), so there is a real potential for deadly combinations. It is also probable that these patients will develop a cross-tolerance to hepatic-metabolized drugs. For instance, persons who develop a tolerance to alcohol have an increased tolerance to diazepam, but not when alcohol and diazepam are taken together. It is not uncommon to hear a patient who is experienced in taking diazepam speak with disdain about typical dosages; for example, "10 mg of Valium doesn't even touch me!" Although it may be true that diazepam alone does not "touch" these patients, diazepam combined with alcohol *will*. The nurse should remind these patients that if they mix diazepam with alcohol, they could die.

Teaching patients

"Patient education must be the initial step in promoting medication adherence" (Forman, 1993). Benzodiazepines have tremendous potential for abuse. Consequently, it is important to teach patients and their families about these drugs. The nurse should teach the following:
- Benzodiazepines are not for the minor stresses of everyday life.
- Over-the-counter drugs may potentiate the actions of benzodiazepines.
- Driving should be avoided until tolerance develops.

- Alcohol and other CNS depressants potentiate the effects of benzodiazepines.
- Hypersensitivity to one benzodiazepine may mean hypersensitivity to another.
- These drugs should not be stopped abruptly.

Withdrawal

Withdrawal from benzodiazepines is similar to that of alcohol and barbiturates, all of which produce their pharmacological effect by binding to GABA receptors. Withdrawal symptoms range from mild dysphoria and insomnia following abrupt discontinuance from therapeutic dosages to convulsions, tremor, vomiting, cramping, and sweating from high dosages taken over a long period of time. See Table 22-3 for a list of potential withdrawal symptoms.

SPECIFIC BENZODIAZEPINES

Diazepam

Diazepam (Valium) is an often-prescribed antianxiety agent. It has multiple uses related to its CNS-depressing effect. Besides anxiety disorders and short-term relief from symptoms of anxiety, diazepam is used preoperatively to relieve presurgery "jitters," for skeletal muscle spasms (e.g., lower back pain), as a drug of choice for status epilepticus, and as an adjunct for endoscopic procedures. In addition, diazepam may be useful for symptomatic relief of alcohol withdrawal.

Alprazolam

Alprazolam (Xanax) is particularly useful for generalized anxiety, adjustment disorders, and anxiety associated with depression. Shelton (1993) reports that alprazolam is effective for the treatment of panic disorder at doses of 2 to 6 mg per day or more. It has been criticized for its potential to cause addiction and dependence, and for reports of alprazolam-caused violent/aggressive behavior (Glod, 1992; Shelton, 1993).

Chlordiazepoxide

Chlordiazepoxide (Librium) is prescribed for anxiety disorders, the relief of the symptoms of anxiety, and acute alcohol withdrawal. It is absorbed well orally.

Clonazepam

Clonazepam (Klonopin) is used most often as an anticonvulsant but also has clinical utility in the treatment of panic disorder. Clonazepam alone or as an adjunct is useful in the treatment of Lennox-Gastaut syndrome (a petit mal variant) and akinetic and myoclonic seizures. Patients with panic disorder taking clonazepam should be slowly tapered off this drug because evidence exists suggesting that abrupt withdrawal can precipitate status epilepticus (Shelton, 1993).

Clorazepate

Clorazepate (Tranxene) is used to treat anxiety and acute alcohol withdrawal and as an adjunct in the treatment of partial seizures.

Lorazepam

Lorazepam (Ativan) is used to treat anxiety disorders. It is available for oral (PO) and parenteral administration. The metabolites of lorazepam are inactive, so the effects of this drug do not persist. Patients with impaired liver function can handle this drug better than they can most other benzodi-

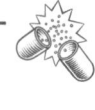

Table 22-3	Symptoms Emerging after Withdrawal from Benzodiazepines	
Neurologic		**Psychiatric**
Convulsions		Anxiety
Insomnia		Irritability
Light-headedness		Cognitive
Involuntary movements		Memory impairment
Headache		Depression
Weakness		Confusion
Gastrointestinal		**Other**
Nausea		Tachycardia
Vomiting		Sweating
Diarrhea		
Weight loss		
Decreased appetite		

azepines because it does not undergo oxidative metabolism.

Oxazepam

Oxazepam (Serax) is similar to lorazepam in that its metabolite is inactive and it is metabolized by conjugative reaction rather than by oxidation. Thus, the drug is effective for a relatively short time (24 hours) and is suitable for persons with liver disorders and for the elderly.

OTHER ANTIANXIETY AGENTS

Buspirone

Buspirone (BuSpar) is not a benzodiazepine but is from the azapirones chemical group. Buspirone does not bind to benzodiazepine recognition sites but probably acts as a serotonin agonist (the same neurotransmitter implicated in depression). The azapirones are considered the first purely anxiolytic agents to be developed. There is considerable interest in buspirone because it causes no sedation and no cross-tolerance with sedatives or alcohol has been demonstrated.

Buspirone's effects help distinguish anxiety control from the sedative and euphoric actions of older benzodiazepines. Buspirone is particularly effective in reducing symptoms of worry, apprehension, difficulties with concentration and cognition, and irritability. Furthermore, there is no evidence that it produces the benzodiazepine effects of dependence, withdrawal, sedation, hypnosis, and muscle relaxation. It does not depress the CNS, and its lack of a sedative effect make buspirone less attractive for abuse (Hollister, 1994). Because there is not abuse potential, busipirone is not a controlled substance.

Buspirone provides relief from anxiety within 7 to 10 days, but maximum therapeutic gain is not achieved until 3 to 6 weeks of treatment. It has a probable half-life of 2 to 11 hours, so it is usually given in divided doses (Lydiard, Roy-Byrne, and Ballinger, 1988). It is extensively metabolized after the first pass. As little as 1% becomes bioavailable. Foods increase its bioavailability by decreasing first-pass metabolism. Side effects include dizziness, nausea, headache, nervousness, light-headedness, and excitement.

Buspirone is a remarkably safe drug. There have been no reports of death from taking buspirone

alone. Dosages as high as 2400 mg per day have been taken without major side effects (Keltner and Folks, 1997). There is no data on the use of buspirone during pregnancy.

There are few drug interactions with buspirone, but haloperidol and MAOIs have been reported to cause some adverse effects when coadministered.

It should be noted that when switching from a benzodiazepine to buspirone that buspirone cannot be substituted immediately for the benzodiazepine. Because of dissimilarities in their pharmacology, the benzodiazepines must be tapered while the buspirone is initiated.

▪ Critical Thinking Question

Why is it preferable to give a benzodiazepine with a shorter half-life to elderly patients?

Propranolol

Propranolol (Inderal) is a beta-blocker that effectively interrupts the physiological responses of anxiety related to social phobia. It is less effective than the benzodiazepines but is relatively safe and has little abuse potential. Most side effects are transient and mild. However, bradycardia, light-headedness, and heart block can occur.

Clomipramine

Clomipramine (Anafranil) is a tricyclic antidepressant that is effective for obsessive-compulsive disorder (OCD) at a dose of approximately 100 to 150 mg per day. Clomipramine is a relative serotonin reuptake inhibitor (SRI), though not as potent as the more traditional selective serotonin reuptake inhibitors (SSRIs). It inhibits norepinephrine, thus possibly accounting for its antiobsessional effect. The major long-term consequence of clomipramine has to do with dental problems associated with reduced production of saliva. The nurse should teach mouth-hygiene techniques to avoid this complication.

Other Tricyclic Antidepressants

Imipramine (Tofranil), in dosages over 150 mg per day, has proven to be effective for panic-anxiety attacks (Beeber, 1989). Desipramine (Norpramin), at higher dosages and for longer trial periods, has also proven effective. Trazodone (Desyrel) has antianxiety properties and has been used to treat cocaine withdrawal. Trazodone has a highly sedative quality and is often prescribed for individuals suffering from anxiety, particularly the elderly, to facilitate sleep.

Selective Serotonin Reuptake Inhibitors

SSRIs are prescribed for OCD, panic attacks, and phobias. SSRIs are considered first-line approaches to OCD. Specifically, fluoxetine (Prozac) and fluvoxamine (Luvox) are approved for treatment of this disorder. SSRIs may be the most effective, as well as the safest, agents for the prophylaxis and long-term treatment of panic attacks (Black, et al, 1993).

Table 22-4 outlines pharmacological interventions for specific anxiety disorders.

■ Critical Thinking Question

What are some approaches to dealing with anxiety without drugs?

■ Key Concepts

1. Antianxiety agents are the most commonly prescribed psychotropic drugs, and benzodiazepines are the most commonly prescribed class of antianxiety agents.
2. Diazepam (Valium) is the prototype and best-known benzodiazepine; however, other benzodiazepines, particularly alprazolam (Xanax) and lorazepam (Ativan), are now used extensively.

TABLE 22-4 Pharmacological Interventions for Specific Anxiety Disorders

Disorder	Pharmacological Treatment
Panic Disorder Manifests as discrete and intense period of anxiety, apprehension, and distress. Associated symptoms include palpitations, sweating, trembling, dyspnea, etc.	SSRIs are perhaps the safest for long term and prophylaxis: sertraline 25 mg qd or fluoxetine 10 mg qod have proven effective. Benzodiazepines: clonazepam (average dose 1.5 mg qd) and alprazolam (average dose 3 mg qd) can provide more immediate relief. TCAs: same dosage as used in treating depressive syndromes, but dosage should be carefully titrated because of the risk of a paradoxical effect.
Phobic Disorder *Agoraphobia* Fear of being away from home or in situations where escape is inhibited	Alprazolam at the relatively high dose of 3 to 6 md qd has proven effective. TCAs: typically between 150 and 200 mg per day. SSRIs and highly serotonergic TCAs, e.g., clomipramine, amitriptyline, and trazodone, are effective for agoraphobia.
Social Phobia Persistent fears of situations in which one is exposed to the scrutiny of others, e.g., stage fright.	Beta-blockers often in combination with antidepressant or benzodiazepine. Propranolol 10 to 20 mg tid or qid. Benzodiazepines alone or in combination with antidepressants. Clonazepam 0.5 mg bid. SSRIs: low doses initially.
Obsessive Compulsive Disorder Obsessions, compulsions, or both	Clomipramine 100 to 200 mg per day. Fluvoxamine 200 to 300 mg per day. Other SSRIs. Venlafaxine.

3. Antianxiety drugs have four basic clinical uses: for treatment of persons with chronic anxiety, for time-limited periods in persons going through crises, for presurgery nervousness, and for the treatment of panic disorder.

4. Antianxiety drugs achieve their effect by depressing the CNS, particularly the reticular activating system, where they mute incoming stimuli.

5. The ability to mute incoming stimuli gives benzodiazepines a great potential for abuse.

6. Benzodiazepines can cause a physical dependence and produce a withdrawal syndrome. Discontinuance should be tapered gradually.

7. Side effects of the benzodiazepines include drowsiness, fatigue, ataxia, and other peripheral and central effects; however, tolerance to side effects occurs.

8. Benzodiazepines are relatively safe drugs when taken alone but can be deadly if mixed with other CNS depressants (e.g., alcohol).

9. Benzodiazepines that are not dependent upon hepatic oxidizing processes for metabolism are more appropriate for the elderly (e.g., lorazepam [Ativan] and oxazepam [Serax]).

10. Buspirone is a nonbenzodiazepine and has gained extensive usage for the treatment of anxiety. It does not produce the typical benzodiazepine side-effect profile (i.e., CNS depression) and does not have an abuse potential.

11. Buspirone is a relatively safe drug that interacts with few other drugs.

🚩 Study Questions

(Answer key is in the back of the book.)

1. Benzodiazepines are abused because:
   a. They increase inhibitions.
   b. They blur reality.
   c. They can be safely mixed with other drugs, such as alcohol.

2. Benzodiazepines are thought to work by:
   a. Exciting the CNS
   b. Depressing the reticular activating system
   c. Increasing inhibitory feelings

3. Benzodiazepines given alone can usually cause all but one of the following:
   a. Dependence
   b. Withdrawal
   c. Death from overdose
   d. Abuse problems

4. Valium interacts with alcohol to cause:
   a. CNS depression
   b. CNS excitement
   c. An increase in tolerance to alcohol
   d. A depletion of neuronal stores

5. Which of the following benzodiazepines is most often prescribed for elderly patients?
   a. Diazepam (Valium)
   b. Lorazepam (Ativan)
   c. Chlordiazepoxide (Librium)

6. Which of the following antianxiety drugs shows no cross-tolerance with CNS depressants and no withdrawal symptoms?
   a. Diazepam
   b. Buspirone
   c. Oxazepam
   d. Alprazolam

7. The major concern(s) when administering flumazenil (Mazicon) is/are:
   a. It does not speed the metabolism of benzodiazepines.
   b. It has a short duration of action.
   c. The patient may respond and then return to the benzodiazepine-induced state.
   d. All of the above

8. Benzodiazepines have been shown to cause fetal abnormalities in pregnant women who take these drugs.
   a. True
   b. False

9. The drug of choice for obsessive-compulsive disorder is:
   a. Imipramine
   b. Clomipramine
   c. Diazepam
   d. Propranolol

REFERENCES

Ayd FJ: The early history of modern psychopharmacology, *Neuropsychopharmacology* 5(2):71, 1991.

Beeber LS: Treatment of anxiety, *J Psychosoc Nurs Ment Health Serv* 27:42, 1989.

Black DW, et al: A comparison of fluvoxamine, cognitive therapy, and placebo in the treatment of panic disorder, *Arch Gen Psychiatry* 50:44, 1993.

Carey KB: Emerging treatment guidelines for mentally ill chemical abusers, *Hosp Community Psychiatry* 40:341, 1989.

Ciraulo DA, et al: *Drug interactions in psychiatry,* Baltimore, 1989, Williams & Wilkins.

Cohen LS: Psychotropic drug use in pregnancy, *Hosp Community Psychiatry* 40:566, 1989.

Forman L: Medication: reasons and interventions for noncompliance, *J Psychosoc Nurs Mental Health Serv* 31(10): 24, 1993.

Garcia RI, et al: Use of lorazepam for increased anxiety after neuroleptic dose reduction, *Hosp Community Psychiatry* 41:197, 1990.

Glod CA: Xanax: pros and cons, *J Psychosoc Nurs Ment Health Serv* 30(6):36, 1992.

Harvey SC: Hypnotics and sedatives. In Gilman AG, Goodman LS, and Rall TW, editors: *The pharmacological basis of therapeutics,* ed 7, New York, 1985, Macmillan.

Hollister LE: New psychotherapeutic drugs, *J Clin Psychopharmacol* 14(1):50, 1994.

Keltner NL and Folks DG: *Psychotropic drugs,* St. Louis, 1993, Mosby.

Lydiard RB, Roy-Byrne PP, and Ballinger JC: Recent advances in the psychopharmacological treatment of anxiety disorders, *Hosp Community Psychiatry* 39:1157, 1988.

Olin BR: *Drug facts and comparisons,* St Louis, 1996, JB Lippincott.

Rapport DJ and Covington EC: Motor phenomena in benzodiazepine withdrawal, *Hosp Community Psychiatry* 40:1277, 1989.

Shelton RC: Pharmacotherapy of panic disorder, *Hosp Community Psychiatry* 44(8):725, 1993.

Shlafer M: The nurse, pharmacology, and drug therapy: a prototype approach, Redwood City, Calif, 1993, Addison-Wesley.

Smith AR, et al: Trends in psychotropic prescribing practice and general medical patients, *Postgrad Med J* 62:637, 1986.

Watsky EJ and Salzman C: Psychotropic drug interactions, *Hosp Community Psychiatry* 42(3):247, 1991.

UNIT FIVE

Milieu Management

CHAPTER 23

Introduction to Milieu Management

BRUCE P. MERICLE

LEARNING OBJECTIVES

After reading this chapter you should be able to:
- Define and describe the therapeutic milieu.
- Describe the goal of milieu management in the care of psychiatric patients.
- Identify the elements of the therapeutic milieu.
- Discuss several ways in which a therapeutic milieu promotes mental health in patients.

Note to the Student: The context in which nurses practice today is very different from even 10 years ago. In the past most professional nurses practiced in hospitals. Today, and in the professional career that lies ahead for you, you are likely to practice in settings other than the hospital. In psychiatric nursing many patients are cared for in day programs (e.g., nonresidential treatment from 9:00 AM to 3:00 PM Monday through Friday), in clinics, in group homes, or while they live with their families. This chapter will aid your understanding of how we as nurses can construct a therapeutic environment within, as well as outside, the hospital.

Note to the Instructor: This unit, "Milieu Management," is intended to assist you in preparing students who will work in care environments both within and outside the hospital. Emphasis is placed on a changing health care system and how principles of milieu may be applied to the inpatient setting and to a variety of nonhospital settings.

The purpose of a therapeutic environment is to help patients recognize and recover from psychiatric problems that led to their current situation. In a rapidly changing health care system that environment may be the person's home, a day program within his community, or at times a hospital inpatient unit. Regardless of the setting, these persons can best recover from their psychiatric problems when all aspects of the environment are focused on their recovery. In such an environment, there is no downtime. All resources of the environment are harnessed to provide optimal psychiatric care for patients. The terms *therapeutic milieu* and *therapeutic environment* are used to describe such an atmosphere. Providing a therapeutic environment is a fundamental activity of psychiatric nursing (Benfer, 1980; American Nurses Association [ANA], 1994).

Because nurses bear the primary responsibility for shaping the therapeutic environment, it is critical that they understand the importance of milieu management. Nurses may provide around-the-clock care

KEY TERMS

Therapeutic milieu The context in which treatment occurs

Milieu management Purposeful manipulation of the environment to promote a therapeutic atmosphere

Here-and-now focus Assisting patients to understand how their current behaviors influence daily living

Community meeting A meeting that occurs within the therapeutic milieu in which joint problem solving by community members is encouraged

Norm An expected behavior for a given therapeutic setting

Limit setting Holding people to established norms with the intent of assisting them to function more constructively and effectively

Balance The process by which patients are helped to strive for independence while conforming to norms

in a variety of settings. Nurses are the managers of the patient milieu.

To the degree that nurses and others are trained and motivated to deliver care, the patient care climate can consistently reflect the philosophy of care. Conversely, the most promising psychiatric model of therapy cannot overcome a poorly trained and poorly motivated nursing staff. Reread the summary of the seminal article "On Being Sane in Insane Places," which is presented again in Box 23-1 to illustrate this point. No doubt a number of individuals in leadership positions within those facilities believed everything was going well!

Nursing staff members are representatives of and for the model of care. In fact, the true test of the philosophy of care of any facility does not occur during a morning team meeting, but at night, when a single staff member interacts with a single patient. The term *representatives* is used advisedly; in a well-functioning therapeutic environment, the nurses are not really representatives. They are partners in the development and implementation of the philosophy of health care.

Wilmer (1981) labels environments in psychiatric facilities much as a journalist might label political groups, referring to them as *left, right,* and *center.* Wilmer views the first two as distortions of what should be. Environments to the *left* are characterized by permissiveness and an antiprofessional stance. Unit staff members work too hard at identifying with their patients. Identification may take the form of staff members using foul language, male staff members being "hip" by wearing long hair and earrings, and so on. Unit leaders have closed minds to new

approaches, suggesting that their approach is the only path to mental health.

Right-leaning environments tend to follow blindly one theoretical model without flexibility, thus helping the staff to gain comfort in their work environment. Wilmer's most interesting comment is that right-leaning milieus have staffs with high morale amid dismal results. The challenge for psychiatric nurses is to develop a balanced therapeutic environment.

The psychiatric environments in the *center* are characterized by their emphasis on the here-and-now and by their recognition of a need for flexibility.

HISTORICAL OVERVIEW

Concepts related to milieu management were first applied to inpatient settings. It is only recently that those concepts have been utilized in other care settings. The discussion in this chapter will focus on milieu as it applies to hospital inpatient settings.

For many years, custodial care was the norm in inpatient settings. Custodial care does not necessarily mean cruel or neglectful care; rather, it refers to a mind-set in which nursing interventions were focused almost exclusively on meeting safety and physical needs. However, even these basic goals were sometimes not reached. In "better," usually private, institutions, custodial care was provided 23 hours of the day, and then for 1 hour the patient was ushered into the presence of the therapist. Less than 5% of the day was spent in a therapeutic situation.

Box 23-1   On Being Sane in Insane Places

Rosenhan wondered whether the "sane" could be distinguished from the "insane." He selected eight pseudopatients (people who pretended to be mentally ill) and instructed them to attempt to gain admission to public mental hospitals. The task was much easier than anyone had anticipated. Twelve hospitals in five states were used. The pseudopatient group consisted of a graduate student in psychology, three psychologists (including Rosenhan himself), a pediatrician, a psychiatrist, a painter, and a housewife. Three were women and five were men. No one in the hospital knew of the deception.

The pseudopatients were trained to do the following:
1. Call the hospital and make an appointment.
2. Upon arriving at the hospital they were to tell the psychiatrist they had been hearing voices.
3. Upon being asked to describe the voices all were to say they were not sure but did remember the words "empty," "hollow," and "thud."
4. Other than giving this false information and false information about their names, occupations, and employers, they were from that point forward to be truthful and "normal."
5. Immediately upon admission the pseudopatients were instructed to cease simulating abnormal behavior and to behave "normally."
6. When asked how they were doing the pseudopatients were trained to respond "fine" and to inform the staff that they were no longer experiencing problems.

Despite behaving normally, none of the pseudopatients were discovered by the staff. However, about 25% of the other patients made comments about the pseudopatients' "sanity" and a few even guessed that the pseudopatients were doing some kind of undercover work. Rosenhan noted a reluctance by the staff to see mental health in their patients. He stated, "Having once been labeled schizophrenic, there is nothing the pseudopatients can do to overcome the tag." Pseudopatient histories were written to support their diagnosis. In other words, psychiatrists saw problems that had never existed.

The pseudopatients were also asked to write down their observations. At first, elaborate precautions were followed to avoid detection. However, they were soon jotting down observations in front of the staff. The pseudopatients had discovered that no one was paying any attention to them.

Another part of the experiment was to determine how much time was spent with patients. This was difficult to measure so a proxy behavior was substituted: time the nurses spent outside of the nurses' station. Nursing attendants had the highest percentage of time outside the station: 11.3%. Rosenhan found it impossible to measure RN time outside of the nurses' station because it occurred so infrequently. Psychiatrists were even worse. They hid behind closed office doors; at least the patients were able to *see* the nurses. Rosenhan concluded, "Those with the most power have least to do with patients, and those with the least power are most involved with them."

Rosenhan decries the powerlessness and the depersonalization experienced by the pseudopatients. He remembered how he was frequently awakened in the hospital where he was admitted: "Come on you m- - - - - f- - - - - s, out of bed."

The pseudopatients were hospitalized on average for 19 days before they were deemed well enough for discharge. The range of stays was from 7 to 52 days.

From Rosenhan DL: On being sane in insane places, *Science* 179:250, 1973.

It was a paternalistic system in that the staff "knew best" what the patient needed and there were few attempts to "allow" the patient to participate in his or her own care planning.

After World War II, several individuals began to be concerned about this "waste" of potentially therapeutic time. Some recognized that institutionalization could be pathological in and of itself, causing patient apathy, lack of interest, and an unwillingness by some to leave the facility. Stanton and Schwartz (1954) noted the discrepancy between "what could be and what was" in the hospital. They believed a better yield from hospitalization could be realized if therapeutic mileage could be gained from all dimensions of care.

The most notable figure of this time was Maxwell Jones. In 1953, Jones wrote his landmark book, *The Therapeutic Community,* in which he described the benefits of an environment that was therapeutic in and of itself. He proposed that patients become involved in decision making, that group meetings be held, that patients participate in planning ward events, and that patients practice self-regulation.

As milieu therapy evolved, the therapeutic benefits of a multidisciplinary staff in the rehabilitation process were more fully recognized (Gutheil, 1985). Nurses, in particular, assumed more "therapeutic territory" as their importance to the therapeutic environment became apparent. By the early 1960s, professional nurses became full partners in these therapeutic efforts. As noted by Pinsker and Vingiano (1988), nurses relinquished their white uniforms and dressed in street clothes, attempting to form a closer bond with patients. This thinking was based on Maxwell's notion that "we are all just people who need to wear clothes." His idea was mined for its full therapeutic value.

Just as the therapeutic environment was being considered as a legitimate psychiatric modality, other forces converged to direct energies away from milieu therapy. (See Chapter 1 for a more detailed recounting of these events.) Psychopharmacology, concern for patients' rights, and reactions to institutional care culminated in the community mental health movement. These forces worked against a basic underpinning of milieu therapy: hospital care for patients. As Gutheil (1985) pointed out, proponents of psychopharmacology viewed hospitalization as a time when patients could be "held still" long enough to be stabilized on medication. If anything beyond stabilization took place, "well and good," but it was not necessary. Community mental health advocates viewed the inpatient staff as psychiatric evangelists in business to "convert" inpatients to outpatients as fast as possible. However, times are changing. Hospitalization and particularly the effective use of the milieu (therapeutic environment) are again being examined.

The pendulum has begun to swing back toward using the therapeutic milieu as an important treatment modality. Reardon (1993) notes that milieu counselors are of such importance today that they should be specially trained and able to advance through an established career-ladder structure. The Society for Education and Research in Psychiatric-Mental Health Nursing (SERPN), in its 1994 position statement, recommends that psychiatric nurses possess knowledge of the "community as milieu as a therapeutic modality." Home health care agencies are utilizing milieu principles when establishing treatment plans for people who are chronically mentally ill and being cared for at home by family members (Hellig, 1993).

The use of the therapeutic milieu now is being extended to the practice of psychiatric nursing in the community setting. Murray and Baier (1993) describe the use of the principles of milieu therapy in a transitional residential facility for chronically mentally ill homeless persons.

Parrish (1990) argues for providing permanent community housing for the severely mentally ill. She envisions homes in which patients (residents) have full access to a variety of mental health services. Peplau (1995) notes that with the movement of nurses into the community they are increasingly responsible for facilitating the therapeutic environment whether it be in a private family home, group home, or among homeless street people.

THERAPEUTIC MILIEU

Florence Nightingale was the first to recognize nursing's responsibility for creating and controlling patients' milieu (Emrich, 1989). In the inpatient setting, psychiatric nursing has 24-hour responsibility for patient care. No other discipline provides this on-site, around-the-clock care. Patients and nurses alike benefit from the recognition of the value of a therapeutic environment. Patients benefit because the use of many resources, including interpersonal interactions, psychotropic drugs, and the environment, help staff members to maintain a consistent focus on and involvement with the recipients of care, the patients.

Nurses benefit because attention and value are brought to a dimension of psychiatric care that is decidedly nursing. June Mellow (1986), an important figure in psychiatric nursing, has said about the milieu:

Certainly nurses, as the chief inhabitants of its terrain, have not emphasized enough its great therapeutic potential, perhaps because so much of the experimental medium is comprised of what are considered mundane activities associated with women's sphere of work—feeding, bathing, dressing, granting privileges, teaching, comforting, scolding, joking, socializing, counseling. Yet it is the often unstructured, unpredictable flow of these activities, compared with the more structured world of verbal therapy, that can be transposed and shaped into a therapeutic modality.

Kahn and White (1989) noted, "[nursing] staff exert a powerful therapeutic effect through their moment-to-moment interactions with the patient." Mellow calls for nurses to recognize the significance of the environment they, and they alone, manage—the significance of milieu management.

Historically, the term *therapeutic milieu* conveyed a broad conceptual approach in which all aspects of the environment were channeled to provide a therapeutic environment for patients. "At its root is the idea that variables in the interaction between person and environment affect behavior" (Emrich, 1989). The milieu could be therapeutic in and of itself (e.g., "milieu therapy" [Jones, 1953]) and could be developed in many settings.

Therapeutic community, on the other hand, has been considered a concept restricted to the inpatient setting in which a patient-led government establishes and enforces community rules. Over the years, the distinction between therapeutic milieu and therapeutic community has all but disappeared, and the terms are now often used synonymously. Regardless of the term used to describe the context in which milieu principles are used, interventions are successful only when the environment is effectively managed. *Milieu management*, then, is a descriptive term that implies the need for purposeful activity by the nursing staff in order to develop a *therapeutic environment*.

Traditionally, the hospital has been the only setting thought to be appropriate for milieu concerns. Today, however, psychiatric nurses expend therapeutic energies on developing a therapeutic environment in residential programs and in home care management, as well as in the hospital setting. Appropriate management of the environment, regardless of the setting, is an important aspect of patient care.

Clinical Example

South of Birmingham in a rural area of the state is a day treatment program for chronically mentally ill individuals. The day treatment program is housed in a large rustic building where persons with chronic mental disorders attend educational and therapy sessions five days a week during the day. Within easy walking distance are two group homes. Emphasis is placed on developing a therapeutic milieu at both the day treatment center and the group home. Days and evenings are structured by trained staff members.

Another example, Rose (1996) emphasizes the need for continuing critical analysis and further research of the needs of family members in their ever-increasing role as primary caregivers for the mentally ill living at home.

Milieu management is the purposeful use of all interpersonal and environmental forces to enhance mental health. According to Talbot and Miller (1966): "An ideal psychiatric hospital is not merely a sanctuary, a cotton-padded milieu that emphasizes the fragility, the incompetence, the helplessness, the bizarreness of patients. Rather it should reflect a sane society by permitting the optimal use of the intact ego capacities through its social organization, its social supports, and its community values."

THE GOAL OF MILIEU MANAGEMENT

The goal of milieu management, regardless of the care setting, is to organize all interpersonal and environmental forces to develop an atmosphere that facilitates patients' growth, rehabilitation, and restoration of health. The effectiveness of milieu therapy is judged by its effectiveness during every 24-hour period. This suggests that all members of the health care team are responsible for understanding and maintaining the therapeutic environment.

In ineffective milieus there is an overabundance of television watching. Hillbrand, Waite, and Young (1998) describe this as a "default" activity and wonder about the effect of indiscriminate TV watching on patients whose condition renders them vulnerable to its negative effects.

Nurses must be active in the therapeutic environment. Patients will be no more active than the nurses (Kahn and White, 1989). Nurses must be available, flexible, and willing to help patients to develop problem-solving skills and coping mechanisms to deal with problems (Leibenluft and Goldberg, 1987). Gunderson (1978) identified three essential features of the therapeutic environment:

1. Distribution of responsibility and decision making
2. High levels of interaction between patients and staff
3. Clarity of the role and leadership of the program

Milieu management in hospital settings achieves these characteristics by establishing community meetings, activity groups, social skills groups, physical exercise programs, psychoeducational programs, transition groups, and work programs. In addition, the therapeutic community is enhanced by staff groups in which milieu status is reviewed and ongoing training occurs.

In community-based programs, achievement is accomplished also through use of community living groups and time management groups, among others.

ELEMENTS OF THE EFFECTIVE MILIEU

For the milieu to be effectively managed, six environmental elements must be present: safety, structure, norms, limit setting, balance, and environmental modification.

Safety

Safety, or *being safe,* implies freedom from danger or harm. It is an important concern in any therapeutic environment and encompasses freedom from both psychological and physical harm. In the therapeutic environment, the safety of all members of the environment is equally important.

Protection from psychological harm is provided by norms that do not permit undue confrontation of one patient by another, or excessive confrontation of patients by others. Patients may be protected also by restricting visitors, including family members, who are known to disparage patients.

Patients who experience severe anxiety may suffer unnecessarily if staff members do not intervene. Interventions to decrease anxiety and promote a feeling of psychological safety may include giving psychotropic medications, assuring patients that a staff member will stay with them, and providing such patients with a nonstimulating environment.

Freedom from physical harm also is important. Safety is ensured by developing unit norms that do not permit physical violence by any community member. Policies and procedures for control of aggression are necessary. Some institutions use "timeout" rooms (the patient's room or a designated but isolated spot on the unit) to which patients who are acting in a threatening way are directed to go until

they are in control. At times, patients must be physically restrained with leather restraints or secluded in a seclusion room until they are more in control. Whenever patients are restrained or secluded, they must be told that they are not being punished, but rather that external controls are being used until they are able to regain control. Consider the following clinical problem.

CLINICAL EXAMPLE

In response to hearing voices, a patient named Tim hits one of the staff nurses. Tim agrees to walk to the seclusion room. At that time, he is given an intramuscular (IM) dose of an ordered medication. Tim is told that the medication is to help him relax, and that he will be kept in seclusion until he indicates, and staff members agree, that he can control his behavior. A staff member is assigned to stay with Tim in order to reaffirm that he is not being punished, but rather that the staff is concerned that he and others on the unit remain safe.

It should be noted by the student that although the above scenario is realistic, giving the prn medication after the hitting incident occurred is somewhat in opposition to the principles presented in Chapter 14. The conceptualization of aggression presented there (the assault cycle) suggests the time to medicate is during the escalation phase—not after the crisis has occurred.

Structure

Structure can be identified as the physical environment, the regulations, and the daily schedule of classes and groups (Emrich, 1989). It is provided by establishing community meetings, activity groups, social skills groups, living skills groups, street skills groups, self-esteem groups, physical exercise programs, psychoeducational programs, transition groups, and work programs. Groups, both formal and informal, in which patients share problems and triumphs are also part of the therapeutic environment. Structure denotes the design of the unit. Space, areas for socializing, and areas for privacy are required. Telephones must be available, and visiting rooms appropriate. Because seclusion rooms often are necessary, their design, location, and furnishings must maintain both safety and dignity. Furnishings, the color of the walls, and so on all communicate facility philosophy to the patients, their families, and the staff. While reviewing "structure" in Chapter 24, the reader should ask: "What is it about a given dimension of unit structure that makes it therapeutic?"

Norms

Norms are those expectations of behavior that pervade the setting. They are intended to promote community living through behaviors that are socially acceptable. For instance, a common norm is that violent behavior is not permitted. A norm of nonviolence provides for physical and emotional security. The following clinical example illustrates how a norm of nonviolence would be implemented.

CLINICAL EXAMPLE

John is angry with another patient and is threatening him with bodily harm. The nurse intervenes by firmly directing John to go to his room. The nurse stays with John and encourages him to talk about what he is feeling rather than to act on his feelings.

"Talking a patient down" avoids potentially violent encounters and provides patients with an opportunity to examine what generated the anger and how they might more effectively resolve the issue (Stevenson, 1991).

Other norms focus on the level of personal control. For example, patients may be required to take psychotropic drugs. However, the time at which they take the medication may be negotiable. Other norms focus on openness, giving and receiving feedback, respect for the patient, privacy, acceptance, independence, and individual responsibility. All these norms attempt to build a climate of universality or shared experience.

Limit Setting

Limit setting is important in inpatient settings as well as other settings and is related to norms. Limits should be set on acting-out behavior, such as self-destructive acts, physical aggressiveness, lack of compliance, use

of alcohol or illicit drugs, use of over-the-counter drugs, and elopement (running away). If patients are likely to engage in any of these behaviors, it is important to discuss the behavior with the patient in an anticipatory fashion, rather than to wait until after the fact (Leibenluft and Goldberg, 1987).

■ Critical Thinking Question

In what ways are the concepts of *norms* and *limit setting* similar? In what ways are they different?

CLINICAL EXAMPLE

Mary, who is attending a partial hospital day program, is very anxious and approaches the nurses' station every 10 minutes, asking to talk with a staff member. Staff members are concerned that they may be encouraging Mary to be too dependent by talking with her each time she approaches. The staff jointly decides to set limits on Mary by telling her that a staff member will meet with her once every 4 hours for a 15-minute period. This encourages the patient to limit her demands on others, and also to meet some of her own needs between the times she meets with a staff member.

Balance

Balance is also an important concept, but it is more difficult to describe and does not lend itself to a concrete list of rules. Perhaps more than any other dimension of milieu management, balance represents the "art" of nursing. Balance is the process of gradually allowing independent behaviors in a dependent situation. Independence is gained in increments because too much independence may overwhelm the patient. Examples best illustrate this point.

In the case of a self-destructive patient, the nurse attempts to balance the patient's (and the nurse's) need for safety (a dependency-creating approach) with the patient's need for self-control and independence. A seemingly different example is patients who are very religious. The nurse may have to balance patients' rights to religious expression with the need for treatment. It is somewhat common for patients to refuse medication on religious grounds, even though they are frankly psychotic. Is this refusal a true representation of religious beliefs, or is it a psychotic manifestation?

Balance is an important concept because it forces the nurse to articulate the opposing forces that are at work. The skillful use of balance comes with an understanding of ethical concerns, legal issues, and psychopathology.

■ Critical Thinking Question

In this chapter, balance is defined as "... the process of gradually allowing independent behavior in a dependent situation." What is meant by a "dependent situation"?

Environmental Modification

Through *environmental modification,* the nurse can facilitate the development of a therapeutic environment and communicate patients' worth. Physical arrangement, safety issues, and orientation features, when addressed, can create an atmosphere in which patients are enabled to maximize their strengths. Ongoing review of environmental norms, rules, and regulations is also an important aspect of milieu modification. Flexibility in maintaining a therapeutic environment is important.

CLINICAL EXAMPLE

A residence norm requires that the television is turned off at 10:00 PM on weeknights. During a morning community meeting, several residents of the home indicate that a special television program, of interest to patients, is scheduled to air from 10:00 PM until midnight. A joint staff-resident decision is made to permit the residents to watch this special show. Temporarily modifying the norm promotes autonomy and allows for individuality, while keeping the basic structure intact.

Together, safety, structure, norms, limit setting, balance, and environmental modification are tools the psychiatric nurse uses to manage the milieu. In an environment where all resources are used, every verbal interaction becomes significant because it is part of a larger process developed to facilitate mental health and personal growth. Each individual re-

action is important but finds even greater meaning within the construct of psychotherapeutic management in the well-managed milieu.

ROLES OF THE PSYCHOTHERAPEUTIC MANAGER

Milieu management requires nurses to serve in multiple roles. Nurses work with patients individually, lead groups, participate in community meetings, coordinate medical care (with physicians), dispense routine medications and make decisions concerning prn medications, make discharge arrangements, and work with families in a variety of health care settings. In addition, they provide leadership in interdisciplinary team meetings and are the professionals who most often implement team decisions.

Teaching is also an important role for nurses involved in the therapeutic milieu. Medication compliance is a major factor in preventing recidivism and often in maintaining a patient in the community. Nurses are actively engaged in teaching patients and their families about the therapeutic use of medications, as well as about the possible side effects.

As psychiatric patients have moved into the community settings over the past several decades, nurses oftentimes are the primary source of information and support for families and other caregivers. These individuals need nurses to provide guidance and education for enhancing the therapeutic effectiveness of the patients' environments.

■ Critical Thinking Question

A 16-year-old boy has been admitted to the adolescent unit of a psychiatric hospital because of recent fighting at school and threatening his parents at home. How do you think the use of a therapeutic milieu as a treatment approach might assist this boy to change his behaviors?

◆ Key Concepts

1. Milieu management is the purposeful use of all interpersonal and environmental forces to enhance the mental health of psychiatric patients through the development of a therapeutic environment.

2. When nursing has 24-hour accountability for patient care, nurses have the major responsibility for shaping the therapeutic environment.

3. Historically, nurses provided only custodial care, but after World War II, Maxwell Jones (1953) and others conceptualized an environment in which all aspects of the psychiatric patient's day would be used to promote mental health.

4. Nurses gained more influence over the care of patients as the result of this emphasis on the environment. However, just as milieu therapy was gaining acceptance as a viable treatment form, other forces converged and changed the locus of psychiatric treatment from a therapeutic inpatient setting to a community mental health setting.

5. Hospitalization and the effective use of milieu management currently are being reconsidered as psychiatric nursing leaders look for more effective ways to treat persons with mental disorders.

6. The goal of milieu management is to organize all interpersonal and environmental forces to develop an atmosphere that is conducive to patients' growth, rehabilitation, and restoration.

7. Three essential features of the therapeutic environment are distribution of responsibility and decision making, high levels of interaction between patients and staff, and clarity of the role and leadership of the program.

8. The effectively managed milieu is composed of six elements: (1) safety, (2) structure, (3) norms, (4) limit setting, (5) balance, and (6) environmental modification.

9. Concepts of managed milieu are increasingly being applied to care settings other than inpatient units.

▼ Study Questions

(Answer key is in the back of the book.)

1. Milieu management is the purposeful use of all interpersonal and environmental forces to enhance mental health.
   a. True
   b. False

2. Twenty-four-hour care for psychiatric patients is traditionally provided by:
   a. Nurses
   b. Psychiatrists
   c. Psychologists
   d. Social workers

3. When psychotropic drugs alone are used to treat patients, this is considered to be:
   a. Custodial care
   b. Milieu management
   c. Psychotherapeutic management
   d. Routine nursing care

4. The first professional to conceptualize the need for all aspects of the patient's environment to be therapeutic was:
   a. Sigmund Freud
   b. Maxwell Jones
   c. Emil Kraepelin
   d. Hildegard Peplau

5. Concepts borrowed from inpatient milieu management settings now are being applied in:
   a. Home-care settings
   b. Outpatient mental health clinics
   c. Shelters for the homeless
   d. Psychiatric crisis centers
   e. All of the above

6. The primary purpose of limit setting is to communicate to patients that:
   a. Behavior must conform to established norms
   b. Inappropriate behavior will be punished
   c. Their behavior is wrong
   d. The nurse is in charge

REFERENCES

American Nurses Association, Council on Psychiatric and Mental Health Nursing: *Statement on psychiatric mental health clinical nursing practice,* Washington, 1994, The Association.

Assey JL: The suicide prevention contract, *Perspect Psychiatr Care* 23(3):99, 1985.

Beckmann R and Baier M: Use of therapeutic milieu in a community setting, *J Psychosoc Nurs Ment Health Serv* 31:10, 1993.

Benfer B: Defining the role and function of the psychiatric nurse as a member of the team, *Perspect Psychiatr Care* 18:166, 1980.

Emrich K: Helping or hurting? Interacting in the psychiatric milieu, *J Psychosoc Nurs Ment Health Serv* 27:26, 1989.

Gunderson JG: Defining the therapeutic processes in psychiatric milieus, *Psychiatry* 41:327, 1978.

Gutheil T: The therapeutic milieu: changing themes and theories, *Hosp Community Psychiatry* 36:1279, 1985.

Hellig K: Psychiatric home care nursing: managing patients in the community setting, *J Psychosoc Nurs Ment Health Serv* 31(12):21, 1993.

Hillbrand M, Waite BM, Young JL: Restricting TV access by forensic patients, *Psychiatric Services* 49(1):107, 1998.

Jones M: *The therapeutic community,* New York, 1953, Basic Books.

Kahn EM and White EM: Adapting milieu approaches to acute inpatient care for schizophrenia patients, *Hosp Community Psychiatry* 40:609, 1989.

Keltner NL: Psychotherapeutic management: a model for nursing practice, *Perspect Psychiatr Care* 23:125, 1985.

Leibenluft E and Goldberg RL: Guidelines for short-term inpatient psychotherapy, *Hosp Community Psychiatry* 38:38, 1987.

Mellow J: A personal perspective of nursing therapy, *Hosp Community Psychiatry* 37:182, 1986.

Murray RB and Baier M: Use of therapeutic milieu in a community setting, *J Psychosoc Nurs Ment Health Serv* 31(10):11, 1993.

Parrish J: Supported housing: A critical component of effective community support, *Psychosoc Rehabil J* 11(4):9, 1990.

Peplau HE: Some unresolved issues in the era of biopsychosocial nursing, *J Am Psychiatr Nurses Assoc* 1(3):92, 1995.

Pinsker H and Vingiano W: A study of whether uniforms help patients recognize nurses, *Hosp Community Psychiatry* 39:78, 1988.

Reardon J: A clinical ladder for milieu counselors, *J Psychosoc Nurs Ment Health Serv* 31:1, 1993.

Rose LE: Families of psychiatric patients: a critical review and future research directions, *Arch Psychiatr Nurs* 10(2):67, 1996.

Society for Education and Research in Psychiatric-Mental Health Nursing (SERPN): *Position statement*, 1994.

Stanton A and Schwartz M: *The mental hospital*, New York, 1954, Basic Books.

Stevenson S: Heading off violence with verbal de-escalation, *J Psychosoc Nurs Ment Health Serv* 29:9, 1991.

Talbot E and Miller SC: The struggle to create a sane society in the psychiatric hospital, *Psychiatry* 29:165, 1966.

Walsh S: Orientation intervention for parents of adolescents after psychiatric hospitalization, *J Psychosoc Nurs Ment Health Serv* 31:7, 1993.

Wilmer HA: Defining and understanding the therapeutic community, *Hosp Community Psychiatry* 32:95, 1981.

CHAPTER 24

Developing the Therapeutic Environment

BRUCE P. MERICLE

LEARNING OBJECTIVES

After reading this chapter you should be able to:

- Understand the implications of the Joint Commission on Accreditation of Healthcare Organizations (JCAHO) guidelines for a therapeutic environment.
- Identify major safety issues related to patient care.
- Describe the various approaches to developing structure.
- Describe the various dimensions of norms.

- Describe common themes of limit setting within and outside the hospital.
- Understand the competing issues involved in balance.
- Identify important measures in environmental modification.
- Describe the use of milieu principles in the community.

Over 40 years ago, Maxwell Jones (1953), the "father" of milieu therapy, observed the remarkable benefits of structuring the environment of a psychiatric unit. He defined treatment as the normal interactions of healthy community life where everyone has a role to play (Murray and Baier, 1993). Nursing has the unique expertise required to develop the therapeutic environment, and has the number of professionals to do so. According to the U.S. Department of Health and Human Services (1992), there are 66,142 psychiatric registered nurses employed in inpatient hospital settings (cited in

Thompson and Strand, 1994). With a workforce of this size, psychiatric nursing has considerable influence on the milieu.

More recently, nurses are in a position to influence the environment in a variety of community-based psychiatric settings. Peplau (1995) notes that community-based care was first instituted with the passage of the 1963 Community Mental Health Centers Act, and today nurses regularly care for psychiatric patients and their families within the home setting. Psychiatric home care has evolved as part of ever-increasing trends toward home care.

KEY TERMS

Feedback   Articulation of one's perception of what another person has said or meant; this process requires at least two people

Milieu therapy   The use of any care environment to promote optimum functioning of a group or an individual

Openness   An atmosphere in which people are free to express their thoughts and feelings without fear of ridicule or censure

Psychoeducation   A strategy of teaching patients and families about disorders, treatments, coping techniques, and resources based on the observation that people can be better participants in their own care if knowledge deficits are removed.

In addition to the obvious investment of time, nursing has an investment in developing the "healthy community life" described by Jones. Kyes and Hofling (1974) astutely observed, "The interpersonal environment in which a patient lives may be therapeutic or non-therapeutic depending almost entirely on the interest and ability of the [nursing] staff." Because patients are incapable of *not* interacting with their environment, the nurse has the potential to shape the environment to cause that inevitable interaction to be therapeutic.

In Chapter 23, milieu building was presented as a process of establishing safety, structure, norms, limit setting, balance, and environmental modification. These, in turn, are derived from practice philosophy and objectives. Those concepts are developed in this chapter.

Standards for management of the environment of care are outlined and described in detail in the JCAHO Comprehensive Manual for Hospitals (JCAHO, 1997). The goal of management of the environment is "to provide a safe, functional, and effective environment for patients, staff members, and other individuals in the hospital." These standards apply also to noninpatient environments, including outpatient clinics and counseling centers.

The environment of care standards (see Box 24-1) requires that facilities be designed and constructed to ensure that the environment is safe and accessible and that the facility is routinely evaluated for ongo-

Box 24-1   JCAHO Environment of Care Standards

Safety

According to JCAHO, environmental safety is attained through:

- Ongoing assessment and maintenance of all equipment
- Hazard surveillance
- Reporting and investigation of safety issues
- Monitoring of safety management techniques and procedures
- Orientation programs that address safety issues

Security

Security of all people, including patients, staff, and visitors, is assured through policies and procedures that prevent harm. A health care facility ensures the security of all people through:

- Mechanisms for addressing security issues
- Provision of appropriate identification for all staff, patients, and visitors
- Security orientation programs
- Mechanisms for handling emergencies
- Mechanisms for interacting with the media

Social Environment

Social environment refers to those attributes of a therapeutic milieu that enhance recognition of patients as unique individuals. The social environment must provide:

- Space for storage of grooming and hygiene articles
- Closet and drawer space for personal property
- Clothing that is suitable for clinical conditions

Physical Setting

The physical setting must provide:

- Adequate privacy to insure respect for patients
- Door locks consistent with program goals
- Availability of telephones that allow for private conversations
- Sleeping rooms with doors for privacy unless clinically contraindicated
- Furnishing suitable to the population served
- Access to the outdoors unless contraindicated for therapeutic reasons

---

ing effectiveness of providing care. Additionally the facility must establish a social environment that supports its basic philosophy, and finally, it must establish and enforce a nonsmoking policy throughout the institution.

SAFETY

Safety overlaps with all dimensions of the therapeutic milieu, but is discussed separately for emphasis. For example, bedrooms must be assigned so that privacy is protected and safety is ensured (a balance issue). For this reason, many units have doors with small windows. This allows the nurse to look in, but broadly protects patients' privacy. The nurse can observe for any difficulties or self-injurious behavior while essentially maintaining patients' modesty.

It can be argued that, without proper regard for safety, little else of what nurses do makes a difference. For example, no matter how therapeutic a unit might be, if safety needs are not met and patients are hurt, the unit will lose creditability in the community. The example of bedroom privacy is quite helpful here. To respect a patient's privacy is good, but to be unobservant to the point that self-destructive behavior is allowed is negligent.

Once a patient is discharged from the hospital to a community setting, safety takes on different characteristics. Nurses must make ongoing assessments to determine that patients are capable of meeting their own need for safety. For example, a patient preoccupied with internal stimuli might be at risk for walking into traffic when leaving a day program. He or she therefore may need to be escorted home to his or her family. Striking a balance between promoting patient independence and providing for patient safety requires skilled observation of patient behaviors when patients are cared for in the community.

STRUCTURE

Structure is the framework around which the therapeutic community, therapeutic milieu, or therapeutic environment revolves and from which it takes direction. Although the concept of structure is most often applied to inpatient units, it is also applicable in other situations.

The goal is not to make a perfect environment, but to develop a nurturing setting that can contain and soothe aggression, frustration, deprivation, disappointment, and loss (Kahn and White, 1989). If all resources in the patient's environment are to be used to achieve this goal, a strategy or structure must be developed to use those resources therapeutically. To enhance the therapeutic environment and to add structure and direction to the treatment program, the psychiatric nurse and other treatment team members often utilize community meetings, activity groups, social skills groups, living skills groups, street skills groups, physical exercise programs, and psychoeducational programs for inpatients.

In an era of managed care when patients are hospitalized only briefly, many of these groups are continued outside the hospital. Of particular importance are groups that focus on living in the community, prevention of relapse, and monitoring of responses to psychopharmacologic agents. McPherson (1996) describes the importance of obtaining an accurate medication history as one aspect of home health care.

Community Meetings

Democratization, reality confrontation, emphasis on social skills learning, and a sense of group cohesion or community are fundamental themes of a therapeutic environment (Murray and Baier, 1993). The community meeting is a group commonly found in settings with a therapeutic environment. The community is a large group, typically consisting of all patients, staff, and students in the treatment setting. It incorporates both small-group dynamics and large-group characteristics. The community meeting can be led by a staff of patients who serve as officers (patients' government) or by the treatment staff. During community meetings, new patients are welcomed, milieu rules are reviewed, patients who serve as government leaders (if appropriate) are identified, staff members are identified, and general announcements are made about the day's activities. The community meeting serves as a forum for patients to voice their opinions of the environment's efficacy, to receive feedback from staff and other patients, and to initiate discussions of community or individual concerns.

For patients newly admitted to a program or for disturbed patients, this businesslike atmosphere may seem threatening; for example, a new patient says, "These people act like 'business as usual,' and my life is coming apart. This is crazy!" But the dominant opposite theme has a more lasting impact; for example, "People with problems are not acting 'crazy.' They are influencing the treatment setting. They are rational." The latter message comforts patients and is conducive to Jones's (1953) hope for "normal interactions of a healthy community where everyone has a role to play." It also encourages patients on several levels and communicates the ability to get on with the business of life.

Community meetings also can be used to plan activities such as program picnics or social gatherings. Patients' assignments, such as housekeeping chores, can be discussed, assigned, or evaluated. Topics such as preparing for life outside the hospital and gaining insight into the reason for hospitalization are appropriate for the community meeting in the hospital (Arons, 1982). Living life in the community is an appropriate topic for noninpatient meetings. Finally, the community meeting provides a forum for exploring the problems of community living. Conflicts between patients or between patients and staff are frequent concerns. Common patient-patient conflicts are over the control of the television, generational issues (e.g., the radio is played too loudly, type of music), and personal hygiene (e.g., someone is not bathing regularly).

Patient-staff conflicts are more delicate, but in the effective community meeting they can be handled skillfully. Common conflicts between patients and staff include issues related to how staff act or fail to act with patients. *Balance,* a concept to be discussed later, is required. Nurses must balance the need to respond to patients' concerns (and all the therapeutic advantages of doing so) with the need to support staff members. Community meetings are not forums for discussing individual treatment needs of patients. The skilled group leader will direct patients to discuss personal issues with an appropriate staff person following the community meeting.

Constitution

A community constitution is a written document that provides the basis for the therapeutic community. The document presents definitions, objectives, meetings, responsibilities of patients who are elected as officers, officer approval or removal procedures, and community response to infractions.

It is a formalized document and not used in all milieu environments.

Step System

A *step system* is a process by which inpatients gain privileges and responsibilities. New patients and acutely disturbed patients in the hospital are designated as "unit status," the most restrictive level. Through various efforts individual patients can earn privileges and responsibilities leading to discharge status. A step system serves to motivate patients and provides content for community meetings. In recent years legislation has reduced the number of privileges that can be withheld and step programs have lost some of their therapeutic appeal. The particulars of this system and even the terminology vary from program to program.

Token Systems

Some inpatient units and partial hospitalization programs use a token system for rewarding patients when they behave in a predetermined acceptable manner. When a patient complies, he or she receives tokens with which items may be purchased at a hospital store. This system is a variant of milieu and is usually reserved for treatment of the more chronically ill patients. Although this is often criticized as an ineffective treatment approach, Corrigan (1995) argues that when administered properly it can be a very effective treatment for this population. For a token system to be helpful, target goals must be clearly identified, target contingencies must be established, and rules for exchange of tokens must be spelled out.

Activity Groups

There are many kinds of activity (remotivation) groups. Nurses may direct these groups, or the groups may be directed by occupational, recreational, or music therapists. The emphasis is on activity. The therapeutic payoff comes from the sense of accomplishment patients achieve by making an item (e.g., a wallet or a belt), the distraction from internal processes, and the socialization experience. As patients focus on matters outside themselves, fewer energies are used in self-defeating, morbid thinking. Structured socialization in a nonthreatening environment can be beneficial to many psychiatric patients.

Social Skills Groups

Social skills groups, as might be expected, represent efforts to help psychiatric patients who are deficient in social skills to learn, practice, and develop them. Skills training might focus on appropriate dress, grooming, or table manners. More advanced efforts address appropriate social and interpersonal verbal skills; for example, meeting new people, initiating conversations, and interviewing for a job. Some persons may tell more about themselves than anyone needs or wants to know within minutes of meeting someone, for example. Such behavior tends to be self-defeating.

Practical living skills can be incorporated into the social skills group. Paying bills, shopping for groceries, cleaning house, and returning an item of purchase are important skills both practically and socially.

Approaches to social skills training

Group sessions need to be structured, with each skill explained simply and demonstrated by the nurse leader. An opportunity for role-playing is essential to learning. Plante (1989) lists 13 role-playing scenarios:

1. Starting a conversation
2. Keeping a conversation going
3. Ending a conversation
4. How to say "no"
5. Asking a favor
6. Giving and receiving compliments graciously
7. Making introductions
8. Interviewing for a job
9. Coping with shyness
10. Telling a joke
11. Developing listening skills
12. Developing nonverbal social skills
13. Asking someone for a date

The opportunity to try out new skills and make mistakes in a safe environment is crucial to learning. Each attempt made by the patients to practice a particular behavior or skill must be acknowledged and praised during and outside the group session. Feedback helps patients to assess their social skills development. Specific skills may need to be taught and demonstrated step-by-step. For example, verbal skills and nonverbal behaviors may be taught and practiced separately, then combined after patients have learned both components.

Many patients living in long-term facilities suffer symptoms associated with clinical depression. Social isolation often exaggerates those symptoms. Morse and Intrieri (1997) propose the use of group inter-action between patients as a means for fostering psychosocial well-being in this population. Interestingly, the authors noted that nonconfused residents sometimes were effective in reorienting a confused resident.

Living Skills Groups

Living skills are related to social skills but are distinct enough to warrant separate mention. An example of this type of group is provided by the West Los Angeles Veterans Affairs Medical Center (VAMC). The hospital staff has developed a training program that covers the following topics for severely mentally ill patients to help them in daily life (VAMC, 1993):

Medication self-management
Symptom self-management
Recreation for leisure
Grooming and self-care
Money management
Finding employment
Food preparation
Personal effectiveness

Street Skills Group

Just as living skills differ from social skills, street skills differ from mainstream living skills. Corrigan and Holmes (1994) emphasize what most people know intuitively: for many patients who will return to urban streets, concentrating on social and living skills is not practical. These patients need to be "street smart." Clinicians may not be street smart themselves nor familiar with the hazards facing the patients they propose to teach about survival. Nonetheless by recognizing this need, efforts to prepare patients can be discussed.

Physical Exercise Groups

Physical health and mental health are linked. As patients become withdrawn, their motivation to exercise decreases. Exercise groups counter this tendency to a degree. If exercise were the key to mental health, however, everyone would want to be a marathon runner. So, even though there is not a direct correlation between exercise and mental health, a certain level of fitness enhances a sense of mental well-being. Physical exercise can also distract patients from stressful thoughts; that is, it takes their minds off themselves. Exercise can provide a bene-fit for psychiatric patients similar to the benefit de-rived by businesspeople who play racquetball during their lunch hours: it provides a distracting physical activity.

Benefits from exercise help all ages. For example, many geropsychiatric patients are being encouraged to participate in exercise groups as a means for im-proving oxygenation to the brain and for promoting social interaction.

Psychoeducational Programs

The term *psychoeducational* refers to teaching people psychological knowledge or skills (Maynard, 1993). Accumulating evidence suggests that such educa-tion accelerates change in the appropriate direction (Dinkmeyer, 1991). Teaching patients has been a focus for some time, but the concept of psychoedu-cation has emerged only recently in the literature because many families feel burdened since the changing health care scene now requires them to ac-cept significant responsibility for the care of men-tally ill family members (e.g., individuals with chronic schizophrenia). Psychoeducational strategies are particularly timely. Future research directions must include looking for ways to provide effective support to the families through such psychoeduca-tional interventions.

Glynn, Pugh, and Rose (1990) found that fam-ilies want information about their family mem-ber's illness. Common themes in psychoeduca-tional groups include the discussion of both physical and psychosocial symptoms and how those symp-toms affect home life, work life, and social life. Theories of etiology—biological, psychosocial, and developmental—are discussed in understandable lan-guage. Treatment approaches, including pharmaco-logical and psychological therapies, are reviewed as well. Side effects of medication are discussed can-didly, and patients are encouraged to share their own experiences. A specific "curriculum" for a group of women with depression is provided in Box 24-2 as an example of the content covered in a targeted psy-choeducational program (Maynard, 1993).

Psychoeducational efforts are based on empirical evidence that understanding mental illness helps patients and their families to cope better with the illness (Dinkmeyer, 1991; Lamb, 1976; Leff, et al, 1982). Psychoeducational programs occasionally

---

> ### Box 24-2 Psychoeducational Issues for Working with Women Who Are Depressed
>
> Depression
> Relationship of Thoughts to Depression
> Role of Social Factors in Depression
> Goal Setting
> Self-Esteem
> Understanding Family of Origin
> Assertiveness
> Stress Management
> Caring for the Body

Modified from Maynard C: A psychoeducational approach to de-pression in women, *J Psychosoc Nurs Ment Health Serv* 31(12):9, 1993.

---

have taken a more rudimentary form. Psychiatric pa-tients who have academic problems with basic arith-metic and reading are taught those skills. Although "three Rs" education is not true psychoeducation, it can benefit patients in a number of ways.

Transition Groups

Newly hospitalized psychiatric patients experience both the crisis of the personal problems that brought them into the hospital, and the crisis of being hos-pitalized. Transition programs can both ease new pa-tients into the unit structure and facilitate successful outpatient treatment.

Work Groups

Work is an adult activity that reinforces a sense of well-being, but many psychiatric patients have expe-rienced one work-related setback after another. In fact, compared to the general population (approxi-mately 5% unemployment), the severely mentally ill are disproportionately unemployed (approximately 85%) (Allen, et al, 1994). Further, unemployment is positively correlated to drug abuse (Bickel, 1994), a significant problem among those with mental disor-ders. Work groups can focus on the social skills needed to gain employment, on work-defeating be-haviors, and on actual work skills (Barter, Queirolo, and Ekstrom, 1984).

Skills related to gaining employment

Many psychiatric patients lack the basic prerequisites even to be considered as candidates for a job. Arriving at work on time, being presentable, and having a history of reliability are basic to the job-seeking process. Group work, including role-playing and videotaping, are helpful approaches to reinforce social competencies.

Work-defeating behaviors

Poor work habits, low self-confidence, lack of motivation, and a negative attitude toward work contribute to keeping psychiatric patients from gaining employment. In addition, some persons have few tangible skills to offer an employer.

Developing work skills

A meaningful work group activity focuses on the development of basic work skills. Orientation to the expectations of the workplace, sharing positive work experiences, tips on getting along with coworkers, and job application and interviewing skills are all helpful if patients anticipate returning to the workplace.

Nursing Students and Group Work

There is less and less reliance on long-term one-on-one relationships with patients. The realities of health care delivery require the use of groups as a means for both assessing patients and responding to their needs. Students enrolled in a psychiatric mental health nursing course can benefit from forming and conducting group experiences. Social skills, exercise, activity and psychoeducational groups are but some of the groups students can conduct as part of their learning experience.

NORMS

Norms can be defined as expectations or as climate. Norms of an inpatient psychiatric unit are listed in Box 24-3. Norms are related to rules and limit setting, but are more abstract.

Norms permeate the atmosphere of the therapeutic environment. To illustrate, two examples are used.

1. First, consider two persons in the same position and work setting who differ in their ex-

pectations of others. One expects to be treated with respect; the other does not expect such treatment. It is not uncommon for each to be treated as they expect to be treated.

2. The second illustration is closer to the topic of psychotherapeutic management. Two psychiatric units may be different in the level of assaultive behavior they experience; yet both, as psychiatric units, seek to eliminate these aggressive behaviors. The difference may be the norms manifested by the unit staff. Norms of nonviolence, physical and emotional security, personal control, openness, giving and receiving feedback, respect for the individual, privacy, acceptance, independence, and individual responsibility build a climate conducive to growth and mental health.

Nonviolence

Interestingly, as large state hospitals have downsized, instances of assaults on staff members have increased (Snyder, 1994). Therefore, it is crucial for the environment to convey a message of nonviolence. A norm of nonviolence means simply that violence is neither expected nor accepted in the environment. Staff members are trained to defuse potentially violent situations and do not let their own need "not to back down" obstruct the therapeutic goal. Levy and Hartocollis (1976) over 20 years ago found that psychiatric units with all-female staff experienced less assaultive behavior than units staffed by both male and female personnel. These researchers suggested

---

Box 24-3 Unit Norms on an Inpatient Psychiatric Unit

Acceptance
Feedback
Independence
Individual responsibility
Nonviolence
Openness
Personal control
Physical and emotional security
Privacy
Respect for the individual

that male staff members allowed their "male egos" to push situations to a crisis.

Physical and Emotional Security

The psychiatric unit should be a safe place, physically and emotionally. Physical safety relates to the norm of nonviolence previously addressed and to the safe administration of medications and treatments (e.g., electroconvulsive therapy). Emotional safety addresses patients' needs to feel accepted as they are. Many experienced psychiatric nurses can attest to the fact that disturbed patients sometimes calm down almost immediately after admission. This phenomenon is related to the asylum or sanctuary concept mentioned in Chapter 1. The fact that new patients know they are emotionally safe is tranquilizing. The freedom to be ill is therapeutic.

Personal Control

The norm of personal control underscores the human need to make decisions about the self. To the degree persons make responsible decisions about themselves, they are moving toward responsible behavior. In the inpatient environment, many daily decisions come under the discretionary control of others (e.g., when to smoke, what to wear, and times for telephone use). As staff members are able to relinquish control, patients are allowed to gain more control over their lives. Menu choices are a good example of personal control that can be emphasized. Even actively psychotic persons can be helped to make these basic decisions. For others, control over medications may be advisable (e.g., dosage schedule). The norm of personal control facilitates maturity and responsibility and defuses remnants of a custodial mentality.

Openness

Openness means an atmosphere in which a free exchange of thoughts and feelings can occur without fear of mockery or retaliation. Feelings and thoughts need not be guarded because of the fear of emotional blackmail. However, an overemphasis on self-disclosure can lead to regressive outpouring of psychotic material that is destructive to patients. The nurse should monitor a *balanced* approach to openness.

Feedback

The process by which one person shares a perception of what another person has meant, or how another person has affected other people, is called *feedback*. Feedback enables people to better understand how they are perceived by others. It is exciting but risky. As patients are able to "hear and respond," they move toward responsible adult behaviors.

Respect for the Individual

Respect is crucial. Without respect, the environment mocks the individual. Even great clinical skill, in the absence of respect, is not adequate for psychiatric nursing. It is a form of elitism to provide care while not respecting the individual.

Privacy

Privacy is a measure of status. The poor, for example, often live some very private moments out in the public—domestic fights and relaxation (sitting outside on a busy street to "get some privacy"). Providing privacy for a patient is also a way of bolstering self-esteem. Privacy on the psychiatric unit conveys respect for human dignity. Knocking before entering a room says one thing to a patient; opening a door without knocking says another.

Acceptance

Acceptance means the ability of the nurse to start in the same place as the individual psychiatric patient. Examples of acceptance are not expecting an anxious person to attend to details when he cannot and not expecting a person with akathisia to sit still. Acceptance of the individual recognizes these less-than-ideal states. The therapeutic tasks in the above examples are to facilitate a decrease in anxiety and to administer prn benztropine for akathisia.

Independence

Independence is related to personal control, but is more far-reaching. Psychiatric treatment facilities foster dependent behaviors. From telling patients when to eat and sleep (in the hospital) to telling them how to be healthy (all settings), these facilities, by definition, create dependency. As independent actions and thinking can be reinforced and supported, patients can begin to test their ideas. Independence is another mark of responsible adult behavior.

Individual Responsibility

In the effective therapeutic environment, patients are given responsibilities and are held accountable for fulfilling them. The step and token systems mentioned under "Structure" usually work toward responsibility. As patients accept and handle greater responsibilities, they move upward through the step system.

These norms or expectations enhance the living environment of psychiatric patients. The nursing staff must embrace these values in order for the norms to permeate the unit. The development and implementation of these norms are a major nursing responsibility.

■ Critical Thinking Question

What are the advantages of openness and feedback on a psychiatric unit? Can you think of any drawbacks? Are the nurses "open" on the unit where you have clinicals?

LIMIT SETTING

Limit setting is the art of clearly identifying acceptable and unacceptable behaviors. Although there is a certain amount of conceptual overlap with structure and norms, limit setting is distinct and warrants special mention. Limits should be identified clearly and early to patients who are prone to "test the system." Self-destructive acts, acts of physical aggression (including offensive language and stealing), noncompliance with treatment plans, use of alcohol or illicit drugs, use of over-the-counter drugs, inappropriate sexual behavior, smoking, and elopement are examples of common behaviors that require limits.

Self-Destructive Acts

Suicides occur more frequently now on psychiatric units than in the past, creating a need for the nursing staff to use every resource to minimize the loss of life and injury (Bultema, 1994). It is important, therefore, to communicate to suicidal patients that self-destructive acts are not permitted and that staff members will do everything within their power to prevent such an act from occurring. Most units have "no harm" or "no self-injury" contracts that patients are asked to sign, in which patients agree to contact the staff if they have an impulse to be self-destructive.

When patients are being treated outside the hospital, the milieu must allow for ongoing assessment of patient risk for suicide. Procedures must be in place for swift readmission of patients who become suicidal.

Physical Aggressiveness Toward Others

Assaultive behavior occurs far too commonly and causes many problems on inpatient units (Dickerson, et al, 1994). Probably the greatest concern most students and nurses have about psychiatric nursing has to do with the potential for violence. About half of all health care professionals will be assaulted during their careers, so this concern is not unwarranted (Vincent and White, 1994). Chapter 14 addresses the aggressive patient.

Within the context of the therapeutic environment, physical aggressiveness (including offensive language) toward others is not allowed. This should be stated clearly, and a contract of nonviolence and appropriate conduct should be developed with these patients.

Theft is always a concern on psychiatric inpatient units, and when it occurs, it is often handled by the patients' government. One approach is to close the unit until the missing item is returned. Although protests are predictable, the process is often successful, and much therapeutic dialogue can transpire.

The psychiatric intensive care unit (PICU)

The PICU is typically a small (15 beds or so), locked unit. Ages of patients range from 18 (children younger than 18 are at risk and create serious liability issues) to 65 (adults older than 65 are at risk). The length of stay typically is determined by individual patient's needs, but court decisions also can affect the length of time a patient stays on the unit. The goal of the PICU staff is to evaluate patients, stabilize their symptoms, and move the patients to a less restrictive environment. Patients who are particularly appropriate for the PICU include patients who are hostile and assaultive, threaten homocide, or threaten suicide but refuse to sign or agree to a "no suicide" contract (Center for Psychiatric Medicine, 1993).

Noncompliance

Noncompliance is a serious problem for many psychiatric patients. Although psychiatric patients are expected to follow the treatment program, the very nature of some disorders (e.g., paranoid thinking) and the type of admission (involuntary) work against this expectation. Nonetheless, the expectation is therapeutic. If an initial agreement can be reached, compliance may be maintained throughout treatment. Compliance with medication regimens is an ongoing problem. As many as 46% of psychiatric inpatients do not take ordered medication consistently and, according to Kelly and Scott (1990), 35% to 65% of outpatients are noncompliant also. They may "cheek" the medication and then spit it out or save it. To counter noncompliance tendencies, liquid medications are often the drug form of choice at the inpatient level and long-acting depot injections the choice for outpatients.

Alcohol and Illicit Drugs

Use of alcohol and illicit drugs by psychiatric patients probably occurs often. Sometimes, "friends" of patients take advantage of the privacy provided and bring drugs in from the outside. In addition to the obvious concern of patients engaging in countertherapeutic activity, drug interactions between psychotropic drugs and mind-altering substances can be harmful.

Over-the-Counter Drugs

Over-the-counter (OTC) drugs can have harmful interactions with psychotropic drugs. Only those OTC drugs approved by the staff should be permitted.

Inappropriate Sexual Behaviors

Historically, sexual behavior by and between psychiatric patients largely has been ignored (Civic, Walsh, and McBride, 1993). This was related to society's reluctance to discuss sexual behaviors and a certain ambivalence about overseeing the sexual behaviors of other adults. Nonetheless, limits must be set on sexual activity on the psychiatric unit to protect patients from uninformed decisions or unwanted sexual activity. Psychiatric patients' sexual behaviors, including the staff's attitudes about those behaviors, have been studied and reported by Civic, Walsh, and McBride (1993). Their study was conducted at a large state hospital. They found that staff members had a generally open view of sexual realities in a state hospital. For instance, staff members found discrete masturbation acceptable but forbade sexual activity between individuals on the unit. Staff members were most concerned about the related issues of victimization and HIV infection potential. The study also revealed what many experienced psychiatric nurses had suspected; sexual behavior in this setting is common and sexual predators take advantage of lower functioning patients.

It is essential that criteria for acceptability are clearly presented so that nurses and patients understand the parameters of sexual behavior. In many states, both heterosexual and homosexual activity between patients must be reported. Reporting may be embarrassing, but it also protects patients.

Smoking

Beginning in the 1980s, an increasing number of psychiatric hospitals banned smoking (Parks and Devine, 1993) and, in 1992, the JCAHO banned smoking altogether in hospital buildings. This action discounted the long-standing belief that psychiatric patients could not tolerate a nonsmoking environment (Beemer, 1993). The prohibitions against smoking were rooted in studies that indicated that smoking was the leading cause of hospital fires and deaths related to fires and was generally unhealthy (Resnick and Bosworth, 1989; Buchanan, Huffman, and Barbour, 1994).

Parks and Devine (1993) wondered whether the negative consequences some clinicians had predicted (e.g., increased agitation and irritability leading to fights and assaults) indeed had occurred. They reviewed the impact of the smoking ban in the 69 state psychiatric hospitals where bans existed and found that, overall, the milieu was perceived as having improved. Eleven hospitals reported having more problems from staff members (no doubt smokers themselves) over this issue than from patients.

Parks and Devine concluded that increases in irritable and assaultive behavior have not occurred and that life can go on inside the psychiatric unit without smoking.

Elopement

Just as suicidal or assaultive patients may be asked to sign a contract, patients who are prone to run away can be asked to sign a contract agreeing to notify the staff before leaving the hospital. Although reasons for elopement are numerous, there are two general causes:

1. Patients believe the treatment is not meeting their needs.
2. Patients do not believe they need treatment.

Rules for the Treatment Setting

A concept closely related to limit setting is the establishment of rules, which must be communicated clearly to patients. Many psychiatric units have rules concerning things such as dress, appearance, group meetings, medication, visiting hours, and telephone use. If there is a dress standard, for example, that prohibits halter tops for women, patients should be informed about it to avoid embarrassing confrontations. Morrison (1987) identified 18 rules on the psychiatric unit that nurses believe to be important. Nine of the rules are social, and nine are therapeutic (Box 24-4).

BALANCE

Psychiatric patients are often in positions of dependency. Patients ask other people to help them to achieve mental health. Comfort is gained initially with dependency because patients hand over their problems to be fixed by the staff. Nurses may also find comfort in this dependency arrangement because they are able to "control the patient," there are fewer risks, and dependency of patients may meet a need nurses have to be "needed." But maintaining dependency is countertherapeutic, and nurses cannot "fix" the problems anyway. Regaining mental health is a process more analogous to recovery from a medical illness than it is to recovery from a surgical procedure. The nurse should foster independence and, as patients progress, they become not only more independent, but also may come to resent the vestiges of dependency. Balance is the careful negotiation of these conflicts.

The patients' rights movement has exposed another dimension of balance. Nurses and physicians are continually balancing patients' rights to make their own decisions with the staff's need to provide treatment that is effective and safe for everyone. All treatment programs must balance the broad issues of freedom vs. restrictions, care vs. self-reliance, and "normal" identity vs. identity as a patient. To better illustrate these concepts, a few relatively common dependency-independency (balance) examples follow.

Box 24-4   Important Inpatient Rules

Social Rules
- Abides by rules regarding smoking and handling of matches
- Listens attentively when others talk in meetings
- Does not dress in a sexually revealing manner
- Does not interrupt conversations
- Uses telephone with consideration for others
- Uses television and stereo with consideration for others
- Eats at designated places and times
- Does not intrude into areas designated off-limits by staff
- Abides by rules regarding visitors

Therapeutic Rules
- Actively participates in setting therapeutic goals for self
- Participates in family therapy and group conferences
- Acknowledges the need for treatment
- Accepts the need for hospitalization
- Participates in individual therapy
- Attends individual therapy as scheduled
- Attends family or group therapy as scheduled
- Seeks out staff to help control psychotic or illness-related behavior
- Examines own progress realistically when considering changes in status

From Morrison EF: Determining social and therapeutic rules for psychiatric inpatients, *Hosp Community Psychiatry* 38:994, 1987.

We have discussed the issue of balance as it pertains to the psychiatric unit. How does the concept of balance affect our personal lives? Have you recently dealt with an issue of balance?

The Suicidal Patient

The nurse must balance patients' needs for safety with patients' needs to regain control over their lives. Should patients be allowed to go to the bathroom alone? Will a patient attempt suicide in the bathroom? To watch a patient use the toilet is unpleasant for the nurse and embarrassing for the patient being watched.

The use of "no suicide contracts" can be helpful in situations in which the nurse is attempting to balance the desire for increasing freedom for a patient with the risk that the patient will attempt to hurt himself. It must be remembered, however, that there is strong evidence that suicide contracts do not work in many situations and that they should never be the sole basis for determining a patient's potential to commit suicide (Egan, et al, 1997). See Chapter 28 for a detailed discussion of the suicidal patient.

CLINICAL EXAMPLE

Maria, a 29-year-old Hispanic woman, entered the bathroom. The nurse waited outside the door. After 3 to 4 minutes, the nurse looked in. Maria was attempting to hang herself on a handrail next to the toilet.

Religious Patients

A patient may be a member of a religious body that prohibits the use of medication, and yet the patient's psychosis requires psychopharmacological intervention. The treatment team must balance patients' rights to practice their religion with their right to be treated.

CLINICAL EXAMPLE

Bill, a 44-year-old man, belongs to a Pentecostal group that does not believe in the use of medication because it is construed as a lack of faith in God. Bill is actively psychotic, yet he, his wife, and his pastor do not want him to be given medication.

The Assaultive Patient

The violent patient frightens other patients and staff members. The nurse must balance the need to protect others by secluding assaultive patients with patients' rights to unencumbrance.

CLINICAL EXAMPLE

A pregnant woman began hitting other patients. Because psychotropic drugs may harm the fetus, the nursing staff had to decide how to protect other patients (and protect the offending patient from retaliation), and yet do nothing that might compromise the pregnancy.

The Dangerous Patient

Sometimes dangerous patients tell nurses or therapists about plans to hurt someone. Patients' rights to confidentiality must be balanced with potential victims' rights to know about threats. The Tarasoff case (1974) was a landmark legal decision that states that psychiatric staff members have a duty to warn potential victims of danger from psychiatric patients (see Chapter 4). Nonetheless, judgment must be used, because indiscriminate warnings violate patients' trust and may cause undue concern to potential victims.

Balance is an important concept because it forces the nurse to articulate what competing interests are at work. The skillful use of balance comes with understanding ethical concerns, legal issues, and psychopathology.

ENVIRONMENTAL MODIFICATION

"An essential goal of psychiatric treatment is to help patients resume their roles as integral members of their community. The physical facility—its architecture and its relationship with its surroundings—can have a major impact on this process" (Gutkowski, Ginath, and Guttmann, 1992).

Attention to the physical environment can make treatment more effective. Treatment modalities can be enhanced by the physical arrangement of furniture, by safety issues, and by orientation strategies embedded within the environment. Treatment may also be enhanced by modification of patient schedules when clinical situations warrant such changes.

Physical Environment

Privacy and adequate room are of major importance in designing the psychiatric unit. Territoriality, proximity, crowding, and density are persistent human themes that need to be anticipated and addressed. Dayroom and dining room areas should be designed so that social, recreational, and occupational therapy events can be conducted with minimal conversion time. Bedrooms should be attractive and private. The nurses' station should offer an unobstructed view of the unit. Seclusion rooms are needed for persons who require isolation, with safety a primary concern. The bed in the seclusion room(s) should be bolted to the floor. No other furniture is warranted. An intercommunication system for audio and or video contact is also a common feature in newer facilities.

In units without these architectural considerations, a number of environmental changes can enhance the milieu. Color is important. Subtle hues most commonly are desired. Paintings, flowers, and inviting furniture add to the overall impression of a norm of civility and caring. Games and cards should be available for socializing. Magazines and books should be available for browsing. Furniture should be arranged in a way that encourages socializing. For example, an arrangement of three or four chairs around a table encourages group seating and lends itself to informal group work.

Orientation Strategies

Persons who are severely disturbed or who are cognitively impaired may not be able to navigate the hospital environment without environmental cues. Environmental cues include large orientation boards on which the date, time, and location of daily events are posted. This serves to keep patients current. Other environmental orientation approaches include public address systems, clearly marked names (e.g., bathroom, bedrooms with patients' names on the doors), and color-coded facilities.

Schedule Modification

Modification of a patient's schedule within the context of the milieu may also be important. Those who are diagnosed with chronic fatigue syndrome, for example, may require daytime rest periods or activities that can be accomplished at a slower pace. (Anderson and Kayner, 1995). Others in the community need to understand that schedule modifications are not a demonstration of preferential treatment but rather consistent with a community member's individual needs.

COMMUNITY-BASED MILIEU

Purposeful structuring of the environment, as initially described by Maxwell Jones (1953), has been used historically as a treatment approach in hospital inpatient units. A rapidly changing health care delivery system now dictates that hospitals be utilized mostly for short-term crisis intervention. Much of the care of psychiatric patients today takes place either in group homes, partial (day) hospitals, or through support offered by nurses to patients and their family members when making home health visits. Throughout this chapter the notion of how and where milieu concepts can and are applied in the community have been incorporated. The use of structured groups, among other milieu ideas, will continue to be increasingly important to the delivery of psychiatric nursing care.

■ Critical Thinking Question

How is milieu utilized in community settings?

Key Concepts

1. Because psychiatric patients are incapable of *not* interacting with their environment, the nurse has the potential to shape the environment in order to cause the inevitable interaction to be therapeutic.
2. The Joint Commission on Accreditation of Healthcare Organizations (JCAHO) mandates that psychiatric facilities invest resources in developing a therapeutic environment.

3. The effectively managed milieu consists of six distinct elements: (1) safety, (2) structure, (3) norms, (4) limit setting, (5) balance, and (6) environmental modification.

4. Safety is nursing's responsibility to protect patients from harm while they are in the hospital. Protecting patients from other patients, falls, medication errors and adverse responses, and self-injurious behavior are major safety considerations.

5. Concepts related to milieu management are increasingly being used in noninpatient settings.

6. Structure provides the framework for the therapeutic environment and includes community meetings, activity groups, social skills groups, life skills groups, street skills groups, physical exercise groups, psychoeducational programs, transition groups, and work groups.

7. Norms are the expectations of behavior that are communicated to patients in both direct and indirect ways and include the norms of nonviolence, physical and emotional security, openness, feedback, respect for the individual, privacy, acceptance, independence, and individual responsibility.

8. Setting limits is the skill of clearly identifying acceptable and unacceptable behavior, including clear communication about self-destructive acts, physical aggressiveness toward others, personal control, noncompliance with treatment plans, use of alcohol and illicit drugs, use of over-the-counter drugs, sexual inappropriateness, smoking, and elopement.

9. Balance is the art of carefully negotiating the competing forces of dependence and independence that are commonly found in the context of psychiatric nursing care.

10. Environmental modification is the purposeful arrangement of the environment and includes attention to the physical environment, safety issues, orientation strategies, and schedule modification.

▌ Study Questions

(Answer key is in the back of the book.)

1. The dimension of the therapeutic milieu that permeates all components is:
   a. Safety
   b. Unit structure
   c. Unit norms
   d. Limit setting

2. The expectation of nonviolence is an example of:
   a. Structure
   b. Norms
   c. Limit setting
   d. Environmental modification

3. When the psychiatric nurse clearly identifies acceptable and unacceptable behavior, he or she is instituting:
   a. Structure
   b. Norms
   c. Limit setting
   d. Environmental modification

4. An example of balance is:
   a. Choosing orange juice for a patient
   b. Articulating the competing forces in deciding whether to go into the bathroom with a suicidal patient
   c. Developing personal interests along with one's professional interests
   d. All of the above

5. Providing a large orientation board for patients is an example of:
   a. Environmental structure
   b. Environmental norms
   c. Limit setting
   d. Environmental modification

6. Bill makes the following statement to John: "John, when you cross your arms each time you speak to me, I feel like I am being treated just like a child." Most specifically, Bill is:
   a. Being open
   b. Providing feedback
   c. Sharing
   d. Confronting

7. Permitting a patient with chronic fatigue syndrome to take rest periods during the day is an example of:
   a. Structure
   b. Schedule modification
   c. Limit setting
   d. Norm development

References

Allen BA, et al: A practical model for a vocational readiness program in a drug treatment setting, *Hosp Community Psychiatry* 45(4):374, 1994.

Anderson JS and Kayner D: Milieu issues in the treatment of a person with chronic fatigue syndrome on an inpatient psychiatric unit, *J Am Psychiatr Nurses Assoc* 1(1):12, February 1995.

Aroian K and Prater M: Transition entry groups: easing new patients' adjustment to psychiatric hospitalization, *Hosp Community Psychiatry* 39:312, 1988.

Arons BS: Effective use of community meetings in psychiatric treatment units, *Hosp Community Psychiatry* 33:480, 1982.

Assey JL: The suicide prevention contract, *Perspect Psychiatr Care* 23:99, 1985.

Baenninger LP and Tang W: Teaching chronic psychiatric inpatients to use differential attention to change each other's behaviors, *Hosp Community Psychiatry* 41:425, 1990.

Barter JT, Queirolo JF, and Ekstrom SP: A psychoeducational approach to educating chronic mental patients for community living, *Hosp Community Psychiatry* 35:793, 1984.

Beemer BR: Hospital psychiatric units: nonsmoking policies, *J Psychosoc Nurs Ment Health Serv* 31(4):12, 1993.

Bickel WK: Employment and addiction, *Hosp Community Psychiatry* 45(2):178, 1994.

Blair DT: Where assault begins, *J Psychosoc Nurs Ment Health Serv* 30(6):4, 1992 (letter, reply).

Buchanan CR, Huffman C, and Barbour VM: Smoking health risk: counseling of psychiatric patients, *J Psychosoc Nurs Ment Health Serv* 32(1):27, 1994.

Bultema JK: Healing process for the multidisciplinary team: recovering post-inpatient suicide, *J Psychosoc Nurs Ment Health Serv* 32(2):19, 1994.

Carey KB: Emerging treatment guidelines for mentally ill chemical abusers, *Hosp Community Psychiatry* 40:341, 1989.

Center for Psychiatric Medicine: *PICU admission criteria*, Birmingham, Ala, 1993, The Center.

Civic D, Walsh G, and McBride D: Staff perspectives on sexual behavior of patients in a state psychiatric hospital, *Hosp Community Psychiatry* 44(9):887, 1993.

Conrad N, Sloan S, and Jedwabny J: Resolving the control struggle on an eating disorders unit, *Perspect Psychiatr Care* 28(3):13, 1992.

Corrigan, PM: Use of token economy with seriously ill patients: criticisms and misconceptions, *Psychiatr Serv* 46(12):1258, 1995.

Corrigan PW and Holmes EP: Patient identification of street skills for a psychosocial training module, *Hosp Community Psychiatry* 45(3):273, 1994.

Cournos F, et al: HIV infection in state hospitals: case reports and long-term management strategies, *Hosp Community Psychiatry* 41(2):163, 1990.

Department of Health and Human Services: *Mental health, United States, 1992*, Rockville, Md, 1992, National Institutes of Health.

Dickerson F, et al: Seclusion and restraint, assaultiveness, and patient performance in a token economy, *Hosp Community Psychiatry* 45(2):168, 1994.

Dinkmeyer D: Mental Health counseling: a psychoeducational approach, *J Ment Health Counseling* 13:37, 1991.

Egan MP, et al: The no suicide contract: helpful or harmful? *J Psychosoc Nurs* 35(3):31, 1997.

Forman L: Medication: reasons and interventions for noncompliance, *J Psychosoc Nurs Ment Health Serv* 31(10):23, 1993.

Glynn SM, Pugh R, and Rose G: Predictor of relatives' attendance at a state hospital workshop on schizophrenia, *Hosp Community Psychiatry* 41:67, 1990.

Greenberg L, et al: An interdisciplinary psychoeducation program for schizophrenia patients and their families in an acute care setting, *Hosp Community Psychiatry* 39:277, 1988.

Gutheil T: The therapeutic milieu: changing themes and theories, *Hosp Community Psychiatry* 36:1279, 1985.

Gutkowski S, Ginath Y, and Guttmann F: Improving psychiatric environments through minimal architectural change, *Hosp Community Psychiatry* 43(9):920, 1992.

Holbrook T: Policing sexuality in a modern state hospital, *Hosp Community Psychiatry* 40:65, 1989.

Hughes JR, et al: Prevalence of smoking among psychiatric outpatients, *Am J Psychiatry* 143:993, 1986.

Joint Commission on Accreditation of Healthcare Organizations: *Accreditation manual for hospitals*, Chicago, 1992, The Commission.

Joint Commission on Accreditation of Healthcare Organizations: *Accreditation manual for hospitals*, Chicago, 1997, The Commission.

Joint Commission on Accreditation of Healthcare Organizations: *The Joint Commission 1994 accreditation manual for hospitals, vol. 1, Standards*, Oak Terrace, Ill, 1993, The Commission.

Jones M: *The therapeutic community*, New York, 1953, Basic Books.

Kahn EM and White EM: Adapting milieu approaches to acute inpatient care for schizophrenic patients, *Hosp Community Psychiatry* 40:609, 1989.

Kelly GR and Scott JE: Medication compliance and health education among outpatients with chronic mental disorders, *Med Care* 28:1181, 1990.

Klose P and Tinius T: Confidence builders: a self-esteem group at an inpatient psychiatric hospital, *J Psychosoc Nurs Ment Health Serv* 30(7):5, 1992.

Kyes G and Hofling C: *Basic psychiatric concepts in nursing*, ed 3, Philadelphia, 1974, JB Lippincott.

Lamb HR: An educational model for teaching living skills to long-term patients, *Hosp Community Psychiatry* 27:875, 1976.

Leff HR, et al: A controlled trial of social intervention in the families of schizophrenic patients, *Br J Psychiatry* 141:121, 1982.

Levy P and Hartocollis P: Nursing aides and patient violence, *Am J Psychiatry* 133:429, 1976.

Maynard C: A psychoeducational approach to depression in women, *J Psychosoc Nurs Ment Health Serv* 31(12):9, 1993.

McPherson ML. Taking an accurate medication history, *Home Health Care Pract* 5(4):35, 1996.

McRae J, et al: What happens to patients after five years of intensive care management stops? *Hosp Community Psychiatry* 41:175, 1990.

Morrison EF: Determining social and therapeutic rules for psychiatric patients, *Hosp Community Psychiatry* 38:994, 1987.

Morrison EF: Tradition of toughness, *Image* 22(1):32, 1990.

Morse JM and Intrieri RC: Patient communication in a long-term care facility, *J Psychosoc Nurs* 35(5):34, 1997.

Munetz MR and Geller JL: The least restrictive alternative in the postinstitutional era, *Hosp Community Psychiatry* 44(10):967, 1993.

Murray RB and Baier M: Use of therapeutic milieu in a community setting, *J Psychosoc Nurs Ment Health Serv* 31(10):11, 1993.

Palmer F: The place of work in psychiatric rehabilitation, *Hosp Community Psychiatry* 40:222, 1989.

Parks JJ and Devine DD: The effects of smoking bans on extended care units at state psychiatric hospitals, *Hosp Community Psychiatry* 44(9):885, 1993.

Pellegrino E: Altruism, self-interest, and medical ethics, *JAMA* 258:1939, 1987.

Peplau HE: Some unresolved issues in the era of biopsychosocial nursing, *J Am Psychiatr Nurse Assoc* 1(3):92, 1995.

Plante TG: Social skills training, *J Psychosoc Nurs Ment Health Serv* 27:7, 1989.

Resnick MP and Bosworth EE: A smoke-free psychiatric unit, *Hosp Community Psychiatry* 40:525, 1989.

Snyder W: Hospital downsizing and increased frequency of assaults on staff, *Hosp Community Psychiatry* 45(4):378, 1994.

Tarasoff v Regents of the University of California, 529 P 2d 553, 1974.

Thompson J and Strand K: Psychiatric nursing in a psychosocial setting, *J Psychosoc Nurs Ment Health Serv* 32(2):25, 1994.

Trygstad LN: The need to know: biological learning needs identified by practicing psychiatric nurses, *J Psychosoc Nurs Ment Health Serv* 32(2):1318, 1994.

Veterans Affairs Medical Center: Living skills training for veterans with serious mental illness, *Hosp Community Psychiatry* 44(10):995, 1993.

Vincent M and White K: Patient violence toward a nurse: predictable and preventable? *J Psychosoc Nurs Ment Health Serv* 32(2):30, 1994.

CHAPTER 25

Roles of the Psychiatric Nurse in the Therapeutic Milieu

BRUCE P. MERICLE

LEARNING OBJECTIVES

After reading this chapter you should be able to:
- Describe the responsibilities of the roles of colleague, team leader, supervisor/trainer, and consultant.
- Describe the roles of other mental health professionals.
- Describe the role of the advanced practice psychiatric nurse as part of the community milieu.
- Identify the two primary types of consulting activities in which the psychiatric nurse participates.

In the preceding two chapters discussion focused on the characteristics of a variety of milieu settings. The overall purpose was to define the *structure* of the treatment environment. In this chapter emphasis is placed on the people who provide care within a milieu structure.

Psychiatric disorders traditionally have been treated in the inpatient setting, using a team approach. The team meeting served as the forum in which caregivers formally met to discuss patient treatment issues. Team participants included psychiatric nurses, psychiatrists, psychiatric social workers, psychologists, therapeutic activity personnel, and others as needed. The team members worked together, within the milieu structure, to foster mental health in patients so those patients might return to their homes and their communities. Today that same treatment approach is being applied to the care of patients living in the community.

Program for Assertive Client Treatment (PACT) teams are an example of professionals working as a unit and charged with the responsibility of intervening before patient problems require hospitalization. PACT teams are in wide use today and are recognized as an important means for delivering psychiatric mental health care in the community (Essock and Kontos, 1995; McFarlane, et al, 1996).

Another major change in health care delivery is the ever-increasing use of advanced practice psychiatric nurses who evaluate patients' response to psychotropic drugs and are certified to prescribe medications in most states (Pearson, 1997). Their presence in the community also is aiding in keeping patients at home, in group homes, and/or attending day programs.

Management of a therapeutic milieu requires leadership ability. Of particular import are working constructively with colleagues, facilitation of team meetings and overall supervision and training of nursing staff. In some settings psychotherapeutic management is accomplished through the consultative process. The focus then of this chapter is on describing four major roles of the psychiatric nurse/psychotherapeutic manager. The psychiatric nursing roles include the following:

1. Colleague
2. Team leader
3. Supervisor and trainer
4. Consultant

COLLEAGUE ROLE

One benefit of working in psychiatry is the opportunity to work collegially with other professionals. Psychiatrists, psychologists, psychiatric social workers, pharmacists, occupational therapists, recreational therapists, and psychiatric nurses are all part of the treatment team. Discussions of treatment issues by the team lends itself to unique input from all disciplines. The nurse is able to share information with fellow team members on the basis of assessment data gathered in settings typically managed by the nursing staff.

Following are basic descriptions of the members of a multidisciplinary team, now commonplace in a variety of health care delivery systems.

Psychiatrist

Certification of a physician (MD) in psychiatry by the American Board of Psychiatry and Neurology requires a 3-year residency, 2 years of clinical practice, and completion of an examination. Psychiatrists are permitted to prescribe psychotropic medications. In recent years, fewer graduating medical students have selected psychiatry as a specialty area, resulting in fewer psychiatrists. This decline in the number of younger psychiatrists in part has led to more opportunities for advanced practice nurses.

Historically, physicians have assumed (and to a large extent had bestowed upon them) an authoritarian role. Today, however, most physicians seek to work collaboratively, developing a more egalitarian style (Klamen, 1994). With input from a variety of professional groups, there is a greater emphasis on comprehensive patient care.

Psychologist

Psychologists who work in the mental health field are called *clinical psychologists*. This designation differentiates clinical psychologists from the varied nonpsychiatric roles of other psychologists. The clinical psychologist has a doctorate (PhD) in psychology and is prepared to practice therapy, conduct research, and administer and interpret psychological tests. The last point is of major significance. Neuropsychological testing is utilized extensively in many psychiatric settings. For example, detecting cognitive decline is important, and several tests can be administered to assess it (Mitrushina, Abara, and Blumenfield, 1994). Psychologists can also administer tests to identify psychosis, depression, anxiety, and other mental disorders. Many psychologists are behaviorally oriented and develop behavior modification programs for individual patients or for the entire milieu.

Psychiatric Social Worker

Most psychiatric social workers are prepared at the master's level (MSW). Social workers are part of the treatment team, and their unique contributions are working with families and mobilizing community support systems. Psychiatric social workers often assume the role of primary therapist. In many settings, the social worker is most knowledgeable about community and financial resources. When patients are not able to return home, or when there is no home to return to, it is typically the social worker who finds suitable placement in the least restrictive environment.

Pharmacist

Pharmacists may work closely with the psychotherapeutic manager both as a clinical resource and as a training resource. The role of the pharmacist is becoming more important with the ever-increasing utilization of both inpatient and community-based psychopharmacology.

Occupational Therapist

Occupational therapy (OT) training emphasizes human occupation and functioning as a baseline for establishing therapeutic goals (Stoeffel, 1994). Emphasis may be placed on both vocational and what might be called prevocational skills. For example, because social, communication, organizational, and cognitive skills are necessary to the independent function of various adult roles, OTs focus on these prevocational skills when appropriate (Center for Psychiatric Medicine, 1993).

OTs work with arts, crafts, and basic psychomotor skills and, through these media, make a unique contribution to psychiatric care. The approach is direct. A therapeutic gain is achieved through the use of accomplishment (i.e., producing something) and distraction (thinking about something other than their problems). Examples of specific OT activities include teaching self-help and employment skills, managing mealtimes, and directing activity/exercise groups. A goal of OT is to introduce activities "... that ensure success and promote feelings of mastery and accomplishment" (Greene, 1993).

Recreational Therapist

The recreational therapist (RT) seeks to increase a person's ability to function in daily activities (Center for Psychiatric Medicine, 1993) and to understand the balance that should exist between work and play. Activities are selected based on their learning value. RTs typically complete a bachelor's degree program, but in some facilities individuals without this special training serve in these roles.

In addition to these distinct categories of psychiatric professionals, one could also add art therapists, substance abuse counselors, marriage and family counselors, dieticians, and others. Each make a unique contribution to the treatment of psychiatric patients.

■ Critical Thinking Question

How is the role of a staff-level psychiatric nurse different from a master's-prepared psychiatric nurse?

TEAM LEADER ROLE

Nurses often assume or share leadership in team meetings. Other disciplines rely on the nursing service to provide an update on patients' status, to report on implementation or treatment team plans, and to provide information regarding patient response to treatment. In a community PACT setting, treatment teams meet with families so that their input may be included (McFarlane, 1996).

"The team meets routinely to discuss the patients' problems, progress, and needs during hospitalization" (Ambrose, 1989). During team meetings, patients are discussed individually, and decisions regarding treatment are developed. In productive team meetings, each discipline recognizes and respects the contributions of the other disciplines. At times, there is an overlapping and conflict of disciplines, but when the welfare of patients is foremost, such distractions can be resolved. When disciplines have "turf wars," patient care is compromised.

If interdiscipline harmony contributes to the therapeutic environment, then it is important to seek such harmony. Interdiscipline relations are enhanced by respect, the desire to help, and understanding. When professionals respect each other, desire to help the patients, and understand the dynamics of interprofessional conflict (e.g., loss of turf, professional jealousy, mistrust), interdiscipline harmony is facilitated. When respect, the desire to help, and understanding are lacking, interprofessional conflict results and undermines the therapeutic environment.

SUPERVISOR AND TRAINER ROLE

An important dimension of psychotherapeutic management is the supervision and training of other members of the nursing staff. The nursing staff is composed of nurses, student nurses, psychiatric technicians, mental health workers, and psychiatric aides. Supervision and training are almost inseparable components of managing the milieu. The nursing staff must strive to consistently represent the agency philosophy and conscientiously implement treatment plans. To do so, individual staff members require training. Supervision reinforces the unit leadership's commitment to these objectives and provides a focus for evaluation. Although nursing faculty are responsible for nursing students, students look to and gain a great deal from interacting with staff serving as role models.

Supervision

In the role of supervisor, the nurse-manager must have staff meetings where concerns can be raised. A hallmark of psychiatric units is the candor with which people interact. The nurse-manager must anticipate the inevitable occurrences of miscommunication. Doing so lessens the sting of miscommunication and facilitates a return to the treatment team's business at hand, avoiding a preoccupation with "who said what," etc. The nurse-manager also should schedule regular meetings with individual nurses he or she supervises. Supervision should be nurturing, supportive, trusting, and open to emotion (Klamen, 1994).

Other nurses

Multiple entry levels into nursing confuse the public, other professionals, and have been the source of intraprofessional conflict. Academic psychiatric preparation varies from several weeks to a semester-long discrete course; therefore, novice psychiatric nurses require supervision and training from more experienced nurses. Student nurses gaining clinical experience on the psychiatric unit are also supervised and trained by unit nurses (albeit this may be done indirectly). It is important that students be given every opportunity to experience meaningful learning situations.

■ **Critical Thinking Question**

Physicians and nurses traditionally get along very well in psychiatry. Why might this be true?

Paraprofessionals

Paraprofessionals are a category of psychiatric health care providers that often serve as "the eyes and ears" for nurses and other team members.

Under most circumstances they are delegated responsibilities by a professional nurse and in turn report to the professional nurse their observations about patients. Those observations may then be used when making decisions about patient care. In some states paraprofessionals attend training programs that last as long as 1 year. Graduates are then licensed by the state in which they practice. In other settings, training is provided by the institution in which the trainee will work. Titles used by this group of health care providers vary widely and may include such names as mental health worker, psychiatric technician, or psychiatric aide.

Training

Training should focus on therapeutic communication (Unit Three), position-appropriate understanding of psychopharmacology (Unit Four), and maintenance of the therapeutic environment (Unit Five), all of which are underscored by a position-appropriate understanding of psychopathology (Unit Six); specialized issues can be taught as necessary (Units Seven and Eight contain some special issues in psychiatric nursing). There are distinct groups among the generic category called nursing staff. Their roles overlap, but this potentially disharmonious situation is easily mitigated by good leadership.

As with any training program, several educational principles apply (Faulkner, 1994):

1. Be clear about what is to be accomplished.
2. Have realistic expectations.
3. Expose trainees to other sources of information.
4. Assign trainees to work with competent nurses.
5. Provide evaluations that guide trainees toward improvement.

Updating medical-surgical nursing skills

It is not uncommon for psychiatric units to admit patients with medical problems. In fact, on some units these patients may represent the difference between financial solvency and operating in deficit.

As mentioned earlier, today's psychiatric nurse often is called upon to care for patients who are also suffering from physical illness. Over the years, psychiatric patients were thought to be medically stable. That assumption no longer holds true. A major contributing factor is the aging of society and the high percentage of hospital admissions in the elderly age group. Dunn (1993) surveyed psychiatric nurses to identify the five skills and five content areas the nurses perceived to be most deficient. The nurses believed they needed updating in the following areas: skills for assessment, intravenous therapy, catheterizations, wound care and dressing, and electrocardiograms; and content related to pharmacology, diabetes mellitus, general disease, interpretation of laboratory values, and the complications and treatments of addictions.

Supervision and training of all nursing staff members are vital to milieu management. The therapeutic environment depends on every member of the team understanding and enhancing the principles described in Chapter 24.

Critical Thinking Question

What are the major contributions to the fact that hospitalized psychiatric patients are more medically ill now than in the past?

CONSULTANT ROLE

Psychiatric nurses who work in a general hospital psychiatric unit may be called upon to consult with other nursing departments. Providing consultation may involve formal or informal processes.

Typically, a "problem" or "disturbed" patient triggers the consultation; that is, a "problem" patient taxes the ability of the unit nursing staff to provide effective care. In the hope that the psychiatric nursing department can help, a consultation is requested. In some hospitals, this is a relatively informal process. In many larger hospitals, the roles of psychiatric liaison and consultant nurse have been developed to provide these services.

Consultation typically takes one of two forms. The psychiatric nurse may work directly with the patient or indirectly by working with the nurse(s) requesting the consultation (consultee). "Problem" patients roughly can be grouped into those who have a history of diagnosable psychiatric disturbances and those who are experiencing disturbances secondary to their current medical problems. The consulting psychiatric nurse uses the nursing process to develop an intervention strategy. Minimal responsibilities for both the consultee and the consultant are found in Box 25-1.

Box 25-1 Responsibilities of the Consultee and Consultant

Consultee Responsibilities
- Identifies (in writing) the need
- Receives approval for consultation from supervisor
- Identifies who should be involved
- If applicable, addresses fees or negotiates payment
- Sets up the time and place for sessions
- Takes action regarding recommendations
- Accepts, rejects, or modifies the consultant's advice
- Evaluates the outcomes of the actions

Consultant Responsibilities
- Ensures that the consultation process and responsibilities are defined clearly and are agreeable
- Assesses whether expertise matches the need
- Clarifies and assesses the stated need
- Facilitates the diagnosis of the problem
- Facilitates recommendations requiring patient, staff, or system actions
- Facilitates or carries out the recommendations
- Follows up on the consultee's response to the recommendations
- Provides a written summary of the process
- Evaluates the process with the consultee

■ Critical Thinking Question

The text noted that multiple entry points into nursing are confusing to the public. Do you agree? If so, what should be done?

▼ Key Concepts

1. Psychiatric nurses serve in multiple roles.
2. In this chapter, four roles of the psychotherapeutic manager are discussed: (1) colleague, (2) team leader, (3) supervisor/trainer, and (4) consultant.
3. The psychiatric nurse most frequently works with the following **colleagues:** psychiatrists, psychologists, psychiatric social workers, pharmacists, occupational therapists, and recreational therapists.
4. The psychiatric nurse usually assumes or shares responsibility for **team leadership.** During the team meeting, patients are discussed, and decisions are developed regarding treatment and discharge or disposition.
5. The **supervision and training** of subordinates is an important function of the psychotherapeutic manager because milieu management is dependent on the contributions of all members of the team. Most training efforts can be subsumed under one of the four components of psychotherapeutic management: therapeutic communication, position-appropriate understanding of psychopharmacology, maintenance of the therapeutic environment, and position-appropriate understanding of psychopathology.
6. Psychiatric nurses often are called upon to fulfill the role of **consultant** to other departments within the hospital or other agencies. Typically the nurse works either directly with patients or indirectly through the nurse/person (consultee) requesting the consultation.

▼ Study Questions

(Answer key is in the back of the book.)

1. Patients are discussed individually and decisions regarding treatment are developed in:
   a. A community meeting
   b. A team meeting
   c. A group meeting
   d. All of the above
2. Which of the following groups do psychiatric nurses typically supervise?
   a. New nurses
   b. Student nurses
   c. Psychiatric technicians
   d. All of the above
3. Advanced practice nurses may prescribe medications in the majority of states.
   a. True
   b. False
4. Which of the following professional groups places an emphasis on functioning when working with patients?
   a. Psychologists
   b. Occupational therapists
   c. Recreational therapists
   d. All of the above
5. Which professional group typically leads team meetings?
   a. Nursing
   b. Psychiatry
   c. Psychology
   d. Social work

References

Ambrose JA: Joining in: therapeutic groups for chronic patients, *J Psychosoc Nurs Ment Health Serv* 27:28, 1989.

Baenninger LP and Tang W: Teaching chronic psychiatric inpatients to use differential attention to change each other's behaviors, *Hosp Community Psychiatry* 41:425, 1990.

Center for Psychiatric Medicine: *Occupational therapy/recreational therapy,* Birmingham, Ala, 1993, The Center.

DeLeon PH, et al: The case for prescriptive privileges: a logical extension of professional practice, *J Clin Chil Psychol* 20(3):254, 1991.

Dunn JR: Medical skills and knowledge: how necessary are they for psychiatric nurses? *J Psychosoc Nurs Ment Health Serv* 31(12):25, 1993.

Essock SM and Kontos N: Implementing assertive community treatment teams, *Psychiatr Serv* 46(7):679, 1995.

Faulkner LR: Ten easy steps to failure of a public training experience, *Hosp Community Psychiatry* 45(2):101, 1994.

Greene S: Occupational therapy intervention with children in school systems, *Hosp Community Psychiatry* 44(5): 429, 1993.

Klamen DL, Ornstein E, and Scofield C: Overcoming obstacles to communication on a psychiatric training unit, *Hosp Community Psychiatry* 45(1):78, 1994.

Libassi MF: *Psychopharmacology in social work education,* Rockville, Md, 1990, US Department of Health and Human Services.

McFarlane WR, et al. A comparison of two levels of family-aide assertive community treatment, *Psychiatr Serv* 47(7):744, 1996.

Mitrushina M, Abara J, and Blumenfield A: The neurobehavioral cognitive status examination as a screening tool for organicity in psychiatric patients, *Hosp Community Psychiatry* 45(3):252, 1994.

Pearson LJ. Annual update of how each state stands on legislative issues affecting advanced nursing practice, *Nurse Pract* 22(1):18, 1997.

Stoeffel VC: Occupational therapists' role in treating substance abuse, *Hosp Community Psychiatry* 45(1):21, 1994.

Ukens C: RPhs expand prescriptive authority but still lagging, *Drug Top* 138(9):16, 1994.

Psychopathology

CHAPTER 26

Introduction
to Psychopathology

NORMAN L. KELTNER

LEARNING OBJECTIVES

After reading this chapter you should be able to:
- Describe the extent of mental illness in the United States.
- Identify the most common mental disorders in the United States.

- List the three requirements for understanding psychopathology.
- Describe several guidelines applicable to all aspects of psychotherapeutic management.

"Telling me that I have a brain disease and that I should take medications does not solve my problems." (Nancy W. Riffer, PhD, former mental patient, 1997)

According to a survey conducted by the National Institute of Mental Health (NIMH), 52 million Americans have some type of mental or chemical-abuse disorder during a given 12-month period (Regier, et al, 1993). As can be seen in the table on the next page, anxiety disorders are the most prevalent, followed by mood disorders (collectively), alcohol disorders, and major depression. This table, also found in Chapter 1 and in each chapter in this unit, lists prevalence rates for a 12-month period. Lifetime incidence of these disorders is slightly higher (Kessler, et al, 1994). Table 26-1 provides the data for lifetime prevalence rates for the most common mental and

chemical-abuse disorders. It is important to note that many individuals have a comorbid status; that is, they may be depressed, anxious, and abuse a chemical. Therefore, psychiatric morbidity is quite concentrated, with approximately 17% of the population having a history of three or more comorbid disorders (Kessler, et al, 1994). Most of these persons do not seek professional help. Kessler (1994) found that less than 60% of persons with a lifetime disorder, and less than 80% of those with a recent disorder, seek professional help. This suggests a great reservoir of unmet mental health needs in the United States.

The incidence of psychopathology is high, and nurses' understanding of psychopathology is basic to effective psychotherapeutic management of mental disorders. Understanding psychopathology requires that knowledge be organized, operational definitions

KEY TERMS

Etiology   The study of the causes of diseases, including both direct and predisposing causes

National Institute of Mental Health (NIMH)   A government organization within the National Institutes of Health concerned with mental health issues in the United States

Nature argument   Etiology is related to biology

Nurture argument   Etiology is related to upbringing, life events, or other stressors

Psychopathology   The systematic study of mental disorders

12-Month Prevalence Rate of Mental Disorders in the United States

Diagnosis	Percentage of Population over 17 Years of Age	Number of Persons
Anxiety disorders	12.6	20,034,000
Phobia disorders*	10.9	17,331,000
Mood disorders	9.5	15,143,000
Alcohol disorders	7.4	11,766,000
Major depression†	5.0	7,950,000
Drug disorders	3.1	4,929,000
Cognitive impairment	2.7	4,293,000
Obsessive-compulsive disorder	2.1	3,339,000
Antisocial disorder	1.5	2,385,000
Panic disorders*	1.3	2,067,000
Bipolar disorder†	1.2	1,908,000
Schizophrenia	1.1	1,749,000
Somatization	0.2	365,000

From Regier DA, et al: The de facto US mental and addictive disorders service system: epidemiologic catchment area prospective 1-year prevalence rates of disorders and services, *Arch Gen Psychiatry* 50:85, 1993.
*Also calculated in anxiety statistics.
†Also calculated in mood disorders statistics.

formed, and criteria for diagnosis developed. Several diagnostic systems have accomplished these tasks: the Feighner criteria (Feighner, et al, 1972); the Research Diagnostic Criteria (RDC) (Spitzer, Endicott, and Robins, 1975); and the *Diagnostic and Statistical Manual of Mental Disorders* (American Psychiatric Association, 1952 [DSM-I], 1968 [DSM-II], 1980 [DSM-III], 1987 [DSM-III-R], and 1994 [DSM-IV]). The DSM-IV, the latest DSM version, is the official diagnostic system used in American psychiatric care, and for that reason it is used in this unit to help convey important concepts related to each mental disorder discussed. In addition, each chapter pre-

sents a discussion of common behaviors, etiology, and psychotherapeutic management.

BEHAVIOR

Patients' behaviors are presented to help the student identify behavioral phenomena. Some behaviors can be observed directly (objective or signs), whereas others must be reported by the patient (subjective or symptoms). Knowledge of these signs and symptoms helps the nurse to anticipate and plan appropriate interventions.

Table 26-1   Lifetime Prevalence Rates for Mental Disorders in the United States

Disorder	Lifetime Prevalence Rate (%)
Anxiety disorders (all)	24.9
Panic disorder	3.5
Agoraphobia with panic disorder	5.3
Social phobia	13.3
Simple phobia	11.3
Generalized anxiety disorder	5.1
Mood disorders (all)	19.3
Major depressive disorder	17.1
Bipolar disorder	1.6
Dysthymia	6.4
Chemical-abuse disorder (all)	26.6
Alcohol abuse without dependence	9.4
Alcohol dependence	14.1
Drug abuse without dependence	4.4
Drug dependence	7.5
Schizophrenia and other psychoses	0.7
Antisocial personality disorder	3.5
ANY MENTAL OR CHEMICAL-ABUSE DISORDER	48

Adapted from Kessler RC, et al: Lifetime and 12-month prevalence of DSM-III-R psychiatric disorders in the United States, *Arch Gen Psychiatry* 51:8, 1994.

ETIOLOGY

For many years psychiatric clinicians have typically fallen into one of two etiological camps: those who believe that mental disorders arise from *nature* (organic, biological, genetic) and those who believe that mental disorders arise from *nurture* (psychodynamic, functional, environmental, due to early life experiences). In recent years, most clinicians have come to recognize that both views provide valuable insights into the complexities of the human mind, and most now embrace a more holistic view of mental illness. Threads of the "nature vs. nurture" argument (or the "biological vs. psychodynamic" argument) are presented in discussions of etiology; however, the overriding theme of this unit is the recognition of the unifying symptoms that point to the contributions of each etiological factor.

PSYCHOTHERAPEUTIC MANAGEMENT

Sections on psychotherapeutic management in each chapter draw on the general intervention strategies presented in Units Three through Five to develop appropriate interventions for each disorder. In addition, a case study and a related nursing care plan (see sample care plan on p. 347) are presented for each disorder. The following rules provide relevant guidelines for all aspects of psychotherapeutic management:

- Provide support for patients. By treating patients with respect, dignity, and as individuals, the nurse helps patients to mobilize their strengths.
- Strengthen patients' self-esteem.
- Treat patients as adults. Do not succumb to the temptation to patronize.
- Prevent failure or embarrassment. Do not involve patients in situations in which they will fail or feel inadequate; for example, competitive games may be inappropriate for some patients. If a patient does something "crazy," like taking off clothes, remove the patient from public view and assist him or her in putting on proper attire.
- Treat patients as individuals. Although patients may be similar to previous patients on the unit, they are unique, and generalizations may damage the nurse-patient relationship.
- Provide reality testing. This rule applies to patients who feel very anxious or unreal, as well as to schizophrenic patients. Reinforce reality.
- Handle hostility therapeutically. Hostile themes are not uncommon on a psychiatric unit. The nurse who is intimidated and frightened by every occurrence is defensive and may be unable to be therapeutic. The ability to be calm and matter-of-fact about norms and limits projects control of oneself and of the situation, and is therapeutic.

■ Critical Thinking Question

You are in this course in order to learn about caring for psychiatric patients. Do you believe people with mental disorders can become completely well? If not, can you justify the necessity of this course?

*C*are *P*lan

NAME: _____   ADMISSION DATE: _____

DSM-IV DIAGNOSIS: _____

ASSESSMENT: **Areas of strength:** _____
_____

Problems: _____
_____
_____

DIAGNOSES: _____
_____
_____

OUTCOMES: **Short-term goals:**   Date met
_____
_____

Long-term goals:
_____
_____
_____

PLANNING/   **Nurse-patient relationship:** _____
INTERVENTIONS: _____

Psychopharmacology: _____
_____

Milieu management: _____
_____
_____
_____

EVALUATION: _____
_____

REFERRALS: _____
_____
_____

THE NURSE'S NEED TO UNDERSTAND PSYCHOPATHOLOGY

"Life was hell in that private hospital. I was heavily medicated, and the staff treated me with indignity. They watched me constantly, even while I was relieving myself and showering. I was permitted only to sit, smoke cigarettes, and play cards with other patients. By the time of my discharge four months later, I had been stripped of my self-esteem. I had lost my confidence; I could not perform even the simplest of tasks." (Jacqueline Chapman, MS, MFCC, former mental patient, 1997)

Nurses cannot gain a true understanding of patients with mental disorders until they understand (or have knowledge about) mental disorders. Psychiatric nursing is more than warm, caring feelings about patients. Although being affirming and kind are wonderful attributes in daily life, more is required of the effective psychiatric nurse. That "more" is based upon an understanding of psychopathology.

The psychiatric nurse can no more effectively plan and provide psychiatric care without an understanding of psychopathology than the medical-surgical nurse can plan and provide care without an understanding of pathophysiology.

In order to understand pathology of mental disorders, the nurse must read journals that utilize medical terminology. Some nurses have gone to elaborate measures to avoid anything resembling the "medical model." This professional provincialism hampers growth.

The avoidance of a common language and a diagnostic system is not new. In the early days of modern psychiatry (1859) Heinrich Neuman stated that mental health professionals ought "to throw overboard the whole business of classification. There is but one type of mental disturbance, and we call it insanity" (Lehman, 1980). The authors of this book obviously disagree and have included chapters on the following mental disorders using the language of the DSM-IV: schizophrenia, mood disorders, anxiety-related disorders, cognitive disorders, personality disorders, sexual disorders, substance-related disorders, dual diagnosis, and eating disorders.

Critical Thinking Question

The biological vs. psychodynamic argument has gone on for a long time. Why is it important to be open to both points of view? Although you may not have used the same words, you probably had a bias one way or the other before you started nursing school. What was your bias?

Key Concepts

1. According to a National Institute of Mental Health survey, 52 million Americans suffer from some type of mental disorder in any given 12-month period.
2. Anxiety disorders are the most common category of mental disorder, followed by mood disorders (collectively), and alcohol disorders.

3. Understanding psychopathology is fundamental to effective psychotherapeutic management. Understanding psychopathology requires organizing knowledge, operationally defining terms, and developing criteria for diagnosis.
4. Several diagnostic systems have been developed to facilitate the understanding of mental disorders and interprofessional and intraprofessional communication.
5. The *Diagnostic and Statistical Manual,* fourth edition, revised (DSM-IV, [American Psychiatric Association, 1994]) is the official diagnostic system used in American psychiatry and emphasized in this textbook.
6. Etiological explanations of mental disorders can be placed under one of two categories: biological (nature or organic causes) and psychological (nurture, psychodynamic, or functional causes).
7. Guidelines appropriate for all aspects of psychiatric care include supportive care, strengthening self-esteem, preventing failure/embarrassment, treating patients as individuals, reinforcing reality, and handling patients' hostility calmly and matter-of-factly.

Study Questions

(Answer key is in the back of the book.)
1. The most common mental disorders are:
   a. Anxiety disorders
   b. Chemical-dependency disorders
   c. Schizophrenia
   d. Mood disorders
2. Approximately what percentage of the population suffers from schizophrenia in any 12-month period?
   a. 10%
   b. 5%
   c. 1%
   d. 0.5%
3. There are several diagnostic systems available for nurses. The system that is most commonly used in the United States is:
   a. Feighner criteria
   b. Research Diagnostic Criteria (RDC)
   c. DSM-IV
   d. ICD-10
4. Signs and symptoms of mental disorders are criteria used by clinicians to establish a diagnosis. When a patient reports hearing voices, the nurse understands this to be a(n):
   a. Objective sign
   b. Subjective symptom
   c. Diagnostic proof of schizophrenia
   d. All of the above

5. When clinicians debate whether schizophrenia is caused by life experiences or by a dopamine imbalance, they are engaging in which of the following arguments?
   ✓ a. Nature vs. nurture
   ✓ b. Organic vs. functional
   ✓ c. Biological vs. psychodynamic
   (d.) All of the above
6. When psychopathology terms are operationally defined, it facilitates:
   ✓ a. Research
   ✓ b. Dissemination of information
   ✓ c. Interdisciplinary communication
   (d.) All of the above

REFERENCES

American Psychiatric Association: *Diagnostic and statistical manual of mental disorders,* ed 4, Washington, DC, 1994, The Association.

Chapman J: The social safety net in recovery from psychosis: a therapist's story. *Psychiatr Serv* 48(10):1257, 1997.

Deegan PE: Recovering our sense of value after being labeled mentally ill, *J Psychosoc Nurs Ment Health Serv* 31(4):7, 1993.

Dincin J: Ending stigma and discrimination begins at home, *Hosp Community Psychiatry* 44(4):309, 1993.

Feighner JP, et al: Diagnostic criteria for use in psychiatric research, *Arch Gen Psychiatry* 26:57, 1972.

Keltner NL: Psychotherapeutic management: a model for nursing practice, *Perspect Psychiatr Care* 23:125, 1985.

Kessler RC, et al: Lifetime and 12-month prevalence of DSM-III-R psychiatric disorders in the United States, *Arch Gen Psychiatry* 51:8, 1994.

Lehman HE: Schizophrenia: history. In Kaplan HI, et al, editors: *Comprehensive textbook of psychiatry,* Baltimore, 1980, Williams & Wilkins.

Regier DA, et al: The de facto US mental and addictive disorders service system: epidemiologic catchment area prospective 1-year prevalence rates of disorders and services, *Arch Gen Psychiatry* 50:85, 1993.

Riffer NW: It's a brain disease, *Psychiatr Serv* 48(6):773, 1997.

Spitzer RL, Endicott J, and Robins E: *Research diagnostic criteria,* New York, 1975, New York State Psychiatric Institute, Biometrics Research.

CHAPTER 27

Schizophrenia and Other Psychoses

NORMAN L. KELTNER

LEARNING OBJECTIVES

After reading this chapter you should be able to:
- Define the term *schizophrenia.*
- Describe the major historical figures, events, and theories that have contributed to the current understanding of schizophrenia.
- Identify Bleuler's four A's.
- Recognize DSM-IV criteria and terminology for schizophrenia.
- Differentiate and describe DSM-IV subtypes, and type I and type II subtypes.
- Recognize and describe objective and subjective symptoms of schizophrenia.

- Identify biological explanations for schizophrenia.
- Describe two theoretical psychodynamic explanations for schizophrenia.
- Develop a nursing care plan for patients with schizophrenia.
- Identify the major drugs used in the treatment of schizophrenia, their mechanism of action, their target symptoms, and their major side effects.
- Evaluate the effectiveness of nursing interventions for patients with schizophrenia.

"There are three inescapable 'facts' about schizophrenia that should be taken into account by any effort to explain it: first, the very high probability that it will become clinically apparent in late adolescence or early adulthood; second, the role of 'stress' in onset and relapse; and third, the therapeutic efficacy of neuroleptic drugs." (Weinberger, 1987, p. 660)

Psychosis is a disruptive mental state in which an individual struggles to distinguish the external world from his internally generated perceptions. This state is complicated by an impaired ability to relate to others. Common symptoms of psychosis include hallucinations, delusions, and difficulty with thought organization. Psychosis can be present in schizophrenia, acute mania, depression, drug intoxication, dementia, and delirium. **Schizophrenia** is one of the most common causes of psychosis.

SCHIZOPHRENIA

While many laypersons are quite sophisticated medically, it is not uncommon to hear the word *schizophrenia* defined as "split personality." By "split

KEY TERMS

Ambivalence   Simultaneous opposite feelings (e.g., love and hate); often expressed as approach-avoidance behavior

Anergia   Absence of energy

Anhedonia   The inability to experience pleasure

Apathy   Lack of feeling, concern, interest, or emotion

Autism   Preoccupation with the self with little concern for external reality; a self-made private world of the schizophrenic

Avolition   Lack of motivation

Blocking   Interruption of thoughts due to psychological factors

Catatonia   Immobility due to psychological causes

Clanging associations   Use of rhyming words

Concrete thinking   The use of literal meaning without the ability to consider abstract meaning (e.g., "Don't cry over spilt milk" might be interpreted as "because the milk is dirty")

Delusions   Fixed, false beliefs of importance to the individual that are resistant to reason or fact

Double-bind   Conflicting demands by significant individuals in a patient's life; unable to meet both demands, the patient is doomed to fail

Echolalia   Repetition of words heard

Echopraxia   Repetitive, meaningless movement

Hallucinations   A false sensory perception unrelated to external stimuli (e.g., seeing things that are not there)

Hebephrenia   An outdated schizophrenic subtype characterized by silliness, delusions, hallucinations, and regression

Ideas of reference   The belief that some events have a special meaning (e.g., people laughing near the patient are perceived as laughing at the patient)

Illusion   Misinterpretation of a real sensory stimulus

Loose association   Thinking characterized by speech in which ideas shift from one subject to another that is unrelated

Mutism   Refusal to speak

Negativism   Motiveless resistance to all instruction

Neologism   A word or expression invented by the patient

Paranoia   Extreme suspiciousness of others and their actions

Premorbid   The state before the onset of a disorder

Psychosis   The inability to recognize reality, complicated by a severe thought disorder and the inability to relate to others

Religiosity   Preoccupation with religious ideas or content

Stereotypy   Persistent repetition of senseless acts or words

Withdrawal   Behaviors designed to avoid interacting with others

Word salad   Randomized set of words without logical connection

---

personality" they mean something akin to a Jekyll and Hyde experience or a multiple personality disorder. This popular depiction does not begin to portray schizophrenia. Schizophrenia is not characterized by a changing personality; it is characterized by a deteriorating personality. Therefore, this popular notion of a dramatic personality change comes far short of capturing the devastating effect schizophrenia has on the life of a person and the person's family. Simply, schizophrenia is one of the most profoundly disabling illnesses, mental or physical, the nurse will ever encounter.

Schizophrenia is a diagnostic term used by mental health professionals to describe a major psychotic disorder. It is characterized by disturbances in thought and sensory perception (e.g., hallucinations, delusions), thought disorders, and by a deterioration in psychosocial functioning. Schizophrenia typically first appears in late adolescence or early adulthood. It affects men and women almost equally, though men usually have an earlier age of onset by about 4 to 6 years, and new onset schizophrenia after age 50 is almost always seen in women (MV Seeman, 1995). It is known that approximately 1% of the population will experience schizophrenia during their lifetime. Though the prevalence rate and symptom presentation for schizophrenia are fairly constant worldwide, inner-city residents, those from lower socioeconomic classes, and individuals who experience difficulties in utero (e.g., mother with influenza) are more likely to be affected and/or diagnosed (American Psychiatric Association [APA], 1997). Economic costs are in the tens of billions of dollars each year (Rice, Kelman, and Miller, 1992;

Twelve-Month Prevalence Rate of Mental Disorders in the United States

Diagnosis	Percentage of Population over 17 Years of Age	Number of Persons
Anxiety disorders	12.6	20,034,000
Phobia disorders*	10.9	17,331,000
Mood disorders	9.5	15,143,000
Alcohol disorders	7.4	11,766,000
Major depression†	5.0	7,950,000
Drug disorders	3.1	4,929,000
Cognitive impairment	2.7	4,293,000
Obsessive-compulsive disorder	2.1	3,339,000
Antisocial disorder	1.5	2,385,000
Panic disorders*	1.3	2,067,000
Bipolar disorder†	1.2	1,908,000
Schizophrenia	**1.1**	**1,749,000**
Somatization	0.2	365,000

From Regier DA, et al: The deFacto US mental and addictive disorders service system: epidemiologic catchment area prospective 1-year prevalence rates of disorders and services, *Arch Gen Psychiatry* 50:85, 1993.
*Also calculated in anxiety statistics.
†Also calculated in mood disorders statistics.

Sex-Based Differences in Schizophrenia

1. Women have later onset of schizophrenia.
2. Women have a less severe course of illness.
3. Women are prescribed 60% of all antipsychotic drugs.
4. Thirty percent of all antipsychotics are prescribed to women during childbearing years (20 to 50).
5. Dopamine receptor decline is slower in women.
6. Women have less cerebral lateralization (may confer greater brain resilience).
7. Women tend to have more positive symptoms and fewer negative symptoms compared to men.
8. Estrogen modulates dopaminergic functions and may play a protective role for women.
9. Women have fewer structural brain abnormalities.
10. Women have a better response to lower doses of conventional antipsychotic drugs.

Adapted from Promedica Research Center: *Women and schizophrenia*, Tucker, Ga, 1997, The Promedica Research Center; Lilly Center for Women's Health: *Sex-based differences in antipsychotic therapy*, Chicago, 1997, The Center.

Wyatt, et al, 1995). The cost in human suffering is incalculable. Box 27-1 outlines the statistical realities of schizophrenia.

Morel was the first to name the psychiatric symptoms of schizophrenia. In 1856, while treating an adolescent boy, he used the phrase *dementia praecox* (precocious senility) to describe the group of symptoms he observed. Kahlbaum (in 1868) and Hecker (in 1870) added to the psychiatric nomenclature with their diagnostic categories *catatonia* and *hebephrenia*, respectively. Kraepelin (1902) added the term *paranoia* and engaged in a rigorous study of what we now call schizophrenia. He found commonalities among these three mental disorders (catatonia, hebephrenia, and paranoia) and, in 1896, grouped them under the diagnostic term that Morel had coined 40 years before, *dementia praecox*. Kraepelin believed that schizophrenia was the result of neuropathology; he envisioned a progressive deteriorating course resulting in disabling mental impairment with little hope of recovery.

It was left to Bleuler in the early 1900s to coin the term *schizophrenia* in a book subtitled "The Group of Schizophrenias." Bleuler believed that schizophrenia does not always follow a course of deterioration (so *dementia* was inappropriate), nor does it always occur early in life (hence, *praecox* was inappropriate). Bleuler broadened Kraepelin's concept by focusing on symptoms rather than on outcomes (Harding, Zubin, and Strauss, 1987). Bleuler identified four primary symptoms that he believed were present in all persons with schizophrenia. All of these classic symptoms begin with the letter "A," which facilitates memorization (Box 27-2).

Adapted from News in mental health nursing, *J Psychosoc Nurs* 35(2):6, 1997; American Psychiatric Association: Practice guidelines for the treatment of patients with schizophrenia, *Am J Psychiatry* 154(4, Supplement):1, 1997.

Box 27-1 Epidemiology of Schizophrenia

1. 1% of the population suffers from schizophrenia.
2. For 95% of sufferers, the disease lasts a lifetime.
3. 75% of taxpayer mental illness expenditures are for schizophrenia.
4. Individuals with schizophrenia occupy 25% of inpatient hospital beds.
5. Approximately one third of all homeless Americans suffer from schizophrenia.
6. 15% of individuals with schizophrenia do not respond to traditional antipsychotic medications, and 70% are only partial responders.
7. 50% experience serious side effects to medications.
8. Unemployment rates reach 70% to 80%, and schizophrenic individuals constitute 10% of all people classified as permanently disabled.
9. Direct health care costs are 2.5% of total health care expenditures.
10. Indirect costs are estimated at $46 billion.
11. 20% to 50% of these individuals attempt suicide, and 10% are successful in killing themselves.
12. Schizophrenic individuals have a 20% shorter life expectancy.

Box 27-2 Bleuler's Four A's

- **Affective disturbance:** inappropriate, blunted, or flattened affect
- **Autism:** preoccupation with the self with little concern for external reality
- **Associative looseness:** the stringing together of unrelated topics
- **Ambivalence:** simultaneous opposite feelings

In recent years, a resurgence of interest in biological research has resulted in renewed respect for Kraepelin's work. In fact, Kraepelin's term *dementia praecox* is again used by some clinicians to provoke powerful images of the deteriorative course associated with approximately 10% of the schizophrenic population (Kopelowicz and Bidder, 1992). Bleuler's work has not enjoyed the same level of regard. His contributions have been viewed as a "softening of the diagnostic criteria" that have served to obscure the deteriorating course of the illness and has led to overdiagnosis. Freud, the father of psychodynamic theories and much better known than Bleuler, cannot escape his critics even in death. Recent works criticizing his psychodynamic models have gone so far as to call him a liar and a fraud (Gray, 1993).

Critical Thinking Question

Why do you think Kraepelin was so pessimistic about the patients he saw with dementia praecox?

DSM-IV TERMINOLOGY AND CRITERIA

The DSM-IV criteria for schizophrenia are found in the box on p. 354. Since the inception of schizophrenia as a diagnostic entity, attempts have been made to divide it into homogeneous subtypes (Kendler, Gruenberg, and Tsuang, 1988). Early attempts to identify homogeneous groups resulted in the subtypes *catatonia, hebephrenia,* and *paranoia.* Bleuler later added *simple* schizophrenia to the nomenclature. This early thinking is still reflected in official diagnostic classifications. The DSM-IV identifies five subtypes of schizophrenia: *paranoid, disorganized, catatonic, undifferentiated,* and *residual* (see the box on p. 354). NANDA nursing diagnoses and the

These two giants of psychiatric history founded two divergent views of schizophrenia. Kraepelin, in using the diagnostic category of dementia praecox, revealed a conceptual alignment between schizophrenia and disorders such as Alzheimer's disease, which have a less optimistic prognosis.

Bleuler, on the other hand, developed a school of thought that was much broader and more optimistic. On the basis of Bleuler's wider grouping, pessimism eased, and some clinicians began to see improvements in their patients. While Kraepelin based his views on biology, Bleuler, influenced by the master analyst Freud and other psychodynamic theorists, sought psychological explanations for schizophrenia. For most of the twentieth century, Freud's psychoanalytic explanations, and by extension, Bleuler's thinking, dominated the understanding of schizophrenia. However, as the limitations of talking cures became more evident, the psychodynamic approach began to lose its grip on mental health professionals.

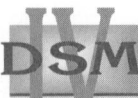

DSM-IV Criteria for Schizophrenia

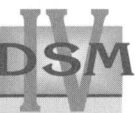

A. Characteristic symptoms (at least two of the following):
  - Delusions
  - Hallucinations
  - Disorganized speech
  - Grossly disorganized or catatonic behavior
  - Negative symptoms

B. Social/occupational dysfunction: work, interpersonal, and self-care functioning is below the level achieved prior to onset

C. Duration: continuous signs of the disturbance for at least 6 months

D. Schizoaffective and mood disorders are not present and are not responsible for the signs and symptoms

E. Not caused by substance abuse or a general medical disorder

Adapted from the American Psychiatric Association: *Diagnostic and statistical manual of mental disorders,* ed 4, Washington, DC, 1994, The Association.

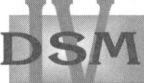

DSM-IV Criteria for Schizophrenic Subtypes

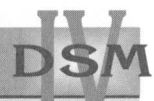

PARANOID: A. Preoccupation with one or more delusions or frequent auditory hallucinations

B. None of the following is prominent: disorganized speech, disorganized behavior, flat or inappropriate affect, catatonic behavior

DISORGANIZED: A. All of the following are prominent: disorganized speech, disorganized behavior, flat or inappropriate affect

B. Does not meet criteria of catatonic type

CATATONIC: At least two of the following are present:

A. Motoric immobility, waxy flexibility, or stupor

B. Excessive motor activity (purposeless)

C. Extreme negativism or mutism

D. Peculiar movements stereotypy of movements, prominent mannerisms, or prominent grimacing

E. Echolalia or echopraxia

UNDIFFERENTIATED: Characteristic symptoms (see box above, criterion A) are present, but criteria for paranoid, catatonic, or disorganized subtypes are not met.

RESIDUAL: A. Characteristic symptoms (criterion A) are no longer present; criteria are unmet for paranoid, catatonic, or disorganized subtypes

B. There is continuing evidence of disturbance, such as the presence of negative symptoms or criterion A symptoms, in an attenuated form (e.g., odd beliefs, unusual perceptual experiences)

Adapted from the American Psychiatric Association: *Diagnostic and statistical manual of mental disorders,* ed 4, Washington, DC, 1994, The Association.

DSM-IV diagnoses related to schizophrenia are listed in the box on p. 355.

Clinical dichotomies were developed over the years as clinicians and researchers attempted to conceptualize better patient groupings. Patients were categorized in an "either/or" fashion, based on onset (acute or insidious), psychological mechanism (reactive or process), prognosis (good or poor), course (acute or chronic), and, most recently,

symptoms (positive or negative) (Kopelowicz and Bidder, 1992).

The authors find the subtyping approach based on positive or negative symptoms most promising because it fits with their clinical observations and can be predictive of medication response. In reality, however, positive vs. negative subtyping is merely another convenient way for the professional to grasp this broad, heterogeneous phenomenon. Most pa-

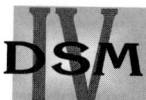 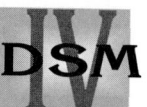

DSM-IV and NANDA Diagnoses Related to Schizophrenia and Other Psychoses

DSM-IV*

Schizophrenia
  Paranoid type
  Disorganized type
  Catatonic type
  Undifferentiated type
  Residual type
Schizophreniform disorder
Schizoaffective disorder
Delusional disorder
Brief psychotic disorder
Shared psychotic disorder

NANDA†

Adjustment, impaired
Anxiety
Communication, impaired verbal
Coping, family potential for growth
Coping, ineffective family compromised
Coping, ineffective individual
Personal identity disturbance
Role performance, altered
Self-care deficit (bathing/hygiene, dressing/grooming)
Self-esteem disturbance
Sensory/perceptual alterations (specify)
Social interaction, impaired
Social isolation
Thought processes, altered
Caregiver role, strained

*American Psychiatric Association: *Diagnostic and statistical manual of mental disorders,* ed 4, Washington, DC, 1994, The Association.
†North American Nursing Diagnosis Association: *NANDA nursing diagnoses: definitions and classifications 1997-1998,* Philadelphia, 1997, The Association.

tients are not either/or, but have a mixture of positive and negative symptoms (Breslin, 1992). This paradigm (positive vs. negative) was first advanced by Strauss, et al (1974) and refined by biologically oriented diagnosticians, such as Andreasen (1982; Andreasen and Olsen, 1982) and Crow (1982), based on clinical findings. Recently a third category, *disorganized,* has been added because careful analysis differentiated it from positive schizophrenia (APA, 1997). Disorganized schizophrenia is characterized by disorganized speech, disorganized behavior, and poor attention (APA).

Positive, or type I, schizophrenia has a different constellation of symptoms than negative, or type II, schizophrenia (Box 27-3). Type I is positive in the sense that symptoms are an embellishment of normal cognition and perception. The symptoms are "additional." Positive symptoms are believed to be caused by a subcortical dopaminergic process (too much dopamine) affecting cortical areas.

CLINICAL EXAMPLE

John is sitting in the dayroom on the psychiatric unit when his eyes begin to dart back and forth and he becomes increasingly anxious. You ask,

"John, are you hearing something that I cannot hear?" "Can't you hear them?" he replies. "They are going to get me." John's auditory hallucination is a positive symptom because it is an exaggeration of a normal perception (he is "hearing" without an auditory stimulus).

Type II is labeled negative because symptoms are essentially an absence or diminution of what should be; that is, lack of affect, lack of energy, and so on. Type II may be a hypodopaminergic process and also caused by cortical structural changes (e.g., cerebral atrophy). Pathoanatomy consistently mentioned in the literature includes decreased cerebral blood flow (CBF), particularly in frontal areas, and increased ventricular brain ratios (VBRs). Decreased frontal blood flow and a hypometabolic state are most pronounced in the dorsolateral prefrontal cortex. Ventricular enlargement can be detected on computed tomography (CT) and magnetic resonance imaging (MRI) film with the naked eye. Other pathoanatomical features observed in some studies that could contribute to negative symptoms include a reduction in brain weight by 5%, a slight decrease in brain length, and neuronal loss in some cortical areas (Roberts, Leigh, and Weinberger, 1993).

Box 27-3　Positive and Negative Symptoms of Schizophrenia

Symptom Category	Symptoms
Positive (Type I) Prognosis: good Precipitating factors: yes Onset: acute Sensorium: dreamlike quality Intellectual impairment: none Pathophysiology: D_2 hyperactivity Pathoanatomy: VBRs normal Response to typical neuroleptics: good Effect of levodopa: increases symptoms	Abnormal thought form Agitation, tension Associational disturbances Bizarre behavior Conceptual disorganization Delusions Excitement Feelings of persecution Grandiosity Hallucinations Hostility Ideas of reference Illusions Insomnia Suspiciousness
Negative (Type II) Prognosis: poor Onset: chronic Family history: more than type I Sensorium: clear Intellectual impairment: yes Pathophysiology: possibly hypodopaminergic, decreased CBF Pathoanatomy: increased VBRs, other changes (see text) Response to typical neuroleptics: varies Response to atypical neuroleptics: good Effect of levodopa: minimal	Alogia Anergia Anhedonia Asocial behavior Attention deficits Avolition Blunted affect Communication difficulties Difficulty with abstractions Passive social withdrawal Poor grooming and hygiene Poor rapport Poverty of speech

From Harris D, Keltner NL: Medication management. In Worley NK, editor: Mental health in the community, St. Louis, 1997, Mosby.

CLINICAL EXAMPLE

Phillip Wilson has a long history of mental problems. He was first diagnosed with schizophrenia in 1963. Mr. Wilson is a patient in the state hospital system. The summary note written by the nursing team leader includes the following observation: "Mr. Wilson is isolative and, for the most part, expressionless. He spends long hours sitting and staring out of the window. Attempts to engage Mr. Wilson in unit activities have not been successful."

An unfortunate side effect of the positive vs. negative subtyping approach has been the tendency by a few professionals to be too pessimistic about the prognosis of type II patients. The outcome of negative schizophrenia is not invariably poor (Soni, et al, 1992). Kopelowicz and Bidder (1992) caution nurses and others against such rash and uninformed thinking. They divide negative symptoms into primary and secondary. The secondary symptoms are therapeutically accessible, particularly early in the course of the illness. These symptoms arise from some of the consequences of a schizophrenic diagnosis: medications, hospitalizations, loss of social supports, and a socioeconomic decline. If assessed early, secondary negative symptoms can be arrested.

Box 27-4   Evolution of Schizophrenic Subtyping

1856   Morel coins the term *dementia praecox*.

1868   Kahlbaum uses the term *catatonia* to describe patients immobilized by psychological factors.

1870   Hecker uses the term *hebephrenia* to describe patients with silly, bizarre, and regressed behaviors.

1896   Kraepelin adds the term *paranoia* to describe highly suspicious patients. He recognizes commonalities among catatonic, hebephrenic, and paranoid individuals. He groups all three categories under the heading *dementia praecox*.

1900s   Bleuler introduces the term *schizophrenia* to describe these mental disorders. He adds the subtype *simple schizophrenia*.

1952   DSM-I: The DSM-I is the first attempt to develop a diagnostic manual for nationwide use. It includes nine subtypes: simple, hebephrenic, catatonic, paranoid, acute undifferentiated, chronic undifferentiated, schizoaffective, childhood, and residual.

1968   DSM-II: The DSM-II is developed in an effort to articulate more efficiently a common diagnostic language. It has a total of 11 subtypes, changing acute undifferentiated to acute schizophrenia, and adding latent schizophrenia and schizophrenia of an unspecified type.

1980   DSM-III: The authors streamline the diagnostic subtypes to five: disorganized, catatonic, paranoid, undifferentiated, and residual.

1982   Andreasen, Crow, and others suggest a new subtyping approach. They categorize schizophrenia, based on symptoms, into positive (type I) and negative (type II).

1987   DSM-III: Revised; same subtypes

1994   DSM-IV: same subtypes as DSM-III

1997   The APA practice guidelines on treating patients with schizophrenia recognizes the addition of the subtype "disorganized" to the positive and negative subtyping concept.

CLINICAL EXAMPLE

Merritt Burgone is a homeless man with a long history of mental illness. He has not seen his family in many years. Although his family was supportive at one time, they simply grew tired of trying to cope with Mr. Burgone. At this point, even modest improvements in his mental health are compromised by his lack of social support.

According to biological theory, typical antipsychotic drugs (drugs that primarily antagonize dopamine D_2 receptors) are likely to be beneficial for positive symptoms because positive schizophrenia is a hyperdopaminergic process (see Box 27-3). Negative schizophrenia, on the other hand, is thought to be more structurally related and possibly a hypodopaminergic process. Dopamine antagonists (i.e., traditional antipsychotics) have relatively less effect and may actually cause the negative symptoms to worsen. Accordingly, the more florid the psychotic symptoms (as in positive schizophrenia), the greater the likelihood of a favorable response to antipsychotics. As was noted in Chapter 20, atypical antipsychotic drugs such as clozapine (Clozaril), risperidone (Risperdal), olanzapine (Zyprexa), and quetiapine (Seroquel) benefit negative symptoms,

apparently because they affect different dopamine receptors. Further, these drugs also antagonize serotonin receptors, which theoretically liberates dopamine in cortical areas "correcting" the hypodopaminergic state. Unfortunately, some of these newer drugs are so expensive that some health maintenance organizations (HMOs) and governments are refusing to pay for them. For example, a 30-day supply of Risperdal costs $240, whereas the same amount of Haldol costs only $2.50 (News, 1997). Box 27-4 provides an overview of the evolution of schizophrenic subtyping.

As is true of all fields, there are special psychiatric terms one must know to communicate effectively with nurses and other professionals. A list of these key terms is provided at the beginning of the chapter.

BEHAVIOR

"My identity began to fragment and seemed to blend with my environment. Rather than just enjoying the wind, for instance, I thought I had merged with it. I had to stare at the sun to appreciate its warmth. Yet gradually I was able to see myself separate from those things. As I neared discharge, I began to feel some stirring of belief in myself.

It was not until much later that I made a conscious effort to develop a sense of control, realizing that I had the power to decide what form my life would take and who I would be." (Leete, 1987)

People who are treated for mental problems come to the attention of mental health professionals in one of two ways. The first way is when patients seek help. Patients who seek help do so because they have experienced such troubling *subjective symptoms* that they want professional intervention. Often, professional help is not sought until patients have exhausted self-help aids, friends, and family. The second way in which people come to the attention of the mental health system is by drawing attention to themselves through behavior that bothers, concerns, or frightens other people. These indicators of a mental disorder are apparent to others and are called *objective signs*. As discussed in the chapter on legal issues, sometimes help is resisted, and the person must be treated on an involuntary basis.

Subjective and objective categories are not as discrete as they may appear at first. Hallucinations, for example, are a subjective phenomenon, but easily may cause objective signs that get the attention of others (e.g., a person who talks back to an auditory hallucination). Nonetheless, dividing the expressions of schizophrenia into subjective symptoms and objective signs is a rational and convenient approach to understanding this mental disorder.

Six significant "alterations" occur in schizophrenia and can be grouped into objective signs or subjective symptoms (Box 27-5). *Alterations in personal relationships* and *alterations of activity* are highly visible to others (objective signs), whereas *altered perception, alterations of thought, altered consciousness,* and *alterations of affect* are more subjective in nature.

Objective Signs

Alterations in personal relationships

Patients with schizophrenia often have altered interpersonal relationships that become apparent to the psychiatric nurses who treat them. Alterations in per-

---

Box 27-5 Objective and Subjective Behavioral Disorders in Schizophrenia

Objective Signs

Alterations in personal relationships
- Decreased attention to appearance and social amenities related to introspection and autism
- Inadequate or inappropriate communication
- Hostility
- Withdrawal

Alterations of activity
- Psychomotor agitation
- Catatonic rigidity
- Echopraxia (repetitive movements)
- Stereotypy (see Key Terms)

Subjective Symptoms

Altered perception
- Hallucinations
- Illusions
- Paranoid thinking

Alterations of thought
- Flight of ideas
- Retardation

- Blocking
- Autism
- Ambivalence
- Loose associations
- Delusions
- Poverty of speech
- Ideas of reference
- Mutism

Altered consciousness
- Confusion
- Incoherent speech
- Clouding
- Sense of "going crazy"

Alterations of affect
- Inappropriate, blunted, flattened, or labile affect
- Apathy
- Ambivalence
- Overreaction
- Anhedonia

sonal relationships take several forms. Often, these problems develop over a long period, well before schizophrenia is diagnosed, and become more pronounced as the illness progresses.

It is not uncommon to hear that a person was asocial, a loner, or a social "misfit" premorbidly.

Frequently, patients become less concerned with their appearance and may not bathe without persistent prodding. Table manners and other social skills may diminish to the point where patients are disgusting to others. These behaviors are related to introspection (autism) and extreme self-absorption. Patients are so focused on internal processes that their external social world collapses. Schizophrenia can cause a diminished energy level (anergia), which also complicates social interactions.

Interpersonal communication becomes inadequate and may be inappropriate. Again, internal processes are at work. Hostility, a somewhat common theme, also distances patients from others. Finally, patients with schizophrenia withdraw, further compromising their abilities to engage in meaningful social interactions.

Alterations of activity

Patients with schizophrenia also display alterations of activity. They may be too active (psychomotor agitation); that is, they are unable to sit still and continually pace, or they may be inactive or catatonic. These signs respond to antipsychotic drugs.

Clinical application: The nurse must be careful in assessing alterations in activity. Restlessness may be caused by akathisia (an extrapyramidal side effect [EPSE] of antipsychotic drugs) and be unrelated to schizophrenia. Rigidity, on the other hand, could be a warning sign of neuroleptic malignant syndrome (NMS), not catatonia. Both EPSEs and NMS are side effects of antipsychotic drugs. Hence accurate assessment is critical: though it is appropriate to administer a prn dose of haloperidol for psychomotor agitation or catatonia, it only serves to intensify akathisia and could prove fatal for patients with NMS.

Subjective Symptoms

Subjective symptoms are, by definition, experienced by patients in a personal way. Patients may hide these symptoms from others. For example, if a pa-

tient suffers from the delusion that he is a famous person, he may be able to keep it to himself. In fact, some clinicians advise patients who resist psychiatric care to "keep your symptoms to yourself, and no one will ever know." Presumably there are persons in society who are not reporting their subjective symptoms to anyone and thus are avoiding psychiatric intervention. For the most part, however, subjective symptoms of schizophrenia spill over into behavior that is noticeable to others. Subjective symptoms can be grouped into the four categories previously mentioned.

Altered perception

Altered perception includes hallucinations, illusions, and paranoid thinking. Hallucinations are false sensory perceptions. They can be auditory, visual, olfactory, tactile, gustatory, or somatic (strange body sensations). Auditory hallucinations are the most common in schizophrenia and often take the form of accusations ("You slut," "Hey, queer") or commands ("Get away from these people"). Visual hallucinations are not as common in schizophrenia. The nurse may suspect a toxic process (drugs, fever) if visual hallucinations are present. Hallucinations are probably caused by a hyperdopaminergic state in the limbic areas.

Illusions are misinterpretations of real external stimuli. For example, a tree might be mistaken for a threatening person. Illusions are often associated with physical illness, as well as schizophrenia.

CLINICAL EXAMPLE

Delirium: While lying in bed with a low-grade temperature, Gladys, a 68-year-old-woman, asked, "Are those cobwebs on the wall?" Her son responded, "No, Mama, those are just shadows from your bedside lamp." Gladys laughed and said, "I guess my mind is going."

CLINICAL EXAMPLE

Schizophrenia: Tim, a patient on the psychiatric unit, mistakes a slipper under his bed for a rat.

Paranoid thinking is manifested by a persistent interpretation of the actions of others as threatening or demeaning. Paranoid themes can color delusions and hallucinations, as well as the ordinary behavior of others. It is important for the student to differentiate paranoid thinking associated with a paranoid personality disorder from paranoid delusions. Paranoid thinking is less severe than paranoid delusions. Paranoid thinking may be "corrected" with facts, whereas paranoid delusions are not.

CLINICAL EXAMPLE

Paranoid Personality: Bill, a voluntary patient on the adult unit, sought help because of trouble on the job and at home. His ability to get along with people has deteriorated to the point where he has no friends. Bill's wife has started divorce proceedings, and he has sought treatment, hoping that she will change her mind. Over the past few years, Bill has been obsessed with the thought that his wife is cheating on him. He follows her when she leaves the house, sometimes listens to her phone calls, and has confronted her with accusations of infidelity. Whenever he finds he is mistaken, he is relieved for a while and apologizes for not trusting her, but soon he begins to have the same paranoid thoughts. His paranoid thinking has caused alterations in his personal relationships.

CLINICAL EXAMPLE

Paranoid Schizophrenia: Fred is a 28-year-old, unemployed laborer. He was recently brought to the emergency department by the police. Fred had been at the downtown bus station preaching loudly to all who passed. He spoke of a conspiracy of blacks and Jews who plan to take over America. Fred told the emergency room nurse that he feared for his life. He went on to explain that he had proof that the FBI was behind President Kennedy's assassination.

A final example of altered perception is based on the observation that the ability to adapt perceptually (or attend selectively) is altered in patients with schizophrenia.

CLINICAL EXAMPLE

A patient was looking out of a seventh-floor window. The nurse approached to look and noticed activity in the yard below. The nurse assumed that the patient was observing the same activity and commented. The patient, however, was not looking beyond the wire mesh screen in the window. He was unable to filter out what for most people would not be a distraction. The inability to filter out extraneous stimuli (ability to attend selectively) is a perceptual problem for some patients.

Alterations of thought

Alterations of thought are common in schizophrenia and are disturbing and frightening at times. Antipsychotic drugs are often beneficial. Often, insomnia diminishes as these symptoms subside, indicating that insomnia may be a secondary symptom. Common thought disorders include flight of ideas, thought retardation, blocking, autism, ambivalence, loose associations, delusions, poverty of speech, and concrete thinking.

Flight of ideas is a rapid process where patients' thoughts are fragmented and move from one unconnected topic to another, stimulated by either external or internal processes. Related phenomena include clanging (rhyming) and punning.

Retardation is a slowing of mental activity. A patient may state, "I just can't think."

Blocking is the interruption of a thought and the inability to recall it. This is very disturbing to patients and, at times, frightening. Blocking may be caused by the intrusion of hallucinations, delusions, or emotional factors. The following is a common example of blocking that could happen to anyone.

CLINICAL EXAMPLE

Joe, a 49-year-old teacher, was in the middle of a lecture when he lost his "train of thought." He could not remember what point he was developing or where to go next. He stalled for time, realizing that he was in a potentially embarrassing situation. Finally, he found his notes and proceeded, a little shaken and distracted, but able to continue.

Autism occurs when patients are so introspective that they are distracted from external events. Patients are preoccupied with themselves and may be oblivious to the reality around them. This results in a personalized view of reality.

Ambivalence is a state in which two opposite, strong feelings exist simultaneously. Patients may be both attracted to and repelled by a person, object, or goal. Ambivalence (e.g., love-hate) toward a domineering parent is common. Another common example is the simultaneous need for and fear of people, resulting in immobilization. Schizophrenic patients may be immobilized by their ambivalence regarding a matter as simple as deciding whether to drink orange juice or apple juice for breakfast. In such cases, it is therapeutic for the nurse to make decisions for patients if the patients will allow this. The following clinical example illustrates ambivalence that occurs in some families and is not meant to depict schizophrenic ambivalence.

CLINICAL EXAMPLE

Joyce, a 38-year-old librarian, has ambivalent feelings toward her father. He still tells her what to do, and she has a hard time standing up for herself. Joyce realizes that her periodic need for financial assistance is partially responsible for her predicament. She finds that she avoids calling her father and, because he calls her excessively to find out what she is doing, she cringes when the phone rings. Although Joyce is not suffering from schizophrenia, she does experience ambivalence. She loves her father but, in her words, "He is driving me crazy."

Loose association is the stringing together of unrelated topics with a vague connection (as opposed to flight of ideas, in which there is no connection). For example, the children's rhyme "Mary had a little lamb" may lead to "Mary was the mother of Christ who was born in a manger. I hate to lie on straw. It makes my skin itch. Have you ever had poison ivy? I have." The patient may even leave out some of the phrases; for example, "Mary had a little lamb. I hate to lie on straw. Have you ever had poison ivy?" but may be able to clarify the connections if asked.

Delusions are fixed, false beliefs and can take many forms. Delusions are described as fixed beliefs because they cannot be changed by logical persuasion. They are described as false because they are not based in reality. Delusional content often relates to life experiences and can include somatic, grandiose, religious, nihilistic, referential, and paranoid content. An example of each type follows:

- *Somatic delusions:* A patient, after medical tests confirm otherwise, still insists, "I have cancer in my stomach."
- *Grandiose delusions:* A patient states, "I am Napoleon."

- *Religious delusions:* A woman attempts to kill her children because she believes the devil wants her to do so: "The devil told me to kill my children."
- *Nihilistic delusions:* A patient states, "I am dead." In response to "If you are dead, how can you talk?" the patient says, "I don't know, but I'm dead."
- *Delusions of reference:* "The TV is talking about me. The guests on 'Oprah' are making fun of me."
- *Delusions of influence:* "I can control her with my thoughts."
- *Paranoid delusions:* "They all think that I am a homosexual."

Related phenomena sometimes found are the schizophrenic delusions that thoughts can be inserted or withdrawn by others: "Other people can read my mind"; "My thoughts are being broadcast so that everyone can hear."

Poverty of speech is manifested by the inability to formulate and articulate thoughts that are relevant to the discussion at hand. Vocabulary is markedly limited in individuals who experience poverty of speech.

Concrete thinking is the inability to conceptualize the meanings of words and phrases. For example, a concrete response to the proverb "People who live in glass houses should not throw stones" might be construed as "The glass would break." Such persons are likely to misinterpret jokes or similes. For example, the meanings of "a diamond in the rough" or "cool as a cucumber" may be lost completely on a person exhibiting concrete thinking.

Altered consciousness

Altered consciousness is perhaps the symptom that is most troubling to patients; fortunately, it is also the most responsive to antipsychotic drugs. Manifestations of altered consciousness include confusion, incoherent speech, clouding, and a sense of "going crazy." The last manifestation of altered consciousness, "going crazy," deserves special mention. Many students are surprised when they enter a psychiatric unit to find that patients are not "crazy." In fact, although by definition psychiatric patients are struggling with mental disorders, psychiatric units are not wild, bizarre environments. Patients can readily differentiate between the "normal struggle" of dealing with a mental disorder and the feeling of "going crazy" (loss of control). The student will observe that patients on the psychiatric unit define a fellow patient who has become "wild" or who is loudly talking to himself or herself as "crazy." In other words, this behavior is unusual—even on a psychiatric unit. Referring to the discussion of incompetence in Chapter 4, the student can appreciate why the designation of "incompetence" is reserved for only a few individuals.

Alterations of affect

Alterations of affect are varied and include inappropriate, flattened, blunted, or labile affects; apathy; ambivalence; and overreaction. For example, responding to bad news with laughter is an affective response that does not match the circumstances and is *inappropriate*. If a patient is unable to generate much affect, and the response to the bad news is weakly appropriate, the **affect** is *blunted* or *dull*. The inability to generate any affective response is referred to as *flattened affect*. *Labile affect* is a condition in which emotional tone changes quickly. A patient may be telling a happy story, suddenly begin to cry, and then quickly return to a happy disposition.

Apathy can be defined as a lack of concern or interest. It is the inability to generate a normal response to people, situations, or the environment.

Ambivalence, discussed earlier, is a condition in which patients are immobilized by the coexistence of opposite feelings. The immobilization can lead to an affective expression that approaches indifference or indecision.

Another alteration of affect is the tendency to **overreact** to events. An analogy is the small child who must put so much energy into closing a car door that the door slams shut, offending the ears and "nerves" of adults nearby. Because of physical limitations, the child has to push as hard as possible to overcome inertia. Because of emotional limitations, schizophrenic patients overreact to normal events to overcome mental and social inertia. And, like the child, these patients may offend the sensitivities of those nearby.

ETIOLOGY

Many authorities suggest that multiple factors must cause schizophrenia, because no single theory satis-

factorily explains the disorder. Explanations can be categorized broadly into biological or psychological (psychodynamic) causes. These two categories parallel the "nature vs. nurture" debate discussed in Chapter 26. Biological theories and psychodynamic theories are discussed here, followed by a vulnerability-stress model, an eclectic approach that seems to capture the major forces at work in the genesis and outcomes of schizophrenia.

Biological Theories

Biological theorists posit that schizophrenia is caused by anatomical or physiological abnormalities. Biological explanations include biochemical, neurostructural, genetic, perinatal risk factors, and other theories. Biological explanations have driven the development of biological interventions, such as psychotropic drugs and somatic therapies.

Some clinicians have been reluctant to endorse biological theories because the exclusive use of biological approaches, such as psychotropic and somatic therapies, excludes interpersonal factors. The psychotherapeutic management model, however, recognizes the importance of both biological and interpersonal interventions.

A positive result of biological theories has been the minimization of the "blaming" that is inherent in other explanations. Just as viewing alcoholism as an illness has helped clinicians, families, and patients to get beyond blaming and on to treatment, biological theories have facilitated the treatment of schizophrenia. To illustrate, just as diabetic or cardiac patients must learn to cope with illness (e.g., change in life-style, threat of death), psychiatric patients must learn to cope with the limitations of their illness.

Biochemical theories

Biochemical theory can be traced to 1952, when Delay and Deniker reported the antipsychotic effects of chlorpromazine. Andreasen and Olson (1982), Crow (1982), and others have postulated that a biochemical process accounts for the positive symptoms of schizophrenia. The prevailing biochemical explanation is referred to as the *dopamine hypothesis*. According to this hypothesis, excessive dopaminergic activity in cortical areas causes acute positive (type I) symptoms of schizophrenia (hallucinations, delusions, and thought disorders). Excessive dopamine could be a result of increased dopamine synthesis, increased dopamine release or turnover, or an increase in the number and activity of dopamine receptors (Brown and Mann, 1985). It is known also that drugs that increase dopamine, such as L-dopa and the amphetamines, can cause a psychotic state. This hypothesis is attractive because it is easy to grasp, and because drugs that block dopamine seem to be very effective in the treatment of schizophrenia. However, these drugs take days, weeks, or months to establish their clinical effectiveness, but the central nervous system (CNS) dopamine receptors are blocked within 20 minutes (Roberts, Leigh, and Weinberger, 1993). Therefore it seems that the dopamine hypothesis is too simplistic and that other factors are involved in the effectiveness of antipsychotic drugs. Table 27-1 outlines the different dopamine receptor subtypes and alerts the nurse to the complexity of brain chemistry.

The dopamine hypothesis, though limited in explanatory power, continues to have great educational value for the following reasons:

1. Dopaminergic drugs (e.g., levodopa, amphetamines) can cause psychotic symptoms.
2. Clinically effective antipsychotic drugs occupy approximately 70% to 80% of D_2 receptors.
3. Postmortem studies of persons with schizophrenia reveal increased numbers of receptors.

Other proposed neurotransmitter contributors to schizophrenia include serotonin, glutamate, and glycine. As early as 1954 Woolley and Shaw suggested a role for serotonin in schizophrenia. Serotonin inhibits dopamine synthesis, therefore serotonin antagonists potentially increase dopamine levels. This is one of the neurophysiological properties that is presumed to cause atypical antipsychotics to be effective. These agents are now referred to as serotonin/dopamine antagonists (SDAs) by some clinicians (and by manufacturers). This degree of certainty (i.e., advertising drugs as SDAs) is not fully embraced by all researchers.

Reduced levels of glutamate, a product of the Krebs' cycle, has also been proposed as a factor in schizophrenia (Kim, et al, 1980). Both glutamate and glycine contribute to regulate N-methyl-D-aspartate (NMDA) receptors, receptors necessary for cognitive processes. When NMDA receptors are normalized, it is suggested that schizophrenic symptoms are reduced (Ereshefsky and Lacombe, 1993). Neither treatment with glutamate nor glycine has proven particularly promising.

Neurostructural theories

The neurostructural theorists propose that schizophrenia, particularly negative (type II) schizophrenia, is a result of pathoanatomy. The three specific neurostructural changes mentioned most often are increased VBRs, brain atrophy, and decreased

---

Table 27-1   Areas of Concentration for Dopamine Receptor Subtypes

D_1—motor neurons in the basal ganglia and may be the principal dopamine-stimulating receptor for motor function.
- It has no direct role in controlling psychotic symptoms
- It does influence D_2 receptor function.

D_2—located in neurons of both the limbic and motor centers. Dopamine stimulation of D_2 receptors activates psychomotor pathways.
- Overactivation thought to be cause of positive symptoms.
- D_2 receptors are modulated when the D_1 receptor is blocked but this does not occur in schizophrenia.

D_3 and D_4—found primarily in limbic centers. Dopamine stimulation of D_3 may suppress behavior; overstimulation of D_3 may be associated with negative symptoms. D_4 receptors are located on neurons that influence thought processes and may be related to positive symptoms.

D_5—found only in the limbic regions including hippocampal gyrus and nucleus accumbens. May be an important dopamine-stimulating receptor for behavior.

From Seeman P: Dopamine receptors as new targets for novel drugs, *Current Approaches to Psychoses*, 4:8, 1995.

Selected Structural Brain Imaging Findings in Schizophrenia

1. Cerebral ventricular enlargement
2. Smaller cerebral and cranial size
3. Hypoplasia of the medial (limbic) temporal structures, especially the hippocampus

Nasrallah HA: Neurodevelopmental pathogenesis of schizophrenia, *Psychiatr Clin North Am* 16(2):269, 1993.

CBF. CT, MRI, positron emission tomography (PET), and single photon emission computed tomography (SPECT) are techniques used to develop images of the brain. CT and MRI provide images of brain structure (i.e., for VBRs and brain atrophy). PET and SPECT provide information on both brain structure and brain activity. Box 27-6 summarizes the most commonly used imaging techniques.

Ventricular brain ratio

The finding that a significant subgroup of persons with schizophrenia have enlarged ventricles according to CT scan was first reported by Johnstone, et al (1976). Persons with enlarged ventricles have a poorer prognosis and exhibit the negative symptoms (type II) noted by Crow (1982); Andreasen, et al (1982); Andreasen, (1985); Rabins, et al (1987); and others.

Box 27-6 Commonly Used Brain Imaging Techniques

1. Computed tomography (CT) is the most widely used x-ray method for imaging the living brain and is approximately 100 times more sensitive than conventional radiography. A number of contrast mediums can be used in conjunction with this procedure to enhance the image. The procedure does not cause pain but does expose patients to radiation.
2. Magnetic resonance imaging (MRI) provides clearer and more complete pictures than a CT scan but is more expensive to perform. In this procedure, patients are surrounded by a strong magnetic field through which pulses of radio frequency irradiation are projected that realign hydrogen atoms. The altered radio frequency caused by the realignment is converted into an image by a computer.
3. Positron emission tomography (PET) is the most sophisticated physiological imaging technique available. PET has a resolution capability of less than 5 mm in the brain. Glucose-containing radioactive atoms are given to the patient, and a computerized image of brain activity can be developed. Because glucose is the primary source of body energy, the extent of metabolic activity in specific brain sites can be traced. PET technology is expensive.
4. Single photon emission computed tomography (SPECT) also uses radioactive atoms that are tagged onto larger molecules. This technology is not as advanced as PET, but it is less expensive. The best SPECT systems have resolution under 8 mm.
5. Brain electrical activity mapping (BEAM) is an advanced form of electroencephalography.

While ventricular enlargement is not peculiar to schizophrenia, anatomical findings are substantially different than those for neurodegenerative disorders such as Alzheimer's disease. Ventricular enlargement in schizophrenia is not associated with a neurodegenerative process (Bogerts, et al, 1993; Casanova, et al, 1993; Marsh, et al, 1994). That is, one would not expect to find a gradual increase in ventricular volume over time in a patient with schizophrenia. In the patient with Alzheimer's disease, however, ventricles continue to increase in volume as brain cells die. It must be noted that not all patients with schizophrenia have abnormally enlarged ventricles. About 50% of these patients fall within the range of control or "normal" subjects (Cannon and Marco, 1994). This overlapping effect has led researchers to study monozygotic twins when one twin suffers from schizophrenia. In documented cases in which the affected twin had ventricles falling within the "normal" range, pathoanatomical deviance could be demonstrated only when contrasted to the ventricles of the unaffected (i.e., nonschizophrenic) twin. Roberts, Leigh, and Weinberger (1993) clearly demonstrate that an otherwise "normal"-appearing ventricle was in actuality enlarged when compared to the "perfect" control—the ventricles of the monozygotic twin.

Brain atrophy

Over 100 years ago Alzheimer described brain cell loss in schizophrenia. Anatomical pathology in cortical and subcortical areas has been suggested by brain imaging techniques and confirmed by postmortem examinations of individuals with schizophrenia. Limbic, hippocampal, thalamic structures, temporal lobes, the amygdala, and the substantia nigra are specific lobes and nuclei found to have neuropathological changes. Selemon, Rajkowski, and Goldman-Rakic (1995) also detected an overall 7% reduction in cortical thickness in individuals with schizophrenia.

Cerebral blood flow

Persons with atrophic changes also have decreased cortical blood flow, particularly in the prefrontal cortex, with a consequent decrease in metabolic activity (Berman, et al, 1987; Ingvar and Franzen, 1974). Cognitive demands, such as organizing, planning, learning from experience, problem solving, introspection, and critical judgment, are compromised (Berman, et al, 1987). A significant subgroup of schizophrenic patients with negative symptoms have decreased brain activity as demonstrated by in vivo studies of CBF and glucose metabolism (Berman et al, 1987; Ingvar and Franzen, 1974).

Genetic theories

Persons with schizophrenia seem to inherit a predisposition to the disorder. Their relatives have a greater incidence of schizophrenia than chance alone would allow. The genetic risk for schizophrenia is shown in Box 27-7. Of particular interest to clinicians is the risk associated with having a parent afflicted with schizophrenia. Though the risk reaches 35% if both parents have schizophrenia (Rosen, 1978), this higher incidence alone does not adequately address the nature (genetics) vs. nurture (upbringing) debate. For instance, a mentally disordered parent may rear children so inadequately that the children are predisposed to schizophrenia on the basis of the parenting skills, not genetics.

To control the "nurture" variable, researchers have studied twins. Both monozygotic (identical) and dizygotic (fraternal) twins have been studied. Monozygotic twins have consistently reported a higher concordance rate (meaning both twins do or do not have symptoms of schizophrenia). Concordance rates are 50% for monozygotic twins. This is 50 times greater than the risk for the general population, and 3 times higher than the risk for dizygotic twins.

These findings seem to establish the genetic or nature basis of schizophrenia; however, there are still extraneous variables that cannot be explained. For instance, many monozygotic twins are dressed alike and often are misidentified; their upbringing may be identical, too. Some argue that it is no wonder that monozygotic twins have a high concordance rate. Unless researchers can control the environment variable, the relative impact of nature and nurture cannot be reported with confidence.

To control for the variable of environment, studies have been conducted of situations in which monozygotic twins have been separated at birth and reared apart. Monozygotic concordance rates remain significantly higher in these studies.

Perinatal risk factors

Some researchers believe that schizophrenia can be linked to the prenatal exposure to influenza, minor malformations developing during early gestation, and complications of pregnancy particularly during labor and delivery (McNeil, 1995). The research about large flu epidemics is far from conclusive, but there is evidence that individuals with schizophrenia are more likely to have been born in the winter months. Research of cohorts conceived during devastating influenza epidemics reveal a meaningfully higher incidence of schizophrenia in products (i.e., children) of conceptions during that time. Other researchers suggest a high incidence of birth trauma and injury among persons with schizophrenia. These studies suggest a relationship between schizophrenia and birth problems, particularly when adverse events occur during the second trimester of pregnancy (Roberts, Leigh, and Weinberger, 1993).

Other biological considerations

In addition to the foregoing, a number of neurological abnormalities, such as motor coordination (e.g., balance, hopping, and finger-thumb opposition), are found among persons with schizophrenia. Eye tracking abnormalities are thought to be a distinguishing biological feature as well.

Psychodynamic Theories of Schizophrenia

Psychodynamic theories of schizophrenia focus on the individual's response(s) to life events. The common theme of these theories is the internal reaction to life stressors or conflicts. These etiological explanations include developmental and family theories.

Developmental theories of schizophrenia

During the early part of the twentieth century, two men—Adolph Meyer and Sigmund Freud—held to

---

Box 27-7	**Genetic Risk for Schizophrenia**	
Identical twin affected		50%
Fraternal twin affected		15%
Brother or sister affected		10%
One parent affected		15%
Both parents affected		35%
Second-degree relative affected		2-3%
No affected relative		1%

Adapted from Roberts GW, Leigh PN, and Weinberger DR: *Neuropsychiatric disorders,* London, 1993, Mosby Europe.

the significance of developmental psychiatry. They believed that the seeds of mental health and illness are sown in childhood, and that to understand the current functioning of individuals, it is important to understand their upbringing or development (Bowlby, 1988). Freud focused on mental processes, on the unconscious forces that influence individuals. The primary difference between the views of the two men was that Freud focused on fantasy and Meyer focused on real-life events. An extension of their arguments is that events in early life can cause problems that are as severe as schizophrenia. Freudian concepts still are used meaningfully in discussions of schizophrenia. These concepts include poor ego boundaries, fragile ego, ego disintegration, inadequate ego development, superego dominance, regressed or id behavior, love-hate (ambivalent) relationships, and arrested psychosexual development.

Two later developmental theorists whose work more directly explains schizophrenia are Erikson (1968) and Sullivan (1953). Erikson theorized an eight-stage model of human development. He saw the first step, "trust or mistrust," as crucial to later interpersonal relationships. The child who is deprived of a nurturing, loving environment, who is neglected or rejected, is vulnerable to mental disturbances. Inadequate passage through this stage predisposes the child to mistrust, isolative behaviors, and other asocial behaviors. Therapeutic intervention focuses on the reestablishment of trust through consistent, anxiety-free relationships.

Sullivan, using different terms, expressed essentially the same ideas. The absence of warm, nurturing attention during the early years blocks the expression of those same affective responses in later years. Without this capacity, persons exhibit disordered social interactions, as well as other disturbances. These persons learn to avoid interpersonal interactions because such interactions are painful.

Family theories of schizophrenia

Family theories of schizophrenia are linked naturally to developmental theories. If early-life experiences are crucial in development, the argument is made that the family—the environment in which most people grow up—is significant to the development of mental health or illness. Lack of a loving and nurturing primary caregiver, inconsistent family behaviors, and faulty communication patterns are thought to be responsible for mental problems in later life.

Outdated and harmful theories specifically tailored to the families of schizophrenics were the *schizophrenogenic mother theory* and the *double-bind theory*. The word *schizophrenogenic* literally means to cause schizophrenia. Perhaps this has been the greatest single disservice of psychodynamic theories. Essentially, this notion stated that the blame for schizophrenia could be placed on the mother. The double-bind theory described family practices in which the child was "damned if he did and damned if he didn't." An example used often was the child who was expected to do well in school but was criticized for taking time away from the family to study.

Geiser, Hoche, and King (1988) called the family theories *blame theories* and described a bias by mental health professionals toward the families of patients with schizophrenia. Families have been viewed as causative agents, saboteurs of treatment, toxic influences, and as patients themselves. Sometimes families have been treated with hostility and distrust. Because families bear the brunt of preprofessional and postprofessional care of these patients, it is important to work with families without alienating them.

Unfortunately, some families are dysfunctional and contribute to later emotional problems. Muenzenmaier, et al (1993) studied chronically mentally ill patients and found that 65 percent had been sexually or physically abused as children. Exactly what that means in the current climate is not known. Many more people, especially women, are coming forward to reveal an abusive childhood. Mental health professionals believe that child abuse, especially sexual abuse, is widespread and underreported (Jaroff, 1993), but it remains unclear whether or not such abuse plays a causative role in schizophrenia. A marginally related issue is the fact that some psychiatric and lay articles now include discussions of the false memory of abuse. This serves to illustrate yet another way in which families can be unfairly maligned.

Vulnerability-Stress Model of Schizophrenia

As stated above, no single etiological theory adequately answers the questions about the genesis of schizophrenia. The vulnerability-stress model addresses the variety of forces that cause schizophrenia in some cases, and in other cases cause the broader schizophrenia-spectrum problems of schizoaffective disorders and schizophrenia-related personality disorders. This model recognizes that both biological and psychodynamic predispositions to schizophrenia, when coupled with stressful life events, can precipitate a schizophrenic process. According to this model, persons with a predisposition to schizophrenia may (but not always) avoid serious mental disorder if they are protected from the stresses of life. Persons with a similar vulnerability may succumb to schizophrenia if exposed to stressors. To illustrate, a wealthy person might be spared the brunt of some stressors because of wealth, whereas a poor member of society, struggling to meet basic needs, finds confrontation with stressors a daily event. According to this model, the second person is more likely to display symptoms of schizophrenia.

"An enduring and consistent finding has been the strong association between schizophrenia and lower socioeconomic status" (Cohen, 1993). Individuals with schizophrenia tend to "drift downward" socioeconomically. This unenviable status enhances their vulnerability by exposing them to constant stressors. In an article entitled "Daily Hassles of Persons with Severe Mental Illness," Segal and Vander Voort (1993) describe some of the daily problems besetting seriously mentally ill persons. Table 27-2 lists some of those daily problems.

Table 27-2   Daily Problems for Schizophrenic Individuals

Daily Problem	Percent of Schizophrenic Individuals Reporting
Rising cost of common goods	48%
Loneliness	45%
Troubling thoughts about the future	42%
Too much time on hands	42%
Crime	40%
Filling out forms	39%
Not enough money for entertainment	39%
Regrets over past decisions	35%
Inability to express self	35%
Fear of rejection	31%
Trouble with reading, writing, and spelling	31%

Adapted from Segal SP and Vander Voort DJ: Daily hassles of persons with severe mental illness, *Hosp Community Psychiatry* 44(3): 276, 1993.

SPECIAL ISSUES RELATED TO SCHIZOPHRENIA

A number of special issues need to be clarified to help the student focus on the breadth of concerns involved in the psychiatric nursing care of patients with schizophrenia.

Families of Schizophrenics

Families, particularly mothers, often have been blamed for the problems of persons with schizophrenia. It is no wonder that many families are suspicious of professionals who may view the family as a villain. Nor is it any wonder that many of these families have little desire to be "studied."

Although research substantiates the state of turmoil in these families, many clinicians argue that dysfunctional families are not the cause of schizophrenia, but rather, the result of having a family member with this illness. Nevertheless, once a family becomes "destabilized," there is a high probability that it will have a negative effect on the schizophrenic member.

Families of persons with schizophrenia tend to have inappropriate family cohesion, and family members may be emotionally overinvolved, hostile, and critical. These families are said to have a high expressed emotion (EE) index (Herz, 1984; de Cangas, 1990). Mothers of persons with schizophrenia are said to "smother instead of mother"; that is, to be overinvolved and overprotective. Fathers are often characterized as cold and distant. These families also demonstrate poor communication patterns. There is a tendency to be unclear, to lack focus, and to participate in incomplete communication. Arguably, many families without a schizophrenic member also have these attributes. What other variables are at work still is not clear. Nonetheless, with education and therapy, families can diminish their negative

Key Objectives for Treating Persons with Schizophrenia

Work with the family.
Treat depression.
Minimize stressful interactions.
Treat substance abuse.
Avoid lengthy, intense verbal interactions.

impact on patients. Breslin (1992) recommends teaching families to interact more constructively with individuals with schizophrenia. When working with a family, it is important for the nurse to avoid any message that places blame on the family.

Persons with schizophrenia, on the other hand, can be a disruptive influence on the family, particularly when they are noncompliant with prescribed medications or use mind-altering drugs. Although there is consensus that the family characteristics described above are present in many families of schizophrenic patients, it should be noted that these families are studied *after* schizophrenia is identified—years after the family may have been disrupted by the illness. This observation leads to the question raised previously: Do disruptive families cause individuals to have schizophrenia, or do individuals with schizophrenia cause families to become disruptive?

Although "blame" may be warranted in some family situations, in most it is not. Blaming the family leads to a sense of alienation between the family and the treatment team. Nurses should remember that families bear the brunt of care outside the hospital. Most discharged psychiatric patients are sent home to live with their families, therefore the family's stake in the patient's care is obvious. As Geiser, Hoche, and King (1988) point out, families become the caregivers and must learn to cope with strange and frightening behaviors, such as apathy, poor personal hygiene, and violence. These researchers add: "Family crises are emotionally draining experiences, and they may escalate into an event involving police or mental health crisis service staff." As time goes on, these families tend to become more and more isolated and to feel more and more frustrated, helpless, and hopeless, even though they care very much about the patient.

Depression and Suicide in Schizophrenia

Depressive symptoms are frequently a part of the psychopathology of schizophrenia (APA, 1997), and 25% of schizophrenic patients experience a postpsychotic (or secondary) depression. These symptoms respond to antidepressants (Mason, Gingerich, and Siris, 1990). A related phenomena is the high incidence of suicide (10%) among schizophrenic patients (Becker, 1988). Suicide is the leading cause of premature death in schizophrenia. There are three explanations for this high prevalence of depression:

1. Depression is a natural part of schizophrenia but is masked during the acute phase of the disorder.
2. Depression is a reaction to schizophrenia in the same way that depression is a reaction to a physical illness. Warnes (cited in APA, 1997) refers to this as a "hopeless awareness of their own pathology."
3. The biological nature of the disorder (schizophrenia is more than a "dopamine" problem) and the drugs used to treat it produce a depressive syndrome.

Relapse

Both clinical opinion and research studies support the observation that many patients with schizophrenia experience relapse and remission of symptoms throughout their illness. A patient in remission described her relapse as having occurred in stages. She reported the following sequence:

"In the first stage, I feel just a bit estranged from myself . . . In the second stage, everything appears a bit

FAMILY ISSUES

Family Issues in Schizophrenia: Support Groups

The National Alliance for the Mentally Ill (NAMI) or an individual state's Alliance for the Mentally Ill (AMI) are groups that help family and friends of the severely mentally ill to understand the illness. NAMI provides support and has become a powerful advocate for the severely mentally ill. This self-help group has influenced mental health legislation, as well as the way society views

the severely mentally ill. For more information families can write:

NAMI
200 N. Glebe Rd, Suite 1015
Arlington, VA 22203-3754
703-524-7600

clouded . . . In the third stage, I believe I am beginning to understand why terrible things are happening to me; others are causing it . . . In the fourth stage, I become chaotic and see, hear, and believe all manner of things. I no longer question my beliefs, but act on them." (Lovejoy, 1984)

Persons most likely to suffer relapse include those exposed to significant stressors and those not taking prescribed antipsychotics. Important prophylatic activities of professionals include developing strategies to ensure compliance with medications and manipulations of the environment (e.g., moving from a crime-ridden neighborhood, remedial three R's).

Stress

According to the vulnerability-stress model, persons with schizophrenia are vulnerable to stress. Common stressors can be categorized as:
1. Biological (e.g., medical illness)
2. Psychosocial (e.g., loss of a relationship)
3. Sociocultural (e.g., homelessness)
4. Emotional (e.g., persistent criticism)

The therapeutic mandate is to minimize the impact of stress on vulnerable persons. Two basic strategies are used:
1. Reduction of stress and stressor accumulation
2. Development of coping skills

Because of their economic and social status, many individuals face major stressors routinely. Stated another way, some of those most vulnerable to stress have more stress to handle. Helping patients learn to identify and avoid stressful events is an important task for the psychiatric nurse.

Substance Abuse among People with Schizophrenia

Substance abuse is the most common comorbid psychiatric condition associated with schizophrenia and seems to be increasing. A high percentage of persons with schizophrenia abuse alcohol and/or other drugs. Alcohol abuse in these patients is thought to be 30% or more (Roeber, 1997). Alcohol, marijuana, and cocaine accounted for most of the drugs abused. Unlike the general population, schizophrenic individuals have little chance of using alcohol in a social manner.

Drug abuse has a negative effect on the treatment of these patients and is associated with poor outcomes. Alcohol, for example, causes a disinhibition effect, aggressiveness, and poor judgment. These symptoms are already present in patients with severe

mental illness. Further, these very symptoms and related lack of social skills hinder patients with schizophrenia from fully benefiting from treatment programs such as Alcoholics Anonymous and Narcotics Anonymous.

Drug abuse may also account for the overrepresentation of schizophrenic persons in jail. Only 5% of the patients with schizophrenia Drake and Wallach (1993) studied could be said to "handle alcohol"; the rest developed problems from drinking including overrepresentation in jail.

■ Critical Thinking Question

Why do you think substance abuse is so high among individuals with schizophrenia?

Work

The lack of work, the inability to work, and the lack of a desire to work are all features of schizophrenia. Because work, or what one does for a living, is a major defining characteristic in this society, the fact that many people with schizophrenia do not work adds to their inability to "fit in." According to Lysaker, et al (1993), the major problem confronting these individuals is not so much a lack of skill, but an inability to cope socially on the job. Such routine behaviors as joking, inviting someone out, or having insight into how one is affecting others are the major obstacles to a productive work life for the schizophrenic population.

Psychosis-induced Polydipsia

Psychosis-induced polydipsia or compulsive water drinking (between 4 and 10 liters per day) associated with hyponatremia occurs in 6% to 20% of patients with psychosis (APA, 1997).

It was recognized as early as the 1930s that patients with schizophrenia urinate twice as much as other patients (Shah and Greenberg, 1992). The desire to drink probably occurs because of thirst and osmotic dysregulation and is manifested by a compulsive approach to water ingestion. Patients report a variety of reasons for polydipsia, including cleansing the body, washing away evil spirits, and relief of dry mouth caused by medication (Snider and Boyd, 1991).

The major concern associated with polydipsia is hyponatremia. Hyponatremia causes light-headedness, weakness, lethargy, muscle cramps, nausea and vomiting, confusion, convulsions, and coma. In a study by Shah and Greenberg (1992), the lowest serum sodium levels averaged 119 mmol/L (n = 31). Treatment includes frequent weighings, restricted fluid intake, sodium replacement, and positive reinforcement (Liberman, et al, 1993). Long-term management has been attempted by prescribing lithium and phenytoin (Dilantin) with some success (APA, 1997).

THE CONTINUUM OF CARE FOR PEOPLE WITH SCHIZOPHRENIA

"Rather than starting to release patients in a few locales and measuring the outcome, officials implemented the policy in cities and counties across the United States virtually simultaneously, based on widespread hope that the new drugs would cure people and the widespread belief in state legislatures that the policy would save taxpayers money." (Torrey, 1997)

By "policy" Torrey means deinstitutionalization and driven by this policy an array of services, or a continuum of care, has developed. Most clinicians agree that a community setting is good for some patients; the institutional setting may be better for others. The continuum of care for persons with schizophrenia includes (APA, 1997):

- Hospitalization for acute symptoms
- Long-term hospitalization for those patients (10% to 20%) who are treatment resistant
- Day hospitalization for those individuals who are acutely psychotic but not at risk of harming self or others
- Day treatment for patients needing ongoing supportive care as they stabilize
- Supportive housing for those individuals who do not or cannot live with their family but who need some level of supervision. Varieties of supportive housing include:
  Transitional halfway houses—providing room and board and social opportunities
  Cooperatives—indefinite living situations with on-site staff
  Crisis community residences—on-site nursing staff who help patients cope with crises
- Foster care
- Board and care home
- Nursing home

Psychotherapeutic Management

"There is a general consensus that structure, medication, a protective nonthreatening environment, and family psychoeducation comprise essential ingredients of any state-of-the-art inpatient treatment package for acute schizophrenic patients." (Mann, et al, 1993)

"Schizophrenic patients are constantly fighting a battle within the brain. If the mind is not divided against itself, these patients are fighting voices, imaginary people, hallucinations, or other terrifying symptoms. Most schizophrenics go on for years struggling alone without anyone to help them become **stronger than their symptoms.**" (Ruocchio, 1989)

Psychotherapeutic management is aimed at helping patients become stronger than their symptoms. The nursing interventions used in the treatment of patients with schizophrenia are derived from the appropriate development of the nursing care plan.

Psychotherapeutic Nurse-Patient Relationship.
The objective of the psychotherapeutic nurse-patient relationship is to build a therapeutic alliance with patients. A long-term relationship in which trust has developed is probably more significant and therapeutic than a particular theory of care. It is known that "insight" therapy has limited usefulness with this population, whereas less invasive modalities such as supportive therapy, problem solving, and reality-adaptive social skills training that focuses on behavior and not "meaning" are more helpful. Long-term, trusting relationships yield better compliance to medications and better outcomes on psychopathology indices (Breslin, 1992).

The objective of this section is to provide basic concepts for working with patients with schizophrenia. The concepts are divided into two sections. First, general **principles** for developing a therapeutic nurse-patient relationship are presented, then basic **intervention strategies** are outlined. In addition, the box on p. 377 lists specific interventions and examples of therapeutic communication for some of these situations.

General principles for developing a therapeutic nurse-patient relationship
- Be calm when talking to patients.
  Rationale: Anxiety is contagious and counterproductive when working with patients who have schizophrenia.
- Accept patients as they are, but do not accept all behaviors.

Rationale: Everyone wants to be accepted. Focusing on behaviors communicates very directly that behaviors can change.
- Keep promises.
Rationale: Dependability builds trust.
- Be consistent.
Rationale: Consistency increases trust.
- Be honest.
Rationale: Honesty increases trust.

Basic intervention strategies for developing a therapeutic nurse-patient relationship
- Do not reinforce hallucinations or delusions.
Rationale: The nurse cannot agree with a hallucination or a delusion. On the other hand, arguing is nonproductive and may make the perceptual disorder stronger. The nurse should simply state his or her perception of reality, voice doubt about the patient's perceptions, and move on to discuss "real" people or events.
- Orient patients to time, person, and place if indicated.
Rationale: Orientation reinforces reality. However, use judgment. To be continually reminded that you are "disoriented" takes an emotional toll.
- Do not touch patients without warning them.
Rationale: Patients who are paranoid may perceive a touch as a threat and retaliate.
- Avoid whispering or laughing when patients are unable to hear all of a conversation.
Rationale: Have you ever wondered whether you were the subject of discussion when around people who whisper or giggle? Suspicious patients will interpret these actions as a personal affront.
- Reinforce positive behaviors.
Rationale: Appropriate reinforcement can increase positive behaviors.
- Avoid competitive activities with some patients.
Rationale: Competition is threatening and can lead to decreased self-esteem.
- Do not embarrass patients.
Rationale: Persons with schizophrenia retain the ability to feel embarrassed and often avoid contacts because they fear embarrassment.
- For withdrawn patients, start with one-to-one interactions.

Rationale: Even in group situations, it is probably most therapeutic for interactions to be a series of nurse-to-patient rather than patient-to-patient interactions. Nurse-to-patient interactions are less threatening to patients and can evolve into a wider circle of social interaction.
- Allow and encourage verbalization of feelings.
Rationale: Patients are helped if they can say what they think without the nurse becoming defensive.

Psychopharmacology
"The discovery of antipsychotic drugs in 1950 is unrivaled as a breakthrough in the treatment of mental illness. The magnitude of this therapeutic advance in psychiatry has been compared to the discovery of insulin for diabetes, antibiotics for infectious disease, and anticonvulsants for epilepsy." (Lieberman, 1997)

The student is encouraged to review Chapter 20, which provides a complete discussion of antipsychotic drugs. Schizophrenic patients need to take psychotropic drugs as prescribed. As many as 46% of psychiatric inpatients and 60% of psychiatric outpatients do not comply with their medication regimens. See the box on the next page for nursing interventions to help assure compliance. A review of major side effects is found in Box 27-8. For a full review of these side effects, the student is referred to Chapter 20.

Milieu Management
"Intensely active, highly staffed units may be disruptively intense for schizophrenic patients, who more often benefit from decreased stimulation and a greater measure of solitude and clear role models." (Simpson and May, 1982)

Milieu management is an important dimension of the psychiatric nursing care of schizophrenic patients. With the dramatic introduction in the 1950s of psychotropic drugs, other forms of treatment were abandoned. Now that psychopharmacologists have had free reign for many years, it is clear that drugs alone are not enough. A therapeutic treatment approach is best developed with all three components of psychotherapeutic management in place.

Environmental manipulation for therapeutic gain can occur both at the inpatient and outpatient levels and helps patients to function better in the

Key Nursing Interventions to Increase Compliance

- Observe patients for side effects and intervene accordingly. Akathisia is a troubling side effect that patients cannot tolerate.
- When giving tablets or pills, make sure patients do not "cheek" the medications (hide the medication in cheeks or mouth) to spit them out or hoard them for later.

- Teach patients and their families about drugs, including side effects, potential interactions, dosage schedules when discharged, and so on.
- Depot drugs are effective for patients who do not comply with drug therapy.

Box 27-8 Review of Major Side Effects of Antipsychotic Drugs

Extrapyramidal side effects (EPSEs) from high-potency drugs
  Parkinsonism
  Akathisia
  Dystonias
  Neuroleptic malignant syndrome
Anticholinergic effects from low-potency drugs
  Dry mouth
  Blurred vision
  Constipation
  Urinary hesitation
  Tachycardia
Tardive dyskinesia
Amenorrhea and galactorrhea
Sedation (associated with low-potency drugs)
Orthostatic hypotension (associated with low-potency drugs)

---

hospital and in the community (Breslin, 1992). General principles that specifically address the environment of schizophrenic patients follow.

Disruptive patients
- Set limits on disruptive behavior.
- Decrease environmental stimuli. Place escalating patients in a low-stimulus environment and give prn medication if indicated.
- Frequently observe escalating patients in order to intervene. Intervention (e.g., medication) before acting out occurs protects patients and others physically and prevents embarrassment for escalating patients.
- Modify the environment to minimize objects that can be used as weapons. Some units use furniture so heavy it cannot be lifted by most persons.
- Be careful in stating what the staff will do if a patient acts out; however, follow through once a violation occurs (e.g., "If you break the window, we will place you in restraints").
- When using restraints, provide for safety by evaluating the patient's status of hydration, nutrition, elimination, and circulation.

Withdrawn patients
- Arrange nonthreatening activities that involve these patients in "doing something"; for example, a walking tour of a park, leather work, and painting.
- Arrange furniture in a semicircle or around a table so that patients are "forced" to sit with someone. Interactions are permitted in this situation but should not be demanded. Sit in silence with patients who are not ready to respond. Some will move the chair away despite the nurse's efforts.
- Help patients to participate in decision making as appropriate (e.g., selecting the menu for next day's meals).
- Provide patients with opportunities for nonthreatening socialization with the nurse on a one-to-one basis.
- Reinforce appropriate grooming and hygiene (assist at first if needed).
- Provide remotivation and resocialization group experiences. Often students work with occupational or recreational therapists to provide these services.
- Provide psychosocial rehabilitation; that is, training in community living, social skills, and health care skills. Occupational and recreational therapists often are involved in these activities.

Suspicious patients
- Be matter-of-fact when interacting with these patients.
- Staff members should not laugh or whisper around patients unless the patients can hear what is said. The nurse should clarify any misperceptions that patients have.

Case Study

Bill, a 25-year-old man, was brought to the hospital by police. He was in a downtown bus station preaching loudly. He stated in the emergency room that he had spoken to God and that God had told him to save San Francisco. He admitted to hearing both God and Satan arguing and was terrified at times. In talking with his family, staff members discover that Bill was a solid student until about a year ago. He began to struggle in school but continued to pass his course work. He dropped out of school 3 months ago. His family believes his problem started when his girlfriend of 4 years broke off their engagement.

Bill began hearing voices a couple of weeks ago, according to his family, but the family lost contact with him until they were notified of this hospitalization. Bill's family is committed to helping him. On admission to the unit, Bill is oriented to time, place, and person, but states: "God has chosen me to be his special angel. I must save the sinners of San Francisco." Bill then stands up and turns his head rapidly from side to side. When asked why, he says: "God and Satan are arguing about what I should do."

See Bill's nursing care plan on page 374.

- Do not touch suspicious patients without warning. Avoid close physical contact.
- Be consistent in activities (e.g., time, staff, and approach).
- Patients who fear being poisoned should be allowed to open a can of food and serve themselves. Obviously, this may be difficult to arrange in some settings.
- Maintain eye contact.
- Do not "slip" medications into juices or foods without talking to patients. "Catching" the nurse in the act of doing this will reinforce their suspicions.

Patients with impaired communication

- Provide opportunities for patients to make simple decisions.
- Be patient and do not pressure patients to make sense.
- Do not place patients in group activities that would frustrate them, damage their self-esteem, or overtax their abilities.
- Provide opportunities for purposeful psychomotor activity (e.g., painting, ceramic work, exercise, and gross motor games).

Patients with disordered perceptions

- Attempt to provide distracting activities.
- Discourage situations in which patients talk to others about their disordered perceptions.
- Monitor television selections. Some programs seem to cause more perceptual problems than others (e.g., horror movies). If staff members cannot censor programs, they should be available to patients for discussion and clarification following programs.

- Monitor for command hallucinations that may increase the potential for patients to become dangerous.
- Have staff members available in the dayroom so that patients can talk to real people about real people or real events.

Disorganized Patients

- Remove disorganized patients to a less stimulating environment.
- Provide a calm environment; the staff should appear calm.
- Provide safe and relatively simple activities for these patients.
- Provide information boards with schedules and refer to them often so patients can begin to use this as an orienting function.
- Help protect each patient's self-esteem by intervening if a patient does something that is embarrassing (e.g., a patient who takes off his or her clothes or becomes overtly sexual).
- Assist with grooming and hygiene.

Patients with altered levels of activity

Hyperactivity

- Allow patients to stand for a few minutes during group meetings.
- Provide a safe environment and a place where patients can pace without inordinately bothering other patients.
- Encourage participation in activities or games that do not require fine motor skills or intense concentration.

Immobility

- Provide nursing care for catatonic or immobile patients in order to minimize circulatory problems and loss of muscle tone.

Care Plan

NAME: Bill Wilson   ADMISSION DATE: _____

DSM-IV DIAGNOSIS: Schizophrenia: undifferentiated type

ASSESSMENT: **Areas of strength:** past accomplishments; past good heterosexual interpersonal relationships (IPRs); alert, oriented to time, place, person; acute symptoms respond to medications; family support.
Problems: religious hallucinations, religious delusions, thought disorder; broken engagement; dropped out of school.

DIAGNOSES:
- Auditory sensory/perceptual alterations related to thought disturbance, as evidenced by hallucinations.
- Anxiety related to disturbed perceptions, as evidenced by fear and extraneous movements.

OUTCOMES: **Short-term goals:**
                                                                    Date met
- Patient will voice freedom from hallucinations. _____
- Patient will report lack of fear of others. _____
- Patient will discuss feelings about loss of girlfriend. _____
Long-term goals:
- Patient will verbalize need for medication and counseling. _____
- Patient will make appointment for outpatient program assessment in mid-July. _____
- Patient will return to school in September. _____

PLANNING/ INTERVENTIONS: **Nurse-patient relationship:** Do not reinforce hallucinations and delusions; voice doubt; encourage identification of strengths and accomplishments; encourage expression of feelings about broken engagement; discuss plans for immediate future.
Psychopharmacology: Haldol 5 mg tid PO (concentrate); Cogentin 1 mg prn for EPSEs.
Milieu management: Provide distracting activities; monitor television, particularly religious programming and movies with satanic themes; encourage participation in self-esteem group and anger-management group.

EVALUATION: Patient responding to Haldol.

REFERRALS: Will see Ms. White, RN, CS, once a week as outpatient. Appt. in 3 weeks with R. Jones for education counseling.

- Provide adequate diet, exercise, and rest.
- Maintain bowel and bladder function and intervene before problems arise.
- Observe patients to prevent victimization (physical and verbal) by others.

OTHER PSYCHOTIC DISORDERS

In addition to schizophrenia, there are several other psychotic disorders described in the DSM-IV with which the student should be familiar. Interventions for these disorders are directed at prominent symptoms and are the same as the interventions used for those symptoms of patients with schizophrenia.

Schizoaffective Disorder

Schizoaffective disorder is a psychosis characterized by both affective and schizophrenic symptoms with substantial loss of occupational and social functioning. Since this disorder is a hybrid of two disorders

*C*ase *S*tudy

A 40-year-old woman with a history of multiple admissions is admitted to the floor. Emma Rice was found wandering downtown incoherent and disheveled. During the assessment interview, Emma is noted to have a flat affect and is withdrawn. She reports not seeing her family for 5 years and cannot remember when she last held a job. There is no history of hallucinatory or delusional thought content in this recent occurrence. The staff knows Emma and knows that, during past admissions,

she has responded to chlorpromazine. On admission, Emma says, "Let me go. Go on, onward, backwards. (pause) Emma hide, died." When asked where she lives, Emma slowly responds, "Over there, somewhere, anywhere, nowhere." Emma's board and care operator knows her well and has indicated that a bed is being held for Emma.

See the next page for Emma's nursing care plan.

thought to have different biochemical origins, it is somewhat of a puzzle to many clinicians. Affective disorders cause people to be very depressed or elated and schizophrenia is expressed as positive, negative, or disorganized symptoms. The fact that patients with affective disorders can experience positive and negative symptoms plus the fact that patients with schizophrenia experience mood changes partially explains the difficulty in diagnosis. Further, patients are not infrequently switched from a diagnosis of schizophrenic to a mood disorder diagnosis or vice versa. The diagnosis of schizoaffective psychosis helps bridge the gap between the affective disorders and schizophrenia and underscores the fluidity of human emotion and behavior (*Harvard Mental Health Letter,* 1996). "The essential feature of schizoaffective disorder is an uninterrupted period of illness during which, at some time, there is a major depressive, manic, or mixed episode concurrent with symptoms that meet Criterion A for schizophrenia" (APA, 1994).

In this disorder, schizophrenic symptoms are dominant but are accompanied by major depressive or manic symptoms. Patients with schizoaffective disorder will have experienced delusions or hallucinations in the absence of a prominent mood disturbance, but symptoms of a mood disorder will be present for a significant period. Substance abuse or a general medical condition must be ruled out before this diagnosis can be made. It should be specified whether the disorder is bipolar (more common in young adults) or depressive (more common in older adults).

This disorder probably occurs more often in women and may be partially accounted for by the differences in brain lateralization between men and women (Crow, 1995). Epidemiological studies indicate the disorder is heritable (Gerson, 1994).

The prognosis for schizoaffective disorder is better than that of schizophrenia but significantly less optimistic than the prognosis for mood disorders (APA, 1994).

Delusional Disorder

Persons with delusional disorder manifest symptoms similar to those seen in patients with schizophrenia. However, substantial differences exist and necessitate a diagnostic differentiation. The following symptoms differentiate delusional disorders from schizophrenic disorders:

- Delusions have a basis in reality.
- The patients have never met the criteria for schizophrenia.
- The behavior of these patients is relatively normal except in relation to their delusions.
- If mood episodes have occurred concurrently with delusions, their total duration has been relatively brief.
- The symptoms are due directly to a substance or to a medical condition.

Brief Psychotic Disorder

The category of brief psychotic disorder includes all psychotic disturbances that last less than 1 month and are not related to a mood disorder, a general medical condition, or a substance-induced disorder (First, et al, 1994). At least one of the following psychotic disturbances must be present: delusions, hallucinations, disorganized speech, or grossly disorganized or catatonic behavior. The DSM-IV cautions against applying these standards to persons from a culture in which they are exhibiting acceptable behavior.

Care Plan

NAME: _Emma Rice_   ADMISSION DATE: _____

DSM-IV DIAGNOSIS: _Schizophrenia, disorganized type_ _____

ASSESSMENT: **Areas of strength:** Board and care operator knows Emma well and wants her back. Staff knows and understands Emma.
Problems: Affective flattening, loose associations, withdrawn, chronic course of illness, no family support.

DIAGNOSES:
- Impaired verbal communication related to thought disturbance, as evidenced by impaired articulation and loose association of ideas.
- Bathing/hygiene self-care deficit related to thought disturbance, as evidenced by inability to maintain appearance at satisfactory level.
- Social isolation related to lack of trust, as evidenced by absence of supportive significant other.

OUTCOMES: **Short-term goals:**   Date met
- Patient will talk in coherent manner.   _____
- Patient will carry out ADLs.   _____
- Patient will participate in nonthreatening activities.   _____
Long-term goals:
- Patient will maintain outpatient program.   _____
- Patient will return to board and care.   _____
- Patient will comply with medication regimen.   _____

PLANNING/ INTERVENTIONS: **Nurse-patient relationship:** Be patient; treat as adult; encourage hygiene and appropriate dress; reinforce positive social behaviors; start with one-to-one interactions with nurse and then encourage independent social behaviors.
Psychopharmacology: Chlorpromazine 150 mg tid PO (concentrate). May need long-acting form on discharge.
Milieu management: Start patient in OT by the end of the week; invite patient to sit with staff and other patients; encourage to make decisions about meals or some other simple tasks; provide resocialization group experience and community living education.

EVALUATION: Patient stabilized on medications.

REFERRALS: Will see Ms. Brown, RN, CS, once a week and will attend outpatient resocialization group five times a week. Board and care operator will monitor drugs (single h.s. dose) and arrange transportation.

Schizophreniform Disorder

Schizophreniform disorder displays symptoms that are typical of schizophrenia and last at least 1 month, but no longer than 6 months. Patients' prognoses should be specified as good or poor. Features of a good prognosis include the onset of psychotic symptoms within 4 weeks of the initial change in behavior, confusion at the height of the psychotic episode, ab- sence of a flat affect, and a history of good social and occupational functioning before the occurrence.

■ Critical Thinking Question

Why do persons with type I schizophrenia often evolve into type II schizophrenia?

Key Nursing Interventions for Developing the Therapeutic Nurse-Patient Relationship

Following are specific interventions and examples for developing a therapeutic nurse-patient relationship, including examples of appropriate responses. These examples are meant to illustrate some of the common situations described in the text. Obviously, each patient is unique, and that uniqueness might necessitate a variation of the response suggested below.

1. Do not argue about delusions.

   Rationale: Arguing tends to reinforce delusions and can make patients angry. Reflect reality and attempt to distract patients in a matter-of-fact manner.

   Patient: The FBI and the Mafia are both after me.

   Nurse: I know your thought seems real to you; however, it does not seem reasonable to me. I also want you to know that you are safe here. Let's go into the dayroom and talk.

   Proceed to talk about occupational therapy efforts (or a similar topic) that focus on the patient's real world.

2. Do not reinforce hallucinations.

   Patient: The voices are calling me terrible names.

   Nurse: I do not hear anything but your voice and mine.

3. If a patient is acting odd and the nurse suspects he or she is hallucinating, the patient should be asked about it.

   Patient's behavior: Looks around the room, eyes darting to the corners of the room.

   Nurse: It looks like you might be listening to something. Are you hearing voices?

4. Help patients to identify the stressors that might precipitate hallucinations or delusions.

   Rationale: This effort might lead to identification and avoidance of triggering events.

   Patient: Nurse, I started hearing the voices last night right after I went to bed.

   Nurse: Tell me about your evening last night. There may be a link between something that happened and your hearing voices again.

5. Focus on real people and real events.

   Rationale: This helps patients to stay in touch with reality.

   Patient: I keep hearing the voices.

   Nurse: I understand, but I want to help you focus away from those voices. Let's go to the dayroom and talk.

   Proceed to bring patients closer to reality by talking about daily life.

6. Be diligent in attempting to understand patients.

   Rationale: It is therapeutic to help patients to communicate what they want to say; however, use judgment. Pushing too hard to understand can be frustrating for the patient.

   Patient: I could have been bitten. It was never a dog's day.

   Nurse: I am not sure what you are saying, but I want to understand. Are you talking about almost being hurt?

7. Attempt to balance siding with inappropriate behavior and crushing a fragile ego.

   Comment: Time and effort help the nurse to learn to negotiate artfully between these potentially negative outcomes.

   Patient: I am going to hit that bastard if he says another word to me.

   Nurse: I know you are upset with him. Let's talk about other ways you can deal with this situation.

Key Concepts

1. The concept of schizophrenia has evolved over the past 100 years as a result of the contributions of early theorists, such as Kraepelin and Bleuler, and modern theorists, such as Andreasen.

2. The DSM-IV identifies five subtypes of schizophrenia: catatonic, disorganized, paranoid, undifferentiated, and residual.

3. Bleuler contributed what he thought to be the four primary symptoms of schizophrenia: affective disturbances, loose associations, ambivalence, and autism (also known as *Bleuler's four A's*).

4. Andreasen (Andreasen and Olsen, 1982), Crow (1982), and others have conceptualized schizophrenia as having only two subtypes: type I (positive symptoms and usually treatable with traditional antipsychotic drugs) and type II (negative symptoms). More recently the subtype disorganized has been added by some researchers.

5. Objective signs of schizophrenia include alterations in personal relationships and activity.

6. Subjective symptoms of schizophrenia include alterations in perception, thought, consciousness, and affect.

7. Etiological explanations for schizophrenia are numerous and include both biological theories (dopamine hypothesis, pathoanatomy, and genetic theories) and psychodynamic theories (developmental theory, family theory).

8. The dopamine hypothesis–the view that schizophrenia is a result of increased bioavailability of dopamine in the brain–is a widely held theory of schizophrenia.

9. Traditional antipsychotic drugs block dopamine receptors and relieve acute symptoms of schizophrenia.

10. Nursing interventions include developing a therapeutic nurse-patient relationship. Several general principles undergird the nurse's interactions with patients who have schizophrenia. These principles include being calm, accepting, dependable, consistent, and honest.

11. In addition to these basic principles, there are several basic interventions that are therapeutic for most patients with schizophrenia. These basic interventions include the following that the nurse should *not* do: do not reinforce hallucinations and delusions, do not touch patients without warning, do not whisper or laugh when patients cannot hear the conversation, do not compete with patients, and do not embarrass patients; and the following that the nurse *should* do: provide reality testing, assist with orientation when appropriate, reinforce positive behaviors, and encourage verbalization of feelings.

12. Psychopharmacology is an important part of the nurse's role in caring for patients with schizophrenia. Understanding therapeutic vs. toxic dosage levels, side effects, interactions, patient teaching issues, use in the elderly, and appropriateness of drugs for use during pregnancy are significant nursing activities.

13. Nurses help shape the milieu of patients with schizophrenia. Strategies for working with disruptive, withdrawn, suspicious, and disorganized patients are crucial for developing a therapeutic environment. Special considerations for patients with impaired communication, disordered perceptions, and altered levels of activity are important.

14. Other psychoses listed in the DSM-IV include schizoaffective disorder, delusional disorder, brief psychotic disorder, and schizophreniform disorder.

▉ Study Questions

(Answer key is in the back of the book.)

1. Schizophrenia may be associated with elevated levels of:
   a. Norepinephrine
   b. Dopamine
   c. Serotonin
   d. Acetylcholine

2. The term *schizophrenia* was coined by:
   a. Morel
   b. Kraepelin
   c. Bleuler
   d. Freud

3. The term *schizophrenia* means:
   a. Splitting of mind and affect
   b. Split personality
   c. Multiple personalities

4. A person brought into the county emergency room is laughing inappropriately, being silly, and not making sense. The patient is dirty, and her clothes are torn. Which DSM-IV diagnostic criteria category would most nearly fit this behavior?
   a. Disorganized type
   b. Catatonic type
   c. Paranoid type
   d. Undifferentiated type

5. Which of the following descriptors does not fit type II schizophrenia?
   a. Cortical
   b. Hyperdopaminergic
   c. Structurally related
   d. Does not respond as readily to drugs

6. A patient states that he hears a voice telling him that he is Jesus. This misperception is called:
   a. Delusion
   b. Hallucination
   c. Illusion
   d. False belief

7. The patient in question 6 believes that he is Jesus. This symptom is called:
   a. Delusion
   b. Hallucination
   c. Illusion
   d. False belief

8. The patient being reviewed during the morning report is described as having bizarre delusions and hallucinations. Based on this limited information, you are:
   a. Optimistic because antipsychotic drugs should help these type I symptoms.
   b. Optimistic because type II symptoms respond well to milieu management
   c. Pessimistic because type I symptoms are slow to respond to antipsychotic drugs
   d. Pessimistic because the bizarre nature of the symptoms indicates a very sick person

9. Mr. Thomas, a single 40-year-old truck driver, is admitted to the psychiatric unit for the first time. He was at a truck stop when he became very agitated, was talking to himself, and frightened people around him. He arrives on the unit in leather restraints with a police es-

cort. He screams, "Get them away from me! Don't let them kill me!" This symptom is best described as:

a. Regression
b. Flight of ideas
c. Hallucination
d. Delusion

10. Mr. Thomas, during his admission processing, tells you that the other truck drivers are against him. He tells you that he has proof that they have bugged his truck. Mr. Thomas's symptoms would probably carry the diagnosis of:

a. Anxiety reaction related to schizophrenia
b. Schizophrenia, paranoid type
c. Schizophrenia, disorganized type
d. Schizoaffective disorder

11. Schizophrenia will affect approximately _____% of the population over their lifetime.

a. 1%
b. 4%
c. 10%
d. 15%

12. Which of the following early scientists had the most pessimistic view of schizophrenia?

a. Bleuler
b. Freud
c. Kraepelin
d. Sullivan

13. Imaging techniques have revealed which of the following anatomical changes in some people with schizophrenia?

a. Increased ventricular brain ratios
b. Decreased cerebral blood flow
c. A hypometabolic process in certain areas of the brain
d. All of the above

14. Rigidity in a person with schizophrenia could be which of the following?

a. Related to drug therapy
b. Catatonic immobility
c. Neuroleptic malignant syndrome
d. All of the above

15. Most professionals no longer subscribe to the schizophrenogenic mother theories of schizophrenia.

a. True
b. False

16. In attempting to distinguish between environmental and genetic etiological factors for schizophrenia, the best population to study is:

a. Fraternal twins
b. Monozygotic twins
c. Unrelated individuals
d. Siblings

17. The major concern associated with water imbalance among patients with schizophrenia is:

a. Hypokalemia
b. Hyponatremia
c. Convulsions
d. Hypomagnesemia

REFERENCES

American Psychiatric Association: *Diagnostic and statistical manual of mental disorders*, ed 4, Washington, DC, 1994, The Association.

American Psychiatric Association: Practice guidelines for the treatment of patients with schizophrenia, *Am J Psychiatry*, 154 (4-Supplement): 1, 1997.

Andreasen NC: Negative symptoms in schizophrenia, *Arch Gen Psychiatry* 39:784, 1982.

Andreasen NC and Olsen S: Negative vs. positive schizophrenia, *Arch Gen Psychiatry* 39:789, 1982.

Andreasen NC: Positive vs. negative schizophrenia: a critical evaluation, *Schizophr Bull* 11:380, 1985.

Andreasen NC: Brain imaging: applications in psychiatry, *Science* 239:1381, 1988.

Andreasen NC, et al: Ventricular enlargement in schizophrenia: relationship to positive and negative symptoms, *Am J Psychiatry* 139:297, 1982.

Becker RE: Depression in schizophrenia, *Hosp Community Psychiatry* 39:1269, 1988.

Berman KF, et al: A relationship between anatomical and physiological brain pathology in schizophrenia: lateral cerebral ventricular size predicts cortical blood flow, *Am J Psychiatry* 144:1277, 1987.

Bick PA and Kinsbourne M: Auditory hallucinations and subvocal speech in schizophrenic patients, *Am J Psychiatry* 144:222, 1987.

Bleuler E: *Dementia praecox or the group of schizophrenias (1908)*, New York, 1950, International Universities (Translated by J Zinkin).

Bogerts B, Lieberman JA, Ashtari M, et al: Hippocampus-amygdala volume and psychopathology in chronic schizophrenia, *Biol Psychiatry* 33(4):236, 1993.

Bowlby J: Developmental psychiatry comes of age, *Am J Psychiatry* 145:1, 1988.

Breslin NA: Treatment of schizophrenia: current practice and future promise, *Hosp Community Psychiatry* 43(9): 877, 1992.

Brown RP and Mann JJ: A clinical perspective on the role of neurotransmitters in mental disorders, *Hosp Community Psychiatry* 36:141, 1985.

Cannon TD and Marco E: Structural brain abnormalities as indicators of vulnerability to schizophrenia, *Schizophr Bull* 20(1):89, 1994.

Casanova MF, et al: A topographical study of senile plaques and neurofibrillary tangles in the hippocampi of patients with Alzheimer's disease and cognitively impaired patients with schizophrenia, *Psychiatry Res* 49(1): 41, 1993.

Cohen CI: Poverty and the course of schizophrenia: implications for research and policy, *Hosp Community Psychiatry* 44(10):951, 1993.

Cohen E and Henkin I: Prevalence of substance abuse by seriously mentally ill patients in a partial hospital program, *Hosp Community Psychiatry* 44(2):178, 1993.

Corrigan PW and Storzbach DM: Behavioral interventions for alleviating psychotic symptoms, *Hosp Community Psychiatry* 44(4):341, 1993.

Crow TJ: Two dimensions of pathology in schizophrenia: dopaminergic and nondopaminergic, *Psychopharmacol Bull* 18:22, 1982.

Crow TJ: The meaning of the morphological changes in the brain in schizophrenia, *Current Approaches to Psychoses*, 4:8, 1995.

Cuffel BJ, Heithoff KA, and Lawson W: Correlates of patterns of substance abuse among patients with schizophrenia, *Hosp Community Psychiatry* 44(3):247, 1993.

Dean SR: Focus on schizophrenia: the role of RISE and the Dean award, *Schizophr Bull* 5:509, 1979.

de Cangas JPC: Exploring expressed emotion: does it contribute to chronic mental illness? *J Psychosoc Nurs Ment Health Serv* 28(2):31, 1990.

Drake RE and Wallach MA: Moderate drinking among people with severe mental illness, *Hosp Community Psychiatry* 44(5):780, 1993.

Ereshefsky L and Lacombe S: Pharmacological profile of risperidone, *Can J Psychiatry* 38(Suppl 3):S80, 1993.

Erikson E: *Childhood and society,* New York, 1968, WW Norton.

First MB, et al: Changes in substance-related, schizophrenic, and other primarily adult disorders, *Hosp Community Psychiatry* 45(1):18, 1994.

Geiser R, Hoche L, and King J: Respite care for the mentally ill patients and their families, *Hosp Community Psychiatry* 39:291, 1988.

Gerson ES: Genetics of schizoaffective disorders, *Current Approaches to Psychoses* 3:8, 1994.

Gray P: The assault on Freud, *Time* 142(23):47, 1993.

Green AI and Salzman C: Clozapine: benefits and risks, *Hosp Community Psychiatry* 41:379, 1990.

Harding CM, Zubin J, and Stauss JS: Chronicity in schizophrenia: fact, partial fact, or artifact? *Hosp Community Psychiatry* 38:477, 1987.

Harvard Mental Health Letter: Schizoaffective disorder. *Harvard Mental Health Letter,* 10:1, 1996.

Hellerstein D, Frosch W, and Koenigsberg HW: The clinical significance of command hallucinations, *Am J Psychiatry* 144:219, 1987.

Herz MI: Recognizing and preventing relapse in patients with schizophrenia, *Hosp Community Psychiatry* 35:344, 1984.

Hornstra RK, et al: The effect of intensive case management on hospitalization of patients with schizophrenia, *Hosp Community Psychiatry* 44(9):844, 1993.

Ingvar DH and Franzen G: Abnormalities of cerebral blood flow distribution in patients with chronic schizophrenia, *Acta Psychiatr Scand* 50:425, 1974.

Jaroff L: Lies of the mind, *Time* 142(23):52, 1993.

Johnstone EC, et al: Cerebral ventricular size and cognitive impairment in chronic schizophrenia, *Lancet* 2:924, 1976.

Jones BE and Gray BA: Problems in diagnosing schizophrenia and affective disorders among blacks, *Hosp Community Psychiatry* 37:61, 1986.

Kane C: The family's response to deinstitutionalization, *J Psychosoc Nurs Ment Health Serv* 22:19, 1984.

Kane CF, et al: Predicting need for long-term hospitalization of severely mentally ill young adults, *Hosp Community Psychiatry* 43(12):1239, 1992.

Kendler KS, Gruenberg AM, and Tsuang MT: A family study of the subtypes of schizophrenia, *Am J Psychiatry* 145:57, 1988.

Kim JS, et al: Low cerebrospinal fluid glutamate in schizophrenia patients and a new hypothesis on schizophrenia, *Neurosci Lett* 20:379, 1980.

Kopelowicz A and Bidder TG: Dementia praecox: inescapable fate or psychiatric oversight? *Hosp Community Psychiatry* 43(9):940, 1992.

Kraepelin E: *Clinical psychiatry: a textbook for students and physicians,* New York, 1902, Macmillan (Translated by AR Defendorf).

Lee DT: Help through Recovery, Inc, *Hosp Community Psychiatry* 44(1):83, 1993.

Leete E: The treatment of schizophrenia: a patient's perspective, *Hosp Community Psychiatry* 38:486, 1987.

Liberman RP, et al: Polydipsia and hyponatremia, *Hosp Community Psychiatry* 44(2):184, 1993 (letter).

Lieberman JA: Atypical antipsychotic drugs: the next generation of therapy, *The Decade of the Brain* 8(3):1, 1997.

Lovejoy M: Recovery from schizophrenia: a personal odyssey, *Hosp Community Psychiatry* 35:809, 1984.

Lysaker P, et al: Work capacity in schizophrenia, *Hosp Community Psychiatry* 44(3):278, 1993.

Mann NA, et al: Psychosocial rehabilitation in schizophrenia: beginnings in acute hospitalization. *Archives of Psychiatric Nursing* 7(3):154, 1993.

Marsh L, et al: Medial temporal lobe structure in schizophrenia: relationship of size to duration of illness, *Schizophr Bull* 11(3):225, 1994.

Mason SE, Gingerich S, and Siris SG: Patient's and caregiver's adaptation to improvement in schizophrenia, *Hosp Community Psychiatry* 41:541, 1990.

McNeil TF: Perinatal risk factors and schizophrenia: selective review and methodological concerns. *Epidemiol Rev* 17(1):107, 1995.

Miller FT and Tanenbaum JD: Drug abuse in schizophrenia, *Hosp Community Psychiatry* 40:847, 1989.

Muenzenmaier K, et al: Childhood abuse and neglect among women outpatients with chronic mental illness, *Hosp Community Psychiatry* 44(7):666, 1993.

Mueser KT and Berenbaum H: Psychodynamic treatment of schizophrenia: is there a future? *Psychol Med* 20:253, 1990.

News: Schizophrenia drug cut off by a California HMO, *J Psychosoc Nurs* 35(3):8, 1997.

Rabins P, et al: Increased ventricle-to-brain ratio in late-onset schizophrenia, *Am J Psychiatry* 144:1216, 1987.

Rawlins RP, Williams SR, and Beck CK: *Mental health-psychiatric nursing*, St Louis, 1993, Mosby.

Rice DP, Kelman S, and Miller LS: The economic burden of mental illness, *Hosp Community Psychiatry* 43(12):1227, 1992.

Roberts GW, Leigh PN, and Weinberger DR: *Neuropsychiatric disorders*, London, 1993, Mosby Europe.

Roeber CR: Schizophrenics who abuse alcohol: dilemmas of treatment, *Clin Care Rev* 9(2):3, 1997.

Rosen H: *A guide to clinical psychiatry*, Coral Gables, Fla, 1978, Mnemosyne.

Ruocchio PJ: How psychotherapy can help the schizophrenic patient, *Hosp Community Psychiatry* 40:188, 1989.

Seeman MV: Schizophrenia in women and men, *Current Approaches to Psychoses* 4:10, 1995.

Seeman P: Dopamine receptors as new targets for novel drugs, *Current Approaches to Psychoses* 4:8, 1995.

Segal SP and Vander Voort DJ: Daily hassles of persons with severe mental illness, *Hosp Community Psychiatry* 44(3):276, 1993.

Selemon LD, Rajkowski G, and Goldman-Rakic PS: Abnormally high neuronal density in the schizophrenic cortex: a morphometric analysis of prefrontal area 9 and occipital area 17, *Arch Gen Psychiatry* 52:805, 1995.

Shah PJ and Greenberg WM: Polydipsia with hyponatremia in a state hospital population, *Hosp Community Psychiatry* 43(5):509, 1992.

Simpson G and May P: Schizophrenic disorders. In Greist J, Jefferson J, and Spitzer R, editors: *Treatment of mental disorders*, New York, 1982, Oxford University.

Snider K and Boyd MA: When they drink too much: nursing interventions for patients with disordered water balance, *J Psychosoc Nurs Ment Health Serv* 29(7):10, 1991.

Soni SD, et al: Differences between chronic schizophrenic patients in the hospital and the community, *Hosp Community Psychiatry* 43(12):1233, 1992.

Strauss J, Carpenter WT, and Bartko J: The diagnosis and understanding of schizophrenia. III. Speculation on the processes that underlie schizophrenic symptoms and signs, *Schizophr Bull* 1:61, 1974.

Sullivan HS: *The interpersonal theory of psychiatry*, New York, 1953, WW Norton.

Teplin LA: The prevalence of severe mental disorder among male urban jail detainees: comparison with the epidemiologic catchment area program, *Am J Public Health* 80:663, 1990.

Torrey EF: The release of the mentally ill from institutions: a well-intentioned disaster, *Chronicle of Higher Education* 43(240):B4, 1997.

Weiss KJ, Valdiserri EV, and Dubin WR: Understanding depression in schizophrenia, *Hosp Community Psychiatry* 40:849, 1989.

Weinberger DR: Implications of normal brain development for the pathogenesis of schizophrenia, *Arch Gen Psychiatry*, 44:660, 1987.

Woolley DW and Shaw E: Biochemical and pharmacological suggestion about certain mental disorders, *Proc Natl Acad Sci USA* 40:228, 1954.

Wyatt RJ, et al: An economic evaluation of schizophrenia—1991, *Soc Psychiatry Psychiatr Epidemiol* 30:196, 1995.

Yesavage JA: Inpatient violence and the schizophrenic patient, *Acta Psychiatr Scand* 67:353, 1983.

CHAPTER 28

Mood Disorders

BARBARA JONES WARREN
NORMAN L. KELTNER

LEARNING OBJECTIVES

After reading this chapter you should be able to:
- Recognize the DSM-IV criteria and terminology for mood disorders.
- Compare the objective and subjective symptoms of major depressive disorder and mania.
- Describe the biological and psychodynamic explanations for mood disorders.
- Describe effective nursing interventions for depressed and bipolar patients.

It is a normal occurrence for every human being to experience different types and levels of moods or emotional states. Brief periods of highs, lows, and sadness occur for everyone because mood is a person's state of mind that is exhibited through feelings and emotions (American Psychiatric Association [APA], 1994). However, mood is considered "disordered" and may be diagnosed as such when an individual has problems with daily functioning because of the presence of exaggerated feelings and emotions. *The Diagnostic and Statistical Manual of Mental Disorders-IV,* or DSM-IV, (APA, 1994) defines a mood disorder as one whose predominant feature is the disturbance in a person's mood. The DSM-IV categorizes mood disorders according to four overarching categories: depressive disorders, bipolar disorders, mood disorder due to a general medical condition, and substance-induced mood disorder. Box 28-1 summarizes criteria for major depressive disorder.

A significant number of patients with mood disorders are not diagnosed or are misdiagnosed because health care professionals lack knowledge regarding the symptoms of these disorders. In addition, findings have indicated that only 16% to 23% of persons who meet the DSM-IV criteria for mood disorders seek treatment from a mental health provider. Consequently, nurses need to be able to apply knowledge regarding the etiology and symptomatology of mood disorders. Doing so will enable them to correctly assess the psychological and physical status of their patients, to develop appropriate interventions and expected outcomes, and to evaluate those interventions and outcomes. The

KEY TERMS

Affect   A person's external response to changing states of moods

Anhedonia   The inability to experience pleasure

Apathy   Lack of feeling, concern, interest, or emotion; inability to be motivated

Atypical depression   Subtype of depression occurring more often among younger individuals and is expressed by "atypical" symptoms; for example increased appetite, weight gain, hypersomnia

Bipolar disorder   Disturbance in mood in which the symptoms of mania have occurred at least one time. An episode of depression may or may not occur.

Clinical depression   Another term for major depressive disorder that defines the disturbance of a person's mood according to DSM-IV criteria

Cortisol   Glucocorticoid hormone formed in the adrenal cortex that participates in carbohydrate and protein metabolism. Cortisol hypersecretion occurs in many depressed individuals. Excretion of this hormone is not suppressed in a significant number of persons with major depression after an injection of dexamethasone.

Cyclothymia   Mood swing that alternates between hypomania and depression

Dexamethasone suppression test [DST]   Diagnostic test for clinical depression that measures the function of the hypothalmic-pituitary-adrenal [HPA] axis

Dysphoria   Disorder of affect characterized by depression, malaise, and anguish

Dysthymic disorder   Disorder resulting in depressed mood with a duration of at least 2 years

Electroconvulsive therapy [ECT]   Form of somatic therapy that uses electrical-induced seizures to relieve a person's intractable depressive symptoms

Euphoria   A subjective, exaggerated feeling of well-being characterized by confidence, elation, and assurance

Hypersomnia   Increased and prolonged sleeping

Hypomania   A milder form of mania that is less intense and severe than mania

Insomnia   Inability to sleep or disrupted sleep patterns

Mania   A person's state of extreme or exaggerated excitement and euphoria that results in accelerated mental and physical activity

Melancholic depression   Subgroup of depression generally occurring in older persons, often misdiagnosed as dementia. More often associated with dexamethasone nonsuppression. Depression usually worse in the morning, early morning awakening occurs, psychomotor retardation or agitation, excessive or inappropriate guilt, and significant anorexia or weight loss are symptoms of melancholia.

Mood   Person's internal state of mind that is exhibited through feelings and emotions

Mood disorder   A disorder whose predominant feature is the disturbance or alteration in a person's mood

Mood disorder due to a general medical condition   Disorder resulting in a disturbance or alteration of a person's mood that is due to a specific medical/physiological consequence

Monoamine oxidase inhibitors [MAOIs]   A classification of antidepressant drugs that inhibit the action of monoamine oxidase. This results in increased levels of norepinephrine, dopamine, and serotonin.

Postpartum depression   Subgroup of depression occurring 30 days or less in the postpartum period

Psychotic depression   Subtype of depression in which a person experiences delusions and hallucinations, often misdiagnosed as schizophrenia or schizoaffective disorder

Seasonal affective disorder   Subtype of depression occurring in late autumn or winter and lasting until spring.

Selective serotonin reuptake inhibitors [SSRIs]   A classification of antidepressants that inhibit the reuptake of serotonin into the presynaptic neuron and increase serotonin in the brain.

Substance-induced mood disorder   Disorder resulting from the disturbance or alteration of a person's mood that is due to the ingestion of a prescribed or nonprescribed drug or medication or exposure to a toxic substance

Tricyclic antidepressants   Drug classification of antidepressants that block the reuptake of norepinephrine and serotonin into the presynaptic neuron

incorporation of this knowledge enhances clinical decision making and improves the quality of patient care. This chapter discusses the etiology and symptomatology of mood disorders with emphasis on major depressive and bipolar disorders. Appropriate interventions for patients who suffer from these disorders is also discussed. Key terms for understanding mood disorders are listed above. DSM-IV and NANDA diagnoses are listed in the box on p. 384.

12-Month Prevalence Rate of Mental Disorders in the United States

Diagnosis	Percentage of Population over 17 Years of Age	Number of Persons
Anxiety disorders	12.6	20,034,000
Phobia disorders*	10.9	17,331,000
Mood disorders	**9.5**	**15,143,000**
Alcohol disorders	7.4	11,766,000
Major depression†	**5.0**	**7,950,000**
Drug disorders	3.1	4,929,000
Cognitive impairment	2.7	4,293,000
Obsessive-compulsive disorder	2.1	3,339,000
Antisocial disorder	1.5	2,385,000
Panic disorders*	1.3	2,067,000
Bipolar disorder†	**1.2**	**1,908,000**
Schizophrenia	1.1	1,749,000
Somatization	0.2	365,000

From Regier DA, et al: The de facto US mental and addictive disorders service system: epidemiologic catchment area prospective 1-year prevalence rates of disorders and services, *Arch Gen Psychiatry* 50:85, 1993.
*Also calculated in anxiety statistics.
†Also calculated in mood disorders statistics.

DSM-IV and NANDA Diagnoses Related to Mood Disorders

DSM-IV*
Bipolar I disorder
Bipolar II disorder
Cyclothymic disorder
Dysthymic disorder
Major depressive disorder

NANDA†
Anxiety
Communication, impaired verbal
Coping, ineffective individual
Grieving, anticipatory
Grieving, dysfunctional

Hopelessness
Injury, potential for
Nutrition, altered
Powerlessness
Self-care deficit
Self-esteem disturbance
Sexual dysfunction
Sleep pattern disturbance
Social isolation
Spiritual distress (distress of the human spirit)
Thought processes, altered
Violence, potential for self-directed

*Adapted from the American Psychiatric Association *Diagnostic and statistical manual of mental disorders,* ed 4, Washington, DC, 1994, The Association.
†North American Nursing Diagnosis Association: *NANDA nursing diagnoses: definitions and classifications 1997-1998,* Philadelphia, 1997, The Association.

DEPRESSIVE DISORDERS

The existence of depression has been documented since biblical times and has been defined by religious writers, philosophers, and scientists (Mahendra, 1986). Historically, we know many important individuals have experienced the devastating symptoms of depression, including King Saul, Job, Elijah, Jeremiah, Mary and Abraham Lincoln, Winston Churchill, and Senator Thomas Eagleton. More recently, Vincent Foster, Mrs. Colin Powell, Mike Wallace, and Governor Lawton Chiles are known to have suffered from this disorder. Of course, normal feelings of sadness are quite appropriate in many

Box 28-1   Key Features of Major Depressive Episodes

At least a 2-week period of maladaptive functioning that is a clear change from previous levels of functioning. At least five of the following symptoms must be present during that 2-week period, one of which must be (1) or (2):
1. Depressed mood
2. Inability to experience pleasure or markedly diminished interest in pleasurable activities
3. Appetite disturbance with weight change (change >5% of body weight within 1 month up or down)
4. Sleep disturbance
5. Psychomotor disturbance
6. Fatigue or loss of energy
7. Feelings of worthlessness or excessive or inappropriate guilt
8. Diminished ability to concentrate or indecisiveness
9. Recurrent thoughts of death or suicidal ideations

The mood disturbance causes marked distress and/or significant impairment in social or occupational functioning.

There is no evidence of a physical or substance-induced etiology for the patient's symptoms or of the presence of another major mental disorder that accounts for the patient's depressive symptoms.

Adapted from the American Psychiatric Association: *Diagnostic and statistical manual of mental disorders,* ed 4, Washington, DC, 1994, The Association.

Table 28-1   Demographic Variables Associated with Mood Disorders (15-54 years old)

Demographic Variable	Most Likely to Have Mood Disorder	Least Likely to Have Mood Disorder
Sex	Female	Male
Age	35-44	15-24
Race	White; hispanic	Black
Income	$0-19,000	>$70,000
Education (years of school)	0-11	13-15
		12
		>16
Urbanicity	Major urban	Rural

Adapted from Kessler RC, et al: Lifetime and 12-month prevalence of DSM-III-R psychiatric disorders in the United States: results from the national comorbidity survey, *Arch Gen Psychiatry* 51:8, 1994.

Table 28-2   Costs Associated with Depression

Excessive absenteeism from work	$11,700,000,000
Reduced worker productivity	$12,100,000,000
Treatment	$12,400,000,000
(Inpatient)	($8,300,000,000)
(Outpatient)	($2,800,000,000)
(Partial care)	($1,200,000,000)
(Miscellaneous)	($100,000,000)
Mortality (deaths related to depression)	$7,500,000,000
TOTAL	$43,700,000,000

Adapted from News and Notes: Costs of depression estimated as nearly $44 billion: time lost from work accounts for largest share, *Hosp Community Psychiatry* 45(1):85, 1994.

situations. In fact, it would be abnormal not to feel sad in certain situations, for example, when a loved one dies or when other losses occur in an individual's life. However, these feelings are typically short lived and do not completely and permanently alter a person's functioning ability.

The DSM-IV categorizes depressive disorders into major depressive disorder [MDD], dysthymic disorder, and depressive disorder not otherwise specified. Depression can manifest itself as a single or recurrent episode and varies somewhat according to age, race, and gender (APA, 1993; 1994). The connection between MDD and suicide is alarming. The suicide rate in the general population with no history of MDD is 1% but swells to 18% for persons diagnosed with MDD (Bourdan et al, 1992). Of the annual 30,000 suicides, 16,000 are attributed to persons diagnosed with MDD, and those rates are highest among single white men under 24 or over 60 years of age (Mellick, Buckwalter, and Stolley, 1992). The cost for society is high, affecting families,

friends, significant others, and work environments. Other demographic factors associated with mood disorders are found in Table 28-1, and economic factors associated with MDD are in Table 28-2.

Criteria and Symptoms of Major Depressive Disorder

MDD involves psychological (e.g., anhedonia; feelings of self-injury, worthlessness, and guilt), biological (e.g., weight changes, insomnia), and social (e.g., passivity, inability to make decisions) symptoms that impair a person's functioning ability and social interactions (Box 28-2). The DSM-IV describes MDD as a mood disorder characterized by symptoms that persist over a minimum 2-week period. A person must have at least five of the nine criteria, one of which must be a depressed mood or anhedonia. The criteria for MDD are:

1. Depressed mood
2. Anhedonia
3. Significant change in weight
4. Insomnia or hypersomnia
5. Increased or decreased psychomotor activity
6. Fatigue or energy loss
7. Feelings of worthlessness or guilt
8. Diminished concentration or indecisiveness
9. Recurrent death or suicidal thoughts

Nurses can be instrumental in the assessment of depression. A variety of instruments may be used for assessment purposes (Table 28-3).

The DSM-IV categorizes MDD into several variants called *specifiers*. These variants include MDD with atypical features, melancholic features, postpartum features, psychotic features, and seasonal patterns (i.e., seasonal affective disorder [SAD]). Overarching symptoms are the same across these subgroups, but variances in expression occur. The DSM-IV description helps define the population, time frame, and/or symptoms for the subgroup. **Atypical** depression is a mood disturbance of depression that generally occurs in younger populations and is expressed by increased appetite or weight gain, hypersomnia, leaden paralysis, and extreme sensitivity to interpersonal rejection. Mood reactivity in which the mood brightens considerably with positive events is another characteristic. **Melan-**

cholic depression is a disturbance of depression occurring most often in older persons and may be misdiagnosed as dementia. It is characterized by anhedonia and an inability to be cheered up. **Postpartum** depression is a mood disturbance that occurs in the first 30 days postpartum. In **psychotic** depression a person has delusions and hallucinations in conjunction with the mood disturbance. And **seasonal affective disorder** (SAD) is a depression occurring in conjunction with a seasonal change most often beginning in fall or winter and remitting in spring (in the Northern Hemisphere).

Adult populations

Depression is one of the most prevalent mental health problems within the United States (Horwath, et al, 1994; Kessler, et al, 1994; U.S. Department of Health and Human Services [DHHS], 1993a). Depressive symptoms are experienced by 9% to 20% of adult persons in the general population, and half of these persons will develop clinical depression within a year (Horwath, et al, 1994). Women's lifetime risk for depression is 10% to 20% compared to men's lifetime risk of 5% to 12% (Nemeroff, 1998). Although depression can occur at any age, the average age of adult onset is in the mid-20s (Bourdan et al, 1992). Some individuals will have a single episode of clinical depression, recover, and never become depressed again. However, about 80% will eventually have recurrent episodes. Ten percent will experience manic phases in addition to depressive ones (about 1.2% of Americans) (Nemeroff, 1998).

Children and adolescents

The occurrence of depression in children and adolescents can be even more devastating than in adults. Children of parents who incur depression are at greater risk to develop the disorder than are children whose parents are not diagnosed with the disorder (Depression Guideline Panel [DGP], 1993). The onset of childhood depression predisposes a child to develop recurrent adult depression (DGP, 1993). Nurses need to be able to assess children and their families for possible symptoms of depression and then develop appropriate interventions for them. Certain events may predispose children and adolescents to develop depressive symptoms or MDD, including (1) loss of parents through divorce,

---

Box 28-2 **Symptoms of Depression**	
Common Symptoms	**Other Symptoms**
Apathy	Fatigue
Sadness	Thoughts of death
Sleep disturbances	Decreased libido
(insomnia or	Ruminations of inadequacy
hypersomnia)	Psychomotor agitation
Hopelessness	Private verbal beratings
Helplessness	of self
Worthlessness	Spontaneous crying without
Guilt	apparent cause
Anger (covert or overt)	Dependency
	Passiveness

Table 28-3   Selected Instruments for Assessment of Adult Depression

Instrument	Resource Area	Purpose
Beck Depression Inventory (BDI)	The Psychological Corp, San Antonio, Tex	Self-report inventory to rate intensity of depressive symptoms; can be used in clinical and nonclinical populations
Center for Epidemiologic Scale (CES-D)	Epidemiology and Psychopathology Research Branch, National Institutes of Health, Rockville, Md	Self-report scale of presence of depressive symptoms in general populations; available in computer format
Diagnostic Interview Schedule (DIS), Version III-R	Lee Robins, Dept of Psychiatry, Washington University, School of Medicine, St Louis, Mo	Structured interview for clinician use regarding diagnosis of depression using DSM-IV criteria; available in computer format
Geriatric Depression Scale (GDS)	T.L. Brink, Redlands, Calif	Structured interview for clinician use in the assessment of nonsomatic symptoms of depression in elderly populations
Schedule for Affective Disorders (SADS)	Jean Endicott, Dept of Research, Assessment and Training, NY State Psychiatric Institute, New York, NY	Structured interview for clinician use in providing information regarding the symptoms of depression, past and current levels
Structured Clinical Interview for Axis I *DSM-IV* Disorders (SCID)	American Psychiatric Assn, Washington, DC	Semistructured interview for clinician use in making Axis I diagnosis, both current and past mood disorders
Hamilton Rating Scale for Depression (HRSD)	Available in Beckham and Leber (1995)	Structured self-report scale to determine current and past presence and levels of depressive symptoms
Taylor's Dysphoria Inventory	Available in Jones (1996)	Self-report scale for determination of the presence and intensity of depressive symptoms in black populations
Zung Self-Rating Depression Scale (SDS)	Available in Beckham and Leber (1995)	Self-report scale for determining the presence and intensity of depressive symptoms

separation, or death; (2) death of other persons close to the child, such as siblings, grandparents, other relatives, or friends; (3) death of a pet; (4) move to another neighborhood or town; (5) academic problems or failure; and (6) physical illness or injury that might require hospitalization and/or prolonged treatment (Hyde, 1993; Kahan, 1993). See Chapter 39 for a further discussion of children and adolescents.

Culture, age, and gender

Little data is available regarding depression in persons from different ethnic, racial, or cultural groups, yet it is known that persons from certain groups may manifest depressive symptoms differently. Depression may be experienced in somatic terms in some ethnic, racial, or cultural groups. Persons from Hispanic, Latino, and Mediterranean groups may describe their sadness or guilt in terms of being nervous or having headaches or stomachaches. Individuals from Asian cultures may describe themselves as being out of balance or feeling weak and nervous. Native American and Asian American groups withdraw for meditation and personal growth as part of their culture so symptoms of depression may be overlooked, ignored, or denied. Please refer to Chapter 17 for more specific information on expression of emotional states in different ethnic, racial, and cultural groups.

Symptoms of depression in children, adolescents, women, and the elderly are also misinterpreted by nurses and other health care providers (McGrath, et al, 1992). For example, depressive symptoms in children and adolescents may mimic normal developmental emotional and physical changes. On the other hand, women's reports of depression may be dismissed as symptoms of nervousness, anxiety, premenstrual syndrome, menopausal symptoms, or chronic fatigue syndrome since these conditions are expressed in ways similar to depression or can occur as comorbid conditions (Beeber, 1996; Kessler, et al, 1994; McGrath, et al, 1992). Finally, recognizing symptoms of depression in elderly populations is particularly challenging since many symptoms of depression are similar to those found in dementia, diabetes, and cardiac conditions (DGP, 1993).

■ Critical Thinking Questions

What factors do you think contribute to the high levels of depression in the United States?

Dysthymic Disorder

Dysthymic disorder is diagnosed when a person has a depressed mood for at least 2 years for more days than not and when three other DSM-IV criteria for depression are met. The distinction between dysthymia and MDD is subtle (e.g., a depressed mood and four other symptoms meet the criteria for MDD), and diagnostic confusion is common. Dysthymic disorder is essentially a disorder of chronicity, whereas severity is the distinguishing factor for MDD (see Box 28-1). These criteria attempt to rule out competing explanations for depression, such as organic and drug-related causes. In addition, because a less severe depression might be expected as a patient is recovering from MDD, the DSM-IV criteria reduce the possibility of confusing a gradual recovery from MDD with the less severe dysthymic disorder.

Behavior

Depression results in both objective and subjective behaviors. Objective signs, such as agitation, can be observed by the nurse. Subjective symptoms, such as hopelessness, are painful but may be hidden by depressed persons. Perhaps more than in schizophrenia, the differentiation between objective and subjective symptoms in depression is difficult to develop. Objective signs are typically extensions of a subjective state. The nurse is encouraged to observe for visible signs of depression and to be aware of, assess for, and expect subjective anguish and anger.

CLINICAL EXAMPLE

Mrs. B. is a 57-year-old woman who presents with dysphoria, tearfulness, suicidal ideation, loss of energy and sexual interest, and insomnia. Although she feels hopeless about the future and worries that she will never get better, Mrs. B. does accept reassurance that her pessimism is exaggerated and is the result of her depression. She feels that she is a great burden on her family and blames herself for letting them down and for not bearing her difficulties with dignified stoicism. Her recent inability to achieve orgasm also convinces Mrs. B. that her sexual life and femininity are a thing of the past (Frances and Hales, 1984).

Objective signs

Depressed patients often demonstrate behavior that is noticeable to others, but these patients may not want to talk to anyone and may seek to be alone. If someone intrudes into the obsessive thinking of their inner world, they may become irritable and aggressive and strike out at the "intruder." Two general areas of objective signs are alterations of activity, including activities of daily living (ADLs), and altered social interactions.

Alterations in activity

Patients may exhibit psychomotor agitation. They may be unable to sit still; they may pace and engage in hand-wringing. They may pull or rub their hair, skin, clothing, or other objects. Tying and retying shoes and buttoning and unbuttoning a shirt or blouse are typical behaviors. Psychomotor retardation is marked by a slowing of speech, increased pauses before answering, soft or monotonous speech, decreased frequency of speech (poverty of speech), and muteness. In addition, a general slowing of body movements occurs. Patients may state they "are tired all the time," even when they are not physically active. For example, a patient may have difficulty getting up from a chair to turn off the television. Even the smallest task may seem impossible.

ADLs suffer as well. Depressed persons often defer basic personal hygiene, such as bathing, shaving, putting on clean clothes, or wiping their mouths after eating. However, these latter objective signs are probably due to more than a lack of energy. Apathy, a lack of feeling, absence of emotion, or an inability to be motivated, plays an important role in these behaviors too. An extreme extension of these anergic symptoms is seen in cases in which depressed persons lie in bed and become incontinent or constipated because of the inability to muster the energy (both physical and psychic energy) to walk to the bathroom.

Depressed persons usually experience a change in eating behaviors that results in either weight loss or gain. Sleeping patterns change as well. Depressed persons may experience insomnia (difficulty falling asleep), middle insomnia (difficulty remaining asleep), or terminal insomnia (early morning awakening). Hypersomnia (increased and/or prolonged sleeping) is an atypical symptom of depression. Depressed persons may deny they are depressed yet spend hours by themselves. Here the nurse should not confuse a request to "go to my room and lie down" with hypersomnia. Many depressed persons want to lie down but do not sleep. There, in the solitude of an empty room, they descend into uninterrupted, self-defeating ruminations.

CLINICAL EXAMPLE

Stan Treback is a 60-year-old white male who has been successful in business for many years. He recently has become "blue" and does not seem to care about anything. He is cooperative and desires treatment. His symptoms are decreased energy, anxiety, agitation, insomnia, and a weight loss over the past year of 54 pounds. He has many somatic complaints.

Altered social interactions

Depressed persons often suffer from poor social skills that are linked directly to other symptoms of depression. Underachievement causes a lack of productivity on the job and at home. The self-absorbing nature of depression causes these individuals to be easily distracted and reduces their interest in people, their ideas, or problems. Depression causes problems with thinking, idea development, and problem solving. In addition, conversations are difficult to main-

tain, and only with great effort can a depressed person sustain a facial expression of interest and concern. Depressed persons are also withdrawn and often seek social isolation over social interaction with others. Hobbies and avocations that were once actively pursued become unimportant and may be abandoned or engaged in half-heartedly. Finally, the body language of depression (e.g., saddened facial expression and a drooping posture) serves as a social barrier.

Subjective symptoms

Alterations of affect

Alterations of affect are the symptoms primarily associated with depression. This is reasonable because these disturbances dominate the internal world of a depressed person. Anger, anxiety, apathy, bitterness, dejection, denial of feelings, despondency, guilt, helplessness, hopelessness, uselessness, loneliness, low self-esteem, sadness, and a sense of worthlessness are all subjective feelings that cause unbearable pain and anguish. Because of this anguish, depressed persons vacillate between sadness and apathy. When the pain becomes too great, they shut down and become apathetic. Finally, although most lay persons consider sadness to be the universal symptom of distress, apathy actually comes closer to being continually present in depressed persons.

The overall affective sense is one of low self-esteem. Guilt may include an overreaction to some current failing or may be associated with an indiscretion in the distant past that cannot be forgiven. Guilt can also take the form of accepting responsibility for occurrences in which the person had little impact. For example, one patient expressed guilt over the death of his son's friend in an automobile accident. The tortured reasoning the man used was as follows: If he had spent more time with the young man, it might have changed the young man's life; if he had changed the young man's life, the young man might have driven more safely. Guilt can also take the form of obsessional preoccupation with "What if I had only. . . ." The person becomes immobilized with "should have's, could have's." An even more morbid extension of guilt is the psychotic delusion of guilt for calamities that happened continents away.

Anxiety is a companion of depression. Depressed persons are filled with anxiousness and dread. A ringing telephone holds the potential for catastrophic news. A siren could mean a loved one has been injured; a child at school might not return. Although these terrible things do happen, most of us go on with life somewhat comforted by the knowledge that they will probably not happen if we do not take unusual risks. But, for many depressed persons, that ringing telephone causes the same anxious reaction each time.

Worthlessness can range from a feeling of inadequacy to total devaluation. Depressed persons may scan the environment for clues to their inadequacy and remark, "I knew I wasn't any good, it just took a while to find out why."

Alterations of cognition

Alterations of cognition include ambivalence and indecision, inability to concentrate, confusion, loss of interest and motivation, pessimism, self-blame, self-depreciation, self-destructive thoughts, thoughts of death and dying, and uncertainty. The inability of depressed persons to make a decision is particularly difficult for others to understand. Faced with even a simple decision, much vacillation is expressed. Once a decision is made, depressed persons may be obsessed with "what if's." Major decisions can be immobilizing.

Alterations of a physical nature

Alterations of a physical nature are common in depressed persons. Almost all parts of the body can be affected. Common physiological disorders include abdominal pain, anorexia, chest pain, constipation, dizziness, fatigue, headache, indigestion, insomnia, menstrual changes, nausea and vomiting, and sexual dysfunction. And, as mentioned in the previous section of this chapter on cultural aspects, some ethnic and racial groups' cultural practices may mimic depressive symptoms, or depression may be expressed somatically in these groups.

These subjective symptoms come to the attention of the nurse because of the numerous somatic complaints of depressed persons. Some persons become so preoccupied with their bodies that every twinge, every body change is greeted with great alarm and dread. One recovering depressed patient joked, "I have had a hundred heart attacks." Monitoring of body functions is not uncommon in the general population and is no doubt related to a variety of factors better addressed by a sociology textbook.

However, overinvestment in self-assessment by depressed persons is pathological and it is the degree of this thinking that sets depressed persons apart. Chest pain, an unusual spot on the face or abdomen, and stomach pain all can precipitate a panic attack in some persons. Panic attacks occur in 15% to 30% of individuals with MDD (APA, 1993).

Alterations of perception

Some depressed persons suffer from altered perceptions. Delusions and hallucinations are typically congruent with the depressed mood (e.g., a delusion of persecution because of a moral mistake). Somatic delusions (e.g., my body is full of cancer) and nihilistic delusions (e.g., my brain is dead) are not uncommon forms of psychotic delusions in depressed persons. Hallucinations tend to be less elaborate than those of schizophrenia and tend to focus on personal faults (e.g., "You are no good. You don't deserve your family.").

Etiology of Depression

The "decade of the brain" has placed great emphasis on the biological causes of depression; however, the biological view of depression is but one of several etiological explanations. Other explanations include psychological and sociological theories (DGP, 1993; McGrath, et al, 1992).

Biological theories of depression

The etiology of depression has been biologically attributed to alterations in neurochemical, genetic, endocrine, and circadian rhythm functions. These alterations produce physical and psychological changes expressed as depression (Warren, 1997). Research findings suggest that a neurochemical depression results when levels of certain neurotransmitters are altered. The biogenic amines norepinephrine and serotonin are most often mentioned, but dopamine, another biogenic amine, is indicated as well. Further, dysregulation of acetylcholine and gamma-aminobutyric acid (GABA) may contribute to the development of biochemical depression too. More specifically, when the levels of these neurotransmitters are altered at receptor sites or when receptor sensitivity changes, a neurochemical depression may result (Asnis, McGinn, and Sanderson, 1995; Beeber, 1996; Haber, 1997; Laraia and Nihart,

1995; Shuchter, Downs, and Zisook, 1996). The serotonergic receptors originate in the raphe nuclei of the brainstem and are located near the midline for most of the length of the brainstem. The more rostral (towards the head) project throughout the cortex. Each serotonergic neuron sends over 500,000 terminals to the limbic system and to the cortex (Dubovsky, 1994). Hence, serotonin contributes to the regulation of many psychological functions (Dubovsky, 1994). Norepinephrine or noradrenergic pathways originate in the locus ceruleus and innervate all areas of the cortex, the hypothalamus, and the hippocampus. As with serotonin, norepinephrine neurons innervate and contribute to regulation of brain areas with a variety of functions (Kandel, Schwartz, and Jessell, 1991).

As appealing as it might be to conceptualize depression as a decreased bioavailability of serotonin and norepinephrine, and as equally appealing to suggest that by increasing the bioavailability of these amines one can successfully treat depression, in doing so we oversimplify both the problem and the solution. Other hypotheses include the sensitivity of both presynaptic and postsynaptic receptors and the modulating effects of acetylcholine and GABA on aminergic systems. It is thought, for example, that beta autoreceptors, which normally inhibit the release of norepinephrine, are down-regulated by antidepressants, thus disinhibiting norepinephrine release (i.e., increasing synaptic norepinephrine). One might think that too many norepinephrine or serotonin receptors would be a positive situation. However, excessive (i.e., up-regulation) receptors indicate insufficient levels of these neurotransmitters. This is an example of the body compensating for decreased monoamine availability (Nemeroff, 1998).

Finally, peptides, dietary practices, and nutritional status are being examined for their biochemical roles in the development of depression since food intake affects the development of precursors (i.e., amino acids) for neurotransmitters. Chapter 21 provides a detailed explanation of antidepressants.

Other researchers have contended that depression may be genetic based and that heredity may predispose persons to develop depression (Kendler, et al, 1993; Shuchter, Downs, and Zisook, 1996). Several studies have been conducted that examined the incidence of depression in twins. Findings have indicated that the concordancy rate for MDD ranges from 32% to 67% in twins where one or both of the biological parents had been diagnosed with MDD (Shuchter, Downs, and Zisook, 1996).

Endocrine changes, in relationship to depression, have also been investigated. Normally, the hypothalmic-pituitary-adrenal (HPA) axis is a system that mediates the stress response. However, in some depressed persons, this system malfunctions and creates cortisol, thyroid, and hormonal abnormalities. Dysregulation of the HPA axis results in hypercortisolemia (in about 40% to 60% of depressed patients), nonsuppression by dexamethasone, and elevated corticotropin-releasing factor (CRF) (Keltner, et al, 1998). The hypersecretion of cortisol is the result of an overexpression of the CRF gene (leading to increased CRF synthesis) and an increase in CRF-producing neurons in the hypothalamus. This, in turn, leads to increased pituitary release of adrenocorticotropic hormone (ACTH) and the subsequent hypersecretion of cortisol by the adrenal glands.

The dexamethasone suppression test (DST) will fail to suppress cortisol in about 40% of depressed patients; however, this test is not conclusive for depression. This malfunctioning and its results are more pronounced in severely depressed patients (Shuchter, Downs, and Zisook, 1996). In addition, the presence of endocrine disease, caused by alterations in the HPA axis, has also been associated with the development of depressive symptoms (Fava, 1994; Maes, et al, 1994; Shuchter, Downs, and Zisook, 1996). For example, women who suffer from bulimia have altered endocrine functioning and a high incidence of MDD. There is controversy regarding the role of genetics and hormonal explanations of depression in women as some researchers have contended that women have a predisposition to develop depressive symptoms and MDD because of fluctuations in hormones (McGrath, et al, 1992). Other researchers have contended that these fluctuations influence the development of MDD through their interaction with neurotransmitters, psychosocial factors, and the stress system (Beeber, 1996; Cockerman, 1992; McGrath, et al, 1992).

Persons experiencing **circadian rhythm changes** are at increased risk for developing depressive symptoms and MDD. These changes may be caused by medications, nutritional deficiencies, physical or psychological illnesses, hormonal fluctuations associated with women's reproductive system, and/or aging (Buysse, et al, 1994; Cartwright and Lloyd, 1994; McEnany, 1995a,b; Warren, 1997). Circadian rhythms are responsible for the daily regulation of wake-sleep cycles, arousal and activity patterns, and hormonal secretions associated with these regulatory mechanisms. In depressed persons these regulatory mechanisms are altered, which leads to shortened rapid eye movements (REM) latency and sleep disturbances such as insomnia, frequent waking, and more intensified dreaming (Shuchter, Downs, and Zisook, 1996).

Psychological theories of depression

The **psychological** explanations for depression flow from psychoanalytic, cognitive, interpersonal, and behavioral perspectives. In addition, related psychosocial/psychodynamic views explain depression from three general themes: adverse early life experiences, intrapsychic conflicts, and/or reactions to life events (i.e., stressors).

Psychoanalytic theorists have contended that depression occurs as a result of a person's ego loss in relationship to early life occurrences (Freud, 1957). Freud viewed depression as the aggressive instinct inappropriately directed at self, often triggered by the loss of a loved person or object. By understanding (i.e., gaining insight into) one's thoughts, feelings, and motives, one can heal. **Cognitive** theorists have contended that depression results when a person perceives all stressful situations as being negative (Beck, 1991; Beck, et al, 1979). In addition, a depressed person reacts to all situations as if they are stressful and sees himself or herself, others, and daily events in a negative light. This reaction to stress is grounded in early childhood losses (e.g., often loss of the parent through death, leaving the home, or divorce) and serves as the basis for how the depressed person makes decisions and sees himself or herself in relationship to other persons and occurrences. Cognitive therapy aims at symptom removal by identification and correction of distorted, negative, moment-by-moment thinking and seeks to prevent recurrence by correcting silent assumptions (DGP, 1993). Some researchers have indicated that when a person has **interpersonal** difficulties, coping with individuals, life events, and life changes can be inordinately stressful and lead to depression (Klerman, 1989). Role dispute, social isolation, prolonged grief reaction, and role transition are major interpersonal themes. Interpersonal difficulties are viewed as either causal, con-

comitant, or exacerbating/maintaining factors for depression (DGP, 1993). According to **behaviorists,** a person develops depression when one develops feelings of helplessness and unworthiness and then learns to use these attitudes to evaluate life outcomes (Abramson, Seligman, and Teasdale, 1978).

Psychological or psychodynamic explanations of depression can be categorized under three general themes: debilitating early life experiences, intrapsychic conflicts, or reactions to life events.

Debilitating early life experiences

According to traditional psychiatric thought, events in early life can lay the foundation for adult depression. The developmental theorists view the early years of life as the foundation of lifelong mental health. Although these theorists use different words to designate life stages, their views of the importance of a solid, nurturing early life environment are similar. Early losses, maternal inconsistency, the giving and withholding of love by the caregiver, and various types of abuse are all explained as causative agents for depression.

Intrapsychic conflict

Intrapsychic conflict refers to the conflicts people have when they have mixed emotions about a behavior, event, or situation. For instance, an individual who has been brought up to refrain from sexual activity, but who also has strong urges to experience sex, has a conflict. To refrain from sexual activity increases sexual frustration and to engage in sexual activity may cause anxiety, guilt, and fear. People are faced with intrapsychic conflicts all the time. Persistent unsuccessful resolution of these conflicts can lead to depression.

Reactions to life events

Most people view depression as a reaction to life stress. Loss is a major theme: of a loved one, of a job, of self-esteem, and of familiar surroundings. Even the loss caused by a psychotic disorder can cause depression (Weiss, Valdiserri, and Dubin, 1989). It is normal to react to loss with grief and sadness; it is abnormal to overreact. However, exactly when normal becomes abnormal is unclear. Klerman (1980) said, "Because clinicians and investigators do not fully agree as to the complete range of affective disorders to be diagnosed as psychopathological, the boundary between normal mood and abnormal depression remains undefined."

CLINICAL EXAMPLE

Elle Jones is a 45-year-old, well-educated, intelligent white female who has been in and out of therapy for a long time (15 to 20 years). She grew up in northern Mississippi with two brothers and a very physically and emotionally abusive father. Elle reports that, when she was quite young, her mother left home and did not return for several years. Elle left home at age 17 and was married twice and divorced shortly after each marriage. She has a history of depression, and she attempted suicide in 1976 when she ran her car off an embankment. After many turbulent years, she started going to bars in hopes "that I might get killed." She refers to this as her "death-hunt days." After emotional and financial collapse, Elle has recently returned to her father's home. He continues to control her life in every way. She has commented that her life is so futile that she would rather be dead.

Sociological theory

Sociological theory incorporates psychoanalytic theory into its explanation for development of depression. In addition, sociological theory uses the medical, social learning, stress, and antipsychiatric models to explain the development of depression. The **medical model** supports the idea that depression is a disease that can be treated through medical interventions such as medications, nutritional therapy, and electroconvulsive shock treatments (Kammeyer, Ritzer, and Yetman, 1992). **Social learning** theorists have indicated that depression occurs when a person learns, through repetitive experiences, to cope with stress in a negative manner (Cockerman, 1992). Proponents of the **stress model** have contended that the development of depression is related to the interactions of a person's experiences, perceptions, social support, biopsychosocial weaknesses, and occurrence of stress (Shuchter, Downs, and Zisook, 1996). The **antipsychiatric model** supports the premise that depression is a person's normal adaptive response to cope with aversive socioeconomic and political situations (e.g., influence of the interaction of political power structures on diverse

populations) and should not be viewed as abnormal (Mechanic, 1983).

Assessment of Depression

Assessment of depression may be accomplished through both nonbiological and biological assessment methods. The Depression Guideline Panel (1993) and Shuchter, Downs, and Zisook, (1996) recommend that patients be examined in a "profile" manner for an accurate diagnosis of depression. The profile should address DSM-IV criteria and biological findings, including:

1. history of onset of symptoms;
2. presence of comorbid substance, alcohol, and medication use (Box 28-3);
3. physical examination to rule out possibility of the presence of medical conditions (Box 28-4 provides a list of medical conditions);
4. the presence of nonmood psychiatric disorders;
5. patient resources and social support systems;
6. interpersonal and coping abilities;
7. level of stressors;
8. presence and/or level of suicidal ideation.

A nurse can be instrumental in the collection of all of this information since he or she is often the health care professional who initially assesses a patient and develops the database for use in the general diagnostic and nursing processes (e.g., development of nursing diagnosis, patient interventions and strategies, expected outcomes, and evaluation guidelines).

Assessment measures are available for use with child, adolescent, and adult populations from various ethnic, racial, and cultural groups. Instrument selection is based upon the nurse's clinical knowledge and experience, as well as the age and mental capacity of the person being assessed. Unfortunately, only limited measures have been developed and normed for use in different ethnic, racial, and cultural groups (Jones, 1996). The lack of measurement specificity for these populations can lead to misdiagnosis or underdiagnosis. Since some researchers contend culturally competent measures predict relevant criteria more accurately than do non–culturally competent measures, this assessment deficiency should be viewed as clinically significant. Routine incorporation of cultural competence facilitates accurate and valid assessment for all patients.

Box 28-3   Drugs and Toxins that May Induce Depression

Analgesics
Pentazocine
Phenacetin

Antibiotics
Aminoglycosides
Chloramphenicol
Sulfonamides

Anticonvulsants
Carbamazepine (rare)
Clonazepam
Phenobarbital
Phenytoin
Primidone
Succinimide

Antihypertensives
Alpha-Methyldopa
Calcium channel blockers (possibly)
Clonidine
Hydralazine (possibly)
Propranolol
Reserpine

Antiinflammatory Agents
Corticosteroids
Indomethacin

Cardiovascular Agents
Digitalis
Disopyramide
Procainamide

Psychotropic and Central Nervous System Agents
Aliphatic phenothiazines
Amphetamines
Appetite suppressants
    Fenfluramine
    Phenmetrazine
Barbiturates
Benzodiazepines
High-potency neuroleptics

Miscellaneous
Baclofen
Choline
Cimetidine
Disulfiram
Phenylephrine
Physostigmine

Antituberculosis Agents
Ethambutol
Isoniazid

Antineoplastic Agents
Asparaginase
Corticosteroids
Nonsteroidal antiinflammatory drugs
Phenylbutazone

Antiparkinsonian Agents
Amantadine
Cycloserine
Levodopa
Vinblastine sulfate

Adapted from Ford CV and Folks DG: Psychiatric disorders in geriatric medical/surgical patients. II. Review of clinical experience in consultation, *South Med J* 78(4):397, 1985.

Cultural issues and the assessment of depression

The reader is referred to Chapter 17 for information regarding cultural competence and cultural influences. However, a few relevant cultural issues regarding depression will be discussed in this chapter. **Culture** is the internal and external manifestation of an individual, group, or community's beliefs, values, and norms that are used as premises for everyday functioning. Tseng and Streltzer (1997)

recommend that clinicians distinguish between normal cultural behavior and psychopathology by using:

1. Cultural competence guidelines and/or a panel of experts (i.e., someone who understands the culture)
2. DSM-IV criteria
3. A functional status measurement
4. The affected person's perception of self and what he or she considers "normal"

Box 28-4 Medical Illnesses Commonly Associated with Depression

Central Nervous System Disorders
Alzheimer's disease (senile and presenile)
Amyotrophic lateral sclerosis
Brain tumor (especially nondominant lobe)
Cerebrovascular accident (stroke)
Chronic subdural hematoma
Multiple sclerosis
Normal-pressure hydrocephalus
Parkinson's disease
Subarachnoid hemorrhage

Infections
Acquired immunodeficiency syndrome
Encephalitis
Hepatitis
Infectious mononucleosis
Influenza
Syphilis
Tuberculosis
Viral pneumonia

Collagen Vascular Disease
Polymyalgia rheumatica
Rheumatoid arthritis
Systemic lupus erythematosus
Temporal arteritis

Neoplastic Disorders
Carcinoma of head of pancreas
Chronic myelogenous leukemia
Lymphoma
Other malignant diseases
Small-cell carcinoma of lung

Toxic-Metabolic Disturbances and Endocrinopathies
Addison's disease
Apathetic hyperthyroidism
Cushing's disease
Diabetes mellitus
Electrolyte disorders
Hypoglycemia
Hypothyroidism
Metal intoxication
Parathyroid disorders
Uremia

Other
Chronic fatigue syndrome
Chronic obstructive pulmonary disease

Adapted from Ford CV and Folks DG: Psychiatric disorders in geriatric medical/surgical patients. II. Review of clinical experience in consultation, *South Med J* 78(4):397, 1985.

Assessment of depression in the elderly

Depression among the elderly is a major health concern (Gomez and Gomez, 1993). The prevalence of MDD has been estimated at 6% to 11.5% within the elderly (DGP, 1993). It is relatively common, but because of the overlapping symptoms of physical illness and the depressive side effects of many medications, diagnosis is complex. To acquaint the nurse with potential confounding variables, a list of depression-causing medications and a list of illnesses that share symptoms with depression are presented (see Boxes 28-4 and 28-5, respectively).

If the depression is related to a treatable medical illness, elimination of the illness often returns the depressed mood to normal. On the other hand, MDD and medical illness can coexist, and in such cases treatment needs to be instituted. The nurse should also be aware that some persons who are di-

agnosed with dementia are, in reality, depressed (referred to as pseudodementia). Hence, it is important to differentiate between depression and dementia. Again, depression and dementia can occur comorbidly, in which case both must be treated. Comorbid MDD and dementia tend to occur early in the course of Alzheimer's disease (DGP, 1993).

Finally, the elderly are at increased risk of suicide. Men are at increased risk over women with elderly white men having the highest risk of suicide in the United States (Mellick, Buckwalter, and Stolley, 1992). Those over the age of 50 years are responsible for 28% of the annual deaths by suicide (Hendin, 1986). In people under 50 years, approximately one out of eight suicide attempts is successful, but for persons over 65 years, one out of two suicide attempts is successful (Gomez and Gomez, 1993). It is estimated that elderly white men will account for

Clinical Features Influencing Treatment of Depression

1. Risk of suicide:
   - People with major depression are at high risk for suicide. Important variables include:
     Social supports
     Access and lethality of suicidal methods
     History of suicide attempts
   - Some patients have more energy to attempt suicide as they improve.
   - It is not possible to predict with certainty whether or not someone will commit suicide.
2. Melancholia: a severe form of major depression with somatic symptoms including hypochondriasis, insomnia, anorexia, anhedonia, and somatic delusions. Responds to somatic therapy.
3. Mild depression: may respond to psychotherapy alone, but may also require medication
4. Recurrent depression: Approximately 50% of depressed patients have a recurrence.
5. Residual symptoms: Approximately 20% to 35% of patients have persistent symptoms that interfere with social or occupational functioning.
6. History of mania: Antidepressants and electroconvulsive therapy (ECT) can provoke a manic or hypomanic episode in these patients.
7. Depression with psychotic features: These patients have a higher risk for suicide. Typical features include delusions and hallucinations. The most common delusions experienced are characterized by persecution, suspiciousness, paranoia, and, somewhat less frequently, guilt, sin, and ideas of reference (Dubovsky and Thomas, 1992). Many patients who have depression with psychotic episodes respond better to amoxapine (Asendin), a metabolite of the antipsychotic drug loxapine (Loxitane).
8. Depression with catatonic features: symptoms include motoric immobility, purposeless motor activity, extreme negativism, and peculiar movements such as posturing and echolalia/echopraxia. ECT is proven to be particularly effective for this type of depression.
9. Atypical depression: symptoms include severe anxiety; reversed vegetative symptoms such as increased sleep, appetite, and weight; marked mood reactivity; sensitivity to emotional rejection; and a sense of severe fatigue such as extreme heaviness of arms and legs. Tricyclic antidepressants (TCAs) are effective only 35% to 50% of the time. Monoamine oxidase inhibitors (MAOIs) are effective in 55% to 75% of these

patients. Fluoxetine and sertraline may have a role to play in atypical depression.
10. Depression complicated by chemical dependency: These patients are more likely to need hospitalization, more likely to attempt suicide, and less likely to comply with treatment.
11. Depression associated with obsessive-compulsive disorder: Clomipramine and the selective serotonin reuptake inhibitors are the drugs of choice.
12. Depression associated with panic disorder and/or anxiety: Panic disorder occurs in 15% to 30% of the cases of major depression. This complicating factor makes recovery more difficult. Although MAOIs seem to be the most effective, there are traditional concerns about MAOI side effects and interactions, and treatment is initiated usually with a TCA.
13. Pseudodementia: Major depression affects cognitive function, particularly in older people. Sometimes depressed older persons appear to be demented. Because depression is a reversible disorder, every effort should be made to correctly diagnose patients with cognitive dysfunction. Differentiating characteristics of these patients include the following:

Patients with Pseudodementia	Patients with Dementia
• Exert little effort in cognitive tasks, but report incapacity ("I can't think.") • Do not have signs of cortical dysfunction	• Do not complain of cognitive problems because they have little insight • Exhibit aphasia, apraxia, agnosia

14. Postpsychotic depression: Approximately 25% of patients with schizophrenia have a complicating depression. Depression in this case is treated by adding an antidepressant to the antipsychotic regimen.
15. Depression during or following pregnancy: The development of pregnancy-related depression causes several concerns for the clinician. Although a direct link between antidepressants and birth defects has not been conclusively established, caution should be observed. The risks vs. benefits must be weighed carefully. ECT may be used because it appears to be safe for both mother and fetus.

Adapted from the American Psychiatric Association Practice guidelines for major depressive disorder in adults, *Am J Psychiatry* (suppl) 150(4):1, 1993.

10,500 suicides annually by the year 2000. Predictor variables include chronic sleep problems, pain, degenerative illness, and clinical depression (Mellick, Buckwalter, and Stolley, 1992).

Nonbiological assessment measures of depression

Nonbiological assessments are comprised of standardized verbal and pen and paper measurement scales. See Table 28-3 for a partial listing of these measures. All of these measures may be given verbally or in writing. However, it is important that nurses follow the directions for each of these instruments so that obtained data is reliable. Obtained data can then be used in conjunction with the DSM-IV criteria and biological assessments to give a more accurate diagnosis regarding MDD.

Biological assessment measures of depression

Some biological measures for depression may be used in child, adolescent, and adult populations, whereas others are solely for use in one of these populations. Various biological measures include the DST, growth hormone secretion, and polysomnographic (i.e., sleep patterns) findings.

The DST is a diagnostic test for clinical depression (i.e., MDD) that measures the function of the HPA axis. Urine and blood samples are collected prior to the test for determination of baseline levels of cortisol. Then a single injection of the drug dexamethasone (e.g., 1 mg for adults and adolescents, 0.5 mg for children) is given to the patient. Urine and blood cortisol levels are monitored for 24 hours. A positive result occurs when cortisol levels do not fall (i.e., are not suppressed) or return to 5 μg/dl or above within 24 hours. Forty percent of severely depressed patients fail to suppress cortisol. The DST has been consistently used in adult populations as an assessment method; however, its appropriateness for use in children and adolescent populations is still being examined (Killeen and Bongarten, 1996). As mentioned above, the DST is not specific for depression as individuals suffering from dementia, alcohol withdrawal, and bulimia do not suppress either.

Growth hormone secretion is often used as a biological assessment measure in childhood depression.

Past research has indicated that some depressed children may have decreased secretion of the growth hormone during the day and increased secretion while asleep. This test is not useful in adolescent and adult populations.

Polysomnographic findings (i.e., examination of sleep patterns) are used in the assessment of depression in adult populations but have not proven valid for children and adolescent populations. The REM stage usually begins within 70 to 100 minutes of a person falling asleep and increases in length throughout the night. However, in depressed adults, the REM latency phase is shortened, which results in frequent night and early morning wakening. Antidepressants can restore the normal pattern of REM sleep.

Psychotherapeutic Management

The nurse utilizes nursing process to develop appropriate nursing interventions and strategies, expected outcomes, and evaluation of the outcomes for depressed patients. The intervention strategy described in this book, psychotherapeutic management, emphasizes the nurse-patient relationship, psychopharmacology, and milieu management. These concepts are discussed in detail in Units Three, Four, and Five, respectively. The case study and care plan presented in this section on depression are geared toward the nursing management of a depressed patient who is residing in a psychiatric hospital environment. However, it is important to realize the majority of psychiatric patients, in the current managed care environment, are hospitalized for short periods of time or may not be hospitalized at all (DGP, 1993). Consequently, nursing management of depressed individuals may occur in medical settings or outpatient clinics. In addition, it is imperative that nurses in any setting be familiar with the DSM-IV criteria of MDD and the information regarding mood disorders presented in this chapter. Finally, it is recommended that the reader refer to Chapter 37 for a detailed explanation of electroconvulsive therapy used in the treatment of depression.

Nurse-Patient Relationship. The objective of this section is to provide specific principles of therapeutic communication for nurses who work with depressed patients.

1. Depressed persons suffer from low self-esteem. The most effective approach to bolster self-esteem is to accept patients as they are (negative attitude and all), to help them to focus on the positive (accomplishments, good points), to provide successful experiences with positive feedback, to keep self-help strategies simple, and to help patients avoid embarrassing social blunders (e.g., smelly clothes, unkempt appearance). (Also see no. 4.)

2. Development of a meaningful relationship in which depressed persons are valued as human beings is important to their sense of personal worth. It is important for the nurse to be honest and to work on developing trust. The "trusting relationship" is developed by doing those things that are in the best interest of each patient. For instance, a patient may wish to tell the nurse something of clinical significance but does not want the nurse to share the information with other staff members. The nurse builds trust by telling the patient that significant information will be shared with those staff members who have a need to know in order to be helpful to the patient. The patient learns to trust the nurse as a professional whose dominant concern is the patient's best interest.

3. The nurse who works effectively with depressed patients must have sincere concern for patients and be empathic. For instance, it is not unusual for a nurse to feel a little sad when working with depressed or suicidal patients. The nurse acknowledges the emotional pain and suffering conveyed by patients and offers to help patients work through the pain. It is important for the nurse to discuss personal feelings with a colleague.

4. It is usually not effective to outline logically why a patient is a worthwhile human being. The nurse does point out even small visible accomplishments and strengths, however (e.g., "I'm glad you combed your hair today"). A patient may agree with everything the nurse says but remain just as depressed. Intellectual understanding does not help severely depressed patients. Cognitive behavior therapists, however, have been successful in helping some depressed persons to learn to "reprogram" negative thoughts (e.g., to progress from "I can't do anything right" to "I can learn from my mistakes").

5. Depressed persons are typically dependent. The nurse may notice that he or she is taking on responsibility for the depression of patients. The nurse should recognize, but not resent, this tendency in depressed persons to become dependent. The nurse should reward even small decisions and independent actions.

6. The nurse should not attempt to "embarrass" patients out of being depressed. For example, pointing out less fortunate persons in the hope that such an action might bring depressed persons to their senses provides, at best, short-lived relief based on the misfortune of others. At worst, it establishes a mind-set that reduces others to object lessons or convinces the patient that the world is unfair and miserable, and increases the patient's guilt.

7. Never reinforce hallucinations, delusions, or irrational beliefs: the nurse cannot agree, and arguing seems to reinforce them. The nurse should state his or her perception of reality, voice doubt about the patient's perceptions, and move on to discuss real people and events.

8. Depressed persons tend to be angry. Sometimes they surprise even themselves with the hateful or hostile things that they say. It is important for the nurse to learn to handle hostility therapeutically by recognizing the anger, not taking it personally, and not retaliating in word, deed, or some passive-aggressive form. Encouraging verbal expressions of anger helps to release patients' tension.

9. The nurse can help withdrawn patients to emerge from their social isolation by spending time with them (even without speaking), by providing a nonthreatening one-to-one relationship, by practicing assertiveness interactions, and by being accepting.

10. Depressed persons can have difficulty in making even simple decisions. It is not therapeutic to badger patients into making a decision, but it is therapeutic to provide decision-making opportunities as patients are able to comply. Initially, the nurse may need to make decisions for patients; for example, "It is time for your bath"; "Here is your apple juice." When possible, the nurse helps to guide patients to appropriate decisions by using problem-solving techniques; that is, identifying options, the advantages and disadvantages of each option, and the potential consequences of each deci-

Key Nursing Interventions for Depressed Patients

The psychiatric nurse should consider the following intervention principles when working with depressed patients.

- Accept patients where they are and focus on their strengths.

   Rationale: Depressed persons have low self-esteem, and this is the best approach to recapturing some sense of value.

- Reinforce decision making by patients.

   Rationale: Depressed patients struggle to make even simple decisions. By reinforcing patients' efforts to make simple decisions, the nurse helps patients move toward health.

- Never reinforce hallucinations or delusions.

   Rationale: Confronting these psychotic symptoms tends to reinforce them. The best approach is for the nurse to state his or her view of reality and to begin discussing real people and events.

- Respond to anger therapeutically.

   Rationale: Depressed persons are typically angry. By understanding that anger is a symptom of depres-

sion, the nurse can focus on the issue at hand and help patients to move toward a more acceptable style of interaction.

- Spend time with withdrawn patients.

   Rationale: Withdrawn patients are aware of their surroundings. By spending time (frequent but brief contact) with these patients, the nurse communicates patients' worth and, consequently, may be available during a time when patients feel comfortable with initiating dialogue.

- Make decisions for patients that they are not ready to make for themselves.

   Rationale: Some patients cannot make a decision. Simply present situations to these patients that do not require decision making (e.g., "It's time to go for a walk").

- Involve patients in activities in which they can experience success.

   Rationale: People can feel good about themselves in several ways. One way to develop self-worth is through accomplishment.

Box 28-5   Important Points for Administering Antidepressant and Antimanic Drugs

- Most antidepressants have a lag time of 1-4 weeks before a full clinical effect occurs. During that time, patients gradually begin to feel better and to have more energy. Suicidal tendencies may be greater as antidepressants increase energy and motivation. Lithium has a lag time of 7-10 days before it takes effect.
- Monitor patients for "cheeking" or hoarding of drugs. At amounts not much greater than the therapeutic amount, TCAs and lithium can become toxic.
- Monitor vital signs of patients who take TCAs and MAOIs. TCAs can cause orthostatic hypotension, reflex tachycardia, and arrhythmias. MAOIs have the potential for triggering a hypertensive crisis. Monitor sexual side effects of SSRIs, e.g. decreased libido, impotence, ejaculatory disturbances occur fairly frequently and can lead to noncompliance.

- Be aware of the drug-drug and food-drug interactions associated with MAOIs.
- Observe for early signs of toxicity:
  - TCAs: drowsiness, tachycardia, mydriasis, hypotension, agitation, vomiting, confusion, fever, restlessness, sweating
  - MAOIs: dizziness, vertigo, fatigue
  - SSRIs: Have low probability for causing toxicity. Symptoms include nausea, vomiting, tremor, myoclonus, and irritability
  - Lithium: diarrhea, vomiting, drowsiness, muscle weakness, ataxia, giddiness, polyuria
- Monitor serum lithium levels. Maintenance levels are 0.6-1.2 mEq/L.

---

sion. Other nursing interventions are found in the box above.

Psychopharmacology.   To understand the range of information required for effective psychopharmacological intervention, the student is encour-

aged to review Chapter 21, which provides a complete discussion of antidepressant and antimanic drugs. A brief review of critical parameters of antidepressant drug administration is given in Box 28-5 and the side effects table on the following page.

Side Effects and Nursing Interventions for Antidepressant and Antimanic Drugs

Side Effects	Interventions
Antidepressants (TCAs, SSRIs)	
Dry mouth	Provide sugarless hard candy, sugarless chewing gum, frequent rinses
Nasal congestion	Over-the-counter decongestants as approved by physician or nurse practitioner
Urinary hesitancy	Running water, privacy, warm water over perineum
Urinary retention	Catheterize for residual fluids and encourage frequent voiding
Blurred vision	Reassurance; this symptom usually subsides; wear sunglasses outside; caution about driving
Constipation	Laxatives as ordered, diet with roughage, fluids
Sedation, ataxia	Caution to avoid dangerous tasks (e.g., driving); advise that alcohol compounds sedation; daytime sedation is minimized if drug is given at bedtime
Confusion	Possibility of anticholinergic-induced delirium; withhold drug and notify physician
Orthostatic hypotension	Instruct patients to rise slowly; if patient is lying down, should sit on side of bed for 1 full minute before rising to walk; instruct to avoid standing in one place too long and to avoid taking hot baths or showers
Arrhythmias, tachycardia, palpitations	Record vital signs; if patient experiences tachycardia, withhold drug
Decreased sweating	Instruct patients to be cautious about strenuous activity in hot weather
Monoamine Oxidase Inhibitors	
Overstimulation such as agitation, hypomania	Withhold MAOIs and notify physician
Blurred vision, hypotension, dry mouth, constipation	See interventions above
Hypertensive crisis related to food-drug or drug-drug interactions	Avoid these food and drug combinations
Lithium	
Confusion, restlessness, sleeplessness	Withhold lithium
Gastrointestinal symptoms	
Nausea	Give lithium with meals
Thirst	Instruct patients to drink 10-12 8-ounce (240 ml) glasses of water each day
Diarrhea	Observe closely for depletion of electrolytes; this can cause higher serum lithium levels
Weight gain	Weigh patients weekly; patients may need to be placed on structured diet
Sedation, blurred vision, arrhythmias, tachycardia, palpitations, dry mouth, constipation	See interventions above

Milieu Management. Milieu management is an important dimension of the psychiatric nursing care of depressed patients. The student is referred to Unit Five for a complete discussion of milieu management. General principles that specifically address the environment of depressed patients are considered below.

Patients with low self-esteem

- Encourage patients with low self-esteem to participate in activities, including group activities, in which they will be able to experience accomplishment and receive positive feedback. Most people develop a sense of self-worth through mastery or accomplishment.

Case Study

Sylvia Green is a 75-year-old married woman with a long history of depression and hospitalizations. She has been on the unit for 6 weeks. She is experiencing insomnia, anxiety, and anorexia. She does not talk to other patients and tries to stay in her bedroom. Improvements, if any, have been slight. She has multiple physical problems, including hypertension, left-sided weakness due to a cerebral vascular accident, and glaucoma. Her 81-year-old husband of 52 years states that he is at his "wit's end," but wants her to "get well and come home." He reports that she has never been this bad before. Mrs. Green lies in bed when her room is open and on the unit furniture at other times. Her verbal complaints include statements such as "I'm weak across the back"; "My head is driving me crazy"; "I can't eat. It goes right through me"; "I'm drawn up in a knot"; "I can't relax"; "My stomach is quivering and I shake all over"; "My head is crawling"; "I have terrible thoughts"; and "I'm so sick I wish I could die."

The nurse finds that Mrs. Green is not suicidal, and the statement "my head is crawling" is not delusional. Mr. Green reports that Mrs. Green has been sick before, but always "does real good" after a month in the hospital. He also relates that she has responded to ECT in the past. Mrs. Green is a pathetic figure and feels absolutely hopeless. See p. 403 for Mrs. Green's nursing care plan.

Simply telling patients that they are "OK" is not convincing. Provide successful experiences, however small.

- Provide assertiveness training. Many depressed persons feel like doormats because of their interactional problems. Their communication history is typically a lifetime of being "taken advantage of," punctuated by periodic outbursts of anger when they become "fed up." Assertiveness training helps these patients to learn to take care of their needs and to express their feelings along the way so that the extremes of "doormat" and "flare-up" are avoided.

- Help patients to avoid embarrassing themselves through socially unacceptable appearance or behavior. Many appearance problems are related directly to depressed persons' preoccupation, apathy, and decreased energy level. For instance, food stains on clothes, food in one's beard, an unattended runny nose, uncombed hair, urine on trousers, and an unzipped fly may be seen among depressed persons who "cannot" pay attention to these hygienic concerns. Help patients to shower and dress appropriately. Remind patients to go to the bathroom. In some cases, it is better to encourage patients to walk with the nurse (e.g., to the bathroom area or to the shower). Some patients become so apathetic that they urinate on themselves.

Withdrawn patients

- Keep contacts with withdrawn patients brief but frequent. Depressed patients often do not want anyone around or, at least, anyone to talk to them. Unfortunately, their wishes are not a good indicator of what should be done. Spending time with patients is constructive; allowing patients to isolate themselves is not. Patients may need to increase physical activity before they are able to verbalize issues.

- Many patients are insistent about going to their rooms to lie down. They may stay there all day if the nurse does not intervene. Locking a patient's room during the day may be required to keep the withdrawn or isolative patient from disappearing for hours at a time. Sitting in silence during an activity is better than ruminating in isolation.

Anorectic patients

- The nursing staff must take responsibility for ensuring that depressed patients eat. It is irresponsible to set a tray down in front of a depressed person, particularly in his or her room, and then leave. The nurse must encourage patients to eat and may even spoonfeed them if required.

- Allow patients to participate in selecting preferred foods from the menu.

- Promote a proper diet, adequate fluids, and exercise. Provide small, frequent meals. Record intake.

- Constipation is a side effect not only of antidepressants, but also of depression. A diet with adequate fiber content and sufficient fluids is important. It is important to monitor and record bowel elimination.

- If patients will eat food brought from home, allow them to have such food.

Care Plan

NAME: Mrs. Sylvia Green   **ADMISSION DATE:** _____

DSM-IV DIAGNOSIS: Major depression, recurrent

ASSESSMENT: **Areas of strength:** Supportive husband, financial security, history of good adjustment between recurrent episodes of depression. Past treatment with ECT was successful. Patient is not suicidal at this time.

Problems: Husband (81 years old) states patient has never been *this* depressed before. Patient is making statements about dying. Husband is worn out. States: "I don't know what to do." Patient is isolative, anorexic, cannot sleep, and wants to die.

DIAGNOSES:
- Hopelessness related to physical complaints, as evidenced by decreased appetite and verbal cues indicating despondency.
- Fatigue related to insomnia, as evidenced by increase in physical complaints and disinterest in surroundings.
- Social isolation related to anxiety, as evidenced by withdrawal and uncommunicative behavior.

OUTCOMES:

Short-term goals: Date met
- Patient will stay out of bed and participate in activities.   _____
- Patient will have low-salt diet, low-tyramine food, and maintain weight.   _____
- Patient will sleep at night.   _____
- Husband will attend unit support group.   _____

Long-term goals:
- Patient will return to home and husband.   _____
- Patient will attend outpatient program.   _____
- Patient will accept psychiatric nursing visits through HHA. _____
- Husband will attend ongoing support group.   _____

PLANNING/ INTERVENTIONS: **Nurse-patient relationship:** Develop a trusting relationship based on honesty and genuine concern for patient. Be empathic with patient as she verbalizes her negative thoughts. Spend time with patient. Reinforce strengths and accomplishments.

Psychopharmacology: Nardil 15 mg bid; monitor BP frequently for both hypotension and hypertensive crisis (from drug-drug and food-drug interactions); Lasix 40 mg q AM; Capoten 25 mg bid.

Milieu management: Minimize patient's tendency to isolate. Lock room and assist patient in some activity. Monitor eating and sleeping, eliminate caffeinated drinks and daytime naps. As tolerated, draw patient into small-group situations. Keep environment safe should patient attempt self-injury. Maintain low-tyramine and low-salt diet.

EVALUATION: Patient still very depressed, isolative, hopeless. Low-salt and low-tyramine diet has been maintained. Some improvement in sleeping behavior.

REFERRALS: Patient may be candidate for ECT. Consult sent to Dr. Jones to evaluate for ECT.

Patients with sleep disturbances
- Depressed persons want to sleep, but many suffer from insomnia. The tremendous fatigue is real to these patients because the sleep they manage to get is usually not restful. Patients often wake up looking and feeling exhausted. The nursing staff should record the amount and quality of patients' actual sleep. Patients who lie down during the day are not necessarily sleeping, but may be isolating themselves.

FAMILY ISSUES

Family Issues: Living with the Depressed Person

Living with a depressed person can be very difficult. The person is often irritable, moody, isolative, and pessimistic. Family members may struggle to get along with the person, coworkers may find the person impossible to please, and children may assume responsibility for their depressed parent's mood. Grunebaum and Cohler (1983) found that children of depressed mothers were more vulnerable to emotional problems than children of mothers with schizophrenia. Schizophrenia, they suggested, manifests in such a clearly abnormal fashion that children can recognize the parent as mentally disturbed (e.g., this behavior is abnormal, this behavior is normal). This level of insight affords some degree of emotional insulation from the parent's disruptive behavior. Grunebaum and Cohler further reasoned that because the depressed parent is not clearly "abnormal," but rather basically unhappy, moody, sad, and irritable, children are less able to set these boundaries. Hence, living with a depressed parent can trigger emotional insecurity and self-doubt, and cause a myriad of intrafamilial communication problems. Two brief clinical examples follow to illustrate the difficulties encountered in families with depressed individuals.

Joan is a 40-year-old college professor. She has been married for 15 years and has two children, a 13-year-old daughter and an 11-year-old son. Joan admits to a few close friends and to her husband that she is depressed. She has never "officially" sought help for her depression, but her physician has ordered a TCA at bedtime for "sleep." The problems her family faces related to her depressed mood are subtle, but beginning to take a toll. Joan is never happy, nor can she become excited about anything the family might do together. She spends much of her time at home either soaking in the bathtub or in her bedroom reading. She seems to have energy for her research at the university, but for little else. She resents her husband for many things; some are real, others are not. She is often critical of her daughter and then feels remorse. Joan has great difficulty talking with her family. Her husband, also a professional, realizes that something is wrong, but is losing patience with his wife. He perceives her lack of interest in sex or even talking with him as signs of a failing marriage. What is not clear is whether the failing marriage precipitated Joan's depressed mood (a reactive depression), whether Joan's depressed mood is causing the marriage to fail (an endogenous depression), or whether there is a synergistic combination of the two.

Harold is a 58-year-old white male who has been hospitalized numerous times over the years for depression. He has not worked for over 12 years. The past 6 years have been punctuated with threats of suicide and suicidal gestures. He talks about suicide often and, at home, has taken out a gun on several occasions while talking about killing himself. Harold is the father of five children, four boys and a girl, ages 15 to 32. Three children still live at home. His wife of 36 years, Molly, does not know what to do. When Harold's "suicide talk" becomes "serious," she either takes him to the hospital or calls the sheriff's office. The hospital staff, the sheriff's deputies, the children, Molly, and even Harold are tired of these frequent emergencies. Every time Molly leaves the house and returns, she admits to a fear of finding Harold dead. She is angry with Harold, but keeps her feelings to herself for fear of precipitating a suicide attempt. The children living at home become very anxious if they do not see their father as soon as they return from school each day. Molly states that she feels like a prisoner in her own home and cannot take it anymore.

An accurate understanding of the amount of sleep being obtained helps the nurse to formulate an intervention strategy.

- For patients taking a sedating tricyclic antidepressant (TCA), combining the daily dose into a single bedtime dose is known to decrease daytime sedation.
- People suffering from insomnia often engage in self-defeating behaviors, such as daytime napping and drinking stimulants (e.g., coffee, colas). Eliminating these behaviors increases the likelihood of nighttime sleep.
- Depressed patients who sleep too much (hypersomnia) should have restricted access to their rooms. The goal of working with patients who cannot sleep or who sleep too much is adequate rest (6 to 8 hours per night). Activities can be substituted for daytime sleeping. Exercise often increases energy levels.

BIPOLAR DISORDERS

Bipolar disorders are classified in the DSM-IV as bipolar I, bipolar II, cyclothymic disorder, and bipolar disorder not otherwise specified (APA, 1994). Epidemiologic research indicates approximately 2 million women and men experience bipolar disorder yearly, and the lifetime prevalence is estimated at 1.2% (Regier, et al, 1993; Simmons-Alling, 1996). Bipolar I disorders appear to be equally common among men and women but with evidence of a difference in order of expression (APA, 1994). In men the first episode is more likely to be a manic episode, whereas in women depression is more likely to be experienced first. There are no reports of differential incidence based on ethnic or racial groupings; however, findings suggest bipolar disorder may occur more commonly in higher socioeconomic groups (Simmons-Alling, 1996). And, as with depressive disorders, many individuals with bipolar disorder do not seek treatment. Sadly, about 10% to 15% of individuals with bipolar I disorder die by suicide (APA, 1994).

Description

Bipolar disorders are those in which individuals experience the extremes of mood polarity. Persons may feel very euphoric or very depressed. Although the term *bipolar* is the accepted diagnostic terminology, many professionals, and much professional literature, still use the term *manic-depressive*. Manic-depressive is the diagnostic equivalent of bipolar, but it is perhaps less precise. The first part of this chapter focuses on depression; this part focuses on bipolar disorders that encompass both extremes of mood. Because depression has been discussed, this section emphasizes manic symptoms.

Bipolar disorder can be traced from earliest recorded history to the present day. Thousands of years ago the Greeks recognized the vacillation between extremes of elation and depression. Other peoples have also observed and recorded wide mood swings for the historical record.

Manic episodes are characterized by an elevated or expansive mood. Symptoms are listed in Box 28-6. Manic episodes usually begin suddenly, escalate rapidly, and last from a few days to several months. Judgment is impaired, social blunders occur, and involvement with alcohol and drugs is common (often as an attempt at self-medication). Onset usually oc-

curs in the early 20s. What has been referred to traditionally as manic-depressive illness (mood swings) is now designated as bipolar illness. Manic episodes also can be part of organic mental disorders, a general medical condition, another psychotic process, or may be substance induced. Mania, as a component of bipolar illness, is the focus of this section. Approximately 1.6% of the adult population has this mental disorder at some point during their lifetime (Kessler, et al, 1994).

Often, mood swings are not severe enough to warrant hospitalization; however, problems with everyday life still occur. *Hypomania* is the term for an elevated state that is less intense than full mania. Fieve (1975), in his highly respected book *Moodswings*, points out that many creative people in our society ride the energy from their manic state to success. Fieve points out that successful producer Joshua Logan *(South Pacific)* and astronaut Buzz Aldrin (first moon landing) used the tremendous energy from their elevated moods to accomplish great things. Unfortunately, for manic-depressive patients, the climb up the emotional ladder does not stop with elation, and excessive energy moves into psychotic thinking and unacceptable behavior. In addition, an equally extreme depression can follow these highs. Both Logan and Aldrin required professional help to restore their moods to normal.

DSM-IV Terminology and Criteria

The DSM-IV defines several variations under the category of bipolar disorders. In order to understand

---

Box 28-6 Symptoms Occurring During Manic Episodes

Common Symptoms	Other Symptoms
Elevated mood	Lack of awareness of
Grandiosity	illness
Irritability	Resistance to treatment
Anger	Labile mood
Insomnia	Depression
Anorexia	Delusions
Flight of ideas	Hallucinations
Distractibility	
Hyperactivity	
Involvement in pleasurable activities	
Loud, rapid speech	

the DSM-IV diagnostic categories, the student must be able to distinguish the basic syndromes presented, such as the manic episode, the hypomanic episode, and cyclothymic disorder. The DSM-IV diagnostic criteria for these syndromes are presented in the box below.

The *manic episode* is the condition Fieve describes so clearly in his book. Individuals experiencing a manic episode have an inflated view of their importance, sometimes reaching grandiosity ("I'm so important that the president needs my advice on international affairs"). The episode presents as an elevated, expansive, or irritable mood. The impairment is sufficiently serious that functioning deteriorates at home, work, school, or in social contexts. Other symptoms include a decreased need for sleep, talkativeness, flight of ideas, and distractibility. The mind races and seems to go faster and faster. Indi-

viduals experiencing a manic episode may engage in risky behavior, such as sexual relationships that are not in keeping with their normal conduct. They may speculate on a risky business venture because they "understand" the big picture of business. People have lost everything in such periods of manic thinking. Excess is common: spending sprees, sexual indiscretions, loud clothing, and excessive make-up often are seen in individuals in a manic state. Hospitalization frequently is required to prevent harm to the person or to others.

CLINICAL EXAMPLE

Mary Bones is a 45-year-old secretary for a small computer software company. She has recently experienced job-related stress and is not coping well. Her boss has forced her to take a couple of days off in

---

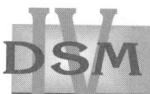 **DSM-IV Criteria for Bipolar Disorders**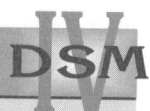

I. Manic episode:
    A. A distinct period of abnormal and persistent elevated, expansive, or irritable mood that lasts at least 1 week (or less if hospitalization is required).
    B. At least three of the following symptoms must occur during the episode (or four if the patient is only irritable).
       1. Inflated self-esteem or grandiosity
       2. Decreased need for sleep
       3. Very talkative
       4. Flight of ideas or subjective feeling that thoughts are racing
       5. Distractibility
       6. Increase in goal-directed activity (social, occupational, educational, or sexual) or psychomotor agitation
       7. Excessive involvement in pleasurable activities that have a high potential for personal problems (e.g., sexual promiscuity, spending sprees, bad business investments)
    C. Mood disturbance severe enough to cause problems socially, interpersonally, or at work, or the person has to be hospitalized to prevent harm to self or others
    D. Not due to a substance

II. Hypomanic episode:
    The person experiencing a hypomanic episode meets most of the criteria for manic episode, with two major exceptions: the symptoms must last at least 4 days and the person must manifest an unequivocal change in functioning that is observable by others. A hypomanic episode is not severe enough to result in significant impairment or to require hospitalization.

III. Bipolar disorders:
    A. Bipolar episodes are divided into bipolar I and bipolar II. There are six categories of bipolar I. In bipolar I, the patient must have a history of a manic episode.
    B. Bipolar II: The patient has experienced major depression and a hypomanic episode (but not a manic episode)

IV. Cyclothymic Disorder:
    For a period of 2 years, the patient has had numerous periods of hypomanic symptoms and numerous periods of a depressed mood. The patient is never symptom-free for more than 2 months at a time. The patient has never experienced major depression.

Adapted from the American Psychiatric Association: *Diagnostic and statistical manual of mental disorders*, ed 4, Washington, DC, 1994, The Association.

order "get herself together." Apparently, Mary was working long hours, but not always efficiently. She had become very irritable and demanding to the point that coworkers avoided her. At other times, she became loud and made suggestive remarks that made most of her coworkers uncomfortable. The final straw for Mary's boss was her insistence that she had a strategy that would put the company on the same level as IBM. Mary's boss was not interested in listening to her "theory," and she became extremely rude and condescending. These behaviors precipitated her "medical leave."

The *hypomanic episode* is similar to the manic episode but denotes a less severe level of impairment. Because the level of severity is somewhat subjective, the DSM-IV has attempted to differentiate manic from hypomanic episodes with more objective criteria. For a hypomanic episode to be diagnosed, the length of the episode must be at least 4 days in duration, but not severe enough to warrant hospitalization. Additionally, the episode is not severe enough to cause *major* problems at home, work, school, or in the social milieu but is observable by others and is distinct from the person's typical behavior.

Cyclothymic disorder is characterized by mood swings that have occurred for at least 2 years without symptom remission for more than 2 months. The swings in either direction are not quite severe enough to warrant the ultimate diagnoses manic episode and major depression. Using a pendulum as a metaphor, the person experiencing cyclothymic disorder swings from one side to the other but never quite reaches the extremes of the arc. The person experiencing a cyclothymic disorder is depressed but does not meet the criteria for major depression. The person is elated and expansive but does not meet the criteria for manic episode. The person experiences numerous hypomanic episodes and numerous dysthymic-level episodes.

The DSM-IV *bipolar diagnoses* are based on an understanding of these definitions. The DSM-IV divides bipolar diagnoses into bipolar I and bipolar II. There are six variants of bipolar I and one type of bipolar II.

The bipolar I diagnosis is based on a single episode subtype and subtypes in which the most recent episode was manic, hypomanic, mixed, depressed, or unspecified (First et al, 1993). The subtypes are:

Bipolar I disorder, single episode
Bipolar I disorder, most recent episode manic
Bipolar I disorder, most recent episode hypomanic
Bipolar I disorder, most recent episode mixed
Bipolar I disorder, most recent episode depressed
Bipolar I disorder, most recent episode unspecified

Bipolar II disorder is similar to bipolar I disorder, with the major exception that the person has never experienced a manic episode. In this disorder, the person has experienced major depression (the depressive side of the pendulum reaches its full arc) but has experienced a hypomanic episode rather than a full manic episode on the other side of the mood continuum. Figure 28-1 visually depicts the subtle differences in the bipolar disorders.

Perhaps an additional word is warranted for the bipolar I, mixed subtype. This disorder is characterized by both manic and depressive symptoms. Secunda, et al (1987) report that a high percentage of bipolar patients fall into this category and believe that a mixed syndrome suggests a lower response to lithium. The term *rapid cycling* refers to a condition in which there are four or more episodes of mania and depression in 1 year (Kuyler, 1988; APA, 1994).

Behavior

Objective behavior

The person experiencing a manic episode appears enthusiastic and euphoric. These behaviors are recognized as excessive by others around the person. Objective behaviors include disturbances of speech; disturbances of the individual's social, interpersonal, and occupational relationships; and disturbances of activity and appearance.

CLINICAL EXAMPLE

A manic patient states that a black attendant is a prejudiced black-power advocate who hates Jews. She proclaims that the attendant hates white people and that he brutalizes patients because of race and religion. She refers to him as a "black bastard" and concentrates on demeaning him and questioning his ability to help her based on his low educational level, lack of articulateness, and presumed prejudice. The nursing attendant, who has presented few overt problems before, becomes increasingly angry with the patient. He begins to avoid talking with her.

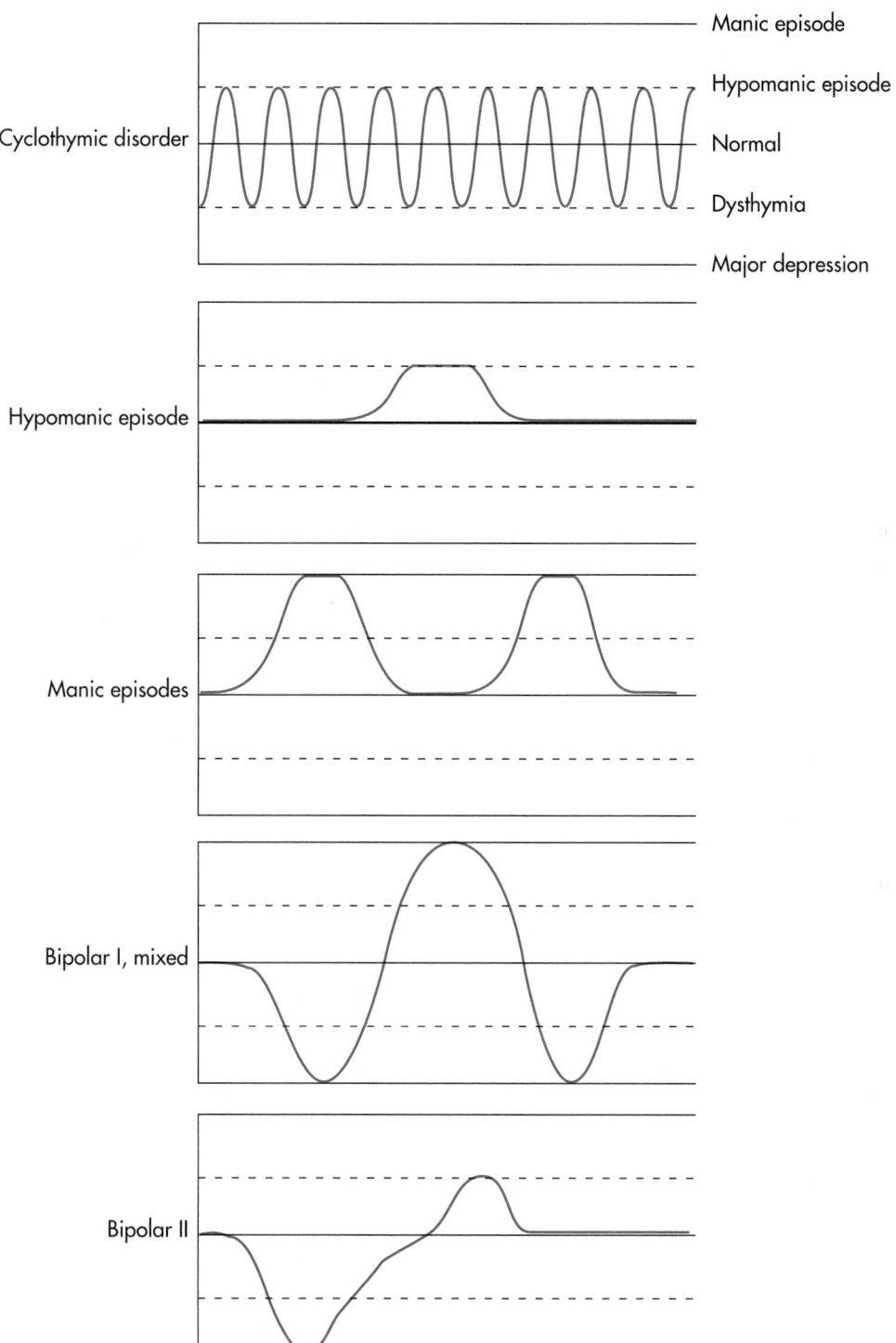

FIGURE 28-1   Differences in the bipolar disorders on the mood continuum. By understanding this table, the student will be able to conceptualize the differences among these bipolar disorders.

At times he begins to refer to her as a "rich bitch." He becomes defensive about his lack of education, wonders why so few black patients are admitted to the ward, and does not know if blacks are being treated fairly at the hospital (Janowsky, Leff, and Epstein, 1970).

Disturbed speech patterns

Manic patients may speak loudly in a rapid-fire fashion. They monopolize the dialogue and deflect attempts by others to contribute. Conversations are filled with jokes and puns. Sarcastic and biting remarks are not uncommon. In fact, even though mental health professionals are aware of this tendency, the ability of manic patients to find a "weak spot" often frustrates, embarrasses, and angers mental health professionals. The tendency to complain often and loudly is also present. Manic patients have the ability to engage staff members in debate and place them on the defensive. Speech is often dramatic, and it is not uncommon for manic persons to burst into song. Speech is often pressured.

These patients also are quite easily distracted. For example, while in the middle of an apparently meaningful discussion, a patient may be distracted by a bird flying outside the window and change the topic of the conversation to flying. This phenomenon, in which patients jump from topic to topic, is referred to as flight of ideas.

Altered social, interpersonal, and occupational relationships

It is not surprising that manic patients irritate others with their fault-finding, anger, and blaming. In a seminal article entitled, "Playing the Manic Game," Janowsky, Leff, and Epstein (1970) identify five tendencies of manic patients.

1. *Manipulation of the self-esteem of others:* Patients use coercive techniques to increase or decrease another's self-esteem. It is easy to fall prey to the manipulation of praise ("No one here really understands me but you"). It is just as easy to feel the ego-deflating wrath when plans are thwarted. Some insightful nurses have disclosed the feeling of "having been played like a yo-yo."
2. *Ability to find vulnerability in others:* Manic patients can exploit weakness in others or create conflicts among staff members.

3. *Ability to shift responsibility:* Through the technique mentioned above, patients somehow shift personal responsibility (e.g., not arriving at breakfast on time) to someone else. Nurses are particularly vulnerable in this area because they are trained to take responsibility for many concerns of their patients.
4. *Limit testing:* Manic patients keep pushing the limits set on the psychiatric unit. If a limit is relaxed, these patients will push it even more.
5. *Alienation of family:* Manic patients drive away their families with their behavior.

Janowsky, Leff, and Epstein (1970) noted the tendencies that cause manic-depressive patients to have difficulty socially, interpersonally, and occupationally. The same behaviors that drive away family also drive away friends, lovers, bosses, coworkers, ministers, and nonpsychiatric health care providers. In a study by the National Depressive and Manic-Depressive Association (NDMDA) and the APA, several sobering trends were noted among bipolar patients who are not adequately treated (News in Mental Health Nursing, 1993). Results from the survey indicate the following:

1. Failed relationships were reported by 59% of poorly treated patients, compared with 32% who received adequate treatment.
2. More than half reported difficulties maintaining long-term friendships.
3. More than one third had been fired when the illness was not well controlled.
4. Among such patients, 56% were forced to change jobs more often than were other people.

Obviously, the effects of bipolar illness permeates all types of relationships. The expansive mood overflows into excesses as well. The otherwise faithful spouse may become sexually promiscuous; the otherwise thrifty homemaker may go on a shopping or spending spree; and the conservative investor may make a dangerously speculative investment.

Alterations in activity and appearance

Manic patients often are hyperactive and agitated. Overt manifestations, such as pacing, flamboyant gestures, colorful dress, singing, and excessive use of make-up, are relatively common. Patients also may dress sloppily and omit personal grooming. They may not need sleep, or perhaps need only a few hours per night. Some have gone for days without sleep, and at one time reports of manic patients dropping from exhaustion were not uncommon. Many manic patients suffer from poor nutrition because they quit eating. They simply do not have the patience, the ability to sit still long enough, or the desire to eat.

Subjective behavior

Alterations of affect

Manic patients experience euphoria and a high regard for the self. The inflated self-image can reach levels of grandiosity. Subjectively, the person going through a manic episode experiences an elevated mood, a feeling of joy, and greatness. A certain sense of invincibility leads to the social, interpersonal, and occupational problems already discussed.

Another significant symptom is a labile or quickly changing affect. For example, a 64-year-old woman was laughing and talking about her personal acquaintance with the president. "You know, my husband's name was Bill." She abruptly began to cry. "He is dead, you know." She quickly returned to the topic of her importance, becoming very excited, with an elevated mood.

Alterations of perception

Delusions and hallucinations occur, and their content is typically consistent with mood. For example, if a patient is grandiose about his importance to the government, a mood-congruent delusion could include paranoid thinking related to being pursued by enemy forces.

■ Critical Thinking Question

What do you think of the following statement? "There are many people in American society who could be diagnosed as hypomanic. Many high-level, 'workaholic' executives are hypomanic and just don't know it."

Etiology

Psychodynamic theories

Family dynamics

At one time most psychiatric professionals believed that bipolar, or manic-depressive, illness was caused by psychological difficulties. Developmental theorists have hypothesized that faulty family dynamics during early life are responsible for manic behaviors in later life. According to this view, the mother (or primary caregiver) enjoys being the "giver of life" and resents autonomy. As the child grows independent, the mother becomes unhappy; to please the mother, the child becomes more dependent; that is, to gain affection, the child at an early age learns to deny his or her own natural tendencies. The unnatural tension between dependence and independence, and the inherent ambivalence in this family environment, can be a causative factor in bipolar illness, according to this view.

Others have suggested that the polar events of childhood are so significant for some people that an adult emotional counterpart to the emotional roller coaster is caused: bipolar disorder; for example, receiving praise (elation) and disapproval (depression), or being breastfed (elation) and being taken away from the breast (depression). Still others have suggested that bipolar disorder is related to an alternating identification with parents: depression with the mother figure and mania with the father figure. Although some of these explanations seem more credible than others, many professionals believe that family dynamics play an important role in the genesis of manic-depressive illness.

Mania as a defense

Another psychodynamic hypothesis explains manic episodes as defense against or massive denial of depression. According to this view, manic-depressive individuals go through life appearing to be independent and excessive to others (too pushy, too talkative, and too manipulative) only to eventually be blocked by someone who no longer tolerates being pushed, talked to, or manipulated. When this happens, the manic individual (who is actually overdependent) may become psychotic.

Biological theories

Although some professionals still hold to the importance of psychological influences, most are aware of the role of biology. Just as depression seems to be caused by neurotransmitter deficiency, manic episodes also seem to be related to excessive levels of norepinephrine, serotonin, and dopamine (Ettigi and Brown, 1977). A related biochemical theory views manic-depressive illness as an imbalance between cholinergic and noradrenergic systems. According to this view, depression is related to increased cholinergic activity, and mania is related to increased noradrenergic activity.

Genetic considerations

It seems clear that genetics has a role in manic-depressive illness (Gershon, et al, 1982; Rosenthal, 1970). Monozygotic twins (identical) have a very high concordancy rate (up to 80% in some studies), whereas dizygotic twins (fraternal) have a higher rate than normal siblings and other close relatives. Siblings and close relatives have a higher incidence of manic-depressive illness than the general population, and cyclothymic characteristics are common among family members of bipolar patients. Approximately 5.8% of first-degree relatives of patients with bipolar illness develop manic-depression, and 15% to 20% develop a primary affective disorder (Packer, 1992). Significant issues arise surrounding family planning counseling for women with bipolar illness, including the heritability of the disease, the stress of parenthood, and the effect an ill parent has on a child (Packer, 1992). Furthermore, teratogenicity of lithium, carbamazepine, and valproic acid is a concern when treating a pregnant woman who has bipolar disorder. Consequently, pregnant women with bipolar disorder should be prescribed these drugs only when the risk of not doing so is greater than the risk of fetal insult.

Psychotherapeutic Management

Nurse-Patient Relationship. The box below lists specific interventions to be used with manic patients.

- Safety: It is important for the nurse to prevent manic patients from hurting themselves or others. Manic patients can become very angry when things do not go their way. This pathological irritability leads to arguments, fights, self-injury (e.g., hitting the wall, not paying attention to the environment), and hurting others. By providing emotional support and responding to patients in a matter-of-fact manner, the nurse conveys both control of the situation and empathy. It is reassuring to patients to realize that the staff will not let them harm themselves or others.
- Clear, concise directions and comments: Working with hyperactive patients who are very talkative, easily distracted, experience flight of ideas, and who have poor judgment and a labile affect is difficult. When the nurse is confronted with very talkative patients, it is not unusual for the nurse to attempt to use familiar skills. For example, most people learn not to interrupt another person until a pause. The pause may never come with manic patients. To be effective, the nurse may need to raise his or her hand and say, "Wait just a minute. I do not want to be rude, but I would like to say something." As a patient starts improving, the nurse may be able to work out a nonverbal signal to indicate when the patient needs to stop and let

Key Nursing Interventions for a Manic Episode

For Patients "Too Busy" to Eat

The nurse should use the following interventions to maintain patients' body weight:

1. Provide patients with foods that can be eaten "on the run" (sometimes referred to as finger foods) because some patients cannot sit still long enough to eat.
2. Provide high-protein, high-calorie snacks for patients. A vitamin supplement may be indicated.
3. Weigh patients regularly (sometimes daily weighings are needed).

For Patients Who Cannot Sleep

Manic patients experience insomnia. The nurse can help patients to maximize the opportunity for sleep by doing the following:

1. Provide a quiet place to sleep.
2. Structure patients' days so that there are fewer stimulating activities toward bedtime.
3. Do not allow caffeinated drinks and provide warm milk before bedtime.
4. Assess the amount of rest patients are receiving. Manic patients are not capable of judging the need for rest, and exhaustion and death have resulted from lack of rest.

someone else speak. Although manic patients are talkative, there is a tendency for the talk to be superficial. When talking to hyperactive patients, the nurse should keep remarks brief and simple. Many patients literally cannot tolerate a lengthy discussion of any subject.

- Limit setting: When the nurse is leading a group, a talkative patient can be disruptive because of the tendencies described by Janowsky, Leff, and Epstein (1970):
  - Manipulation of the self-esteem of others
  - Ability to find vulnerability of others
  - Ability to shift responsibility to others
  - Limit testing

These patients have the ability to damage the self-esteem of other patients, to ridicule the nurse, to blame others, to pick fights, to create problems between patients, and to manipulate others. The nurse needs to protect vulnerable patients and to keep them from being drawn into the anger that manic patients feel. When the nurse is able to remain calm instead of becoming angry, it helps manic patients and the other patients in the group. This calmness should be based on an understanding of psychopathology; otherwise, it may be simply an unhealthy defense by the nurse (i.e., "You cannot bother me; you are not important enough"). The nurse absolutely does not want to convey that she is engaged in an adult version of the childish behavior of plugging the ears and saying, "I can't hear you." It is also very important to avoid arguing with patients about unit rules and limits. Do not debate these issues with patients. Simply state the unit policy and move on. Debating and arguing reinforces the tendencies mentioned above.

- Reinforcement of reality: Manic patients also experience disturbances in perception. The intervention strategies outlined for other patients with disturbed perceptions are recommended for manic patients also.
- Provide a homogeneous group if possible: Pollack (1993) found that working with a group of inpatients with exclusively bipolar disorder was beneficial. The patients found the group to be helpful and they felt "understood." In addition, the topics were focused into an area of relevance for this group of patients. While this homogeneity may not always be possible or even desirable, Pollack's early work provides a challenge for the psychiatric nurse to continue to explore avenues for working with bipolar patients.

Psychopharmacology. Lithium is the most prescribed drug for manic patients. The starting dose is

Case Study

Mr. Casey Tubbs, a 44-year-old electrician, was admitted to the unit with the diagnosis of bipolar I disorder, manic type. He was brought in by police after starting a fight with three Hispanic men in a bar. He had been drinking heavily. He was hyperactive, distractible, irritable, talkative, and demanding upon admission. He demonstrated flight of ideas and was verbally hostile concerning a Hispanic coworker, whom he accused of sleeping with his wife. Mr. Tubbs has vowed to get even. He made several comments about Hispanics in general while looking at Mr. Azteca, a Hispanic nurse.

This is Mr. Tubbs's third hospitalization. The first occurred 12 years ago when he contracted a *Candida* infection after having sexual intercourse with his wife. The second hospitalization occurred in 1995. No precipitating event was recorded; nor does Mr. Tubbs recollect anything unusual about the second admission.

Mr. Tubbs has responded well to lithium in the past, and during his other hospitalizations also was given chlorpromazine because of his agitation. Between hospitalizations Mr. Tubbs has functioned well and is considered a good worker. His perfectionistic tendencies are appreciated by his boss. Mrs. Tubbs states that Mr. Tubbs has not slept in 3 days and has not stopped to eat for some time (the actual length of time is not clear). She reports a good marriage until Mr. Tubbs stops taking his lithium, which he says he will no longer take. She wants him to "get better and come home." The head nurse decides to streamline the admission process because of Mr. Tubbs's agitated state. He is taken to a quiet area and provided with peanut butter crackers and milk.

Mr. Tubbs's nursing care plan is given on the next page.

Care Plan

NAME: __Casey Tubbs__   ADMISSION DATE: _____

DSM-IV DIAGNOSIS: __Bipolar I disorder, most recent episode manic__

ASSESSMENT: **Areas of strength:** Patient's marriage is solid between hospitalizations. Patient's boss likes him and is eager for him to return to work. Good adjustment between hospitalizations. He has responded well to lithium in the past.

Problems: Patient is threatening and irritating others. Patient has legal problems from bar fight. Patient is threatening to get even with his wife's alleged lover. Patient has not complied with medication regimen recently and states that he will not take lithium.

DIAGNOSES: • Violence, high risk for, related to manic dyscontrol and delusions, as evidenced by irritability and verbal hostility.
• Fatigue related to insomnia, as evidenced by lack of sleep for 3 days.
• Nutrition, altered: less than body requirements related to anorexia and hyperactivity, as evidenced by lack of interest in food.

OUTCOMES: **Short-term goals:**   Date met
• Patient will not hurt anyone while in hospital.   _____
• Patient will comply with medication regimen.   _____
• Patient will become less agitated.   _____
• Patient will comply with unit norms and limits.   _____
Long-term goals:
• Patient will remain free of manic episodes.   _____
• Patient will continue to take lithium on outpatient basis.   _____
• Patient will resolve legal problems.   _____
• Patient will join manic-depressive support group.   _____

PLANNING/ INTERVENTIONS: **Nurse-patient relationship:** Talk to patient in matter-of-fact tone and clearly indicate that aggressive behaviors are not acceptable. Set firm, clear limits. Do not engage in debates over unit policy, limits, etc. Keep comments brief and simple. Do not respond to sarcastic remarks with anger. Reinforce good behavior and confront (carefully) unacceptable behavior.

Psychopharmacology: Lithium carbonate, 600 mg tid, PO (concentrate); chlorpromazine, 200 mg tid, PO (concentrate); chlorpromazine, 50 mg, IM, q 2 hr prn for agitation.

Milieu management: Provide quiet room and decrease stimuli. Do not include in group activities for a few days. Provide opportunities for rest and monitor sleep. Provide finger foods and weigh daily. Set limits.

EVALUATION: Mr. Tubbs is less agitated and is taking lithium on schedule. Patient is beginning to talk less about his wife's alleged infidelity. Has not lost weight. Patient continues to test limits.

REFERRALS: Schedule outpatient appointment and give patient and wife phone number for manic-depressive support group.

usually 600 mg tid. The typical maintenance dose is 900 to 1200 mg a day. Maintenance blood levels are 0.6 to 1.2 mEq/L. Approximately 10% to 20% of patients who take lithium are resistant to it and are not helped. The two most beneficial alternatives to lithium are carbamazepine and valproic acid. A full discussion of these drugs is found in Chapter 21.

Milieu Management.   Milieu management is an important dimension of the nursing care of manic patients because they test the unit perhaps more than any other group of patients.

1. Because manic patients tend to create conflict, to pick on vulnerable persons (patients and staff), to blame others, to test limits, and to shift responsibility to others, the nurse must carefully develop a plan of care. Nursing and other staff members should meet often to defuse conflict and clarify communication. All staff members should be aware of intervention strategies and agree to abide consistently by team decisions. Inexperienced staff members must guard against falling prey to esteem-building statements that tend to split the staff, for example, "You're the only one who understands."

2. Because manic patients are hyperactive, talkative, irritable, and angry, it is important to decrease environmental stimuli. Patients are distractible and respond to all sorts of environmental cues, so it is important to modify the environment as much as possible. Helpful environmental modifications include private (if possible), quiet rooms; limited activities with others and scheduled rest periods; gross motor activities (e.g., walking, sweeping, and aerobics) to discharge some of the need to be active; and a public room free from a television or stereo.

3. Manic patients can become hostile and aggressive. It is important for the staff to deal with this aggressiveness in a calm, confident manner. For patients who are escalating, an antipsychotic drug, such as haloperidol, can be administered to prevent physical aggressiveness, and potential weapons (e.g., chairs, pool cues) can be removed. Limits and the consequences of violating those limits should be reviewed. Do not include limits that are not significant. It is countertherapeutic to defend a poor policy, and it is also countertherapeutic to allow patients to debate a unit issue. It is therapeutic to follow through with appropriate action should a patient violate a unit norm.

SUICIDE AND MOOD DISORDERS

Hardin (1996) proposes that suicide is the outcome of a person's inability to deal with catastrophic stress resulting from biological or psychological illnesses, including mood disorders. Suicide is a complex phenomenon, influenced by a person's cultural beliefs, values, and norms. Suicide may occur in children, adolescent, and adult populations. Nurses need to assess a patient's **suicidal ideation** level; suicidal ideation includes a person's thoughts regarding suicide as well as suicidal gestures and threats. **Suicidal gestures** are a person's nonlethal self-injury acts, including cutting or burning of skin areas or the ingestion of small amounts of drugs. Often others see these gestures as "attention-getting" measures and do not consider them serious problems that may lead to a suicide attempt or completion. **Suicidal threats** are a person's verbal statements that may declare their intent to commit suicide. Threats often precede an actual **suicidal attempt,** the actual implementation of a self-injurious act with the express purpose of ending the person's life.

Suicide is a significant cause of death in the United States. Suicide is the ninth leading cause of death in the United States (Pearson, 1998) and is among the three leading causes of death for those aged 15 to 34 years (Mann, 1998). The overall ratio of attempted to completed suicide is approximately 7:1 (DHHS, 1993b). The annual number of suicides in this country is about 12.5 per 100,000, or roughly 30,000 individuals (News and Notes, 1994).

The prototypical suicide victim is an unemployed white man, living alone, who has made a serious suicide attempt in the past. Men are 4 times as likely as women, and whites are twice as likely as blacks, to successfully complete a suicide attempt (Cugino, et al, 1992; News and Notes, 1994). Seventy-three percent of all suicides are committed by white men (Pearson, 1998).

The overall suicide rate for the general adult population in the United States is high, but it is still considerably lower than for persons with psychiatric disorders. Psychiatric diagnosis is the most reliable risk factor for suicide (DHHS, 1993b). Approximately 90% of all suicides are performed by individuals with a diagnosable mental or substance abuse disorder according to one study (Pearson, 1998). Clark et al (1987) estimate that over a period of 10 to 15 years, 10% to 15% of all patients with depression, schizophrenia, or alcoholism will die by suicide. Approximately 10% of all deaths of persons with schizophrenia are from suicide (APA, 1994). Table 28-4 compares the suicide rates by diagnostic entity of the general population with those for mentally disordered persons (Clark, et al, 1987). Box 28-7 provides a list of other risk factors that have been related empirically to suicide (DHHS, 1993b).

The death by suicide of psychiatric patients is of particular importance to the nurse because of opportunities for assessment and intervention. The psychiatric nurse continually must assess for suicide potential among all patients, but especially among schizophrenic, depressed, and alcoholic patients.

Although Table 28-4 provides separate suicide rates for schizophrenics, the depressed, and alcoholics, Hendin (1986) points out that when schizophrenics kill themselves, they are typically in a depressed phase, and the act typically is not a product of psychosis. Alcoholics kill themselves usually in response to loss (divorce, separation, being fired) and when they have been drinking. Hendin makes the point that suicide most often is the result of depression, diagnosed or not. Drake, et al (1984) depict the most vulnerable psychiatric patients as "young patients with chronic relapsing illness, good educational backgrounds, high-performance expectations,

painful awareness of illness, fear of further mental disintegration, and hopelessness about the future."

The major themes of suicidal patients are loss, unbearable psychic pain, helplessness, hopelessness, loneliness, and abandonment ("nobody cares"). These themes complement the common suicidal expressions of a loss of self-esteem, a cry for help, or suicide as a threat (see Box 28-8 for a more complete list of suicidal expressions). Hendin (1986) underscores that suicidal patients view and utilize death differ-

---

Box 28-7   Risk Factors for Completed Suicide

Hopelessness
General medical illness
Severe anhedonia
Male
Caucasian and Native American
Living alone
Prior suicide attempts
Age 60 and older
Unemployed or financial problems

Table 28-4   Clinical Risk Factors for Suicide in the United States

Population	Suicides per 100,000
Adult general public	15-19
Schizophrenic	140
Depressed	230
Alcoholic	270

Box 28-8   Common Expressions of Suicidal Individuals

Cry for help	Admission of inability to handle problem.
Escape	"I can't put up with this mess any longer" (especially with embarrassing or traumatic situations).
Heroic	To gain respect; some cultures view suicide as a manly alternative to failure; occasionally a male patient who is ambivalent about suicide has been taunted into showing he is a real man.
Loss of self-esteem	Failure in an area of great personal investment. On 7/18/89, Donnie Moore, a major league baseball pitcher, committed suicide. His former teammates felt it was related to a home run he gave up in a play-off game.
Manipulation	This is a coercive measure. "You had better come back to me or I will kill myself." An attempt to control
Martyrdom	"Nobody cares about me. Everyone would be better off without me."
Rebirth	Fantasy of getting a new start in life. "Heaven has got to be better than this."
Redemption	An attempt to make up for some wrong; for example, a man responsible for the death of a child might kill himself.
Relief of pain	"I can't stand the pain (emotional or physical) any longer" (especially with terminal illness).
Retaliatory	Suicide is viewed as getting even. "I'll show them."
Reunion	Joining a loved one in heaven. "I can't live without her."

ently from other people. There is a tendency for suicidal patients to use their own death to control others and to maintain control over their own lives. Hence, death is viewed as a means of ensuring control.

Critical Thinking Question

Why do you think the prevalence of suicide is higher in whites than in other races?

The Impact of Guns on Suicidal Behavior

Approximately 18,000 suicides per year are related to self-inflicted gunshot wounds (Frierson, 1989). Guns are used to commit 64% of male suicides and 36% of female suicides (Frierson, 1989). See Box 28-9 for a sobering summary of the impact of guns on American life.

Suicide and the Elderly

While suicide rates among the general population are 12.5 per 100,000 (total population) and 15 to 19 per 100,000 (adult population), the rate for men over age 65 is 28.8 per 100,000 (News and Notes, 1994). This age group has a high attempt-to-completion ratio that is accounted for probably by the seriousness of the intent and the lethality of the means (Mellick,

Box 28-9   **What's the Leading Cause of Gun Deaths? Homicide? Guess Again.**

Suicides, not homicides, are the leading cause of gun deaths in this country. Fifty-seven percent of all gun deaths in 1990 were caused by suicide. This translates into 19,000 gun-caused suicides that year. "Furthermore, suicide rates for 15 to 19 year olds has quadrupled between 1950 and 1988 making suicide the third leading cause of death in that age group." According to the National Center for Health Statistics, a youth between the ages of 10 and 19 committed suicide with a gun every six hours—1,436 in 1991.

Adapted from Hallinan J: What's the leading cause of gun deaths? Homicide? Guess again, *The Birmingham News*, 14A, March 6, 1994.

Buckwalter, and Stolley, 1992). Whereas the general attempt-to-completion ratio is 8:1, in the elderly it is 2:1 (Gomez and Gomez, 1993). Although the upsurge in recent years of suicide among the young has resulted in much media coverage, the suicide rate among the elderly is more widespread. Young persons may use the suicide gesture as a cry for help; elderly persons may just want to die. They often do.

Assessment of Suicidal Patients

It is important for the nurse to be able to assess the suicidal potential of mentally disordered patients because those patients are at a higher risk of suicide. Most facilities provide the nurse with a format for evaluating suicidal lethality. The crucial variables are the plan, the method, and the provision for rescue.

Plan

The more developed the plan, the greater the risk of suicide. Persons who have developed a suicidal plan carefully are more serious about suicide and present a greater risk. Although impulsive suicide attempts can result in death, generally they are less often lethal because the lack of planning sometimes foils the effort.

Method

Some methods of attempting suicide are more lethal than others. Accessibility of the means to commit suicide is important also. Having three bottles of pills on hand is more lethal than having to make an appointment with a doctor to ask for a prescription. A crucial factor in determining the lethality of a particular method is the amount of time between initiation of the suicide method and delivery of the lethal impact of that method. For instance, the person using a gun has no opportunity to avoid the bullet once the trigger is pulled. On the other hand, sitting in the garage with the motor running affords some time to choose an alternative to self-destruction, as does taking an overdose of certain drugs. Lethal methods of suicide include the use of guns, jumping from high places, hanging, drowning, carbon monoxide poisoning, and overdose with certain drugs (e.g., barbiturates, alcohol, and several central nervous system [CNS] depressants). Methods that are less likely to be lethal include wrist cutting and overdosing on aspirin or Valium.

Rescue

The person who deliberately attempts to deceive would-be rescuers has a high lethality potential. For instance, a person who says she is going to the ocean for the weekend and then drives to the mountains makes it difficult for family and friends to intervene. A person who leaves a note or makes a telephone call before making an attempt is more likely to be rescued.

In summary, the more detailed the *plan,* the more lethal and accessible the *method,* and the more effort that is exerted to block *rescue,* the greater the likelihood of the suicidal effort being successful. However, impulsive efforts of suicidal persons with rescuers in sight have proved fatal, particularly when a lethal method (e.g., a gun) has been selected.

Intervention

Face-to-face

In working face-to-face with suicidal patients, several general guidelines are useful to the nurse. (Also see the box below.)

1. Suspect suicidal ideation in most depressed patients (DHHS, 1993b).
2. Ask patients if they plan to hurt themselves. It is important for the nurse to understand the following:

A. Talking to patients about their suicidal intentions will not drive them to suicide. Asking patients directly provides useful information and often provides patients with a sense of relief (e.g., "Finally, someone hears me").

B. Many persons have died from suicide who did not mean to die. They tragically miscalculated. It can be said accurately that many persons who die from suicide die accidentally. The nurse must take all suicidal threats seriously.

3. If a patient is considering suicide, the nurse should ask about the plan (when and where), method, and how the patient intends to accomplish the suicide. (Is the plan to frustrate rescue attempts?) If the patient wants to use a gun, ask someone at the patient's home to remove the gun. If the patient plans to overdose, ask someone in the home to throw away the pills. Do not offer a weekend pass to this patient. Some clinicians believe that if the method of choice can be blocked, many suicidal patients will not use another method. For example, a woman who might use a drug overdose would not consider jumping off a building.

4. Ask about previous suicide attempts. Ask about the "when" and the "how." How did the patient feel concerning rescue? How was the response to treatment? Previous attempts put persons at a higher risk.

Key Nursing Interventions for Suicidal Patients

- Evaluate patients for suicidal risk.
    Rationale: Risk is based on plan, method, and rescue prevention. By knowing the risk, the nurse can establish a reasonable plan of care.
- Suspect suicidal ideation in most depressed patients.
    Rationale: Suspecting suicidal ideation prevents the nurse from overlooking a potentially suicidal patient.
- Inquire directly about frequency and content of suicidal ideation.
    Rationale: The nurse will not provoke suicide by asking patients about it. In fact, the nurse will convey concern, the worth of the patient, and a sense of understanding. Furthermore, the nurse needs this information to plan care.
- Ask patients about the advantages and disadvantages of suicide.
    Rationale: This information enables the nurse to understand how patients see their situations.

- Evaluate patients' access to a means of suicide.
    Rationale: If a patient has a means of suicide, the nurse should arrange to have that means blocked. For some patients, if the method of choice is blocked, they will not use another method.
- Develop a formal "no suicide" contract with patients.
    Rationale: Many patients will honor the contract; hence, the nurse has one more tool to prevent patients from self-injury.
- Advise patients to discontinue drugs and/or alcohol.
    Rationale: Drugs and alcohol significantly increase the risk of suicidal behavior.
- Support patients' reasons to live.
    Rationale: As the nurse is able to align with the healthy part of each patient's personality, the nurse gains a therapeutic ally.

From the Department of Health and Human Services: *Depression in primary care: vol 2, treatment of major depression,* Washington, DC, 1993b, DHHS.

5. Evaluate patients for depression, recent loss or threat of loss, self-destructive hallucinations, and alcohol or drug use, all of which place persons at a higher risk for suicide.

6. Once patients are hospitalized, many units protect them by using one of two levels of suicide prevention:

   A. Level 1 is used for patients who are not considered to be at immediate risk of suicide. The nursing staff provides periodic observation (every 15 minutes) and monitors drug taking, eating utensils, shaving gear, and other potentially dangerous devices in the environment. The staff communicates concern and control with this close observation of patients and their environment. Patients are asked to sign a contract with the staff stating that they will not harm themselves during hospitalization and will seek out a staff member should they begin to contemplate self-injurious behavior. Clinicians are divided in their view of the efficacy of "no-suicide" contracts (Valente, 1997).

   B. Level 2 is used for patients who present an immediate and serious threat of suicidal behavior. Level 2 also may be initiated for patients who refuse to sign a "no suicide" contract. Restraints may be used occasionally, as can neuroleptic drugs. Continuous observation is another alternative. This is an expensive use of manpower but provides the needed control and human interaction. Patients at serious risk usually are confined to the unit and have restrictions on visitors, where meals are taken, and so on. Harmful objects are removed from the environment.

Over the telephone

Former patients frequently call the psychiatric unit or outpatient clinic where psychiatric nurses work. Helpful guidelines for nurses who work with suicidal persons over the telephone follow (Green and Wilson, 1988).

1. Express genuine concern and a desire to work with callers. ("Let's see what we can do.") Give callers your full attention.

2. Acknowledge how difficult and painful recent losses must be. ("It's been a tough time for you lately.")

3. Assess lethality, especially if the suicidal attempt has begun.

4. Focus on the healthy side of callers. ("You called for help. That tells me you want help, and that's what we want to do.")

5. Ask about alcohol or drug use. If present, these substances increase the lethality level.

6. Ask callers for their ideas about immediate solutions to the current situation. Assess feasibility, appropriateness, and availability. Suggest alternatives if needed.

7. Obtain each caller's name, telephone number, address, and whereabouts during the call. Ask callers how they want to be addressed. ("Your name is Mr. Robert Smith. What would you like for me to call you?")

8. If other staff members are available, the nurse may need to direct them to call the police or an ambulance. Ask for consent to do so or, at least, inform the caller of the plan.

9. Ask if anyone is with the caller. If so, ask to speak to that person to obtain assistance in planning instructions.

10. If family members can be reached, they should be asked to go to the caller and intervene if it is safe to do so (ask for caller consent).

11. Refer callers to walk-in crisis services or a regular outpatient counselor.

12. If a caller refuses further help, give the telephone number of a crisis center or a suicide-prevention hotline.

■ Critical Thinking Question

Do you think doctors have the right to help terminally ill patients end their lives? Should adults in their right minds be allowed to commit suicide?

⚑ Key Concepts

1. Mood disorders are divided into depressive disorders (e.g., major depression, dysthymia) and bipolar disorders (e.g., bipolar disorder, hypomania, and cyclothymia).

2. The DSM-IV defines major depression as an episode of depression (apathy, weight changes, sleep changes, psychomotor changes, fatigue, feelings of worthlessness or guilt, decreased cognitive ability, and recurrent thoughts of death) without a history of manic episodes.

3. Reacting to a disappointment or loss with sadness, guilt, or "depression" is normal; however, if any of these reactions persist too long, then a diagnosable condition (either dysthymia or major depression) exists.

4. Objective signs of depression include alterations in activity and social interactions.
5. Subjective symptoms of depression include alterations in affect, cognition, physical nature (somatic concern), and perception.
6. Biological explanations for depression include neurotransmitter deficiency, genetics, and endocrine dysfunction. Psychodynamic explanations concern debilitating early life experiences, intrapsychic conflicts, and reaction to life events.
7. Psychotherapeutic management includes developing a therapeutic nurse-patient relationship, administering antidepressant drugs when appropriate, and providing a well-managed milieu with particular emphasis on safety.
8. The psychiatric nurse should suspect suicidal ideation in most depressed patients because suicide is a prevalent theme among this population.
9. Manic episodes are characterized by an elevated or expansive mood that usually begins suddenly, escalates rapidly, and lasts from a few days to several months.
10. Objective signs of bipolar illness include altered speech patterns; altered social, interpersonal, and occupational relationships; and altered activity and appearance.
11. Subjective symptoms of bipolar illness include alterations in affect and perception.
12. Psychodynamic theories of bipolar illness include theories about family dynamics and psychoanalytical explanations that view manic behavior as a defense against overwhelming feelings of depression.
13. Biological explanations of bipolar disorder include excessive levels of neurotransmitters (norepinephrine, serotonin, and dopamine) and genetics (80% concordancy rates among identical twins in some studies).
14. Lithium is the drug of choice for the treatment of bipolar disorders. Carbamazepine (Tegretol) and valproic acid (Depakene) are used when a patient does not respond to lithium.

◆ Study Questions

(Answer key is in the back of the book.)

1. Which of the following classifications of mood disorders most accurately reflects the DSM-IV?
   a. Reactive vs. endogenous depression
   b. Primary vs. secondary depression
   c. Unipolar vs. bipolar depression
   d. Psychotic vs. neurotic depression
   e. Major depression vs. dysthymia
2. Which of the following classifications of mood disorders best explains the effectiveness and appropriate use of antidepressants?
   a. Reactive vs. endogenous depression
   b. Primary vs. secondary depression
   c. Unipolar vs. bipolar depression

d. Psychotic vs. neurotic depression
   e. Major depression vs. dysthymia
3. *Subjective* symptoms of major depression include:
   a. Alterations in activity
   b. Alterations in social interactions
   c. Alterations in affect
4. Pessimism, self-blame, and self-deprecating thoughts are examples of:
   a. Alterations in affect
   b. Alterations in cognition
   c. Alterations in activity
   d. Alterations in perceptions
5. Chest pain, constipation, dizziness, and fatigue are examples of:
   a. Alterations in affect
   b. Alterations of a physical nature
   c. Alterations of perceptions
   d. Alterations of cognition
6. Delusions and hallucinations are examples of:
   a. Alterations in affect
   b. Alterations of a physical nature
   c. Alterations in perceptions
   d. Alterations in cognition
7. Most depression is a reaction to loss or failure.
   a. True
   b. False
8. Psychodynamic theories of depression include all of the following *except:*
   a. Debilitating early life experiences
   b. Nonsuppressor status on the DST
   c. Intrapsychic conflict
   d. Reaction to life events
9. Ms. Long is taking lithium and has a lithium serum level of 1.5 mmol/L. Which of the following is expected, based on an understanding of appropriate lithium serum levels?
   a. Some manic behavior
   b. Appropriate symptom control
   c. Mild symptoms of toxicity
10. The important parameters for suicidal patients are:
    a. Whether or not they mean to hurt themselves
    b. Whether they have a plan, have chosen a lethal method, and have attempted to block rescue efforts
    c. Whether the suicidal attempt is a cry for help or represents a manipulation
11. Marilyn is a 73-year-old white female who recently lost her husband of 40 years and was just admitted to the unit. Her daughter reports that she will not eat, does not sleep, and seems a little confused at times. The most important concern is about:
    a. Starting her on the correct antidepressant
    b. Differentiating between depression and dementia
    c. Addressing her basic needs (e.g., sleep, food, and proper elimination)
    d. All of the above

12. John, who is 70 years old, is admitted to the unit for depression. He has been a successful businessman for many years. He complains of weight loss, early morning awakening, fatigue, slowed gait, pain, and feeling sad for several months. He cannot think of anything that has happened that would make him so depressed. John should be told that:
    a. Depression can occur "out of the blue" without precipitating life events
    b. Depression is a symptom of old age
    c. Many people feel sad
    d. The depression will probably stop within 2 months
13. Flight of ideas, insomnia, delusions of grandeur, and intense irritability are symptoms that could be attributed to:
    1. Bipolar I disorder, single episode
    2. Bipolar I disorder, most recent episode manic
    3. Bipolar I disorder, most recent episode hypomanic
    4. Bipolar I disorder, most recent episode depressed
    5. Bipolar II disorder
        a. 1, 2
        b. 2, 3
        c. 1, 2, 3
        d. 1, 4, 5
        e. All of the above

REFERENCES

Abramson LY, Seligman ME, and Teasdale JD: Learned helplessness in humans: critique and reformulation, *J Abnorm Psychol* 87:48, 1978.

American Psychiatric Association: Practice guidelines for major depressive disorder in adults, *Am J Psychiatry* (suppl) 150(4):1, 1993.

American Psychiatric Association: *Diagnostic and statistical manual of mental disorders,* ed 4, Washington, DC, 1994, The Association.

Asnis GM, McGinn S, and Sanderson WC: Atypical depression: clinical aspects and noradrenergic function, *Am J Psychiatr Nurs* 6(5):257, 1995.

Beck AT: *Depression: causes and treatment,* Philadelphia, 1991, University Press.

Beck AT, et al: *Cognitive therapy of depression,* New York, 1979, Guilford.

Becker RE: Depression in schizophrenia, *Hosp Community Psychiatry* 39:1269, 1988.

Beckham E and Leber WR, editors: *Handbook of depression,* ed 2, New York, 1995, Guilford.

Beeber LS: Depression in women. In McBride AB, and Austin JS, editors: *Psychiatric mental-health nursing: integrating the behavioral and biological sciences,* Philadelphia, 1996, WB Saunders.

Bourdan KH, et al: Estimating the prevalence of mental disorders in US adults from the Epidemiological Catchment Area Survey, *Public Health Rep* 107(6):663, 1992.

Brown DR, et al: Major depression in a community sample of African Americans, *Am J Psychiatry* 152(3):373, 1995.

Buysse DJ, et al: Do ECG sleep studies predict reoccurrence in depressive patients treated with psychotherapy? *Depression* 2:105, 1994.

Cartwright RD and Lloyd SR: Early REM sleep: a compensatory change in depression, *Psychiatry Res* 51:245, 1994.

Clark DC, et al: A field test of Motto's risk estimator for suicide, *Am J Psychiatry* 144:923, 1987.

Cockerman WC: *Sociology of mental disorder,* ed 3, Englewood Cliffs, NJ, 1992, Prentice-Hall.

Cugino A, et al: Searching for a pattern: repeat suicide attempts, *J Psychosoc Nurs Ment Health Serv* 30(3):2326, 1992.

Department of Health and Human Services: Depression in primary care: detection, diagnosis, and treatment, *J Psychosoc Nurs Ment Health Serv* 31(6):19, 1993a.

Department of Health and Human Services: *Depression in primary care, vol 2, Treatment of major depression,* Washington, DC, 1993b, DHHS.

Depression Guideline Panel: *Depression in primary care, vol 1, Detection and diagnosis,* DHHS Pub No 93-0550, Washington, DC, 1993, US Government Printing Office.

Drake RE, et al: Suicide among schizophrenics: who is at risk? *J Nerv Ment Dis* 172:613, 1984.

Dubovsky SL: Beyond the serotonin reuptake inhibitors: rationales for the development of new serotonergic agents, *J Clin Psychiatry* 55:2(suppl):34, 1994.

Dubovsky SL and Thomas M: Psychotic depression: advances in conceptualization and treatment, *Hosp Community Psychiatry* 43(12):1189, 1992.

Elkin I, et al: National Institute of Mental Health Treatment of Depression Collaborative Research Program, *Arch Gen Psychiatry* 46:971, 1989.

Ettigi PG and Brown GM: Psychoneuroendocrinology of affective disorder: an overview, *Am J Psychiatry* 134:493, 1977.

Fava GA: Affective disorders and endocrine disease: new insights from psychosomatic studies, *Psychosomatic* 35(4):341, 1994.

Fieve RR: *Moodswings,* New York, 1975, Bantam.

First MB, et al: DSM-IV in progress: changes in mood, anxiety, and personality disorders, *Hosp Community Psychiatry* 44(11):1034, 1993.

Frances A and Hales RE: Determining how a depressed woman's personality affects the choice of treatment (treatment planning), *Hosp Community Psychiatry* 35:883, 1984.

Freud S: *Mourning and melancholia,* standard ed, vol 14, London, 1957, Hogarth Press.

Frierson RL: Women who shoot themselves, *Hosp Community Psychiatry* 40:841, 1989.

Gershon ES, et al: A family study of schizoaffective, bipolar I, bipolar II, unipolar, and normal control probands, *Arch Gen Psychiatry* 39:1157, 1982.

Gomez GE and Gomez EA: Depression in the elderly, *J Psychosoc Nurs Ment Health Serv* 31(5):28, 1993.

Green LW and Wilson CR: Guidelines for nonprofessionals who receive suicidal phone calls, *Hosp Community Psychiatry* 39:310, 1988.

Grunebaum H and Cohler B: Children of parents hospitalized for mental illness. I. Attentional and interactional studies. In Frank M, editor: *Children of exceptional parents,* New York, 1983, Haworth.

Haber J: Mood disorders. In Haber J, et al: *Comprehensive psychiatric nursing,* ed 5, St. Louis, 1997, Mosby.

Hardin SB: Catastrophic stress. In McBride AB and Austin JK, editors: *Psychiatric mental-health nursing: integrating the behavioral and biological sciences,* Philadelphia, 1996, WB Saunders.

Hendin H: Suicide: a review of new directions in research, *Hosp Community Psychiatry* 37:148, 1986.

Hirschfeld RMA, Russell JM: A synopsis of the assessment and treatment of suicidal patients. *Decade of the Brain* 8(4):7, 1998.

Holinger PC, Offer D, and Ostrov E: Suicide and homicide in the United States: an epidemiologic study of violent death, population changes, and the potential for prediction, *Am J Psychiatry* 144:215, 1987.

Horwath EM, et al: What are the public implications of subclinical depressive symptoms? *Psychiatr Q* 65(4):323, 1994.

Howland RH: Chronic depression, *Hosp Community Psychiatry* 44(7):633, 1993.

Hyde MS: Childhood depression, *Guidelines* p. 1, spring 1993.

Janowsky DS, Leff M, and Epstein RS: Playing the manic game, *Arch Gen Psychiatry* 22:252, 1970.

Jones RL, editor: Handbook of tests and measurements for black populations, vols 1, 2, Hampton, Va, 1996, Cobb & Henry.

Kahan BB: Not just another stage, *Insight* 14(2):7, 1993.

Kammeyer KCW, Ritzer G, and Yetman NR: *Sociology: experiences changing societies,* ed 5, Houston, 1992, Allyn and Bacon.

Kandel ER, Schwartz JH, Jessell TM: *Principles of neural science,* ed 3, Norwalk, Conn, 1991, Appleton & Lange.

Keltner NL: Drugs for treatment of depression and mania. In Shlafer M and Marieb E, editors: *The nurse, pharmacology, and drug therapy,* Redwood City, Calif, 1993, Addison-Wesley.

Keltner NL, Folks DG, Palmer C, Powers RE: *Psychobiological foundations of psychiatric care,* St. Louis, 1998, Mosby.

Keltner NL and Folks DG: Alternatives to lithium in the treatment of bipolar disorder, *Perspect Psychiatry Care* 27(2):36, 1991.

Kendler KS, et al: The lifetime history of major depression, *Arch Gen Psychiatry* 50:863, 1993.

Kessler RC, et al: Lifetime and 12-month prevalence of DSM-III-R psychiatric disorders in the United States: results from the national comorbidity survey, *Arch Gen Psychiatry* 51:8, 1994.

Killeen MR and Bongarten CF: Caring for depressed children and adolescents. In McBride AB and Austin JS, editors: *Psychiatric mental-health nursing: integrating the behavioral and biological sciences,* Philadelphia, 1996, WB Saunders.

Kizilay PE: Predictors of depression in women, *Women's Health* 27(4):983, 1992.

Klerman GL: Overview of affective disorders. In Kaplan HI, Freedman AM, and Sadock BJ, editors: *Comprehensive textbook of psychiatry III, vol 2,* Baltimore 1980, Williams & Wilkins.

Klerman GL: The interpersonal model. In Mann JJ, editor: *Models of depressive disorders,* New York, 1989, Plenum Press.

Kuyler PL: Rapid cycling bipolar I illness in three closely related individuals, *Am J Psychiatry* 145:114, 1988.

Laraia MT and Nihart MA: *Psychopharmacology for psychiatric nurses: case studies and the ANA guidelines.* Invited paper presented at Contemporary Forums Tenth Anniversary Conference on Psychiatric Nursing, Boston, May 1995.

Loving RT and Kripke DF: Daily light exposure among psychiatric inpatients, *J Psychosoc Nurs Ment Health Serv* 30(11):1519, 1992.

Maes M, et al: A further investigation of basal HPT axis function in unipolar depression: effects of diagnosis, hospitalization, and dexamethasone administration, *Psychiatry Res* 51:185, 1994.

Mahendra B: *Depression: the disorder and its associations,* Boston, 1986, MTP Press Limited.

Mann JJ: Brain biology influences the risk for suicide. *The Decade of the Brain,* Arlington, Va, NAMI 8(4):3, 1998.

McEnany GW: *Neuropsychiatric disorders: dementia versus depression versus drug intoxication.* Invited paper presented at Contemporary Forums Tenth Anniversary Conference on Psychiatric Nursing, Boston, May 1995a.

McEnany GW: *Restless nights: understanding and treating sleep disturbances.* Invited paper presented at Contemporary Forums Tenth Anniversary Conference on Psychiatric Nursing, Boston, May 1995b.

McGrath E, et al: *Women and depression: risk factors and treatment issues,* Washington, DC, 1992, American Psychological Association.

Mechanic D: Handbook of health, health care, and the health professions, New York, 1983, The Free Press.

Mellick E, Buckwalter KC, and Stolley JM: Suicide among elderly white men: development of a profile, *J Psychosoc Nurs Ment Health Serv* 30(2):29, 1992.

Metcalfe M: The personality of depressive patients. In Coppen A and Walk A, editors: *The psychology of depression: contemporary therapy and research,* New York, 1974, John Wiley & Sons.

Nemeroff CB: The neurobiology of depression, *Sci Amer* 278(6):42, 1998.

News and Notes: Cost of depression estimated at nearly $44 billion: time lost from work accounts for largest share, *Hosp Community Psychiatry* 45(1):85, 1994.

News in Mental Health Nursing: Prompt diagnosis of manic-depression improves quality of life, *J Psychosoc Nurs Ment Health Serv* 31(9):46, 1993.

News in Mental Health Nursing: Screening identifies individuals with untreated depression, *J Psychosoc Nurs Ment Health Serv* 32(1):45, 1994.

Packer S: Family planning for women with bipolar disorder, *Hosp Community Psychiatry* 43(5):479, 1992.

Pearson J: Suicide in the United States, *The Decade of the Brain,* Arlington, Va, NAMI 8(4):1, 1998.

Pollack LE: How do inpatients with bipolar disorder evaluate diagnostically homogeneous groups? *J Psychosoc Nurs Ment Health Serv* 31(10):26, 1993.

Regier DA, et al: The de facto US mental and addictive disorders service system: epidemiologic catchment area prospective 1-year prevalence rates of disorders and services, *Arch Gen Psychiatry* 50:85, 1993.

Rosenthal D: *Genetics and abnormal behavior,* New York, 1970, McGraw-Hill.

Shuchter SR, Downs N, and Zisook S: *Biologically informed psychotherapy for depression,* New York, 1996, Guilford Press.

Secunda SK, et al: Diagnosis and treatment of mixed mania, *Am J Psychiatry* 144:96, 1987.

Simmons-Alling S: Bipolar mood disorders. In McBride AB and Austin JS, editors: *Psychiatric mental-health nursing: integrating the behavioral and biological sciences,* Philadelphia, 1996, WB Saunders.

Tseng W and Streltzer J: *Culture and psychopathology: a guide to clinical assessment,* New York, 1997, Brunner/Mazel, Inc.

Valente SM: Preventing suicide among elderly people, *Am J Nurse Pract* 1(4):15, 1997.

Warren BJ: Depression, stressful life events, social support, and self-esteem in middle class African American women, *Arch Psychiatr Nurs* 11(3):107, 1997.

Weiss KJ, Valdiserri EV, and Dubin WR: Understanding depression in schizophrenia, *Hosp Community Psychiatry* 40:849, 1989.

CHAPTER 29

Anxiety-Related Disorders

CAROL E. BOSTROM
LEE H. SCHWECKE

LEARNING OBJECTIVES

After reading this chapter you should be able to:
- Recognize the special terms related to anxiety disorders, somatoform disorders, and dissociative disorders.
- Describe DSM-IV criteria for these disorders.
- Describe objective and subjective symptoms of these disorders.

- Develop nursing care plans for individuals with these disorders.
- Evaluate the effectiveness of nursing interventions for individuals with these disorders.
- Recognize issues related to the care of individuals with these anxiety-related disorders.

The anxiety-related disorders discussed in this chapter include disturbances in which felt anxiety (subjective) or expressed anxiety (objective) is a major symptom. The disorders are classified in the DSM-IV as anxiety disorders, somatoform disorders, and dissociative disorders. Interventions for each disorder are included. First, to understand anxiety-related disorders, it is crucial to understand *what* anxiety is, *where* it comes from, *why* it is difficult to deal with, and *how* individuals normally cope with it. See Chapter 13 for a conceptualization of the dynamics of anxiety-related disorders. To understand these dynamics and to provide effective treatment, it is important to understand the concepts of *primary gain* and *secondary gain*. Primary gain refers to the individual's desire to relieve anxiety in order to feel better and more secure. Secondary gain refers to the attention or support the individual derives from others because of illness. For example, "If I am sick, I cannot leave home to go grocery shopping, so I will call my husband at work and tell him to stop at the grocery store on his way home to buy the needed items." The assistance from the husband is a secondary gain.

Sometimes the attention or the benefit of the secondary gain becomes more important than reducing the anxiety. This phenomenon immeasurably complicates the treatment of these patients.

KEY TERMS

Primary gain   Relief or expression of anxiety through symptoms of disorder

Secondary gain   Support received from others while one is ill

Flashbacks   Cognitive, emotional, and physical reexperiencing of traumatic events

Derealization   Feelings of unreality

Depersonalization   Feeling detached from oneself

Dissociation   Removal from conscious awareness of painful feelings, memories, thoughts, or aspects of identity

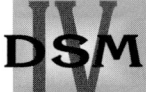

DSM-IV and NANDA Diagnoses Related to Anxiety-Related Disorders

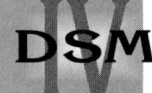

DSM-IV*
A. Anxiety disorders
   Generalized anxiety disorder
   Panic disorder with or without agoraphobia
   Agoraphobia without panic disorder
   Specific phobia
   Social phobia
   Obsessive-compulsive disorder
   Acute stress disorder (ASD)
   Posttraumatic stress disorder (PTSD)
   Anxiety disorder due to a general medical condition
B. Somatoform disorders
   Somatization disorder
   Pain disorder
   Hypochondriasis
   Conversion disorder
C. Dissociative disorders
   Dissociative amnesia
   Dissociative fugue
   Depersonalization disorder
   Dissociative identity disorder (Multiple personality disorder)

NANDA†
Adjustment, impaired
Anxiety
Body image disturbance
Breathing pattern, ineffective
Communication, impaired verbal
Coping, ineffective family
Coping, ineffective individual
Decisional conflict
Fear
Injury, potential for
Pain, chronic
Posttrauma response
Powerlessness
Role performance, altered
Self-esteem disturbance
Sensory/perceptual disturbance
Sleep pattern disturbance
Social interaction, impaired
Social isolation
Spiritual distress
Thought processes, altered
Violence, potential for, self-directed or directed at others

*From the American Psychiatric Association: Diagnostic and statistical manual of mental disorders, ed 4, Washington, DC, 1994, The Association.
†From the North American Nursing Diagnosis Association: NANDA nursing diagnoses: definitions and classifications 1997-1998, Philadelphia, 1997, The Association.

ANXIETY DISORDERS

GENERALIZED ANXIETY DISORDER

In generalized anxiety disorder (GAD), anxiety is directly felt and expressed. The anxiety or worry is excessive and concerns everyday events, such as work or school. These individuals have great difficulty in controlling the anxiety. Patients with GAD are admitted to the hospital usually for relief of their intense symptoms of anxiety, which is their immediate concern. The anxiety causes significant distress and impairment in interpersonal, social, and/or occupational functioning. Feelings of depression can also be experienced by these patients because of the sense of helplessness that results from the anxiety.

12-Month Prevalence Rate of Mental Disorders in the United States

Diagnosis	Percentage of Population over 17 Years of Age	Number of Persons
Anxiety disorders	12.6	20,034,000
Phobia disorders*	10.9	17,331,000
Mood disorders	9.5	15,143,000
Alcohol disorders	7.4	11,766,000
Major depression†	5.0	7,950,000
Drug disorders	3.1	4,929,000
Cognitive impairment	2.7	4,293,000
Obsessive-compulsive disorder	2.1	3,339,000
Antisocial disorder	1.5	2,385,000
Panic disorders*	1.3	2,067,000
Bipolar disorder†	1.2	1,908,000
Schizophrenia	1.1	1,749,000
Somatization	0.2	365,000

From Regier DA, et al: The de facto US mental and addictive disorders service system: epidemiologic catchment area prospective 1-year prevalence rates of disorders and services, *Arch Gen Psychiatry* 50:85, 1993.
*Also calculated in anxiety statistics.
†Also calculated in mood disorders statistics.

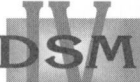 **DSM-IV Criteria for Generalized Anxiety Disorder**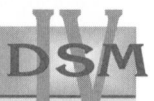

1. Excessive worry and anxiety
2. Difficulty in controlling the worry
3. Anxiety and worry are evident in:
   Restlessness
   Fatigue and irritability

Decreased ability to concentrate
Muscle tension
Disturbed sleep

Adapted from the American Psychiatric Association: *Diagnostic and statistical manual of mental disorders,* ed 4, Washington, DC, 1994, The Association.

Frequently, patients have used alcohol or other drugs to the point of dependence in an attempt to control anxiety. The box above lists the DSM-IV criteria for GAD.

When anxiety is caused by or related to a medical condition, the diagnosis of *anxiety disorder due to a general medical condition* is used. Presumably successful treatment of the medical illness will result in a reduced level of anxiety.

Psychotherapeutic Management

Nurse-Patient Relationship. The first step in the nurse-patient relationship is for the nurse to assist patients in reducing their level of anxiety. Anxiety must be reduced before problem solving can occur. The nurse's ultimate goal is to assist patients with developing adaptive coping responses.

Initially, patients need support and reassurance from the nurse. The nurse promotes trust through acceptance of patients' positive and negative feelings and acknowledgment of their discomfort. Conveying empathy tells patients that the nurse is concerned and understanding and does not minimize the level of distress. For example, the nurse might say, "This must be uncomfortable and painful for you." To help patients manage and reduce their level of anxiety, the nurse should use the interventions found in the box at the top of p. 425.

After the anxiety level is reduced to a more manageable and comfortable level, the nurse should begin to assist patients in examining their coping

Key Nursing Interventions to Reduce Anxiety

1. Provide a calm and quiet environment.

   Rationale: to identify and reduce stimulation, which includes exposure to situations and interactions with other patients that could provoke anxiety.

2. Ask patients to identify what and how they feel.

   Rationale: to help patients to increase their recognition of what is happening to them.

3. Encourage patients to describe and discuss their feelings with you.

   Rationale: to help patients to increase their awareness of the connection between feelings and behaviors.

4. Help patients to identify possible causes of their feelings.

   Rationale: to assist patients in connecting their feelings with earlier experiences.

5. Listen carefully for patients' expressions of helplessness and hopelessness.

   Rationale: to assess for self-harm; patients could be suicidal because they want to escape their pain and do not think that they will ever feel better.

6. Ask patients if they feel suicidal or have a plan to hurt themselves.

   Rationale: same as above, and to initiate suicide precautions if necessary.

7. Plan and involve patients in activities such as going for walks or playing recreational games.

   Rationale: to help patients to release nervous energy and to discourage preoccupation with the self.

Key Nursing Interventions in Problem Solving

1. Discuss with patients their present and previous coping mechanisms.

   Rationale: to reinforce effective adaptive behaviors.

2. Discuss with patients the meaning of problems and conflicts.

   Rationale: to help patients appraise stressors, explore their personal values, and define the scope and seriousness of their problems.

3. Use supportive confrontation and teaching.

   Rationale: to increase patients' insight into the negative effects of their maladaptive and dysfunctional coping behaviors.

4. Assist patients with exploring alternative solutions and behaviors.

   Rationale: to increase adaptive coping mechanisms.

5. Encourage patients to test new adaptive coping behaviors through role-playing or implementation.

   Rationale: to provide an opportunity for patients to practice new behaviors.

6. Teach patients relaxation exercises.

   Rationale: to reduce the level of anxiety. These techniques help patients to manage or control anxiety on their own.

7. Promote the use of hobbies and recreational activities.

   Rationale: to help patients deal with routine feelings of stress and anxiety.

behaviors. Through the use of problem-solving methods, adaptive coping skills can increase. The nurse should use the interventions found in the box above.

The process of helping patients to learn to use adaptive coping behaviors requires patience and the awareness that individuals learn and change at their own pace. The nurse must also be aware of his or her own verbal and nonverbal behavior when working with these patients, because anxiety is contagious. The nurse should manage his or her own stress and anxiety so that the work between the nurse and patients is not compromised. The nurse educates the patient about the illness, including the effects of anxiety on the patient's life and also on the members of the family (Thompson, 1996).

Psychopharmacology. Benzodiazepines, such as lorazepam (Ativan) and alprazolam (Xanax) are used for patients with GAD. These medications usually are ordered on a scheduled basis. Additional doses also are given on a prn basis, depending on the need of the patient and the severity of the anxiety. Benzodiazepines improve somatic symptoms and help patients to feel better physically. Patients with alcohol or substance abuse problems are not generally treated with benzodiazepines because of the potential for abuse, although oxazepam (Serax) is sometimes used (Thompson, 1996). Buspirone (BuSpar), a nonbenzodiazepine, is effective for the cognitive symptoms of anxiety. If depression is also present, patients can benefit from an antidepressant.

Milieu Management. The patient with GAD can benefit from a variety of milieu activities. Recreational activities help to reduce tension and anxiety. The use of relaxation exercises and tapes helps to decrease bodily tension and promotes relaxation and comfort.

Groups that focus on stress management, problem solving, self-esteem, assertiveness, codependency, and goal setting are helpful with stress. Depending on the issues and concerns of each patient, a variety of groups can be beneficial.

PANIC DISORDER

Patients with panic disorder experience recurrent panic attacks and are worried about having more attacks. A panic attack is accompanied by intense fear or discomfort and lasts from minutes to approximately an hour. Symptoms of anxiety can last for hours after an attack. These panic attacks are severe, frightening, and incapacitating to patients who experience them. A panic attack usually develops suddenly, often with no obvious precipitating factor, and reaches a peak in approximately 10 minutes. In addition to somatic symptoms, patients who experience panic attacks fear they are losing control over themselves, "going crazy," having a heart attack, or dying. Panic attacks can occur during sleep, resulting in exhaustion. The box below lists the DSM-IV criteria for panic attack.

According to the DSM-IV, panic attacks are (1) unexpected, occur "out of the blue," or occur spontaneously, or (2) are situationally bound, meaning that they occur in anticipation of or upon exposure to a trigger situation. Panic attacks that occur in response to a situation or trigger are related to social and specific phobias.

Patients become preoccupied with their health after experiencing panic attacks because of the physical symptoms they experience. Thinking that cardiac, neurological, or gastroenterological problems may be present, patients often consult with medical specialists before being diagnosed with panic disorder (Federici and Tommasini, 1992).

Panic disorder can result in agoraphobia because patients fear having a panic attack in a place where embarrassment could occur, where help might not be available, or where escape is impossible. Patients who have panic disorder with agoraphobia restrict their activities outside of the home or require another person to be with them when outside the home. Thus, they become agoraphobic due to the fear of having an attack outside the home. Treatment for agoraphobia is discussed later in this chapter. Agoraphobia affects about one third of all people with panic disorder and is diagnosed approximately twice as often in females as in males (Grinspoon, 1996a). Feelings of depression can occur because patients feel helpless and hopeless about getting better. Patients with panic disorder who have an additional axis I diagnosis of major depression may attempt suicide. Some may abuse alcohol (Grinspoon, 1996b). The DSM-IV box on p. 427 lists the DSM-IV criteria for panic disorder.

Etiology

Panic disorder may be genetically transmitted. Genetic factors, coupled with environmental factors, may be associated with vulnerability to this disor-

---

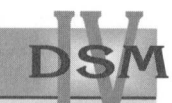

DSM-IV Criteria for Panic Attack

1. Increased heart rate, palpitations, or chest pain
2. Chills or hot flushes, sweating, trembling, dizziness, or light-headedness
3. Feeling of choking, smothering, or shortness of breath
4. Nausea or abdominal distress
5. Numbness or tingling
6. Fear of dying, "going crazy," or losing control
7. Derealization or depersonalization

Adapted from the American Psychiatric Association: *Diagnostic and statistical manual of mental disorders,* ed 4, Washington, DC, 1994, The Association.

der while brain and biochemical factors may account for its development. Bursts of activity in the raphe nuclei (serotonin) and the locus ceruleus are thought to play a role in anxiety formation. Abnormalities in the brain's benzodiazepine receptors are also implicated in the etiology of anxiety disorders. In patients with panic disorder, panic attacks can be induced with caffeine, carbon dioxide, and sodium lactate (Grinspoon, 1996a). Patients are less likely to panic when informed about the symptoms they will experience. This suggests a psychological as well as a biological component to panic disorder.

Psychotherapeutic Management

Nurse-Patient Relationship. The therapeutic relationship between the nurse and patients with panic disorder is centered on the same issues and interventions discussed for patients with GAD. Interventions specific to patients experiencing a panic attack are described in the box below. The rationale for the interventions is to help patients to get through the panic attack safely with as little discomfort as possible. With the nurse's assistance, patients' anxiety can be reduced to more manageable levels.

The nurse educates patients about panic disorder to reassure them that they are not losing their minds or dying during an attack. Patients experience relief when given information about the disorder and about medications that can block symptoms (Wakefield and Pallister, 1997). The nurse should help patients realize that attacks are time limited and that symptoms will abate. Cognitive restructuring helps the patient to reinterpret and reappraise beliefs regarding the danger of an event or bodily sensations (Wakefield and Pallister, 1997).

Psychopharmacology. The selective serotonin reuptake inhibitors (SSRIs) are the drugs of choice for treating panic disorder (Keltner, et al, 1998). An antidepressant such as imipramine (Tofranil), a benzodiazepine such as alprazolam (Xanax) or clonazepam (Klonopin), or a monoamine oxidase

---

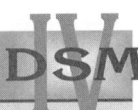

DSM-IV Criteria for Panic Disorder

1. Recurrent, unexpected panic attacks
2. Panic attacks are followed by a month or more of worry about having additional attacks, worry about

the results of the attacks, and behavior changes related to the attacks

Panic disorder can be accompanied by agoraphobia

Adapted from the American Psychiatric Association: *Diagnostic and statistical manual of mental disorders,* ed 4, Washington, DC, 1994, The Association.

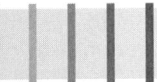

Key Nursing Interventions for Panic Attack

1. Stay with the patient who is having a panic attack and acknowledge the patient's discomfort.
2. Maintain a calm style and demeanor.
3. Speak in short, simple sentences, and give one direction at a time in a calm tone of voice.
4. If the patient is hyperventilating, provide a brown paper bag and focus on breathing with the patient.
5. Allow patients to pace or cry; this enables the release of tension and energy.
6. Communicate to patients that you are in control and will not let anything happen to them.
7. Move or direct patients to a quieter, less stimulating environment. Do not touch these patients; touching can increase feelings of panic.
8. Ask patients to express their perceptions or fears about what is happening to them.

    Rationale: to help patients reduce anxiety to a more manageable and comfortable level.

Case Study

Sandra Johnson, a 41-year-old white woman, is being admitted to the psychiatric unit of a general hospital. She is accompanied by her husband and is coming from the emergency room. Her presenting symptoms in the emergency room were shortness of breath, hyperventilation, palpitations, chest pain, and fear of dying. She stated that these symptoms had occurred unexpectedly while she was cooking dinner. She thought that she was having a heart attack.

These attacks had happened three times before. The first attack occurred 2 months ago. After the first attack, she went to her family physician, who gave her an electrocardiogram, a stress test, and a complete physical examination. All results were negative for any physiological causation of the symptoms. After the second attack, Mrs. Johnson stated that she took 2 weeks off from work because she was worried about having another attack. She had been employed for 5 years as a secretary for a small insurance agency. Just before she was about to return to work, she experienced another attack. After this third attack, she decided not to return to work and quit her job. She was unable to leave the house to go grocery shopping, to drive the children to activities, and to

go out socially with her friends. Her husband, who is 42 years old, stated that he and their three daughters, aged 15, 12, and 9 years, were very concerned about her and had been helping her with daily tasks.

After her husband leaves, Mrs. Johnson begins to cry and states that she is letting her family down. They have tried to help her and she cannot do anything at home, cannot work, and cannot even leave the house because she is so afraid of not being able to control the possibility of another "attack." She does not understand what is happening to her and wants medication to help her feel better.

On the third day of her hospitalization, Mrs. Johnson tells the nurse that she is upset because her husband has not visited her since her admission. As she talks more about her husband, she starts to cry and states that she is afraid of losing him. She reports that 2 or 3 months ago she noticed a change in her husband. He was less affectionate and was spending more time away from home. He suddenly had more business trips. She is afraid he is having an affair. She says: "What am I going to do if he leaves? I can't support myself and my children alone. I don't even have a job. I can't go out of the house. I've lost contact with my friends."

---

inhibitor (MAOI) such as phenelzine (Nardil) can be used to block the symptoms or to reduce panic attacks (Keltner, et al, 1998; DuPont, 1997).

Patients with panic disorder may resist drug therapy because it may mean a loss of control at a time when they are struggling to maintain control over themselves and their symptoms (Katon, Sheenan, and Uhde, 1992). Some fear medications and their side effects (DuPont, 1997). A good, simple explanation of the disorder and its biological components often can convince patients that medication is helpful and not a sign of "weakness."

The nurse must be able to differentiate symptoms of increased anxiety levels from medication side effects. Anxiety symptoms increase when pertinent issues are addressed or stressors are present. When symptoms of anxiety remain constant, or decrease just prior to the next dosage of medication, the symptoms are probably related to the medication. Anxiety-reduction strategies (e.g., relaxation exercises) may help patients to manage anxiety.

Milieu Management.   As a patient's anxiety decreases from the panic level to other levels of anxiety, gross motor activities, such as walking, jogging, basketball, volleyball, or the use of a stationary bicycle, are appropriate to help decrease tension and anxiety. Other milieu interventions are located in the section about GAD.

OBSESSIVE-COMPULSIVE DISORDER

According to the DSM-IV, obsessions are recurrent and persistent thoughts, ideas, impulses, or images that are experienced as intrusive and senseless. (See the box on p. 430.) Persons with obsessive-compulsive disorder (OCD) recognize that the thoughts are products of their own minds. They know that the thoughts are trivial, ridiculous, or morbid but cannot stop, forget, or control them. The thoughts are distressful and anxiety provoking. An example of a morbid obsession is a woman experiencing an obsession to kill

Care Plan

NAME: Sandra Johnson   ADMISSION DATE: _____

DSM-IV DIAGNOSIS: Panic disorder with agoraphobia

ASSESSMENT: **Areas of strength:** Managing her role as mother, homemaker, and secretary; was socially active with her friends; in relatively good health

Problems: Fear of dying related to fear of heart attack; unable to leave the house; afraid of losing her husband; feelings of inadequacy

DIAGNOSES:
- Anxiety: panic related to life stress, as evidenced by somatic symptoms and fear of dying.
- Self-esteem disturbance related to feelings of helplessness, as evidenced by inability to function.
- Fear related to avoidance, as evidenced by inability to leave home.

OUTCOMES: **Short-term goals:**   Date met
- Patient will discuss fears, her sense of inadequacy and helplessness, and anger.   _____
- Identify relationship between anxiety and physiological responses.   _____
- Develop strategies for reducing anxiety, such as relaxation techniques. _____
- Use problem-solving techniques for life stresses.   _____

Long-term goals:
- Patient will meet with husband and social worker to discuss marital issues. _____
- Schedule appointment with outpatient therapist for systematic desensitization or self-exposure training.   _____
- Identify schedule for attending an agoraphobia support group.   _____

PLANNING/ INTERVENTIONS: **Nurse-patient relationship:** Empathy and supportive-suppressive techniques to keep anxiety at a minimum; encourage ventilation of feelings and issues; help patient to identify relationships among stress, anxiety, and physiological responses; assist with adaptive coping strategies.

Psychopharmacology: Xanax, 1 mg q 4 hr prn; Prozac 20 mg q AM

Milieu management: Decrease stimuli and provide quiet, calm atmosphere; monitor anxiety level to prevent escalation; encourage recreational and diversional activities; use quiet room if necessary; later encourage problem-solving, assertiveness, communication, problem-centered, self-esteem, and stress management groups.

EVALUATION: Patient reports being less anxious for the past 2 days. Met with husband and social worker.

REFERRALS: Outpatient appointments for cognitive therapy and self-exposure training.

---

her child. An example of a silly obsession is the rhyme "Sticks and stones may break my bones but words will never hurt me."

Compulsions can be defined as repetitive behaviors that are performed in a particular manner in response to an obsession. The compulsions are performed to prevent discomfort and to bind or neutralize anxiety. Individuals with OCD experience anxiety if they try to resist the obsessions or the compulsions. Some examples of compulsions are repetitive hand washing, checking the locks on doors, counting, and touching. These persons know or recognize that their actions are absurd, but they are compelled to perform the rituals to avoid an extreme

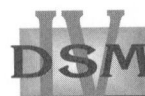 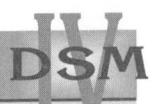

DSM-IV Criteria for Obsessive-Compulsive Disorder

A. Obsessions
1. Intrusive, inappropriate, recurrent, and persistent thoughts, impulses, or images that are distressful or produce anxiety
2. Unsuccessful attempts to ignore or neutralize thoughts or impulses by other thoughts or actions
3. Recognition that obsessions are produced by own thoughts

OR

4. Not simply excessive worry about real-life problems

B. Compulsions
1. Repetitive behaviors, such as hand washing, or mental acts, such as counting, are performed in response to an obsession
2. Excessive behaviors or mental acts are used to reduce distress or prevent dreaded events

C. Recognition that obsessions or compulsions are unreasonable or excessive

D. Obsessions or compulsions cause distress, are time-consuming, and interfere with usual daily functioning

Adapted from the American Psychiatric Association: *Diagnostic and statistical manual of mental disorders,* ed 4, Washington, DC, 1994, The Association.

increase in tension and anxiety. These individuals have a great need to control themselves, others, and their environment. Some find it difficult to express emotions and to be introspective. Depression is a feature associated with this disorder because of its impact on self-esteem and self-worth. Avoidance of anxiety is employed in this disorder, along with the defense mechanisms reaction-formation, isolation, and undoing.

An important feature to remember about OCD is that the obsessions or compulsions are so severe that they significantly interfere with the patient's normal routine and are so time consuming that they interfere with occupational and social functioning. The obsessions and compulsions also interfere with these patients' interpersonal relationships because they do not have time to relate to others—they are too busy thinking or doing. Persons who experience *magical thinking* believe that thinking *equals* doing.

CLINICAL EXAMPLE

John is watching a football game on television. As his favorite player prepares to attempt a field goal, John experiences severe anxiety because he thinks the player will miss the field goal attempt. John is afraid that his thinking will cause the player to miss.

Thinking processes in individuals with OCD may also be rigid, and these persons may be task oriented.

Relaxation is very difficult. Patients with OCD are extremely overcontrolled persons and have a strong sense of right and wrong.

In our society, value is placed on performing well in school and at work. Being responsible and perfectionistic is often rewarded by the boss or by family members. Thus, at times, anyone may be "compulsive." Generally, however, people do not allow their compulsiveness to rule their lives. They are able to maintain a balance between work and play, between role expectations and performance. There is a difference between having characteristics or traits and having an illness. Occasional brooding, rumination, or steadfastness to a task is not usually considered ridiculous or excessively bothersome. These thoughts and feelings do not rule most people's lives.

Etiology

Current views concerning the etiology of obsessive-compulsive disorder point to genetic transmission. OCD may run in families (Grinspoon, 1995a). Biological findings in OCD identify increased brain activity in the frontal lobe and basal ganglia (Glod and Cawley, 1997). Clinical trials have also supported the hypothesis that serotonin dysregulation is involved in the formation of OCD (Glod and Cawley, 1997). This may account for the effectiveness of clomipramine (Anafranil) and the SSRIs.

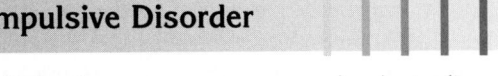

Key Nursing Interventions for Obsessive-Compulsive Disorder

1. Ensure that basic needs of food, rest, and grooming are met.

     Rationale: Patients are too busy to attend to these tasks. Reminders and specific directions are usually necessary.

2. Provide patients with time to perform rituals.

     Rationale: Patients need to keep anxiety in check. Later, work to decrease the rituals by setting limits, but never take away a ritual, or panic may ensue.

3. Explain expectations, routines, and changes.

     Rationale: to prevent an increase or escalation of anxiety.

4. Be empathic toward patients and aware of their need to perform rituals.

     Rationale: to convey acceptance and understanding.

5. Assist patients with connecting behaviors and feelings.

     Rationale: to promote the ability to identify and understand feelings.

6. Structure simple activities, games, or tasks for patients.

     Rationale: to help patients focus on alternatives to their thoughts and actions.

7. Reinforce and recognize positive nonritualistic behaviors.

     Rationale: to increase patients' self-esteem and self-worth.

■ Critical Thinking Question

A patient with OCD washes her hands after each time she touches anything. Her skin is cracked and bleeding. She states to the nurse, "I'm afraid that my hands are terribly infected, and what will happen if I have to have them amputated?" The patient reaches a state of panic when she attempts to wash her hands because of the fear of amputation. What would you say and do when this patient approaches the sink to wash her hands?

Psychotherapeutic Management

Nurse-Patient Relationship. Basic nursing interventions for hospitalized patients with OCD are listed in the box above.

Therapeutic work involves the nurse increasing patients' abilities to verbalize feelings, solve problems, and make decisions concerning stressors and problems. The nurse focuses on teaching and helping patients to develop adaptive coping behaviors to deal with anxiety. Patients need to learn to substitute positive, anxiety-reducing behavior for obsessions and rituals. A variety of positive behaviors can include physical exercise such as walking or using a stationary bicycle. Positive coping behaviors are slowly introduced into each patient's schedule, allowing time for rituals as well as normal activities. The nurse supports patients and positively reinforces nonritualistic behavior. Hobbies and social activities are introduced slowly as patients are able to handle them.

Psychopharmacology. The antidepressant clomipramine (Anafranil) is the medication of choice for the treatment of OCD. Clomipramine is related to the tricyclic antidepressants (TCAs) and helps to decrease obsessions and alleviate rituals. The SSRIs fluoxetine (Prozac), sertraline (Zoloft), and fluvoxamine (Luvox) are also effective in treating OCD (Glod and Cawley, 1997). Patients tolerate the SSRIs better than clomipramine (Anafranil) because of a better side effect profile (Kaplan, 1997). Monoamine oxidase inhibitors have been found to be helpful in treating OCD if there is a history of panic attacks. While benzodiazepines may relieve anxiety in this condition, they do not seem to affect the core symptoms of OCD.

Milieu Management. A variety of milieu activities and groups are beneficial to patients after anxiety decreases and the need for obsessions and compulsions starts to decrease. Of particular importance are stress management groups, recreational or social skills groups, cognitive therapy, problem-solving groups, and communication or assertiveness training groups. Care is always based on the individual needs of patients.

Behavior treatment is effective for patients with OCD. Patients can perform in vivo exposure treatment on an outpatient basis. They are encouraged to contact feared stimuli and then to resist the urge to perform rituals. Exposure treatment is explained in Chapter 36 on behavior therapy. A form of cognitive therapy such as thought stopping can be used. When an intrusive thought occurs, the patient says "stop" and snaps a rubber band on the wrist (Grinspoon, 1995b).

PHOBIC DISORDERS

Phobic disorders are intense, irrational fear responses to an external object, activity, or situation. Anxiety is experienced if the person comes into contact with the dreaded object or situation. Like all anxiety disorders, a phobia is a response to experienced anxiety. It is characterized by a persistent fear of *specific* places or things, as opposed to GAD, in which the anxiety is free-floating; thus, anxiety is displaced or externalized to a source outside the body.

Phobias persist even though phobic persons recognize that they are irrational. Persons can control the intensity of anxiety simply by avoiding the object or situation they fear.

In the DSM-IV, phobias are categorized into three types:

1. Agoraphobia without history of panic disorder: a fear of being in public or open spaces, places, or situations where escape could be difficult or help might not be available; for example, if the person should faint.
2. Social phobia: fear of being humiliated, scrutinized, or embarrassed in public; for example, choking while eating in front of others or stumbling while dancing in view of others.
3. Specific phobia: fear of a specific object or situation that is not either of the above. Examples are a fear of animals, flying, or heights.

Exposure to the stimulus results in an anxiety response. It is common to have some fears or phobias about certain objects or situations. Some people are afraid of public speaking, while some may be afraid of elevators or heights. However, these fears do not ruin most people's lives to the extent that they can never leave home. Most people are still able to function and fulfill role expectations, responsibilities, and relationships. Phobic symptoms become phobic disorders when they cause severe distress and impair functioning.

Etiology

Research has led to theories that specific individual factors, environment, family environment, and genetic factors underlie phobic disorders (Kendler, et al, 1992). Types of phobias develop based on the influence of environment and genetic predisposition.

Psychotherapeutic Management

Nurse-Patient Relationship. Patients with phobic disorders usually are treated on an outpatient basis. If the phobia incapacitates a patient to a severe extent, as in panic disorder with agoraphobia, the patient may be hospitalized. Another example in which hospitalization is indicated is the case of a person who has a phobia about germs and may not eat or drink. Some interventions useful for persons experiencing phobic disorders are the following:

1. Accept patients and their fears with a noncritical attitude.
2. Provide and involve patients with activities that do not increase anxiety but will increase involvement rather than avoidance.
3. Help patients with physical safety and comfort needs.
4. Help patients to recognize that their behavior is a method of coping with anxiety.

Psychopharmacology. Behavior therapies are the most successful treatments of phobic patients, and drugs traditionally have no effect on avoidant behaviors. Medication that reduces or blocks panic attacks or reduces depression is used if those features are present. Examples are imipramine (Tofranil), alprazolam (Xanax), clonazepam (Klonopin) and phenelzine (Nardil) (Marshall and Schneier, 1996).

Milieu Management. Assertiveness-training and goal-setting groups are beneficial. Social skills groups and other milieu activities help patients to redevelop social skills and decrease avoidance.

Behavior therapy, such as systematic desensitization, flooding, exposure, and self-exposure treatments, is most therapeutic for phobic patients. Self-exposure treatment is being used more often in order to avoid frequent therapy sessions (see Chapter 36).

ACUTE STRESS DISORDER AND POSTTRAUMATIC STRESS DISORDER

Acute stress disorder (ASD) and posttraumatic stress disorder (PTSD) are somewhat different from the other anxiety disorders. ASD and PTSD are disorders that can develop after exposure to a clearly identifiable traumatic event that threatens the self, others, resources, and/or a sense of control or hope. Some of the traumatic stressors that may precipitate the development of ASD and PTSD are war, community violence, torture, natural and man-made disasters, bombings, major fires, accidents, catastrophic illness, injury to self or others, chronic abuse, rape, assault, and major personal or business losses (Brandt, et al, 1997; Bremner, et al, 1996; Clark, 1997; Stein, et al, 1997). Various studies report that 50% to 70% of Americans have suffered at least one

such traumatic event in their lifetimes (Solomon and Davidson, 1997). Anyone experiencing such events would be distressed, probably with intense fear, horror, and a sense of helplessness. (The box below lists the criteria for ASD and PTSD). To an extent, the type and degree of the initial and later reactions to trauma depend on the individual's preexisting characteristics and conditions, usual coping style and defense mechanisms, personal and social resources, previous exposure to trauma, and the meaning of the event to the individual.

The diagnosis of ASD is made when an individual has dissociative symptoms *during or immediately after* the distressing event: amnesia, depersonalization, derealization, decreased awareness of surroundings, numbing, detachment, and/or lack of emotional response. The diagnosis of PTSD is not made because of any initial reactions at the time of the trauma but is based on the characteristic symptoms

---

DSM-IV Criteria for Acute Stress Disorder and Posttraumatic Stress Disorder

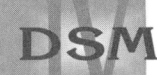

Acute Stress Disorder

1. Exposure to a traumatic event involving threat of death/injury to self or others, or actual injury to self or others
2. Responses of horror, helplessness, and/or fear
3. Dissociative symptoms during or immediately after the event:
   Absence of emotions, numbing, detachment
   Decreased awareness of surroundings (in a "daze")
   Derealization and/or depersonalization
   Amnesia
4. Avoidance of stimuli related to trauma: feelings, thoughts, people, conversations, places, and activities
   Distress when exposed to reminders of the event
5. Increased arousal or anxiety: sleep disturbance, hypervigilance, startle response, irritability, restlessness, decreased concentration
6. Reexperiencing or reliving the traumatic event: distressing thoughts, dreams, flashbacks, illusions
7. Impairment or distress in functioning: occupational, social, or other important area

8. Onset: within 4 weeks after the event
9. Duration: 2 days to 4 weeks

Posttraumatic Stress Disorder

1. Same criteria as ASD
2. Same criteria as ASD
3. Numbing of responsiveness
   Restricted affect, such as not being able to love
   Sense of "foreshortened future" (lack of expectations about the future)
   Inability to recall aspects of the event
4. Same criteria as ASD, plus
   Decreased participation/interest in activities
   Estrangement and detachment from others
5. Same criteria as ASD, plus
   Outbursts of anger
6. Same criteria as ASD, plus
   Hallucinations
7. Same criteria as ASD
8. Acute: within 6 months after the event
   Delayed: 6 months or more after the event
9. Acute: 1-3 months
   Chronic: 3 months or more

Adapted from the American Psychiatric Association: *Diagnostic and statistical manual of mental disorders*, ed 4, Washington, DC, 1994, The Association.

that occur *one month or more after* the trauma. It is common for PTSD to be unrecognized for years, sometimes even 10 to 20 years. This is due in part to the major characteristic of both ASD and PTSD: "numbing of responsiveness" to or reduced involvement with the external world. There is a persistent attempt to avoid situations, activities and, sometimes, persons that evoke memories of the trauma. These efforts include trying to avoid thoughts and feelings related to the event.

Denial, repression, and suppression are common, especially in PTSD. A constricted or blunted affect, or a limitation in the range of feelings, may occur, such as not being able to show affection. Patients may feel detached or estranged from family and friends. An inability to trust and to love may lead to a withdrawal. There is often a loss of interest in activities, even those unrelated to the traumatic event. There also may be a change in the individual's perceptions about the future—a kind of hopelessness; for example, hopelessness about having a family or a career.

A second major characteristic of ASD and PTSD is the reexperiencing of the traumatic event in some way. This may occur as intrusive, unwanted memories; upsetting dreams or nightmares; illusions; or suddenly feeling as if the event were reoccurring (flashbacks). With PTSD, there may be hallucinations with content related to the traumatic event. It is not known precisely why these unpleasant, frightening experiences begin to break through the denial, repression, or suppression. The triggers for the reexperiencing episodes may have obvious connections to the trauma or may not resemble the original situation at all. In the latter case, patients may try to avoid activities and people in an effort to prevent reexperiencing the flashback.

CLINICAL EXAMPLE

Three days after an earthquake had destroyed her home and seriously injured her son, Joan Marin was found wandering around the hospital in which her son was a patient. She was not injured but complained of nightmares and irritability. She said she could not bear to see her son because he "just wanted to talk about what happened—things I can't remember." Joan had not been to work since the earthquake. She was taken to the crisis unit and diagnosed with acute stress disorder.

Other criteria of ASD and PTSD include increased arousal, anxiety, restlessness, irritability, disturbances in sleep, and impairment in memory or concentration. Especially with PTSD, there may be occasional outbursts of anger or rage and "survivor guilt," that is, guilt about surviving or the actions taken in order to survive. For example, disaster victims or combat soldiers may feel they survived because of cowardly acts; rape victims may feel guilty for not resisting their attacker. Up to 75% of the nurses in Vietnam developed some posttraumatic symptoms, including guilt about not having saved more lives (Bille, 1993; Furey, 1991; Stanton, et al, 1996).

Another consequence of ASD and PTSD can be psychological and physiological symptoms that develop during exposure to situations resembling the original trauma, such as anxiety or panic attacks. Psychophysiological illnesses (e.g., gastrointestinal disorders, headache) may develop (Solomon and Davidson, 1997). It is sometimes difficult to differentiate ASD and PTSD from other disorders.

Persons experiencing posttraumatic symptoms may develop problems with depression, suicidal ideations and attempts, anxiety-related disorders, and substance abuse (Grinspoon, 1998; Solomon and Davidson, 1997). Patients may appear avoidant, schizoid, schizophrenic, paranoid, or even manic. These symptoms complicate treatment, especially if the ASD and PTSD are ignored and only the other diagnoses are treated.

Preexisting psychiatric disorders, including personality disorders, can increase the risk of developing ASD and PTSD after a traumatic event (Barton, Blanchard, and Hickling, 1996). A history of previous traumas, including childhood abuse, rape, and abuse by a partner, leads to an increased risk for PTSD after later traumas (North and Smith, 1992). On the other hand, events later in life may trigger previously unrecognized PTSD. For example, some World War II and Korean veterans have not shown PTSD symptoms until after experiencing retirement, losses, and other processes associated with aging (Snell and Padin-Rivera, 1997). Activation and reactivation of PTSD symptoms has also been reported in veterans following the Persian Gulf War and in people who survived the Oklahoma City bombing (Moyers, 1996).

There may be difficulties such as arrests, unemployment, homelessness, abusiveness, divorce, and paranoia toward authority figures or other persons whom patients perceive as directly and indirectly responsible for not helping with the original traumatic situation. Mistrust, isolation, abandonment fears, workaholism, focusing on the needs of others, feelings of inadequacy, anger toward God, unresolved grief, and fear of losing control of emotions are common (Bille, 1993).

The family members of individuals with ASD or PTSD may develop problems as well (see the box below). In some cases, family members experience the same trauma (e.g., a major fire, war, or disaster) and develop symptoms themselves. The family, particularly the partner, may react directly or indirectly to the trauma itself or to the behaviors of the trauma victim and develop his or her own problems as a result especially if there is violence or verbal abuse by the partner with PTSD (Nelson and Wright, 1996). The family may or may not be able to help in the treatment of their family member with ASD or PTSD. The whole family or selected members may need treatment.

Following a community disaster, many people may experience acute stress or posttraumatic symptoms and initially find it difficult to get support from others. When the danger is over, small groups of victims may gather for mutual support and assistance with grieving (Samter, et al, 1993). Disaster personnel often encourage and facilitate debriefing in groups, including groups of emergency personnel. Fear, concern, uncertainty, frustration, anger, and humor are all to be expected (Dahl and O'Neal, 1993).

■ Critical Thinking Question

Ron Jenkins's workplace was severely damaged by a tornado. He was found staring at the cars in the parking lot and repeating that he had to find his car and wife. He could not give his address or say where his wife would be at that time of day. He refused to be treated for cuts and bruises until he could find his wife. What interventions would you use at the scene? What referrals and recommendations would you make to prevent ASD and PTSD?

Neurochemical Basis of Acute Stress Disorder and Posttraumatic Stress Disorder

It is proposed that fear conditioning, a failure of extinction (of the fear/anxiety response), and behavioral sensitization may be important in the development of ASD and PTSD symptomatology following exposure to a traumatic event (Charney, et al, 1993; van der Kolk, 1997). It has been shown that *fear conditioning* to auditory and visual stimuli can last for years and produce relatively indelible emotional and visceral memories. If *extinction* of fear responses does not occur, the responses continue even when the traumatic event is absent. Normally, associations leading to the conditioned response would be "erased," or new associations would "mask" the response-producing associations over time. Conditioned fear responses, after being dormant for years, can be reactivated by trauma-associated stimuli. *Sensitization* is the increased magnitude of response to

FAMILY ISSUES

Family Issues with Acute Stress Disorder and Posttraumatic Stress Disorder

Family members of patients with ASD or PTSD need to be assessed along with patients. Issues to be addressed include the following:

1. Assessing whether any or all members of the family have been exposed to the same trauma as the patient and, if so, if family members may be experiencing symptoms of ASD or PTSD as well.
2. Assessing whether any or all of the family members are having reactions to the behaviors of the member with ASD or PTSD.

3. Teaching family members about the causes, symptoms, and treatment of ASD and PTSD.
4. Educating family members about ways to help the member(s) with ASD or PTSD.
5. Referring family members to a support group for families of ASD or PTSD survivors or a related group, if available.
6. Referring members for couple or family counseling if needed.

one stimulus, but especially to repeated traumatic stimuli. This behavioral sensitivity produces increased arousal *(hyperarousal)* and stress sensitivity that can endure for a long time. *Cross-sensitization* can occur so that there is overreaction to other, even minor, stimuli that resemble the original traumatic stimulus (Charney, et al, 1993; van der Kolk, 1997; Friedman, 1997).

Avoidance (behavioral), numbing (emotional), autonomic hyperarousal (somatic), and reexperiencing of the trauma (cognitive, emotional, somatic, and behavioral) are characteristic symptoms of ASD and PTSD. Avoidance and numbing (in response to fear conditioning and behavioral sensitization) are likely to be related to increased endogenous opiate release (Friedman, 1997), producing emotional blunting, physical analgesia, and depersonalization. Autonomic hyperarousal (also in response to fear conditioning and behavioral sensitization) is related to increased noradrenergic and dopaminergic system activity and decreased serotonergic activity, causing fear, anxiety, and "fight or flight" readiness. Reexperiencing the trauma (in response to fear conditioning and failure of extinction) is related to activation of the amygdala, locus ceruleus, thalamus, and hippocampus, which enhances encoding of traumatic memories, and sensory and cognitive memory retrieval (Charney, et al, 1993; van der Kolk, 1997; Friedman, 1997). Prolonged stress eventually results in down-regulation of the corticotropin-releasing factor (CRF) and adrenergic receptors, and decreased adrenocorticotropin-releasing hormone (ACTH) release, so that the fear/anxiety response may become blunted and desensitization induced (van der Kolk, 1997; Friedman, 1997).

Hyperarousal may cause memories to be dissociated, repressed, or stored as bodily sensations that are not available at a conscious level. Fragments of these memories may appear later as physiological reactions, nightmares, flashbacks, and emotional reenactments of the trauma (van der Kolk, 1997). ASD and PTSD patients typically have more psychophysiological symptoms, sleep disturbances, and altered immune function than individuals who do not have ASD and PTSD (van der Kolk, 1997).

Genetic susceptibility to posttraumatic symptoms has been suggested by one identical vs. fraternal twin study of Vietnam era veterans. Data were obtained on symptoms of reexperiencing trauma, heightened arousal, avoidance of activities, emotional numb-

ness, feeling that life was empty, feeling that people were distant, and levels of combat experience. It was found that heredity accounted for 13% to 34% of the individual differences in the categories of symptoms after adjusting for the level of combat exposure. The severity of posttraumatic symptoms, especially in the category of reexperiencing, rose as the level of combat increased (Grinspoon, 1994).

The incidence of alcohol, opiate, and benzodiazepine abuse in those with posttraumatic symptoms may be related to attempts to reduce those symptoms that result from increased noradrenergic and dopaminergic activity. Conversely, "addiction" to trauma (compulsively exposing oneself to traumatic events) may in part be explained by the recurrent increase in endogenous opiates. Those with posttraumatic symptoms also have an exaggerated response to amphetamines and cocaine because of their preexisting hyperarousal. After taking these drugs, individuals with posttraumatic symptoms are more vulnerable to paranoia and psychosis (Bremner, et al, 1996).

Psychotherapeutic Management

The treatment of patients experiencing ASD or PTSD must be individualized according to the predominant symptoms and the associated problems, such as depression, suicidal ideation, or substance abuse. (See Chapter 34 for working with dually diagnosed patients.)

Principles of critical incident debriefing (adapted from the military) are often applied to natural and man-made disaster situations where the development of posttraumatic symptoms in some victims is likely. These principles include treatment (1) at the site; (2) as soon as the stress reaction develops; (3) with an expectation of recovery; and (4) after replenishment, rest, and debriefing. This conveys that the stress reaction is "simple, temporary, and expected" and that recovery is possible in a relatively short period (McDuff and Johnson, 1992). The overall goal, whether with groups or individuals, is to prevent or decrease PTSD (Samter, et al, 1993; Friedman, 1997) and ASD.

If either disorder develops, the goal is progressive, intensive review of the traumatic experiences and then integration of the feelings and memories, often from the least to the most painful. This involves moving from a victim status to a survivor status, from "I can't go on because of this" to "I have learned from it and can go on with my life." As with any crisis, there is a potential for growth and the development of improved coping skills, appreciation of the value of life, and enhanced relationships (Hierholzer, et al, 1992).

Nurse-Patient Relationship. The first priority in the relationship with patients experiencing ASD or PTSD is the development of trust. This may be difficult because these patients have a tendency to be withdrawn, to feel alienated, and to be suspicious of others. It is sometimes difficult for patients to seek help or to accept it when offered. When a patient is aware of the current influence of the trauma, there is often a tendency for him or her to believe that "No one can understand what I've been through unless they have been through it too." Therefore, the nurse needs to be nonjudgmental, honest, empathic, and supportive. The nurse can convey the message, "I haven't been through what you have, but the more you tell me, the better I will understand what you have been and are experiencing." It is important to acknowledge any unfairness or injustices that were part of the trauma.

These patients also need to hear that they are not "crazy" but that they are having typical reactions to a serious trauma. Teaching about the dynamics of PTSD (Snell and Padin-Rivera, 1997; Foa, 1997) and ASD is often appropriate. Depending on the nature of the trauma, the nurse must be prepared to hear "horror stories" about hideous injuries, unpredicted behaviors, and gross destruction. If the nurse cannot tolerate the stories of atrocities, patients are not free to process all of the losses and changes that have occurred in their lives as a result of the trauma. Nurses may need help themselves to avoid vicarious victimization or burnout when working with trauma victims (Blair and Ramones, 1996).

It may take time for patients to recognize the relationship between current problems and the original traumatic event. When patients are not initially aware of the connection between the original trauma and current feelings and problems, the nurse should gently clarify those connections as they emerge.

Patients need to evaluate their past behaviors according to the original context of the situation, not by current values and standards (Foa, 1997). For example, a rape victim who did not resist her knife-wielding attacker needs to judge her behavior in the context of the life-or-death situation, not by an acquaintance's comment that she "must have asked for it." Another example is the Vietnam veteran who must evaluate his experience of killing a woman who was holding a grenade within the context of war, not by society's current view of that war as immoral. It is not always easy for patients to develop a new perspective on the original trauma, and it involves clarification of facts, feelings, and values.

A particular approach with PTSD that is currently being studied is eye movement desensitization and reprocessing (EMDR) (Herbert, 1995; Shapiro, 1995). EMDR alternately stimulates the left and right brain hemispheres by having the patient's eyes follow the therapist's fingers as these move back and forth rapidly at the same time the patient is focusing on a traumatic event. Patients also replace negative beliefs about the event with positive ones; this process may activate and then positively alter the neurological network by which the traumatic memory was stored. Patients report improvements in their cognitions, emotions, and physical sensations (Hinkle, 1997).

Patients need significant help in safely verbalizing feelings, particularly anger, that often have been ignored or repressed. This is especially true if there have been destructive outbursts and/or patients are trying desperately to remain in control. Writing in a journal is often helpful. Expressive therapy (psychodrama, art, music, and poetry) can facilitate externalizing painful emotions that are difficult to verbalize (Hines-Martin and Ising, 1993; Clark, 1997.)

As patients struggle through the sometimes lengthy process of reexperiencing, reintegrating, and processing memories of and feelings about trauma experiences, patients need empathy and reassurance that they will be safe and not overwhelmed with anxiety (Foa, 1997). It is also important to take "time-outs" to focus on emergent problems and potential solutions. These problems, such as finances, housing, divorce, and their associated feelings, can be as stressful as the original event.

Patients need to be involved in problem solving, decision making, and taking specific actions toward

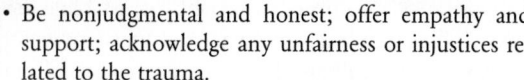

Key Nursing Interventions for Patients with Acute Stress Disorder and Patients with Posttraumatic Stress Disorder

- Be nonjudgmental and honest; offer empathy and support; acknowledge any unfairness or injustices related to the trauma.
   Rationale: Building trust may be difficult for patients.
- Assure patients that their feelings and behaviors are typical reactions to serious trauma.
   Rationale: Patients often feel they are "going crazy."
- Help patients to recognize the connections between the trauma experience and their current feelings, behaviors, and problems.
   Rationale: Patients often are unaware of these connections.
- Help patients to evaluate past behaviors in the context of the trauma, not in the context of current values and standards.
   Rationale: Patients often have guilt about past behaviors and are judgmental of themselves.
- Encourage safe verbalization of feelings, especially anger.

   Rationale: Feelings are and/or have been repressed or suppressed.
- Encourage adaptive coping strategies, exercise, relaxation techniques, and sleep-promoting strategies.
   Rationale: Patients may have been using maladaptive or dysfunctional coping to avoid dealing with feelings and issues.
- Facilitate progressive review of the trauma and its consequences.
   Rationale: Review helps patients to integrate feelings and memories, and to begin the grieving process.
- Encourage patients to establish or reestablish relationships.
   Rationale: Relationships (needed for assistance and support) may have been affected by patients' suspiciousness or fear of asking for help.

---

overcoming these stresses. Patients' adaptive coping skills and use of relaxation strategies need to be encouraged, while dysfunctional ones, especially avoidance of responsibility for one's actions and the abuse of alcohol and drugs, are discouraged. For patients plagued by intrusive thoughts, it may be helpful to have them imagine the word "stop" or to snap a rubber band on their wrist to interrupt these thoughts (Clark, 1997).

Patients also need to try to establish or reestablish relationships that provide support and assistance. Couple or family education and counseling may be recommended if appropriate (Nelson and Wright, 1996). Hospitalization of ASD and PTSD patients is normally necessary only if they are suicidal, homicidal, self-mutilating, or unable to function in daily activities. The box above lists additional nursing interventions to use with ASD and PTSD.

Psychopharmacology. Medications for patients experiencing ASD or PTSD are used generally for short-term therapy during the acute crisis or for intensive counseling periods to prevent or reverse neurochemical fear conditioning and sensitization. The choice of medications depends on the primary symptoms.

Benzodiazepines (GABA-ergic antagonists) may be prescribed to reduce levels of conditioned fear and anxiety symptoms. These medications also may help patients with sleep disturbances and nightmares. Of course, there is a risk of dependence, especially with patients who are already abusing alcohol or drugs. Benzodiazepines are usually prescribed on a prn basis rather than on a fixed schedule.

Clonidine (noradrenergic inhibitor) and *propranolol* (beta-blocker) may produce responses similar to those of the benzodiazepines. Propranolol can help to diminish the peripheral autonomic response associated with fear.

Lithium carbonate is sometimes given to patients who are experiencing explosive outbursts and intense feelings of being out of control. It can help decrease hyperarousal, startle response, and nightmares.

SSRIs (fluoxetine, fluvoxamine) may reverse continued emergency responses and decrease repetitive behaviors, images, and somatic states.

TCAs are used if depression, anhedonia, and sleep disturbances are primary problems. TCAs, especially amitriptyline, usually are given in one dose at bedtime.

Case Study

Billy Craig was 19 years old when he spent a year in heavy combat in Vietnam. Although he was upset when his buddies were killed, he was secretly relieved when his wounds got him sent home. He studied forestry and became a ranger in a national forest. He was viewed as a loner and showed no interest in marriage. He had never talked about his experiences in Vietnam with anyone.

During the television coverage of Desert Storm operations, Billy began to have nightmares and flashbacks about killing Vietcong and about a friend who was dis-membered. Billy became angry more frequently and startled easily. After a month of not seeing him, other rangers found Billy in his cabin, very depressed and surrounded by old guns and grenades. He kept repeating that he should have died in Nam too. He admitted that he was intending to shoot himself. With effort, the rangers convinced him to come with them to the mental health center, where he was admitted and diagnosed with delayed posttraumatic stress disorder and major depression.

MAOIs may be used for patients with severely constricted affect and may help decrease flashbacks and nightmares.

Antipsychotics are used if patients also have psychotic thinking. These may be used for hyperarousal in acute crisis periods. Low doses of thioridazine *(Mellaril)* can help to decrease flashbacks and nightmares (Bloche and Eisenberg, 1993; Charney, et al, 1993; Davidson, 1997; Famularo, 1997; Friedman, 1997).

Milieu Management. Patients experiencing ASD or PTSD can benefit from many inpatient or outpatient milieu activities. Social activities can help to rebuild social skills that have been damaged by suspiciousness and withdrawal. Recreational and exercise programs can help to reduce tension and promote relaxation. Groups that may be useful are those that focus on self-esteem, decision making, assertiveness, stress management, and relaxation techniques. Victims of a variety of traumas may benefit from group meetings that focus on the similarities in their reactions and feelings, such as mistrust, helplessness, fear, guilt, numbing, detachment, nightmares, and flashbacks.

Community resources. A particularly useful therapeutic aid for patients experiencing ASD and PTSD is group therapy or self-help groups with others who have experienced the same or a similar trauma. A community may have a veterans outreach center for Vietnam veterans and their spouses, as well as groups for victims of rape, incest, or torture and their family members. The community may hold meetings for victims after a community disaster. There also may be a victim's assistance program for crime victims.

ADJUSTMENT DISORDERS

This separate group of adjustment disorders is *not* part of the anxiety disorders category but is included here because of its contrasts with ASD and PTSD. The diagnosis of adjustment disorder may be made when symptoms develop within 3 months after an identifiable life event and the reaction is not severe enough to fit the criteria of ASD or PTSD. Common events or circumstances that may precipitate an adjustment disorder are divorce, moving, marriage, retirement, illness or disability, financial problems, or difficulties in child rearing.

The symptoms of maladaptive reactions to a stressful event or circumstances are not defined as specifically as those for ASD and PTSD, but they are still considered more severe than a "normal" stress response or grief reaction. The reaction interferes with functioning but lasts no longer than 6 months after the stressor and its consequences have ended. The diagnosis of adjustment disorder is based on subcategories according to the predominant feature of the patient's maladaptive stress reaction. The major feature may be a mood disturbance of *anxiety* or *depression*. It may be a disturbance with *mixed anxiety and depressed mood*. There may be a *disturbance of conduct:* interpersonal or social impairment, or work (or academic) inhibition. There is a subcategory of *mixed disturbance of emotions and conduct.*

The psychotherapeutic interventions for patients with adjustment disorders are generally similar to those used for patients experiencing ASD and PTSD. The major goals are to recognize the relationship between the stressful situation and current problems and to review and reintegrate feelings and memories of the original situation.

Care Plan

NAME: Billy Craig   **ADMISSION DATE:** _____

DSM-IV DIAGNOSIS: Axis I posttraumatic stress disorder, delayed; major depression

ASSESSMENT: **Areas of strength:** Intelligent, enjoys his work, has supportive coworkers.
Problems: Suicidal ideation, flashbacks of and anger about Vietnam, disturbed sleep, lives in an isolated area.

DIAGNOSES:
- Potential for self-directed and other-directed violence related to suicidal ideation, anger, as evidenced by suicidal behavior and statements.
- Sleep pattern disturbance related to nightmares, as evidenced by interrupted sleep, increasing irritability.
- Posttrauma response related to war experiences, as evidenced by reexperience of traumatic events in flashbacks and nightmares.

OUTCOMES: **Short-term goals:**   Date met
- Patient will state that he is no longer suicidal and will appropriately verbalize feelings of anger and sadness. _____
- Patient will describe his experiences in Vietnam. _____
Long-term goals:
- Patient will schedule outpatient appointments at the veterans outreach center and the mental health center. _____

PLANNING/ INTERVENTIONS: **Nurse-patient relationship:** Assess and monitor suicidal ideations. Assist patient with identification and verbalization of feelings, especially anger. Assist patient in describing Vietnam experiences and their connection to current issues.
Psychopharmacology: Fluoxetine (Prozac) 20 mg 8 AM and 12 noon; thioridazine (Mellaril) 5 mg tid and hs; lorazepam (Ativan) 1 mg q 4 hr prn.
Milieu management: Groups focusing on stress and anger management, relaxation techniques, social skills, and self-esteem.

EVALUATION: Patient verbalizes that he is no longer suicidal. Patient is beginning to verbalize his anger and sadness about Vietnam and the loss of his buddies.

REFERRALS: His appointment at the veterans center is on 1/12; his appointment at the mental health center is on 1/25.

SOMATOFORM DISORDERS

The major characteristic of somatoform disorders is that patients have physical symptoms for which there is *no known organic cause or physiological mechanism.* Evidence is present or a presumption exists that the physical symptoms are connected to psychological factors or conflicts. These patients are not in control of their symptoms, which are unconscious and involuntary. Patients express conflicts through bodily symptoms and complaints using the defense of somatization.

Patients with these disorders repeatedly seek medical diagnosis and treatment, even though they have been told that there is no known physiological or organic evidence to explain their symptoms or disability.

Traditional views concerning somatoform disorders consider repression, denial, and displacement as defense mechanisms used in these disorders. Repression occurs in reference to feelings, conflicts, and unacceptable impulses. Denial of psychological problems is present even though these patients have been told that there is no physiological

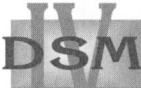

DSM-IV Criteria for Somatoform Disorders

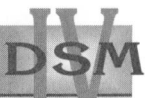

Somatization disorder: many physical complaints over several years, resulting in treatment being sought or impairment in functioning

Pain disorder: pain in one or more areas of the body that is severe enough to seek treatment; causes impairment in functioning or significant distress

Conversion disorder: one or more symptoms or deficits affecting voluntary motor or sensory function that suggest a neurological or general medical condition

Hypochondriasis: preoccupation with fear of having, or the idea that one has, a serious disease, includes misinterpretation of bodily symptoms; preoccupation persists despite medical evaluation and reassurance

Adapted from the American Psychiatric Association: *Diagnostic and statistical manual of mental disorders*, ed 4, Washington, DC, 1994, The Association.

cause or basis for their symptoms. Displacement occurs when the anxiety is transformed into bodily symptoms.

Current research suggests that genetic, developmental-learning, personality, and sociocultural factors can predispose, precipitate, and maintain somatoform disorders. Stressful life events can also precipitate bodily concerns and somatization (Lipowski, 1986). Persons with somatoform disorders often appear to be needy and dependent on others.

The somatoform disorders discussed here are somatization disorder, pain disorder, hypochondriasis, and conversion disorder. The box above presents a definition of each disorder according to the DSM-IV.

SOMATIZATION DISORDER

According to the DSM-IV, the main characteristic of somatization disorder is that these individuals verbalize recurrent, frequent, and multiple somatic complaints for several years without physiological cause. It usually begins before the age of 30. Research findings indicate that this disorder occurs with similar clinical characteristics in men and women (Golding, Smith, and Kashner, 1991). These patients see many physicians through the years and may even have exploratory and unnecessary surgical procedures. Impairment in social and occupational functioning may be present. DSM-IV criteria for somatization disorder are found in the box on p. 442.

PAIN DISORDER

The chief complaint in pain disorder is severe pain in one or more anatomical sites that causes significant distress or impairment in functioning (American Psychiatric Association [APA], 1994). The location or complaint of the pain does not change, unlike the complaints voiced in somatization disorder. Psychological factors play a role in the development and maintenance of pain disorder. There is no organic basis for this disorder.

There may be underlying psychological factors related to pain disorder that patients may not recognize consciously. For example, feelings connected with the loss of a job or status may occur prior to the development of pain disorder. This type of pain disorder is classified as *pain disorder associated with psychological factors*. In some cases, the pain may allow patients to avoid something that they do not want to do; for example, a woman's chest pain may prevent her from going to work.

Sometimes there is a physiological disorder, but the amount of pain or impairment is greatly exaggerated or out of proportion. For example, a patient who has experienced a mild myocardial infarction (MI) is now convinced that he can no longer engage in recreational activities such as bicycling or swimming, due perhaps to feelings of inadequacy or fear of suffering another MI. This pain disorder would be classified as *pain disorder associated with both psychological factors and a general medical condition*.

Patients with pain disorder are often "doctor shoppers" and may use analgesics excessively

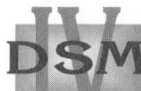 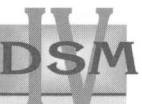

DSM-IV Criteria for Somatization Disorder

A. Multiple physical complaints beginning before age 30
B. The following symptoms that are not due to a medical condition must occur, or the complaints or impairment are in excess of what is expected.
  1. Four pain symptoms in four different bodily sites or functions (e.g., head, chest, during sexual intercourse, or during urination)
  2. Two gastrointestinal symptoms occur other than pain (e.g., nausea, diarrhea, intolerance to several different foods)
  3. One sexual or reproductive symptom other than pain (e.g., erectile or ejaculatory problems, irregular menses, excessive menstrual bleeding)

4. One pseudoneurological symptom or deficit that suggests a neurological disorder (e.g., blindness, deafness, paralysis, seizures, difficulty swallowing or breathing, and dissociative symptoms such as amnesia)

These patients may be anxious or depressed. They may feel nervous, have sleep disturbances, and experience suicidal ideation because they experience hopelessness about ever getting better.

Adapted from the American Psychiatric Association: *Diagnostic and statistical manual of mental disorders,* ed 4, Washington, DC, 1994, The Association.

without experiencing any relief from their pain. These patients are often anxious about their symptoms and depressed about ever getting better.

HYPOCHONDRIASIS

Hypochondriacs are worried about having, or believe that they have, a serious disease based on the misinterpretation of bodily signs and sensations (APA, 1994). Medical evaluation and reassurance does not help dispel the fear. These patients displace anxiety onto their bodies and misinterpret bodily symptoms. Hypochondriacs "check" for reassurance from physicians or friends in ways that are similar to the compulsive behavior of patients with obsessive-compulsive disorder. Hypochondriacs are afraid that they have a disease, whereas patients with OCD fear getting an illness and constantly check for germs. Like patients with OCD, hypochondriacs constantly check for reassurance about illness (Fallon, Klein, and Liebowitz, 1993).

CLINICAL EXAMPLE

Roberta is worried about having an ulcer. She experiences acid ingestion on occasion after dinner. The uncomfortable feeling in her stomach causes her to fear that her stomach acid will burn a hole in the stomach lining. After each episode, Roberta visits her doctor for a physical examination. Based on the negative results from examinations and tests, the doctor has repeatedly told her that she does not have an ulcer.

Hypochondriasis by itself is rare; it is seen more often in conjunction with other disorders, such as major depression, OCD, and GAD.

CONVERSION DISORDER

The major characteristic of conversion disorder is a deficit or alteration in voluntary motor or sensory function that suggests a neurological or medical condition (APA, 1994). Psychological factors, conflicts, or stressors are associated with or precede the development of this disorder. The most common conversion symptoms suggest neurological disease such as paralysis, blindness, or seizures. As mentioned earlier, primary gain refers to the alleviation of anxiety that the disorder provides because conflict is kept out of conscious awareness. Secondary gain is the gratification received as a result of how people in these patients' environment respond to their illness.

Another characteristic of this disorder is that the symptom often is determined by the situation that produced it. For example, a soldier suddenly devel-

*C*ase *S*tudy

William Robinson, a 62-year-old white man, was admitted to the psychiatric inpatient unit on June 15 at 10 AM. He walked onto the unit limping and supported by his wife, Harriet. He stated that he was experiencing horrible pain in his left leg and foot. Anger and irritability were evident in his voice.

Mr. Robinson's pain started suddenly about 7 months ago. Since that time, he has seen numerous physicians to obtain treatment and relief from his pain. He was told by the last physician that the pain was due to stress, and it was recommended that he be hospitalized to obtain treatment from a doctor who was trained to manage stress-related disorders. The patient stated that he hoped this doctor would know what to do, and that none of the others did.

Mrs. Robinson brought her husband's medications to the hospital. The nurse found that a number of analgesics had been prescribed, along with sleeping medication. Mr. Robinson said that he took what he wanted, when he wanted it, and that it was better than not taking anything at all.

The next day, after visiting her husband, Mrs. Robinson told the nurse that Mr. Robinson needed a lot of help with everything. In fact, she had been so physically tired that she had called their only daughter, Sheila, for assistance. Sheila lives 400 miles away and they had not seen her for 3 years. Their daughter was so concerned about her parents that she had come to help for 2 weeks last month.

As the conversation continued, Mrs. Robinson told the nurse that her husband had been in good health, ex-cept for an occasional cold, until about 8 months ago, when he suddenly started to complain about awful pain in his leg and foot. He had never in all of his years working for a cabinet manufacturer experienced anything like this before. Mrs. Robinson did not know why all of this pain was happening now, especially since her husband had retired 9 months earlier. He had been forced to retire early because the company he worked for had not been doing well and all employees aged 60 and over were forced to retire. She stated that her husband had never said too much about it, and she thought that now they would have time to travel and take fishing trips, which her husband had always enjoyed. They had taken many fishing trips as a family while their daughter was growing up and had enjoyed them immensely. Periodically, her husband went fishing with some friends. Since the onset of her husband's pain, they had not done anything socially, together or with friends.

From the time he was admitted to the hospital, Mr. Robinson refused to do anything but sit in a lounge chair in the community room. He needed much assistance from staff members to walk to the dining room and to the restroom. At times, his food was brought to him in the community room because he refused to walk to the dining room.

Interactions with the nurse centered on his pain and on requests for pain medication. He described his pain in detail and would talk of little else.

Mr. Robinson was getting Darvon for pain, and an antidepressant as ordered by his physician.

---

ops paralysis of his hand. As a result, he can no longer engage in combat because he cannot pull the trigger on his gun. The symptom is related to the conflict. This soldier can discuss combat, but he cannot connect his feelings about fighting to the development of his paralysis.

This patient also may have an attitude of *la belle indifference,* meaning that he expresses little concern or anxiety about his distressing disorder. This occurs because his symptom binds his anxiety so that it is not behaviorally expressed. It may seem as though patients with conversion disorder minimize their illness.

Traditional views of this disorder consider repression and conversion as the primary defense mechanism used. Today, patients with conversion disorder are seen infrequently in inpatient settings.

Psychotherapeutic Management

Nurse-Patient Relationship. The focus of the nurse-patient relationship is to improve patients' overall levels of functioning by building adaptive coping behaviors. Patients with somatoform disorders often are not able to identify and express their feelings, needs, and conflicts. Teaching them how to appropriately verbalize feelings helps to eliminate or diminish the need for physical symptoms.

Patients need time to understand their need for physical symptoms. Awareness and insight develop slowly as they begin to verbalize their needs. For some patients, this awareness and insight take longer to develop, and they may have only begun to work on this area by the time they are discharged from an inpatient unit.

Care Plan

NAME: William Robinson   **ADMISSION DATE:** _____

DSM-IV DIAGNOSIS: Pain disorder

ASSESSMENT: **Areas of strength:** Enjoyed fishing and traveling; had been in good health; wife is very supportive; had worked for many years.
Problems: Experiencing pain in his left leg and foot; social functioning has declined; focus with staff is about his pain; secondary gains maintain his sick role.

DIAGNOSES:
- Ineffective individual coping related to anger, as evidenced by complaints of physical pain.
- Chronic pain, related to low self-esteem, as evidenced by inability to verbalize feelings.
- Anxiety: severe, related to dependency, as evidenced by inability to care for self.

OUTCOMES: **Short-term goals:**   Date met
- Patient will verbalize feelings and needs.   _____
- Patient will verbalize underlying anger due to early retirement.   _____
- Patient will verbalize awareness about connecting conflict with physical symptoms.   _____
- Patient will develop adaptive coping behaviors.   _____

Long-term goals:
- Patient will assume responsibility for self-care and independent functioning.   _____
- Patient will schedule appointments for joint counseling with his wife.   _____
- Patient will identify plans to volunteer in his community.   _____
- Patient will plan leisure activities.   _____

PLANNING/ INTERVENTIONS: **Nurse-patient relationship:** Convey interest and support focus on assisting the patient to verbalize feelings and needs related to anxiety, self-esteem, and anger, give positive feedback when the patient focuses on issues other than pain; set limits on need for attention and medication.
Psychopharmacology: Decrease the use of analgesics. Paxil 20 mg q AM.
Milieu management: Encourage participation in assertiveness and communication groups, as well as problem-solving, discharge-planning, and social skills groups, diversional occupational therapy and recreational activities.

EVALUATION: Patient's focus on pain is decreasing and is able to assume self-care activities with little assistance.

REFERRALS: Appointments for outpatient group therapy and counseling with wife.

The physician or psychiatrist orders tests and laboratory workups to thoroughly assess patients physically for the presence of any physiological or organic disease or causation (if this has not been done prior to admission). The absence of any relevant medical findings strongly suggests that somatization is present.

The nursing interventions used for patients with somatoform disorders are described in the box on p. 445.

Psychopharmacology. Because patients with somatoform disorders may be using too much medication and taking a variety of drugs before they are admitted to the hospital, medication should be used temporarily and sparingly.

Milieu Management. For patients with conversion disorder, hypnosis may be used to help to identify the source of the conflict. Psychological testing and relaxation exercises also may be helpful.

Key Nursing Interventions for Somatoform Disorders

1. Use a matter-of-fact, caring approach when providing care for physical symptoms.

   Rationale: to decrease secondary gains and to decrease focusing on physical symptoms

2. Ask patients how they are feeling and ask them to describe their feelings.

   Rationale: to increase the use of verbalization about feelings (especially negative ones), needs, and anxiety rather than about somatization.

3. Assist patients with developing more appropriate ways to verbalize feelings and needs.

   Rationale: to increase adaptive coping through assertiveness.

4. Use positive reinforcement to increase noncomplaining behavior, and set limits by withdrawing attention from patients when they focus on physical complaints or make unreasonable demands.

5. Be consistent with patients and have all requests directed to the primary nurse providing care.

   Rationale: to decrease attention-seeking or manipulative behaviors.

6. Use diversion by including patients in milieu activities and recreational games.

   Rationale: to decrease rumination about physical complaints.

7. Do not push awareness of or insight into conflicts or problems.

   Rationale: to prevent an increase in anxiety and the need for physical symptoms.

Relaxation exercises and behavior modification may help patients with other somatoform disorders. Assertiveness, decision-making, goal-setting, stress-management, and social skills groups often benefit these patients.

Outpatient therapy is also necessary for most patients. Because patients with somatoform disorders are usually overusers of medical care, some hospitals and clinics provide psychotherapy groups as part of the medical care. These groups focus on underlying psychosocial needs, not on physical needs. The success of this type of treatment approach can result in decreasing hospital costs while providing more appropriate patient care. It is hoped that the efficacy of such groups will be recognized and, thus, used in more hospitals to provide optimal and appropriate patient care.

DISSOCIATIVE DISORDERS

Dissociation is the removal from conscious awareness of painful feelings, memories, thoughts, or aspects of identity. It is an unconscious defense mechanism that protects an individual from the emotional pain of experiences or conflicts that have been repressed. This "splitting off" helps these individuals to endure and survive intense emotion and/or physical pain.

Dissociation occurs in extreme stress or trauma, such as war or abuse in childhood and adulthood. "Dissociation is a fight to maintain stability" (O'Reilly-Knapp, 1996). Everyone uses dissociation at times. For example, a person may be so engrossed in a book or a movie that they do not hear anything or anyone around them. This is not pathological. Everyone forgets things or daydreams. However, this does not indicate an illness. Abnormal dissociative states are the dissociative disorders when identity, memory, or consciousness are disturbed or altered. Dissociative disorders in the DSM-IV are dissociative amnesia, dissociative fugue, depersonalization, and dissociative identity disorder (multiple personality disorder). The box on p. 446 summarizes the main characteristics of dissociative disorders.

DISSOCIATIVE AMNESIA

Amnesia is the loss of memory or the inability to recall important personal information. Recent amnesia can occur immediately after a traumatic event such as a car accident. *Remote amnesia* can occur regarding past traumatic events such as childhood abuse. Some patients experience both recent and remote amnesia. It is important to remember that patients are sometimes found by the police; these patients wander aimlessly and are confused and disoriented. They may be taken to a hospital and may be frightened and perplexed. The precipitant is usually something that causes severe psychosocial stress, such as the threat of physical injury or death.

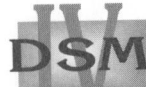
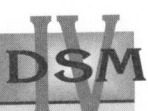

DSM-IV Criteria for Dissociative Disorders

Dissociative amnesia: loss of memory of important personal events that were traumatic or stressful in nature

Dissociative fugue: sudden, unexpected travel away from home or work with a loss of memory about the past; confusion about identity or assumption of partial or completely new identity is present

Depersonalization: experiences of feeling detached from, or an outside observer of, one's body or mental processes; reality testing is intact

Dissociative identity disorder: presence of two or more identities or personalities that take control of the person's behavior; loss of memory for important personal information

Adapted from the American Psychiatric Association: *Diagnostic and statistical manual of mental disorders,* ed 4, Washington, DC, 1994, The Association.

The DSM-IV describes dissociative amnesia as one or more episodes of the inability to recall important personal information that is beyond ordinary forgetfulness. The information is usually stressful or traumatic in nature. The amnesia does not occur only during the course of dissociative identity disorder, nor is it due to a substance (drug or medication) or a medical condition such as head trauma (APA, 1994). Two subgroups of amnesia have been identified: amnesia related to trauma such as abuse, and a rarer form of amnesia that develops during or as a result of overwhelming psychological conflict (Lowenstein, 1991). Memory gaps can occur for a specified amount of time; for example, not remembering what occurred during first and second grade or before the age of 8. Amnesia may also be chronic and recurrent in relation to later traumas or conflicts.

DISSOCIATIVE FUGUE

The major feature of dissociative fugue is sudden, unexpected travel away from home or locale with the assumption of a new identity (partial or complete) or a confusion about one's identity. The travel and behavior appear normal to casual observers, so the person does not seem to be wandering in a confused state.

Fugue states last from a few hours to several days. They are usually accompanied by amnesia, so patients do not remember what happened during the fugue state. Sometimes depression is also present.

Dissociative fugues usually follow severe psychosocial stress, such as marital quarrels, personal re-jections, military conflict, or natural disaster. The fugue state then allows escape or flight from an intolerable event or situation.

DEPERSONALIZATION

According to the DSM-IV, depersonalization is included in this group of disorders because the sense of one's reality is changed, but the person is oriented to time, place, and person. In depersonalization, persons feel detached from parts of their body or mental processes. It involves an altered sense of self so that persons feel unreal or strange or feel that danger is not happening to them but to someone else. Therefore, as a response to overwhelming stress, these persons are protected from overwhelming anxiety. Depersonalization is rare and occurs usually as a symptom in other disorders (Coons, 1996). It can also involve feeling like a robot or feeling as though one is in a dream. Depersonalization is often accompanied by symptoms of derealization in which persons feel that the outside world is changed or unreal. For example, buildings may appear to be leaning, or everything may seem gray and dull.

A diagnosis of depersonalization is made only when the prevalence or intensity of the disorder causes marked distress, interferes with daily functioning, and occurs in the absence of other disorders. Depersonalization disorder is rare and is often chronic, with remissions and exacerbations.

There is preliminary evidence that depersonalization may be due to biological as well as psychological mechanisms. Serotonergic dysfunction may account for the obsessive preoccupation with depersonalization symptoms and compulsive scrutiny to check out feelings of unreality, as in obsessive-compulsive disorder. A degree of response to treatment with SSRIs, such as fluoxetine (Prozac), also lends credence to the involvement of biological mechanisms (Simeon and Hollander, 1993). There is no pattern of inheritance for those with depersonalization disorder (Coons, 1996).

DISSOCIATIVE IDENTITY DISORDER

The major feature of dissociative identity disorder is the existence of two or more identities or personalities that take control of the person's behavior (APA, 1994). The person, or "host," is unaware of the other personalities, but the other personalities may be aware of each other in varying degrees.

Traditional views of this disorder consider dissociation to be a defense against extreme anxiety that is aroused in highly painful and emotionally traumatic situations, such as physical, emotional, and sexual abuse. The "splitting off" of these painful events allows the person to survive the trauma but leaves an impaired personality with disconnected parts or "alters." The alter personalities contain feelings and behaviors associated with the trauma. They may be helpful or destructive (Stafford, 1993).

Each personality is quite different from the others and from the original personality. Each personality has its own name, behavior traits, memories, emotional characteristics, and social relations. The most common personality is a fearful, terrified child, and the next most common is a persecutor personality modeled on the abuser(s).

A shy, quiet woman may have alternate personalities that are promiscuous or flamboyant, childlike, and aggressive. A woman may awaken one morning and find the living room of her apartment littered with toys or strewn with empty alcohol bottles and leftover food. She does not remember what happened because she has amnesia for the span of time when another personality has taken over or "come out."

Sometimes a switch to another personality is preceded by a headache, or persons may cover their face and eyes with their hands. For example, the patient or original personality may state that he or she hears voices talking to one another in his or her head. This could be misdiagnosed as auditory hallucinations, and the disorder misdiagnosed as schizophrenia.

These patients are admitted to inpatient psychiatric units when they are suicidal, meaning that an alter personality is trying to harm or kill one of the other personalities for revelations, or when mutilation or uncontrollable impulses to harm the self are present. Severe anxiety or depression related to the coming out of upsetting alters also may be a reason for admission (Kluft, 1991). Sometimes the safe structure of a hospital setting provides emotional security when working with difficult or overwhelming material.

Some patients experience numerous hospitalizations with different diagnoses before they are finally and accurately diagnosed with dissociative identity disorder. The array of symptoms these patients present may be one reason for inaccurate diagnoses. Another reason may be that patients do not recognize their symptoms or know what they mean. Patients may think that they are "going crazy" or "losing their minds" because they do not understand what their symptoms mean or represent. Thus, they might delay seeking treatment until their disorder severely interrupts their functioning in life. Others around them, such as family members, may not understand what is occurring, may not know how to help, or may want to keep the disorder a secret, especially if the perpetrator of abuse is among them.

■ Critical Thinking Question

A patient with dissociative identity disorder is admitted to the inpatient unit because of self-mutilating behavior. Prior to admission, the patient has stated to a friend, "I'll kill you and kill myself." The patient refuses to sign a "no-harm" contract. Design an initial care plan, including types of precautions.

Psychotherapeutic Management

Nurse-Patient Relationship. The nurse's relationship with persons experiencing amnesia and fugue includes interventions to establish trust and support. Patients have physiological and neurological workups to rule out organic causations. The nurse assists with gathering data regarding feelings, conflicts, or situations that patients experienced prior to the amnesia or fugue state. Patients also may have sessions under hypnosis or amobarbital sodium (Amytal) to gather data about forgotten material. The nurse should slowly help patients to deal with anxiety and conflicts in their lives.

Patients with depersonalization disorder usually are not found in an inpatient setting unless they have become suicidal, extremely anxious, or depressed. Nurses may work with these patients in outpatient settings.

The treatment goal of dissociative identity disorder is to ultimately integrate the personalities or memories, if possible, so that they can survive or coexist in the original personality. Therapy, combined with hypnosis and amobarbital sodium, assists in this process.

The nurse works with patients to establish trust because the relationships of these patients with authority figures may have been inconsistent, rigid, and unpredictable (Stafford, 1993). A contract should be initiated for patients' safety and to reduce self-harm and violence. An alter may be homicidal because of revelations concerning abuse. Self-mutilation and suicidal behaviors also may be present when overwhelming anxiety or depression occurs. The nurse also must be alert to "splitting" by staff members regarding patients' diagnoses. The staff may divide into groups of believers and nonbelievers regarding the validity of patients' diagnoses. Education about diagnoses; management of feelings, especially anger and rage; and consistency of approach assist the staff with developing a caring, supportive environment for patients so that trust increases and a predictable positive learning environment ensues.

Psychopharmacology. The symptoms of the dissociative identity disorder are not alleviated by medication. Patients' response to medication may be partial, and alters' response to medication may be different and inconsistent (Kluft, 1991). If symptoms of pain, somatoform disorders, anxiety, and depression are present in these patients, medication may not alleviate them.

Because of the rarity of depersonalization disorder, little is known about its treatment. As mentioned earlier, there has been some success with fluoxetine (Prozac) (Simeon and Hollander, 1993).

Milieu Management. The nurse assumes an important role in the care of patients who are hos-

pitalized in an inpatient psychiatric unit because of suicidal or uncontrollable attempts to harm themselves. Provisions for a safe environment and a trusting relationship are basic to helping these patients, who usually have not had trusting relationships with anyone. Assisting with therapy sessions, providing emotional security, acceptance, support, and helping patients to cope with daily living are all involved in nursing care.

For patients with dissociative identity disorder, ongoing process-oriented groups may be nontherapeutic when patients reveal too much and overwhelm the group or regress. Individual therapy should be in progress and may have been initiated prior to hospitalization. Task-oriented groups are beneficial. Occupational therapy and art therapy provide patients with a means of nonverbal expression to reveal material that cannot be verbally accessed. Attendance at milieu meetings decreases isolation from the community. Patients should attend activities that they and their alters can cooperate and participate in appropriately.

Prior to discharge, a safety plan and no-harm contract may be necessary, as well as initiating or continuing a system of support for the patient. Self-help support groups provide outpatients the opportunity to learn social skills and problem solving to develop a sense of empowerment and control (Dallam and Manderino, 1997).

Key Concepts

1. The issues of primary and secondary gains are important to patients because primary gain relieves discomfort, while secondary gain may encourage patients to maintain their sick role.
2. Patients' anxiety must be reduced to a mild or moderate level before the nurse can work with them on problem solving and adaptive coping.
3. In the category of anxiety disorders, symptoms of anxiety are directly felt or expressed.
4. With somatoform disorders, anxiety is expressed through physical symptoms.
5. In dissociative disorders, anxiety is "split off" (or removed) from conscious awareness, which helps patients to survive extreme emotional pain.
6. Uncovering and linking feelings with conflicts and managing feelings are important aspects of recovery and nursing care plans.

Study Questions

(Answer key is in the back of the book.)

1. Secondary gain refers to:
   a. The benefits received from others while sick
   b. Decreasing and relieving anxiety
   c. Increased ability to cope with anxiety in the future
   d. The benefit received from medication

2. Before patients with anxiety-related disorders can solve problems and develop adaptive coping responses, the nurse must first:
   a. Confront patients with their maladaptive behaviors
   b. Assist patients with managing and reducing anxiety
   c. Administer prn lorazepam (Ativan) to eliminate subjective symptoms of discomfort
   d. Help patients to develop insight into their illness

Match each of the following disorders with its appropriate description.

3. Panic disorder C
4. Phobic disorder a
5. Obsessive-compulsive disorder b
   a. Characterized by a persistent fear of specific places and things; anxiety is displaced or externalized
   b. Neutralizes anxiety by performing repetitive behaviors or experiencing recurrent, persistent thoughts that cannot be controlled or stopped
   c. Spontaneous attacks of intense fear and discomfort

6. The characteristic symptom of acute stress disorder and posttraumatic stress disorder that distinguishes them from other anxiety-related disorders is:
   a. Severe depression
   b. Suspiciousness of others
   c. Lack of interest in family and activities
   d. Reexperiencing the trauma in nightmares and flashbacks

7. Which intervention would be *least* appropriate in planning care for patients with a somatoform disorder?
   a. Push insight or awareness to connect conflict with the need for physical symptoms
   b. Set limits by withdrawing attention from patients when they persist in complaining about physical symptoms
   c. Encourage patients to verbalize negative and positive feelings
   d. Decrease patients' focus on physical complaints by involving them in milieu activities

REFERENCES

American Psychiatric Association: *Diagnostic and statistical manual of mental disorders*, ed 4, Washington, DC, 1994, The Association.

Barton KA, Blanchard EB, and Hickling EJ: Antecedents and consequences of acute stress disorder among motor vehicle accident victims, *Behav Res Ther* 34(10):805, 1996.

Bille DA: Road to recovery, posttraumatic stress disorder: the hidden victim, *J Psychosoc Nurs Ment Health Serv* 31(9):19, 1993.

Blair DT and Ramones VA: Understanding vicarious traumatization, *J Psychosoc Nurs Ment Health Serv* 34(11):24, 1996.

Bloche MG and Eisenberg C: The psychological effects of state-sanctioned terror, *Harvard Mental Health Letter* 10(5):4, 1993.

Brandt GT, et al: Psychiatric morbidity in medical and surgical patients evacuated from the Persian Gulf War, *Psychiatr Serv* 48(1):102, 1997.

Bremner JD, et al: Vietnam vet's PTSD experience, *J Psychosoc Nurs Ment Health Serv* 34(6):48, 1996.

Charney DS, et al: Psychobiologic mechanisms of posttraumatic stress disorder, *Arch Gen Psychiatry* 50(4):294, 1993.

Clark C: Posttraumatic stress disorder, *Am J Nurs* 97(8):27, 1997.

Coons P: Depersonalization and derealization. In Michelson L and William R, editors: *Handbook of dissociation theoretical, empirical, and clinical perspectives*, New York, 1996, Plenum Press.

Dahl J and O'Neal J: Stress and coping behaviors of nurses in Desert Storm, *J Psychosoc Nurs Ment Health Serv* 31(10):17, 1993.

Dallam S and Manderino MA: "Free to be" peer group supports patients with MPD/DD, *J Psychosoc Nurs Ment Health Serv* 35(4):22, 1997.

Davidson JRT: Biological therapies for posttraumatic stress disorder: an overview, *J Clin Psychiatry* 58(9):29, 1997.

DuPont R: Panic disorder and addiction: the clinical issues of comorbidity, *Bull Menninger Clinic* 61(2):A54, 1997.

Fallon B, Klein B, and Liebowitz S: Hypochondriasis: treatment strategies, *Psychiatr Ann* 23(7):374, 1993.

Famularo R: What are the symptoms, causes, and treatments of childhood posttraumatic stress disorder? *Harvard Mental Health Letter* 13(7):8, 1997.

Federici C and Tommasini N: The assessment and management of panic disorder, *Nurse Pract* 17(3):20, 1992.

Foa EB: Trauma and women: course, predictors, and treatment, *J Clin Psychiatry* 58(9):25, 1997.

Freud S: *The problem of anxiety*, New York, 1936, WW Norton.

Friedman MJ: Posttraumatic stress disorder, *J Clin Psychiatry* 58(9):33, 1997.

Furey JA: Women Vietnam veterans: a comparison of studies, *J Psychosoc Nurs Ment Health Serv* 29(3):11, 1991.

Glod C and Cawley D: Psychobiology perspectives: the neurobiology of obsessive–compulsive disorders, *J Am Psychiatr Nurses Assoc* 3(4):120, 1997.

Golding J, Smith R, and Kashner M: Does somatization disorder occur in men? *Arch Gen Psychiatry* 48(3):1991.

Grinspoon L, editor: Heredity and environment in post-traumatic stress reactions, *Harvard Mental Health Letter* 10(7):7, 1994.

Grinspoon L, editor: Obsessive compulsive disorder. Part I, *Harvard Mental Health Letter* 12(5):1, 1995a.

Grinspoon L, editor: Obsessive compulsive disorder. Part II, *Harvard Mental Health Letter* 12(6):1, 1995b.

Grinspoon L, editor: Panic attacks and panic disorder. Part I, *Harvard Mental Health Letter* 12(10):1, 1996a.

Grinspoon L, editor: Panic attacks and panic disorder. Part II, *Harvard Mental Health Letter* 12(11):1, 1996b.

Grinspoon L, editor: PTSD and depression, *Harvard Mental Health Letter* 14(7):7, 1998.

Herbert JD: What is EMDR?, *Harvard Mental Health Letter* 12(2):8, 1995.

Hierholzer R, et al: Clinical presentation of PTSD in World War II combat veterans, *Hosp Community Psychiatry* 43(8):816, 1992.

Hines-Martin VP and Ising M: Use of art therapy with post-traumatic stress disordered veteran clients, *J Psychosoc Nurs Ment Health Serv* 31(9):29, 1993.

Hinkle LK: Eye movement desensitization and reprocessing, (unpublished), 1997.

Kaplan A: OCD "expert guidelines" address critical treatment need, *Psychiatr Times* 14(7):24, 1997.

Katon W, Sheenan D, and Uhde T: Panic disorder: a treatable problem, *Patient Care* 81, 1992.

Keltner N, et al: Anxiety disorder. In *Psychobiological foundations of psychiatric care*, St. Louis, 1998, Mosby.

Kendler K, et al: The genetic epidemiology of phobias in women, *Arch Gen Psychiatry* 49(4):273, 1992.

Kluft RP: Hospital treatment of multiple personality disorder, *Psychiatr Clin North Am* 14(3):695, 1991.

Lipowski ZJ: Somatization: a borderland between medicine and psychiatry, *Can Med Assoc J* 135:609, 1986.

Lowenstein RJ: Psychogenic amnesia and psychogenic fugue: a comprehensive review. In Sasman A and Goldfinger SM, editors: *American Psychiatric Press review of psychiatry*, Washington, DC, 1991, American Psychiatric Press.

Marshall R and Schneier F: An algorithm for the pharmacotherapy of social phobia, *Psychiatr Ann* 26(4):210, 1996.

McDuff DR and Johnson JL: Classification and characteristics of army stress casualties during Operation Desert Storm, *Hosp Community Psychiatry* 43(8):812, 1992.

Moyers F: Oklahoma City bombing: exacerbation of symptoms in veterans with PTSD, *Arch Psychiatr Nurs* 10(1):55, 1996.

Nelson BS and Wright DW: Understanding and treating post-traumatic stress disorder symptoms in female partners of veterans with PTSD, *J Marital Fam Ther* 22(4):455, 1996.

North CS and Smith EM: Posttraumatic stress disorder among homeless men and women, *Hosp Community Psychiatry* 41(10):1010, 1992.

O'Reilly-Knapp M: From fragmentation to wholeness: an integrative approach with clients who dissociate, *Perspect Psychiatr Care* 32(4):5, 1996.

Regier DA, et al: The de facto US mental and addictive disorders service system: epidemiologic catchment area prospective 1-year prevalence rates of disorders and services, *Arch Gen Psychiatry* 50:85, 1993.

Samter J, et al: Debriefing: from military origin to therapeutic application, *J Psychosoc Nurs Ment Health Serv* 31(2):23, 1993.

Shapiro F: *Eye movement desensitization and reprocessing,* New York, 1995, Guilford.

Simeon D and Hollander E: Depersonalization disorder, *Psychiatr Ann* 23(7):382, 1993.

Snell FI and Padin-Rivera E: Group treatment for older veterans with post-traumatic stress disorder, *J Psychosoc Nurs Ment Health Serv* 35(2):10, 1997.

Solomon SD and Davidson JRT: Trauma: prevalence, impairment, service use, and cost, *J Clin Psychiatry* 58(9):5, 1997.

Stafford L: Dissociation and multiple personality disorder: a challenge for psychosocial nurses, *J Psychosoc Nurs Ment Health Serv* 31(1):15, 1993.

Stanton MP, et al: Shared experiences of military nurse veterans, *Image J Nurs Sch* 28(4):343, 1996.

Stein MB, et al: Full and partial post-traumatic stress disorder: findings from a community survey, *Am J Psychiatry* 154(3):1114, 1997.

Thompson P: Generalized anxiety disorder treatment algorithm, *Psychiatr Ann* 26(4):227, 1996.

van der Kolk BA: The psychobiology of posttraumatic stress disorder, *J Clin Psychiatry* 58(9):16, 1997.

Wakefield M and Pallister R: New hope for a disabling condition: cognitive-behavioral approaches to panic disorder, *J Psychosoc Nurs Ment Health Serv* 35(3):12, 1997.

CHAPTER 30

Cognitive Disorders

RENEE WILSON SAUL
NORMAN L. KELTNER

LEARNING OBJECTIVES

After reading this chapter you should be able to:
- Differentiate dementia and delirium.
- Recognize DSM-IV criteria for delirium, dementia, amnestic, and other cognitive disorders.
- Describe the primary symptoms of dementia.
- Understand theories that explain the psychopathology of Alzheimer's disease and other dementias.

- Develop a nursing care plan for a patient with dementia.
- Evaluate the effectiveness of nursing interventions for patients with dementia.

Intellectual functioning is highly valued by all persons because of the importance of the ability to think rationally. The ability to think and to reason is one of the distinguishing features of a human being. Cognitive abilities, including memory, reasoning, orientation, perception, and attention, are processes that allow the person to make sense of experience and to interact productively with the environment. Memory is the foundation of these cognitive processes. Memory is an important cognitive process, as one must remember past experiences to exercise judgment, make decisions, and orient to time and place. Loss of memory is devastating, leaving the affected person in a state of confusion, unable to understand experience, and unable to relate

current or past events. Impairment of any of these functions indicates a cognitive disorder.

The terms *organic brain syndrome, organic mental disorder,* and *organic mental syndrome* have been used interchangeably in the past to describe the cognitive disorders. These terms are no longer used because they are not specific and because they include implications of prognosis and suggest that other mental disorders do not have an organic component (First, et al, 1994). The American Psychiatric Association has replaced the former with the more specific categories of delirium, dementia, amnestic, and other cognitive disorders. A discussion of the differences between and among these terms is presented to facilitate the student's

KEY TERMS

Alzheimer's disease More correctly referred to as dementia of the Alzheimer type (DAT). DAT is the most common type of dementia. The characteristic symptoms are amnesia, aphasia, apraxia, and agnosia (the four As).

Cognitive disorder A disorder that affects consciousness, memory, and other cognitive processes.

Dementia A cognitive disorder that causes pronounced memory and cognitive disturbances. Typically, dementias are gradual in onset and progressive in course.

Delirium A disorder with alterations in consciousness and changes in cognition that are usually caused by a general medical condition or are substance induced. Typically, deliria develop over a short period of time and are treatable.

Vascular dementia (formerly multiinfarct dementia) Dementia resulting from interruption of blood to the brain, which causes anoxia, ischemia, and subsequent infarction.

12-Month Prevalence Rate of Mental Disorders in the United States

Diagnosis	Percentage of Population over 17 Years of Age	Number of Persons
Anxiety disorders	12.6	20,034,000
Phobia disorders*	10.9	17,331,000
Mood disorders	9.5	15,143,000
Alcohol disorders	7.4	11,766,000
Major depression†	5.0	7,950,000
Drug disorders	3.1	4,929,000
Cognitive impairment	**2.7**	**4,293,000**
Obsessive-compulsive disorder	2.1	3,339,000
Antisocial disorder	1.5	2,385,000
Panic disorders*	1.3	2,067,000
Bipolar disorder†	1.2	1,908,000
Schizophrenia	1.1	1,749,000
Somatization	0.2	365,000

From Regier DA, et al: The de facto US mental and addictive disorders service system: epidemiologic catchment area prospective 1-year prevalence rates of disorders and services, *Arch Gen Psychiatry* 50:85, 1993.
*Also calculated in anxiety statistics.
†Also calculated in mood disorders statistics.

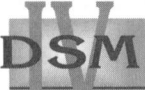 ## DSM-IV Criteria for Delirium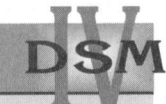

Delirium is characterized by:
1. Disturbances of consciousness (i.e., reduced clarity of awareness of the environment) with reduced ability to focus, sustain, or shift attention.
2. Change in cognition (such as memory deficit, disorientation, language disturbance, perceptual disturbance).
3. Development over a short period of time (usually hours to days) and with a tendency to fluctuate during the course of the day.

Adapted from the American Psychiatric Association: *Diagnostic and statistical manual of mental disorders,* ed 4, Washington, DC, 1994, The Association.

understanding and appreciation of this and other psychiatric literature.

DSM-IV TERMINOLOGY AND CRITERIA

The Diagnostic and Statistical Manual of Mental Disorders, fourth edition, (DSM-IV), of the American Psychiatric Association (1994) makes the following distinctions:

- *Deliria.* Delirium is characterized by a change in cognition and a disturbance of consciousness, which manifests as a reduced ability to focus, sustain, or shift attention. Delirium tends to develop over a short period of time and tends to fluctuate during the course of the day. Typically the cause can be determined from either history, physical examination, or laboratory findings. Deliria can be further subdivided into those caused by a general medical condition such as dehydration, those caused by substances (e.g., benztropine [Cogentin], alcohol), and those caused by several factors (e.g., a fever and a medication). See the box on p. 452 for DSM-IV criteria.
- *Dementias.* Dementia is characterized by the development of multiple cognitive deficits manifested by both memory impairment (amnesia) and at least one of the cognitive disturbances of aphasia, apraxia, agnosia, or disturbance in planning, sequencing, and abstracting. See the box below for DSM-IV criteria. The course is gradual in onset with an unabated cognitive decline. The cognitive deficits cause significant impairment in social and/or occupational functioning that are clearly less adaptive when compared to the person's previous level of functioning. Prog-

nosis is typically poor. Several classifications of dementias exist, including dementia of the Alzheimer's type (DAT) and vascular dementias (American Psychiatric Association [APA], 1994).
- *Amnestic disorders.* Amnestic disorders refer to the development of memory impairment as manifested by inability to learn new information or the inability to recall previously learned information. Etiologically related data can be obtained from the history, laboratory findings, or physical examination (including physical trauma). The impairment may be transient or chronic and is not associated with delirium or dementia (APA, 1994).
- *Other cognitive disorders.* The DSM-IV provides a category for cognitive disorders that do not meet the criteria of the above cognitive disorders. Mild cognitive disorder is an example of a cognitive disorder that does not meet other criteria.

According to Pieri, Cumin, and Hinzen (1989), dementia is one of the most prevalent disorders of later life. Among the dementias, the most common form is DAT followed by vascular or multiinfarct dementia (MID). The morbidity of dementias is as follows:

DAT–52% (up to 75% [APA, 1997])
MID–17%
DAT combined with MID–14%
Brain tumors, Huntington's disease, Pick's disease, Creutzfeldt-Jakob (CJ) disease–7%
Parkinson's disease–2%
Acquired immunodeficiency syndrome (AIDS) dementia–1%
Other–7%

Following is a discussion of the two broad classifications, delirium and dementia, which then proceeds to a discussion of the degenerative dementias

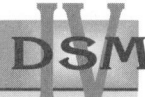

DSM-IV Criteria for Dementia

Dementia is characterized by the development of multiple cognitive deficits manifested by:
1. Memory impairment (amnesia)
2. At least one of the following cognitive disturbances:
   a. Aphasia (language disturbance)
   b. Apraxia (inability to carry out motor activities despite intact motor function)

c. Agnosia (failure to recognize or identify objects despite intact sensory function)
d. Disturbance in executive functioning (i.e., planning, organizing, sequencing, abstracting)

Dementia is further characterized by a significant impairment in social or occupational functioning that is noticeably different from prior levels of functioning.

Adapted from the American Psychiatric Association: *Diagnostic and statistical manual of mental disorders,* ed 4, Washington, DC, 1994, The Association.

of Alzheimer's disease (AD), Parkinson's disease (PD), diffuse Lewy body disease (DLBD), Huntington's disease, Pick's disease, and Creutzfeldt-Jakob (CJ) disease. Vascular or multiinfarct dementia (MID), alcoholic dementia, and transient ischemic attacks (TIAs) will also be examined. Psychotherapeutic management of these organically based disorders will conclude the chapter. A list of DSM-IV and NANDA nursing diagnoses related to organic mental disorders is in the box below. In addition to DSM-IV and NANDA criteria, the recently published APA "Practice Guidelines for the Treatment of Patients with Alzheimer's Disease and Other Dementias of Late Life" (1997) will be utilized.

DELIRIUM

Delirium is a common condition, particularly in the elderly (Batt, 1989). It is estimated that between

24% and 65% of acutely hospitalized elderly patients become delirious at some time during their hospitalization (Levkoff, et al, 1991). Approximately 30% of elderly patients in surgical or cardiac intensive care unit (ICU) and 40% to 50% of those recovering from hip fracture surgery will have an episode of delirium (Cameron, et al, 1987).

Delirium has a sudden onset, often starting at night. When the causative factor is identified and treated, its duration is usually brief, about 1 week. It is rare for delirium to persist for more than 1 month.

Objective and Subjective Behavior

The diagnostic features of delirium are noted in the DSM-IV box on p. 452. The cerebral dysfunction associated with delirium not only causes subjective symptoms but also causes visible signs. For instance, the patient with delirium may be incontinent of urine and feces and may have psychomotor agita-

---

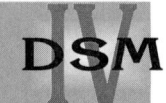

DSM-IV and NANDA Diagnoses Related to Cognitive Disorders

DSM-IV*
Delirium due to a general medical condition
Substance-induced delirium
Delirium due to multiple etiologies
Dementia of the Alzheimer's type
Vascular dementia
Dementia due to HIV disease
Dementia due to head trauma
Dementia due to Parkinson's disease
Dementia due to Huntington's disease
Dementia due to Pick's disease
Dementia due to Creutzfeldt-Jakob disease
Dementia due to other general medical conditions
Substance-induced persisting dementia
Dementia due to multiple etiologies
Amnestic disorder due to a general medical condition
Substance-induced persisting amnestic disorder

NANDA†
Anxiety
Bowel incontinence

Communication, impaired verbal
Coping, ineffective family: compromised
Coping, ineffective individual
Diversional activity deficit
Fear
Fluid volume deficit, potential
Health maintenance, altered
Home maintenance management, impaired
Injury, potential for
Mobility, impaired physical
Role performance, altered
Self-care deficit
   Bathing/hygiene, feeding, dressing/grooming, toileting
Sensory/perceptual alterations (specify)
   Visual auditory, kinesthetic, gustatory, tactile, olfactory
Skin integrity, potential impaired
Sleep pattern disturbance
Social interaction, impaired
Social isolation
Thought processes, altered
Trauma, potential for

*From the American Psychiatric Association: *Diagnostic and statistical manual of mental disorders,* ed 4, Washington, DC, 1994, The Association.
†From the North American Nursing Diagnosis Association: *NANDA nursing diagnoses: definitions and classifications 1997-1998,* Philadelphia, 1997, The Association.

tion, including tremors and choreiform (irregular) movements (Wills, 1986; Gomez and Gomez, 1987; Patkar and Kunkel, 1997).

The essential features of delirium are impaired consciousness with global cognitive impairment. This manifests as reduced awareness of and attentiveness to the environment, disorganized thinking, and rambling, irrelevant, or incoherent speech. The syndrome also involves memory impairment, disturbances of the sleep-wake cycle (typically a reversal), disturbances in the level of psychomotor activity, and sensory misperceptions, as when a patient listens to a public address system and thinks that God is talking to him or her. Box 30-1 presents the clinical features of delirium.

Etiology

Delirium may be caused by chronic or acute physical illnesses and by chemical agents, such as drugs and alcohol. The most common physical illnesses associated with delirium are congestive heart failure, pneumonia, uremia, malnutrition, dehydration, can-

cer, and cerebrovascular accidents. Other factors include vascular disease, brain damage or disease, impaired vision and hearing, sleep loss, and fatigue. Fever may or may not be associated with these physical illnesses, since the elderly can have a substantial infection with much less change in temperature than younger persons.

Prescription drug intoxication is probably the most frequent single cause of delirium. Several medications may be implicated, even when administered in therapeutic doses. They include anticholinergic drugs, such as when combinations of the following drugs are prescribed: amitriptyline (Elavil, an antidepressant), antihistamines, antispasmodics, analgesics, steroids, sedatives, cardiovascular drugs (especially digoxin and diuretics), and cimetidine (Tagamet) (Lipowski, 1989).

The central cholinergic system, necessary for memory, learning, attention, and wakefulness, is aggravated by the use of anticholinergic medications. Delirium is most likely when several drugs with anticholinergic properties are prescribed at the same time. Therefore polypharmacy (the prescribing of multiple drugs) should be avoided as much as possible, and the nurse attending the patient should be aware of these dangers. Table 30-1 lists the relative anticholinergic effects of often prescribed psychotropic medications compared to benztropine.

Treatment

Patkar and Kunkel (1997) describes a twofold management of delirium by identifying and correcting the underlying condition or conditions and by controlling behavioral symptoms by judicious use of medications and environmental manipulation. The patient should be cared for in a well-lighted room with a visible clock and calendar. If the delirious state is thought to be caused by physical illness, it is important to first treat the primary problem. For instance, measures for correction of anemia, dehydration, nutritional deficiencies, or electrolyte imbalance should be undertaken. These measures include close monitoring of vital signs, pulse oximetry, nutrition, and fluid electrolyte balance. For those patients suspected of alcohol withdrawal, thiamine and folate should be administered. Any nonessential medications should be discontinued or dose reduced.

Although most cases of delirium are reversible, persistent cognitive deficits are common. The reversal

---

Box 30-1 Clinical Features of Delirium

Prodrome* (restlessness, anxiety, sleep disturbance, irritability)
Rapidly fluctuating course
Decreased attention (easily distractible)
Altered arousal and psychomotor abnormality
Disturbance of sleep-wake cycle
Impaired memory (cannot register new information)
Disorganized thinking and speech
Disorientation (time, place, and [very rare] person)
Altered perceptions (misperceptions, illusions, delusions [poorly formed], and hallucinations)
Neurological abnormalities
  Dysphagia
  Apraxia
  Aphasia
  Motor abnormalities (tremors, myoclonus, and reflex and tone changes)
  EEG abnormalities (almost always global slowing)
Other features (sadness, anger, euphoria, or other affects)

From Wise MC and Brandt GT: Delirium. In Yodofsky SC and Hales RE, editors: *The American Psychiatric Press textbook of psychiatry,* ed 2, Washington, DC, 1992, American Psychiatric Press.
*Prodrome = An early manifestation of an impending disease before specific symptoms begin.

TABLE 30-1 Anticholinergic Effect of Frequently Prescribed Psychotropic Drugs Compared to Trihexyphenidyl

Drug	Equivalent in Milligrams	Typical Use
Atropine	0.5	Given before surgery
Benztropine (Cogentin)	1.0	Antiparkinson
TRIHEXYPHENIDYL (ARTANE)	2.5	Antiparkinson
Biperiden (Akineton)	1.0	Antiparkinson
Amitriptyline (Elavil)	10	Antidepressant
Doxepin (Sinequan)	30	Antidepressant
Nortriptyline (Pamelor)	60	Antidepressant
Imipramine (Tofranil)	75	Antidepressant
Desipramine (Norpramin)	150	Antidepressant
Amoxapine (Asendin)	600	Antidepressant
Clozapine (Clozaril)	15	Antipsychotic
Thioridazine (Mellaril)	50	Antipsychotic
Chlorpromazine (Thorazine)	370	Antipsychotic
Diphenhydramine (Benadryl)	50	Antihistamine

According to this table, 50 mg of thioridazine has the same anticholinergic effect as 1 mg of benztropine.
Adapted from de Leon J, et al: A pilot effort to determine benztropine equivalents of anticholinergic medications, *Hosp Community Psychiatry* 45(6):606, 1994.

of an episode of delirium does not necessarily imply a good prognosis. There is a high short-term mortality of patients with delirium. Increased mortality also exists at 1-year follow-up after an episode of delirium (Francis, Martin, and Kapoor, 1990).

Distinguishing between delirium and dementia is an extremely important, yet difficult, task. It is difficult to make this distinction because about one third of hospitalized demented patients also experience delirium. Of course, even when delirium is successfully treated, the dementia remains. Box 30-2 differentiates delirium and dementia.

CLINICAL EXAMPLE

Mrs. Wilson is a 70-year-old widow who lives alone and is still active and able to drive her car for short distances for shopping. She also is able to visit her friends and children. During the winter months she developed a fever, chills, and other "flulike" symptoms. She was taken to her granddaughter's home to be cared for. She was initially treated with over-the-counter cold medications. She continued these medications until her symptoms of fever and weakness worsened. She also was confused and disoriented to time and place. Her family rushed her to the hospital, and she was admitted for pneumonia. Her medical condition deteriorated. Mrs. Wilson was dehydrated by the fever and at times incoherent and delirious. The family was distraught by her rapid physical and mental decline. At the hospital she was started on antibiotics and intravenous fluids for rehydration. As the antibiotic therapy began to control the infectious process and as the rehydration strategy began to work, Mrs. Wilson's delirium lifted, and she soon returned to her normal state.

DEMENTIA

Dementia is broadly defined as an altered mental state secondary to cerebral disease. It is usually an irreversible mental state characterized by a decreased intellectual function, personality change, impaired judgment, and often a change in affect. Dementia is the result of a disease or an abnormal condition, such as a vascular injury. The symptoms are severe enough to interfere with the patient's activities of daily living, work, or social relationships. More than 20 illnesses can cause dementia (Geldmacher and Whitehouse, 1997).

Objective and Subjective Behavior

The primary symptoms of dementia are cognitive (e.g., problems with orientation, judgment, atten-

Box 30-2	**Differential Diagnosis of Delirium and Dementia**	
Feature	Delirium	Dementia
Onset	Acute, often at night	Insidious
Course	Fluctuating, with lucid intervals, during day; worse at night	Stable over course of day
Duration	Hours to weeks	Months or years
Awareness	Reduced	Clear
Alertness	Abnormally low or high	Usually normal
Attention	Lacks direction and selectivity; distractibility; fluctuates over course of day	Relatively unaffected
Orientation	Usually impaired for time; tendency to mistake unfamiliar for familiar place and persons	Often impaired
Memory	Immediate and recent memory impairments	Recent and remote memory impairments
Thinking	Disorganized	Impoverished
Perception	Illusions and hallucinations (usually visual) are common	Often absent
Speech	Incoherent, hesitant, slow or rapid	Difficulty in finding words
Sleep-wake cycle	Always disrupted	Fragmented sleep
Physical illness or drug toxicity	Either or both present	Often absent, especially in Alzheimer's disease

From Lipowski ZJ: Delirium (acute confusional states), *JAMA* 258:1789, 1987.

tion, intellect, memory). These subjective experiences can be objectively observed by the nurse in several ways. The lost patient, the confused patient, and the frustrated patient all demonstrate behaviors that are evidence of their neuropathological state. For instance, impaired judgment commonly manifests itself through the purchase of unneeded or worthless items. Impaired attention span may disrupt the patient's ability to communicate satisfactorily. The disinhibiting effect of dementia may lead to social blunders, such as sexually inappropriate behavior or inappropriate language. Many objective manifestations of cognitive degeneration could be listed. The following cognitive disturbances are the fundamental symptoms of dementia.

Alterations in memory

The most prominent symptom of dementia is the impairment of short-term and long-term memory, compounded by significant alterations in reasoning, language, and personality. In mild dementia there is moderate memory loss, characterized by forgetting telephone numbers, conversations, or events of the day. In more severe cases, only highly learned material, such as one's own name or previous occupation, is retained, and new information is quickly forgotten. Events that occurred many years ago tend to be remembered better than those events that have occurred more recently, although this pattern of loss is variable. In advanced cases of dementia, memory impairment can be so severe that the person forgets his or her own name, age, and occupation or the names of close relatives.

Alterations in abstract thinking

Impairment of abstract thinking is noted in reduced capacity for generalization, differentiation, concept formation, and logical reasoning. The patient has difficulty defining words and cannot organize concepts around familiar themes (e.g., if shown a picture in which the task is to identify similar pictures, the patient with dementia would have difficulty). If asked to give the meaning of proverbs such as "don't cry over spilled milk," the patient responds that the milk was dirty. The diminished ability for abstract thinking results in more and more self-preoccupation. Frequently people with dementing illnesses can be demanding and appear to be self-centered, which may be a reversal of their former caring and responsible self (Mace and Rabins, 1991).

Alterations in judgment

Patients with dementia cannot make the same adequate judgments that they formerly made. For instance, planning may become impossible for them. If a well-intentioned person were to find a stamped envelope near a mailbox, he or she would most likely put the letter into the mailbox. A well-intentioned person with dementia might not have the good judgment to do so.

Alterations in perception

Hallucinations are sensory experiences that occur without external stimulus; they may involve all senses but are predominant in the auditory and visual spheres. Patients with dementia have hallucinations. Abnormal behavior as a result of hallucinations may occur when patients act on these visual and auditory hallucinations (Lucas, Steel, and Bognanni, 1986).

Delusions are present at times in relation to a dementia syndrome, although they usually arise out of a reaction to a cognitive deficit. For example, patients are unable to remember where they put a specific item and will accuse others of stealing from them.

Illusions are common in patients with dementia syndromes and are described as misrepresentations of sensory perceptions triggered by environmental stimuli. For example, a tree outside a window may be misperceived as a person standing outside the window. It is important to distinguish an illusion from a hallucination, as the environmental stimuli can be manipulated to decrease stimulation associated with illusions. Accurate observation and documentation can distinguish between a visual illusion and a visual hallucination and can determine the correct intervention strategy.

Reversible Dementia

Reversible dementia is a term used in the medical literature to describe a dementia that has a specific treatable cause. In the past, dementia has implied a progressive or irreversible course. Potentially reversible dementia syndromes include those arising from inflammatory processes (e.g., encephalopathy caused by systemic lupus erythematosus [SLE]); infections such as syphilis; or toxic conditions (e.g., alcohol abuse) that produce memory loss and abnormal frontal lobe functions (Cummings, 1987). Metabolic-related dementia, such as hypothyroidism or hyperthyroidism, and nutritional syndromes, such as vitamin B_{12} and folate deficiencies, may also be reversible with appropriate therapy (Geldmacher and Whitehouse, 1997). It is estimated that 30% to 40% of persons with memory disturbances have a reversible and, therefore, treatable dementia. Although most of the patients will have physical disorders, psychiatric disturbances such as depression are a significant challenge in the differential diagnosis. Treatment of such conditions as depression, drug-induced dementia, infections, and metabolic disturbances leads to complete restoration of functioning. With prompt diagnosis and appropriate treatment, the dementia can be reversed.

Nonreversible Dementia

When a reversible cause of intellectual impairment cannot be identified, the clinical diagnosis is presumed to be a nonreversible dementia. Many diseases can produce a progressive and nonreversible dementia. Most of these are rare and can affect adults of all ages with older individuals more likely to be affected. When dementia does occur in a younger person, it has been associated with suicide (Margo and Finkel, 1990). The most common nonreversible dementias occur in AD, PD, Huntington's disease, Pick's disease, CJ, and MID. TIAs are included in this category because they can lead to a disabling cerebral infarction. All of these dementias are progressive, and treatment must evolve with time to address each new issue. At each stage the nurse should help the patient and family anticipate future symptoms and the care likely to be required (APA, 1997).

ALZHEIMER'S DISEASE

Description and Incidence

Alzheimer's disease (AD), or dementia of the Alzheimer's type (DAT), is the form of dementia most commonly seen in the elderly. It is the most prevalent of all nonreversible dementias, accounting for about 50% to 75% of all diagnosed cases of dementia (APA, 1997). It is defined as an age-related, progressive disorder of the central nervous system, characterized by chronic cognitive dysfunction. The cause of AD is unknown (Cohen, 1990). The disorder eventually leads to pronounced impairment in activities of daily living, and patients may require total care. Figures 30-1 and 30-2 provide examples of both gross and microscopic changes associated with AD.

AD usually begins after the age of 65, and new data suggest a greater prevalence than formerly thought.

CLINICAL EXAMPLE

Mr. Wallace is a 79-year-old man who has cared for his wife with AD for 12 years, 6 years at home and 6 years at a nursing home. During the first year, Mr. Wallace noticed her forgetfulness. "She would forget what happened 10 minutes ago but could recall things that happened years ago, to the letter." But over the next couple of years, things progressed to the point that she could not find her way to old once-familiar places. She was unable to dress and feed herself. In the months before she was placed in a nursing home, Mrs. Wallace would get up at night and open and rearrange dresser drawers. Once she wandered outside and was not found until the next morning, several blocks from their home. Mr. Wallace could no longer manage her at home by himself.

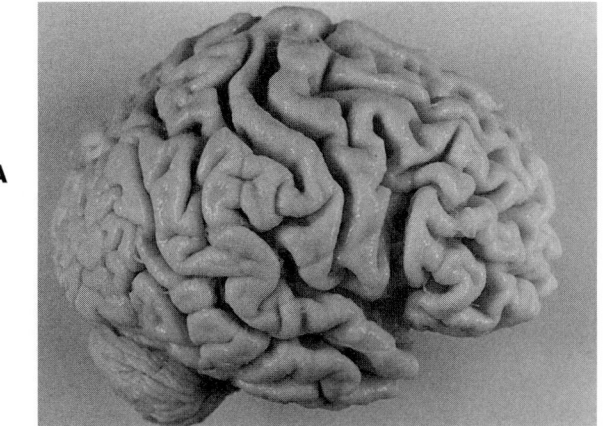

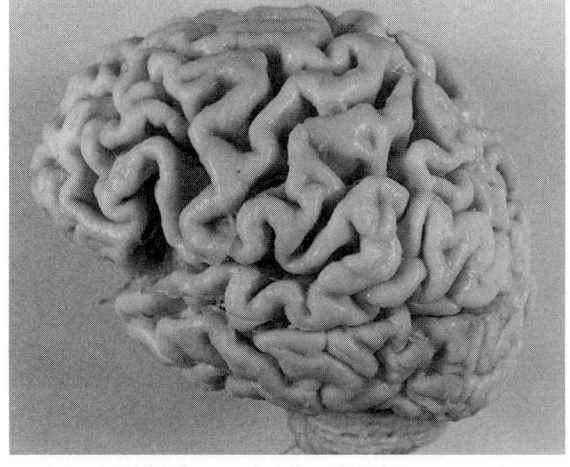

FIGURE 30-1 A, Right side of brain of patient with Alzheimer's disease. Note narrow gyri and larger sulci. **B,** Left side of same brain demonstrating even narrower gyri and larger sulci. (A to D photographed by Berto Tarin, Western University of Health Sciences.)   *Continued*

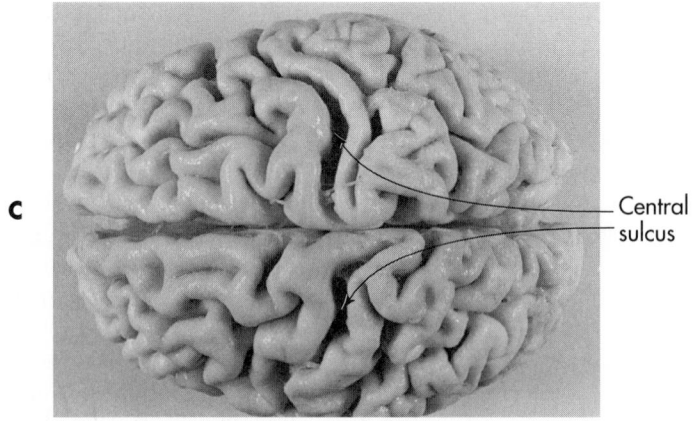

C

Central
sulcus

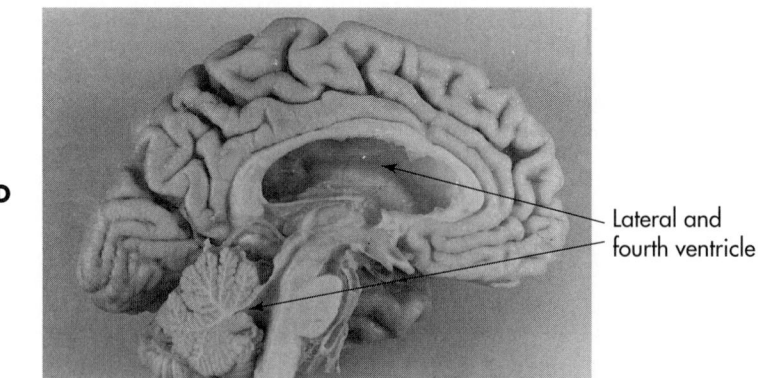

D

Lateral and
fourth ventricle

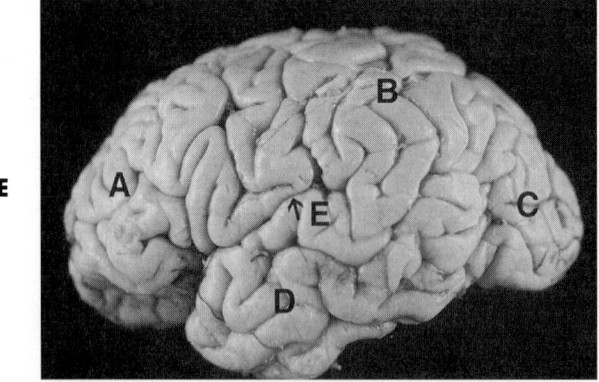

E

FIGURE 30-1, cont'd   C, Superior view. Central sulcus is very wide. **D,** Midsagittal view of left hemisphere. Note the greatly enlarged lateral and fourth ventricles. (A to D photographed by Berto Tarin, Western University of Health Sciences.) **E,** Normal brain, *a,* frontal lobe; *b,* parietal lobe; *c,* occipital lobe; *d,* temporal lobe; *e,* lateral fissure. (E courtesy of Dr. Richard E. Powers, University of Alabama at Birmingham Brain Resource Program [UAB-BRP].)

Mr. Wallace is retired, and he visits his wife daily at the nursing home. Most days she does not recognize him. The Wallaces have two children who live in distant cities. He describes the children as "supportive" but absent for any real decision making and assistance. Friends from his church and work are available, but he describes his main support system as friends that he has made over the last few years through AD support groups.

Mr. Wallace talks about guilty feelings that he has associated with care decisions and his wish for the disease to be over. He admits to praying for his wife's death.

Alois Alzheimer, a German neuropathologist, first described the condition that later assumed his name in 1907 after he detailed the characteristic neurological changes in the brains of affected persons. One of his patients was a 51-year-old woman with symptoms of memory loss, disorientation, hallucinations, and profound dementia. She died 4½ years after the onset of the disease. Postmortem examination revealed brain atrophy and distortions in the

cortical neurofibrils. These distortions were named Alzheimer's tangles and are now referred to as neurofibrillary tangles (see Figures 30-3 and 30-4).

The syndrome affects about 5% to 8% of people over age 65, 15% to 20% of those over age 75, and 25% to 50% of individuals over age 85 (APA, 1997). AD has become the most common dementing illness among older adults and afflicts between 3 and

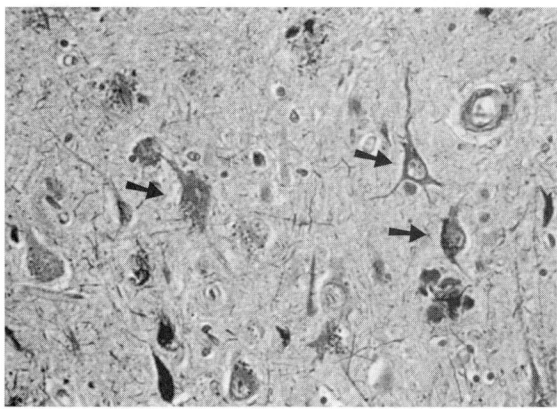

FIGURE 30-3 The dark flame-shaped objects are neurofibrillary "tangles" or dead neurons. Tangles are twisted fibrils inside the neuron that disrupt cellular processes and eventually kill the cell. (Courtesy Dr. Richard E. Powers, UAB-BRP.)

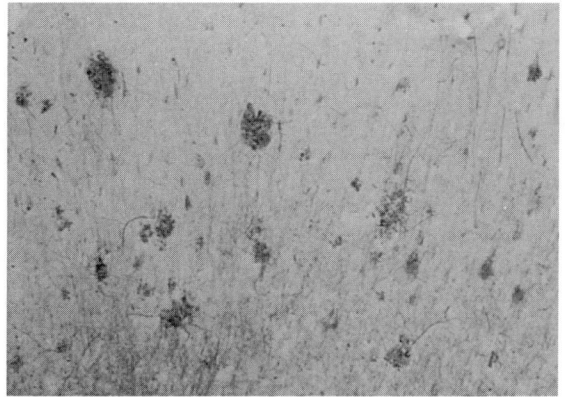

FIGURE 30-4 The darker objects are plaques, one of the two microscopic findings in AD (the other are the tangles seen in Figure 30-3). Since plaques can be found in about 50% of elderly persons over age 70, it is the quantity of plaques in relation to the person's age that is significant. (Courtesy Dr. Richard E. Powers, UAB-BRP).

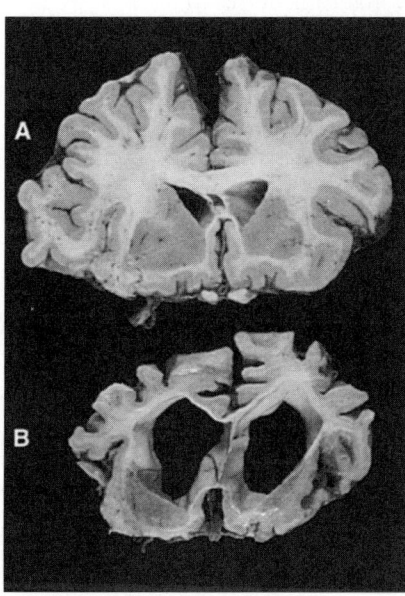

FIGURE 30-2 A, This brain is normal; the sulci and gyri are not atrophied. **B,** This brain shows the effects of AD: widened sulci and narrowed gyri. Additionally, the lateral ventricles of this brain are increased in size because of the decrease in brain mass associated with AD. (Courtesy Dr. Richard E. Powers, UAB-BRP.)

5 million individuals in the United States at a cost of $100 billion per year (Keltner, et al, 1998; Ernst and Hay, 1994). AD is believed to be the fourth leading cause of death in persons over 65 years of age and accounts for about 120,000 deaths per year. AD is slightly more common in women than in men, and a definite diagnosis can be made only on autopsy. The disease progresses slowly, with the average victim living between 8 and 10 years from onset of symptoms to death (APA, 1997).

Progression of the Disease

AD is difficult to diagnose, especially in the early stages when it resembles many other disorders. Over time there are progressive changes in language, learned motor performance, memory, abstraction, and visuospatial function (Box 30-3 presents the 4 As of AD). AD progresses from mild to moderate to severe.

Language disability progresses from expressive aphasia to receptive aphasia to mindless repetition of words.

Behavior progresses from indifference to agitation.

Memory dysfunction progresses from recent memory loss to recent/remote memory loss and can reach the point where the patient does not know his or her own name.

Interestingly, motor function is spared except in advanced AD.

In the last stage, the patient eventually becomes emaciated, helpless, and bedridden. The most frequent cause of death is pneumonia and other infections, with malnutrition and dehydration as contributing factors (Kermis, 1986; Williams, 1986). Table 30-2 summarizes the impairments in activities of daily living (ADLs) associated with various stages of the disease. The box below lists the DSM-IV criteria for AD.

CLINICAL EXAMPLE

It is important for nurses to teach other health care workers about the progression of memory loss to prevent frustration and specifically to prevent overreaction to patients based on that frustration. For example, a patient with AD may not remember what he ate for breakfast 10 to 30 minutes ago but may remember with surprising clarity events of 10 to

---

Box 30-3 Four As of Alzheimer's Disease

1. Amnesia: inability to learn new information or to recall previously learned information.
2. Agnosia: failure to recognize or identify objects despite intact sensory function.
3. Aphasia: language disturbance that can manifest in both understanding and expressing the spoken word.
4. Apraxia: inability to carry out motor activities despite intact motor function (e.g., ability to grab a doorknob but not knowing what to do with it).

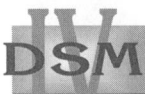 **DSM-IV Criteria for Dementia of the Alzheimer's Type**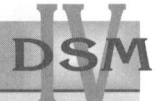

Alzheimer's disease presents with multiple cognitive deficits manifested by:
1. Memory impairment (amnesia)
2. At least one of the following cognitive disturbances:
   a. Aphasia (language disturbance)
   b. Apraxia (inability to carry out motor activities despite intact motor function)
   c. Agnosia (failure to recognize or identify objects despite intact motor function)
   d. Disturbance in executive function (i.e., planning, organizing, sequencing, abstracting)

It is characterized by gradual onset and continuing cognitive decline.

There is a significant impairment in social or occupational functioning, which represents a significant decline from previous levels of functioning.

Cognitive deficits cannot be attributed to any of the following:
1. Central nervous system conditions that cause progressive deficits in memory and cognition
2. Systemic conditions that are known to cause dementia
3. Substance-induced conditions

Adapted from the American Psychiatric Association: *Diagnostic and statistical manual of mental disorders,* ed 4, Washington, DC, 1994, The Association.

30 years ago. To many people who just want to apply "common sense" to caring for AD patients, this does not make sense. This progressive trajectory of brain degeneration has everything to do with the area of the brain first affected by AD. Hence, recent memory is lost before remote memory is lost. Further, nurses and others should understand that the progression of language loss does not always make sense either. For example, a patient who has expressive aphasia (a left-brain function) may be able to sing or curse (the musical and emotional component of speech is a right-brain function). The caretaker ignorant of these specific localized functions may consider an AD patient purposely uncooperative rather than biologically impaired.

Etiology

The presence of senile plaques and neurofibrillary tangles (NFTs) are definitive diagnostic criteria for Alzheimer's disease, and the numbers of both tangles and plaques correlate strongly with the degree of dementia (Alafuzoff, 1992; Iqbal and Wisniewski, 1983). In fact, most people over age 65 have a small number of senile plaques, with NFTs being less common in normal aging. The structural changes in the brain of the patient with AD do not cause the disease. They are the result of something else, and several theories exist regarding what might cause plaques and NFTs.

Other diagnostic phenomena that can be observed microscopically in AD are dystrophic neurites (thickened, swollen neuronal processes) and abnormal amyloid deposits within the senile plaques and around blood vessels. Amyloid may be neurotoxic and may precipitate neuronal damage. It is thought that the amyloid neurotoxic process develops in a specific manner. Amyloid is part of a neuronal repairing process in which it is broken down and eliminated after its "work" is finished. For patients with AD this does not occur and the remnants of incomplete amyloid breakdown, amyloid derived diffusable ligand (ADDL), is toxic to brain cells. Inflammatory chemicals in the brain affect the development of ADDLs and this fact helps explain the effectiveness of the use of long term nonsteroidal antiinflammatory drugs (NSAIDs), discussed later in the chapter (Kotulak, 1998).

Several models or theories have been proposed to explain the etiology of AD. A brief discussion of those models follows.

Table 30-2   Impairment in Activities of Daily Living Based on the Stage of Alzheimer's Disease

Mild Impairment:
The patient has difficulty with:
Balancing a checkbook
Preparing a complex meal
Managing a difficult medication schedule

Moderate Impairment:
The patient has difficulty with:
Simple food preparation
Household cleanup
Yardwork
Some aspects of self-care: e.g., needs reminding to use the bathroom, help with fasteners, help with shaving, etc.

Severe Impairment:
The patient needs considerable assistance with:
Personal care
Feeding
Grooming
Toileting

Profound Impairment:
The patient is oblivious to surroundings and almost totally dependent on caregivers

Terminal Phase:
The patient is bed-bound, requiring constant care.

Adapted from the American Psychiatric Association: Practice guidelines for the treatment of patients with Alzheimer's disease and other dementias of late life, *Am J Psychiatry* 154(5)(suppl):1, 1997.

Genetic model

The genetic model researches the possibility that there may be one or more faulty genes responsible for AD. It is hypothesized that there is some factor in the genetic makeup that renders a person vulnerable to some factor in the environment. In some families several members representing four to five generations have developed a dementia of the Alzheimer's type (DAT) (Burnside, 1988). Familial AD accounts for 10% to 15% of all AD cases (Roberts, Leigh, and Weinberger, 1993). Mohs, et al (1987) suggest a morbidity rate of 50% by age 90 for first-degree relatives of AD victims. They use what is called a "life table method," which accounts for family members who die before age 90 by non-AD causes. The fact that individuals with Down's syndrome develop the characteristic pathology of AD is also suggestive of genetic influence (Roberts, Leigh, and Weinberger, 1993). The gene for amyloid, which is overabundant in AD, is found on the long arm of chromosome 21, the disordered chromosome in Down's syndrome. Genetic studies within families have linked familial AD to mutations of chromosomes 1, 14, 19, and 21 (Schellenberg, et al, 1992). For example, the depositing of the supposedly neurotoxic amyloid is facilitated by the cholesterol-bearing protein apolipoprotein E4 (Apo-E4). The presence of Apo-E4 on chromosome 19 is a risk factor for AD (Corder, et al, 1993).

Toxin model

The toxin model is based on the belief by some researchers that the salts of aluminum may be contributing to the development of AD. These salts may be released by aluminum cans, antiperspirants, and utensils or may be added to food and drugs, such as processed cheeses, antacids, and buffered acids. Several researchers have reported higher concentrations of aluminum in the brains of patients with AD than in those of older persons without dementia. Current researchers are divided on the role of aluminum in AD. Some research suggests that aluminum brain concentrations are a result and not a cause of AD, whereas other research continues to implicate aluminum as an etiological factor (Davis, 1994). To date, no data have been presented regarding the efficacy of aluminum chelator therapy in patients with AD (Gottfries, 1992).

Infection model

The infectious agent model was an early hypothesis arising from suggestions that AD was caused by a slow-growing virus. However, research has not isolated a virus, and there is no current evidence that AD can be transmitted from person to person (Cohen and Eisdorfer, 1986).

Cholinergic deficit model

The cholinergic hypothesis is based on the direct relationship between the loss of cholinergic neurons in the brain, primarily in the nucleus basalis of Meynert, and the degree of cognitive impairment in AD (Zubenko, et al, 1988; Sparks, et al, 1992). Biochemical abnormalities such as reductions in choline acetyltransferase (ChAT), acetylcholinesterase (AChE), and acetylcholine (ACh) biosynthesis and metabolism are strongly associated with the degree of cognitive dysfunction and memory loss observed in AD (Cummings, 1992a; Sparks, et al, 1992). The combination of acetyl coenzyme A and choline to form ACh occurs in cholinergic presynaptic neurons by the action of the enzyme ChAT. These metabolic processes are required for normal cholinergic transmission. ACh binds to cholinergic receptors located at postsynaptic neurons and stimulates those receptors (causing a cholinergic response). AChE is responsible for the metabolism of ACh. As will be discussed later, current efforts to treat AD are focused on decreasing the levels of AChE to slow the metabolism of ACh.

Marked decreases in the activity of the cholinergic enzyme ChAT and reductions in AChE activity have been observed in AD cases. Overall reductions in choline metabolism and marked decreases in the release and synthesis of ACh have all been found in patients with AD (Nordberg, 1992). Further, supportive evidence of the importance of ACh is derived from investigations in which powerful cholinergic antagonists such as scopolamine and atropine have been found to impair cognitive abilities. This information represents strong evidence for the cholinergic hypothesis. It should be noted that significant reductions in norepinephrine, serotonin, gamma-aminobutyric acid (GABA), substance P, corticotropin-releasing factor, and other transmitters also occur in AD. These neurotransmitter reductions may partially explain other symptoms frequently seen in AD patients, for example, depression, sleep-wake disturbances, and motor dysfunction. Intense research efforts to determine the causes of AD and what preventive steps, if any, can be taken continue and are a high national research priority.

Psychiatric Symptoms of AD

Behavioral symptoms of AD have a profound impact upon care both in the home and in the institutional setting (Box 30-4). Often, it is the severity of these symptoms that creates the need for institutionalization. Often families that can absorb the demands associated with cognitive impairment find they cannot adjust to behavioral deviance.

Treatment

New drugs for AD and new information about genetic links offer hope for individuals with this progressively debilitating disease. The recently released AChE inhibitor donepezil (Aricept) and the slightly older tacrine (Cognex) have worked well for many patients with mild-to-moderate disease. These drugs inhibit cholinesterase (or AChE) and by doing so enhance cholinergic function. This action is thought to be responsible for the modest improvement found in some victims of early-stage AD who can tolerate the drugs.

There is no evidence that these drugs alter the course of the underlying process of dementia. Patients who benefit usually improve to the level of function they had the previous year. There is a relatively high incidence of side effects with tacrine. It is potentially hepatotoxic, and liver aminotransferase (ALT, also known as SGPT) must be closely monitored. Tacrine therapy also requires the patient have a well-established diagnosis of AD, normal liver function, and a caregiver who is willing to administer the drug 4 times a day (Keltner, et al, 1998).

Donepezil, unlike tacrine, allows once-daily dosing, causes fewer side effects, and is not associated with hepatotoxicity or tolerance. Although the specific long-term effects of these cognitive-enhancing drugs have not been established, there is some indication that the drugs will favorably affect the course of AD. Families must be discouraged from expecting major improvements and encouraged to hope for sustained patient functions that help to maintain independence (Keltner, et al, 1998). Finally, the long-term use of nonsteroidal antiinflammatory drugs (NSAIDs) or steroids may prevent or slow the onset of AD (Breitner, et al, 1994). These findings are consistent with previous observations that an inverse relationship exists between AD and rheumatoid arthritis when arthritic patients are treated with these drugs.

Vitamin E and other antioxidants are thought to be of potential benefit in the treatment of Alzheimer's disease. The antioxidant qualities of these vitamins combats the oxidation process that synthesizes cytotoxic free radicals. The American Psychiatric Association (1997) reports a delay in neg-

---

Box 30-4	**Behavioral Symptoms Associated with Alzheimer's Disease**

Hallucinations
Delusions
Dysphoria and depression
Fearfulness
Repetitive purposeless acts
Avoidance behavior
Motor restlessness
Apathy
Verbal and physical aggression
Resistance to interventions:
   Hygiene
   Nutrition
   Safety

Adapted from Borson S and Raskind MA: Clinical features and pharmacologic treatment of behavioral symptoms of Alzheimer's disease, *Neurology* 48(suppl 6):S17, 1997.

---

ative outcomes such as death and institutionalization with moderately impaired Alzheimer's patients when they are treated with antioxidants.

■ Critical Thinking Question

When assessing patients and their families with cognitive disorders, what skills of the nurse are the most essential?

Family Considerations

Approximately 80% of the care of AD patients is provided by members of the patient's family (Haley, 1997; Office of Technology Assessment, 1987). The median length of care in the home before placement in a nursing home is roughly 6.5 years, with the average family providing about 60 hours of care per patient per week (Aneshensel, et al, 1995; Max, Webber, and Fox, 1995). This service the family provides is valued at $34,000 and obviously saves third-party payers, including the government, a great deal of money (Max, Webber, and Fox, 1995). No wonder taking care of an AD patient at home has been described as the toughest job in the world. For families facing this daunting task the nurse can recommend

FAMILY ISSUES

Family Issues: Strategies for Coping with Alzheimer's Disease and Dementia

Be informed. The more you know about the nature of dementing illnesses, the more effective you will be in devising strategies to manage behavior problems.

Share your concerns with the patient. When a person is mildly impaired, he can take part in managing his problems. Together you may be able to devise memory aids that will help the patient remain independent.

Try to solve your most frustrating problems one at a time. Day-to-day problems often seem to be the most insurmountable. Getting the person to take his bath or getting a meal prepared, eaten, and cleaned up can become daily ordeals. If you are at the end of your rope, single out one thing that you can change to make life easier and work on that.

Get enough rest. One of the dilemmas families often face is that the caregiver may not get enough rest. This can make the caregiver less patient and less able to tolerate irritating behaviors.

Use your common sense and imagination. Adaptation is the key to success. If a thing cannot be done one way, ask yourself if it must be done at all. For example, if a person can eat successfully with his fingers but cannot use a fork

and spoon appropriately, don't fight the problem; serve as many finger foods as possible.

Maintain a sense of humor. The sick person is still a person. He needs and enjoys a good laugh too. Sharing your experiences with other families will help you.

Try to establish an environment that allows as much *freedom* as possible but also offers the *structure* that confused people need. Establish a regular, predictable, simple routine for meals, medication, exercising, bedtime, and other activities.

Remember to talk to the confused person. Speak calmly and gently. Avoid talking about him in front of him, and remind others to avoid this also.

Have an ID necklace or bracelet made for the confused person. This is one of the single most important things you can do. Many confused people get lost or wander away, and an ID can save you hours of frantic worry.

Keep the impaired person active but not upset. Activity helps to maintain physical well-being and may help to prevent other illnesses and infections. Being active helps the ill person to continue to feel that he is involved in the family and that his life has meaning.

From Mace NL and Rabins PV, editors: *The 36-hour day,* Baltimore, 1991, Johns Hopkins University Press.

---

the book *The 36-Hour Day.* The Family Issues box in this chapter provides important excerpts from this book.

PARKINSON'S DISEASE

Description and Incidence

Parkinson's disease (PD), a hypokinetic disorder, is a progressive, chronic, degenerative disease involving an area of the brain called the extrapyramidal system. The extrapyramidal system is associated with involuntary movements; when compromised, as in PD, it will cause an individual to experience tremor, bradykinesia, and rigidity and a host of associated symptoms. The major cause of extrapyramidal system malfunction is a deficiency in the neurotransmitter dopamine and a subsequent decrease in dopamine transmission to the basal ganglia.

Dopamine is primarily produced in a pigmented area of the midbrain called the substantia nigra. In PD the substantia nigra loses its pigmentation and consequently its ability to produce dopamine (see Figure 30-5).

Nigrostriatal decline does not occur in isolation. Cholinergic and adrenergic systems are affected as well. Consequently, dementias and depressions occur in PD patients. Dementia develops in 15% to 20% of patients with PD, and approximately 40% of these patients suffer from depression (Cummings, 1992a; Stacy and Jankovic, 1992). Chapter 19 provides a more complete review of the overall pathology associated with PD, and that detail is not repeated here.

PD occurs worldwide and was first described by its namesake, Dr. James Parkinson, in 1817. The incidence of the disease is increasing in the United States in large part due to greater public awareness and better diagnostic capabilities. Incidence rates in the United States and Europe show figures close to 20 new cases per 100,000 per year (Tanner, 1992). Approximately 2% of the U.S. population over age 65 suffers from PD (Montgomery, 1995). Onset is usually in the fifth and sixth decades of life and affects men and women equally. Life expectancy for patients with untreated PD is reduced.

Progression of the Disease

PD is predominantly a motor disorder, characterized by slowness and weakness of voluntary movement, rigidity, and tremor. Usually there is no clear sign showing when the disease begins. Tremor is usually the initial symptom, beginning on one side of the body in an upper extremity. The tremor often spreads to both sides of the body, and there is a general tendency to move more slowly and to experience difficulty in performing activities of daily living. The slowdown in voluntary movement may be so severe that the person becomes unable to initiate movement. The patient has increased difficulty in walking and resorts to short, quick steps or a shuffling of the feet. Older persons have difficulty with balance and may have frequent falls. They often have trouble bathing and dressing themselves, getting in and out of bed, and turning themselves in bed. Handwriting may become illegible. The patient may have an expressionless face with monotonous speech, excessive salivation, and limited ocular mobility. The patient with PD may become confused, depressed, disoriented, delusional, and hallucinatory.

It is important for patients with PD to remain as physically, socially, and intellectually active as possible. Exercise programs and increased activity are important to maintain optimal performance. The current treatment for PD includes the administration of antiparkinson drugs (see Chapter 19).

Etiology

The disease is degenerative, affecting the basal ganglia and the extrapyramidal nervous system. The basal ganglia contain short anatomical pathways that connect the basal ganglionic structures to the cerebral cortex. This system has an important role in modifying posture for cortically induced movements. As noted above, there is a loss of dopamine-

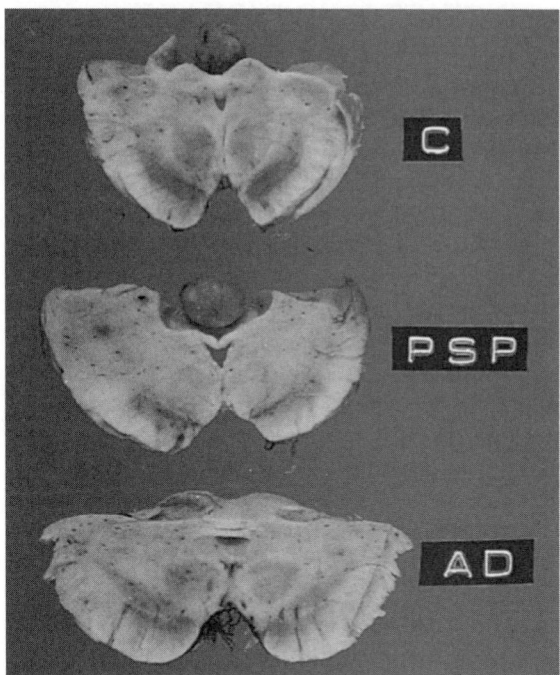

FIGURE 30-5   Contrast of the midbrains of three persons: *C,* control subject; *PSP,* person with a Parkinson-like disease; and *AD,* person with Alzheimer's disease. Note that the substantia nigra (source of dopamine) is more pigmented in *C* than in *PSP* or *AD.* (Courtesy Dr. Richard E. Powers, UAB-BRP.)

generating cells in the substantia nigra, which is located in the midbrain. These cells are rich in dopamine, and cell loss decreases dopamine levels, leading to the symptoms of PD (Matteson and McConnell, 1988).

DIFFUSE LEWY BODY DISEASE

Diffuse Lewy body disease (DLBD) is becoming recognized as a significant cause of dementia. DLBD is similar to AD but typically occurs earlier in life and is associated more often with hallucinations and extrapyramidal symptoms. It evolves more rapidly as well (APA, 1997). The pathological features are the presence of multiple Lewy bodies (eosinophilic cytoplasmic inclusions) in cortical and subcortical neurons (Keltner, et al, 1998). DLBD may account for 7% to 26% of all dementia cases.

HUNTINGTON'S DISEASE

Huntington's disease, formerly called Huntington's chorea, involves both motor and cognitive changes. It is almost the kinetic opposite of PD (i.e., it is a hyperkinetic disorder). The disease is characterized by uncontrollable quick, jerky, and purposeless writhing movements. Disturbances of gait and slurred speech are noted in the beginning and progress into neurological and intellectual deterioration. These actions can be mistaken for alcoholism, as the victims resemble drunks in their movement and speech. The symptoms include memory loss, paranoia, irritability, impaired impulse control, and lack of tongue and breathing control.

The onset of Huntington's disease usually begins between the ages of 25 and 45, with an average duration of 15 to 20 years. It is a hereditary (autosomal dominant) but fairly *rare* disorder, occurring in 5 of every 100,000 persons in the United States with no gender preference. Children of an affected parent have a 50% chance of inheriting the disease. It does not skip a generation, so unaffected parents cannot pass it on to their children. The only available medical treatment is the administration of drugs to manage the symptoms and decrease choreiform movements. Nursing care and physical, occupational, and speech therapy can help slow the problems of dysphagia, malnutrition, impaired communication, functional disabilities, and behavioral abnormalities. Cognitive decline progresses to dementia, and psychologically, depression and psychotic manifestations are expressed. Death usually results from heart failure or pulmonary complications caused by asphyxiation or aspiration of food.

PICK'S DISEASE

The onset, course, and clinical presentation of Pick's disease are similar to those of AD and are usually treated in the same manner. This disease is almost exclusively associated with aging and is without race or gender bias. It usually occurs between the ages of 50 and 60 (APA, 1997). Onset is slow, and the disease progresses until death, with an average duration of 5 to 7 years (Matteson and McConnell, 1988).

Symptoms include progressive impairment of cognition, memory, and orientation, which are similar to those of Alzheimer's disease. Neuropsychiatric problems include hallucinations, delusions, and personality changes. Language disorders, apathy, and depression are also noted. Treatment is aimed toward management of the symptoms, as there is no cure. There is no known genetic component to the disease.

Pick's disease is differentiated from AD in several ways post mortem. Whereas AD is characterized by involvement of higher brain structures, Pick's disease is characterized by shrinkage of the frontal lobes. Neurons decrease in number in Pick's disease, and the preponderance of senile plaques, amyloid deposits, and neurofibrillary tangles found in AD is not found at postmortem examination.

CREUTZFELDT-JAKOB DISEASE

Creutzfeldt-Jakob (CJ) disease (also known as a prion disease) is a noninflammatory dementia that accounts for fewer than 1% of all cases of dementia. A prion is an infectious particle, smaller than a virus. There is no gender, racial, or socioeconomic predisposition for the infectious disease. Approximately 10% of cases are familial (Keltner, et al, 1998). It is a rapidly progressive disorder of the central nervous system involving severe neurological impairment with marked dysfunction. This disease affects the cerebral cortex through cell destruction. Symptoms include early vision and hearing disturbances, impaired cognition, myoclonus, ataxia, muscle wasting, tremor, hallucinations, and illusions. This fatal brain disorder resembles scrapie, a disease found in sheep and cattle (i.e., mad cow disease). Box 30-5 presents the health problems associated with mad cow disease in Britain.

CJ disease is rare, with approximately one case per 1 million population. It is distinguished clini-

---

Box 30-5 Mad Cow Disease

As of late summer 1997, 22 people in Britain had contracted mad cow disease, a variant of Creutzfeldt-Jakob disease. The latest victim was a vegetarian, which adds to concerns related to disease containment. Twenty people have died. Other European countries have responded by banning British beef exports.

Adapted from *Birmingham News*, p. 12A, August 23, 1997.

cally by a rapid onset. There is no known cure, and death occurs within 9 months to 1 year after the onset of symptoms (Brown, Preece, and Will, 1992). CJ disease is of interest because it can be passed from person to person, and antimicrobial and antiviral medications are not effective for prion-mediated diseases. Most cases of CJ disease occur spontaneously in the population; scientists are unsure how an infected person contracts the prion. Some health care professionals have contracted the disease through neurosurgical or autopsy contamination. There is no evidence that nursing personnel are at increased risk for developing the disease, but standard universal precautions should be observed (Keltner, et al, 1998).

VASCULAR OR MULTIINFARCT DEMENTIA

Vascular dementia, also referred to as multiinfarct dementia (MID), is identified as being a vascular disorder in which there are multiple large and small cerebral infarctions. Cerebrovascular disease may be the leading cause of acquired intellectual impairment in the age 85 and older population (Skoog, et al, 1993).

Two criteria increase the probability that a patient is suffering from a MID (Butler, et al, 1994):

1. The first symptoms of dementia appear within the first year of focal neurologic symptoms or signs.
2. The patient has known risk factors for vascular disease.

Risk factors include hypertension, hyperlipidemia, atrial fibrillation, diabetes, history of smoking, and a sedentary life-style. Public health considerations mandate health teaching and health interventions aimed at prevention and early treatment. Numerous options are considered when a person is asymptomatic but at high risk. These include treatment of hypertension, elevated cholesterol, and atrial fibrillation, as well as smoking cessation, exercise, and dietary changes.

The diagnosis of MID is made by clinical history, physical assessment, neurological examination, and brain imaging studies. There is no blood or spinal fluid test that distinguishes MID from other types of dementia (Keltner, et al, 1998). Although there is no specific treatment for MID, anticoagulants such as aspirin and warfarin (Coumadin) may help. Manage-

ment of patients with high-risk factors by correcting underlying medical problems (e.g., controlling hypertension) may slow the progression of the disease. For patients with advancing MID, treatment focuses on preventing further cardiovascular damage and managing related symptoms, such as depression (Butler, et al, 1994).

ALCOHOLIC DEMENTIA

Dementia related to alcoholism accounts for between 1% and 10% of all cases of dementia in patients over age 65. Alcoholic dementia typically occurs after 15 to 20 years of continuous drinking. Alcoholic dementia has three primary causes:

1. Alcohol is directly toxic to neurons.
2. Alcoholism causes a destructive nutritional deficit.
3. Alcoholism causes end organ failure such as cirrhosis and cardiomyopathy which, in turn, affect the central nervous system.

Cognitive problems include amnesia, slowness of thinking, and impaired judgment. Wernicke's encephalopathy and Korsakoff's psychosis are the diagnostic terms used to identify specific neurodegenerative processes. Prominent features include confusion and short-term memory loss. Alcohol also worsens the cognitive function in the elderly who are afflicted with other types of cognitive disorders; for example, alcohol worsens the cognitive state of a patient with Alzheimer's disease.

TRANSIENT ISCHEMIC ATTACKS

Transient ischemic attacks (TIAs) are brief episodes of focal neurologic dysfunction that are entirely reversible and without any residual deficit; they last less than 24 hours, usually less than 20 minutes. TIAs may recur with striking uniformity or may vary considerably. The two main types of TIAs are vertebrobasilar ischemic attacks and carotid ischemic attacks. The chief importance of a TIA is as a precursor of a major stroke, myocardial infarction, or death (Kane-Carlsen, 1990).

This syndrome is caused by a microembolism to the brain from atherosclerotic plaques in the aortocranial arteries in about 90% of the persons who have TIAs. In the remaining 10%, TIAs are caused by mural thrombi, valvular diseases of the heart, vegetation on the heart valve, polycythemia, or some other blood clotting disorder (Harrell, 1988).

Specific symptoms of TIAs vary, depending on the vessel involved, the degree of obstruction of the vessel, and the collateral blood supply. If the posterior (vertebrobasilar) system is involved, symptoms may include tinnitus, vertigo, facial weakness, ataxia, diplopia, and falling without loss of consciousness. If the anterior (carotid) system is involved, the patient may experience ipsilateral blindness, monocular blurring, flashes of light, and headaches.

An elderly person who has a TIA may ignore an attack as the symptoms completely resolve; however, a physician should be consulted to prevent a possible disabling stroke (Harrell, 1988).

Psychotherapeutic Management

Nurse-Patient Relationship. In a nurse-patient relationship the highest priority of nursing care for a patient with **delirium** is given to interventions that will maintain life. If the patient is unable to attend to basic physiological needs, nursing care must be planned to meet these needs. In a patient with **dementia** the highest priority should be given to providing nursing care to maintain an optimal level of functioning. This will be different for each individual. Often the attitude of hopelessness evolves in those who work with chronically ill persons. This can result in stereotyping and decreased ability to see and appreciate the individuality of each person. Searching for this individuality can be a challenge for the nurse working with patients who have cognitive disorders. Ongoing assessment should include periodic monitoring every 4 to 6 months for the development and evolution of cognitive and noncognitive psychiatric symptoms and their response to intervention (APA, 1997).

The nurse should learn as much as possible about the background and life-style of the patient. This information will enable the nurse to individualize a care plan for each patient. The nurse should address the patient on a one-to-one basis by using the title and last name. However, it should be noted that there are exceptions to this level of formality, and being less formal is often therapeutic as well. Use praise, touch, and affection whenever possible. The patient should be dressed in his or her own clothing during the day with his or her hair combed. Women should wear makeup, and men should be shaved. These and other actions will promote self-confidence and self-esteem in the patient, as well as improve communication between the nurse and the patient. Although independence in all ADLs is fostered, all patients and families should be informed that the risk of accidents is much higher in these individuals. The APA (1997) guidelines urge that moderately and severely impaired individuals stop driving (see Table 30-2 for other areas of impairment).

Psychopharmacology. In general, antipsychotics are recommended for psychotic symptoms, antidepressants for depression, and benzodiazepines for anxiety and insomnia.

Antipsychotics. Antipsychotic medications or neuroleptics are often effective in treating psychotic symptoms such as agitation, hallucinations, delusions, wandering, and assaultiveness. They are of little value in the treatment of apathy or withdrawal and may worsen cognitive-related behavioral deterioration such as incontinence (Borson and Raskind, 1997). Little is known about the optimal use of these drugs in the elderly. Selection of an antipsychotic is typically based on side effect avoidance. The low-potency agents such as chlorpromazine (Thorazine) cause sedative, anticholinergic, and antiadrenergic effects to which the older individual is particularly sensitive. On the other hand, high-potency agents such as haloperidol (Haldol) cause the neurological extrapyramidal effects to which people with neurodegenerative processes are very sensitive as well. Typically, given the need to address psychotic symptoms, the high-potency drugs are more often prescribed. The newer atypical agents such as clozapine (Clozaril) and risperidone (Risperdal) may be the best option.

Antidepressants. Antidepressants are used to treat depression associated with cognitive disorders. Not nearly as many studies have been completed in the cognitively impaired with antidepressants as have been conducted with antipsychotics. Since cognition is compromised when acetylcholine is blocked, antidepressants with significant anticholinergic properties are best avoided. A tricyclic antidepressant (TCA)-induced delirium due to their anticholinergic effects is relatively common among elderly patients receiving these drugs. Patients with diagnosed cognitive impairment are at even greater risk. The best TCAs for this population include the secondary amines nortriptyline (Pamelor) and desipramine (Norpramin). The newer selective serotonin reuptake inhibitors (SSRIs) may be the drug of choice, however, even when psychotic features are prominent, because of the widespread influence of the serotonin system on mood and behavior (Borson and Raskind, 1997).

Antianxiety agents. Benzodiazepines continue to be used for agitation, anxiety, and sleep disturbances, though the Omnibus Budget Reconciliation Act (OBRA) restricts their use in some situations. In the cognitively impaired patient, benzodiazepines may exacerbate confusion and produce agitation, particularly at night. When benzodiazepines are used, those that are conjugated rather than oxidized are preferable (see Chapter 22). Lorazepam (Ativan) and oxazepam (Serax) are favored over drugs such as diazepam (Valium) and chlordiazepoxide (Librium). The nonbenzodiazepine buspirone (BuSpar) is a very safe drug and not subject to OBRA restriction. It is known to be effective in the treatment of anxiety. The SSRIs can be used successfully as well.

Treatment of cognitive impairment. Other than the cholinergic enhancers previously mentioned in the discussion of AD, several other chemical approaches have been or are being studied. The oldest group are the **metabolic enhancers/vasodilators.** Of this group, Hydergine, a compound of ergoloid mesylates, is approved for the treatment of dementia. Studies have not found a benefit to the use of this compound. **Nootropic agents** are used to enhance neuronal metabolic activity and through this process increase cholinergic transmission.

Milieu Management. Patients with cognitive disorders require a milieu in which they are neither overstimulated nor understimulated. They should be in a safe environment; free from injury, stress, and anxiety. The nurse should maintain an environment free of misleading and frightening stimuli. Though environmental considerations such as television, a public address system, pictures of animals, and large group activities can be positive, they can also confuse and frighten the cognitively impaired patient. Good judgment based on understanding the perceptual and conceptual deficits of the cognitively impaired should guide the nurse. Patients should have a warm, caring atmosphere that will fa-

cilitate their developing a trusting interpersonal relationship with the caregivers and other patients. The nurse should develop a routine the patient can follow daily. Close supervision should be provided during bathing, eating, and other activities. All hot or sharp objects or other hazardous materials should be removed from the patient's surroundings. The doors of the facility should be monitored to prevent escape. Through these and other management efforts the patient should be able to live in a relatively comfortable and safe environment. To achieve these goals, the nursing staff must be aware of three milieu-related issues: stress, safety, and wandering.

Stress. Stress has been shown to be a cause of anxious behavior in demented persons. If the level of stress continues or increases, dysfunctional or catastrophic behavior follows. Hall (1988) lists five types of stressors that produce dysfunctional behavior in the cognitively impaired person. Any combination of these stressors will cause the cognitively impaired person to perform at a lower level of functioning than would occur with the cognitive disability alone. In other words, in order to help the cognitively impaired patient perform at his or her highest potential, the nurse needs to structure the environment to minimize these stressors. Following is a concise discussion of these stressors and examples of milieu management.

1. Fatigue
2. Change of environment, routine, or caregiver
3. Overwhelming or competing stimuli
4. Demands that exceed capacity to function
5. Physical stressors

Fatigue. Patients fatigue rapidly from performing basic daily functions and frequently require rest periods both morning and afternoon. These short rest periods should be scheduled in a comfortable chair, such as a recliner, so as not to confuse the patient with going to bed.

Change of environment, routine, or caregiver. A change of environment, routine, or caregiver can be stressful for patients because of their altered ability to plan, initiate, and carry through voluntary activities. Patients will express frustration at trying to initiate and complete simple tasks and may refuse to attempt any activity they feel they cannot complete. Many patients (and nursing staff) compensate for this by developing a consistent routine.

Overwhelming or competing stimuli. Overwhelming or competing stimuli are easily misinterpreted by patients. Elimination of such stimuli as high noise levels, multiple activities, and crowds of people will minimize anxious behavior.

Demands that exceed capacity to function. Demands that exceed patients' functional capacity can be devastating. Some families and staff members think that frequent testing of patients to determine the amount of memory loss is important. However, being asked questions they cannot answer and being told they are wrong can be very frustrating. Reality orientation is generally helpful to patients with mild cognitive impairments. However, if memory loss is severe, reality orientation probably will not succeed. For these patients, reality orientation seems only to deepen their anxiety. Burnside (1988) states that reminiscence group therapy can be used successfully with severely demented patients because it reinforces identity, acknowledges what was significant and enduring in the person's life, and often compensates for the dullness of the present.

Physical stressors. Physical stressors are identified as anything that causes physical discomfort, such as pain, acute illness, and other psychological alterations. Caffeine is one of the most commonly used physical stressors, and its use should be eliminated. Other common stressors are impacted bowels, full bladder, infections, influenza, and medication reactions and interactions. Patients exhibiting stress-related behavior should be given a physical assessment to determine the presence of any physical stressors.

Safety. Safety is an important area that must be addressed in planning care for the patient. As the disease progresses, patients are unable to consider their own safety needs and risks. Disoriented patients may try to run away, resulting in injuries to themselves or others. Falls are a safety problem, and the nurse should make an evaluation of the environment to eliminate obstacles, slippery floors, throw rugs, and inadequate lighting.

Key Nursing Interventions for Wandering

Possible Causes for Wandering
- Confusion
- Restlessness
- Boredom
- Need for exercise

Interventions
- Safety first
- Identification
- Medic Alert bracelets
- Motion or sound detectors
- Alternative outlet for energy
- Medications

*C*ase *S*tudy

Nancy Moore, age 74, has been diagnosed with Alzheimer's disease for 4 years. Initially she was able to function at home with the help of her husband. After his death she went to live with her daughter. While at her daughter's home her memory and cognitive function deteriorated rapidly. She became more and more withdrawn during the day and began staying awake at night and was found wandering in the yard several times. She became less and less socially interactive and started refusing food and water. After several weeks her daughter could no longer manage her and went to her family doctor to discuss her mother's condition. Mrs. Moore was examined at the office and found to have a 20-lb weight loss and to be severely dehydrated. She was admitted to the hospital for fluids and nutritional support. In the hospital environment she continued to deteriorate, and it became necessary to feed her with a nasal feeding tube and then to place a gastric feeding tube for more permanent access. It was her family's desire to continue to care for her at home for as long as possible, so a home health referral was made and a home teaching program was initiated. During this hospitalization Mrs. Moore's family has had their attention focused on just how serious her care needs and the family's responsibilities have become. On the one hand they want to give the very best care to their mother, but now they are faced with the decision of where and how that care can best be delivered. They hope to keep her in the home setting for as long as possible, but they now realize that this may not be a realistic solution.

Other hazards include such objects as razors and electrical devices, which should be used under supervision. Anything that might harm the patient should not be left at the bedside. Substances that could be ingested, such as toiletries, cleaning solutions, and plants, should be monitored carefully. All caregivers should be aware of and trained to recognize potential hazards to assure a safe environment for the patient. Soft restraints should not be used indiscriminately and should be used only when all other nursing interventions have been unsuccessful in protecting the patient.

Wandering.   Patients who wander inadvertently or who try to escape present a problem for caregivers, whether at home or in an institution. These patients must be identified and plans made to minimize the risks. The patient's clothing must carry some markings to identify him or her, and a photograph should be on file to be used in locating the individual. Special alarms should be installed to alert staff if the patient attempts to leave the facility. A number of risks are involved when a patient wanders, ranging from simple exposure to being the potential victim of crime. Possible causes of wandering and intervention strategies are presented in the box on p. 472.

Care Plan

NAME: _Nancy Moore_   **ADMISSION DATE:** _____

DSM-IV DIAGNOSIS: _Dementia, Alzheimer's type_

ASSESSMENT: **Areas of strength:** Supportive family who wishes to provide care at home for as long as possible.
Problems: Severe confusion, recent and remote memory loss. Wandering behavior. Sensory aphasia. Has had recent placement of gastric feeding tube to meet nutritional needs.

DIAGNOSES:
• Self-care deficit related to cognitive impairment, as evidenced by wandering, confusion, and inability to take care of her own nutritional needs.
• Impaired social interaction, related to communication barriers and altered thought processes, as evidenced by observed discomfort in different social settings.
• Impaired verbal communication, related to sensory aphasia, as evidenced by disorientation and inability to communicate her needs.

OUTCOMES: **Short-term goals:**   Date met
• Patient will remain safe and free of injury.   _____
• Family will learn feeding requirements of the patient.   _____
Long-term goals:
• Patient will remain active and as independent as possible.   _____
• Patient's nutritional and other physical needs will be met in the home
  setting.   _____

PLANNING/ **Nurse-patient relationship:** Provide a set routine for care.
INTERVENTIONS: Have family return-demonstrate appropriate care while feeding the patient.
Psychopharmacology: Monitor medication side effects. Teach family.
Milieu management: Monitor and provide safe care in all ADLs; monitor home setting for indicators of stress overload in family members as well as patient.

EVALUATION: Patient remains safe and secure; patient will gain 1 to 2 lb per month until at ideal body weight.

REFERRALS: Contact home health nurse. Give family phone number for AD support group.

■ Critical Thinking Question

Decisions regarding the need for placement in a long term care facility depend upon the degree to which the patient's needs can be met in the home. What is the first priority for consideration when moving to long-term care or another type of facility?

■ Key Concepts

1. In delirium there is sudden but usually temporary widespread cerebral dysfunction.
2. The primary symptoms of dementia are cognitive symptoms that interfere with daily functioning. Dementia is gradual in onset but progressive, hence a poor prognosis.
3. Alzheimer's disease (AD) is a chronic, nonreversible form of dementia, most commonly seen in the elderly. The four As of AD are amnesia, aphasia, agnosia, and apraxia.
4. Other cognitive disturbances include alterations in abstract thinking, judgment, and perceptions.
5. Parkinson's disease (PD) is a degenerative motor disorder related to the loss of dopamine-generating cells in the substantia nigra.
6. Huntington's disease is a rare hereditary disorder involving deterioration of both motor and cognitive functions.
7. Priority nursing interventions with delirium are those that maintain life. Priority nursing interventions with dementia are those that maintain an optimal level of functioning.
8. Medications prescribed for cognitive disorders depend on the predominant type of symptoms, but all are used cautiously with the elderly.
9. Patients with cognitive disorders require a caring, structured milieu that minimizes stress, provides for safety, and reduces the possibility of wandering.

■ Study Questions

(Answer key is in the back of the book.)

1. The major symptoms of delirium include:
   a. Primarily cognitive disturbances developing gradually with age
   b. A widespread cerebral dysfunction affecting thinking, attention, perception, memory, consciousness, and activity level
   c. Transient pathological, neurological symptoms such as ataxia and diplopia
   d. Changes in motor functioning, rigidity, and tremor

2. The major symptoms of dementia include
   a. Depression, aphasia, restlessness, and wandering
   b. Vision and hearing disturbances and ataxia
   c. Impaired intellectual function and judgment and changes in personality and perceptions
   d. Disturbances in reflexes, memory, and impulse control

Match each of the following cognitive disorders with its primary characteristics:

3. ____ Alzheimer's disease (AD)
4. ____ Parkinson's disease (PD)
5. ____ Huntington's disease

   a. Neurological disorder causing tremor, rigidity, and weakness in voluntary movement
   b. Deterioration of neurological, motor, and intellectual functions
   c. Progressive nonreversible CNS disorder affecting cognitive function

Mark questions 6 and 7 true or false.

6. ____ Antipsychotic medications are not particularly effective in treating symptoms of delirium and dementia.
7. ____ The primary goal of nursing care for a patient with dementia is an individualized approach that maintains an optimal level of functioning.
8. The percentage of the American population over age 17 that has a cognitive disorder is approximately:
   a. 1%
   b. 3%
   c. 5%
   d. 10%
9. The incidence of AD in the U.S. population over the age of 65 is:
   a. Less than 1%
   b. About 5%
   c. About 10%
   d. About 30%
10. Tacrine is classified pharmacologically as a:
    a. Cholinomimetic
    b. Cholinesterase inhibitor
    c. MAO-B inhibitor
    d. Antipsychotic
11. Over the age of 85 about what percentage of the U.S. population develops AD?
    a. 5%
    b. 10%
    c. 25%
    d. 50%
12. A serum enzyme that can elevate when using tacrine is:
    a. ChE
    b. CPK
    c. ALT
    d. MAO

13. Lesions related to AD can be found in all of the following brain sites except the:
    a. Hippocampus
    b. Cerebral cortex
    c. Nucleus basalis of Meynert
    d. All of the above

REFERENCES

Adem A: Putative mechanisms of action of tacrine in Alzheimer's disease, *Acta Neurol Scand* 139(suppl):69, 1992.

Alafuzoff I: The pathology of dementias: an overview, *Acta Neurol Scand* 139(suppl):8, 1992.

American Psychiatric Association: *Diagnostic and statistical manual of mental disorders,* ed 4, Washington, DC, 1994, The Association.

American Psychiatric Association: Practice guidelines for the treatment of patients with Alzheimer's disease and other dementias of late life, *Am J Psychiatry* 154(5)(suppl):1, 1997.

Aneshensel CS, et al: *Profiles in caregiving: the unexpected career,* San Diego, 1995, Academic Press.

Batt LJ: Managing delirium, *J Psychosoc Nurs Ment Health Serv* 27:22, 1989.

Borson S and Raskind MA: Clinical features and pharmacologic treatment of behavioral symptoms of Alzheimer's disease, *Neurology* 48(suppl 6):S17, 1997.

Breitner JC, et al: Inverse association of anti-inflammatory treatments and Alzheimer's disease: initial results of a co-twin control study, *Neurology* 44:227, 1994.

Brown P, Preece MA, and Will RG: "Friendly fire" in medicine: hormones, homografts, and Creutzfeldt-Jakob disease, *Lancet* 340:24, 1992.

Burnside IM: Dementia and delirium. In Burnside IM, editor: *Nursing and the aged: a self-care approach,* ed 3, New York, 1988, McGraw-Hill.

Butler RN, et al: Vascular dementia: an updated approach to patient management, *Geriatrics* 49:39, 1994.

Cameron DJ, et al: Delirium: a test of the Diagnostic and Statistical Manual III criteria on medical inpatients, *J Am Geriatr Soc* 35:1007, 1987.

Cohen D and Eisdorfer C: Dementia disorders. In Calkins E, Davis PJ, and Ford AB, editors: *The practice of geriatrics,* Philadelphia, 1986, WB Saunders.

Cohen GD: Alzheimer's disease: clinical update, *Hosp Community Psychiatry* 41:496, 1990.

Corder EH, et al: Gene dose of alipoprotein E type allele and the risk of Alzheimer's disease in late-onset families, *Science* 261:828, 1993.

Cummings JL: Dementia syndromes: neurobehavioral and neuropsychiatric features, *J Clin Psychiatry* 48(suppl):3, 1987.

Cummings JL: Clinical diagnosis of dementia of the Alzheimer type. In Miner GD, et al, editors: *Caring for Alzheimer's patients: a guide for family and healthcare providers,* New York and London, 1991, Plenum Press, Insight Books.

Cummings JL: Depression and Parkinson's disease, *Am J Psychiatry* 149(4):443, 1992a.

Cummings JL: Neuropsychiatric aspects of Alzheimer's disease and other dementing illnesses. In Yodofsky SC and Hales RE, editors: *The American Psychiatric Press textbook of neuropsychiatry,* ed 2, Washington DC, 1992b, American Psychiatric Press.

Davis WM: The status of therapy for Alzheimer's disease, *Drug Topics* 138(9):96, 1994.

Dawson P, et al: Preventing excess disability in patients with Alzheimer's disease, *Geriatr Nurs* 7:299, 1986.

de Leon J, et al: A pilot effort to determine benztropine equivalents of anticholinergic medications, *Hosp Community Psychiatry* 45(6):606, 1994.

Ernst R and Hay J: The US economic and social cost of Alzheimer's disease, *Am J Public Health* 84:1261, 1994.

Farlow M, et al: A controlled trial of tacrine in Alzheimer's disease, *JAMA* 268:365, 1992.

First MB, et al: Changes in substance-related, schizophrenic, and other primarily adult disorders, *Hosp Community Psychiatry* 45(1):18, 1994.

Foreman MD: Acute confusional states in hospitalized elderly: a research dilemma, *Nurs Res* 35:34, 1986.

Francis J, Martin D, and Kapoor W: A prospective study of delirium in hospitalized elderly, *JAMA* 263:1097, 1990.

Geldmacher DS and Whitehouse PJ: Differential diagnosis of Alzheimer's disease, *Neurology* 48(suppl 6):S2, 1997.

Gomez GE and Gomez EA: Delirium, *Geriatr Nurs* 8:330, 1987.

Gottfries CG: Review of treatment strategies, *Acta Neurol Scand* 139(suppl):63, 1992.

Haley WE: The family caregiver's role in Alzheimer's disease, *Neurology* 48(suppl 6):S25, 1997.

Hall GR: Alterations in thought process, *J Gerontol Nurs* 14:30, 1988.

Hall GR and Buckwalter KC: Progressively lowered stress threshold: a conceptual model for care of adults with Alzheimer's disease, *Arch Psychiatr Nurs* 1:399, 1987.

Harrell JS: Age related changes in the cardiovascular system. In Matteson MA and McConnell ES, editors: *Gerontological nursing concepts and practice,* Philadelphia, 1988, WB Saunders.

Heim KM: Wandering behavior, *J Gerontol Nurs* 12:4, 1986.

Iqbal K and Wisniewski HM: Neurofibrillary tangles. In Reisberg B, editor: *Alzheimer's disease: the standard reference,* New York, 1983, Free Press, Macmillan Publishing.

Kane-Carlsen PA: Transient ischemic attacks: clinical features, pathophysiology and management, *Nurse Practit* 7:9, 1990.

Keltner N: Tacrine: a pharmacological approach to Alzheimer's disease, *J Psychosoc Nurs Ment Health Serv* 32(3): 37, 1994.

Keltner NL, et al: *Psychobiological foundations of psychiatric care*, St Louis: Mosby, 1998.

Kermis MD: Mental health in late life: the adaptive process, Boston, 1986, Jones & Bartlett.

Kotulak R: Protein find could lead to anti-Alzheimer's drug, *Birmingham News*, 5/28/98, p. 11A, May 23, 1998.

Levkoff SE, et al: Epidemiology of delirium: an overview of research issues and findings, *Int Psychogeriatr* 3(2): 149, 1991.

Lipowski ZJ: Delirium in the elderly patient, *N Engl J Med* 320:578, 1989.

Lucas MJ, Steel C, and Bognanni A: Recognition of psychiatric symptoms in dementia, *J Gerontol Nurs* 12:11, 1986.

Mace NL and Rabins PV, editors: *The 36-hour day,* Baltimore, 1991, Johns Hopkins University Press.

Margo GM and Finkel JA: Early dementia as a risk factor for suicide, *Hosp Community Psychiatry* 41:676, 1990.

Matteson MA: Age-related changes in the neurological system. In Matteson MA and McConnell ES, editors: *Gerontological nursing concepts and practice,* Philadelphia, 1988, WB Saunders.

Matteson MA and McConnell ES, editors: *Gerontological nursing concepts and practice,* Philadelphia, 1988, WB Saunders.

Max W: The economic impact of Alzheimer's disease, *Neurology* 43(suppl 4):S6, 1993.

Max W, Webber P, and Fox P: Alzheimer's disease: the unpaid burden of caring, *J Aging Health* 7:179, 1995.

McDowell FH: Other neurologic diseases of the elderly. In Calkins E, Davis PJ, and Ford AB, editors: *The practice of geriatrics,* Philadelphia, 1986, WB Saunders.

Mohs RC, et al: Alzheimer's disease: morbid risk among first-degree relatives approximates 50% by 90 years of age, *Arch Gen Psychiatry* 44:405, 1987.

Montgomery EB: Heavy metals and the etiology of Parkinson's disease and other movement disorders, *Toxicology* 97:3, 1995.

Nordberg A: Biological markers and the cholinergic hypothesis in Alzheimer's disease, *Acta Neurol Scand* 139(suppl):54, 1992.

Office of Technology Assessment: Losing a million minds: confronting the tragedy of Alzheimer's disease and other dementias, Washington, 1987, US Government Printing Office.

Patkar AA and Kunkel EJ: Treating delirium among elderly patients, *Psychiatr Serv* 48:1, 1997.

Pieri L, Cumin R, and Hinzen DH: Nosological and epidemiological aspects of Alzheimer's disease, *Dis Neurol Psychiatry* 2:248, 1989.

Roberts GW, Leigh PN, and Weinberger DR: *Neuropsychiatric disorders,* London, 1993, Wolfe Publishing.

Schellenberg GD, et al: Genetic linkage evidence for a familial Alzheimer's disease locus on chromosome 14, *Science* 258:668, 1992.

Skoog I, et al: A population-based study of dementia in 85-year olds, *N Engl J Med* 328:153, 1993.

Sparks DL, et al: Monoaminergic and cholinergic synaptic markers in the nucleus basalis of Meynert(nbM): normal age-related changes and the effect of heart disease and Alzheimer's disease, *Ann Neurol* 31:611, 1992.

Stacy M and Jankovic J: Differential diagnosis of Parkinson's disease and the parkinsonism plus syndromes, *Neurol Clin* 10(2):341, 1992.

Tanner CM: Epidemiology of Parkinson's disease, *Neurol Clin* 10(2):317, 1992.

Williams L: Alzheimer's: the need for caring, *J Gerontol Nurs* 12:21, 1986.

Wills R: Cognitive changes of normal aging and the dementias. In Carnevali DL and Patrick M, editors: *Nursing management for the elderly,* ed 2, Philadelphia, 1986, JB Lippincott.

Young SH, Muir-Nash J, and Ninos M: Managing nocturnal wandering behavior, *J Gerontol Nurs* 14:6, 1988.

Zisook S and Braff DL: Delirium: recognition and management in the older patient, *Geriatrics* 41:67, 1986.

Zubenko GS, et al: Bilateral symmetry of cholinergic deficits in Alzheimer's disease, *Arch Neurol* 45:255, 1988.

CHAPTER 31

Personality Disorders

CAROL E. BOSTROM

LEARNING OBJECTIVES

After reading this chapter you should be able to:
- Recognize characteristics of each personality disorder.
- Describe behaviors of persons with personality disorders.
- Describe nursing interventions for patients with personality disorders.
- Recognize issues related to the care of patients with personality disorders.

This chapter focuses on patients with personality disorders hospitalized in the inpatient psychiatric setting or treated in outpatient programs. Except for the patient with a borderline disorder, these patients are not usually hospitalized because of their personality disorders but because of other mental disorders diagnosed on axis I. The interventions focus primarily on the nurse-patient relationship unique to each personality disorder, and this chapter does not repeat the general nurse-patient interventions described in Chapter 7. Neither milieu issues nor psychopharmacology will be addressed for each disorder because milieu and pharmacological interventions are not appropriate for all disorders. Medication may be given if the patient has an axis I diagnosis or a symptom severe enough to interfere with functioning, such as severe anxiety or depression.

All of us have personality traits and characteristics that make us unique and interesting human beings. Our traits are exhibited in the way we think about ourselves and others and in how we behave. When traits are inflexible and dysfunctional, we generally have problems in functioning and experience subjective distress. Patients with personality disorders suffer lifelong, inflexible, and dysfunctional patterns of relating and behaving. These dysfunctional patterns and behaviors usually cause distress to others. However, individuals with personality disorders do not find their behaviors distressing to themselves. They become distressed because of other people's reactions or behaviors toward them. This affects them by causing immense emotional pain and discomfort. The nurse conveys acceptance of the individual and empathy for emotional pain regardless of the patient's behavior.

Personality disorders are listed on axis II. Axis II can also be used to designate developmental disorders, personality traits, or habitual use of particular defense mechanisms. For example, compulsive traits are not the same as obsessive-compulsive personality disorder, which, in turn, is not the same as obsessive-compulsive disorder. Many high-functioning people have compulsive traits, whereas only a few have compulsive personality disorders. Patients benefit

KEY TERMS

Dissociation   Separation of mental or behavioral processes from the rest of the person's consciousness or identity

Idealization   Viewing others as perfect, exalting others

Devaluation   Criticism of others, which defends against own feelings of inadequacy

Splitting   Inability to integrate good and bad aspects of self and others; viewing self and others as all good or all bad

Projective identification   Placement of feelings on another to justify own expression of feelings

12-Month Prevalence Rate of Mental Disorders in the United States

Diagnosis	Percentage of Population over 17 Years of Age	Number of Persons
Anxiety disorders	12.6	20,034,000
Phobia disorders*	10.9	17,331,000
Mood disorders	9.5	15,143,000
Alcohol disorders	7.4	11,766,000
Major depression†	5.0	7,950,000
Drug disorders	3.1	4,929,000
Cognitive impairment	2.7	4,293,000
Obsessive-compulsive disorder	2.1	3,339,000
Antisocial disorder	**1.5**	**2,385,000**
Panic disorders*	1.3	2,067,000
Bipolar disorder†	1.2	1,908,000
Schizophrenia	1.1	1,749,000
Somatization	0.2	365,000

From Regier DA, et al: The de facto US mental and addictive disorders service system: epidemiologic catchment area prospective 1-year prevalence rates of disorders and services, *Arch Gen Psychiatry* 50:85, 1993.
*Also calculated in anxiety statistics.
†Also calculated in mood disorders statistics.

from the fact that some nurses may have compulsive traits, for example, rechecking labels, dressings, and drainage tubes.

GENERAL ETIOLOGY

Traditional Views

Some psychoanalytical theorists, developmentalists, behaviorists, and social learning theorists believe that personality disorders originate in early childhood experiences. Psychoanalytical and developmental theorists agree that unsuccessful mastery of tasks in early stages of development leads to anxiety and the resultant use of defense mechanisms. The exclusive use of rigid and dysfunctional defense mechanisms characterizes personality disorders.

Behavioral and sociocultural factors reinforce and maintain dysfunctional social behavior exhibited by people with personality disorders. Responses of others reinforce personality tendencies and traits. Children develop personality characteristics by learning, through social experiences. They model their actions after persons around them, particularly their parents. Children repeat actions that bring them rewards and avoid actions that incur punishment. Behavior that has been consistently rewarded from infancy, before the development of understanding, cognition, and language, is the most difficult to unlearn or modify.

Contemporary Views

The development of personality disorders is related to a combination of biological, psychological, and

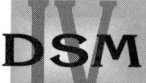

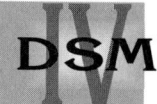

DSM-IV and NANDA Diagnoses Related to Personality Disorders

DSM-IV*

Cluster A—Odd, Eccentric Behaviors
Paranoid personality disorder
Schizoid personality disorder
Schizotypal personality disorder

Cluster B—Dramatic, Emotional, Erratic Behaviors
Antisocial personality disorder
Borderline personality disorder
Histrionic personality disorder
Narcissistic personality disorder

Cluster C—Anxious, Fearful Behaviors
Avoidant personality disorder
Dependent personality disorder
Obsessive-compulsive disorder

NANDA†
Altered family processes
Anxiety
Defensive coping
High risk for self-mutilation
High risk for violence: self-directed or directed at others
Hopelessness
Impaired verbal communication
Ineffective individual coping
Powerlessness
Self-esteem disturbance
Social isolation

*From the American Psychiatric Association: *The diagnostic and statistical manual of mental disorders,* ed 4, Washington, DC, 1994, The Association.
†From the North American Nursing Diagnosis Association: *NANDA nursing diagnoses: definitions and classifications 1997-1998,* Philadelphia, 1997, The Association.

social risk factors (Paris, 1993). These risk factors include genetic components, life experiences, and the influence of the environment. The interaction of these risk factors determines whether or not strong personality traits develop into personality disorders. Biological factors alone are not totally responsible for the occurrence of these disorders. Twin studies indicate that specific traits rather than disorders are inherited.

The social environment coupled with psychological vulnerability strongly influences the individual. The effects of societal changes, a stressful environment, and negative childhood experiences, along with biological factors, are important in the genesis of personality disorders.

PERSONALITY DISORDER CLUSTERS

According to the DSM-IV, the personality disorders are grouped into three clusters on the basis of descriptive features. Cluster A includes the schizoid, schizotypal, and paranoid disorders characterized by odd or eccentric behaviors. Cluster B includes the narcissistic, histrionic, antisocial, and borderline disorders characterized by dramatic, emotional, or erratic behaviors. Cluster C includes the dependent, avoidant, and obsessive-compulsive disorders characterized by anxious or fearful behaviors (American Psychiatric Association [APA], 1994).

When a person exhibits features of more than one specific personality disorder or does not meet the full criteria for any one disorder, the classification of "personality disorder not otherwise specified" is used. DSM-IV diagnoses and potential NANDA nursing diagnoses for personality disorders are listed in the box above.

CLUSTER A: ODD/ECCENTRIC

PARANOID PERSONALITY DISORDER

Suspiciousness and mistrust of people characterize the person with a paranoid personality disorder. They interpret the actions of others as personal threats. This interpretation results in an increase in anxiety and the need to scan the environment. They are hypersensitive to other people's motives but externalize their own feelings by projecting their own desires and traits to others. They feel vulnerable because they think others treat them unfairly. Persons with paranoid personality disorders are unable to laugh at themselves and are often humorless and serious. Speech is logical and goal directed, although the bases of arguments are false due to their suspiciousness. Other symptoms include prejudice and sometimes ideas of reference. Their affect is blunted, and they may appear to be cold, but they are capable of close relationships with a select few. However, they may be suspicious of those close to them. For example, they may unjustifiably believe their spouse is having an affair. The DSM-IV criteria box below presents the diagnostic criteria for this disorder.

Unlike persons with paranoid schizophrenia, these people do not have fixed delusions or hallucinations. Transient psychotic symptoms may be precipitated by extreme stress. People with paranoid personality disorders are hospitalized when their behavior is out of control in response to a threat perceived as overwhelming or immediate. Because they are quick to respond with anger or rage if they feel severely threatened, these patients may be brought to the hospital because of their loss of control and potential for violence.

Unique Etiology

There is some evidence that the paranoid personality disorder tends to occur in biological relatives of identified schizophrenic patients and is diagnosed more often in men than in women (APA, 1994).

CLINICAL EXAMPLE

James Sneed is admitted to the hospital accompanied by a female friend. Mr. Sneed states, "My neighbor is taking my land. He built a fence on my property instead of his." The female friend states that James had barricaded himself in his house surrounded by his collection of shotguns and was threatening to "blow away" his neighbor.

SCHIZOID PERSONALITY DISORDER

People with schizoid personalities do not want to be involved in interpersonal or social relationships. These persons rarely have close friends and appear uncomfortable interacting with others. They could be thought of as hermits because of their shyness and introversion. They respond with short answers to questions and do not initiate spontaneous conversation. Cold or neglectful early parenting is often seen in their histories (Gunderson, 1988). As a result, these persons have learned to withdraw because they do not view relationships as beneficial.

The defense mechanism of intellectualization is being used when these patients describe emotional and interpersonal experiences in a matter-of-fact and impersonal manner (Millon, 1986). They can function at work successfully especially if little verbal interaction is required. They are reality oriented, but fantasy and daydreaming may be more gratifying than real persons and situations. For additional characteristics, see the DSM-IV criteria box on p. 481.

If a person with schizoid personality disorder is hospitalized, initially the nurse-patient relationship will focus on building trust followed by the identification and appropriate verbal expression of feelings. At first the patient may be able to participate only on the fringe of unit activities due to discomfort and anxiety. Slowly involving the patient in milieu and group activities may help increase social skills.

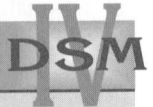

DSM-IV Criteria for Paranoid Personality Disorder

A. Suspicious of others
B. Doubt trustworthiness of others
C. Fear of confiding in others
D. Fear personal information will be used against them
E. Interpret remarks as demeaning or threatening
F. Hold grudges toward others
G. Become angry and threatening when they perceive they are attacked by others

Adapted from the American Psychiatric Association: *Diagnostic and statistical manual of mental disorders*, ed 4, Washington, DC, 1994, The Association.

SCHIZOTYPAL PERSONALITY DISORDER

Persons with schizotypal personality disorder look similar to patients with schizophrenia with the major exception that psychotic episodes are infrequent and less severe. These patients have problems in thinking, perceiving, and communicating. Their outward appearance may be eccentric and their behavior odd. They are sensitive to the behaviors of others, especially rejection and anger. Fantasies about imaginary relationships may be substituted for real relationships. The DSM-IV diagnostic criteria for this disorder are listed in the box on the bottom of this page.

Schizotypal personality disorders are more common in the biological relatives of schizophrenics (APA, 1994). Genetic studies indicate that patients with this disorder show disturbances (behaviors) similar to those found in people with schizophrenia.

When a person with schizotypal personality disorder is hospitalized, interventions offering support, kindness, and gentle suggestions will help the patient become involved in activities with others. It is essential for the nurse to help the patient improve interpersonal relationships, social skills, and appropriate behaviors. Social situations are uncomfortable and cause discomfort and anxiety because of the reactions of others to the patient's appearance and behavior. These patients can benefit from socializing experiences if those experiences are carefully orchestrated. Vocational counseling and assistance with job placement increase the patient's opportunity for success. Low doses of neuroleptic drugs may decrease the severity of symptoms exhibited in the transient psychotic state in relation to thinking, perception, and anxiety.

Psychotherapeutic Management

Nurse-Patient Relationship.   The most important psychotherapeutic task centers on dealing with trust issues. A professional demeanor coupled with honesty and nonintrusiveness will assist with the development of some trust. Low doses of phenothiazines may be prescribed to manage anxiety and other symptoms, however the patient may resist taking medication if basic trust has not been developed (Gunderson, 1988). Clear, simple explanations and requests will reduce the patient's feelings of being threatened or controlled. Patients with paranoid personality disorders do not tolerate group therapies that expect or involve confrontation or much emotional involvement.

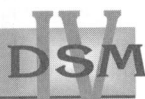

DSM-IV Criteria for Schizoid Personality Disorder

A. Lacks desire for close relationships or friends
B. Chooses to be alone
C. Lack of sexual experiences
D. Avoids activities
E. Appears cold and detached

Adapted from the American Psychiatric Association: *Diagnostic and statistical manual of mental disorders,* ed 4, Washington, DC, 1994, The Association.

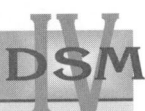

DSM-IV Criteria for Schizotypal Personality Disorder

A. Ideas of reference
B. Magical thinking or odd beliefs
C. Unusual perceptual experiences, including bodily illusions
D. Peculiar thinking
E. Vague, stereotypical, overelaborate speech
F. Suspiciousness
G. Blunted or inappropriate affect
H. Eccentric appearance or behavior
I. Few close relationships
J. Uncomfortable in social situations

Adapted from the American Psychiatric Association: *Diagnostic and statistical manual of mental disorders,* ed 4, Washington, DC, 1994, The Association.

CLUSTER B: DRAMATIC/ERRATIC

ANTISOCIAL PERSONALITY DISORDER

The main feature of antisocial personality disorder is a pattern of disregard for the rights of others, which is usually demonstrated by repeated violation of the law. Before age 15, these behaviors are diagnosed as conduct disorder. Affected persons engage in unlawful behavior as evidenced by driving while intoxicated and engaging in spouse or child abuse. They are promiscuous and have no guilt about hurting others. Lying, cheating, and stealing are common. Their criminal behavior places them within the court and prison system more than the mental health system. Not all criminals, however, have antisocial personality disorders.

The diagnosis of the antisocial personality disorder is based on history of disordered life functioning rather than on mental status. These individuals may experience distress and anxiety because of others' hostility toward them, but they see the problem as being within others and not themselves. People with an antisocial personality disorder may appear to be charming and intellectual. They are smooth talkers and deny and rationalize their behavior. Expected anxiety over their predicament is absent. Guilt, sorrow for offenses, or loyalty is nonexistent as if they do not have a conscience. These individuals do not behave as responsible, mature, and independent adults. See the DSM-IV box below.

Unique Etiology

Both genetics and the environment are known to influence the development of antisocial personality disorder (APA, 1994). Parents establish an environment where unstable parent-child relationships exist, resulting in delinquency in their children. Genetic studies of twin or adoptive siblings and family history data provide significant evidence that suggests a genetic predisposition to this disorder (Siever, et al, 1983). In other words, children inherit traits that may lead to the development of an antisocial personality disorder. Substance abuse and dependency problems are highly correlated with the antisocial personality disorder. Electroencephalogram (EEG) abnormalities also exist in adults with antisocial personality disorder and their parents. This disorder is seen more often in males than females (APA, 1994).

Psychotherapeutic Management

Nurse-Patient Relationship. Long-term treatment in a therapeutic milieu is necessary for any type of lasting changes to occur. With short-term hospitalization the nurse can initiate the therapeutic process by setting firm limits. These patients try to manipulate staff and bend rules for their wants and needs. The nurse must be steadfast and consistent in confronting behaviors and enforcing rules and policies. Consequences of behavior, both for the unit and for the patient's life, are also a point of focus. Helping the patient to be aware of consequences is a concrete way to assist the patient in realizing what the results of behaviors are or will be. Pointing out the effects that the patient's behaviors have on others is also part of the therapeutic process. The patient needs to begin to understand how others feel and react to his or her behaviors and why they react the way they do. The nurse avoids moralizing and assists the patient in identifying and verbalizing feelings that may reflect anxiety and depression. Group membership can help the patient feel accepted as a person even if the patient's behaviors are not acceptable. Groups of

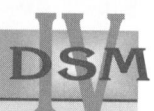

DSM-IV Criteria for Antisocial Personality Disorder

A. Violates rights of others
B. Engages in illegal activities
C. Aggressive behavior
D. Lack of guilt or remorse

E. Irresponsible in work and with finances
F. Impulsiveness
G. Recklessness

Adapted from the American Psychiatric Association: *Diagnostic and statistical manual of mental disorders,* ed 4, Washington, DC, 1994, The Association.

other individuals with this same diagnosis can be effective in confronting inappropriate and manipulative behavior because these individuals are "experts" in spotting smooth talking, rationalizing, and lying. These groups can be very effective in helping the antisocial patient. In summary, the keys to working with the antisocial patient are consistency by the nursing staff and accountability by the patient.

■ Critical Thinking Question

A patient with antisocial personality disorder is verbally threatening to the staff when limits are set on his manipulative behaviors. How would the nurse manage the patient's threatening behavior?

BORDERLINE PERSONALITY DISORDER

Of all personality disorders, the borderline personality disorder (BPD) is the most commonly treated. However, since the full range of symptoms and behaviors is typically not manifested during one short-term inpatient hospitalization, it is often difficult to fully appreciate the complexity of these individuals' mental disorder. These patients usually require hospitalization when they are in a crisis or exhibit self-mutilating or suicidal behaviors.

The patient with a BPD has problems with identity, self-image, relationships, thinking, mood, and behaviors (Salzman, 1996). Identity problems are apparent in the patient who is uncertain about his or her self-image, career goals, personal values, and sexual orientation. Interpersonal relationship problems exist in choosing unhealthy relationships and in short-term intimate relationships. The patient alternates between overidealization and devaluation of

individuals. For example, this BPD "falls in love" with the perfect person and shortly thereafter can find no redeeming qualities in the formerly idealized person. The person with BPD cannot appreciate the "mixed-bag" of qualities most people have.

Manipulation and dependency commonly occur. This patient has great difficulty in being alone and therefore seeks intense but brief relationships. Mood disturbances are exhibited in symptoms of depression, intense anger, and labile mood. Projective identification is used to protect the self. Patients displace their angry feelings onto others to justify their own feelings. Blaming others helps the patient to deal with feelings even though it is dysfunctional and inappropriate. Intense emotional pain contributes to mood shifts, which range from euphoria to crying to acting-out behaviors such as displays of temper and physical fights. Impulsiveness is manifested in repetitive self-destructiveness such as self-mutilation, suicidal behaviors, use of substances, and anorexia/bulimia. Other relatively common impulsive activities include overspending, promiscuity, compulsive overeating, and unhealthy risk taking and decision making. DSM-IV criteria for this disorder are listed in the box below.

Recent research findings indicate that as many as 75% of individuals with BPD are women and victims of childhood sexual abuse (Hampton, 1997). This finding is significant because it suggests the possible dynamics of BPD behaviors, which in turn, impact nursing interventions. The dissociation used by a child sex abuse victim may result in "splitting", which is found in the BPD. The defense mechanism of "splitting" is defined as the inability to view both self and others as having both good and bad qualities. Therefore self and others are viewed as either all good or all bad. Splitting helps the individual to avoid the pain and feelings associated with

---

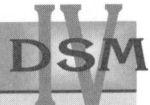

DSM-IV Criteria for Borderline Personality Disorder

A. Frantic avoidance of abandonment; real or imagined
B. Unstable and intense interpersonal relationships
C. Identity disturbances
D. Impulsivity
E. Self-mutilating behavior

F. Suicidal behavior
G. Rapid mood shifts
H. Chronic feelings of emptiness
I. Problems with anger
J. Transient dissociative and paranoid symptoms

Adapted from the American Psychiatric Association: *Diagnostic and statistical manual of mental disorders*, ed 4, Washington, DC, 1994, The Association.

past abuse and/or current situations involving threat of rejection or abandonment. The complexity of behaviors associated with BPD can include severe symptoms of posttraumatic stress disorder and dissociative disorder (Figueroa and Silk, 1997). See Chapter 38 on victims of violent behavior and Chapter 29 on anxiety-related disorders for related discussions.

On admission to an inpatient psychiatric unit, the person with a BPD may exhibit a need for attention and affection by contradictory behaviors of manipulation, dependency, or acting out. Frustration on the part of the staff may be seen as rejection. This perception by the patient can lead to increased anger and withdrawal. Shifts between depression, anxiety, euphoria, and anger are seen in the patient's labile mood. Under stress the patient regresses to immature behaviors and is unable to cope with conflict (Millon, 1986). The patient vacillates between clinging and disengaged behaviors, as demonstrated by desiring the staff to solve all problems or by the patient viewing the inpatient treatment as unnecessary and meaningless. When progress seems to be occurring, the patient with a BPD may suddenly exhibit opposite behaviors, and it may seem as if the staff will need to start over from the beginning.

Unique Etiology

The development of the borderline personality disorder may be due to a combination of biological, environmental, and stress-related factors. "Biological studies show inadequate regulation of serotonin, dopamine, and other neurotransmitters" (Salzman, 1996). Abnormalities of the serotonin system as seen in impulsive behaviors and abnormalities of cholinergic and adrenergic systems predispose individuals to dysphoria, emotional lability, and hyperreactivity related to environmental stimuli (Figueroa and Silk, 1997).

Environmental factors include a traumatic home environment, such as emotional discord in the family, neglect of the child's feelings and needs, and/or verbal, emotional, physical, and sexual abuse (Zanarini and Frankenburg, 1997).

Stress-related events may trigger the individual's vulnerable temperament and create misery and frustration. The individual is reminded of earlier stress or trauma, which results in the development of the borderline symptoms and condition (Zanarini and Frankenburg, 1997).

According to the concepts of Mahler, et al (1975) regarding normal development, by the end of the separation-individuation phase (age 2), the child is able to see self and others as separate. The "normal" child can retain the images of nurturing figures when they are absent. He or she can integrate the possibility of good and bad coexisting. The child who is developing a BPD fails in this developmental task. The parent may cling to the child and prevent autonomy and individuation, or the parent may withdraw attention and support, leaving the child with feelings of confusion, rage, and abandonment that continue throughout life. The person with a BPD, in response to his or her unmet need for love, dismisses safety and becomes self-destructive in his search for attention and love (Lynch and Lynch, 1977).

The conflict between abandonment and domination brings negative feedback from others in response to the person's ambivalent needs for attachment and detachment. Attachment is evident in clinging, dependency, and idealization behaviors, while detachment is displayed through anger, pouting, depression, and devaluation (Melges and Swartz, 1989). Intense moods of anger and depression are accompanied by chronic feelings of emptiness.

Persons with a BPD may become suicidal when blocked, frustrated, or stressed. The risk of suicide is substantial. Suicide completion is more likely in younger patients, with the risk declining as patients age (APA, 1994).

Typically, recurrent self-mutilation is a cry for help; an expression of intense anger, helplessness, or guilt; or a form of self-punishment. It is also a means to block psychological pain by inducing physical pain, which is a means to validate that the person is still alive and can still feel physical pain when experiencing emotional feelings of numbness and unreality. Research findings have suggested an inverse correlation between serotonergic activity and the severity of self-mutilation (Favazza and Rosenthal, 1993). This may have implications for use of medications.

■ Critical Thinking Question

A 22-year-old woman is admitted to the unit with major depression and borderline personality disorder. She self-mutilates and is anorexic. What would be the nurse's priorities in establishing a care plan for this patient?

Psychotherapeutic Management

Nurse-Patient Relationship. The use of empathy by the nurse is important in establishing a relationship with the patient diagnosed with BPD. The nurse acknowledges the reality of the patient's pain, offers support, and empowers and works with the patient to understand, control, and change dysfunctional behaviors. The patient is ultimately in control of his or her own behaviors even when the behaviors seem out of control (Wester, 1991). With the nurse's assistance, the patient can identify and verbalize feelings, control negative behaviors, and slowly begin to replace them with more appropriate actions.

The patient is usually in a crisis situation when hospitalized because of suicidal ideation or behavior, self-mutilation, acute personality disorganization, and/or inability to function. The nurse provides a safe environment to decrease self-harm but then works with the patient to find alternatives to express anger and rage. Alternatives may include ventilation and discussion of feelings, punching pillows, and the use of foam bats. In order for self-harm behaviors to diminish, the nurse helps the patient identify feelings and verbally express them appropriately so the patient can understand that his or her actions are habitual responses to handling emotions (Gallop, 1992). Recognizing behavioral and emotional cues can help the patient decrease impulsive and self-harm behaviors. Reducing the frequency of suicide attempts is vital to transition to the outpatient setting (Hampton, 1997). The use of a behavioral contract to decrease self-mutilation in inpatient and outpatient settings provides the patient with clear expectations of behavior, alternative behavior, and coping strategies (Dyckoff, 1996).

Patients can be helped with understanding themselves and their feelings by writing in a notebook on a daily basis. In sharing the journal with the nurse, the patient gains an understanding of self and a sense of autonomy and responsibility (Gallop, 1992). This technique can be useful for many patients with BPD.

Patients with BPD who are victims of abuse need to talk about their trauma in a safe environment. The nurse should acknowledge their pain and convey empathy and the appropriateness of their feelings (Perry, et al, 1990). When patients understand current behaviors are linked to past trauma, they can learn to recognize and then work toward changing dysfunctional actions towards self and others. See Chapter 38 on victims of violent behavior for more detailed interventions.

The patient with BPD is often manipulative. Consistency, limit setting, and supportive confrontation are necessary interventions to provide clear expectations regarding patient behaviors. These patients are adept at sidestepping rules, avoiding consequences, and at pitting staff members against each other all for the sake of getting what they want. Enforcing unit rules, providing clear structure, and placing the responsibility for appropriate behaviors on the patient though vigorously resisted will benefit the person with a BPD. The need to help the patient develop realistic short-term goals must be part of the treatment plan if the patient's responsibility for self is to increase.

The psychiatric nurse is in a perfect position to help the patient with BPD with the daily give-and-take issues of life that create so many problems for this patient. The nurse should work with the patient on appropriate verbal expression of feelings and assertiveness even though the nurse's ability to be empathetic, nonjudgmental, and therapeutic is sometimes severely tested by the patient's behaviors. The nurse may feel frustrated and ineffective as a caregiver because of the patient's behaviors and defenses. Hence, it may be less frustrating and "safer" to offer superficial solutions to problems, point out rules, and interact superficially. However understanding and working with the patient therapeutically can result in a positive experience for the nurse and be of lasting import to the patient.

Psychopharmacology. Psychopharmacology is generally not used, nor is it therapeutic for patients with BPD. Transient psychotic states due to overwhelming stress are treated with low-dose neuroleptics for 3 to 12 weeks to decrease symptoms. Lithium, valproic acid, and carbamazepine are used for rapid mood swings (Salzman, 1996). Benzodiazepines are used cautiously for anxiety, sleep disorders, and restlessness. The selective serotonin reuptake inhibitors (SSRIs) are useful in reducing anger, impulsiveness, and mood instability (Salzman, 1996).

Milieu Management. Interventions mentioned in the nurse-patient relationship discussion regarding firm limits, consistency, and clear structure are basic to the milieu for the BPD patient. The patient's manipulation of other patients must be confronted since the BPD patient can mobilize others against the staff. Consistent communication among staff members is essential to minimize the patient's attempts to divide the staff.

Group sessions including assertiveness training, problem solving, stress management, anger management, and victimization are some therapeutic activities important for these patients.

Referral to self-help groups where applicable for alcohol and drug problems, eating disorders, and victimization is also important. Vocational counseling and training are important to foster autonomous and independent functioning. Residential treatment may need to be considered particularly for patients with chronic self-destructive behavior (Stone, 1990).

NARCISSISTIC PERSONALITY DISORDER

The patient with a narcissistic personality disorder displays grandiosity about his/her importance and achievements. This grandiosity is unlike the delusions of grandeur found in schizophrenia or bipolar disorders. The grandiosity of the narcissistic personality disorder is based somewhat in reality but is distorted, embellished, or convoluted to meet the patient's needs of self-importance. For example, the patient may say that he was a star football player in high school and could have played for the Indianapolis Colts. He does not tell the nurse that he barely made the second-string football team in high school.

The narcissistic patient overvalues himself, is arrogant, and seems indifferent to the criticism of others. Those around this person are often viewed as superior or inferior. For example, the patient views the nurse who is understanding and supportive as competent or superior, whereas the nurse who questions or confronts is viewed as incompetent or inferior.

The patient may appear nonchalant or indifferent to criticism while hiding feelings of anger, rage, or emptiness. Relationships with others seem shallow but may be meaningful if the patient's self-esteem is positively enhanced. The feelings of others are not understood or considered. These persons use others selfishly to meet their own needs but do not reciprocate. This type of patient has a sense of entitlement and expects special treatment. The patient uses rationalization to blame others, makes excuses, and provides alibis for self-centered behaviors (Millon, 1986). See the box below for DSM-IV criteria.

CLINICAL EXAMPLE

The patient has been admitted to the unit and insists on a private room with a telephone and television because he needs to keep up with the reports on the financial news network.

Unique Etiology

Studies of biological and genetic factors in the narcissistic personality disorder have not been done. Some theorists believe that the self-centered person is arrested at an early developmental stage because "parents do not provide adequate empathetic experiences or adequate exposure to disillusioning realities" (Gunderson, 1988). The parents fail to mirror what is appropriate or inappropriate back to the child (Gunderson, 1988). Consequently the child

---

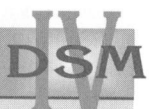

DSM-IV Criteria for Narcissistic Personality Disorder

A. Grandiose self-importance
B. Fantasies of unlimited power, success, or brilliance
C. Believes he or she is special
D. Needs to be admired
E. Sense of entitlement (i.e., deserves to be favored or given special treatment)

F. Takes advantage of others for own benefit
G. Lacks empathy
H. Envious of others or others are envious of him or her
I. Arrogant

Adapted from the American Psychiatric Association: *Diagnostic and statistical manual of mental disorders,* ed 4, Washington, DC, 1994, The Association.

develops without any feedback about his or her behaviors.

Psychotherapeutic Management

Nurse-Patient Relationship. If this patient is hospitalized, the nurse must deal with decreasing the constant recitation of self-importance and grandiosity. The nurse must mirror what the patient sounds like, especially if contradictions exist, and help the patient focus on the identification and verbal expression of feelings. Supportive confrontation is used to point out discrepancies between what the patient says and what actually exists to increase responsibility for self. Limit setting and consistency in approach are used to decrease manipulation and entitlement behaviors. Realistic short-term goals focused on the here and now are important to decrease the patient's use of fantasy and rationalization and to increase responsibility for self. The patient needs to be taught that no one is perfect and that one has worth even if one makes mistakes and has imperfections.

HISTRIONIC PERSONALITY DISORDER

The patient with the histrionic personality disorder dramatizes all events and draws attention to self. This patient is extroverted and thrives on being the center of attention. Behavior is silly, colorful, frivolous, and seductive. Speech is vague, descriptive, superficial, and overembellished but lacking in detail, insight, and depth. The patient seems to be in a hurry and restless. Temper tantrums and outbursts of anger are seen, as well as overreaction to minor events. This patient may use somatic complaints to avoid responsibility and support dependency. Dissociation is a common defense to avoid feelings. Therefore this patient cannot deal with his or her own true feelings. The patient views relationships with others as special or possessing greater intimacy than is real. Recently met individuals are thought of as being dear friends (Pfohl, 1991). The box below presents additional DSM-IV criteria.

The causes of histrionic personality disorder are unknown but are probably due to many factors. In the early mother-child relationship the mother negates the child's inner feelings. The child then turns to his or her father for nurturance, and the father responds to the child's dramatic emotional behaviors (Gunderson, 1988).

Positive reinforcement in the form of attention, recognition, or praise is given for unselfish or other-centered behaviors. Because the patient needs much reassurance and feels helpless, the nurse works to provide support to facilitate independent problem solving and daily functioning. Since the patient is unaware of and does not deal with feelings, the nurse must help clarify what the patient's true feelings are and help the patient learn how to express them appropriately. Working with this type of patient can be frustrating for the nurse, since the patient needs time to internalize the meaning of what the nurse is trying to accomplish.

CLUSTER C: ANXIOUS/FEARFUL

DEPENDENT PERSONALITY DISORDER

The main characteristic of the dependent personality disorder is a "pervasive and excessive need to be taken care of that leads to submissive and clinging behaviors and fears of separation" (Hirschfeld, Shea, and Weise, 1991). Dependent persons want others to

---

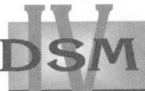 **DSM-IV Criteria for Histrionic Personality Disorder**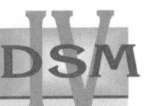

A. Needs to be center of attention
B. Displays sexually seductive or provocative behaviors
C. Shallow, rapidly shifting emotions
D. Uses physical appearance to become center of attention
E. Uses speech to impress others but is lacking in depth
F. Dramatic expression of emotion
G. Easily influenced by others
H. Exaggerates degree of intimacy with others

Adapted from the American Psychiatric Association: *Diagnostic and statistical manual of mental disorders,* ed 4, Washington, DC, 1994, The Association.

make everyday decisions for them, for example, type of clothes to wear and type of job to seek. They need direction and reassurance. These individuals feel inferior and cling to others excessively because they are afraid they will be left alone. Avoiding responsibility and expressing helplessness, the patient maintains the need to rely on others.

CLINICAL EXAMPLE

The patient has been telling the nurse about her alcoholic, abusive husband. She has been married to him for 16 years. She expresses sadness and frustration about her marriage but states, "How could I leave him? What would I do? Who will take care of me? I could never live alone."

Dependent persons also expect that if they perform good deeds for others, they will be rewarded by someone doing something for them. An intimate relationship with a spouse who is abusive, unfaithful, or an alcoholic is tolerated so as not to disturb the sense of attachment and should be rewarded by a change in the person. Passivity and concealing of sexual feelings and anger are a means of avoiding conflict. DSM-IV criteria are listed in the box below.

Biochemical and genetic factors have not been correlated with dependent personality disorders. Psychosocial theories consider culture to be the basis of the development of this disorder. Certain cultures dictate that females should maintain a dependent role. Parents or society may believe that the child should not exhibit certain autonomous behaviors and the child in turn may believe disapproval or loss

of attachment are consequences of these behaviors. Individuals with dependent personality disorder assume a passive role regarding self but do for others to foster attachment.

Psychotherapeutic Management

Nurse-Patient Relationship. The nurse slowly works on decision making with the patient to increase responsibility for self in day-to-day living. The patient needs assistance with managing anxiety since it will increase as the patient assumes more responsibility for self. Assertiveness is an important area of the nurse's teaching so that the patient can clearly state his or her own feelings, needs, and desires. Verbalization of feelings and how to cope with them is essential.

AVOIDANT PERSONALITY DISORDER

Patients with the avoidant personality disorder are timid, socially uncomfortable, withdrawn, and hypersensitive to criticism. Although they are fearful and shy, they desire relationships and challenges. To keep their anxiety at a minimum level they avoid situations where they might be disappointed or rejected. (Grinspoon, 1996). When interacting with someone, this person sounds uncertain and lacks self-confidence. This person is afraid to ask questions or speak up in public. They withdraw from social support and convey helplessness (Vollrath, et al, 1996). See the box on page 489 for the DSM-IV criteria for this disorder.

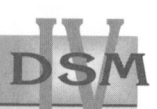

DSM-IV Criteria for Dependent Personality Disorder

A. Unable to make daily decisions without much advice and reassurance
B. Needs others to be responsible for important areas of life
C. Seldom disagrees with others because of fear of loss of support or approval
D. Problem with initiating projects or doing things on own because of little self-confidence

E. Performs unpleasant tasks to obtain support from others
F. Anxious or helpless when alone because of fear of being unable to care for self
G. Urgently seeks another relationship for support and care after a close relationship ends
H. Preoccupied with fear of being alone to care for self

Adapted from the American Psychiatric Association: *Diagnostic and statistical manual of mental disorders,* ed 4, Washington, DC, 1994, The Association.

Few biological, genetic, and psychological studies have been conducted. The nurse helps the patient gradually confront what he or she fears. Discussing the patient's feelings and fears before and after that person does something he or she is afraid to do is an essential part of the relationship. The nurse supports and directs the patient in the accomplishment of small goals. Helping the patient to be assertive and to develop social skills is necessary. The nurse includes the patient in interactions with others and then progresses to small groups as the patient is able to tolerate them. Because of the patient's anxiety, relaxation techniques are taught to enable the person to be successful in interactions. The nurse will give positive feedback to the patient for any real success or attempt to engage in interactions with others to promote self-esteem.

OBSESSIVE-COMPULSIVE PERSONALITY DISORDER

Persons with obsessive-compulsive personality disorder are perfectionistic and inflexible. These patients are overly strict and often set standards for themselves that are too high, so that their work is never good enough. They are preoccupied with rules, trivial details, and procedures. They find it difficult to express warmth or tender emotions. There is little give and take in their interactions with others, and they are rigid, controlling, and cold. The patient is serious about all of his or her activities, and it is difficult for that person to have fun or to experience pleasure. Because the person is afraid of making mistakes, he or she can be indecisive or will put off decisions until all the facts are accumulated. The person's affect is constricted and he or she may speak in a monotone. See the box on p. 490 for DSM-IV criteria.

Early parent-child relationships around issues of autonomy, control, and authority may predispose a person to this disorder. Recent genetic studies indicate that this malady and the more severe obsessive-compulsive disorder may be inherited.

The nurse needs to support the patient in exploring his or her feelings and in attempting new experiences and situations. The nurse helps the patient with decision making and encourages follow-through behavior. At times, there is a need to confront the patient's procrastination and intellectualization. The nurse teaches the patient the importance of leisure activities and explores interests in this area. Because the patient lacks awareness of how he or she affects others, the patient needs to look at and understand how others view him or her. Teaching the patient that he or she is human and that it is all right to make mistakes helps decrease irrational beliefs about the necessity to be perfect.

■ Critical Thinking Questions

Staff on the unit are frustrated and angry with a patient who is attempting to split staff on the various shifts against each other. They are even beginning to be angry with each other for the inconsistencies occurring with this patient's care. What strategies should the head nurse employ to help the staff and ultimately the treatment of the patient?

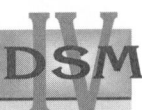

DSM-IV Criteria for Avoidant Personality Disorder

A. Avoids occupations involving interpersonal contact due to fears of disapproval or rejection
B. Uninvolved with others unless certain of being liked
C. Fears intimate relationships due to fear of shame or ridicule
D. Preoccupied with being criticized or rejected in social situations
E. Inhibited and feels inadequate in new interpersonal situations
F. Believes self to be socially inept, unappealing, or inferior to others
G. Very reluctant to take risks or engage in new activities due to possibility of being embarrassed

Adapted from the American Psychiatric Association: *Diagnostic and statistical manual of mental disorders*, ed 4, Washington, DC, 1994, The Association.

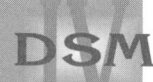

DSM-IV Criteria for Obsessive-Compulsive Personality Disorder

A. Preoccupied with details, rules, lists, organization
B. Perfectionism that interferes with task completion
C. Too busy working to have friends or leisure activities
D. Overconscientious and inflexible
E. Unable to discard worthless or worn-out objects

F. Others must do things his or her way in work- or task-related activity
G. Reluctant to spend and hoards money
H. Rigid and stubborn

Adapted from the American Psychiatric Association: *Diagnostic and statistical manual of mental disorders*, ed 4, Washington, DC, 1994, The Association.

Case Study

Sherry Morgan, a 27-year-old woman, is brought to the psychiatric inpatient unit from the emergency room. Both wrists were bandaged after suturing. She is complaining of nausea and heartburn. She vacillates between being angry and crying. Sherry states, "I know I am bad. I should not have done it. I do not want to die, but I am tired of the hassles." She has brought with her three suitcases filled with her belongings. During the admission interview the nurse finds that Sherry has had three previous admissions to this inpatient unit during the past 8 years. Sherry states that she refuses to return to work because her boss accuses her of bothering the other employees instead of doing her own work. She states her boss is falsely accusing her of using alcohol and drugs and does not accept her reasons for being absent from work. This morning she called her outpatient therapist, whom she had not seen in a year and a half but who agreed to see her at 3 PM. When she called the therapist

back at noon and found he was at lunch, she used her scissors to cut her wrists. "I used to think he understood me, but now I know he doesn't care." Her parents are on vacation out of state, and her only close friend is busy going through a divorce. She had taken some of her mother's Valium, but it did not help calm her down. She has averaged only 3 to 4 hours of sleep each night for the past 5 days and has been unable to eat regular meals. Her attempts to clean her parents' house were never completed. She could not even finish watering her mother's plants. A male acquaintance of 2 weeks was no longer calling her, so she was frequenting several bars and inviting men home. She never heard from these men again, even though she thought that their relationships were sexually satisfying.

Sherry completed 2 years of college and is dressed attractively. She enjoys reading romance novels and has brought five of her favorite books with her.

◤ Key Concepts

1. Personality traits are enduring approaches to the world expressed in how the person thinks, how the person feels, and what the person does. Traditionally these traits have been viewed as being driven by unconscious processes.
2. When personality traits become rigid, dysfunctional, and cause distress in self and others, they may be diagnosed as a personality disorder. Personal discomfort arises primarily from others' reactions to or behaviors toward that person.
3. The odd/eccentric cluster of personality disorders includes the following:
    a. Paranoid, characterized by suspiciousness and mistrust

    b. Schizoid, characterized by hermitlike life-style, aloneness
    c. Schizotypal, characterized by symptoms similar to but less severe than those of schizophrenia
4. The dramatic/erratic cluster includes the following:
    a. Antisocial, characterized by disregard of others' rights without guilt
    b. Borderline, characterized by problems with self-identity, interpersonal relationships, mood shifts, and self-destructiveness
    c. Narcissistic, characterized by overevaluation of self, arrogance, and indifference to the criticism of others
    d. Histrionic, characterized by dramatic behaviors, attention seeking, and superficiality

Care Plan

NAME: Sherry Morgan   **ADMISSION DATE:** _____

DSM-IV DIAGNOSIS: Axis I major depression
Axis II borderline personality disorder

ASSESSMENT: **Areas of strength:** Well-groomed, neat and clean, intelligent, enjoys reading.
Problems: Self-mutilating behavior, absence of support systems, loss of job, decreased sleeping and eating, irresponsible and impulsive sexual behavior.

DIAGNOSES:
- High risk for self-mutilation related to absence of support systems as evidenced by cutting wrists.
- Defensive coping related to low self-esteem as evidenced by angry and labile emotions.

OUTCOMES: **Short-term goals:**   **Date met**
- Patient will eliminate self-mutilating behavior and appropriately verbalize feelings of anger and sadness.   _____

Long-term goals:
- Patient will schedule outpatient appointment and meeting with boss regarding job problems.   _____

PLANNING/ INTERVENTIONS: **Nurse-patient relationship:** Monitor and set limits on acting-out behaviors. Assist patient with identification and verbalization of feelings. Discuss fears about accepting responsibility for self and decision making. Discuss behaviors interfering with job performance.
Psychopharmacology: Prozac 20 mg q AM, Desyrel 50 mg q hs.
Milieu management: Groups focusing on self-esteem, stress and anger management, assertiveness training, social skills, problem-solving skills, discharge planning.

EVALUATION: Patient has not engaged in self-mutilating behavior. Patient beginning to verbalize feelings of anger and sadness.

REFERRALS: Appointment weekly with Mrs. Taylor MSN, RN, CS, outpatient mental health clinic after discharge.

---

5. The anxious/fearful cluster includes the following:
   a. Dependent, characterized by submissiveness, helplessness, fear of responsibility, and reliance on others for decision making
   b. Avoidant, characterized by timidity, social withdrawal behavior, and hypersensitivity to criticism
   c. Obsessive-compulsive, characterized by indecisiveness, perfectionism, inflexibility, and difficulty expressing feelings
6. Nursing interventions for persons with personality disorders help the patient focus on specific behaviors distressing to self or others or both and awareness of dysfunctional and self-defeating patterns.

🚩 Study Questions

(Answer key is in the back of the book.)
1. Individuals with personality disorders
   a. Experience discomfort because of others' reactions toward them
   b. Receive psychotropic medication to eliminate their personality disorder
   c. Are flexible in how they relate with others
   d. Are usually hospitalized for their personality disorder
2. Which nursing approach is most appropriate for a patient with a paranoid personality disorder?
   a. Involve the patient in groups as much as possible.

b. Use a light-hearted manner in interacting with the patient.

c. Confront the patient's use of projection and need to control.

d. Use clear, simple explanations when making requests.

3. A patient with a borderline personality disorder uses self-mutilation:

a. As a means to get attention

b. To express intense feelings of anger or frustration

c. To express feelings of autonomy

d. As a means to manipulate staff

4. Mrs. Cannon withdraws from everyone on the unit. She refuses to go to activities because no one will like her, and she feels she is unable to initiate conversation with others. The nurse would:

a. Escort Mrs. Cannon to her activity and leave her there

b. Tell the patient that she should rest in her room until she feels more comfortable with others

c. Include Mrs. Cannon when the nurse initiates a conversation with the patient's roommate

d. Suggest to the patient that she discuss these difficulties with her doctor

5. Mr. Brand constantly bends rules to meet his needs and then gets angry when other patients and staff confront him on his behavior. He threatens patients and manipulates staff to get what he wants. Which is the best nursing approach to use with Mr. Brand?

a. Administer prn medication every time Mr. Brand does not follow the rules.

b. Ignore his behavior and privately tell the other patients to let Mr. Brand switch the television channels as much as he wants.

c. Encourage the other staff to take turns watching Mr. Brand.

d. Set firm limits for Mr. Brand and be consistent in confronting behaviors and enforcing unit rules.

REFERENCES

American Psychiatric Association: *Diagnostic and statistical manual of mental disorders,* ed 4, Washington, DC, 1994, The Association.

Dyckoff D, et al: The investigation of behavioral contracting in patients with borderline personality disorder, *J Am Psychiatr Nurses Assoc* 2(3):71, 1996.

Favazza AR and Rosenthal RJ: Diagnostic issues in self-mutilation, *Hosp Community Psychiatry* 44:2, 1993.

Figueroa E and Silk K: Biological implications of childhood sexual abuse in borderline personality disorder, *J Pers Disord* 11(1):71, 1997.

Gallop R: Self-destructive and impulsive behavior in the patient with a borderline personality disorder: re-thinking hospital treatment and management, *Arch Psychiatr Nurs* 6:3, 1992.

Grinspoon L, editor: Personality disorders: the anxious cluster. Part I, *Harvard Mental Health Letter* 12(8):1, 1996.

Gunderson JG: Personality disorders. In Nicholi A, editor: *The new Harvard guide to psychiatry,* Cambridge, Mass, 1988, The Belknap Press.

Hampton M: Dialectical behavior therapy in the treatment of persons with borderline personality disorder, *Arch Psychiatr Nurs* 11(2):96, 1997.

Hirschfeld RM, Shea MT, and Weise R: Dependent personality disorder: perspectives for DSM-IV, *J Pers Disord* 5:2, 1991.

Lynch V and Lynch M: Borderline personality, *Perspect Psychiatr Care* 15:72, 1977.

Mahler MS, Pine F, and Bergman A: *The psychological birth of the human infant symbiosis and individuation,* New York, 1975, Basic Books.

Melges T and Swartz M: Oscillations of attachment in borderline personality disorder, *Am J Psychiatry* 146:1115, 1989.

Millon T: *Personality prototypes and their diagnostic criteria: contemporary directions in psychopathology toward the DSM-IV,* New York, 1986, Guilford Press.

Paris J: Personality disorders: a biopsychological model, *J Pers Disord* 7:3, 1993.

Perry JC, et al: Psychotherapy and psychological trauma in borderline personality disorder, *Psychiatr Ann* 20:1, 1990.

Pfohl B: Histrionic personality disorder: a review of available data and recommendations for DSM-IV, *J Pers Disord* 5:2, 1991.

Salzman C: What drug treatments are available for borderline personality disorder? *Harvard Mental Health Letter* 13(3):8, 1996.

Sebastian L: Promoting object constancy: writing as a nursing intervention, *J Psychosoc Nurs Ment Health Serv* 29:1, 1991.

Siever L, Insel T, and Uhde T: Biogenic factors in personalities. In Frosch J, editor: *Current perspectives in personality disorders,* Washington, DC, 1983, American Psychiatric Press.

Stone MH: Personal reflections: borderline personality disorder—contemporary issues in nosology, etiology, and treatment, *Psychiatr Ann* 20:1, 1990.

Vollrath M, et al: Coping in DSM-IV options personality disorders, *J Pers Disord* 10(4):335, 1996.

Wester JM: Rethinking inpatient treatment of borderline clients, *Perspect Psychiatr Care* 27:2, 1991.

Zanarini M and Frankenburg F: Pathways to the development of borderline personality disorder, *J Pers Disord* 11(1):93, 1997.

CHAPTER 32

Sexual Disorders

CAROL E. BOSTROM

LEARNING OBJECTIVES

After reading this chapter you should be able to:
- Recognize the importance of the nurse's role in assessing patients' sexual concerns and problems.
- Describe the categories of sexual dysfunctions, sexual disorders, and gender identity.
- Identify the issues related to the care of patients with sexual disorders.
- Demonstrate an understanding of the need for referral for in-depth assessment and treatment of patients with sexual disorders.

This chapter presents an overview of sexual disorders and sexual dysfunctions. It does not include normal sexuality or sexual preference issues, such as homosexuality.

Individuals engage in a wide range of sexual activities, resulting in a wide range of sexual responses. Sexual activity may focus on objects or people; it is unacceptable legally when it involves a nonconsenting individual, a child, or the use of objects in a way that could interfere with healthy relationships. Sexual activity is unacceptable morally when it violates the norms, standards, and values of the culture. Sexual activity should be evaluated according to its effects on the individual and others, such as the level of functioning, self-esteem, and relationships with others.

It is important to consider coercion vs. consent between sexual partners. An individual's rights and needs should never be violated. Power and control issues affect the definition of consent and the degree of coercion. For example, some clinicians believe that a sexual relationship between a powerful political figure and a young female office worker, though apparently consensual, is actually coercive at its core.

DSM-IV CRITERIA AND TERMINOLOGY

The DSM-IV (American Psychiatric Association [APA], 1994) categorizes sexual disorders according to sexual dysfunctions, the paraphilias, and gender identity disorders. Sexual dysfunctions are characterized by the inhibition of sexual appetite or psychophysiological changes that compromise the sexual response cycle. Paraphilias are characterized by intense sexual urges focused on (1) nonhuman objects, (2) the suffering or humiliation of oneself or one's partner, or (3) children or other nonconsenting persons. Gender identity disorders are characterized by a discomfort with one's biological sex or the desire to have the characteristics of the other sex.

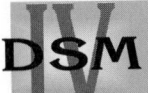 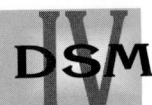

DSM-IV and NANDA Diagnoses Related to Sexual Disorders

DSM-IV*	NANDA†
Sexual dysfunction disorders	Altered family process
Paraphilias	Altered sexuality patterns
Gender identity disorders	Anxiety
	Ineffective individual coping
	Knowledge deficit
	Potential for violence: self-directed or other
	Sexual dysfunction
	Social isolation

*From the American Psychiatric Association: *Diagnostic and statistical manual of mental disorders,* ed 4, Washington, DC, 1994, The Association.
†From the North American Nursing Diagnosis Association: *NANDA nursing diagnoses: definitions and classifications, 1997-1998,* Philadelphia, PA, 1997, The Association.

> ### Box 32-1   Initial Nursing Assessment of Sexual Concerns
>
> Describe any difficulties you have experienced with sexual performance or satisfaction.
> What are your feelings and concerns about sexuality?
> How satisfied are you with your sexual relationship?
> What kind of changes would you like to make in your sexual relationship?
> What kind of negative sexual experiences have you had?

SEXUAL DYSFUNCTIONS

As part of the admission interview, the nurse assesses each patient for potential or actual problems with sexual functioning. Box 32-1 lists initial questions the nurse may use to assess the patient's feelings and concerns about sexuality. Potential or actual problems can occur as a result of emotional and/or physiological factors. Medications and/or chemicals can also alter sexual desire and functioning. A more thorough assessment or evaluation is necessary for appropriate referral and treatment. Treatment is individualized according to the cause or combination of causes. For example, the individual who becomes impotent due to a medical illness and/or a medication side effect may also have diminished self-esteem and self-confidence that compounds the problem. Therefore, treatment would focus on both the physiological aspects and emotional needs of the individual.

The phases of human sexual activity have been called the *sexual response cycle.* There are four phases: the desire phase, the excitement phase, the orgasm phase, and the resolution phase. Freud may have been the first to observe the similarity between the sexual response cycle and aggression. The assault cycle presented in Chapter 14 closely parallels these phases. Sexual dysfunctions are grouped into disorders that compromise one of these phases. Sexual desire disorders effectively stop the sexual response cycle from beginning. Sexual arousal disorders sidetrack the sexual response cycle at the excitement phase. Orgasm disorders arrest the progression of the cycle in the orgasm phase. Finally, sexual pain disorders can abort the sexual response cycle at any phase.

Sexual Desire Disorders

Individuals with these disorders have little or no sexual desire or have an aversion to sexual contact.

Sexual Arousal Disorders

Individuals with these disorders cannot maintain the physiological requirements for sexual intercourse. Women cannot maintain the lubrication-swelling response of sexual excitement, and men cannot maintain an erection.

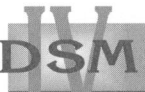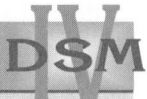

DSM-IV Criteria for Paraphilias

Exhibitionism
- Recurrent, intense sexually arousing fantasies, sexual urges, or behaviors involving exposing one's genitals to unsuspecting strangers.

Fetishism
- Recurrent, intense sexually arousing fantasies, sexual urges, or behaviors using nonliving objects.

Frotteurism
- Recurrent, intense sexually arousing fantasies, sexual urges, or behaviors involving touching and rubbing against a nonconsenting person.

Pedophilia
- Recurrent, intense sexually arousing fantasies, sexual urges, or behaviors that involve sexual activity with a child or children generally 13 years of age or younger.
- The person is at least 16 years of age and at least 5 years older than the child or children involved.

Sexual Masochism
- Recurrent, intense sexually arousing fantasies, sexual fantasies, urges, or behaviors involving the act of being humiliated, beaten, restrained, or otherwise made to suffer.

Sexual Sadism
- Recurrent, intense sexually arousing fantasies, urges, or behaviors involving acts in which the psychological or physical suffering of the victim is sexually exciting to the person.

Voyeurism
- Act of observing an unsuspecting person who is naked, in the process of disrobing, or engaging in sexual activity.

The paraphiliac activities last over a period of 6 months and cause distress or impairment in social, occupational, or other important areas of functioning.

Adapted from the American Psychiatric Association: *Diagnostic and statistical manual of mental disorders,* ed 4, Washington, DC, 1994, The Association.

Orgasm Disorders

Individuals with these disorders cannot complete the sexual response cycle because of the inability to achieve an orgasm. In premature ejaculation, a man reaches orgasm with minimal sexual stimulation, frustrating both himself and his partner.

Sexual Pain Disorders

Individuals with these disorders suffer genital pain (dyspareunia) before, during, or after sexual intercourse. Vaginismus—involuntary spasm of the outer third of the vagina—interferes with sexual intercourse.

PARAPHILIA

Paraphilia is a condition in which the sexual instinct is expressed in ways that are socially prohibited or unacceptable or are biologically undesirable.

Individuals with paraphilia may seek inpatient treatment because of a distinct axis I diagnosis that does not reflect a sexual disorder. The nurse on an inpatient unit may encounter individuals admitted with major depression and suicidal ideation who may be trying to avoid criminal prosecution or to obtain a minimized sentencing by seeking psychiatric treatment. Therefore, the nurse intervenes with behaviors reflective of the axis I diagnosis rather than specifically addressing the paraphilia.

Treatment for pedophilia, exhibitionism, and voyeurism generally occurs on an outpatient basis. Information about paraphiliacs comes from individuals who have been arrested and incarcerated, and from their victims (Kaplan and Sadock, 1989). Outpatient treatment programs and programs for incarcerated individuals also provide information about assessment and treatment.

Paraphiliacs may be male or female, and paraphiliac activity may be limited to a period of stress rather than following a chronic or repetitive pattern. Generally, chronic paraphiliacs have a large number of victims. Paraphiliac behaviors may increase with symptoms of depression (APA, 1994). See the box above for DSM-IV criteria for the various paraphilias.

Pedophilia

Pedophilia involves recurrent intense sexual urges and sexually arousing fantasies involving sexual activity with children. The individual acts on the urges or is distressed by them (APA, 1994). By definition, the victim of pedophilia must be younger than 13 years of age and the pedophile 16 years or older, and at least 5 years older than the victim. Pedophilic behavior can be expressed for opposite sex children, same sex children, or both. It also can be limited to incest. Fondling and oral sex are typical pedophilic behaviors. Vaginal and anal penetration are usually found in incest.

Much controversy exists regarding the personality profiles of sex offenders against minors. It is impossible to state accurately the personality characteristics that are present in all sex offenders. Some of the characteristics reported are shyness, sensitivity, and isolation in social situations, low self-esteem, dependency, depression, low self-confidence, use of alcohol and drugs, and a history of being sexually abused. In order to compensate for feelings of powerlessness, the pedophile may need to feel power over the victim through control and domination. Some sex offenders are nonaggressive; others use aggression in the form of trickery or bribery. The threat of violence may be used to encourage the victim's silence. The use of physical violence may indicate that the offender is a child rapist. The pedophile may seek an occupation that provides easy access to children. Typical occupations are teaching school, working in a day care setting, coaching, or scout leadership.

Incest

Incest is pedophilia with child relatives. It involves relationships by blood, marriage (step-parents), or live-in partners. Incest is so traumatic to children because they are victimized by someone they depend upon and trust and are unable to escape their victimization.

The characteristics of the perpetrator of incest are as varied as those of the pedophile. There is agreement that families in which incest occurs are generally disorganized and exhibit disturbed relationships (Ames and Houston, 1990). Sex is always involved between the perpetrator and the victim, but the perpetrator turns to the child for gratification, intimacy, emotional fulfillment, power, and control. Unlike pedophiles, perpetrators of incest do not typically select occupations for access to potential victims because their victims are easily accessible.

Exhibitionism

The primary characteristic of exhibitionism is sexual pleasure derived from exposing one's genitals to an unsuspecting stranger. The stereotypical offender is a young man in a raincoat who "flashes" women while walking down the street. No other sexual activity is attempted. The exhibitionist is stimulated by the effect of shocking his victims. The exhibitionist usually has satisfactory sexual relationships with adult partners. Emotional conflict or excessive free time may stimulate exhibitionist activity (Kaplan and Sadock, 1989).

Fetishism

The primary characteristic of fetishism is the sexual pleasure derived from inanimate objects. Common fetish objects are bras, underpants, stockings, and shoes. Less common fetish objects include urine-soaked and feces-smeared items. The individual with fetishism often masturbates while holding or rubbing these items.

Frotteurism

The primary characteristic of frotteurism is sexual pleasure derived from touching or rubbing one's genitals against a nonconsenting individual's thighs or buttocks. The individual with frotteurism may also attempt to fondle the person's breasts or genitals. Frotteurism usually occurs in a crowded place where escape into the crowd is possible.

Sexual Masochism

The primary characteristic of sexual masochism is the sexual pleasure derived from being humiliated, beaten, or otherwise made to suffer. Some sexually masochistic persons enjoy being urinated or defecated on and may pay prostitutes to do so. Hypoxyphilia is the act of enhancing sexual arousal by strangulation or other oxygen-depleting activities. Apparently, sexual response is heightened by these activities. People have died in their search for enhanced orgasms.

Sexual Sadism

The primary characteristic of sexual sadism is sexual pleasure derived from inflicting psychological or physical suffering on another. Partners can be consenting or masochistic. Sadistic behaviors include spanking, whipping, pinching, beating, burning, and restraining. Some sadistic individuals derive great pleasure from torturing or even killing their victims, and may be sadistic rapists. The so-called snuff films, found in the underground of the pornography world, apparently show the actual rape, torture, and murder of women and children for the convenient viewing of sadistic individuals in our society.

Voyeurism

The primary characteristic of voyeurism is sexual pleasure derived from observing unsuspecting persons who are naked or undressing, or who are engaged in sexual activity. The voyeur is commonly referred to as a "peeping Tom." The voyeur may masturbate during peeping or upon returning home.

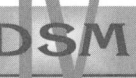 **Critical Thinking Question**

A patient with pedophilia attends a self-esteem group on the inpatient unit. Three members of the group are victims of childhood sexual abuse. What would you discuss with the patient regarding how he could benefit from the group without upsetting the other members?

GENDER IDENTITY DISORDER

Gender identity disorder in adults involves discomfort with one's sex or the gender role of that sex. In adults, this disorder can include the desire to live as the other sex or can involve feelings and reactions of the other sex (APA, 1994). See the box below for DSM-IV criteria for gender identity disorder. Another characteristic is a preoccupation with getting rid of primary and secondary sexual characteristics. These individuals believe that they were born as the wrong sex, and they desire hormones and surgery to become the opposite sex. Transsexualism is another name for this disorder.

Sexual reassignment surgery is not undertaken immediately upon request. The individual must be thoroughly assessed for the presence of other psychiatric disorders that could involve problems with gender identity. The individual desiring sexual reassignment is generally in psychotherapy for 6 to 12 months. Some gender identity programs require a written second opinion from another physician or psychologist before proceeding with surgical reassignment. Hormonal treatment, and living and relationship changes, are slowly made over months while the individual is in therapy. During this time, the individual's attitudes toward sexual reassignment may change and sexual reassignment surgery is not chosen. Those who do choose surgery can be helped to live more comfortable and productive lives.

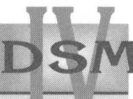

DSM-IV Criteria for Gender Identity Disorder

A. A strong and persistent cross-gender identification
   1. In children:
      a. Stated desire or insistence that he or she is the other sex
      b. In boys, dressing in female attire; in girls, wearing only masculine clothing
      c. Make-believe play or fantasies of being the other sex
      d. Desire to participate in games and pastimes of other sex
      e. Prefers playmates of other sex
   2. In adolescents and adults:
      a. Stated desire to be the other sex
      b. Frequently passes as the other sex
      c. Desires to be treated as the other sex
      d. Conviction that he or she has typical feelings and reactions of other sex.

B. Feelings of discomfort with own sex or inappropriateness in gender role of own sex

Adapted from the American Psychiatric Association: *Diagnostic and statistical manual of mental disorders,* ed 4, Washington, DC, 1994, The Association.

Psychotherapeutic Management

Nurse-Patient Relationship.   The nurse must have an accepting, empathic, and nonjudgmental attitude if patients are to be comfortable enough to disclose problems with sexuality. This comes about only after the nurse has reconciled and accepted his or her own feelings related to sexuality. The nurse's discomfort with sexual issues and sexuality may be interpreted by patients as disapproval of them and of their sexual issues and concerns. A private area in which to discuss fears or concerns about sexuality and victimization helps patients to disclose and discuss their feelings. The nurse discusses options for dealing with sexual issues and problems. Clarification and education may be needed about sexual functioning, effective communication, and healthy relationships. The nurse may also need to intervene to discuss self-esteem issues, anxiety, guilt, and empathy for victims.

It is necessary to help patients who are perpetrators deal with physical and emotional dimensions. Physical dimensions may include anorexia, insomnia, and weight loss. Emotional dimensions may include guilt, helplessness, shame, and relief about getting caught (Schella and Stern, 1994). Setting limits on how much the patient discloses in a group setting, especially if other group members may be victims of sexual assault, must be discussed.

The nurse is involved in the planning of patients' care regarding what issues and problems are addressed during an inpatient stay vs. what is addressed in outpatient treatment. The nurse also collaborates with social workers and chaplains, if patients choose, about feelings and religious views. The nurse is legally obligated to report suspected and actual sexual abuse of children to police and/or appropriate agencies. All states have mandatory child abuse reporting statutes. The nurse discusses possible referrals with patients and family members and refers patients to sex therapists if necessary. Referrals to outpatient treatment programs or therapy groups for specific disorders may be necessary. Individual, group, and family treatment for incest and support groups for perpetrators and victims may be appropriate.

▪ Critical Thinking Question

Outline the issues that you would discuss about sexual disorders in a staff education session.

Psychopharmacology.   Patients with axis I diagnoses are prescribed psychotherapeutic medication for their specific disorders. The nurse assesses all medications for side effects that affect sexual performance or dysfunction. The use of pharmacological agents for the treatment of sexual disorders is controversial, and effectiveness is variable. Men with paraphilias can be treated with agents to lower testosterone levels, which reduces their sex drive. Antiandrogen therapy with oral and parenteral preparations has been shown to reduce recidivism rates in male sexual aggressors (Bradford, 1995). Lower oral doses diminish sexual arousal with fewer side effects than parenteral doses (Grinspoon, 1997). The use of selective serotonin reuptake inhibitors (SSRIs), including fluoxetine (Prozac) and sertraline (Zoloft), are being used for paraphiliac and related disorders (Kafka, 1996). As the activity of serotonin increases, sexual appetite decreases along with depression and anxiety, which often accompany these disorders (Grinspoon, 1997).

Milieu Management.   Patients with sexual disorders and dysfunctions benefit from groups dealing with self-esteem, assertiveness, anger management, social and relationship skills, sex education, and stress management. Referrals may be indicated as mentioned previously. Self-help groups such as Sex Addicts Anonymous can benefit those with paraphilias. A multidimensional treatment plan using a combination of education and cognitive, behavioral, and family intervention must be used to reduce recidivism for sexual offenders (Dwyer, 1997). Longitudinal research studies will eventually help to determine which treatment factors are effective in reducing recidivism rates (Hanson, 1997).

▪ Critical Thinking Question

A patient with insulin-dependent diabetes states: "After I leave the hospital, I'm going to use only half of the prescribed insulin because I heard insulin might affect my sexual performance." What are your interventions with this patient?

▼ Key Concepts

1. Sexual dysfunctions may occur as the result of psychological, physiological, and pharmacological factors.
2. Paraphilias involve sexual activity with objects, children, and consenting or nonconsenting adults.

*C*ase *S*tudy

Bill Wood, 62 years old, has been admitted to the inpatient unit. His wife died 2 years ago; he has one daughter and three grandchildren. Bill is presently employed, but has few friends or hobbies. He visits his daughter and grandchildren approximately once a month, does not date, and does not have any female companions. For the past year, he has noticed an increase in sexual fantasies concerning children. He did not act on the fantasies until a week ago when he was babysitting for his youngest grandchild, 8-year-old Stephanie. He admits to fondling Stephanie's breasts, but denies other sexual contact with her. Bill states to the nurse, "I never thought I would be capable of such a horrible thing. I deserve to die. I even thought of killing myself."

*C*are *P*lan

NAME: Bill Wood   ADMISSION DATE: _____

DSM-IV DIAGNOSIS: Major depression
Pedophilia

ASSESSMENT: **Areas of strength:** Employed, visits daughter and grandchildren, remorse for contact with child, first offense.
Problems: Death of wife, few friends, disturbing sexual fantasies, suicidal ideation.

DIAGNOSES:
- Potential for self-directed violence related to guilt, as evidenced by suicidal ideation.
- Sexual dysfunction related to lack of significant other, as evidenced by fondling child.
- Social isolation related to lack of social support, as evidenced by loneliness.

OUTCOMES: **Short-term goals:**   Date met
- Patient will state he no longer has thoughts of suicide.   _____
- Patient will discuss sexual concerns and needs, and methods to satisfy
  these needs.   _____
  Long-term goals:
- Patient will contact support groups and senior citizen organizations.   _____
- Patient will schedule outpatient appointment for further assessment of
  sexual disorder   _____

PLANNING/
INTERVENTIONS: **Nurse-patient relationship:** Instruct patient to approach staff when suicidal thoughts occur. Discuss feelings of guilt, remorse, anger, loneliness, and low self-esteem. Discuss the patient's beliefs and values about sexuality with him. Discuss and help the patient to identify sexual concerns, needs, and methods to satisfy needs.
Psychopharmacology: Prozac 20 mg q AM.
Milieu management: Groups focusing on self-esteem, stress and anger management, assertiveness training, social skills, and discharge planning.

EVALUATION: Patient reports he is no longer suicidal.

REFERRALS: He will attend senior citizen activities at his church with a friend. Appointment scheduled at a sexual disorders clinic.

3. Efforts to achieve sexual pleasure do not give individuals the right to violate the rights of others through coercion and control.
4. Gender identity disorder in adults involves persistent discomfort with one's biological sex.
5. The nurse's role in the treatment of sexual disorders is primarily one of referral.

Study Questions

(Answer key is in the back of the book.)

1. During the admission interview, a patient states to the nurse that she has no interest in sexual intercourse with her husband. The nurse first:
   a. Advises the patient to talk to her doctor about this
   b. Tells the patient not to worry about it now
   c. Directs the patient to discuss another subject
   d. Further questions the patient about this concern
2. A patient states to the nurse, "I feel so guilty because I fondled my daughter's 7-year-old friend." Which of the following responses is most appropriate?
   a. "We can't do anything about that now."
   b. "Tell me more about what happened."
   c. "Your guilt will lessen after your medication starts to work."
   d. "Does your wife know about this?"
3. A patient is an incest perpetrator. In a discussion with the patient's wife, the nurse:
   a. Tells the wife to divorce her husband
   b. Explains that the husband alone needs treatment
   c. Recommends a support group for the wife
   d. Advises the wife to call the police about her husband's activity
4. A patient with major depression is also a known pedophile. The nurse includes which of the following strategies in the plan of care?
   a. Isolate the patient in his room as much as possible.
   b. Help the patient to discuss his feelings about himself and his problems.
   c. Tell the patient that he ought to be ashamed of himself.
   d. Advise the patient to discuss his problems openly with other patients on the unit.

REFERENCES

American Psychiatric Association: *Diagnostic and statistical manual of mental disorders*, ed 4, Washington, DC, 1994, The Association.

Ames A and Houston D: Legal, social, and biological definitions of pedophilia, *Arch Sex Behav* 19(4):333, 1990.

Bradford JMW: Pharmacological treatment of the paraphilias. In Oldham JM and Riba MB, editors: *American Psychiatric Press review of psychiatry*, vol 14, Washington, DC, 1995, American Psychiatric Press.

Dwyer SM: Treatment outcome study: seventeen years after sexual offender treatment, *Sexual Abuse: A Journal of Research and Treatment* 9(2):149, 1997.

Grinspoon L, editor: How are drugs used in the treatment of paraphilic disorders, *Harvard Mental Health Letter* 14(3):8, 1997.

Hanson RK: How to know what works with sexual offenders, *Sexual Abuse: A Journal of Research and Treatment* 9(2):129, 1997.

Kafka M: Therapy for sexual impulsivity: the paraphilias and paraphilia-related disorders, *Psychiatric Times*, June 1996.

Kaplan H and Sadock B: *Comprehensive textbook of psychiatry*, ed 5, Baltimore, 1989, Williams & Wilkins.

Schella RA and Stern PN: Falling apart: a process integral to the remodeling of male incest perpetrators, *Arch Psychiatr Nurs* 8(2):91, 1994.

CHAPTER 33

Substance-Related Disorders

GORDON I.G. PUGH
NORMAN L. KELTNER

▲   ▲   ▲   ▲   ▲   ▲

LEARNING OBJECTIVES

After reading this chapter you should be able to:
- Recognize the personal and societal toll of substance abuse.
- Recognize DSM-IV criteria and terminology for substance-related disorders.
- Recognize and describe objective and subjective symptoms of substance dependence and abuse.
- Describe physiological, emotional, and interpersonal theoretical explanations for the development of substance-related disorders.

- Develop a nursing care plan for substance abuse/ dependence patients.
- Evaluate the relative effectiveness of nursing interventions for patients with substance-related disorders.
- Understand the contributions of nonmedical interventions in recovery from substance-related disorders.

"The news is not good. Even though total casual use remains stable, more kids are using drugs than last year, especially more marijuana. . . .

Crack cocaine users, burned out on the drug's stimulating effects, are turning to opiates. Heroin dealers are luring them, as well as first-time drug users, by packaging the drug for snorting and smoking. Hardcore drug users are continuing to commit crimes, drive health-care costs upward, and give dealers more reasons to fight over drug market turf, often with violent and terrible consequences.

Even though there is less casual drug use today than in years past, the increase in use among the nation's youth adds another ingredient to the volatile mix of drug trends that already threaten the Nation's stability." (National Drug Control Strategy, 1995)

Note to the Student: The student will find it helpful to know that *chemical dependency, substance abuse, drug problem, addiction, alcoholism,* and other terms are frequently used interchangeably. We generally follow the DSM-IV designations for substance-related disorders. Such phrases eliminate the use of more cumbersome, albeit technically correct, terminology.

This is a revision of a chapter revised by Virginia M. Spaulding, originally written by MaryLou Scavnicky-Mylant.

KEY TERMS

Abstinence syndrome   Physical signs and symptoms that occur when the addictive substance is reduced or withheld; also referred to as withdrawal

Abuse   Excessive use of a substance that differs from societal norms

Blackouts   A period of time in which the drinker functions socially but for which there is no memory

Cirrhosis   Disease of the liver typically caused by abuse of alcohol

Codependency   Stress-related preoccupation with an addicted person's life, leading to extreme dependence on that person

Dependence   A state in which a drug abuser must take a usual or increasing dose of a drug in order to prevent the onset of abstinence symptoms/withdrawal

Metabolic tolerance   Occurs when the body is more efficient at metabolizing the substance

Pharmacodynamic tolerance   Occurs when higher blood levels are required to produce a given effect

Tolerance   The need for increasing amounts of a substance to achieve the same effects.

Withdrawal   Physical signs and symptoms that occur when the addictive substance is reduced or withheld; also referred to as an abstinence syndrome

12-Month Prevalence Rate of Mental Disorders in the United States

Diagnosis	Percentage of Population over 17 Years of Age	Number of Persons
Anxiety disorders	12.6	20,034,000
Phobia disorders*	10.9	17,331,000
Mood disorders	9.5	15,143,000
Alcohol disorders	**7.4**	**11,766,000**
Major depression†	5.0	7,950,000
Drug disorders	**3.1**	**4,929,000**
Cognitive impairment	2.7	4,293,000
Obsessive-compulsive disorder	2.1	3,339,000
Antisocial disorder	1.5	2,385,000
Panic disorders*	1.3	2,067,000
Bipolar disorder†	1.2	1,908,000
Schizophrenia	1.1	1,749,000
Somatization	0.2	365,000

From Regier DA, et al: The de facto US mental and addictive disorders service system: epidemiologic catchment area prospective 1-year prevalence rates of disorders and services, *Arch Gen Psychiatry* 50:85, 1993.
*Also calculated in anxiety statistics.
†Also calculated in mood disorders statistics.

Also, please note that AOD is a common abbreviation for *"alcohol and/or other drugs."*

A BRIEF INTRODUCTION TO SUBSTANCE-RELATED DISORDERS

While drug abuse statistics are important, they vary from time to time and from culture to culture. Because of the enormity of these numbers, we find it difficult to grasp the human touch and the individual suffering produced by substance abuse and dependence. The authors hope that the content of this chapter will help the nurse understand the deeply personal aspects of substance abuse and dependence. Even the genocidal Joseph Stalin recognized that people can easily be inoculated from the shock of many deaths by the overwhelming magnitude of the numbers. Nevertheless, he noted, "A single death is a tragedy; a million deaths is a statistic." Substance abuse and dependence have many costs, but one person's pain is tragic. The vignettes of patients you will meet in these pages and others like them reveal the real people who make up these "statistics." The effects of their pain because of drug and alcohol abuse are magnified innumerable times, have a tremendous ripple effect on society, and touch everyone to some degree.

We know that human beings have used mood-altering substances at least since the beginning of recorded history. The first recorded use of alcohol occurred as early as 3500 BC, and ancient Chinese writings make reference to marijuana. In the United States during the 1820s, per capita alcohol consumption was 5 times what it is today (Forbes, 1997). Whether using Far Eastern opium, South American cocaine, North American peyote, French wine, or modern pharmaceuticals, human beings have consistently found ways to alter their mood. Often these effects are therapeutically beneficial—even with the substances just mentioned—and add a certain legitimacy to their use. Only in relatively recent times have we been able to provide pain relief beyond drinking copious amounts of alcohol or biting a bullet. But even a good thing can be taken to extremes, often with dire consequences. This chapter concentrates on maladaptive uses of alcohol and other drugs—both legal and illegal—commonly referred to as "drug abuse."

The information in this chapter is important for you to know for at least two reasons. *First*, maladaptive use of mood-altering substances leads to diverse complications that you need to be aware of professionally. When a patient presents "hearing voices," for example, knowing the patient's substance abuse history (if any) could make the difference between trying to treat schizophrenia and treating alcohol withdrawal (or intoxication). These conditions require significantly different therapeutic interventions and such diagnostic dilemmas are not at all uncommon. (Chapter 34 deals specifically with the problems of dual diagnoses.) A *second* reason is that abuse of alcohol and other drugs is a widespread concern with broad social ramifications (e.g., drunk driving or drug-related crime) and personal consequences (e.g., a friend or family member who contracts hepatitis or human immunodeficiency virus [HIV] by sharing a needle, or a child who is abandoned—or worse—because the parents are too busy using drugs to provide attentive child care). Table 33-1 outlines the extent of drug use in a given month.

You probably know people who suffer from substance abuse issues and who have experienced some

Table 33-1 The Numbers Game

Substance	Number Who Used in Past Month
Heroin	200,000
Amphetamines	800,000
Cocaine/crack	1,500,000
Marijuana	10,000,000
Alcohol	11,000,000 (abusers)
Nicotine	61,000,000
Caffeine	130,000,000

Adapted from Nash JM: Addicted: why do people get hooked?, *Time*, p 68, May 5, 1997.

of the problems associated with them. Perhaps you know someone in this position and are not even aware of the fact. As a nurse, you will see patients suffering from the consequences of substance abuse. You will probably know other people who are suffering from it as well. The key is to be able to recognize this possibility and to be able to help with appropriate referrals and/or interventions. You could be the only professional to whom they will turn when they realize their use has become problematic. We hope you take the time to study this information carefully and diligently. The patient's care begins with the initial assessment.

CLINICAL EXAMPLE

Robert had an average childhood and made good grades in school. He grew up in a home with both parents and with other siblings. His parents were active in the community. In high school, he was particularly talented in sports and was popular among his peers. Robert was, and is, an immensely likable fellow. He began drinking beer when he was 15 years old, with his baseball teammates. After graduation from high school with honors, he went to college on a baseball scholarship. In college he was known to smoke some marijuana, but "never let it get in the way" of his sports or his studies. He was good at hiding his drug use. It would never have occurred to him that he "had a problem," not even later when his self-destruction was blatantly apparent to everyone else in his life except himself. Robert has since learned, however, that he suffers from addiction and has learned how to manage his condition.

At first he stayed out a little too late one night before a big game, and he had a bad game or two because of his slightly decreased performance. Eventually he was introduced to cocaine, discovered intravenous (IV) use ("mainlining"), lost his promising sports career, was divorced by his wife, stole from people, lied to his family, tried to kill himself, and spent time in prison. While he was incarcerated, he realized how self-destructive his drug use had become, and he vowed to do whatever it would take to become and remain drug free. He reasoned that he had been willing to do a great many things in his search for dope, so he ought to be willing to exert the same amount of energy in his search to break free from its grip on his life. Robert had been hospitalized for detoxification in the past but "wasn't ready." When he attended a small treatment group at the county jail, however, he was ready to listen and learn.

Today Robert is in his early 30s, has earned his bachelor's degree, has a good job, makes a good salary, is no longer on parole, plays ball with a local community league, is married to a wonderfully supportive spouse, and—most importantly—remains drug free. Robert's life did not get back together overnight, however. It took several years to undo most of the damage that his drug use caused. *Some damage can never be repaired*, but he is far better off now than he was before he could see the extent of the problems caused by his drug use.

Assessment Strategies for Chemical Dependency

As a component of every patient assessment, the nurse should inquire about the amount and type of the patient's use of prescribed medication as well as alcohol and other mood-altering substances. Helping to save lives is a good reason to seek accuracy. Significant underreporting is common by AOD users; however they have a great need to be accurately assessed. The nurse should be acutely aware of the potential pitfalls of self reporting among these patients. The nurse should always ask how much alcohol the patient drinks or how much prescription medication the patient actually takes (not simply how it is prescribed to be taken). Many people abuse prescription medications. If one pill once a day is good, then two pills twice a day must be even better, a drug abuser will reason. The patient might also be asked if there are or ever have been medical problems associated with AOD use by any family member. Furthermore, because many substance abusers tend to minimize their level of AOD use (as well as the consequences of their use), many facilities routinely use a blood or urine drug screen to get objective information. Urine screens are typically believed to be more reliable in detecting trace amounts of substances because of the higher concentration of metabolites in the urine. Galletly, Field, and Prior (1993) found that about one fourth of the psychiatric patients admitted to a state hospital underreported their level of alcohol or drug use. The importance of such objective data cannot be overemphasized. The authors have found it helpful to estimate underreporting of around 40% to 60% during an initial interview. Many addicted patients will not readily reveal in an initial interview more than what one can already discover by other means. Someone who is referred to treatment because alcohol use has led to problems with the legal system, for example, is often unwilling to admit cocaine or marijuana use until it is detected by objective means. Even then, some patients will deny use of the substance detected.

Far more insidious, however, is the phenomenon of denial (Box 33-1). Denial occurs when the dependent person is unable to see how destructive AOD use has become, even though it is blatantly obvious to others. Denial is associated with an inability to link the problems in one's life causally with the AOD use. Denial is one manifestation of active defense mechanisms and is quite strong in most chemically dependent persons. This inability to see self-destructive behavior and attitudes, or to link life problems with AOD use, is a primary symptom of substance dependence (Koop, et al, 1996).

Urinalysis will often provide a more objective report of recent drug use (Table 33-2). Blood levels are perhaps best used to detect recent use and trigger treatment protocols. Hair toxicology is highly effective in determining long-term patterns of use but is not thought to be as cost-effective as analysis of blood or urine. Hair samples of Henri Paul, the driver of the car in which Diana, Princess of Wales, was killed in 1997, were subjected to such a test in an attempt to find objective evidence about his actual long-term AOD use (Sancton, 1997). Some hair toxicology kits are available in the retail market, designed for parents to test the hair of children they suspect may be using drugs. One problem, however, is that blonde hair does not seem to accumulate certain drugs such as cocaine as effectively as darker hair (Muha, 1997).

√

Box 33-1 Defense Mechanisms at Work: Denial

An intoxicated 60+-year-old Madison, Wisconsin, woman, who was dressed as a clown on her way to entertain children at a birthday party, tried to kill her 83-year-old mother-in-law over a beer. "I've had 40 years of hell because of you," she is reported to have told the victim. When asked about her long-standing alcohol problem, she indicated that she has no "problem," except for the mother-in-law.

Adapted from "Whatdyaknow," Wisconsin Public Radio, June 4, 1994. The story is from *USA Today,* p 10A, June 3, 1994. (Chris Bannon, the producer of "Whatdyaknow," is available at Bannon@VILAS.uwex.edu or (608) 262-3970.)

Interview Approaches

Since underreporting can lead to misdiagnosis, it is important for the nurse to approach the patient in a manner that encourages forthrightness. The nurse should be rather matter-of-fact and nonjudgmental while eliciting information that might carry with it some feelings of shame for the patient. Most nurses are not prepared for the defensiveness displayed by the chemically dependent person, but some genuine concern for the patient can help overcome this barrier. Furthermore, since many nurses themselves have been personally affected by drugs and alcohol, it is important for nurses to be in touch with their own feelings regarding people involved in substance dependence and not to allow these attitudes to be projected onto the patient. Phrases such as "problem with drinking" or "difficulties with drug use" might be more palatable than the labels "addict" or "alcoholic," but these, too, may not elicit the accurate information the nurse seeks.

Imagine trying to elicit accurate clinical information from the woman in Box 33-1 about whether or not she is intoxicated. It may also be helpful initially to focus more on legally or culturally accepted substances such as caffeine and nicotine. The patient's consumption should be evaluated in more detail if the initial assessment data identify the patient as being more at risk for chemical dependence. The authors suggest using the terms "problems because of drinking" or "using more than intended" as more accurate and diagnostic, less threatening, and more likely to link patients' AOD use with the problems in their lives. This factor is important both in effective care planning and in providing the patient with good internal motivation.

Table 33-2 Period of Time after Ingestion That Drugs Can Be Detected in the Urine

Drug	Detection Period
Opioids	
Heroin	2-4 days
Morphine	2-4 days
Meperidine (Demerol)	2-4 days
Methadone	2-4 days
Fentanyl	can be <1 hour
Depressants	
Barbiturates	12 hours to 3 weeks
Benzodiazepines	Up to 1 week
Stimulants	
Amphetamines	2-4 days
Cocaine	2-4 days
Hallucinogens	
Marijuana	3 days to <1 month
PCP	1 day to 1 month

Adapted from Sullivan E, Bissell L, and William E: *Chemical dependency in nursing,* Redwood City, Calif, 1988, Addison-Wesley.

Various assessment guides are available to the nurse, including both subjective interviews and objective assessment instruments. Early diagnosis of substance-related disorders is often missed due to misdiagnosing or underdiagnosing related to misunderstandings about AOD disorders and/or inadequate training (Alcohol and Health, 1990). Selected instruments will be covered later in this chapter.

Substance abuse is widespread in North America and demands the attention of psychiatric nurses both as a singular phenomenon and as a variable in other psychiatric disorders. For example, it is estimated that one third to one half of all patients undergoing psychiatric treatment abuse alcohol and/or drugs (Carey, 1989; Ananth, et al, 1989). Substance abuse is the most common comorbid psychiatric condition associated with schizophrenia (Cuffel, Heithoff, and Lawson, 1993), with some studies indicating as many as 64.7% of these patients abusing drugs or alcohol (Kovasznay, et al, 1993). It is also common among patients with dissociative disorders (Kolodner and Frances, 1993) and affective disorders (Brown, et al, 1995). Comorbidity, or when patients have a dual diagnosis, is such an important issue that a separate chapter addresses that subject.

It is also believed that the use and abuse of alcohol and drugs among the general population is one of the most significant social issues of our times. In addition to the statistics quoted in professional journals related to substance abuse, almost every issue of our newspapers and news magazines carries accounts of national and international problems related to the abuse of alcohol and other drugs. Economic problems associated with substance abuse are staggering. One report estimates that the annual cost to the American economy is $161.3 billion (National Foundation for Brain Research [NFBR], 1992).

Because of the significance of the problem, this chapter addresses the general issues surrounding substance abuse. In order to treat the substance-abusing person's condition effectively, the nurse must understand three areas important to effective intervention:

1. The DSM-IV criteria used to assess substance-related disorders
2. The nature of the substance(s) being abused

Box 33-2   Controlled Substances: Uses and Effects

Drugs/CSA Schedules		Trade or Other Names	Medical Uses	Dependence	
				Physical	Psychological
Narcotics					
Opium	II III V	Dover's Powder, Paregoric Parapectolin	Analgesic, antidiarrheal	High	High
Morphine	II III	Morphine, MS Contin, Roxanol, Roxanol-SR	Analgesic, antitussive	High	High
Codeine	II III V	Tylenol w/Codeine, Empirin w/Codeine, Robitussin A-C, Fiorinal w/Codeine	Analgesic, antitussive	Moderate	Moderate
Heroin	I	Diacetylmorphine, horse, smack	None	High	High
Hydromorphone	II	Dilaudid	Analgesic	High	High
Meperidine	II	Demerol, Mepergan	Analgesic	High	High
Methadone	II	Dolophine, methadone, Methadose	Analgesic	High	High-low
Other narcotics	I II III IV V	Numorphan, Percodan, Percocet, Tylox, Tussionex, fentanyl, Darvon, Lomotil, Talwin*	Analgesic antidiarrheal, antitussive	High-low	High-low
Depressants					
Chloral hydrate	IV	Noctec	Hypnotic	Moderate	Moderate
Barbiturates	II III IV	Amytal, Butisol, Florinal, Lotusate, Nembutal, Seconal, Tuinal, phenobarbital	Anesthetic, anticonvulsant, sedative, hypnotic, veterinary euthanasia agent	High-mod.	High-mod.
Benzodiazepines	IV	Ativan, Dalmane, diazepam, Librium, Xanax, Serax, Valium, Tranxexe, Verstran, Versed, Halcion, Paxipam, Restoril	Antianxiety, anticonvulsant, sedative, hypnotic	Low	Low
Methaqualone	I	Quaalude	Sedative, hypnotic	High	High
Glutethimide	III	Doriden	Sedative, hypnotic	High	Moderate

From *Federal Register* 55(159):33590, Washington, DC, Aug 16, 1990.

3. The treatment of patients with substance-related disorders

Drugs of abuse fall into four classes: alcohol and other central nervous system (CNS) depressants, opioids, stimulants, and hallucinogens (Box 33-2).

DSM-IV CRITERIA

The DSM-IV specifies criteria for classifications of substance dependence, substance abuse, substance intoxication, and substance withdrawal (First, et al, 1994). Dependence is often marked by physiological need for the substance, usually in increasing amounts to gain the same effect; a persistent desire to cut down, which is met with little success; and a continued substance use even though physical, social, and emotional processes are compromised. Regardless of the substance, behavior patterns that meet these criteria indicate a problem. The term *dependence* has generally replaced the term *addiction* for describing compulsive drug use because it more

Tolerance	Duration (hours)	Usual Method of Administration	Possible Effects	Effects of Overdose	Withdrawal Syndrome
Yes	3-6	Oral, smoked	Euphoria, drowsiness, respiratory depression, constricted pupils, nausea	Slow and shallow breathing, clammy skin, convulsions, coma, possible death	Watery eyes, runny nose, yawning, loss of appetite, irritability, tremors, panic, cramps, nausea, chills and sweating
Yes	3-6	Oral, smoked, injected			
Yes	3-6	Oral, injected			
Yes	3-6	Injected, sniffed, smoked			
Yes	3-6	Oral, injected			
Yes	3-6	Oral, injected			
Yes	12-24	Oral, injected			
Yes	Variable	Oral, injected			
Yes	5-8	Oral	Slurred speech, disorientation, drunken behavior without odor of alcohol	Shallow respiration, clammy skin, dilated pupils, weak and rapid pulse, coma, possible death	Anxiety, insomnia, tremors, delirium, convulsions, possible death
Yes	1-16	Oral			
Yes	4-8	Oral			
Yes	4-8	Oral			
Yes	4-8	Oral			

Continued

Box 33-2 Controlled Substances: Uses and Effects—cont'd

Drugs/CSA Schedules		Trade or Other Names	Medical Uses	Dependence	
				Physical	Psychological
Depressants—cont'd					
Other depressants	III IV	Equanil, Miltown, Noludar, Placidyl, Valmid	Antianxiety, sedative, hypnotic	Moderate	Moderate
Stimulants					
Cocaine	II	Coke, flake, snow, crack	Local anesthetic	Possible	High
Amphetamines	II	Biphetamine, Delcobese, Desoxyn, Dexedrine, Obetrol	Attention deficit disorders, narcolepsy, weight control	Possible	High
Phenmetrazine	II	Preludin	Weight control	Possible	High
Methylphenidate	II	Ritalin	Attention deficit disorders, narcolepsy	Possible	Moderate
Other stimulants	III IV	Adipex, Cylert, Didrex, Ionamin, Melfiat, Plegine, Sanorex, Tenuate, Tepanil, Prelu-2	Weight control	Possible	High
Hallucinogens					
LSD	I	Acid, microdot	None	None	Unknown
Mescaline and peyote	I	Mexc, buttons, cactus	None	None	Unknown
Amphetamine variants	I	2.5-DMA, PMA, STP, MDA, MDMA, TMA, DOM, DOB	None	Unknown	Unknown
Phencyclidine	II	PCP, angel dust, hog	None	Unknown	High
Phencyclidine analogues	I	PCE, PCPy, TCP	None	Unknown	High
Other hallucinogens	I	Bufotenine, ibogaine, DMT, DET, psilocybin, psilocin	None	None	Unknown
Cannabis					
Marijuana	I	Pot, Acapulco Gold, grass, reefer, Sinsemilla, Thai sticks	None	Unknown	Moderate
Tetrahydrocannabinol	I II	THC, Marinol	Cancer chemotherapy antinauseant	Unknown	Moderate
Hashish	I	Hash	None	Unknown	Moderate
Hashish oil	I	Hash oil	None	Unknown	Moderate

From *Federal Register* 55(159):33590, Washington, DC, Aug 16, 1990.

precisely defines the condition. Heroin addiction and alcoholism are therefore correctly referred to as drug dependencies.

In 1987 the American Medical Association declared all drug dependencies to be diseases. When chemical dependencies are viewed as diseases, their treatment and understanding are facilitated. Such a view also reduces the guilt and blame traditionally associated with chemical dependency. Although not all psychiatrists and psychiatric nurses embrace

Tolerance	Duration (hours)	Usual Method of Administration	Possible Effects	Effects of Overdose	Withdrawal Syndrome
Yes	4-8	Oral			
Yes	1-2	Sniffed, smoked, injected	Increased alertness, excitation, euphoria, increased pulse rate & blood pressure, insomnia, loss of appetite	Agitation, increase in body temperature, hallucinations, convulsions, possible death	Apathy, long periods of sleep, irritability, depression, disorientation
Yes	2-4	Oral, injected			
Yes	2-4	Oral, injected			
Yes	2-4	Oral, injected			
Yes	2-4	Oral, injected			
Yes	8-12	Oral	Illusions and hallucinations, poor perception of time and distance	Longer, more intense "trip" episodes, psychosis, possible death	Withdrawal syndrome not reported
Yes	8-12	Oral			
Yes	Variable	Oral, injected			
Yes	Days	Smoked, oral, injected			
Yes	Days	Smoked, oral, injected			
Possible	Variable	Smoked, oral, injected, sniffed			
Yes	2-4	Smoked, oral	Euphoria, relaxed inhibitions, increased appetite, disoriented behavior	Fatigue, paranoia, possible psychosis	Insomnia, hyperactivity, and decreased appetite occasionally reported
Yes	2-4	Smoked, oral			
Yes	2-4	Smoked, oral			
Yes	2-4	Smoked, oral			

the disease concept of drug dependence, there are convincing arguments for accepting it. Using alcoholism as an example, Ohlms (1991) points out that it (1) causes the person to function abnormally, (2) has a characteristic chain of symptoms reflecting specific stages of the disease that are both reliable and predictable, and (3) has the inevitable outcome of death if drinking continues. These three criteria are in concert with a disease model. Further, Blum and Trachtenberg (1988) discuss the effects of how a

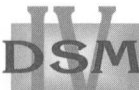
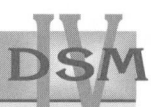

DSM-IV Criteria for Substance-Related Disorders

Substance Dependence
A. A maladaptive pattern of substance use as manifested by three or more of the following:
1. Tolerance
2. Withdrawal
3. A need for more of the substance than was intended
4. Inability to stop using even when wanting to do so
5. A great deal of time is spent in acquiring the substance or in recovering from its effects
6. Substance use causes social, occupational, or recreational problems
7. Continued substance use despite knowledge that the substance is causing physical or psychological problems

Substance Abuse
A. A maladaptive pattern of substance use leading to clinically significant impairment or distress as manifested by one or more of the following:
1. Failure to fulfill major role obligations at work, school, or home
2. Recurrent substance use in hazardous situations

3. Recurrent substance-related legal problems
4. Continued substance use despite problems
B. Has never met the criteria for substance dependence for this class of substance.

Substance Intoxication
A. The development of a substance-specific syndrome due to a recent ingestion of a substance
B. Clinically significant maladaptive behavioral or psychological changes due to the effect of the substance on the central nervous system
C. Not due to a general medical condition and not better accounted for by another mental disorder

Substance Withdrawal
A. The development of a substance-specific syndrome due to the cessation of or reduction in the intake of a substance
B. The substance-specific syndrome causes clinically significant distress or impairment
C. Not due to a general medical condition and not better accounted for by another mental disorder

Adapted from the American Psychiatric Association: *Diagnostic and statistical manual of mental disorders,* ed 4, Washington, DC, 1994, The Association.

lack of naturally occurring opiate-like substances in the body at brain receptor sites can produce a craving for alcohol, a condition that can be treated chemically to alleviate the craving. The fact that a purely physiological intervention can produce change lends further credibility to the disease model concept.

Some professionals use a working definition of chemical dependency that is less rigid than the criteria outlined in the DSM-IV. They define use of substances as a problem when the effects of such use interfere with and disrupt family, work, or social relationships. If those areas of a person's life are being adversely affected, then the person is seen as having a problem and as being in need of treatment.

ABUSED SUBSTANCES

ALCOHOL ABUSE

Alcohol abuse is the primary drug problem in North America and is addressed separately because of the enormity of the problem it poses. The cost to

the United States in health problems, lost work hours, family disruption and disintegration, and criminal activity (Box 33-3) is estimated at more than $90.1 billion annually (NFBR, 1992). An estimated 17 million Americans (6.8%) manifest symptoms of alcoholism (Bucholz, 1992), and after cardiovascular disease and cancer, alcoholism ranks third among the causes of death and disability in the United States (Whitfield, Davis, and Barker, 1986). Alcoholics have a death rate 2 to 4 times higher than nonalcoholics. Approximately 98,000 deaths each year are directly related to alcohol. Cirrhosis, the tenth leading cause of death (Smart and Mann, 1992), other medical problems, homicides (50% alcohol related), and suicides (25% alcohol related) are directly linked to alcohol use (see Box 33-3). Furthermore, accidental deaths such as motor vehicle accidents (50% alcohol related), fires and burns (47% alcohol related), drownings (34% alcohol related), and falls (28% alcohol related) are examples of the different ways alcohol use is lethal (Cherpitel, 1992). In motor vehicle accidents where pedestrians are killed, 40% of the pedestrians are under the influence (Feldman, 1994).

Etiological Theories

Psychodynamic theories

A number of psychological theories have attempted to explain how people become substance dependent. People who are alcohol dependent have often been viewed as individuals who easily succumb to the escape provided by alcohol. Psychoanalytic theory describes people with alcohol dependency as having strong oral tendencies related to unresolved needs for early attachments (Frosch, 1985). Drinking alcohol is thought to be an attempt to satisfy unconscious oral needs. More recent theories have described people likely to become alcohol dependent as more phobic and inferior-feeling than social drinkers. Over time the search for an "alcoholic personality" has given way to a multivariate model that incorporates the biopsychosocial components of addiction. Current researchers believe that many of the stereotypical characteristics found among alcohol-dependent people such as dependency, low self-esteem, passivity, and introversion are the result of and not the cause of substance dependence. Psychodynamically oriented treatment tends to emphasize behavioral management techniques and reject the disease model of substance dependence.

Biological theories

Heredity as an etiological factor has been studied for many years and continues to provide insight into understanding the genesis of alcoholism. Genetic predisposition is considered to be the single most significant piece of information in identifying alcoholism (Ohlms, 1991). We have known for a quarter of a century that children of alcoholic parents, even if raised in an alcohol-free environment, are more likely to become alcoholics than are the children of nonalcoholic parents (Goodwin, et al, 1973). Though studies indicate different degrees of effect, hereditary explanations at the very least provide a good basis for understanding one's vulnerability to alcohol dependency. But predisposition means neither fatalism nor determinism. Even patients who are genetically predisposed to certain types of cancer, for example, can take steps to minimize their risk.

> ### Box 33-3   Alcohol and Crime
>
> The statistics are striking. Sixty percent of convicted homicide offenders drank just before committing the offense. Sixty-three percent of adults jailed for homicide had been drinking before the offense. Sixty percent of prison inmates drank heavily just before committing the violent crime for which they were incarcerated. The relationship between poverty and homicide is stronger in neighborhoods with higher rates of alcohol consumption than in those with average or below-average rates. Numerous studies report a strong association between sexual violence and alcohol, finding that "anywhere between 30 and 90 percent of convicted rapists are drunk at the time of the offense." Juveniles, especially young men, who drink to the point of drunkenness are more likely than those who do not drink to get into fights, get arrested, commit violent crimes, and recidivate later in life. Alcohol-dependent male factory workers are more than three times as likely to physically abuse their wives than are otherwise comparable, non–alcohol-dependent counterparts. The high incidence of drinking among convicted criminals does not necessarily prove that drinking stimulates crime; it may be nearer to being evidence that criminals who drink are more likely to get caught and convicted than those who do not. But it is important not to discount or deny the probable, and in some cases patently obvious, connections between [alcohol use], disorder, and crime.

From Dilulio JJ Jr: Broken bottles: alcohol, disorder, and crime, *Brookings Review* (The Brookings Institution), p 14, Spring 1996.

Pharmacokinetics of Alcohol

Metabolism

The chemical name for alcohol is ethanol (CH_3CH_2OH). The United States Navy produced an educational film some years ago that points out that the combination of the elements in two ethanol molecules could produce the compound ethyl ether (($C_2H_5)_2O$) and water (H_2O), in its attempt to demonstrate why it is important to think of alcohol as a drug through a comparison of alcohol with ether. Alcohol is primarily metabolized in the liver. The oxidation process can be described chemically as follows:

$$CH_3CH_2OH \rightarrow CH_3CHO + H_2 \rightarrow CH_3-C-OH-O \rightarrow CO_2-H_2O$$

(ethanol)   (acetaldehyde)   (acetic acid)   (carbon dioxide)   (water)

At each step of the metabolizing process an enzyme breaks down the chemical. Ethanol is broken down by alcohol dehydrogenase to acetaldehyde and hydrogen. The hydrogen molecule causes the liver to bypass normal energy sources (the hydrogen from fat) and to use the hydrogen from ethanol. Fat accumulates and leads to fatty liver, hyperlipemia, hepatitis, and cirrhosis. Acetaldehyde is toxic to the body; it compromises normal cell function in the liver. If the metabolism of acetaldehyde is impaired, it accumulates in the liver, causing cell death and necrosis. Liver cell loss contributes to cirrhosis. Acetaldehyde also interferes with vitamin activation. Aldehyde dehydrogenase breaks down acetaldehyde to acetic acid, which is an innocuous substance. When enzymatic action on acetaldehyde is blocked by the aldehyde dehydrogenase blocker disulfiram (Antabuse), acetaldehyde accumulates, causing severe sickness.

Research confirms an age-old suspicion that women become intoxicated more easily than men, even when studies are controlled for size differences. Frezza, et al (1990) discovered that the gastrointestinal tissue of women and of alcohol-dependent men contains little alcohol dehydrogenase. The alcohol dehydrogenase in the gastrointestinal tissue of non–alcohol-dependent men oxidizes a significant amount of ethanol in the gut before it enters the bloodstream. The inability of women's bodies to make this "first-pass metabolism" accounts for their enhanced vulnerability to alcohol.

Absorption

Alcohol is absorbed partially from the stomach but mostly from the small intestine. If it is ingested by a person with an empty stomach, alcohol is in the bloodstream within 20 minutes. The rate of absorption is affected by the form of alcohol consumed. Alcohol in beer and wine is absorbed more slowly than alcohol in liquor. This may be due partially to dilution. Beer contains 4% ethanol; wine, 12% ethanol; whiskey, 40% to 50% ethanol. However, slower absorption cannot be totally accounted for by dilution of the alcohol in its beverage medium. Food also slows alcohol absorption. Ethanol is distributed equally in all body tissue according to water content. Larger persons (who have greater amounts of body water) can therefore ingest more alcohol than smaller persons, who have less body water. Alcohol affects the cerebrum and cerebellum before it affects the spinal cord and the vital centers because the former

areas contain more water. The rate of absorption largely determines how quickly a person will become intoxicated, but one's metabolic rate largely determines how long alcohol will affect the body. The healthy body can metabolize 10 ml of alcohol (1 oz of whiskey or one 12-oz can of beer) about every 90 minutes. In persons who drink alcohol frequently over a number of years, hepatic drug-metabolizing levels are increased to hasten alcohol metabolism (metabolic tolerance). Hot coffee, "sweating it out," and other home remedies do not increase alcohol metabolism, nor do they speed the sobering-up process. Attempts by scientists to develop a pill to prevent or decrease intoxication have been unsuccessful. In late-stage alcoholism, tolerance decreases as the abused liver finally can no longer adequately metabolize the alcohol.

Tolerance to alcohol occurs and is probably related to elevated hepatic enzyme levels and to cellular adaptation (pharmacodynamic tolerance). Where the normal drinker might be noticeably drunk after 10 to 12 drinks, the long-term drinker with pharmacodynamic tolerance might seem unaffected by drinking the same amount. "Drinking someone under the table" is therefore more of an indicator of "practice" than of virility.

Physiological Effects

People generally begin consuming alcohol because it causes a reaction they desire. Disinhibition, impaired judgment, and fuzzy thinking are initial responses to alcohol ingestion. These signs represent cerebrum intoxication. In many situations this mental relaxation is pleasant. Alcohol also depresses psychomotor activity. Alcohol has been described as a social lubricant because it relaxes self-imposed barriers that inhibit sociability. Anxiety and tension are relieved, usually for a couple of hours after a drink is taken. Eventually, at least for the alcoholic, drinking becomes defensive; that is, the alcoholic often drinks to avoid the effects of many years of drinking. For instance, once the anxiety-reducing effect wears off, more tension and anxiety are caused, so the drinker must consume more alcohol to regain the "anxiety-free" state. Many alcohol-dependent people, even after drinking all they "can hold," are not able to quell the rebound psychomotor upheaval caused by years of alcohol-related CNS irritation. The presenting complaint of many of those who seek treatment for alcohol dependence is "nervousness" or "depression."

The adverse effects of alcohol can be categorized as central or peripheral. Central nervous system (CNS) effects are related to sedation and toxicity. As the vital centers become affected, a slowed, stuporous-to-unconscious mental state develops. Large amounts of alcohol can cause sleep, coma, deep anesthesia, and death. Other common symptoms of intoxication include slurred speech, a short retention span, loud talk, and memory deficits. Blackout is a period in which the drinker functions socially but for which the drinker has no memory.

Historically the brain damage associated with alcoholism was thought to be caused by alcohol-related nutritional deficiencies. Alcohol-dependent people do eat poorly, and no doubt such behavior leads to pathological change. It is now known, however, that brain damage occurs with drinking even when a nutritious diet is maintained. In fact, all alcohol-dependent drinkers will have some brain cell loss.

Increased psychomotor activity as a consequence of alcohol is called the alcohol-withdrawal syndrome. Sedation is the predominant effect of alcohol, but as sedation wears off, psychomotor activity increases. This is referred to as a rebound phenomenon. As the CNS becomes more irritated, the normal drinker feels sick and irritable (a hangover) but lives through it, perhaps vowing "never again." The heavy drinker and the alcoholic have to drink again to "resedate" the psychomotor system. Eventually the alcohol-dependent person has to drink larger amounts in order to feel somewhat "normal." Some drinkers reach the point where they cannot drink enough alcohol, and CNS irritability is not "sedatable." Then alcoholic tremors, sweating, palpitations, and agitation occur. Most often these symptoms occur when alcohol ingestion has stopped, but in some cases they occur while the alcohol-dependent person is drinking.

Alcoholic hallucinosis, a state of auditory hallucinations, is a phenomenon that alcohol-dependent people can sometimes experience. The brain begins to "invent" sensory input. Alcoholic hallucinosis usually begins 48 hours or so after drinking has stopped. Usually within the context of a clear sensorium, frightening voices or sounds are heard.

The ultimate level of CNS irritability is delirium tremens (DTs). In DTs the body not only invents sensory input but also has extreme motor agitation. Hallucinations become visual (e.g., the proverbial pink elephants), and the sufferer is tremulous and terrified. Tonic-clonic seizures (grand mal) can occur.

Wernicke-Korsakoff syndrome is a mental disorder characterized by amnesia, clouding of consciousness, confabulation (falsification of memory) and memory loss, and peripheral neuropathy. This disorder results from the poor nutrition of the alcoholic (specifically, inadequate amounts of thiamine and niacin in the diet) and from the neurotoxic nature of alcohol.

Peripheral effects are varied and cause great suffering. For a complete discussion of these various processes the reader is directed to a medical-surgical textbook. Cirrhosis and peripheral neuritis are the physical health problems most commonly associated with alcohol. As the alcohol-dependent person's liver functions become impaired, he or she is less able to "tolerate" alcohol. The person who once boasted of drinking exploits becomes drunk after only a few beers. Physical consequences of cirrhosis include obstructed blood flow (which leads to portal hypertension, ascites, and finally esophageal varices) and decreased liver cell function, low serum albumin levels, high ammonia and high bilirubin serum levels, and clotting problems. Peripheral neuritis causes numbness and subsequent injury in the legs, as well as changes in gait.

Alcohol is also an irritant. It burns the mouth and throat and prompts the stomach to secrete more hydrochloric acid. Gastric ulcers are caused and then worsened by alcohol. Alcoholics can experience ulcers, gastritis, bleeding, and hemorrhage in the stomach. Ulcers can eventually perforate, creating a life-threatening situation.

The pancreas is affected by alcohol in many direct and indirect ways. Pancreatitis and diabetes are not uncommon consequences of alcoholism. A malabsorption syndrome is caused by irritation of the intestinal lining. This seems to affect B vitamins generally and to lead to a deficiency of vitamin B_1 (thiamine) in particular. Thiamine deficiency contributes to peripheral neuritis. Alcohol also has a direct effect on muscle tissue, a condition known as alcoholic myopathy. Other organs affected by alcohol include the eyes (loss of peripheral and night vision), the heart (hypertension, enlarged left ventricle), and reproductive organs. As a depressant, alcohol can cause impotence. Further, prolonged drinking shrinks the testicles and decreases testosterone. Sexual potency is further compromised by a failing liver that is unable to detoxify female hormones, thus increasing the level of those hormones and adding to the male's sexual decline.

CLINICAL EXAMPLE

Anthony is a 36-year-old suffering from alcohol abuse with physiological dependence. As alcohol predominates, a primary diagnosis of polysubstance dependence is not appropriate. He has a long history of presentations at the emergency room for suicidal ideations. Alcohol and other drugs are always found in his system. He presents at a local treatment facility saying, "I just can't keep it up any more. I've been drinking for 23 years and my life is falling apart. Everyone I know hates me. I can't keep a job. No one trusts me. I have to have some help." First Anthony needed detoxification. He then went through a 28-day treatment program. He attends AA 5 times each week and has a sponsor, someone in whom he can confide and from whom he can "learn to live life on life's terms." He also attends an aftercare treatment group 3 times per week to focus on dealing with his shame. After 108 days of sobriety, Anthony began to think that he was cured and no longer needed his sobriety support system. He drank again. Just before he was pulled over for driving under the influence, he managed to throw away the cocaine he had just bought. Five months later, the consequences of his past life-style are catching up with him. He is considered a habitual offender and has been offered 20 years in prison by the district attorney. Now, instead of trying to run from his obligations, he is prepared to go to prison, if necessary. "I did it. I don't want to go to prison, but if that's what God has in mind for me because of my foolish decisions, then so be it. Maybe there's somebody out there who needs to hear my story. I can share my experience, strength, and hope, and let them know that God is a way-maker."

Nursing Issues

Overdose

People die from overdoses of alcohol because it depresses the CNS. Vital centers become anesthetized, compromising breathing and heart rate and leading to a comatose state or death. Gastrointestinal bleeding or hemorrhage can occur. As a vasodilator, alcohol also leads to heat loss, and many people have succumbed to hypothermia in colder climates. People consistently underestimate the potency of alcohol, and deaths have occurred simply because individuals have drunk too much. Almost every year newspapers report the death of a college student by alcohol poisoning. Although alcohol alone can kill, most overdose-related deaths are the result of combining alcohol with other CNS depressants.

Disulfiram

Disulfiram (Antabuse) inhibits the breakdown of acetaldehyde by the enzyme aldehyde dehydrogenase. Because acetaldehyde is toxic to the body, the person who drinks alcohol while taking disulfiram will become ill (as evidenced by sweating, flushing of the neck and face, tachycardia, hypotension, a throbbing headache, nausea and vomiting, palpitations, dyspnea, tremor, and/or weakness). This combination can also cause arrhythmias, myocardial infarction, cardiac failure, seizures, coma, and death. The unpleasant response to alcohol is intended to help reinforce the alcoholic's efforts to stop drinking alcohol. Basically, the patient taking disulfiram only has to make one decision a day about drinking. Once the pill is taken the patient dare not drink. Disulfiram is usually started with a single 500-mg dose at bedtime. After 1 or 2 weeks the dose is reduced to a maintenance dose of 250 mg per day. Anecdotal accounts note that some alcoholics will experience an ostensibly spontaneous relapse episode that coincides with their "forgetting" to take disulfiram for a couple of weeks before their return to alcohol use. Disulfiram is most effective in patients with significant internal motivation for long-term change.

Naltrexone hydrochloride

Naltrexone hydrochloride (ReVia) is an opioid-receptor antagonist, formerly used to treat narcotic dependence. It was approved by the Food and Drug Administration (FDA) in 1995 for the treatment of alcohol dependence. In one study in which 54% of subjects treated with placebo relapsed, roughly half that many (23%) of the subjects treated with ReVia did. Naltrexone is purported to increase abstinence and reduce alcohol craving when used as a part of "a comprehensive treatment plan." It works by interfering with opioid functioning. It has been known to cause liver toxicity if taken at higher than recommended levels, and it is contraindicated for patients who have abused narcotics within 7 to 10 days (*FDA Consumer,* 1995).

Interactions

Alcohol taken with other CNS depressants causes profound CNS depression, often leading to death. For instance, diazepam, which is seldom lethal when taken alone, even in large doses, can lead to death if it is combined with alcohol. Alcohol should be avoided when a person is taking barbiturates, antipsychotic drugs, antidepressants, benzodiazepines, and other sedatives. Chloral hydrate and lorazepam (Ativan) have been associated with intentional sedating of unsuspecting persons in bars. A chloral hydrate and alcohol combination (the legendary "knockout drops") was used years ago to "recruit" men for ship duty or for robbery. An updated version with Ativan replacing chloral hydrate has been used by young women to rob men who thought they were going out for a good time.

Use by the elderly

Alcohol use in the elderly is underreported, frequently unrecognized, and rarely treated (Box 33-4). As the population of older adults has grown, so have the substance-related problems many of these people bring with them. People with impaired liver function do not metabolize alcohol efficiently and therefore can tolerate little of the drug alcohol. Decreased liver function is a product of aging, and, consequently, many older persons cannot drink much alcohol without becoming inebriated, confused, and sedated. The nurse should be particularly watchful for combinations of alcohol with other CNS depressants among patients in this age group.

Fetal alcohol syndrome

Pregnant women who drink alcohol run the risk of seriously harming their unborn child. Fetal alcohol syndrome (FAS) is the result of alcohol's inhibiting fetal development during the first trimester. FAS is the third most commonly recognized cause of men-

tal retardation and the only one that is preventable. Characteristic signs of FAS include microcephaly and an associated severe mental retardation. The risk of FAS is directly related to the amount of alcohol the mother drinks during pregnancy.

Withdrawal and detoxification

Withdrawal from alcohol can be painful, scary, and even lethal (Table 33-3). As the person abstains from alcohol, he or she begins to reap the consequences of the CNS irritation caused by alcohol: tremulousness, nervousness, anxiety, anorexia, nausea and vomiting, insomnia and other sleep disturbances, rapid pulse, high blood pressure, profuse perspiration, diarrhea, fever, unsteady gait, difficulty concentrating, exaggerated startle reflex, and a craving for alcohol or other drugs. As the withdrawal symptoms become more pronounced, hallucinations can occur. The body is undergoing alcohol toxicity and needs detoxification. Mueller and Ketcham (1987) identify the three crucial elements, or the three Ss, of the detoxification process: secure environment, sedation, and supplements. A calm, secure environment is important, since the physical experience of withdrawal can be dramatically influenced by emotional and psychological distress. Sedation can be used to slow and thus ameliorate the withdrawal process and to calm the anxious, hallucinating, or delirious patient. Chlordiazepoxide (Librium) is

---

Box 33-4   Older Alcoholics

Older alcoholics are divided into two groups. About two-thirds are "early-onset" drinkers who have abused alcohol much of their lives and have survived into an unhealthy, unhappy old age. The second group—about one-third of all drinkers over age 60—is unlike the general alcoholic population. This is the "late-onset" group, which has an excellent chance for recovery.

"They are not as impaired physically, emotionally or cognitively as the early-onset drinkers . . . With abstinence, proper diet and time, recovery can be complete."

Heavy drinking in the late-onset group is usually triggered by traumatic loss. The deterioration is very rapid, covering in a year or two the progression seen in alcoholics who have been drinking for 20 to 40 years.

From Robertson N: The intimate enemy: will that friendly drink betray you?, *Modern Maturity,* 35(1):28, Feb-March 1992.

TABLE 33-3 Courses of Withdrawal from Addictive Drugs

Drugs	Length of Acute Detoxification	Common Detoxification Agents	Withdrawal Signs and Symptoms
CNS Depressants			
Alcohol	3-5 days	Librium Serax, Valium, Vistaril, alcohol*	Anxiety, sweats, tremors, flushed face irritability, sleeplessness, confusion, seizures, delirium
Valium	Slow drug taper, up to 2 weeks	Librium, Valium	
Phenobarbital	Slow drug taper, 2-4 weeks	Librium, phenobarbital	
Narcotics			
Heroin	3-5 days	Methadone or other tapering opiate or nonopiate withdrawal regimens†	Yawning, dilated pupils, gooseflesh, vomiting, diarrhea, runny nose and eyes, sleeplessness, anxiety, irritability, elevated blood pressure and pulse, craving for narcotics
Morphine	3-5 days		
Demerol	3-5 days		
Methadone	2 weeks +		
Stimulants			
Amphetamines	3-5 days	Drug intervention usually not required	General fatigue, apathy, depression, drowsiness, irritability, paranoia
Cocaine	3-5 days		
Hallucinogen			
Marijuana	2-3 days (metabolites remain in the body up to 2 weeks)	Drug intervention usually not required	Few signs of withdrawal, craving for marijuana, general anxiety and restlessness

From Mueller LA and Ketcham K: *Recovering: how to get and stay sober,* New York, 1987, Bantam Books.
*Low-dose alcohol withdrawal: Traditionally, alcohol was used by laymen to taper a drunk off a binge. With the advent of sedative medication, this practice was discouraged. The use of general sedatives was thought to be more "clinical" and to achieve better control with less toxicity. In recent years, however, the alcohol withdrawal model has been revived. Leading the way in this detox method is Walter Gower, MD, of the North Central Alcohol Research Foundation, Inc, Fort Dodge, Iowa. *Treatment Regimen:* 1/2 oz vodka (80-100 proof) with $\frac{1}{2}$ oz water every 1-6 hours for detox control. Indications for use are the same as for sedative interventions. This can be used alone or in combination with sedatives such as Librium. (Patients with seizure histories are better protected during withdrawal with the combined regimen.) (*Transition,* "A half-ounce prevention for the DT's," was presented in September, 1983. The relationship of ethanol to the occurrence of delirium tremens with prophylactic and therapeutic considerations was presented by Dr. Gower at the National Alcoholism Forum, 1979; *Alcoholism Update* 2(3), Aug-Sept 1979 [abstract].)
†Other-opiate-withdrawal protocol:
Darvon N-100: 1-2 every 4-6 hrs to control detox signs and symptoms; taper to discontinue in 3-4 days.
Catapres: 0.1 mg initially; repeat in 1 hr if needed, then 0.1-0.2 every 6-8 hrs as long as blood pressure is no lower than 90/60. This can be used for 7-14 days to control opiate withdrawal symptoms.

effective in the treatment of alcohol withdrawal (Holister, et al, 1993). A dose of 50 to 100 mg followed by repeated doses as needed (up to 300 mg per day) is given for acute alcohol withdrawal. Nutritional supplements are also recommended during and up to 4 months after detoxification. Supplements include a multivitamin, B-complex, vitamin C, calcium, and magnesium. See the case study and care plan for the alcoholic patient on p. 517.

BARBITURATES— CNS DEPRESSANTS

Barbiturates are relatively new pharmacological agents. Barbiturates were first used medicinally as sedatives in the last half of the nineteenth century. It was not until 1950 that researchers were able to confirm their ability to produce physical dependence. CNS depressants decrease the awareness of

Case Study

E.F., a 28-year-old white man, was brought to treatment by his wife following his third driving-under-the-influence offense in which he ran off the road and into a neighbor's mailbox. He has a history of alcohol and drug use since age 14. Though neither of his parents drank, he had a grandfather who died from cirrhosis of the liver and bleeding esophageal varices.

E.F. has been in counseling twice before in an effort to salvage his previous marriage. Following the breakup of the marriage, he lost his business. He became very depressed, but when he drank he became belligerent and at one point threatened his ex-wife and child, forcing her to file for sole custody of their son. It was during this period that he also began gambling in an effort to make quick money.

E.F. says that he is willing to enter treatment at this time so that he does not lose his wife and because he fears the men to whom he owes gambling debts. He knows that he will be safe in the hospital until he can figure out what to do. He does not believe that he has a problem with alcohol, drugs, or gambling and attributes his misfortunes to the ill will of others. He denies suicidal ideation at this time. Blood level alcohol on admission was 0.02%.

E.F.'s current life-style involves hunting and doing things with his wife and two step-children, Ann, 4, and Steve, 6. He misses his 2-year-old, who lives with his ex-wife.

Care Plan

NAME: __E.F._____   ADMISSION DATE: _____

DSM-IV DIAGNOSIS: __Alcohol dependence (or alcoholism)_____

ASSESSMENT: **Areas of strength:** Has no medical problems and denies suicidal ideation. Has also been in counseling twice and enjoys hunting and doing things with his family.
Problems: Has a genetic history of chemical dependency and long-time use of alcohol and drugs. Denies that alcohol is a problem in his life despite family and occupational problems.

DIAGNOSES:
- Ineffective individual coping related to alcohol abuse as evidenced by legal and financial problems.
- Ineffective family coping: disabled related to alcohol abuse as evidenced by potential marriage separation and financial difficulties.

OUTCOMES: **Short-term goals:**   Date met
- Patient will state that his marital and occupational problems are due to
  drinking.   _____
Long-term goals:
- Patient will remain chemical free on monthly testing, which will be
  assessed through urine testing by his probation officer.   _____

PLANNING/ INTERVENTIONS: **Nurse-patient relationship:** Recognize initial need to use denial; discuss the natural consequences of his drinking and the need for total abstinence; educate regarding the diagnosis concept, offering hope for long-term recovery; encourage attendance at AA meetings.
Psychopharmacology: No caffeine or sugar, multivitamin daily.
Milieu management: Family treatment; encourage ADLs.

EVALUATION: E.F. is sober after 1 month according to probation officer.

REFERRALS: Refer to AA and make appointment with substance abuse counselor.

The Cost of Drug Abuse

The true cost of drug abuse may be incalculable. The National Foundation for Brain Research (1992) estimates current costs to be $71.2 billion per year. The cost, though crippling to the economy, can measure only economic losses. The cost in human terms, including crime, vicious murders, lost human potential, and wrecked lives seems to be destroying the nation. The pervasiveness of drug abuse is such that most Americans will be affected by it. In 1986 there were a little over 19,000 drug-related murders in the United States, about 3.9% of all U.S. murders. In 1993, that number approached 25,000, or 5.2% of all U.S. murders that year.

From Drug use and its consequences, National Drug Control Strategy (Executive Office of the President)

and response to sensory stimuli. Antipsychotic drugs and antianxiety agents, which also depress the CNS, are discussed elsewhere.

Barbiturates are used to relieve anxiety or to produce sleep. They have a narrow therapeutic index, the lethal dose being only slightly higher than the therapeutic dose. These drugs produce both physical and psychological dependence. Barbiturates are classified according to their duration of action: ultrashort (30 minutes to 3 hours), short (3 to 4 hours), intermediate (6 to 8 hours), and long (10 to 12 hours). Uses range from anesthesia (ultrashort-acting barbiturates such as thiopental) to long-term use in epilepsy (long-acting barbiturates such as phenobarbital).

Metabolism

Barbiturates are usually taken orally. They are metabolized by the liver and excreted by the kidneys. When barbiturates are combined with alcohol, dangerous levels of CNS depression can occur.

Physiological Effects

Barbiturates cause CNS depression, thus decreasing awareness of external stimuli, shortening the attention span, and decreasing intellectual ability. Regular sleep patterns are changed, with a loss of rapid eye movement (REM) sleep.

Barbiturates are used to treat insomnia, to soften withdrawal from heroin, and as anticonvulsants.

Drug abusers take barbiturates to maintain a state of relatively anxiety-free living. These drugs are also taken to counteract the effects of amphetamines, "to come down," or in place of heroin when it is not available. The acutely intoxicated person will have an unsteady gait, slurred speech, and sustained nystagmus. Chronic users can have mental symptoms that include confusion, irritability, and insomnia. Persons who regularly use barbiturates develop a tolerance to them.

Nursing Issues

Overdose

The toxic dose of barbiturates varies, but in general an oral dose of 1 g results in serious poisoning, and doses of 2 to 10 g can be fatal. Acute overdose is manifested by CNS and respiratory depression. Coma and death are possible. Treatment is supportive.

Interactions

Barbiturates interact with many other drugs, but the most significant are those that increase CNS depression. Other CNS depressants such as alcohol, sedatives, tranquilizers, and antihistamines can cause serious CNS depression.

Use by the elderly

Barbiturates frequently cause excitement in the elderly. The elderly are also more prone to confusion caused by barbiturates.

Use during pregnancy

Barbiturates can cause fetal abnormalities. These drugs cross the placental barrier and fetal serum levels approach maternal blood levels. Infants born to mothers who take barbiturates during the last trimester of pregnancy can experience withdrawal symptoms.

Withdrawal and detoxification

Symptoms of withdrawal from barbiturates are severe and can cause death. Symptoms usually begin 8 to 12 hours after the last dose. Minor withdrawal symptoms include anxiety, muscle twitching, tremor, progressive weakness, dizziness, distorted visual perception, nausea and vomiting, insomnia, and orthostatic hypotension. More serious withdrawal symptoms include convulsions and delirium beginning approximately 16 hours after the last dose and lasting up to 5 days. Untreated, withdrawal symptoms may not decline in intensity for some time. Detoxification requires a cautious and gradual reduction of these drugs. One approach is to reduce the patient's regular dose by 10% each day.

INHALANTS

There are three basic forms of inhalants: hydrocarbon solvents (gasoline and glues), aerosol propellants (the propellants in spray cans), and anesthetics (chloroform, nitrous oxide). Inhalants usually depress the CNS and increase hilarity. They are particularly dangerous because the amount inhaled cannot be controlled. Deaths from asphyxiation have been reported. Inhalants cross the blood-brain barrier quickly. Common side effects include mouth ulcers, gastrointestinal problems, anorexia, confusion, headache, and ataxia. Because of their accessibility, children are at a special risk of coming into contact with substances in this category.

OPIOIDS (NARCOTICS)

Note to student: Though a distinction can be made between the terms *opioids* (technically endogenous) and *opiates*, the authors use the term *opioids*. Opioids include opium, morphine, codeine, heroin, hydromorphine, Demerol, and methadone.

Opioids are widely abused. Until the "cocaine crisis," the general public viewed heroin as the most significant drug of abuse. Although heroin abuse has been relegated to a lower status for some time, it is again becoming the focus of attention as drug users find it less expensive than cocaine and less devastating. Using cocaine and heroin together ("speedballing") is growing in popularity. Illicit drugs can be swallowed, smoked, snorted, injected into soft tissue ("skin popping"), and "mainlined" (injected intravenously).

Parenteral use of heroin, for example, involves (1) "cooking" the substance in a spoon or bottle cap,

(2) filtering it with a cotton ball, (3) "sterilizing" a needle with a match, and (4) injecting the drug into a vein. Initially veins in the antecubital space are used, but as vein membranes break down and sclerose (form "tracks"), they "get used up" and other veins are selected for injection. The needle is frequently passed from one user to another. Infections, including acquired immunodeficiency syndrome (AIDS), have been relatively common. Because of AIDS, snorting is increasing in popularity as a route of administration. Morphine is the prototype drug of this class and will be discussed in more depth.

CLINICAL EXAMPLE

Terry is a 39-year-old opioid-dependent registered nurse whose presentation in treatment is precipitated by the state nursing board. Nursing was Terry's life, and her identity centered around being a nurse. Reporting that it was not uncommon to "share medication" with patients, Terry told of how easy it was at first to document giving the maximum prn pain medications in a patient's chart, but not always giving them to the actual patient. "I never let one of my patients be in pain, though," Terry reported.

Terry's supervisor did not suspect a problem until medication became unaccounted for. Terry thought that all areas had been covered but was eventually caught, not by stupidity, but by the kind of impaired judgment that results from drug use.

Terry's nursing license was put on probationary status. Most facilities were not willing to hire a nurse on probation—the limitations placed by the board were strict. Terry cannot work the night shift and cannot hold the keys to the medication storage. Without a job, Terry cannot begin to fulfill the conditions of the probation.

Terry was hired as a nurse at a treatment facility and has 6 months remaining until another hearing date can be set.

Metabolism

Morphine is metabolized in the liver and is excreted by the kidneys. It is not absorbed well in the gut but is readily metabolized there and in the liver. It can be given orally but is usually given parenterally. Drugs that compete for liver metabolism increase the effect of morphine.

Physiological Effects

Opioids relieve pain by increasing the pain threshold and by reducing anxiety and fear. They do this by stimulating opioid receptor sites in the brain. There are three major classes of opioid receptors, *mu, delta,* and *kappa.* Morphine, heroin, and methadone act primarily through the *mu* receptors. The naturally occurring neurotransmitters, the endorphins, among other responses, mediate pain and regulate mood. The opioids are endorphin agonists. It is their effect on mood (a feeling of euphoria) that attracts drug abusers. Drug abusers frequently refer to the euphoric mood created by morphine and heroin as "better than sex." In addition to the euphoria, an overall CNS depression occurs. Drowsiness or "nodding" and sleep are common effects.

Heroin has a higher abuse potential than morphine because it more readily passes the blood-brain barrier. Once heroin enters the brain, its chemical structure is changed to that of morphine so it becomes "trapped" in the brain. This property of heroin causes a more sustained high. CNS effects of opioids include respiratory depression related to decreased sensitivity to carbon dioxide stimulation by the medullary center for respiration. Respiratory depression is the primary cause of death among opioid abusers. PNS effects include constipation; decreased gastric, biliary, and pancreatic secretions; urinary retention; hypotension; and reduced pupil size. Pinpoint pupils are a sign of opioid overdose. Morphine also causes vomiting.

Nursing Issues

Overdose

At therapeutic doses prescribed and administered by professionals, morphine is a helpful and safe analgesic. Drug abusers can rarely be sure of the amount of opioid they are taking, however. Street purchases are not standardized, and occasionally users obtain "purer" drug than they anticipated. Inadvertent overdose may thus occur. The primary effect of overdose is respiratory depression. A respiratory rate below 12 per minute is cause for concern. A recognizable symptom pattern for overdose is documented:

- The person becomes stuporous and then sleeps.
- The skin is wet and warm.
- Next, a coma develops, accompanied by respiratory depression and hypoxia.
- The skin becomes cold and clammy.

- The pupils dilate.
- Death quickly follows at this point.

Provision of adequate airway and assisted ventilation, if needed, are treatment priorities. A narcotic antagonist is administered to reverse the effects of opioids.

Narcotic antagonists

The opioids are the only class of commonly abused drugs that have a specific antidote. Naloxone (Narcan), a narcotic antagonist, is the intervention of choice if opioid overdose is suspected. Naloxone blocks the neuroreceptors affected by opioids, so the patient responds in a few minutes to an IV injection of naloxone. Respiration improves, and the patient consciously responds. However, since most opioids have a longer lasting effect than naloxone has, it is often necessary to repeat the antagonist to maintain adequate respiration. The nurse who administers naloxone must carefully observe the patient to determine whether additional antagonist will be needed. Nalorphine (Nalline) is also a narcotic antagonist. Narcotic antagonists do not interrupt the effects of nonnarcotics.

CLINICAL EXAMPLE

A hospice team member told the following story: The patient was a 70-year-old man suffering from prostate cancer with painful bone metastases. A nursing concern is maintaining a balance between the need for pain management and the risk of respiratory suppression. The patient built up tolerance to his pain medication. His family members were afraid that he was becoming an "addict," so they decided to reduce his medication intake without consulting the physician. Cutting in half and administering a time-release pain pill (a synthetic morphine that lost its "time release" characteristic when broken), they quickly noticed that Dad was not very responsive. He was taken to the hospital, and Narcan was administered. Because it blocks the opioid receptor sites, there was no effective pain relief for this patient. The man was in extreme physical pain, because his family was afraid of the legitimate medical uses of pain medication.

Interactions

The effects of opioids are increased when they are combined with other CNS depressants. Since the use of multiple drugs is common among drug abusers, the potential for deadly combinations is real. If it is known that heroin was taken and naloxone does not reverse CNS depression, it can be safely assumed that other depressants (e.g., barbiturates) were taken also. In such cases supportive nursing care is indicated.

Use by the elderly

Elderly persons are particularly at risk for decreased pulmonary ventilation associated with opioids.

Use during pregnancy

Women who abuse opioids give birth to babies who suffer withdrawal symptoms. These drugs can cross the placental barrier and produce respiratory depression in neonates.

Withdrawal and detoxification

The unassisted withdrawal from alcohol or barbiturates can be fatal, but the unassisted withdrawal from opioids is rarely fatal, though often painful. The term "kicking the habit" comes from the leg spasms associated with the withdrawal from opioids. Withdrawal symptoms are related to the degree of dependence and the abruptness of the discontinuance. Maximum intensity is reached within 36 to 72 hours and subsides in 5 to 10 days. Withdrawal symptoms can be categorized into early, intermediate, and late appearing. Early symptoms of withdrawal include yawning, tearing, rhinorrhea, and sweating. Intermediate symptoms include flushing, piloerection, tachycardia, tremor, restlessness, and irritability. Late-appearing symptoms include muscle spasm, fever, nausea, diarrhea, vomiting, repetitive sneezing, abdominal cramps, and backache. Treatment is primarily symptomatic and supportive.

Specific Drugs

Drugs related to morphine include hydromorphone (Dilaudid), a more potent derivative of morphine; levorphanol (Levo-Dromoran), a drug whose action is identical to that of morphine but used for less severe pain; meperidine (Demerol), a synthetic narcotic analgesic; pentazocine (Talwin), which has weaker analgesic effects than other narcotic drugs, is less addicting, and is not supposed to cause eupho-

ria; and several related drugs such as oxymorphone (Numorphan), alphaprodine (Nisentil), anileridine (Leritine), butorphanol (Stadol), and nalbuphine (Nubain). Fentanyl (Sublimaze), an anesthetic, is similar to but 100 times stronger than morphine and 20 to 40 times stronger than heroin.

Methadone

Methadone (Dolophine), although an opioid similar to morphine, is used specifically to prevent withdrawal symptoms. Methadone is given orally and is poorly metabolized in the liver. Accordingly, it has a much longer half-life (15 to 30 hours) than morphine (1½ to 2 hours). Because of the long half-life, once-a-day dosing is effective and conducive to outpatient care. When used to aid in lessening physiological dependence on opioids, methadone is of great benefit.

Heroin

Heroin is derived from morphine and is referred to as a semisynthetic drug. It was originally thought to be a cure for morphine addiction but proved to be more addictive than morphine.

Codeine

Codeine is used primarily as a cough suppressant. Its abuse preceded the general drug abuse of the mid to late 1960s because it was easily available in over-the-counter cough syrups. Ease of access was eliminated at about the same time that drug abuse became recognized as an emerging national problem. It is not a drug of choice for many substance abusers today.

STIMULANTS

Use of stimulants containing caffeine such as soda pop, coffee, tea, and nicotine is widespread. Many people feel sluggish if they do not start their day with a cup of coffee. Should they remain caffeine free all day, they experience symptoms associated with stimulant withdrawal: headache, nausea, and vomiting. Tobacco is a stimulant but is not discussed in this chapter.

CLINICAL EXAMPLE

Gladys is a 32-year-old woman who suffers from cocaine dependence and was referred to outpatient treatment through the legal system because of a possession charge. After her second group therapy session she requests an individual session with her counselor. There she reveals that one month earlier, she was raped by other "customers" at the local crack house that she has frequented. She is frightened and embarrassed. Her urge to escape the emotional pain she feels by using is mitigated by her traumatic experience at the crack house. Although she says that she has a supportive family, she is further ashamed and terrified because she thinks that she is pregnant. In her helplessness, she experiences some suicidal ideation. Gladys talks about aborting the pregnancy. After she is calm, she agrees to consult with her physician. After she does not return to treatment, no one answers the telephone, and there is no response to letters sent, she is lost to contact. Six months later Gladys calls her counselor to say that she laid aside her shame and talked with her pastor, her mother, and her 12-year-old daughter. She reports that all is going well, although the baby was stillborn. She has not used since.

Cocaine

Coca plants grow high in the Andes mountains and the Incas chewed coca leaves long before the Spanish explorers arrived. Note that this is not cocoa, from which we get chocolate, but coca. It is still in legitimate use today in some parts of Andean South America. Used as a mild tea, it can help bring relief for altitude sickness. Cocaine is extracted from the coca plant. It is a fine, white, odorless powder with a bitter taste. It was introduced to Western medicine as an anesthetic in 1858. Sigmund Freud was known to use cocaine and believed it to be a remedy for morphine addiction. He reported on its effects in his book, *Cocaine Papers*. It was once used in some cola drinks and advertisements extolled the ability of cola as well as of other "brain tonics" to "refresh." After the Pure Food and Drug Act was passed in 1906, cocaine was eliminated from these beverages. Cocaine and its offspring crack have caused a major drug problem today. A downturn in crack use was noted in the early 1990s at the height of the "drug war," but use has begun increasing again. The list of famous and not-so-famous persons struck down in their youth by this stimulant is lengthy. The problems associated with cocaine extend to every level of society.

Metabolism

Cocaine passes the blood-brain barrier quickly, causing an instantaneous high. When administered IV (mainlining), cocaine is rapidly metabolized by the liver, so the "rush," though exhilarating, does not last long. Cocaine exerts both CNS and peripheral nervous system (PNS) effects because of its ability to block norepinephrine and dopamine reuptake into presynaptic neurons. It depletes these neurotransmitters. Cocaine can also be swallowed (but is poorly absorbed this way) and snorted. Snorting, in which cocaine is absorbed through the nasal mucosa, was the preferred route of administration especially glamorized in the 1980s. With the discovery of smoking an adulterant-free cocaine crystalline base, freebasing became popular and paved the way for the advent of "crack" or "rock" cocaine. Crack is a less cost-prohibitive way of using cocaine than snorting or mainlining, primarily because it is sold and marketed in smaller packages—most commonly as $10 or $20 rocks.

Crack is purported to be the most addictive drug on the streets today. It is produced in a relatively uncomplicated procedure (mixed with baking soda and water, heated, and hardened) and then smoked. It is reported to produce an instantaneous high and almost as instantaneous a "crash." An intense desire to smoke again is produced. Crack is cheap on a per-dose basis, but the user wants more immediately, so it is not an inexpensive drug to use. It is also easy to find. When the user's money is gone, however, the crash often gives way to cocaine-induced depression. This depression is sometimes so severe that users attempt suicide. Tolerance to CNS and PNS effects develops quickly because neuronal norepinephrine stores are depleted, causing a need to increase drug amounts to create the desired effect. Tolerance develops to otherwise lethal amounts.

Physiological effects

Cocaine and its derivatives are addicting stimulants. Cocaine's exhilarating effect is related to its ability to block dopamine reuptake, particularly in the nucleus accumbens pleasure center in the brain (see Chapter 5). Although physical dependence is less severe than with opioid abuse, psychological dependence is intense. Abusers become tongue-tied when attempting to describe the sensations of this drug. Euphoria, increased mental alertness, increased strength, anorexia, and increased sexual stimulation are desired effects of these drugs. Increased motor activity, tachycardia (up to 200 bpm), and high blood pressure are PNS effects. Sensory and motor nerve endings are numbed, causing blood vessels to contract. Decreased stimulation occurs. CNS effects include stimulation of the medulla resulting in deeper respirations, euphoria, increased mental alertness, dilated pupils, anorexia, and increased strength. The cocaine user can be loquacious and stimulated sexually (libido is increased, ejaculation retarded). This latter characteristic no doubt adds to the drug's overall appeal. Intense paranoia is common. It is this paranoia, in combination with other factors such as decreased inhibitions, that explains, at least in part, why many drug deals "go bad" and result in someone being murdered.

Less common reactions are specific hallucinations and delusions. Cocaine users report "bugs" crawling beneath the skin (formication) and foul smells. Nasal septum perforation is associated with snorting cocaine and is due to extreme vasoconstriction, which impedes blood supply to this area and thus causes nasal necrosis. Death from cocaine is linked to metabolic and respiratory acidosis and hyperthermia associated with prolonged seizures (Holister, et al, 1993). Tachyarrhythmias have also led to death.

■ Critical Thinking Question

The older generation of former cocaine abusers seem to be turning to heroin as they have grown older. Can you think of a reason why this might be so?

Amphetamines

Amphetamines were developed in 1887. They have medicinal uses, such as short-term treatment of obesity, attention-deficit disorders in childhood, and narcolepsy. Amphetamines, sometimes referred to as speed or crank, are widely abused. They are sometimes called the poor person's cocaine. Speed produces a longer high than cocaine and is typically less expensive. It is frequently used as an adulterant of cocaine.

Metabolism

Amphetamines are taken orally and are well absorbed from the gastrointestinal tract. They are excreted basically unchanged by the kidney and continue to have an effect until cleared. Therapeutic parenteral administration is illegal in the United States, but many speed users self-administer amphetamines intravenously.

Physiological effects

Amphetamines (speed) are indirect-acting sympathomimetics that cause the release of norepinephrine from nerve endings. Amphetamines also block norepinephrine reuptake in presynaptic nerve endings. As with cocaine, amphetamines also have a profound effect on the subcortical structure and the nucleus accumbens. Amphetamines block dopamine reuptake but also stimulate excess release of dopamine and retard its enzymatic breakdown. CNS effects include wakefulness, alertness, heightened concentration, energy, improved mood to euphoria, insomnia (sometimes desired, sometimes not), and amnesia. The most common side effects of amphetamine use are restlessness, dizziness, agitation, and insomnia. PNS effects are palpitations, tachycardia, and hypertension. Respirations also increase because, like cocaine, the amphetamines stimulate the medulla. A psychiatric side effect of amphetamine use is amphetamine-induced psychosis. In the emergency room this psychotic presentation can be almost indistinguishable from paranoid schizophrenia.

Nursing Issues

Overdose

Cocaine and amphetamine "overdose" has resulted in a number of deaths, primarily due to arrhythmias and respiratory collapse. Smoked cocaine adds to the problem because large amounts reach the system quickly. Toxic levels of amphetamines cause tachycardia, severe hypertension, cerebral hemorrhage, seizures, and coma. Treatment includes induction of vomiting, acidification of the urine, and forced diuresis. In patients with amphetamine psychosis related to toxic levels of these drugs, chlorpromazine or haloperidol given intramuscularly will antagonize the amphetamine effect.

*C*ase *S*tudy

J.R. is a 25-year-old unemployed carpenter who lives with his aunt. One night he began tearing the house apart then locked himself in the bathroom yelling that he was going to kill himself. His aunt called the police, who delivered J.R. to the emergency room of the local hospital. The emergency room examiner noted that J.R. was suicidal and having auditory hallucinations, delusions of persecution, disorganized thinking, anorexia, insomnia, anxiety, and agitation. He had been threatening to the police and continued to be extremely agitated and threatening the emergency room personnel. Following some history from the aunt, the diagnosis of cocaine intoxication was made.

J.R.'s aunt stated that she had been concerned about possible drug use for the past couple of years but had never pursued the issue with J.R. He was often belligerent and was fired from his job until he could get "cleaned up." She had noticed things missing around the house but never questioned J.R. about this.

The emergency room physician decided to keep J.R. in the emergency room until his thinking cleared and to monitor him for tachycardia, cardiac arrhythmia, and seizure activity. The physician ordered 5 mg of diazepam (Valium) to be given IV for 2 to 3 minutes every 10 to 15 minutes if needed for seizures and propranolol (Inderal) IV (0.1 to 0.15mg/kg at a rate of 0.5 to 0.75 mg every 1 to 2 minutes) should the patient experience cardiac arrhythmias. J.R. was transferred to the psychiatric unit following 4 hours of observation in which there was no seizure activity or cardiac abnormalities.

Upon arrival at the unit J.R. was noticeably irritable, agitated, anxious, and complained of a headache. His responses to questions indicated continuing difficulty in concentration and some disorganized thinking. The care plan on the following page was developed.

Interactions

The effects of cocaine and amphetamines are augmented when they are combined with other CNS stimulants. Many over-the-counter products such as hay fever medications and decongestants contain stimulants. Urinary alkalinizing agents such as sodium bicarbonate decrease the elimination of amphetamines, whereas urinary acidifying agents increase the elimination of amphetamines.

Use during pregnancy

Amphetamines should be used during pregnancy only if clearly needed because harm to the fetus has been demonstrated. Cocaine-addicted mothers give birth to addicted babies with multiple problems, withdrawal and physical problems of the neonate being only the beginning of a lifetime of resulting effects. About 400,000 infants born each year in the United States are exposed to cocaine in the womb (Clinical News, 1998). As "crack babies" have reached school age, impaired neurological development of the exposed fetus has become apparent and is associated with an explosion of children with behavior and learning problems in special education programs.

Withdrawal and detoxification

Although cocaine and amphetamines are highly addictive, physical withdrawal is relatively mild. Psychological withdrawal is severe, however, because the drugs are so pleasurable. For persons withdrawing from amphetamines under medical supervision the withdrawal process is gradual and safe. "Cold turkey" withdrawal without medical supervision causes agitation, irritability, and severe depression, frequently with suicidal ideation. As a rule of thumb, the "low" of withdrawal will be inversely proportional to the "high" experienced. Withdrawal from cocaine causes intense craving for the drug. A number of approaches are used, all aiming to restore depleted neurotransmitters. Amino acid catecholamine precursors such as tyrosine and phenylalanine, tricyclic antidepressants, and the dopamine agonist bromocriptine are three approaches used to increase the availability of neurotransmitters.

HALLUCINOGENS

Hallucinogen use is on the rise again, especially among young people. Also referred to as psychotomimetics or psychedelics, hallucinogens alter perception. There

*C*are *P*lan

NAME: __J.R._____   ADMISSION DATE: _____

DSM-IV DIAGNOSIS: __Substance intoxication/dependence__

ASSESSMENT: **Areas of strength:** Young (25 years old); lives with aunt who wants him to return once he begins to feel better; previous employer would hire him if he gets "clean."
Problems: Suicidal ideation, hallucinations (auditory), delusions that someone wants to kill him, thinking disorganized (has difficulty completing thought), anorexia, insomnia, anxious (has exaggerated startle reflex), agitated.

DIAGNOSIS: • Potential for self-directed violence related to substance abuse or CNS agitation as evidenced by history of suicide attempt.
• Alterations in perception related to substance abuse or CNS agitation as evidenced by suicidal ideation, disorganized thinking, and hallucinations and delusions.
• Alteration in nutrition: less than body requirements related to anorexic effect of cocaine as evidenced by loss of weight.

OUTCOMES: **Short-term goals:**   **Date met**
• Patient will not experience physical injury during hospitalization.   _____
• Patient will not experience symptoms of cocaine withdrawal.   _____
• Patient will sleep 6 to 8 hours per night.   _____
• Patient will admit that cocaine is a problem in his life.   _____
Long-term goals:
• Patient will maintain optimal levels of nutrition and maintain at least
90% of normal weight.   _____
• Patient will attend outpatient Cocaine Anonymous meetings.   _____
• Patient will practice abstinence from psychoactive drugs.   _____
• Patient will verbalize and show some evidence of developing non–drug-
using friends.   _____

PLANNING/   **Nurse-patient relationship:** Develop a contract with patient to report to nurse if suicidal
INTERVENTIONS: thoughts occur. Establish trusting relationship with patient. Provide reality-based conversation. Accept patient. Set limits on behavior; confront the patient with inconsistencies; and do not allow patient to manipulate. All staff must be consistent. Allow patient to verbalize anxiety and fear. Teach patient the effects of drugs on his body. Encourage independence in self-care and reinforce examples of self-denial and delayed gratification.
Psychopharmacology: Desipramine 50 mg bid for cocaine withdrawal for 2 weeks (last dose 0800). Haldol 5 mg po q4h prn agitation; Cogentin 2 mg po with first dose of Haldol on the days it is given. Tylenol tabs 2 q4h prn headache.
Milieu management: Provide patient with a quiet room to decrease stimulation and agitation. Provide safe environment, including frequent observation by staff, monitoring of smoking, assess vital signs prn. Monitor the environment for dangerous objects such as glass, razors, and belts. Provide foods the patient likes to increase interest in food. Provide group setting for patient to explore the issues of substance abuse with other patients and to help the patient get past the notion that no one understands his problems. Orient to surroundings.

EVALUATION: Patient has not experienced significant cocaine withdrawal; appetite is returning. Beginning to sleep better (4 to 6 hours). Patient has not attempted self-injury and denies suicidal intent.

REFERRALS: Outpatient treatment for after care, including Cocaine Anonymous meetings and random urine screens for increased accountability.

are two basic groups of hallucinogens: natural and synthetic. Natural hallucinogenic substances include mescaline (peyote [from cactus]), psilocybin (psilocin [from mushrooms]), and marijuana (*Cannabis sativa*). Synthetic or semisynthetic substances include lysergic acid diethylamide-25 (LSD); 2,5-dimethoxy-4-methylamphetamine (STP), phencyclidine (PCP), N,N-dimethyltryptamine (DMT), and 3,4-methylenedioxyamphetamine (MDA). In general, hallucinogens can heighten awareness of reality or can cause a terrifying psychosis-like reaction. Users report distortions in body image and a sense of depersonalization. Particularly frightening is a loss of the sense of reality. Hallucinations depicting grotesque creatures, such as a "dog with a snake for a tongue," can be extremely frightening. Emotional consequences of such effects are panic, anxiety, confusion, and paranoid reactions. Some persons have experienced frank psychotic reactions after minimal use. In the jargon of the hallucinogens, such an experience is a "bad trip."

Mescaline (STP, DMT, MDA)

Mescaline (peyote) is derived from cactus plants found in America. Native Americans harvested peyote "buttons" from cacti and used them in their religious ceremonies. This religious practice was protected by law as part of their worship until 1990, when the U.S. Supreme Court ruled that states can prohibit its use. STP, DMT, and MDA are synthetic forms of mescaline.

Metabolism

Mescaline, whether naturally occurring or synthetically produced, is taken orally and is quickly absorbed. Its site of action is probably the norepinephrine synapses. Mescaline passes the blood-brain barrier and usually takes effect within 30 to 40 minutes. Its effects last up to 12 hours. It is excreted in the urine.

Physiological effects

With mescaline, colors are vivid, music more beautiful, and sounds more intense. When users close their eyes, colors and images can be seen. A distorted sense of space and time occurs. A young person who drove his car after taking peyote stated that it seemed to take an eternity to reach a stop sign no more than 50 feet away. The experience is directly related to preingestion expectations. "Good" experiences include hilarity and joy. The user may feel especially insightful. The answers to such questions as those involving the "meaning of life" may seem clear. Such insights can easily add to a sense of an almost "religious" experience. If the conversation were recorded and replayed later, however, the users would not be so impressed with their having encountered what they believed to be ultimate truth (this is also true of marijuana). "Bad" trips are the side effects of concern. Although peyote is less potent than LSD, it still can cause panic, paranoid thinking, and anxiety if the trip is too intense. Dependence does not occur in the strict sense, yet users enjoy the experience and seek to repeat it. Pupil dilation and tremors sometimes occur.

Psilocybin, Psilocin

Psilocybin is derived from mushrooms (*Psilocybe mexicana*).

Metabolism

Psilocybin is taken orally. Once in the stomach it is converted to psilocin by enzymatic action. Psilocybin decreases the reuptake of serotonin in the brain. Onset of action is experienced in 25 to 40 minutes. Its effects last up to 8 hours.

Physiological effects

Hallucinations and time, space, and perceptual alterations are experienced and are the sensations that caused some Native American groups to continue its use. Psilocybin dilates the pupils and increases heart rate, blood pressure, and body temperature. Tingling of the skin and involuntary movements can occur. As with other hallucinogens, a sense of unreality can occur. An inability to concentrate may add to feelings of anxiety and lead to panic and paranoia. Hallucinations and illusions may occur. Although no deaths due to psilocybin toxicity have been reported, deaths related to perceptual distortions have occurred.

Marijuana

Cultivation of marijuana has taken place for over 5,000 years (Schlosser, 1994). Marijuana is the drug most widely used illegally in the United States. Mar-

Marijuana Makes People Inattentive and Stupid

Former "Drug Czar" Dr. William J. Bennett tells the following story: He was invited to "Alaska—where personal possession of marijuana was legal" and was asked "to weigh in on behalf of a new initiative seeking to recriminalize possession of marijuana. Not surprisingly, the percentage of high school students using dope in Alaska was much higher than in the rest of the nation." He continues, "When I accepted the invitation, the prolegalization forces went into action. The 'pothead lobby,' as I called it, distributed fliers in Anchorage and Fairbanks saying 'Confront the Drug Bizarre.' But when I arrived, there was very little opposition. . . . It later became apparent why. When the 'pothead lobby' passed out fliers announcing my visit, they had put the wrong date on them. I had been saying for a long time that marijuana makes people inattentive and stupid. I rested my case."

Bennett WJ: *The de-valuing of America: the fight for our culture and our children,* New York, 1992, Summit Books.

Fanning the Flames about the Medical Use of Marijuana Produces More Heat than Light

Proponents say it is "natural." Critics point out that lead, radiation, and hemlock are also natural. Three primary medical benefits are noted: (1) It eases the extreme nausea associated with many treatments, such as with chemotherapy. Critics point out that wine is commonly prescribed for this purpose. (2) It reduces intraocular pressure associated with glaucoma. Critics point out that the synthetic form of the drug has the same benefits. (3) Pain management (e.g., with migraine headaches) is purported to be superior to more established medications. Critics point out that alternatives are available that do not run the risk associated with smoking marijuana (the preferred route of administration for most of these patients), including the inhalation of smoke and fungal spores, tar ("resin") and other negative side effects.

ijuana and other related drugs (hashish and tetrahydrocannabinol) come from an Indian hemp plant. Marijuana is difficult to categorize. Placement with the hallucinogens seems appropriate, but other categorizations can be defended also.

Metabolism

The active ingredient in marijuana is Δ-6-3,4-tetrahydrocannabinol (THC). THC is changed to metabolites in the body and is stored in fatty tissues. It remains in the body for up to 6 weeks after it is smoked and can be detected in blood and urine from 3 days to about 4 weeks, depending on level of use (see Table 33-2). The effects of smoked marijuana last between 2 and 4 hours. If marijuana is ingested, effects may last up to 12 hours.

Physiological effects

Marijuana produces a sense of well-being, is relaxing, and alters perceptions. Euphoria results and is the cause of drug-seeking behaviors. Increased hunger ("the munchies") is an effect that makes it useful for anorexic persons (e.g., chemotherapy cancer patients). Marijuana's antiemetic properties make it useful for treating nausea and vomiting as-

sociated with chemotherapy. There is an FDA-approved synthetic version of THC under the trade name Marinol, but many patients prefer smoking marijuana over the capsule form, ostensibly because they believe it to be "more effective." (Brazaitis, 1995)

Balance and stability are impaired for up to 8 hours after marijuana use. Short-term memory, decision making, and concentration are also impaired. Dry mouth, sore throat, increased heart rate, dilated pupils, conjunctival irritation, and keener sight and hearing are physical responses to marijuana. It has been thought to be amotivational, but not all research supports this thinking.

Other effects associated with the use of marijuana include harmful pulmonary effects (bronchitis), weakening of heart contractions, immunosuppression, and reduction of serum testosterone and sperm count. Some males who are chronic users of marijuana have been known to alter their hormones to the point of growing breasts and producing milk (Ohlms, 1993). Anxiety, impaired judgment, paranoia, and panic are not uncommon reactions to marijuana. These experiences may culminate in some health-compromising behavior. Flashbacks, more commonly associated with LSD, have also been reported. A flashback is a spontaneous reliving of feelings experienced during a "high."

If you believe that marijuana is benign, would you want your neurosurgeon to "take the edge off" by taking a few tokes just before surgery to remove your mother's brain tumor? Yes or no? Explain and justify your answer.

LSD (Lysergic Acid Diethylamide)

Metabolism

LSD stimulates the sympathetic nervous system by inhibiting the reuptake of serotonin. It is taken orally and onset of action occurs within 30 to 40 minutes. Effects are experienced for up to 12 hours. Rather small amounts of LSD, usually only 50 to 300 μg (micrograms, or "mikes"), produce these effects.

Physiological effects

LSD causes a phenomenon known as synesthesia. Synesthesia is the blending of senses (e.g., smelling a color or tasting a sound). Expectations and environment govern the "quality" of the LSD "trip." LSD causes an increase in blood pressure, tachycardia, trembling, and dilated pupils. CNS effects include a sense of unreality, perceptual alterations and distortions, and impaired judgment (Box 33-5). Another problem with LSD is flashbacks. Flashbacks are scary

Box 33-5   Research Gone Wrong!

The 40-year-old remains of a scientist who fell to his death after he was given LSD in a CIA experiment were found in good condition when they were exhumed . . . A government commission investigating the CIA indicated that the agency had experimented with LSD and other hallucinogens in the early 1950s and that a number of experiments were conducted on unwitting federal employees, including [the] civilian biochemist involved in biological warfare research. . . . Forensic experts plan to analyze hair, brain tissue, fingernails and bones . . . for toxins and drugs, including LSD and other hallucinogens.

From the Associated Press: *Los Angeles Times,* p A-4, June 5, 1994.

and can heighten a sense of "going crazy." Bad trips from LSD cause anxiety, paranoia, and acute panic. Some persons have suffered psychotic "breaks" from LSD and have never fully recovered. A number of persons have killed themselves while under the influence of LSD.

PCP (Phencyclidine)

PCP, a synthetic drug, traditionally has been used as an animal tranquilizer. Many emergency room nurses are familiar with this drug because PCP-intoxicated persons are often brought to the emergency room. Their unpredictable outbursts of violent behavior are legendary. They literally change from coma to violent behavior and back. Caution must be exercised when one is providing care to these patients because of their unpredictable behavior.

Metabolism

PCP is taken orally, intravenously, is smoked, and snorted. PCP is well absorbed by all routes. Effects last for 6 to 8 hours.

Physiological effects

The PCP user experiences a high. Euphoria and a peaceful, easy feeling can occur and are sought after. Perceptual distortions are common. Undesired effects of PCP can be serious. Blood pressure and heart rate are elevated. Other PNS effects include ataxia, salivation, and vomiting. A catatonic type of muscular rigidity alternating with violent outbursts is particularly frightening to bystanders. Psychological symptoms include hostile, bizarre behavior, a blank stare, and agitation.

Nursing Issues

Overdose

High doses of mescaline are not generally toxic, but high doses of STP and MDA can cause hyperexcitability. Deaths have occurred because of these drugs. Psilocybin overdose has not been associated with any deaths, and usually a calm environment is all that is needed to assist withdrawal. LSD- and PCP-related deaths are not uncommon. Deaths can be caused by overdose but are more likely to be associated with perceptual disorientation and unresponsiveness to environmental stimuli. Confusion and acute panic can result from an overdose of marijuana, LSD, and other hallucinogens. Diazepam (Valium) can be administered for psilocybin, LSD, and mescaline overdoses and is known to terminate panic attacks caused by these drugs (Holister, et al, 1993). PCP presents greater problems. Diazepam may be given for seizures and agitation, and haloperidol (Haldol) for psychotic behavior. Acidifying the urine to a pH of 5.5 accelerates its excretion. Urine screening is the best means of identifying abused substances.

Interactions

Mescaline, psilocybin, and LSD can potentiate sympathomimetics. Marijuana should not be used with alcohol, because marijuana masks the nausea and vomiting associated with excessive alcohol consumption. Respiratory depression, coma, and death can occur.

Use during pregnancy

A number of birth defects have been associated with these drugs.

Withdrawal and detoxification

Hallucinogens do not produce physical dependence, so there are no withdrawal symptoms. Symptoms of withdrawal from marijuana can include extreme irritability, insomnia, restlessness, and hyperactivity. One of the biggest concerns for the nurse is development of an approach for dealing with the intoxicated person. Basically, the nurse should provide a calm, reassuring environment.

CLINICAL EXAMPLE

Bill Waters was a 48-year-old house painter. He was an alcoholic and though he was not as productive as he had been in years past, he still made a good living until recently. In the past 6 months his alcoholism began to have more and more of an effect on his work. He lost one important job because he could not meet the deadlines he had established. His home life had been dysfunctional for years. Weekends were only a blur as he drank beer continuously

and watched television. His wife Wanda made sure the bills were paid and took care of all the children's needs. Bill never interfered but occasionally would spend money on alcohol before Wanda could pay a bill. In recent years, however, Wanda had caught on to all of Bill's tricks, and he rarely had an opportunity to spend household money. When Bill was too hung over to go to work, Wanda called and made up the excuses. Wanda covered for Bill at church and in other situations in which his heavy drinking would be an embarrassment. Wanda alternated between protecting Bill and blaming him for their problems. Her life now revolved around Bill and his problems. After Bill lost an important paint contract, Wanda insisted upon treatment. Bill attended a 6-week inpatient treatment program. Upon his return he was ready to reestablish himself as the husband and father, but Wanda was not ready to trust him. In essence, what had happened and what happens in many such families is that Wanda had to take over responsibilities of making decisions and she was not willing to give them up without long-term proof of Bill's sobriety and responsibility. He had promised to stay sober many times before and failed. Bill, on the other hand, had a clear head for a change and wanted to be the "man of the house" again. Although neither could articulate the new problems with which they were struggling, they did recognize emotions they could not control. Bill and Wanda soon divorced. A marriage that could withstand alcoholism could not withstand recovery.

THE TREATMENT OF SUBSTANCE-RELATED DISORDERS
FAMILY ISSUES

Although the substance-dependent person is the designated patient, all family members are affected. In some cases where the family has been so affected, the "well" family member may alternate between rescuing (or enabling) the abuser and blaming the abuser. Examples of rescuing include the following: (1) Making excuses for the abuser, (2) lying for the abuser, and (3) doing things that the abuser should have done. Oddly enough, sometimes a recovering addict or alcoholic can be more difficult to live with than when he or she was actively using (see previous clinical example). Most chemical dependency units have a number of classic stories in which, after abstinence was achieved, the abuser was "encouraged" to start again, or the spouse separated from the abuser. The clinical example about Bill represents a situation in which a family resists role changes. Sometimes the family gets well, but the addicted person does not. It is sometimes difficult for these people to hold their family members accountable, but they reason that it is better to know that their loved one is in jail than to hear the dreaded words from the police, "Your loved one is dead."

TREATING THE CHEMICALLY DEPENDENT PERSON

The most common goal of treatment for the chemically dependent person is abstinence from alcohol and/or drugs. It is thought that the person who is dependent upon one substance can easily become dependent on another. The term *cross-dependence* describes this condition. Professionals working with chemically dependent persons realize their vulnerability and usually refrain from thinking of anyone as being "cured." Conversely, they tend to view treatment as an ongoing, lifelong process in which the person abstaining from formerly abused substances is "recovering." The term *recovering* indicates a current and dynamic process but also indicates the ever-present possibility of "slipping."

DIAGNOSTIC TOOLS FOR CHEMICAL DEPENDENCY

Many tools exist for the evaluation of chemical dependency. Criteria set forth in the DSM-IV are among the most helpful in diagnosing a person with chemical dependence. The DSM-IV is a valuable tool. Other instruments such as the Twenty Question List developed at Johns Hopkins University (George, 1990) and the MAST can help the clinician identify substance dependency.

Early diagnosis can mean a better treatment prognosis. Misdiagnosis can lead to unsuspected withdrawal and/or drug interactions. Ultimately, accurate diagnosis may mean the difference between life and death. It is most important that the nurse look for behavioral and physical clues when making diagnostic evaluations with the treatment team.

Alcohol

Several screening questionnaires have been developed to assist the health care professional in diagnosing alcohol dependency. Among the easiest are the MAST and the CAGE. Other tools, such as the Adolescent Alcohol Involvement Scale, the Problem Drinking Scale, the Alcohol Use Inventory, the Comprehensive Drinker Profile, the Drinking and You self-report, and the Addiction Severity Index can also aid in assessing the severity of substance abuse problems (George, 1990).

Michigan Alcoholism Screening Test

The MAST, or Michigan Alcoholism Screening Test, is a good screening tool that can help the unconvinced patient gain insight into at least the possibility of a problem if questions are answered honestly. It can also aid the clinician in diagnostic assessment. It can be easily modified to identify other drug problems.

The CAGE questionnaire

The CAGE questionnaire is another valid instrument. Even easier to administer, and possibly perceived as less accusatory than the MAST, the following four questions comprise this tool:

1. Have you ever felt you should *C*ut down on your drinking?
2. Have people *A*nnoyed you by criticizing your drinking?
3. Have you ever felt bad or *G*uilty about your drinking?
4. Have you ever had a drink first thing in the morning to steady your nerves or get rid of a hangover (*E*ye-opener)?

Two positive responses are suggestive of alcoholism, and three or four positive responses are diagnostic (Whitfield, Davis, and Barker, 1986). Schofield (1988) points out that questions 1 and 3 assess introspection and reflection on personal drinking, and question 2 provides reinforcement of this introspection by external cues. Question 4 reflects a change in behavior.

Drugs

Alcohol abuse and drug abuse have many similarities; however, there are several significant differences: alcohol is typically legal, whereas many drugs of abuse are typically illegal (or taken out of accordance with the law); stages of drug abuse tend to advance more rapidly; and drugs can produce their desired effect almost instantly. See the box below for a list of appropriate NANDA diagnoses.

The problem with most screening tests, particularly for drug abusers, has been their susceptibility to faking and denial on the part of the patient (Creager, 1989). The MacAndrew Scale (MacAndrew, 1965), made up of appropriate items from the Minnesota Multiphasic Personality Inventory (MMPI) (Allen, Eckardt, and Wallen, 1988), and the Substance Abuse Scale have been developed to identify the tendency of substance abusers towards denial and lying. The

---

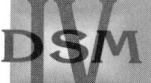

DSM-IV and NANDA Diagnoses Related to Chemical Dependency

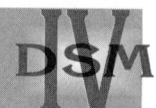

DSM-IV*
Alcohol dependence
Alcohol abuse
Alcohol intoxication
Alcohol intoxication delirium
Alcohol withdrawal
Amphetamine (or related substance) dependence
Amphetamine (or related substance) abuse
Amphetamine (or related substance) intoxication
Amphetamine (or related substance) withdrawal
Caffeine intoxication
Cannabis dependence
Cannabis abuse
Cannabis intoxication
Cocaine dependence
Cocaine abuse
Cocaine intoxication
Cocaine withdrawal
Hallucinogen dependence
Hallucinogen abuse
Hallucinogen intoxication
Hallucinogen persisting perception disorder
Inhalant dependence
Inhalant abuse
Inhalant intoxication
Nicotine dependence
Nicotine withdrawal
Opioid dependence
Opioid abuse
Opioid intoxication
Opioid withdrawal
Phencyclidine (or related substance) dependence
Phencyclidine (or related substance) abuse
Phencyclidine (or related substance) intoxication
Sedative, hypnotic, or anxiolytic dependence
Sedative, hypnotic, or anxiolytic abuse

Sedative, hypnotic, or anxiolytic intoxication
Sedative, hypnotic, or anxiolytic withdrawal
Polysubstance dependence
Other (or unknown) substance dependence
Other (or unknown) substance abuse
Other (or unknown) substance intoxication
Other (or unknown) substance withdrawal

NANDA†
Growth and development, altered
Infection, potential for
Injury, potential for
Nutrition, altered
Pain
Self-care deficit
Sensory-perceptual alteration
Sexual dysfunction
Sleep pattern disturbance
Knowledge deficit
Noncompliance
Thought processes, altered
Anxiety
Communication, impaired verbal
Coping, ineffective individual
Family processes, altered
Fear
Growth and development, altered
Parenting, altered
Self-esteem disturbance
Social isolation
Violence, potential for
Grieving, dysfunctional
Hopelessness
Powerlessness
Spiritual distress

*From the American Psychiatric Association: *Diagnostic and statistical manual of mental disorders,* ed 4 Washington, DC, 1994, The Association.
†From North American Nursing Diagnosis Association: *NANDA nursing diagnoses: definitions and classifications 1997-1998,* Philadelphia, 1997, NANDA.

Box 33-6   Motivation

Whether external coercion is a positive influence on treatment outcome is a matter of disagreement. Participants who voluntarily seek treatment are more compliant with their therapists than those coerced into treatment. Participants who are coerced into treatment may be compliant only while the coercive influence is present, and may be compliant only with behaviors specified by the coercive agent. [One example would be the client who does not drive after drinking, but insists on continuing alcohol use which has proven to contribute to problems in other areas of life.] Data are contradictory about whether coerced and voluntary participants have different treatment outcomes.... [One measure] found that external motivation was related to a positive treatment outcome only when internal motivation was also present. . . .

Internal sources of motivation [included] spouse/family (28.5%), increasing problems with alcohol/wants to stop but can't (17.1%), and mental health affected by drinking (15.9%). Of the 19 participants with external sources of motivation, 18 (90%) were coerced by their spouses to seek treatment.

Steinberg ML, et al: Sources of motivation in a couples outpatient alcoholism treatment program, *Am J Drug Alcohol Abuse* 23(2): 191, May 1997.

Substance Abuse Scale requires only 10 minutes to complete and claims 90% accuracy of diagnosis (Creager, 1989).

Psychotherapeutic Management

Alcoholism is highly treatable. Success of treatment for abuse of other chemical substances varies, but all chemical dependencies can be helped. The success of treatment, however, depends first on the patient's motivation (Box 33-6) and then on the clinician's skill in interpreting data and implementing treatment strategies. The importance of understanding the role of each of the three psychotherapeutic management interventions is crucial. In working with these individuals, the nurse must realize that milieu management has the potential to be more important for this group of patients than for other types of patients. With these ideas in mind, it is important to note that two dominant but divergent general philosophies inform the treatment most professionals will provide. In their broadest sense, the two umbrella treatment philosophies are (1) the behavioral model and (2) the disease model. The disease model is predicated on the notion that there is a physical link (usually portrayed as a biological predisposition) where addiction is concerned.

The behavioral model defines *addiction* as "an ingrained habit that undermines your health, your work, your relationships, your self-respect, but that *you feel you cannot change*" (emphasis added) (Peele and Brodskey, 1991). Adherents of this model point to research that seems to indicate that two brief counseling sessions with a problem drinker's physician can lead to sustained, significantly reduced alcohol consumption (Manissa Communication Group, 1997). In one study, although medical inpatient hospitalization days were reduced, there was no decrease in number of presentations to the emergency department (Van Meter, 1987).

The disease model points to physiological effects and explanations. Supporters cite sources indicating drugs that decrease the function of gamma-aminobutyric acid (GABA) receptors have been known to reduce alcohol consumption by rats (Roberts and Koob, 1997). They believe that "not even the most hard-core behaviorists would say" of some very severely addicted patients, "Gee, you don't have a disease. Your liver's falling out, you've got brain damage, you've got organ damage, you've been drinking a fifth a day for the last 12 years, you are nearly dead and in an intensive case unit. Let's set up our little experimental drinking bar in your room and teach you how to drink in a controlled manner" (Gorski, 1996).

One mediating approach of the behavioral model is "moderation management." It distinguishes between heavy drinkers, who can control their use, and AOD dependent persons, who cannot (Manissa Communications Group, 1996). One Australian study found that almost 75% of participating treatment facilities thought that controlled drinking is a clinically appropriate goal, but reported that fewer than one quarter of their patients had such a goal in their care plans. Community- and hospital-based programs were more likely to endorse a moderation management approach than residential or private providers (Donovan and Heather, 1997).

The two camps vehemently disagree. They do agree, however, that substance dependence frequently manifests itself in self-destructive behavior of the users. Most professionals are legitimately concerned about this self-destruction and want to be a part of relieving the negative results of AOD use among this population. The authors see validity with both perspectives and believe that a proper approach lies somewhere between the philosophical poles. A person's initial exposure to AOD use seems to be influenced by both genetic and environmental factors, but it also seems that, once ingested, the substance is able to "encourage its continued use through direct action on the nerve cells in the brain" (Roberts and Koob, 1997).

Nurse-Patient Relationship. Since most addicted people are experiencing a problem in many areas of their lives at the time they seek treatment, understanding positive motivators will help in establishing new goals and directions for the patient's life. The patient's ability to function at work, at home, in society, and in his or her many roles has been compromised by alcohol and drugs. Stated another way, no one (or hardly anyone) comes to treatment because life is going well. The converse is almost always true; the boss is going to fire him or her, the spouse is going to leave, the judge is sending the person to jail. Treatment for chemically dependent people is usually initiated out of a crisis. To the degree treatment can help the patient replace ineffective behaviors with new coping skills, the patient has a better chance of getting and staying sober. Coping skills worthy of nursing effort include work skills and habits, job search skills, homemaking, parenting, financial management, family communication, family role responsibilities, and exploration of leisure activities (Stoffel, 1994).

Establishing a trusting therapeutic relationship with the patient in which the rules for treatment are consistently applied is the benchmark for working with chemically dependent individuals. Genuineness is the single most important quality of this relationship. Expressing empathy and providing a safe environment that minimizes anxiety are also important, especially in the early stages of treatment while the patient is going through the painful withdrawal process. Engendering feelings of hope for the future is also necessary as the patient begins to establish new life goals (George, 1990).

Group treatment. Contrary to the assertions of Fox television's Hank King, treatment is not "all about Witchcraft, Pills, and Molestation" (Jacobs, 1997). Since denial is the most predominant defense of the alcoholic, treating it appropriately is important. A group therapy setting seems to provide the best avenue for treatment because groups are especially effective in breaking down the denial process through confrontation as well as support of group members who share a common struggle. Confrontation includes telling a patient what is observed through supportive, but reflective listening techniques, irrespective of the strength of a patient's denial.

Examples of confrontation include the following:

"You say you have not been drinking (or using drugs), but I can smell alcohol on your breath (or cocaine was detected in your urine sample)"; or "I hear you saying that you are in treatment because you believe you need help; so help me understand how you see your need, given your absence from treatment all week without a medical excuse."

What seems to be most effective is when the peers of the patient provide appropriate confrontation, as when Lloyd reported to the group that he had not used alcohol in the past 3 months.

Lloyd's peer, Christy, had used the group well for support earlier that session to process her own recent relapse episode. Christy was able to confront Lloyd directly about his lying, because she had happened to see him at the same club herself the previous weekend!

Personal responsibility. It is important to help the patient learn to foster personal responsibility for recovery. The nurse must cultivate an awareness that responsibility for change lies within the patient himself or herself. Further, while expressing support and concern for the patient in recovery, the nurse must not shield the patient from the negative consequences of the patient's own addictive behavior.

Conscience development. Paradoxically, one of the most effective means for placing responsibility with the patient is in a group that fosters responsibility for another patient in the group. Essentially, in such groups, patients are directly told that they have done such a poor job of guiding their own lives that such a level of personal responsibility is incomprehensible. However, perhaps they would be able to guide and be responsible for someone else. Such an idea is novel and intriguing to most patients until a crisis moment occurs. For example, the program has a rule that no one can drink alcohol on pass. Joe is responsible for Bill. Bill drinks over the weekend, and Joe is punished. Punishment can range from a loss of coffee privileges to dismissal from the treatment program. Joe, who has perhaps lied, stolen, and connived for years in order to pursue his dependency, is speechless at the "unfairness" of such a decision. Bill, on the other hand, while feeling some sense of relief at first because he escapes "his punishment," soon begins to feel the anger of other group members for causing the "innocent" Joe to be punished. Bill, who may have perpetrated all kinds of dastardly things in his life with little remorse (a limited internal conscience), begins to have all sorts of feelings because the group is his conscience now (external). Such groups are effective, particularly when occupational or legal consequences are dependent on program completion.

Life-style issues. Teach the patient the effects of chemical abuse on the body and provide for the physical and special nutritional needs of the patient. Exercise is crucial to increase mental and physical vitality as are relaxation, avoidance of stress, and rest. A balanced diet and vitamin and mineral supplements are also essential parts of treatment and recovery.

Psychopharmacology. Treatment for chemical dependency using medication is becoming more important as we know more about brain biochemistry. Major categories of chemical dependency and pharmacological approaches to those dependencies will be briefly addressed.

Medications used to treat alcohol dependence. Long-acting benzodiazepines (BZs) such as chlordiazepoxide (Librium), diazepam (Valium), and lorazepam (Ativan) are useful for treatment of alcohol withdrawal. The principle behind this treatment is the rapid substitution of the benzodiazepine for the alcohol to suppress withdrawal symptoms. BZs apparently bind to the GABA-benzodiazepine receptor sites, so the effectiveness of BZs makes sense (Zorumski and Isenberg, 1991). The next step is a gradual tapering of BZs over several days. Some clinicians prefer barbiturates for alcohol withdrawal but respiratory depression and safety concerns dissuade most prescribers.

All patients being treated for alcoholism should be given thiamine. Thiamine specifically prevents the development of Wernicke's encephalopathy, its characteristic ataxia, nystagmus, and mental status changes. Disulfiram (Antabuse), an inhibitor of the enzyme aldehyde dehydrogenase, is effective in preventing drinking because of the severe symptoms it causes when combined with alcohol. Naltrexone (ReVia) functions as an opioid-receptor antagonist that is used to reduce alcohol craving. Other compounds show promise of helping reduce cravings. Animal experiments with daidzin and daidzein, two herbal extracts from kudzu, a vine prolific in the American South, reduced alcohol consumption by 50%. Chinese studies with human subjects indicate that 80% of participants report that alcohol cravings disappeared (Manissa Communication Group, 1993). A combination of fluoxetine (Prozac) and tiapridal has also been prescribed for the treatment of alcoholism (Sancton, 1997).

Medications used to treat opioid dependence. Drugs used to treat opioid dependence can be divided into those for opioid overdose and those for long-term treatment. Naloxone (Narcan) (see previous discussion) blocks the neuroreceptors affected by opioids. In case of an opioid overdose, naloxone can be given to reverse the CNS depression caused by the opioid. Though improvement occurs rapidly in the patient who has taken an overdose, due to naloxone's short half-life, its effect is short lived and the patient may return to the prenaloxone state. Maintenance treatment of opioid dependence is accomplished with methadone (Dolophine). Methadone is an opioid with a much longer half-life than the prototype opioid, morphine, and can be given in once-per-day doses. It relieves the "drug hunger" associated with opioid abuse. Typically, no more than 40 mg per day is prescribed. An alternative to methadone is LAAM, a long-acting methadone cogener with a half-life of 96 hours. It can be given on an every-other-day schedule.

Medications used to treat stimulant dependence. A number of medications have been used to treat stimulant dependency. Dopaminergic drugs such as amantadine (Symmetrel) and bromocriptine (Parlodel), anticonvulsants such as carbamazepine (Tegretol), tricyclic antidepressants such as desipramine (Norpramin), and amino acid catecholamine precursors such as tyrosine and phenylalanine have all been associated with successful treatment of stimulant dependency (Keltner and Folks, 1997).

Medications used to treat hallucinogen dependence. Diazepam has been found to be effective in terminating episodes of panic, violence, and paranoid ideations induced by LSD and other hallucinogens (Hollister, et al, 1993). Initial doses ranged from 10 mg to 50 mg.

Milieu Management. The six dimensions of milieu management are all important when shaping the milieu of the chemically dependent inpatient. Some of these dimensions are significant for the patient who receives outpatient care as well. Safety issues such as a drug-free environment are critical. Nurses and others must be vigilant to protect the environment from those who would bring drugs into the milieu. Psychiatric units are not necessarily drug-free places. Multiple avenues exist for illicit contraband. Other safety issues such as suicide prevention, thwarting inappropriate sexual behavior, and so forth continue to be the responsibility of nursing staff. Structure considerations such as an active, meaningful schedule provide for less downtime. People who abuse alcohol, for instance, often structure their day around planning to drink alcohol, drinking alcohol, and being under the influence of alcohol (Stoffel, 1994). Structure then attempts to replace the old structure with a new, therapeutic structure. Effective unit structure maximizes what the milieu has to offer the patient. Norms of nonviolent behavior, openness, feedback, and the prohibition of nonprescribed drugs is critical to an effective treatment program. As noted above, confrontation is a useful technique for working with chemically dependent individuals. Many patients will have never truly been held accountable. They certainly will rarely have experienced an environment in which direct and sometimes painful comments are expected to be absorbed and digested. Strong norms reinforce the expectation of a reasoned, nonviolent response to such comments.

Limit setting is perhaps the most important and most challenged milieu management technique the nurse will use. Limit setting can be characterized as providing an environment that protects the patient from himself and from other patients.

Therefore the nurse needs to recognize the symptoms of a still actively addicted mind–substance seeking, stubbornness, belligerence, mood swings, and violent and aggressive behavior–and then set limits on those behaviors. Urine drug screens are also a dimension of limit setting because these tests reinforce the no-drug policy (see Table 33-2). If drugs are found, the patient must be confronted and held accountable.

Balance and environmental modification also play significant roles in the well-managed milieu for the chemically dependent patient. Balance is especially important, for example, when using the technique of confrontation. Although confrontation is important and therapeutic, in the hands of some less skilled staff and some patients it can become little more than a heavy-handed counterpart to the physical abuse visited upon patients years ago. It requires sensitivity to confront without crushing or totally alienating the patient.

OTHER INTERVENTIONS

A number of programs exist for the treatment of chemical dependency. The fact that these various programs exist gives testimony to the complexity and seriousness of chemical dependencies in North America.

Alcoholics Anonymous

The best known intervention programs are Alcoholics Anonymous (AA) and Narcotics Anonymous (NA). These programs use a self-help, support group model made up of fellow users in various stages of "recovery" (Box 33-7). Philosophically, AA and NA view psychosocial problems as stemming from substance abuse and generally reject the idea that an underlying psychopathology is responsible for substance use. AA has established the twelve suggested steps (Box 33-8), which start with a person's admitting personal powerlessness over alcohol and end with that person's being available, night or day, to another alcoholic in need. The popular bumper sticker slogan "Easy does it" reflects a philosophy of taking life one day at a time and avoiding a frenetic life-style. AA and NA subscribe to the belief that only total abstinence can free the chemically dependent person from the bondage of alcohol and drugs, because, they maintain, "A drug is a drug is a drug," meaning that if one is addicted to one substance, one is by definition addicted (at least potentially) to all. AA's relationship with physicians and mental health professionals has become more cooperative over the past few years (*Harvard Mental Health Letter,* August, 1996).

While AA in particular has a program that has helped many people, it does not appeal to everyone. Reasons vary, but some professionals believe that the spiritual nature of AA is a deterrent to some individuals' seeking help (Satel, Becker, and Dan, 1993).

Box 33-7 Self-Help Groups for People Recovering from Substance Abuse

ALCOHOLICS ANONYMOUS—for individuals recovering from alcoholism. Founded in 1935

AL-ANON—for families of alcoholics

ALATEEN—for teenagers 12-20 years of age who have been affected by someone else's drinking problem (usually a parent)

ASSOCIATION OF RECOVERING MOTORCYCLISTS—support group for motorcyclists who are recovering from alcohol or drug addiction

CALIX SOCIETY—Catholic alcoholics who are maintaining sobriety through affiliation with and participation in AA

CHRISTIAN ADDICTION REHABILITATION ASSOCIATION—provides support for individuals with a ministry to addicts

COCAINE ANONYMOUS—for men and women who are recovering from cocaine addiction. A 12-step program

DRUG-ANON FOCUS—for families and friends of persons addicted to mind-altering drugs. A 12-step program

DRUGS ANONYMOUS—for persons addicted to drugs. A 12-step program

DUAL DISORDERS ANONYMOUS—for people with both alcohol or drug addiction and mental or emotional disorders. A 12-step program

FAMILIES ANONYMOUS—for parents, relatives, and friends of drug addicts

GAY AA—provides support for gay and lesbian alcoholics

IMPAIRED PHYSICIAN PROGRAM—provides assistance to physicians and their spouses who have problems with alcohol, drugs, or codependence

INTERNATIONAL NURSES ANONYMOUS—for nurses, nursing students, and former nurses who are involved in a 12-step recovery program

NARANON—provides assistance to drug-dependent individuals and their families

NARCOTICS ANONYMOUS—for individuals recovering from drug abuse. A 12-step program

RATIONAL RECOVERY SYSTEMS—uses rational emotive therapy (vs. a spiritual approach) to assist people in their recovery from substance abuse

---

Box 33-8 The Twelve Steps of Alcoholics Anonymous

1. We admitted we were powerless over alcohol—that our lives had become unmanageable.
2. Came to believe that a power greater than ourselves could restore us to sanity.
3. Made a decision to turn our will and our lives over to the care of God *as we understood Him.*
4. Made a searching and fearless moral inventory of ourselves.
5. Admitted to God, to ourselves, and to another human being the exact nature of our wrongs.
6. Were entirely ready to have God remove all these defects of character.
7. Humbly asked Him to remove our shortcomings.
8. Made a list of all persons we had harmed, and became willing to make amends to them all.
9. Made direct amends to such people whenever possible, except when to do so would injure them or others.
10. Continued to take personal inventory, and when we were wrong, we promptly admitted it.
11. Sought through prayer and meditation to improve our conscious contact with God *as we understood Him,* praying only for knowledge of His will and the power to carry that out.
12. Having had a spiritual awakening as the result of these steps, we tried to carry His message to alcoholics, and to practice these principles in all our affairs.

The Twelve Steps are reprinted with permission of Alcoholics Anonymous World Services, Inc. Permission to reprint this material does not mean that AA has reviewed or approved the contents of this publication. AA is a program of recovery from alcoholism *only*—use of the Twelve Steps in connection with programs and activities that are patterned after AA, but that address other problems, does not imply otherwise.

Specifically, the concept of a higher power, the expectation that one "tell one's story" publicly, and the notion of making a "searching and fearless moral inventory" and then making amends when needed is incongruent with some people's belief system. AA continues to be an important treatment alternative for thousands of individuals suffering from alcoholism. Other programs, developed by more traditionally oriented mental health professionals, may view underlying problems, such as depression or bipolar illness, as the cause of substance abuse. The goal of this therapy is to treat the underlying problem. Its proponents believe that successful treatment of the underlying problem facilitates resolution of the chemical dependency. Such programs may use a group format or individual therapy format. Boxes 33-9 and 33-10 provide contrasting views of AA.

Another Self-Help Support Group

AA and NA are the best known self-help groups, but other, less well known self-help groups are used by

---

Box 33-9 AA Works!

The research builds a convincing argument that AA in combination with professional treatment is the most effective form of help. The difference is observable from the very start. Fifty to 60 percent of the alcoholics attending only AA will drop out within the first ninety days. The dropout rate is cut in half for patients referred to AA as a part of their professional treatment. AA members who are also active in counseling and therapy relapse less frequently and achieve more comfort and peace of mind in sobriety than those who only attend AA.

AA has no position for or against professional therapy, but many AA members have benefited from using both. For instance, Bill Wilson, one of the founders of AA, participated in psychiatric treatment for depression after he got sober.

From Gorski TT: *Understanding the twelve steps,* New York, 1992, Simon & Schuster.

Box 33-10 Maybe AA Does Not Work

At least four studies...have found no differences between groups of alcoholics assigned to Alcoholics Anonymous and no treatment at all.... Consistently negative findings have also come from controlled studies of insight-oriented psychotherapies, antipsychotic drugs, confrontational counseling, most forms of aversion therapy, educational lectures, group therapy, psychedelics, and hospitalization. One sample of something which seems to work is BRIEF INTERVENTION. According to William Miller, "Studies show conclusively that very brief treatment, if designed properly, is highly successful against even moderately severe addictions."

The article continues, "'We found this one out the hard way,' he recalls. In 1976, in one of his studies of controlled drinking, Miller separated his subjects into two groups. The treatment group got a variety of treatments, including counseling and disulfiram (Antabuse). The control group was given only a brief self-help manual and told to go home, read it, and do their best.'

'To our amazement, people in the control group did just as well as the treatment group. We thought we had really messed up the study so we repeated it twice again and got the same results.

'Then we went looking for what was really happening. We gave one group the manual and another group no manual. The manual turned out to be the variable that was the potent treatment. But why? We knew it wasn't the effect of our initial interview with the subjects, or some difference in the patient groups.'

'The key was that we had inadvertently motivated the control group and in spite of our expectations, the addicts changed and moderated their drinking. Simply giving them the manual, saying to them that we believed they could help themselves, could handle it, you can do this, was enough.'"

Since then, Miller and other therapists have refined and modified "motivational interviewing" and brief-intervention therapy. More than 30 studies in 14 countries have affirmed the value of its key components, dubbed FRAMES: **F**eedback—specific and tailored to the individual, not general; **R**esponsibility—it's up to you, your choice, you are not the helpless victim of a disease; **A**dvice—firm and clear recommendations; **M**enu—there are different ways to work this out; **E**mpathy—the best therapists have this and are neither pushy nor confrontational, but supportive and warm; and **S**elf-efficacy—you can do it; empowerment.

Rodgers JE: Addiction: a whole new view, *Psychology Today* 27(5):77, Sept/Oct 1994.

thousands of people. A self-help group by definition is composed of people with something in common. In the case of substance-abuse self-help groups, the commonality is substance-related issues. Self-help groups work because the new member recognizes that others in the group have been where he or she is and truly understand the situation. One group, which offers itself as a "nonspiritual" alternative to AA, is Rational Recovery (RR). RR is particularly offended by the AA suggestion that one submit one's egocentric will to a "Higher Power." They are supported legally somewhat since some state and federal courts have maintained that AA is equivalent to a religion under the First Amendment's Establishment Clause (Brodsky and Peele, 1991).

■ Critical Thinking Question

The founders of AA were clear that the recovery process was a spiritual journey. However, we now live in a day when most are reluctant to speak of spiritual things for fear of offending others or of imposing their views on others. Do you think that in our efforts not to "offend" people we have deemphasized an important part of psychiatric nursing?

EVALUATION, RELAPSE, AND FOLLOW-UP CARE

Evaluation

Since abstinence is the overarching goal of most treatments, and since so many people in treatment are referred by the criminal justice system, accurate information is often difficult to come by. Another complicating factor is deciding just which criteria

Box 33-11 Antecedents to Relapse		
Event	Cocaine Group	Alcohol Group
Being around users	87%	40%
Severe craving	67%	25%
Stopping AA/NA	48%	75%
Not expressing feelings	20%	75%
Major emotional crisis	33%	50%

From Rawson R, Obert J, and McCann M: *The neurobehavioral treatment manual,* Beverly Hills, Calif, 1990, Matrix Institute on Addictions. Quoted in Corrie D, editor: *CWASAINT trainee notebook,* Atlanta, 1993, Child Welfare Institute.

are significant. Unfortunately, there are more questions than answers. Is self-reported abstinence after 6 months, or 1 year, or 5 years best? Is self-report believable? Should police records be consulted for AOD-related arrests? Outcome evaluations for substance dependence are often among the most confusing of statistics.

Relapse

Not only must the chemically dependent person recover from the dependency or addiction, but also the potential for relapse must be addressed. This can best be done by helping the person to see the danger signs of relapse. Rawson, Obert, and McCann (1990) described five antecedents to relapse (Box 33-11).

Gorski (1989) has identified the phenomenon of post–acute withdrawal (PAW), whose symptoms include difficulty in thinking clearly, managing feelings and emotions, avoiding accidents, managing stress, remembering things, or sleeping restfully. PAW is often a natural part of the recovery process, but its presence can bring about a "stuck point," inducing stress and beginning the relapse process. Danger signs are the changes of attitude that precede actual return to use.

Follow-Up Care

Follow-up care is essential for preventing relapse. Patients and nurses need to be aware that recovery has only begun when an inpatient or outpatient program is completed. The few months immediately following completion of a treatment program can be dangerous for the chemically dependent person. This is when relapse is most common. The nurse should confirm that arrangements for aftercare, outpatient counseling, and self-help support group meetings are made before discharge.

■ Critical Thinking Question

Is the "Drug War" worth fighting? Justify your answer.

▼ Key Concepts

1. Chemical dependency is a major physical and mental health problem in North America, and most nurses, whether they want to or not, will take care of chemically dependent people.

2. Drugs of abuse can be categorized into four basic groups: alcohol and other CNS depressants, opioids (e.g., morphine, heroin), stimulants (e.g., amphetamines, cocaine, crack, crank), and hallucinogens (e.g., mescaline, marijuana, LSD, PCP).

3. The DSM-IV distinguishes between substance dependence and substance abuse, with substance dependence indicating more severe problems with a substance.

4. Alcohol is the no. 1 drug problem in North America; it exacts a high price economically from our society and is responsible for great suffering and death.

5. Alcohol causes disinhibition and impaired judgment, and it is relaxing when first used. The primary concern with respect to alcohol overdose is severe and often fatal CNS depression. Withdrawal causes tremors, nausea, vomiting, tachycardia, diaphoresis, seizures, anxiety, and depression. Withdrawal can be fatal.

6. Other CNS depressants include barbiturates (downers, reds, blues, rainbows), benzodiazepines such as Librium (green and whites), antipsychotic drugs, methaqualone ('ludes), and inhalants (gasoline, cement for model airplanes).

7. Depressants cause relief from anxiety, euphoria, disinhibition, and drowsiness. The primary effect of overdose is respiratory depression. Withdrawal from CNS depressants can be life threatening.

8. Opioids (narcotics) come from the juice of the opium poppy, with opium being the natural product and morphine, codeine, and the semi-synthetic heroin being easily derived from the poppy juice. Synthetic preparations such as meperidine (Demerol), pentazocine (Talwin), propoxyphene (Darvon), and methadone (Dolophine) have been developed in the vain search for a pain reliever with no addicting qualities.

9. Opioids are taken intravenously, orally, intramuscularly, and subcutaneously (skin popping). Overdose can be fatal, with respiratory depression being the most serious side effect. Withdrawal, while miserable (flulike symptoms), is not particularly life threatening.

10. Naloxone (Narcan) is a narcotic neuroreceptor blocker and is given in emergency rooms to treat opioid overdose. Naloxone causes an opioid-abstinence syndrome.

11. Stimulants include amphetamines and cocaine. Stimulants cause elation, grandiose thinking, talkativeness, and other less pleasant effects. The primary concerns in the event of overdose are agitation, tachycardia, cardiac arrhythmias, and convulsions. Withdrawal from stimulants, while miserable, is not particularly serious.

12. Hallucinogens include mescaline, marijuana, LSD, and PCP. Hallucinogens cause illusions, hallucinations, diminished ability to perceive time and distance, anxiety, and paranoid thinking. The primary effects of hallucinogenic overdose are intense "trips," psychotic reactions, and panic. Withdrawal from hallucinogens can cause anxiety, fear, and panic. However, physical withdrawal has not been found to be particularly serious.

13. While several treatment approaches are effective, the therapeutic goal for most approaches is abstinence from the substance—although the patient might still be seeking a way to engage in "controlled use." (If the patient were able to do that, he or she probably would not qualify as "dependent" in the first place.)

14. Nursing interventions include group work, education, confrontation, tough love (really, simply not allowing oneself to be a participant in the patient's self-destruction), providing for physical and nutritional needs, and helping the patient become involved in AA and NA.

◼ Study Questions

1. The primary drug problem in North America is with:
   a. Alcohol
   b. Cocaine
   c. Heroin
   d. Marijuana

2. Constricted pupils indicate use of:
   a. Mescaline
   b. Psilocybin
   c. Alcohol
   d. Opioids

3. Drug use accounts for approximately how many murders per year in the United States (in 1993)?
   a. 25,000
   b. 100,000
   c. 200,000
   d. 1,000,000

4. Alcohol is metabolized at about what rate?
   a. 10 ml every 90 minutes
   b. 10 g per 10 kg of body weight per hour
   c. 5 g per 10 kg of body weight per hour
   d. None of the above

5. Alcohol is classified as a(n):
   a. CNS stimulant
   b. CNS depressant
   c. Opioid
   d. Hallucinogen

6. Which of the following is the best example of denial?
   a. The patient states that she does not drink.
   b. The patient claims to drink only on the weekend.
   c. The patient states that he "can take it or leave it alone" when it comes to alcohol
   d. None of the above

7. A common effect of CNS stimulants is:
   a. Hypotension
   b. Anorexia

c. Sedation
d. All of the above

8. In which of the following ways does crack cocaine differ from "regular" cocaine?
   a. More rapid high
   b. Stronger effect
   c. Is less expensive per purchase
   d. All of the above

9. Which of the following are opioids?
   a. Opium
   b. Morphine
   c. Heroin
   d. All of the above

10. Opioids are best classified as:
    a. CNS depressants
    b. CNS stimulants
    c. Agonists
    d. Antagonists

11. Overdose of heroin is more lethal than withdrawal from heroin.
    a. True
    b. False

12. Death from opioids usually occurs from:
    a. Hypertension
    b. CNS stimulation
    c. Respiratory depression
    d. Cardiac arrhythmia

13. Withdrawal from barbiturates is:
    a. About as severe as withdrawal from stimulants
    b. About as severe as withdrawal from opioids
    c. More severe than withdrawal from heroin

14. If opioid overdose is suspected, the patient can be given:
    a. Antabuse
    b. Narcan
    c. Elavil
    d. Librium

15. Which of the following short-term effects have often been found in users of hallucinogens?
    a. Dystonia
    b. Time distortion
    c. Sexual preoccupation
    d. None of the above

16. Deaths related to PCP are usually due to:
    a. Overdose
    b. Perceptual distortions
    c. The pain-producing quality of the drug

17. The combined cost to our economy of both alcohol and drug abuse is estimated to be
    a. $50 billion
    b. $100 billion
    c. $160 billion
    d. $500 billion

REFERENCES

Alcohol and health: an overview, Seventh special report to the US Congress on alcohol and health, Rockville, Md, 1990, US Department of Health and Human Services.

Allen JP, Eckardt MJ, and Wallen J: Screening for alcoholism: techniques and issues, *Public Health Rep* 103:6, 1988.

Ananth J, et al: Missed diagnosis of substance abuse in psychiatric patients, *Hosp Community Psychiatry* 40:297, 1989.

Berridge KC and Robinson TE: The mind of an addicted brain: neural sensitization of wanting versus liking, *Curr Dir Psychol Sci*, p 71, June 1995.

Blum K and Trachtenberg MC: Alcoholism: scientific basis of a neuropsychogenic disease, *Int J Addict* 23:781, 1988.

Brazaitis T: The illegal wonder drug, *Plain Dealer* (Cleveland, Ohio), p 1-C, July 2, 1995.

Brodsky A and Peele S: AA Abuse, *Reason*, p 39, Nov 1991.

Brown SA, et al: Alcoholism and affective disorder: clinical course of depressive symptoms, *Am J Psychiatry* 152:(1):45, 1995.

Bucholz KK: Alcohol abuse and dependence from a psychiatric epidemiologic perspective, *Alcohol Health Res World* 16(3):197, 1992.

Burman S: A model for women's alcohol and drug treatment, *Alcohol Treat Q* 9(2):87, 1992.

Caetano R: Relationship between two ways of measuring alcohol dependence, *Addict Behav* 17:237, 1992.

Carey KB: Emerging treatment guidelines for mentally ill chemical abusers, *Hosp Community Psychiatry* 40:341, 1989.

Cherpitel LJ: The epidemiology of alcohol-related trauma, *Alcohol Health Res World* 16(3):191, 1992.

Clinical News: Cocaine exposure in utero, *A J Nurs* 98(6):9, 1998.

Collins AC: Inheriting addictions: a genetic perspective with emphasis on alcohol and nicotine. In Milkman HB and Shaffer HJ, editors: *The addictions*, Lexington, Mass, 1985, Lexington Books.

Creager C: SASSI test breaks through denial, *Professional Counselor*, p 65, July-Aug 1989.

Cuffel BJ, Heithoff KA, and Lawson W: Correlates of patterns of substance abuse among patients with schizophrenia, *Hosp Community Psychiatry* 44(3):247, 1993.

Donovan M and Heather N: Acceptability of the controlled-drinking goal among alcohol treatment agencies in New South Wales, Australia, *J Stud Alcohol* 58(3):253, May 1997.

DSM-IV Task Force: *DSM-IV draft criteria*, Washington, DC, 1993, American Psychiatric Association.

Estes N, Smith-Dijutio K, and Heinemann ME: *Nursing diagnosis of the alcoholic person*, St Louis, 1980, Mosby.

FDA Consumer: Drug approved to treat alcoholism, *FDA Consumer* 29(3):2, 1995.

Feldman M: "Whadyaknow," Wisconsin Public Radio, June 4, 1994.

First MB, et al: Changes in substance-related, schizophrenic, and other primarily adult disorders, *Hosp Community Psychiatry* 45(1):18, 1994.

Forbes S: Speech before Iowans for Tax Relief, as broadcast on C-Span, Oct 27, 1997.

Frezza M, et al: High blood alcohol levels in women, *N Engl J Med* 322(2):95, 1990.

Frosch WA: An analytic overview of addictions. In Milkman HB and Shaffer HJ, editors: *The addictions,* Lexington, Mass, 1985, Lexington Books.

Galletly CA, Field CD, and Prior M: Urine drug screening of patients admitted to a state psychiatric hospital, *Hosp Community Psychiatry* 44(6):587, 1993.

George R: Counseling the chemically dependent: theory and practice, Englewood Cliffs, NJ, 1990, Prentice-Hall.

Goodwin DW, et al: Alcohol problems in adoptees raised apart from alcoholic biological parents, *Arch Gen Psychiatry* 28:238, 1973.

Gorski TT: Passages through recovery: an action plan for preventing relapse, New York, 1989, Harper Collins.

Gorski TT: Alcoholism: disease or addiction?, *Professional Counselor,* p 15, Oct 1996.

Harrell AV and Wirtz PW: Screening adolescents for drinking problems. Paper presented at the 1988 National Alcoholism Forum, Arlington, Va, April 1988.

Herman R: To your health, *Washington Post,* Health section, p 10, April 6, 1993.

Hollister L, et al: Clinical uses of benzodiazepines, *J Clin Psychopharmacol* 13(6):1S, 1993.

Hough ESE: Alcoholism: prevention and treatment, *J Psychosoc Nurs Ment Health Serv* 27(1):15, 1989.

Jacobs AJ: The hills are alive, *Entertainment Weekly,* p 17, Oct 17, 1997.

Keltner NL and Folks DG: *Psychotropic drugs,* St Louis, 1997, Mosby.

Kolodner G and Frances R: Recognizing dissociative disorders in patients with chemical dependency, *Hosp Community Psychiatry* 44(11):1041, 1993.

Koop CE, et al: *Alcoholism at time of diagnosis,* New York, 1996, Time Life Medical, Patient Education Media, Inc.

Kovasznay B, et al: Substance abuse and onset of psychotic illness, *Hosp Community Psychiatry* 44(6):567, 1993.

Lacks HE and Leonard CA: Fear of feeling: addressing the emotional process during recovery, *Alcohol Treat Q ,* p 69, Fall 1986.

Lester L: The special needs of the female alcoholic, *Soc Casework* 63:451, 1982.

MacAndrew C: The differentiation of male alcoholic outpatients from non-alcoholic psychiatric outpatients by means of the MMPI, *Q J Stud Alcohol* 26:238, 1965.

Manissa Communication Group: Extract from kudzu vine curbs alcohol desire. *The Addiction Letter* 9(12):4, 1993.

Manissa Communication Group: What do you say when a client wants to cut back, not abstain? *The Addiction Letter* 12(3):1, 1996.

Manissa Communication Group: US trial confirms value of physician advice to reduce drinking. *The Brown University of Addiction Theory and Application* 16(8):4, 1997.

Midanik LT and Room R: The epidemiology of alcohol consumption, *Alcohol Health Res World* 16(3):183, 1992.

Mueller LA and Ketcham K: *Recovering: how to get and stay sober,* New York, 1987, Bantam Books.

Muha L: Home drug tests: what concerned parents must know, *Good Housekeeping,* p 137, July 1997.

National Drug Control Strategy: Drug use in America, Social Issues Resources Series 6:17, 1995.

National Foundation for Brain Research: The cost of disorders of the brain, Washington, DC, 1992, The Foundation.

Noble J: Working paper: projections of alcohol abusers, 1980, 1985, 1990, Washington, DC, 1985, NIAAA, Department of Biometry and Epidemiology.

Ohlms D: The disease of alcoholism, 1991, Gary Whitaker Corp, (videotape).

Ohlms D: Marijuana in the '90's, 1993, Gary Whitaker Corp, (videotape).

Peele S and Brodsky A with Arnold M: *The truth about addiction and recovery,* New York, 1991, Simon and Schuster.

Peyser HS: Alcohol and drug abuse: underrecognized and untreated, *Hosp Community Psychiatry* 40:221, 1989.

Piazza NJ and Wise SL: An order-theoretic analysis of Jellinek's disease model of alcoholism, *Internat J Addictions* 23(4):387, 1988.

Powers JS and Spickard A: Michigan alcoholism screening test to diagnose early alcoholism in a general practice, *South Med J* 77:852, 1984.

Rawson R, Obert J, and McCann M: *The neurobehavioral treatment manual,* Beverly Hills, Calif, 1990, Matrix Institute on Addictions. Quoted in Corrie D, editor: *CWA SAINT trainee notebook,* Atlanta, 1993, Child Welfare Institute.

Roberts A and Koob GF: The neurobiology of addiction, *Alcohol Health Res World* 21(2):101, 1997.

Sancton T: The dossier on Diana's crash, *Time,* p 50, Oct 13, 1997.

Satel SL, Becker BP, and Dan E: Reducing obstacles to affiliation with Alcoholics Anonymous among veterans with PTSD and alcoholism, *Hosp Community Psychiatry* 44(11):1061, 1993.

Schlosser E: Reefer madness, *Atlantic Monthly,* p 45, Aug 1994.

Schofield A: The CAGE questionnaire and psychological health, *Br J Addict* 83:761, 1988.

Scott EM: Who decides if there's a pink elephant, *Alcohol Treat Q* 9(2):101, 1992.

Smart RG and Mann RE: Alcohol and the epidemiology of liver cirrhosis, *Alcohol Health Res World* 16(3):217, 1992.

Smolowe J: Choose your poison, *Time* 142(4):56, 1993.

Stoffel VC: Occupational therapists' roles in treating substance abuse, *Hosp Community Psychiatry* 45(1):21, 1994.

Vaillant G, et al: Prospective study of alcoholism treatment, *Am J Med* 75:455, 1983.

Van Meter RA: Physician advise for problem alcohol drinkers, *J Fam Pract* 45(1):17, July 1987.

Wallace J: *Alcoholism: new light on the disease,* Newport, RI, 1985, Edgehill Publications.

What do you say when a client wants to cut back, but not abstain?, *The Addiction Letter* 12(3):1, March 1996.

Whitfield C, Davis J, and Barker L: Alcoholism. In Barker LR, Burton JR, and Zieve PD, editors: *Principles of ambulatory medicine,* Baltimore, 1986, Williams & Wilkins.

Zorumski CF and Isenberg KE: Insights into the structure and function of GABA-benzodiazepine receptors: ion channels and psychiatry, *Am J Psychiatry* 148(2):162, 1991.

CHAPTER 34

Dual Diagnosis

CAROL E. BOSTROM

LEARNING OBJECTIVES

After reading this chapter you should be able to:
- Define the term *dual diagnosis.*
- Describe major perspectives related to etiologies for dual diagnosis.
- Understand issues related to treatment of dual-diagnosis patients.

Traditional psychiatric treatment has divided patients into distinct categories based upon the thinking that one type of illness or disorder is primary, or more urgent, than another. Historically, patients were categorized as having either a mental illness or a substance-abuse/dependency problem. The mental illness or the substance problem was treated without recognition that another diagnosis was appropriate, or that there were important issues underlying the substance abuse. Today there is a growing movement to view patients more holistically.

Based on research and experience, it is now known that all diagnoses are important and need to be addressed. With this recognition, additional or more comprehensive therapeutic approaches have been developed. The complexity of patients' problems and diagnoses requires individual case management as well as programming for groups of patients with common needs. Part of this effort is to reduce frequent hospitalization, or the "revolving-door syndrome."

This chapter discusses issues related to patients with dual diagnoses rather than focusing on specific interventions for this population of patients. Three issues in this area will be addressed: the concept of dual diagnosis, etiology, and treatment.

DUAL DIAGNOSIS DEFINED

Dual diagnosis usually refers to the presence of at least one psychiatric disorder in addition to a substance-abuse or dependency problem. The psychiatric disorder may be a mental illness and/or a personality disorder. Research studies indicate a range of about 10% to 80% of selected patient populations qualify for dual diagnosis (Ortman, 1997; Ries, 1993). The treatment team can expect that approximately 50% of patients will be dually diagnosed. Having multiple diagnoses does not meet the criteria for dual diagnosis. For example, a patient with the diagnoses of major depression and dependent personality disorder is not considered a dual-diagnosis patient. An example of a patient with a dual diagnosis is an individual with chronic schizophrenia and marijuana abuse. Another example is a patient with alcohol dependency and antisocial personality disorder. Box 34-1 provides examples of dual-diagnosis combinations. Considering the

Box 34-1 **Examples of Dual Diagnoses**	
Axis I	Schizophrenia
	Alcohol abuse
Axis I	Cocaine abuse
Axis II	Antisocial personality disorder
Axis I	Major depression
	Anxiolytic dependency
Axis I	Major depression
	Marijuana abuse
Axis II	Borderline personality disorder

number of axis I and axis II diagnoses, a multitude of combinations is possible. Therefore, patients with dual diagnoses are a heterogeneous group.

ETIOLOGY

The etiologies for diagnoses are discussed in the chapters specific to the disorders. One of the issues that mental health professionals traditionally deal with is which comes first: the mental illness or the substance problem. Because of this dilemma, the treatment of patients has been affected and has followed specific patterns. From the perspective that the mental illness occurred first, many reasons could account for the development of a substance problem. As is true for mental illnesses, heredity and biological factors may predispose an individual to problems with substances. Some persons may be predisposed to develop both a mental illness and substance abuse. The largest category of dual-diagnosis patients includes those who have a primary psychiatric disorder and a primary substance-use disorder with separate etiologies (Hein, et al, 1997).

Many patients indicate that the use of a substance helps them feel calmer. For patients experiencing psychotic symptoms, self-medicating with alcohol or drugs can help them feel better, less anxious, and can decrease the intensity of hallucinations. Furthermore, using substances does not result in bothersome and uncomfortable side effects when compared with antipsychotics. Patients can also experience some degree of social acceptance when they drink alcohol or use drugs (Carey, 1996). With the decision to use a substance, the feeling of autonomy or power results in a temporary increase in self-esteem. Problems or issues are avoided, and patients feel better and temporarily in control of themselves.

From the perspective that the substance abuse precedes mental illness, it follows that brain chemistry can be altered, that is, neurotransmitter imbalance or depletion. Chemicals can induce acute and chronic psychiatric problems. Substance-induced psychosis, schizophrenia, depression, and mania can occur in vulnerable individuals. Substance abuse can also lead to feelings of guilt, depression, and altered self-esteem.

Substance-abuse issues are often present in the population of persons with personality disorders, particularly those with antisocial personality disorder or Cluster B disorders (borderline, narcissistic, histrionic) with antisocial traits (Walker, 1992; Schubert, et al, 1988). Some traits or behaviors of substance abusers are the same as those of persons with personality disorders. Regardless of which disorder or problem came first, the existence of a substance problem, a mental illness, and/or a personality disorder complicates diagnosis and treatment, prolongs rehabilitation, and increases the incidence of relapse (Ries, 1993). The complexity of these patients' problems requires a holistic, multifaceted approach.

TREATMENT ISSUES

Traditional models of treatment have focused on one issue at a time or on the most acute problem first. One model assumed when mental illness was stabilized, substance use would subside. Another idea suggested stabilization of the mental illness would enhance patient participation and benefit from substance-abuse treatment. Some clinicians believed detoxification from chemical substances had to occur before other treatment was possible (Grinspoon, 1995). All of these assumptions were valid for some patients, some of the time. For example, the severely psychotic patient needs antipsychotic medication before being able to participate in treatment groups. However, many problems exist with these models of treatment. For example, treatment was disrupted when patients had to be transferred from one unit or facility to another. Separate agencies/facilities with different treatment responsibilities did not coordinate and could not provide the multiple modalities needed in treatment for patients with dual diagnoses (Tsuang, et al, 1997). Continuity of care was difficult to maintain, resulting in gaps in treatment. Consequently, follow-up care was sporadic and care of patients was not managed effectively or adequately.

Another problem area arises from traditional differences between mental health and substance abuse programs and staff philosophies. A substance-abuse program may discourage the use of all psychotropic medications, while the psychiatric unit may strongly encourage medication compliance. Confrontational groups on substance-abuse units differ greatly from support groups found in psychiatric units. For example, patients with religious delusions, preoccupations, and distortions find it difficult to participate and work in the 12-step recovery program in Alcoholics Anonymous and like groups.

In the past, education and training for many staff members focused on the type of unit where they would be working. As a result, staff members were often unprepared to treat patients with other problems. The lack of understanding of dual-diagnosis patients resulted in the staff having unrealistic expectations of what patients could accomplish during a specific time frame. Within the past 10 years, programs integrating treatment for mental illness and substance use have been increasing. Research is showing that integrated treatment programs have positive results—e.g., remission of substance use, improvement in mental health (Drake, et al, 1996).

Problems Affecting Program Development

Given the heterogeneity of dual-diagnosis patients, many issues have to be considered regarding program development. In working with these patients, the difficulty lies not so much with individual counseling, but with group programming. Treatment programs must identify which issues pertain to the majority of patients and can be dealt with in large groups and which issues should be addressed in smaller groups. Unique or very personal issues are more appropriately handled on a one-to-one basis. For example, education about the disease concept of alcoholism or nutrition may be applicable to an entire group of patients. Education about the side effects of specific antidepressants may be appropriate for a select group of patients. A patient may want to discuss his or her feelings about acquired immunodeficiency syndrome (AIDS) on a one-to-one basis

before talking in a group. On a given day, changes in a patient's mental status may affect his or her ability to participate in a large group. Therefore, staff members need to be flexible in assigning patients to specific groups.

Patients with dual diagnoses also need flexibility regarding the length of treatment rather than being assigned a fixed number of treatment days, sessions, or appointments. A program that is open-ended, occurs in stages, and provides support and empowerment may be necessary for patient compliance with treatment. For some patients, abstinence from a substance should be a goal of treatment and not a prerequisite (Carey, 1996). For example, a chronic schizophrenic patient may be able to quit smoking marijuana with the nurse's help in developing assertiveness skills. For a patient with antisocial personality disorder, abstinence from alcohol may be required prior to beginning treatment.

Staff need to be aware of and prepared for dealing with issues and conflicts inherent in this population. In groups and in the milieu setting, patients with personality disorders may try to manipulate more regressed members. Depending on the substances abused, conflict may arise around degrees of addiction and drugs of choice ("Cocaine is worse than alcohol"; "My addiction is worse than yours"). Because most of these patients experience difficulties in concentration and memory, education groups must be structured with concrete concepts, simplified material, and repetition of material. Handouts and homework assignments may be helpful to practice and apply key treatment concepts.

Often, some patients in this group are perpetrators of violence, and others are victims. As a result, victims may find it difficult to participate in or even attend a group with perpetrators. In dealing with dual-diagnosed patients, it is evident that there are more issues and questions than answers. Continued work and development of models and strategies are necessary for these patients. The hope is that patients ultimately will benefit from more appropriate programming.

■ Critical Thinking Question

What benefits could a patient receive from dual-diagnosis treatment?

Psychotherapeutic Management

Effective treatment for patients with dual diagnoses must be multifaceted and multidisciplinary. Box 34-2 summarizes treatment components. Individual case management for social, medical, and emotional needs requires professional staff to integrate their knowledge on addictions and mental illness. Communication, cooperation, and collaboration among professional staff responsible for assessing, diagnosing, and treating patients are required.

Nurse-Patient Relationship. In working with dual-diagnosis patients, the nurse must use interventions specific to patients' individual needs, mental illness, and substance problem. The nurse deals with all of these areas simultaneously.

Trust between the nurse and patients develops if patients feel that the nurse is knowledgeable, skilled, nonjudgmental, and empathic. This is especially important with the short length of inpatient hospitalization.

Box 34-2   Treatment Components for Patients with Dual Diagnoses

Case management
Individual therapy
Group therapy
Skills training
Education groups
Vocational counseling
Referrals to community resources
Self-help groups

Monitoring patients for symptoms of withdrawal is ongoing. (Specific interventions for the relevant mental illness and chemical dependency are found in other chapters.) The nurse is involved in teaching patients about the effects of alcohol and drugs on the mind and body. Patients need education about their mental illness, and help with recognizing the signs of relapse regarding their specific mental illness and substance problem. Strategies for relapse prevention are based on each patient's individual needs.

■ Critical Thinking Question

A young male patient with schizophrenia abuses alcohol. How do the behaviors of these individual illnesses complicate treatment?

Psychopharmacology. Medication is specifically prescribed for patients according to their mental illness. Compliance with prescribed medication is supported by the nurse. Assistance with interferences to medication compliance are addressed, such as lack of money or transportation to purchase medications. The nurse teaches patients about side-effect management and about potential problems resulting from using alcohol or other substances with medication. (Refer to chapters on psychopharmacology for specific information.) Caution is used in prescribing anxiolytics, which cause dependence (e.g., benzodiazepines).

Milieu Management. Enforcing the rules of the unit or program and setting limits provide structure and clear expectations for patients. This helps

---

*C*ase *S*tudy

Barbara Abel is a 28-year-old patient who was transferred from CCU because of imipramine (Tofranil) overdose and alcohol withdrawal. She is weak, shaky, and needs assistance with ambulation. Her diagnoses are major depression and alcohol abuse. Barbara states to the nurse, "I only wanted to sleep, have some peace, and forget my problems. I was so tired and couldn't eat, or get out of bed. Ending it all would be better. I'd be happy again and like myself."

Barbara's husband divorced her 3 months ago because "he didn't understand that I needed to have a few drinks to sleep and forget my problems." She is an RN and was employed as a unit manager. She recently lost her job due to absenteeism. Barbara moved in with a friend who is employed as an accountant. Her friend occasionally uses cocaine to "stay on top of things" at work. Two of Barbara's co-workers encouraged her to seek treatment, but she was too tired to make an appointment with her psychiatrist.

Care Plan

NAME: Barbara Abel

ADMISSION DATE: _____

DSM-IV DIAGNOSIS: Alcohol abuse

ASSESSMENT: **Areas of strength:** RN who has nursing and leadership skills. Has basic knowledge about her illnesses because of her education. Was medication compliant prior to overdose. Two co-workers are supportive of her.

Problems: Suicide attempt with overdose, alcohol abuse, insomnia, anorexia, recently divorced, no place to stay, unemployed, drug-using friend.

DIAGNOSES:
- High risk for violence: self-directed related to depressed mood as evidenced by suicide attempt.
- Low self-esteem related to divorce and job loss as evidenced by statement of not liking self.
- Risk for injury related to imipramine overdose and alcohol withdrawal as evidenced by weakness and shakiness.
- Altered nutrition: less than body requirements related to depressed mood as evidenced by anorexia.
- Sleep-pattern disturbance related to stress as evidenced by insomnia.

OUTCOMES: **Short-term goals:**   Date met
- Patient will verbalize plans for the future.   _____
- Patient will sleep 6 to 8 hours per night.   _____
- Patient will eat three balanced meals per day.   _____
- Patient will recognize and describe problems associated with drinking alcohol and depression.   _____
- Patient will make plans to live with a friend who does not use drugs or at halfway house.   _____

Long-term goals:
- Patient will practice abstinence from alcohol.   _____
- Patient will attend self-help groups like Double Trouble or Alcoholics Anonymous.   _____
- Patient will attend outpatient treatment.   _____
- Patient will be medication compliant.   _____
- Patient will live at halfway house or with a friend who does not abuse drugs.   _____
- Patient will participate in impaired nurse program through the state nurses' association.   _____

PLANNING/
INTERVENTIONS: **Nurse-patient relationship:** Contract with patient to report to nurse if suicidal thoughts occur. Convey empathy and encourage verbalization of feelings. Reinforce strengths and accomplishments. Teach patient personal signs of relapse and relapse prevention for depression and alcohol abuse. Offer nutritious snacks. Assist patient with ambulation and ADLs when necessary and encourage independence when patient is able to perform own ADLs.

Psychopharmacology: Trazodone (Desyrel) 50 mg tid
                                        Multivitamin 1 qd

Milieu management: Invite and encourage patient to attend groups on assertiveness, stress management, alcohol, mental illness, medication education, and relapse prevention.

EVALUATION: Patient denies suicidal ideation. She is expressing interest in employment and making alternative living arrangement. She is sleeping 6 hours per night and is eating three balanced meals per day. The patient is able to identify some positive characteristics of self and past accomplishments.

REFERRALS: Patient to attend weekly Double Trouble meetings and appointments for dual diagnosis treatment at a mental health clinic.

to decrease manipulation and conflict among patients on the unit and in group sessions. Treatment groups focus on education about substances, mental illness, and medication. Stress management, assertiveness, and community living skills are also a focus of treatment. The staff must be flexible in assigning patients to groups because of possible changes in mental status due to withdrawal from substances and/or exacerbation of mental illness symptoms. Supportive, gentle confrontation techniques are more effective than intense confrontation.

Attendance at self-help group meetings such as Alcoholics Anonymous, Narcotics Anonymous, and Double Trouble (for dual-diagnosis patients) begins while patients are on the inpatient unit, if possible. Referral to and involvement with outpatient programs, self-help groups, halfway houses, and vocational counseling is completed prior to discharge. Sometimes self-help groups are not attended until later in outpatient treatment when the patient feels more able and capable of participating (Noordsy, et al, 1996). Continuity of treatment is necessary to prevent relapse and decrease recidivism.

CONTINUUM OF CARE

An outpatient integrated treatment model has led to decreased utilization of inpatient services, a reduction or elimination of substance use, and improvement in other areas of life (Drake, et al, 1996). Treatment that occurs in stages, is open ended, empowers individuals, and extends beyond weeks or months can be beneficial for individuals with dual diagnoses. The following five-step model conceptualized by Kate Carey (1996) combines mental-health and substance-abuse treatment.

- *Step 1 Establish a working alliance.* Establish trust with the individual so that he or she is able to express fears and concerns about changing behaviors.
- *Step 2 Evaluate costs and benefits of continued substance abuse.* Discuss the use of substances and their effects on the individual's life. Raise awareness of consequences due to substance use rather than its causes. Establish goals, such as obtaining employment, and focus on goal achievement (usually requires a reduction in substance use). Discuss costs and benefits of substance use.

- *Step 3 Individual goals for change.* Reduce the use of substances when the individual is willing and able instead of requiring complete abstinence. This enhances involvement in treatment with the ultimate goal of abstinence.
- *Step 4 Build an environment and life-style supportive of abstinence.* Working on family and social supports is necessary. Day treatment or frequent appointments may be needed early in treatment. Assistance with time structuring and encouragement to attend self-help groups are necessary for success.
- *Step 5 Coping with crises.* Plan for and manage crises such as relapse and symptom management.

Key Concepts

1. *Dual diagnosis* can be defined as the comorbid presence of a substance disorder and a mental illness or personality disorder.
2. The population of dual-diagnosis patients is heterogeneous.
3. There are many issues to be addressed in treating dual-diagnosis patients because of their diverse abilities and needs.
4. Patients with dual diagnoses can benefit from treatment that integrates substance-use and mental-health services.

Study Questions

(Answer key is in the back of the book.)
1. The nurse, in planning care for a patient with dual diagnoses, knows that these patients:
   a. All have the same needs and require the same interventions
   b. Require interventions relevant to individual needs and their specific mental illness and substance problems
   c. Should be treated for the mental illness only
   d. Should be referred to a substance-dependency unit for their alcohol problems
2. A patient with dual diagnoses is being admitted to the unit. Which of the following diagnoses would the nurse expect the patient to have?
   a. Chronic paranoid schizophrenia and dependent personality disorder
   b. Major depression with suicide attempt
   c. Undifferentiated schizophrenia and alcohol dependence
   d. Major depression and borderline personality disorder

3. The nurse is leading a group with patients who have dual diagnoses. The nurse:
   a. Uses supportive and gentle confrontation
   b. Is intensely confrontational with all patients
   c. Expects all patients to participate in every meeting
   d. Requires all patients to attend every meeting

4. In teaching patients about medication compliance, which of the following would be inappropriate for the nurse to teach?
   a. That patients should take all medication as prescribed by the psychiatrist
   b. Issues regarding the management of medication side effects
   c. That patients should inform the nurse and psychiatrist of any side effects that might produce noncompliance with medication
   d. That patients should stop the medication if they want to drink alcohol or use street drugs

5. A patient with chronic schizophrenia and marijuana abuse will be discharged from the hospital in 2 weeks. The nurse:
   a. Tells the patient that follow-up treatment will not be necessary
   b. Arranges for outpatient treatment with the help of the social worker
   c. Tells the patient to ask his doctor about discontinuing haloperidol (Haldol)
   d. Informs the patient that smoking a little marijuana now and then is safe

REFERENCES

Carey K: Substance use reduction in the context of outpatient psychiatric treatment: a collaborative, motivational, harm reduction approach, *Community Ment Health J* 30(3):291, 1996.

Drake R: Substance use reduction among patients with severe mental illness, *Community Ment Health J* 32(3):311, 1996.

Drake R, et al: The course, treatment, and outcome of substance use disorder in persons with severe mental illness, *Am J Orthopsychiatry* 66(1):42, 1996.

Grinspoon L, editor: Treatment of drug abuse and addiction: part II, *Harvard Mental Health Letter* 12(3):1, 1995.

Hein D, et al: Dual diagnosis subtypes in urban substance abuse and mental health clinics, *Psychiatr Serv* 48(8): 1058, 1997.

McKelvy MJ, et al: Substance abuse and mental illness: double trouble, *J Psychosoc Nurs Ment Health Serv* 25:20, 1987.

Noordsy D, et al: The role of self-help programs in the rehabilitation of persons with severe mental illness and substance use disorders, *Community Ment Health J* 22(1):71, 1996.

Ortman D: *The dually diagnosed,* Northvale, NJ, 1997, Jason Aronson Inc.

Ries R: Clinical treatment matching models for dually diagnosed patients, *Psychiatr Clin North Am* 16:1, 1993.

Schubert DSP, et al: A statistical evaluation of the literature regarding the associations among alcoholism, drug abuse, and antisocial personality disorder, *Int J Addict* 23(8):797, 1988.

Tsuang J, et al: Dual diagnosis treatment for patients with schizophrenia who are substance dependent, *Psychiatr Serv* 48(7):887, 1997.

Walker R: Substance abuse and B-cluster disorders. I. Understanding the dual diagnosis patient, *J Psychoactive Drugs* 24(3):223, 1992.

CHAPTER 35

Eating Disorders

LINDA K. HINKLE

▲ ▲ ▲ ▲ ▲ ▲

LEARNING OBJECTIVES

After reading this chapter you should be able to:
- Recognize the criteria and terminology used in the DSM-IV for eating disorders.
- Recognize and describe objective and subjective symptoms of eating disorders.
- Describe etiological explanations for eating disorders.

- Describe treatment issues with eating disorders.
- Develop nursing care plans for patients with eating disorders.
- Evaluate the effectiveness of nursing interventions for patients with eating disorders.

There is little question that our culture has a preoccupation with food, eating, weight, and fitness. It is quite common for men and women to structure their daily schedules around health-club and exercise programs in pursuit of the desired appearance. More books on diets, nutrition, and fitness are being sold than ever before. The media almost exclusively features female models who are slender. In increasing numbers, however, this preoccupation with and quest for the perceived ideal body is developing into life-threatening eating disorders. In this chapter the clinical examples, case studies, and nursing care plans focus on patients with the specific eating disorders of anorexia nervosa and bulimia nervosa.

ANOREXIA NERVOSA

DSM-IV Criteria

The DSM-IV diagnostic criteria for anorexia nervosa are found in the box on page 551. The major characteristics include a refusal to maintain a normal body weight; an intense fear of gaining weight or becoming fat, even though the individual is underweight; the absence of at least three consecutive menstrual cycles; and a body image disturbance that most commonly manifests itself in patients' perceptions of themselves as overweight, when in fact, they are emaciated. Some studies suggest it is not necessarily a distortion of body image, but rather a "weight phobia" that is present in anorectic patients (Pumariega, et al, 1993; Hsu and Sobkiewicz, 1991). Besides size overestimation, weight or shape may be the most important influence on the person's sense of worth, or they may simply deny the problematic nature of their underweight status.

Postpubertal anorectic females who are not taking hormone supplements experience amenorrhea for at least 3 months. It is common for menstruation to cease early in the illness, before any significant weight loss has taken place. One theory for the cause of amenorrhea suggests the lack of nourishment significantly slows the functioning of the pituitary glands, which are fundamental to the menstrual

KEY TERMS

Amenorrhea   The absence of menstruation

Anorexia nervosa   A disorder characterized by restrictive eating resulting in emaciation, amenorrhea, disturbance in body image, and an intense fear of becoming obese

Binge   Eating an unusually large amount of food in a relatively short period of time

Bulimia nervosa   A disorder characterized by binge eating, compensatory behavior, and overconcern with body shape and weight

Emaciated   Made excessively thin by the lack of nutrition

Lanugo   A fine, soft hair covering almost all parts of the body

Obesity   An abnormal increase in the proportion of fat cells, mainly in the viscera and subcutaneous tissues of the body

Purge   To attempt to compensate for calories consumed via self-induced vomiting or abuse of laxatives, diuretics, or enemas

---

DSM-IV Diagnostic Criteria for Anorexia Nervosa

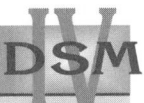

A. Refusal to maintain body weight at or above a minimum normal weight for age and height

B. Intense fear of gaining weight or becoming fat, even though underweight

C. Disturbance in the way in which one's body weight or shape is experienced, overvaluing of shape or weight, or denial of seriousness of low weight

D. In females, the absence of at least three consecutive menstrual cycles

Restricting type: during an episode of anorexia nervosa, persons do *not* engage in recurrent episodes of binge eating or purging

Binge-eating/purging type: during an episode of anorexia nervosa, persons engage in recurrent episodes of binge eating or purging

Adapted from the American Psychiatric Association: *Diagnostic and statistical manual of mental disorders,* ed 4, Washington, DC, 1994, The Association.

---

cycle (Weiner, 1983). Another theory argues that women must maintain approximately 17% body fat to menstruate (Johnson, Sansone, and Chewning, 1992). Fat levels below this amount result in amenorrhea, with accompanying reduction of hormone levels and blunting of some secondary sexual characteristics. In anorectic males, low sex drive and low testosterone may be the equivalent of amenorrhea in female patients (Beumont, 1995).

Anorexia is less common than bulimia, affecting from 0.1% to 0.6% of the general population, with a somewhat higher rate in adolescent girls (Grinspoon, 1997). Females account for approximately 90% of the reported cases of anorexia nervosa. Although the age of onset can range from 10 to 40 years, it is primarily a disorder of adolescence, with the average age of onset at 16 years (Johnson, Sansone, and Chewning, 1992). From 8% to 18% of anorectic pa-

tients die as a result of their affliction (Zerbe, 1992), which is greater than the rate of death associated with any other psychiatric disorder.

The DSM-IV specifies two types of anorexia nervosa: the *restricting type,* in which persons do not regularly engage in binge-eating or purging behavior; and the *binge-eating/purging type,* in which persons do regularly engage in binge-eating or purging behaviors.

Behavior

The onset of anorexia can often be considered insidious (not readily apparent) because the typical adolescent girl who becomes a victim usually portrays an image of being the "perfect little girl," never causing problems for anyone. As dieting and fad foods are such common themes in adolescence, it usually is not until the young woman has lost a significant amount of weight that anyone takes notice. The most common premorbid personality profile is that of a perfectionistic and introverted girl with problems with self-esteem and peer relationships (Beumont, 1995). These girls are typically high achievers, often earning outstanding grades and other honors.

CLINICAL EXAMPLE

Fourteen-year-old Annie seemed like "just one of the girls" to her parents. She was becoming increasingly concerned about her developing body, especially about the weight she was gaining. She began dieting, as "her friends were." She insisted on eating only salads and/or tofu for all meals and gradually began to decrease the size of these portions. Eventually, she was eating no breakfast at all, three bites of salad for lunch, and a minimal portion of salad and tofu for dinner. One day in school, Annie fainted in her physical education class. Upon examination, her physician discovered her emaciated state.

The term *anorexia* is a misnomer because anorectic patients may or may not lose their appetites. If they are hungry, they suppress their appetite in an effort to remain thin or to get thinner.

Objective signs

The most obvious observable behavior of anorexia nervosa is deliberate weight loss. Patients have such a preoccupation with food and such a need to control their weight that their eating behaviors change significantly. Patients with anorexia nervosa are in two groups: the dieters and the vomiters/purgers. The dieters are more often young women who are in the normal weight range for height and build before the eating disorder begins. This group views losing weight as more probable if they simply eat less and avoid social situations in which eating is expected. Consequently, these young women often isolate themselves socially, and others note that they increasingly alienate themselves from their friends and families, often withdrawing into their rooms. It is not uncommon for these young women to be competitive and obsessive about their activities. They also are often observed participating in rigid exercise programs to help reduce their weight.

CLINICAL EXAMPLE

Kristin, age 16, was in the normal weight range when she joined the school volleyball team with her friends. The first time they donned their uniforms, one of Kristin's friends called her "piano legs." Kristin was horrified and began to diet. In addition, she asked her parents to join the local health club so she could exercise to "keep in shape" for the team. Her entire day revolved around preparation and participation on the team, to the extent that she forfeited all other social opportunities. She often did not arrive home until after 9:00 PM, as she went to the health club to exercise after a volleyball game or practice. Kristin lost 21 lb before anyone noticed.

Vomiters and purgers are more often overweight before the eating disorder begins. Their weight tends to fluctuate. These young women are more prone to dangerous methods of weight reduction, such as the induction of vomiting or excessive use of laxatives. This group of anorectic patients commonly denies concerns about weight and typically eat normally in social situations. After the meal, they retreat to the nearest bathroom and purge themselves of the consumed food. Dental problems frequently occur in these patients because the acidic vomitus decays the enamel on their teeth. This group also may be susceptible to times when they binge eat, or uncontrollably eat large amounts of food, rather than being able to maintain dietary restriction.

CLINICAL EXAMPLE

Tina was always a chubby child. When she was 13 years old, her parents sent her to a residential summer camp. Tina told no one that she decided summer camp was a good opportunity to lose weight. It was not too long before Tina's counselors noticed she went to the bathroom after every meal or snack and did not return after a reasonable amount of time. When one counselor eventually followed her, she found Tina vomiting.

Because the intake of nutrients, and thus energy, is so low in anorectic patients, their bodies try to adjust by using less energy. Consequently, other physiological processes are affected. Constipation, hypotension, bradycardia, and hypothermia are commonly reported. In addition, the skin is often dry, and lanugo appears. Many patients have delayed gastric emptying. Dehydration is also common, which can lead to irreversible renal damage (Goldbloom and Kennedy, 1995). Pitting edema occurs in a smaller number of anorectic patients, most often after attempts to gain weight by eating more food. When the young woman notices the swelling, she immediately stops trying to increase her weight and may even be motivated to use diuretics, further complicating the problem. Many anorectic patients become hyperactive and are unable to relax. It is not uncommon for them to complain of insomnia and to be seen taking early morning walks. In addition, osteopenia or osteoporosis may develop with prolonged amenorrhea (De Zwaan and Mitchell, 1993). This loss of bone mass may not be reversible. Moreover, studies have found ventricular dilatation in anorectic patients. (De Zwaan and Mitchell, 1993). Also of great concern are decreases in the thickness of the left ventricular wall, the size of the cardiac chambers, and myocardial oxygen uptake. This can lead to life-threatening cardiac arrhythmias.

As a consequence of semistarvation, anorectic patients often become preoccupied with food and eating (Beumont, 1995). This preoccupation seems to involve all aspects of life. Patients are often found reading multiple materials on food and dieting and sometimes attempt to take control of family meals because they believe they are the resident authority on nutrition in the household. They may engage in bizarre behavior regarding food and eating, such as hoarding food, preparing elaborate meals for others and then not eating the food themselves. They may feel compelled to go through elaborate rituals before they eat.

Subjective symptoms

One of the most outstanding features of anorexia nervosa is the conscious fear these patients have of losing control over the amount of food they eat and of becoming fat. They are very concerned about their bodies, feeling obese, and losing weight or preventing weight gain. Some even say they would rather be dead than fat (Beumont, 1995). It is this fear that motivates them to begin the diet. The fear may have been triggered by one event that seemed trivial in the minds of many, or one event that was traumatic. It is an exaggeration of the concern about weight and dieting in our society (Beumont, 1995). These patients may have felt abandoned or inadequate, which can precipitate an overall feeling of helplessness (Grinspoon, 1997). They try to combat this feeling of helplessness by taking control of what they can control, i.e., their weight and the amount of food they eat. Consequently, most of their energy becomes invested in this effort.

Besides problems with eating behavior and weight concern, anorectic persons often have other psychological symptoms, many of which are known to be consequences of semistarvation (Beumont, 1995). These patients exhibit depression, irritability, social withdrawal, loss of sex drive, and obsessional symptoms. These symptoms often improve with weight gain.

> ## ■ Critical Thinking Question
>
> A 17-year-old girl remarks to you that she feels fat and repulsive. You do not observe that the patient is particularly overweight. How do you begin to assess if the patient is suffering from an eating disorder?

Etiology

The psychiatrist Hilde Bruch (1973) believed anorexia was caused by a number of specific disturbances. Today, most experts agree eating disorders causation is multifactorial with significant variance among individuals. Suggested contributing factors include biological, sociocultural, family, cognitive, behavioral, and psychodynamic factors.

Biological factors

Earlier in this century physiological disturbances were postulated as causative in anorexia. Currently, researchers believe the physiological abnormalities found in anorectic patients are mostly a result of semistarvation and purging behavior rather than the cause of disordered eating (Fairburn, 1995a). An exception may be increased serotonin levels. Studies have found that, even after long-term weight restoration and recovery, anorectics have increased cerebrospinal fluid (CSF) levels of 5-hydroxyindoleacetic acid (5-HIAA), the major metabolite of serotonin. Serotonin activity is known to have inhibitory effects on a number of areas and may lead to food restriction due to inhibited appetite, as well as to the rigid, inhibited, anxious, and obsessional behaviors seen in anorectics (Kaye, 1995).

In addition, researchers have found premorbid obesity to be a risk factor for anorexia, although this may be a general risk factor for dieting in general rather than for anorexia in particular. Moreover, it has been shown that approximately 47% of anorectics have severe gastrointestinal problems in their early feeding history, suggesting the possibility early feeding problems contribute to the development of the disorder (Z. Cooper, 1995).

Sociocultural factors

Feminist theorists highlight the role of Western philosophical, political, and cultural history in the development of eating disorders. It is recognized that the increased incidence of eating disorders in this century has corresponded to an increasingly and unrealistically thin beauty ideal for women (Wilfley and Rodin, 1995). In addition, our culture has advanced the notion that body weight is a matter of personal choice and that shape can be changed at will. This leads to dieting, which, it is widely agreed, is a major predisposing factor to both anorexia nervosa and bulimia nervosa (Striegel-Moore, 1995).

Another factor is the relational orientation of women, which creates a vulnerability to the opinions of others, particularly during adolescence (Striegel-Moore, 1995). In addition, our culture stresses the importance of physical attractiveness in obtaining approval, and, because of the thin beauty ideal, girls believe the way to get approval is to try to be thinner. Lack of approval is interpreted as related to a less than ideal body size.

Family factors

Family and twin studies have found evidence for familial aggregation of eating disorders and for a higher concordance rate for anorexia in monozygotic than in dizygotic twins, suggesting a heritable component (Strober, 1995). Family environment may also play a role. Emotional restraint, enmeshed relationships, rigidity in the organization of the family, and avoidance of conflict are other etiological factors (Vandereycken, 1995; Strober, 1995; Grinspoon, 1997). Odd eating habits and strong concerns about appearance and weight also have been described. As Z. Cooper (1995) points out, however, it cannot be determined how much the observed problems in the families of anorectics are consequences

of the disorder as opposed to causal factors. (Also see box later on p. 557 for a discussion of anorectic families.)

Cognitive and behavioral factors

The role of distorted cognition has been less emphasized in anorexia than it has in bulimia. Behavioral theorists, however, hold that anorectic behavior develops and is maintained as a function of environmental contingencies. Rejecting food and losing weight, for example, may be positively reinforced by attention from others. Behavioral treatments, although they have not been adequately evaluated, are widely used and are thought to be highly beneficial for the anorectic. This treatment involves use of reinforcement and punishment contingent on changing eating behaviors and weight gain.

Psychodynamic factors

Freud believed human beings have two basic drives: sexual and aggressive. Not surprising, then, is his interpretation of anorexia nervosa. Freud postulated that appetite is an expression of the libido (sexual drive). Both eating and sexual drive are appetites. Therefore, when patients deny having an appetite for food, their sexual drive is absent as well. According to Freud, food and eating are symbols of nurturing and love. Anorectics reject nurturing. Therefore, anorectic patients do not eat because food and sex are perceived as repulsive.

Modern psychoanalytic theorists have stressed the role of sexuality in anorexia nervosa. In addition, some clinicians have suggested that eating disorders may be related to an early history of sexual abuse. Overall, however, research finds the rate of sexual abuse histories among persons with eating disorders is similar to that found in the general psychiatric population. Sexual abuse, therefore, may predispose one to psychiatric disorders in general, rather than eating disorders in particular (Palmer, 1995).

In addition, some have suggested that anorexia involves a regression to a prepubertal state, so that the adolescent does not mature physically or emotionally. This regression is reinforced by the adolescent having dependency needs met in this situation. The conscious fear of becoming fat is thought to be the symbolic expression of becoming bigger, or growing up, which is supposedly the real, unconscious fear of the anorectic. Other psychoanalytic theorists suggest that the drive for thinness may be an attempt to reduce the control of an overcontrolling maternal figure, that is, by trying not to look like the mother (Johnson, 1995).

Another theory describes anorexia nervosa as an obsession with weight stemming from a fear of being out of control. In response to this fear, patients, via reaction formation, attempt to organize their lives with a set of rules and regulations for everything they do. They experience a tremendous amount of anxiety if one of their rules is broken and attempt to regain control by tightening the rules. Eating behavior appears to be the most available area of life through which these patients can achieve their goals.

Conclusion

There is widespread agreement among experts that the etiology of anorexia nervosa is multifactorial. Biological, sociocultural, family, cognitive, behavioral, and psychodynamic factors all may play a role. However, the factors leading up to dieting may differ from factors leading to the onset of actual eating-disordered behavior (Z. Cooper, 1995). In addition, the factors contributing to the maintenance of anorexia may also be different than those that lead to its development. Today, most research focuses on factors contributing to the onset of dieting. Greater emphases on factors contributing to the maintenance of eating disorder behavior may yield a better understanding of this disorder.

Psychotherapeutic Management

Psychotherapeutic management is geared toward the following three major objectives:
1. Increasing self-esteem so patients do not need the artificial perfection they believe thinness provides
2. Increasing weight to at least 90% of the average body weight for the patient's height and age

3. Helping patients reestablish appropriate eating behavior. When patients are in the starvation phase of the illness, and malnutrition has become a serious medical problem, treatment usually occurs in a medical environment where appropriate supplies and equipment, such as intravenous and feeding-tube apparatuses, are readily available. When the medical crisis is resolved, patients are transferred to a psychiatric unit or are seen on an outpatient basis, where psychotherapeutic intervention can occur effectively.

Nurses may encounter anorectic patients either on an inpatient basis in a medical or psychiatric unit, or on an outpatient basis in a physician's office. In any setting, a multidisciplinary treatment approach is crucial. Members of the treatment team should include a physician, a nurse, a dietitian, and a psychotherapist specializing in the treatment of eating disorders. These patients need medical monitoring, nutritional education and counseling, and psychotherapy.

Working with anorectic patients usually presents a challenge to the psychotherapeutic team, as patients continue the struggle to maintain control. When the treatment team requires weight gain, patients perceive themselves as losing control, which in turn triggers the unconscious feeling of helplessness. Consciously, patients once again experience the fear of becoming fat. This fear underlies the need to gain more control, restarting the vicious cycle. Nursing interventions for patients with eating disorders are listed in the box below.

Nurse-Patient Relationship. Because most anorectic patients are in treatment under duress, it is usually a challenge for the nurse to develop a therapeutic alliance. Patients primarily believe that the nurse is there simply to make them gain weight, so the nurse is perceived as an enemy rather than as an ally. Specific principles of therapeutic communication helpful in facilitating the nurse-patient

Key Nursing Interventions for Patients with Eating Disorders

- Monitor daily caloric intake
- Observe patients for signs of purging
- Monitor activity level
- Weigh daily
- Plan for dietitian to meet with patients to (a) provide accurate information on nutrition and (b) discuss a realistic and healthy diet
- Regularly monitor electrolyte status

relationship with anorectic patients are presented below.

- Convey warmth and sincerity to patients. Patients need to believe the nurse genuinely cares about and understands their effort to overcome the ambivalence about being in treatment. Increasing the patients' self-esteem is a primary objective in recovery.
- Listen empathically. Although patients are likely to deny weight is a problem, they do admit to feeling extremely lonely and tired of striving to be perfect all the time.
- Be honest. Patients enter treatment basically distrustful of everyone. Honesty is imperative for a trusting relationship to occur.
- Set limits. Because of control needs, patients may attempt to manipulate the nurse. A clear contract must be established between the nurse and each patient to help establish trust and to minimize power struggles.
- Assist patients in identifying positive qualities about themselves. Because self-esteem is low, patients need to see concrete evidence of redeeming qualities.
- Collaborate with patients. To elicit cooperation engage patients in the planning process. This should foster trust and a sense of control.
- Teach patients about their disorder. The more information patients receive about anorexia, the harder it is for them to deny their problems and the easier for them to understand what is happening to their bodies.
- Determine the patients' ability to view weighing. Often, anorectics need to be weighed with their backs to the scale. The overall therapeutic goal is to help patients reduce their focus on body weight.
- Initiate a behavior modification program that rewards weight gain with meaningful privileges. Although the idea of gaining weight is stressful to patients, it is crucial to recovery. As soon as a safe weight is attained, allow patients to regulate their own progression and program.
- Teach and model social skills. Acquiring social skills, particularly expressing emotion assertively, is crucial for anorectic patients.
- Help patients identify and express bodily sensations and feelings. Typically, anorectic patients have little bodily awareness, other than a distorted perception of their size.
- Identify patients' non–weight-related interests. If reactivated, these interests can reduce anxiety as patients invest their energies in areas that do not deal with eating.

Psychopharmacology. Although considerable research is currently being conducted, no specific psychopharmacological agent alleviates anorexia nervosa (Kaye, et al, 1991; Kennedy and Goldbloom, 1991). Management of anxiety, depression, and somatic disturbances can be achieved with appropriate medications.

Milieu Management
- In preparation for inpatient-outpatient treatment, provide the patient with a tour of the setting. This can reduce irrational fears about treatment (Fichter, 1995).
- Provide a warm, nurturing atmosphere. It is important for patients to feel support to reduce anxiety and increase self-esteem.
- Closely observe patients. Eating behaviors need to be identified to plan appropriate interventions. Common eating behaviors include hiding food in a paper napkin to be discarded later, leaving bread crusts on the plate and discarding the rest, discarding food into plants or out of the window, and holding food in the mouth to be discarded when the patient brushes her teeth. Respond to such behaviors with nonjudgmental confrontation, conveying understanding of fears of weight gain and other related issues. Neither pity nor punitiveness will be helpful (Fichter, 1995).
- Encourage patients to approach a team member when feeling the urge to purge. Expression of feelings reduces anxiety, and patients might discover another alternative to vomiting.
- Involve families in treatment. Unless parents, particularly of minors, provide emotional support, treatment efforts are futile. Families need to understand the disorder and how to deal with it in order for patients to recover. (See family issues box on p. 557.) Family therapy of anorectic adolescents is a crucial treatment component.
- Be consistent. Whatever behavior modification program or treatment regimen is implemented must be adhered to by the entire staff at all times. Otherwise, patients quickly discover an area to manipulate.

FAMILY ISSUES

Family Issues in Anorexia: Family Dynamics

From the time anorexia nervosa was first identified, common familial patterns have been observed. First, most of the families are in the upper-middle-income level, and able to devote both emotional and financial attention to their daughters. Parents may be seen as smothering, intrusive, and overprotective. Anorectics do not wish to be the center of attention, but frequently are. Their refusal of food is thought to be, in part, a form of rebellion against their parents and soon becomes a central issue for the family.

In the early stage of the illness, when the patient begins to refuse food, the family initially tries to coax her to eat. Because the mother is typically the primary provider of the family meals, the conflict seems to intensify between her and the patient. When the coaxing fails, the mother may begin to cook and serve the patient's favorite foods and to stress that eating together as a family is one way in which they can express love to each other. Guilt, therefore, becomes a prominent issue because the patient hears the message that, if she really loves her parents, she will eat for them.

As the disorder progresses, the family speaks of little but the eating behavior. The patient is confronted with the issue constantly and attends meals more often and eats minute amounts in an effort to relieve some of the parental pressure. It is not long, however, before emaciation becomes obvious, and the family realizes the need to provide immediate medical attention.

Case Study

Sarah, a 17-year-old girl, was brought to the hospital by her parents and her outpatient therapist, whom she had been seeing on a weekly basis for 1 month. Sarah and the therapist had a contract that agreed to a 2-lb weight gain every week. Sarah, however, had continued to lose weight. On admission, she was 5 feet 5 inches tall and weighed 86 lb. She was strongly opposed to her hospitalization.

Sarah is the youngest of three daughters, ages 27, 24, and 17. She was a late addition to her upper-middle-class family. Her parents admitted she had been steadily losing weight for the past 6 months. At first they believed that Sarah was "just dieting" as teenagers frequently do, but they soon began to see her ribs and vertebrae through her nightgown and became gravely concerned.

Sarah recently was named valedictorian of her high school class. She was active in many school activities and was described as a "teacher's dream." Although she appeared to have many friends, Sarah claimed she only had two real friends.

Sarah said her obsession with weight began approximately 6 months ago when the family went to visit the oldest daughter, whom Sarah had always idolized. One afternoon, the three sisters went berry picking, and the oldest told Sarah, "Don't eat all the berries, or you'll grow into a *real* chub!" Sarah interpreted this to mean that her sister thought she was fat *then*. She became obsessed with food, suddenly deciding to become a vegetarian. She took over the role of planning the menus and educating the family on proper nutrition. When the mother attempted to intervene, Sarah would have a temper tantrum and scream that she knew what she was doing and she was tired of being treated like a baby. If the mother attempted further control over Sarah's eating behavior, she refused to eat at all. The situation in the home deteriorated until there was little communication between any of the family members, particularly with Sarah. The family watched helplessly as she engaged in her irrational rituals and lost a dangerous amount of weight. At this point, they persuaded Sarah to seek help; however, her outpatient experience was not successful.

Sarah is a charismatic young lady; many of the other adolescents in the hospital were attracted to her and wanted to be her friend. However, they quickly noticed her odd eating habits, such as mixing cornflakes in vanilla pudding and pouring cranberry juice over other cereals. Sarah always dressed in baggy overalls and often wore oversized sweaters. When the other patients asked her if she was cold, she quietly told them that she did not want them to stare at her fat body.

During break times, Sarah was found writing morbid poetry, which often contained subtle suicidal messages. She preferred to be alone and became irritable and rude when asked to participate in group therapy sessions. Sarah tried to be a "good girl," as she was accustomed to doing; however, the lack of control she experienced in the hospital made this difficult.

Care Plan

NAME: Sarah Hopkins   ADMISSION DATE: _____

DSM-IV DIAGNOSIS: Anorexia nervosa

ASSESSMENT: **Areas of strength:** intelligence; past achievements; likableness; past healthy interpersonal relationships; good personal hygiene; insight into reasons for hospitalization; family support.
Problems: low weight, disturbed body image, low self-esteem, depression, lack of accurate knowledge regarding nutrition, manipulativeness.

DIAGNOSES:
- Alteration in nutrition: less than body requirements, related to not eating enough nutrients, as evidenced by continued weight loss and inappropriate eating habits.
- Disturbance in body image, related to feeling fat when actually underweight, as evidenced by inappropriate dress and comments about body fat.
- Disturbance in self-esteem, related to feeling as if she is not a "good girl," as evidenced by suicidal messages in poetry and by withdrawal.
- Knowledge deficit in proper nutrition, related to eating imbalanced diet, as evidenced by odd eating habits and refusal to eat certain foods.

OUTCOMES: **Short-term goals:**   Date met
- Patient will gain 2 lb per week.   _____
- Patient will identify three positive qualities about herself.   _____
- Patient will discuss feelings of losing control.   _____

Long-term goals:
- Patient will gain at least 35 lb within 6 months.   _____
- Patient will verbalize knowledge of illness and proper nutrition.   _____
- Patient will identify alternative coping mechanisms to feeling out of control. _____
- Patient will verbalize an increased feeling of self-esteem.   _____

PLANNING/   **Nurse-patient relationship:** Establish a contract to meet at least 3 times a week to discuss
INTERVENTIONS: feelings; express concern for the patient; encourage verbalization of feelings about depression and/or lack of control; encourage patient to identify positive qualities about herself.
Milieu management: Encourage patient to attend meals and sit with peers; encourage participation in group therapy to discuss feelings with peers; encourage patient to share positive qualities of herself with peers; maintain consistency of unit rules and make certain patient is adhering to them.

EVALUATION: Patient gained 3 lb in the first 10 days of hospitalization; attending all unit activities; attending individual therapy with Ms. Mills, RN.

REFERRALS: Patient has been given information about an eating disorder support group in her community.

- Involve the dietitian in the treatment plan. Proper nutrition can be taught while providing patients with an opportunity to select menus.
- Group therapy. Providing an opportunity for patients to participate in a group with peers helps them to see that they are not alone in having difficulty expressing their feelings.

Nurse-led support groups encourage patients to share issues, feelings, and fears (Owen and Fullerton, 1995).
- Psychotherapeutic groups and individual psychotherapy with a qualified therapist also are recommended and may be particularly beneficial following significant weight gain (Fichter,

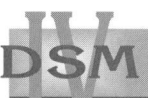

DSM-IV Diagnostic Criteria for Bulimia Nervosa

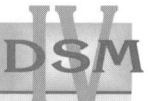

A. Recurrent episodes of binge eating

B. A feeling of lack of control over eating behaviors during the eating binges

C. Recurrent inappropriate compensatory behavior in order to prevent weight gain, such as self-induced vomiting, use of laxatives or diuretics, strict dieting or fasting, vigorous exercise, or taking diet pills

D. Binge eating and inappropriate compensatory behaviors both occur, on average, at least twice a week for 3 months

E. Self-evaluation is unduly influenced by body shape and weight

Purging type: Regularly engages in self-induced vomiting or the use of laxatives, diuretics, or enemas

Nonpurging type: Uses strict diet, fasting, or vigorous exercise, but does not regularly engage in purging

Adapted from the American Psychiatric Association: *Diagnostic and statistical manual of mental disorders,* ed 4, Washington, DC, 1994, The Association.

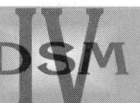

DSM-IV and NANDA Diagnoses Related to Eating Disorders

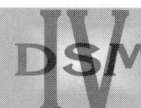

DSM-IV*

Anorexia nervosa
Bulimia nervosa
Eating Disorder NOS

NANDA†

Altered nutrition: less than body requirements
Powerlessness
Fluid volume deficit
Ineffective individual coping
Disturbance in body image
Anxiety

*From the American Psychiatric Association: *Diagnostic and statistical manual of mental disorders,* ed 4, Washington, DC, 1994. The Association.
†From the North American Nursing Diagnosis Association: *NANDA nursing diagnoses: definitions and classifications,* 1997-1998, Philadelphia, 1997, The Association.

1995). Prior to weight restoration, the patient may have difficulty benefiting from psychotherapy due to impaired cognitive processing.

• If the patient is hospitalized, facilitate transition to outpatient treatment providers following discharge. Anorectic patients may relapse or even die because of lack of appropriate outpatient follow-up (Fichter, 1995).

■ Critical Thinking Question

Some theorists contend adolescent eating disorders are an expression of ambivalence toward becoming an adult. Explain how this thought might have some validity.

BULIMIA NERVOSA

DSM-IV Criteria

The DSM-IV diagnostic criteria for bulimia nervosa are found in the box at the top of this page.

NANDA diagnoses that are appropriate for eating disorders are listed in the box above. There are three core features of the bulimic patient (Fairburn and Beglin, 1990):

1. Recurrent episodes of uncontrolled binge eating (eating an unusually large amount of food in a short period of time).

2. Various behaviors designed to control shape and weight; that is, extreme dieting, excessive exercising, self-induced vomiting, taking laxatives or diuretics, use of diet pills, or abuse of enemas/suppositories

3. Persistent overconcern with body shape and weight

The DSM-IV reports bulimia nervosa usually begins in adolescence or early adult life, primarily in females. The prevalence of bulimia among adolescents and young adult women is thought to be approximately 1% in the general population, and 4% among young adult women (Grinspoon, 1997). The usual course of the disorder is chronic and intermittent over a period of many years. Most commonly, the binge periods alternate with periods of restrictive eating.

Behavior

The word *bulimia* literally means to have an insatiable appetite. It is often used to describe massive overeating and is used interchangeably with *binge eating* or *binging*. Other names, such as *bulimarexia*, have also been associated with binge and vomiting behaviors.

Until recently, bulimia nervosa was considered to be a part of anorexia nervosa because almost half of those diagnosed with anorexia were observed to have binge-eating episodes. Bulimia nervosa is now accepted as a separate disorder. The true prevalence of bulimia nervosa is unknown because many patients hide their eating-disordered behaviors. Only those who seek medical attention (which usually is for gastrointestinal or menstrual disturbances) or psychotherapy are actually identifiable.

The onset of the illness is usually between the ages of 15 and 24 years. It may develop after anorexia nervosa but almost always occurs following a period of dieting (Beumont, 1995). The dieting predisposes the individual to binge eating, and purging develops as a means of attempting to compensate for the calories ingested during the binge and to attempt to prevent weight gain. The individual continues restrictive eating during the disorder, which continues to precipitate binge eating.

CLINICAL EXAMPLE

Stacy, age 15, was a popular girl with a very active social life. Although approximately 15 lb overweight, Stacy used her sense of humor to hide any serious concern she had about her appearance. When she was with her close friends during the day, Stacy casually told them that she was dieting and ate less food than they did. When she arrived home after school, however, Stacy found herself secretly opening the refrigerator and making herself several sandwiches before dinner. Despite feeling guilty over her uncontrolled "snacking," Stacy arrived at the dinner table on time to eat with her family. After dinner, feeling uncomfortably full, Stacy retreated to the bathroom, where she vomited until she felt empty. She vowed to herself to try harder to diet the next day, only to have a similar experience.

It is important to distinguish overeating from binge eating. In order to meet DSM-IV diagnostic criteria for a binge episode, the eating behavior has to qualify for what Fairburn and Cooper (1993) describe as an "objective bulimic episode." That is, the person consumes an unusually large amount of food in a relatively short period of time (e.g., less than 2 hours). The amount of food eaten is considered by others to be atypically large for the particular social situation. Also, there is a feeling of lack of control over eating during the binge.

Objective signs

Most bulimic patients are secretive about their behavior. A variety of foods may be eaten during a binge, but the most common is high-calorie, high-carbohydrate food that is easily ingested in a short period of time. Some bulimics visit several different fast food restaurants during a binge so that no one knows how much they are eating at once. Some have been caught shoplifting food. Most binges occur in the evening or at night. The amount of calories consumed during a binge varies, but it may be as much as 30 times the recommended daily allowance (Beumont, 1995). There is a tendency to eat rapidly during the binge.

The bulimic episode usually ends when the patient begins to induce vomiting, is physically exhausted, suffers from painful abdominal distension, is interrupted by others, or has simply run out of food (Fairburn, Cooper, and Cooper, 1986). Following a binge, patients usually promise themselves they will adhere to a strict diet, vowing never to binge again. Many actually resume their usual schedules as if they had never been interrupted. The frequency of binges varies greatly, depending on the patient. Some patients report having several episodes a day, others report losing control 2 or 3 times a week.

Medical complications in bulimic patients depend on the form and frequency of purging. De Zwaan and Mitchell (1993) described mechanical irritation and dilatation of the stomach due to binge eating. Fluid and electrolyte abnormalities may result from self-induced vomiting or abuse of laxatives or diuretics and may include dehydration, hyponatremia, hyphochloremia, hypokalemia, and/or metabolic alkalosis/acidosis. Self-induced vomiting and laxative abuse can both cause mechanical irritation and injuries to the gastrointestinal tract. Abuse of laxatives, diuretics, and diet pills can result in addiction. Laxatives can lead to reflex constipation and both laxatives and diuretics are associated with rebound edema.

Use of ipecac syrup to induce vomiting is particularly dangerous; it can be toxic and cause fatal cardiomyopathy. Bulimics often have menstrual irregularities and/or enlarged salivary glands, particularly the parotid glands. Erosion of the dental enamel from chronic vomiting often occurs (De Zwaan and Mitchell, 1993). Pancreatitis also has been reported in bulimics (Mitchell, 1995).

Subjective symptoms

Although most bulimic patients have a normal body weight, they are gravely concerned about their body shape and weight. Loss of control over their eating causes them great distress and like anorectic patients, they express a fear of becoming fat.

Moods vary considerably among bulimic patients. Some have reported feeling weak and constrained before a binge, followed by either continued anxiety or relief from tension during the binge (Palmer, 1995). Abraham and Llewellyn-Jones (1987) found that most women report feeling anxious, lonely, bored, or having an uncontrollable craving for food before the binge. The anxiety present before the binge is often replaced with guilt after the binge. If the anxiety is not relieved after the binge, patients feel angry and agitated; many become depressed. Because depression is common in bulimic patients, it is discussed in a separate section later in this chapter. Substance abuse and anxiety disorders also occur at a higher than normal rate among bulimics.

Most identified bulimic patients induce vomiting to allay the fear of becoming fat. Many begin to self-induce vomiting by sticking their fingers, a toothbrush, or an eating utensil down their throats. Over time, vomiting usually becomes easier and may require only abdominal pressure or drinking water at the end of the binge. (De Zwaan and Mitchell, 1993). As mentioned above, use of ipecac syrup to induce vomiting is a very dangerous practice with serious health risks. Some bulimics eat a "marker" food at the beginning of the binge and then vomit until this food comes back up. This practice is ill-founded because food is quickly mixed in the stomach. Furthermore, although many bulimics believe self-induced vomiting rids them of all binge calories, researchers have determined that only a partial amount

of calories consumed can be regurgitated (Fairburn, Marcus, and Wilson, 1993). Also, abuse of laxatives or diuretics primarily causes fluid loss, rather than a reduction in absorbed calories (Fairburn, Marcus, and Wilson, 1993).

Other forms of compensatory behavior may include the neglect of insulin requirements in patients with diabetes mellitus, misuse of saunas, excessive use of enemas or suppositories, chewing and spitting, rumination (chewing, swallowing, regurgitating, and then chewing and swallowing again), and breast feeding babies for an excessively long time (De Zwaan and Mitchell, 1993).

Etiology

As with anorexia, the etiology of bulimia nervosa is thought to be multifactorial, with biological, sociocultural, family, cognitive, behavioral, and psychodynamic contributing factors. Many of the factors thought to precipitate anorexia are also thought to be involved in the etiology of bulimia. The focus of this discussion, therefore, will be on the proposed causes of bulimia that are different than those postulated for anorexia.

Biological factors

One biological theory of bulimia suggests a hypothalamic dysfunction (the hunger center) causing a hormonal irregularity (Matthews, 1991). Injury or stimulation to the hypothalamus affects metabolism of fat, carbohydrates, and water. Other studies indicate decreased hypothalamic glucose utilization resulting in the urge to increase food intake.

Another theory proposes a satiety center disturbance resulting in increased carbohydrate intake (National Institute of Mental Health, 1993; Agras and Kirkley, 1986). When more carbohydrates than proteins are consumed, changes occur in the plasma amino acid levels. This causes an increased amount of tryptophan in the brain, which in turn causes an increased synthesis of serotonin. The serotonin enables the person to eat more protein and less carbohydrate at the next meal. The carbohydrate craving occurs again. The person continues to eat in response to these confusing physiological demands, then vomits in an effort to restrict intake.

Similarly, it has been proposed that, as in depression, there is generally lowered serotonin activity in the brains of bulimics (Pirke, 1995). Binge eating is then seen as a form of self-medication to raise the levels of serotonin.

Sociocultural factors

These factors are thought to be the same as those involved in anorexia nervosa (see discussion earlier in this chapter).

Family factors

As with anorexia nervosa, a heritable component for bulimia has been proposed. Twin studies have found a higher concordance rate for bulimia in monozygotic than in dizygotic twins (Strober, 1995). In addition, mood disorders and substance-use disorders are found at a high rate in the families of bulimics (Strober, 1995), which may be due to both biological and environmental factors.

From self-report studies, bulimics tend to view their families as having a great deal of conflict and as disorganized, lacking in nurturance, and noncohesive (Vandereycken, 1995). Observations of family interactions yield similar data. In addition, observers often view bulimics as resentfully submissive to parents who are hostile and neglect them (Vandereycken, 1995). Bulimics tend to remember their early childhood as involving a lack of care by both parents but particularly by their mothers. Fathers are seen as being more overprotective and as controlling without care and concern (Vandereycken, 1995).

Cognitive and behavioral factors

Christopher Fairburn and his colleagues (1993) have pioneered work on cognitive-behavioral theory for the maintenance of bulimia nervosa after its onset. According to this theory, bulimia nervosa is maintained by cycles of low self-esteem, extreme concerns about body shape and weight, strict dieting, binge eating, and compensatory behavior, which interact and affect each other. Thus, bulimia is maintained by the behaviors of dieting, binging, and purging, which in turn are both affected by and contribute to distorted and negative cognitions about the self and the body. This theory has led to the development of the highly successful cognitive-behavioral therapy for bulimia nervosa (Fairburn, Marcus, and Wilson, 1993), which targets both eating-disordered behaviors and cognitions.

Psychodynamic factors

According to Tobin (1993), the psychodynamic understanding of bulimia nervosa depends on the underlying personality structure of the individual. He draws a particular distinction between psychosis and borderline personality, narcissistic personality, and neurotic personality structure, and states that research has shown a variety of personality structures among bulimics. Psychoanalytic theories specific to each of these personality structures is then applied to bulimics in addition to all others with these personality structures. Emphasis is placed on the role of the unconscious in the formation of symptoms.

Some psychodynamic theorists have placed particular emphasis on ambivalent feelings of self-esteem in bulimics. The binge-eating/purging behavior is thought to express the ambivalence patients feel toward themselves. On one hand, they believe they are worthy of the nurturing they lack, and, because food is a symbolic form of nurturing, they binge. On the other hand, they feel unworthy of nurturing, so they purge.

Conclusion

As in anorexia nervosa, the specific factors contributing to the development of bulimia nervosa in an individual may vary, and the factors leading to the onset of bulimia may differ from the influences that maintain it.

Bulimia and Depression

There are some who have postulated that bulimia nervosa is a variant of a mood disorder. The reasons for this are fourfold. First, there is a high rate of mood disorders, particularly depression, among bulimics (P.J. Cooper, 1995). Second, bulimics often have the same reaction on the dexamethasone suppression test as depressed patients do. Next, there is a high rate of mood disorders in the families of bulimics. Last, as discussed below, treatment with an antidepressant medication has been shown to be helpful in reducing bulimic symptoms.

The relationship between bulimia and depression may be that one causes the other, or there may be independent contributing factors to both. Experts in the field are doubtful that depression causes bulimia because depression most often develops after the onset of the eating disorder, and depression in bulimia nervosa differs from major depressive disorder (P.J. Cooper, 1995). It also has been suggested that low serotonin and/or low self-esteem may contribute to both disorders (Z. Cooper, 1995). Studies of the families of depressive patients, however, have failed to show an unusually high incidence of eating disorders. This argues against a common pathogenesis (P.J. Cooper, 1995). Most experts believe depression is secondary to the erratic eating habits and the feeling of lack of control (P.J. Cooper, 1995).

Psychotherapeutic Management

As in the treatment of anorexia nervosa, medical stabilization of the bulimic patient is the initial treatment goal (De Zwaan and Mitchell, 1993). Following medical stabilization, psychotherapy is the treatment of choice. Cognitive-behavioral therapy has the greatest research support, although there is limited evidence suggesting interpersonal psychotherapy may have similar long-term effectiveness (Fairburn, 1995b; McGown and Whitbread, 1996). Pharmacotherapy is used as an adjunct to psychotherapy when indicated (Walsh, 1995).

Similar to the treatment of anorexia, nurses may encounter bulimics in an inpatient setting or as outpatients seen for medical monitoring in a physician's office. Overall, they are less likely than anorectics to be inpatients. A multidisciplinary approach, involving physicians, nurses, dietitians, and psychotherapists, is also recommended with bulimics.

Nurse-Patient Relationship. Bulimic patients differ from anorectic patients in the sense that the former usually want help. They enter therapy of their own volition and are eager to please, behaving so that therapists will like them. In this effort to please, bulimic patients have a tendency to become manipulative and may tell half-truths regarding their problem. The desire to be helped is usually the greatest strength of these patients. Specific therapeutic communication techniques helpful for these patients follow.

- Create an atmosphere of trust. Bulimic patients have a difficult time with this. The nurse must be honest at all times and follow through with what is said.
- Help patients identify feelings associated with the binge-purge behavior. Once the feelings

are identified, patients can begin to explore alternative ways of coping with them.
- Accept patients as worthwhile human beings. Bulimic patients are often ashamed of their behavior and are embarrassed to discuss it. When they realize no negative repercussions are forthcoming, they are more comfortable discussing problems.
- Encourage patients to discuss positive qualities about themselves in order to improve self-esteem.
- Teach patients about bulimia nervosa. Knowledge can affect behavior and sense of control.
- Encourage patients to explore their interpersonal relationships. Many bulimics complain of loneliness. They need to be encouraged to examine the nature of such problems so that they may be resolved.

Psychopharmacology. Recent studies have shown that certain antidepressants, such as imipramine (Tofranil), desipramine (Norpramin), fluoxetine (Prozac), and the MAOIs, significantly reduce the frequency of binge eating (Kennedy and Garfinkel, 1992; Fluoxetine Bulimia Nervosa Collaborative Study Group, 1992). These drugs also have been shown to have greater effect than placebo on associated mood disturbances and preoccupation with shape and weight (Walsh, 1995).

Interestingly, antidepressants appear to be equally effective in both depressed and nondepressed patients with bulimia nervosa. These results suggest that the mechanism of the drug action may not be "antidepressant," but rather direct central effects on neurotransmitter systems, particularly serotonin and norepinephrine. It should be noted, however, that although antidepressants have beneficial effects in the short term, this improvement does not appear to be maintained long term. Furthermore, the amount of improvement with cognitive-behavior therapy appears to be greater than that obtained with antidepressants (Fairburn, 1995b). Generally, a course of psychotherapy is recommended prior to a trial of an antidepressant (Walsh, 1995). Antidepressants are considered when the patient has failed to respond adequately to psychotherapy alone, or when there is comorbidity with severe clinical depression.

Milieu Management. Although bulimic patients are typically seen on an outpatient basis, Abraham

Case Study

Polly, a 19-year-old woman, lives at home with her mother, stepfather, and two sisters, 15 and 12 years of age. Polly's brother, age 22, is away at college. Polly was ready to graduate from a community college and decided to enter treatment because she wanted to go away for her last 2 years of college and knew her eating behavior would cause significant problems for her.

Polly was 5 feet 6 inches tall and weighed 150 lb. There were times in the last 5 years when she weighed as much as 225 lb. She admitted to hating herself when she was "fat" and was concerned about becoming fat again.

Polly always felt she was not as good as her brother and sisters. She saw herself as less attractive, less intelligent, and less coordinated. She described herself as the "ugly duckling." She has never been on a date and has had few girlfriends. She thought people tolerated her, but did not really like her.

Polly began to binge around the age of 15. She would come home from school and eat continually until time for dinner, which she then ate with her family. When everyone went to bed, Polly would go into the kitchen and eat again. Polly states she would easily eat a loaf of bread, 2 lb of cheese, a gallon of ice cream, a jar of peanut butter, a box of cookies, and a half-gallon of milk at one sitting. These episodes occurred approximately 2 or 3 times a week. When Polly reached 225 lb at the age of 17, she entered a diet program and lost 80 lb. It was soon after this weight loss that Polly felt the urge to binge. Rather than endure a great deal of weight gain again, Polly began to induce vomiting after binging. This behavior continued for the past year and a half.

and Llewellyn-Jones (1987) imply reasons to hospitalize a bulimic:

- To treat a psychiatric or medical crisis, such as suicidal feelings or a serious fluid-electrolyte imbalance
- To provide order to an otherwise chaotic life
- To allow patients to examine their living situations
- To provide treatment to patients who live in an area far away from other services

Fairburn (1995b) has recommended a "stepped care" approach to treatment, wherein patients first participate in a simple treatment, such as guided self-help or a psychoeducational group. Individuals who do not respond are then referred for cognitive-behavior therapy. Those who do not adequately improve from this are then referred for a more intensive form of treatment, such as interpersonal psychotherapy, partial/full hospitalization, and/or antidepressant medication.

Some principles for management of the bulimic patient follow.

- For inpatients, encourage patients to adhere to the meal and snack schedules of the hospital. Regularization of eating prevents the precipitation of binge eating by dieting or restrictive eating practices. Encourage all patients to follow the advice of dietitians regarding normalization of eating.
- Encourage patients to approach a staff member when they have the urge to binge and purge. Patients then have the opportunity to identify and express the feelings that precipitate such episodes and to explore alternative ways of coping.
- Encourage patients to attend group therapy sessions for persons with eating disorders. This not only provides support to patients, but also facilitates their experiencing and resolving the problems they have with relating to others.
- For young bulimic patients living at home, encourage family therapy. Communication within families needs to be improved so that these relationships may be strengthened.
- For inpatients, encourage participation in art, recreation, and occupational therapy. These modalities provide and teach patients alternative ways to express their feelings.
- Encourage patients to participate in individual psychotherapy, particularly with a therapist who is familiar with cognitive-behavior therapy for bulimia nervosa.
- As with anorectic patients, determine bulimic patients' ability to view weighing.

EATING DISORDERS IN MALES

The incidence of eating disorders among males is currently about 10% of the eating disorder population, with speculation that this figure will increase (Zerbe, 1992; Farrow, 1992). Although diagnosis, etiology,

*C*are *P*lan

NAME: _Polly Samuels_   ADMISSION DATE: _____

DSM-IV DIAGNOSIS: _Bulimia nervosa_

ASSESSMENT: **Areas of strength:** Desire for treatment, sense of humor, past achievements, intelligence, history of self-control long enough to lose 80 lb, family support.

         Problems: Low self-esteem, disturbed body image, not able to control binge-vomiting behavior, unable to establish intimate relationships, feels defeated and depressed.

DIAGNOSES:
- Powerlessness, related to feeling not in control of eating habits, as evidenced by concern about gaining weight and by overeating and binging/vomiting behavior.
- Disturbance in self-esteem, related to feeling not as worthy as others, as evidenced by negative statements about herself in comparison to others and inability to establish intimate relationships.
- Disturbance in body image, related to feeling overweight, as evidenced by negative statements about body image and overeating and binging/vomiting behavior.

OUTCOMES: **Short-term goals:**   **Date met**
- Patient will establish and adhere to contract on eating behavior.   _____
- Patient will approach the staff when she feels the urge to binge or vomit.   _____
- Patient will participate in all unit therapies, including group, art, recreational, and occupational therapy.   _____

         Long-term goals:
- Patient will maintain present weight without binging or vomiting.   _____
- Patient will participate in physical activity, such as jogging, when she feels anxious.   _____
- Patient will express several positive qualities about herself.   _____

PLANNING/ INTERVENTIONS: **Nurse-patient relationship:** Establish a contract that addresses specific eating behavior; be honest and genuine in all contracts with the patient; encourage the patient to identify when she feels the need to binge; help the patient make association between her feelings and her eating behavior.

         Milieu management: Encourage the patient to attend meals and snacks with peers; encourage the patient to express her feelings in a group setting; encourage the patient to approach the staff when she is feeling out of control; provide diversional activities when patient is feeling anxious.

EVALUATION: Patient has maintained her body weight with only one episode of vomiting; attending occupational and recreational therapies consistently, attending feelings group inconsistently; meeting with individual therapist, Ms. O'Donnell, regularly.

REFERRALS: Patient has information about an eating disorder support group in her community.

---

and treatment of males and females with eating disorders are similar, there appear to be some differences with respect to medical assessment in males. For example, males are more likely to be involved in athletics and to have a history of obesity before the onset of symptoms of an eating disorder. Dieting may be a response to teasing about weight or a desire to build a lean body for participation in sports (Farrow, 1992).

Although controversial, some research has shown male patients with eating disorders exhibit a high frequency of concerns about gender or sexual identity, homosexual orientation, and asexuality (Grinspoon, 1992; Carlat and Camargo, 1991; Zerbe, 1992). It should be noted, however, that although approximately 21% of eating disordered males have a homosexual orientation, this is still a minority of cases (Andersen, 1995).

Treatment for males with eating disorders is similar to that of females. From a psychotherapeutic management standpoint, the following three areas need particular focus with males:

1. Body image and the excessive attention that adolescent boys often place on attaining a masculine physique
2. Healthier dietary habits to promote health, fitness, and muscle mass
3. The ability to express feelings, especially if the patient has an underlying sexual identity concern

Although many adolescents with eating disorders have difficulty expressing their feelings, boys seem to have more difficulty than girls. A therapeutic nurse-patient relationship can be instrumental in the recovery of these young men.

OBESITY

The issue of whether or not obesity is an eating disorder has been professionally debated for some time. The controversy stems from the concept that eating disorders, such as anorexia and bulimia, have physiological components; however, these are not as significant as the psychological components. The reverse seems to be true of obesity. Today, most experts agree that, although obesity has psychological components, it is primarily a genetic or metabolic disorder. The DSM-IV does not include obesity as a psychiatric disorder. Consequently the reader is referred to a textbook on pathophysiology for more information about obesity.

BINGE-EATING DISORDER

The DSM-IV does provide a category for eating disorders that do not fit clearly into the diagnostic criteria for anorexia nervosa or bulimia nervosa (Eating Disorder NOS). Examples of such disorders include the situation where all criteria for anorexia nervosa

are met except for amenorrhea, or a regular pattern of vomiting after normal eating for the purpose of weight control, without underweight status or binge eating. The most frequent disorder to fit this category, however, is binge-eating disorder (BED), which involves regular binge eating in the absence of compensatory behavior. Research has shown that this disorder occurs in approximately 20% of persons seeking help for weight control (Fairburn and Walsh, 1995). The value of BED as a separate diagnostic category is still debated among researchers in the field.

Key Concepts

1. Anorexia nervosa is characterized by a refusal to maintain body weight at or above a minimally normal weight for age and height, an intense fear of becoming fat, a distorted body image, and amenorrhea.
2. Anorectic dieters often begin in a normal weight range, tend to isolate themselves socially, alienate themselves from others, are competitive, and exercise excessively.
3. Bulimia is characterized by episodes of binge eating, a feeling of a lack of control of eating, use of compensatory behavior, and overconcern with body shape and weight. Depression commonly coexists with bulimia.
4. Anorectic and bulimic patients suffer a variety of physiological problems that can cause death. Personality and emotional changes are also evident in these patients.
5. The cause of eating disorders is thought to be multifactorial, including biological, sociocultural, familial, cognitive, behavioral, and psychodynamic factors.
6. Cognitive-behaviorial therapy has the most research support in the treatment of bulimia nervosa.
7. The incidence of eating disorders in males is increasing, with speculation that this trend will continue.
8. Nursing interventions with anorectic patients require caring, supportive relationships; limit setting; a behavior-modification program; and a consistent milieu. Family involvement, individual psychotherapy, and group therapy are also essential. Hospitalization with a structured milieu and antidepressant medications may or may not be needed.

Study Questions

(Answer key is in the back of the book.)
Fran, age 15, enrolled exclusively in honors classes for her sophomore year, including home economics as an elective. Although she was always an excellent student, her parents were concerned about the amount of stress she was imposing upon herself. Fran's social life declined. She invested all of her energies into her studies, particularly home economics. At mealtimes, Fran began to lecture

the family about proper nutrition, although her mother noticed that Fran was eating less and less. At the end of 5 months, Fran's weight had dropped from 105 to 87 pounds. She had missed her periods for the last 3 months.

1. The most appropriate diagnosis for Fran might be:
   a. Bulimia Nervosa
   b. Anorexia Nervosa
   c. Eating Disorder NOS
   d. None of the above
2. Based on the information given, an appropriate nursing diagnosis for Fran would be:
   a. Disturbance in body image related to feeling fat, when she is actually underweight
   b. Disturbance in self-esteem, related to feeling as if she is not a good girl
   c. Alteration in nutrition: less than body requirements, related to not eating enough nutrients
   d. Knowledge deficit in proper nutrition, related to eating an imbalanced diet
3. An appropriate short-term goal for Fran is to:
   a. Gain 2 lb per week
   b. Be able to state two positive qualities about herself
   c. Be able to identify two available support systems
   d. Participate in a group therapy session 3 times per week
   e. All of the above
4. Which of the following behaviors should the nurse employ to most effectively facilitate a nurse-patient relationship with Fran?
   a. Concern and sympathy
   b. Control and challenge
   c. Approval and agreement
   d. Warmth and sincerity

Pat, age 22, graduated from a local college and left home for the first time to accept a position as an assistant editor for a small magazine. Not only did she need to adjust to the demands of her new job, but also to the demands of living on her own. Although her new colleagues were friendly at work, none approached Pat for a social relationship. Pat became increasingly lonely and anxious in all of her new roles and responsibilities. She began dieting, but soon found herself binging during her idle hours at home alone. After consuming large quantities of food, she induced vomiting so that she would not gain a lot of weight. When her binge-purge behaviors began to interfere with her concentration at work, she made an appointment at the local community mental health center for help.

5. Upon the initial interview with Pat, it is a priority that the nurse assess the level of Pat's:
   a. Anxiety
   b. Boredom
   c. Depression
   d. Loneliness

6. The treatment approach that is most likely to lead to the greatest amount of improvement for Pat is:
   a. Cognitive-behavior therapy
   b. A support group
   c. Family therapy
   d. Psychopharmacology
7. One nursing diagnosis that has been established for Pat is "powerlessness, related to not being in control of eating." An effective nursing action that addresses this problem is to:
   a. Encourage Pat to weigh herself daily
   b. Formulate a structured meal and snack schedule with Pat and a dietitian
   c. Remind Pat that excessive vomiting can cause an electrolyte disturbance
   d. Encourage Pat to call home weekly
8. The group of medications that have been found to be effective in the short-term with bulimic patients are:
   a. Antipsychotic
   b. Anxiolytic
   c. Antiparkinsonian
   d. Antidepressant

REFERENCES

Abraham S and Llewellyn-Jones D: *Eating disorders: the facts,* ed 2, Oxford, 1987, Oxford University.

Agras WS and Kirkley BG: Bulimia: theories of etiology. In Brownell KD and Foreyt JP, editors: *Handbook of eating disorders,* New York, 1986, Basic Books.

American Psychiatric Association: *Diagnostic and statistical manual of mental disorders,* ed 4, Washington, DC, 1994, The Association.

Andersen AE: Eating disorders in males. In Brownell KD and Fairburn CG, editors: *Eating disorders and obesity,* New York, 1995, Guilford.

Beumont PJV: The clinical presentation of anorexia and bulimia nervosa. In Brownell KD and Fairburn CG, editors: *Eating disorders and obesity,* New York, 1995, Guilford.

Bruch H: *Eating disorders,* New York, 1973, Basic Books.

Carlat DJ and Camargo CA: Review of bulimia nervosa in males, *Am J Psychiatry* 148:831, 1991.

Cooper PJ: Eating disorders and their relationship to mood and anxiety disorders. In Brownell KD and Fairburn CG, editors: *Eating disorders and obesity,* New York, 1995, Guilford.

Cooper Z: The development and maintenance of eating disorders. In Brownell KD and Fairburn CG, editors: *Eating disorders and obesity,* New York, 1995, Guilford.

De Zwaan M and Mitchell JE: Medical complications of anorexia nervosa and bulimia nervosa. In Kaplan AS and Garfinkel PE, editors: *Medical issues and the eating disorders: the interface,* New York, 1993, Brunner/Mazel.

Fairburn CG: Physiology of anorexia nervosa. In Brownell KD and Fairburn CG, editors: *Eating disorders and obesity*, New York, 1995a, Guilford.

Fairburn CG: Short-term psychological treatments for bulimia nervosa. In Brownell KD and Fairburn CG, editors: *Eating disorders and obesity*, New York, 1995b, Guilford.

Fairburn CG and Beglin SJ: Studies of the epidemiology of bulimia nervosa, *Am J Psychiatry* 147:401, 1990.

Fairburn CG and Cooper L: The eating disorder examination, ed 12. In Fairburn CG and Wilson GT, editors: *Binge eating: nature, assessment, and treatment*, New York, 1993, Guilford.

Fairburn CG, Cooper Z, and Cooper PJ: The clinical features and maintenance of bulimia nervosa. In Brownell KD and Foreyt JP, editors: *Handbook of eating disorders*, New-York, 1986, Basic Books.

Fairburn CG, Marcus MD, and Wilson GT: Cognitive-behavioral therapy for binge eating and bulimia nervosa: a comprehensive treatment manual. In Fairburn CG and Wilson GT, editors: *Binge eating: nature, assessment, and treatment*, New York, 1993, Guilford.

Fairburn CG and Walsh BT: Atypical eating disorders. In Brownell KD and Fairburn CG, editors: *Eating disorders and obesity*, New York, 1995, Guilford.

Farrow JA: The adolescent male with an eating disorder, *Pediatr Ann* 21(11):769, 1992.

Fichter MM: Inpatient treatment of anorexia nervosa. In Brownell KD and Fairburn CG: *Eating disorders and obesity*, New York, 1995, Guilford.

Fluoxetine Bulimia Nervosa Collaborative Study Group: Fluoxetine in the treatment of bulimia nervosa: a multicenter placebo-controlled double-blind trial, *Arch Gen Psychiatry* 49:139, 1992.

Goldbloom DS and Kennedy SH: Medical complications of anorexia nervosa. In Brownell KD and Fairburn CG, editors: *Eating disorders and obesity*, New York, 1995, Guilford.

Grinspoon L: Eating disorders: part I, *Harvard Mental Health Letter* 9(6):1, 1992.

Grinspoon L: Eating disorders: part I, *Harvard Mental Health Letter* 14(4):1, 1997.

Hsu GLK and Sobkiewicz TA: Body image disturbance: time to abandon the concept in eating disorders? *Int J Eat Disord* 10:15, 1991.

Johnson C: Psychodynamic treatment of bulimia nervosa. In Brownell KD and Fairburn CG, editors: *Eating disorders and obesity*, New York, 1995, Guilford.

Johnson CJ, Sansone RA, and Chewning M: Good reasons why young women would develop anorexia nervosa: the adaptive context, *Pediatr Ann* 21(11):731, 1992.

Kaye WH: Neurotransmitters and anorexia nervosa. In Brownell KD and Fairburn CG, editors: *Eating disorders and obesity*, New York, 1995, Guilford.

Kaye WH, et al: An open trial of fluoxetine in patients with anorexia nervosa, *J Clin Psychiatry* 52:464, 1991.

Kennedy SH and Garfinkel PE: Advances in diagnosis and treatment of anorexia nervosa and bulimia nervosa, *Can J Psychiatry* 37(5):309, 1992.

Kennedy SH and Goldbloom DS: Current perspectives on drug therapies of anorexia nervosa and bulimia nervosa, *Drugs* 41:367, 1991.

Matthews JR: *Eating disorders: library in a book*, New York, 1991, Facts on File.

McGown A and Whitbread J: Out of control! The most effective way to help the binge-eating patient, *J Psychosoc Nurs Ment Health Serv* 34(1):30, 1996.

Mitchell JE: Medical complications of bulimia nervosa. In Brownell KD and Fairburn CG, editors: *Eating disorders and obesity*, New York, 1995, Guilford.

National Institute of Mental Health: *Decade of the brain. Eating disorders*, Washington, DC, 1993, NIH.

Owen SV and Fullerton ML: A discussion group in a behaviorally oriented inpatient eating disorder program, *J Psychosoc Nurs Ment Health Serv* 33(11):35, 1995

Palmer RL: Sexual abuse and eating disorders. In Brownell KD and Fairburn CG, editors: *Eating disorders and obesity*, New York, 1995, Guilford.

Pirke KM: Physiology of bulimia nervosa. In Brownell KD and Fairburn CG, editors: *Eating disorders and obesity*, New York, 1995, Guilford.

Pumariega AJ, et al: Clinical correlates of body-size distortion, *Percept Mot Skills* 76:1311, 1993.

Striegel-Moore RH: A feminist perspective on the etiology of eating disorders. In Brownell KD and Fairburn CG, editors: *Eating disorders and obesity*, New York, 1995, Guilford.

Strober M: Family-genetic perspectives on anorexia nervosa and bulimia nervosa. In Brownell KD and Fairburn CG, editors: *Eating disorders and obesity*, New York, 1995, Guilford.

Tobin DL: Psychodynamic psychotherapy and binge eating. In Fairburn CG and Wilson GT, editors: *Binge eating: nature, assessment, and treatment*, New York, 1993, Guilford.

Vandereycken W: The families of patients with an eating disorder. In Brownell KD and Fairburn CG, editors: *Eating disorders and obesity*, New York, 1995, Guilford.

Walsh BT: Pharmacotherapy of eating disorders. In Brownell KD and Fairburn CG, editors: *Eating disorders and obesity*, New York, 1995, Guilford.

Weiner H: The hypothalamic-pituitary-ovarian axis in anorexia and bulimia nervosa, *Int J Eat Disord* 2:109, 1983.

Wilfley DE and Rodin J: Cultural influences on eating disorders. In Brownell KD and Fairburn CG, editors: *Eating disorders and obesity*, New York, 1995, Guilford.

Zerbe KJ: Eating disorders in the 1990's: clinical challenges and treatment implications, *Bull Menninger Clin* 52(2):167, 1992.

Special Therapies in Psychiatric Nursing

CHAPTER 36

Behavior Therapy

LEE H. SCHWECKE

LEARNING OBJECTIVES

After reading this chapter you should be able to:
- Identify three techniques for increasing a behavior.
- Describe two schedules of reinforcement.
- Identify three techniques for decreasing a behavior.
- Understand the principles of a token economy.

- Discuss two techniques for helping patients deal with disturbing stimuli.
- Explain the nursing process using behavioral modification principles.

Behavior therapy is a distinctive approach to influencing interactions between persons, and between persons and their environment. The principles used in behavior therapy were derived from research in conditioned reflex and operant conditioning. Applications of behavior therapy principles are common and effective in psychiatric nursing, especially in helping patients deal with anxiety and change their behaviors. It is typically combined with other models of therapy and with psychotropic medications (Blair, 1996). Discussion of classical conditioning, operant conditioning, applications of behavioral techniques, and behavioral interventions with nursing process are presented in this chapter.

---

*This is a revision of a chapter originally written by Sue Main.

CLASSICAL CONDITIONING

The origin of classical conditioning is credited to Pavlov (1927) and his research on reflexes in laboratory animals. Pavlov was involved in studying reflexes and the various aspects of the secretion of gastric juices in dogs when he discovered that the dogs began salivating before they were presented with food.

$$\underset{\text{(Eliciting stimulus)}}{\text{S (food)}} \longrightarrow \underset{\text{(Respondent)}}{\text{R (salivation)}}$$

He then simultaneously presented food and the sound of a metronome. After several repetitions, the metronome alone was found to elicit the secretion of saliva. *Respondent conditioning* is the process of pairing a neutral stimulus with an eliciting stimulus so that, ultimately, the neutral stimulus alone elicits the response.

S (food) + (metronome) ——→ R (salivation)
(Eliciting stimulus plus neutral stimulus)   (Respondent)

CS (metronome) ——→ R (salivation)
(Conditioned stimulus)   (Respondent)

In an experiment with a young child, Albert, and a white rat (a neutral stimulus), Watson and Rayner (1920) paired the presence of the rat with a loud noise that had been observed to elicit a fear response in Albert. After the noise and the rat were presented simultaneously seven times, the rat alone elicited the fear response in Albert. The fear response was also elicited by stimuli with characteristics similar to those of the rat (rabbit, dog, fur). This process, in which a fear response is elicited by stimuli with similar characteristics, is called *generalization*. Watson and Rayner's research is one of the classics that has become the foundation for behavioral treatment of phobias.

OPERANT CONDITIONING

The basis of the operant learning theory was derived from numerous controlled experiments with animals and was reported originally by B.F. Skinner (1938, 1953, 1956). Attention is directed to the events that immediately precede and follow a person's specific behavior. Theoretical inner causes of behavior, such as psychological, neurological, or conceptual states, are not included in this approach. The existence of such inner states is not denied; however, they are not viewed as relevant to the analysis of behavior.

A response is any movement or observable behavior. The *operant response* (the behavior being analyzed) can be described and measured (frequency, duration, magnitude) (Goisman, 1997). A *stimulus* is an event that immediately precedes or follows a behavior. Three types of stimuli are listed below.

1. A *discriminative stimulus* is an event, immediately preceding a behavior, that predicts or indicates that a response will be followed by reinforcement. Discriminative stimuli may be observed, heard, felt (tactile), or smelled. Examples include pain, subtle verbal or facial expressions, tone of voice, posture, dress, a specific person or situation.
2. A *neutral stimulus* is an event that is not associated with reinforcement or that has no effect on changing the probability of behavior.

3. A *reinforcing stimulus* is an event, following a behavior, that strengthens that behavior and increases the probability of the behavior occurring (e.g., hugs, smiles, attention, an opportunity to play, a paycheck, a chicken dinner).

Primary reinforcers are events of biological importance (e.g., food, water, sexual contact, coat on a cold day, bed for sleeping). *Secondary* or *generalized reinforcers* are events that have been paired repeatedly with a primary reinforcer (e.g., money, tickets, diplomas, attention of others).

DS ——————→ R ——————→ RS
(Discriminative   (Response)   (Reinforcing
stimulus)   stimulus)

For example, a patient in a hospital room wants the nurse's attention. The patient presses a button labeled "nurse" on the paging apparatus. The voice of the nurse ("This is Mrs. White. May I help you?") is heard.

DS ——————→ R ——————→ RS
(Presence of button   (Pressing the   (Voice of the
labeled "nurse")   button)   nurse)

Other buttons labeled "fire," "emergency," or "TV" are neutral stimuli. When a voice responds immediately and consistently following the pressing of the button, *learning* occurs. If the nurse's voice does not immediately follow pushing the button, *extinction* occurs. The button-pushing behavior predictably decreases, and emotional behavior may occur (e.g., yelling loudly for the nurse). If the patient receives a painful electrical shock when pushing the button and the response is suppressed, *punishment* has occurred. The patient may then exhibit an aggressive response (e.g., throwing the paging apparatus against the wall).

APPLICATION OF BEHAVIOR THERAPY IN PSYCHIATRIC NURSING PRACTICE

Behavior therapy is used with children, adolescents, groups, couples, and families. Behavior modification has been used in inpatient and outpatient settings and in skills-training programs. The use of behavior therapy with specific problematic behaviors has been reported in the treatment of anxiety, sexual disorders, posttraumatic stress disorder (PTSD), and addictions. Also, behavioral principles form the basis of self-control treatment programs, such as those used for changes in behaviors such as eating, exercise, or assertive communication.

Behavior Modification: Helping Patients Change Behavior

When patients' problem behaviors are reinforced or maintained by consequences of the behavior, operant conditioning, commonly called *behavior modification,* is the model used. Functional analysis involves a behavioral and reinforcement history (Corrigan, Yudofsky, and Silver, 1993). Contingencies that can be controlled by the therapist, patients, or families are altered to create a change in the problematic behaviors.

Increasing the probability that a behavior will recur

Conditioning

Conditioning is the strengthening of a response by reinforcement. *Positive reinforcement* follows a behavior with a reinforcing stimulus that increases the probability that the behavior will recur. For example, asking for help in an assertive way occurs more frequently when followed by attention and suggestions (reinforcement) in a communication-skills group (specific discriminative stimulus). *Negative reinforcement* is the process of removing a stimulus from a situation immediately after a behavior occurs, which increases the probability of the behavior occurring. For example, when a person steps into an uncomfortably hot shower and turns the dial to reduce the water temperature, the behavior (turning the dial) is reinforced. The stimulus (uncomfortably hot water) is removed.

The timing of reinforcement is important. *Superstitious behavior* is a term used for behavior that has been reinforced by accident. Athletes provide common examples of superstitious behaviors when they display peculiar mannerisms such as tapping a shoe with the bat before stepping up to home plate or tapping their fingers on the strings of a tennis racket before receiving a serve. When reinforcers are presented according to a time schedule (rather than being contingent on a particular response), any behavior immediately preceding the reinforcer is strengthened.

Premack principle

When a person is observed often enjoying a particular activity, the opportunity to engage in that activity can be used as a reinforcer for other behaviors that occur less frequently (Premack, 1962). For example, the opportunity to watch television might be used as a reinforcer for cleaning the living area.

Shaping

Shaping is a process of reinforcing successive approximations of responses to increase the probability of a behavior. For example, to increase the probability of a patient saying "no" in an assertive way, each time the patient makes a response that approximates the target response (or gets closer to the target response), reinforcement is presented until that response occurs at a high frequency. Then reinforcement is withheld until the next response more closely approximates the target behavior, and so on until the target behavior is performed. The selective reinforcement of each behavior that more closely approximates the target response is called *differential reinforcement.*

Schedules of reinforcement

Schedules are the planned sequences for the presentation of reinforcing stimuli.

Continuous reinforcement

Continuous reinforcement is the presentation of reinforcing stimuli following each occurrence of the selected response. Continuous reinforcement is used primarily during the initial phases of conditioning or shaping a behavior, and results in a high rate of behavior, such as when a professional provides reinforcement each time a patient uses appropriate comments during a role-play of conflict-management skills.

Intermittent reinforcement

Intermittent reinforcement is the presentation of the reinforcer following the target response according to a selected number of responses (ratio schedule). An example would be after every fifth target response or according to a selected time period (interval schedule) of 5 minutes after every target response. Schedules may vary as well.

Intermittent schedules of reinforcement result in behavior that is more resistant to extinction than behavior that has been reinforced on a continuous schedule. The comparison of inserting coins into vending machines with inserting coins into slot machines illustrates the difference. Normally, inserting coins into a vending machine is reinforced (with food) every time the behavior occurs. When the reinforcer stops (no food is delivered), the act of inserting coins into that particular machine stops rather quickly. Inserting coins into a slot machine, however, is reinforced with tokens or money on an intermittent schedule, not each time. The act of inserting coins into a slot machine continues for a considerable time, even though reinforcers are not presented.

Decreasing the probability that a behavior will recur

Differential reinforcement of other behavior

Differential reinforcement is a technique used to decrease the frequency of a behavior. When the goal of treatment is to decrease a behavior, another behavior, incompatible with the target behavior, can be reinforced. Target behavior, if emitted, is not reinforced. To decrease the soft speaking of a patient in a group, attention of the group is available only when the patient speaks in a normal, audible voice. The soft speaking voice, incompatible with a normal voice, is ignored.

Extinction

Extinction is the gradual decrease in the rate of responses when reinforcement is no longer available. The rate of responses may increase for a short time, then begin to decrease gradually. Emotional responses characteristically occur during extinction. A familiar example is the behavior that occurs when one pushes the "up" button to ride an elevator. When the elevator door fails to close, repeated and sometimes rapid button-pushing behavior occurs for a short period, then stops. Banging or pulling on the elevator door (an emotional response) may occur during this time. *Social extinction* involves the withdrawal of attention, such as when a patient acts inappropriately (Corrigan, Yudofsky, and Silver, 1993).

Negative consequence

Negative consequence is the presentation of an event immediately following a response that decreases the probability of that response recurring, for example, putting a child in his or her room immediately after seeing him or her playing in the street. Another example is having a patient apologize to other patients and mop the floor after throwing food (Grinspoon, 1991). Negative consequence results in the immediate suppression of that response. For inpatients, a common form of this is to withdraw privileges or withhold passes as a consequence of acting-out behaviors. Negative consequence may result in emotional behavior or aggressive responses (Stilling, 1992). It is used when other techniques are not effective in decreasing the frequency of a particular response, or in combination with other procedures.

Time out

Time out is a negative-consequence technique in which the person is removed from a setting where ongoing reinforcers are available. When a patient is exhibiting aggressive behavior that is followed by social reinforcement from other patients, the patient may be moved to another room where no social reinforcement is available (Corrigan, Yudofsky, and Silver, 1993).

Response cost

Response cost, another negative-consequence technique, is the removal of a reinforcer that is contingent on a specific behavior. Secondary reinforcers, such as points or tokens that were presented for desired behaviors, are removed for inappropriate behaviors (Corrigan, Yudofsky, and Silver, 1993). In outpatient settings, the response-cost technique might involve having patients pay a sum of money at the beginning of therapy and returning small amounts contingent on the patient's exhibition of a specific, desired behavior. The money is withheld when inappropriate behavior, such as noncompliance with the treatment contract, is exhibited.

Skills training

When behavioral responses are not appropriate for a person's age and life situation, new behaviors are acquired through the use of social-skills training and problem-solving procedures. Positive reinforcement and shaping are the basis for these programs; *modeling* and *imitation* are also used. Nurses often make individual assessments of the social skills of patients and form small groups to conduct training of skills that are appropriate for the patients but have not

	S	M	T	W	T	F	S
Get up on time	X	X	X				
Make bed		X					
Complete ADLs	X	X	X				
Go to group on time	X	X	X				
Participate in group			X				
Do own laundry	X						

FIGURE 36-1 Expected outcomes for Mr. Tom Day.

been used in the hospital situation. An example is assertiveness training in which assertiveness is defined, described, and compared to passive and aggressive responses. Assertive responses are modeled. The patients then practice these responses and use them in role-play and homework assignments (Goisman, 1997). Reinforcement is given when assertiveness is appropriately demonstrated (Corrigan, Yudofsky, and Silver, 1993).

Contingency contracting

Contingency contracting is the arrangement of conditions so that patients are able to participate in setting target behaviors and selecting reinforcers. The therapist and the patients jointly specify what, how, when, and where behavioral change will occur. Criteria for the delivery of reinforcement are defined. The type, amount, and schedule of reinforcement are specified. For example, a contract specifying that if the patient approaches the nurse to ask for his or her medications at the scheduled time, he or she can go for a walk with the nurse after dinner (Corrigan, Yudofsky, and Silver, 1993).

Self-control

The direct management of behavioral contingencies by a therapist usually is not practical for adult patients in an outpatient treatment setting. A more frequently used approach is the development of a self-control program with contingency contracting in which patients do the assessment, change their behaviors, provide their own reinforcement, and evaluate the results.

Token economy

Token economy is the term used to describe the use of operant principles in the management of behavior with groups of patients in inpatient or outpatient partial hospital programs (Ayllon and Azrin, 1968).

Tokens (tangible conditioned reinforcers) are presented to patients contingent on specific target behaviors (Goisman, 1997). A simple example is presented in Figure 36-1. Tokens can be exchanged for positive reinforcers, such as privileges and favorite foods.

■ Critical Thinking Questions

1. Jennifer O'Conner inflicts superficial cuts on her wrists when she receives negative consequences for seductive behavior with male patients. Positive reinforcement for opposing behaviors, social extinction, and "time out" have not been successful. What behavioral approaches would you plan instead?
2. One of the patients in your problem-solving group is silent most of the time. Using contingency contracting principles, describe the gradual progression of desired behaviors you would like for the patient to exhibit and the types and schedules of reinforcements you would use.

Respondent Conditioning: Helping Patients Cope with Disturbing Stimuli

When patients' problem behaviors are related to particular stimuli situations such as those related to phobias and PTSD, respondent conditioning is the model used. Treatment may involve making changes in stimuli situations or in control of problematic behaviors.

Reciprocal inhibition

The process of strengthening alternative responses to fear or anxiety associated with a stimulus is called *reciprocal inhibition* or *counterconditioning* (Yates, 1970). Relaxation techniques, for instance, can be taught to highly anxious patients. A person cannot be relaxed and anxious simultaneously. Techniques often taught are positive, affirming self-talk; deep breathing; progressive muscle relaxation; and positive imagery (Manderino and Brown, 1992). For example, the patient is instructed to tense and relax specific muscle groups, in a sequence, until relaxation is achieved. Several sessions of practice are usually carried out with the therapist, audiotape prompts, and/or written instructions.

Systematic desensitization

Originally developed by Wolpe (1958) for the treatment of anxiety, *systematic desensitization* is the planned progressive exposure to stimuli that elicit fear or anxiety while the fear response is suppressed (Goisman, 1997). Hierarchies of the fear-eliciting stimuli are constructed through a detailed assessment. For example, a patient with a fear of being in open and crowded places that limits appropriate shopping behavior may report a hierarchy of fear-eliciting situations as follows: standing in the doorway of the house; standing outside several feet from the house, then two blocks away, then several blocks away; being in a small, empty store; being in an empty department store; being in an empty shopping center; being in a small, crowded store, a crowded department store, then a crowded shopping center. The stimulus least likely to evoke fear or anxiety is introduced initially, followed by gradual exposure to more fearful stimuli.

In traditional desensitization procedures and other prolonged exposure models (Foa, 1997), presentation or imaging of the fearful stimuli is done while an incompatible response, such as relaxation, is used to inhibit the fear or anxiety. A biofeedback program may also be used to reach and maintain a state of relaxation (Hahn, et al, 1993).

Other respondent conditioning techniques

In live (in vivo) exposure, patients actually place themselves, systematically, in the least to the most fearful situations. Usually patients conduct this self-exposure while using incompatible competing responses to fear, such as relaxation. In using these techniques, the therapist carefully assists patients to experience a gradual decrease of the fear or anxiety response in the presence of the eliciting stimulus. *Flooding* or *implosion* is a process in which patients imagine or place themselves in the fearful situation; that is, they immerse themselves in the feared stimuli (Goisman, 1997). For example, an individual with a fear of elevators would stand in an elevator until his or her anxiety subsides.

■ Critical Thinking Question

What phobias, besides the ones mentioned in the text, might systematic desensitization be successful in overcoming?

BEHAVIORAL INTERVENTION WITH THE NURSING PROCESS

The behavioral nursing process consists of the following:

1. Making an *assessment* of behavior and related contingencies
2. Formulating a behavioral nursing diagnosis
3. *Outcome identification*, and *planning* and *implementing* an intervention program to have an impact on this behavior
4. *Evaluating* the results of the intervention

This series of steps meshes quite naturally with steps of the nursing process (Box 36-1). Occasions for conducting this process occur in day-to-day interactions with patients. These interactions focus on providing a well-structured therapeutic milieu (Corrigan, Yudofsky, and Silver, 1993), assisting patients with here-and-now living problems, and helping them to learn behavioral patterns related to emotional health (Maxfield and Pennington, 1996).

Guidelines for Behavioral Nursing Intervention

The following example illustrates the use of a behavioral approach for skills training in a group of patients with chronic psychiatric disorders who were hospitalized in a facility that used a modified token-economy system.

Baseline Observations (Assessment)
1. Appropriate behavior present
2. Inappropriate behavior present
3. Age-appropriate behavior absent
   Assessment of these behavioral categories includes:
   a. Frequency or duration of each response or both
   b. Description of the stimulus conditions that precede responses and follow the behavior
   c. Validation of potential reinforcers

Problem Specification (Behavioral Nursing Diagnosis)
1. Select the response to be changed
2. Define the response so everyone can recognize it
3. Gather baseline data (frequency, duration of behavior, discriminative and reinforcing stimuli)

Formulation of Treatment Plan (Outcome Identification)
1. State the specific response to be changed
2. State how the response is to be changed; include the present status and the target status of the response:
   a. Increase the rate of the response
   b. Decrease the rate of the response
   c. Teach a new response
3. Identify the discriminative and reinforcing stimuli available for use
4. Select and write the intervention plan in detail (with rationales)

Intervention
1. Implement the treatment plan as written
2. Provide reinforcers for those persons implementing the plan

Evaluation
1. State the outcome of the intervention
2. Determine whether the response changed as planned
3. Specify what additional changes are required
4. State techniques for maintaining the desirable change

Baseline observation and assessment

As part of the treatment program, each patient carried a behavioral rating card that listed specific expected behaviors (self-care activities, management of personal items and living area, attendance at prescribed treatment events). When the patients demonstrated these behaviors, a staff member rated the behavior and initialed the card. At the end of each week each patient's ratings on the behavior cards were tallied, and reinforcement was presented contingent on the score for the week. Examples of the reinforcements were opportunities to engage in the purchase of items at the hospital store, participation in hospital social events, privileges to leave the hospital unit, and home visits. The skills-training groups consisted of four to six patients who met weekly. The sessions began with a brief orientation period and an introduction of specific skills relevant to that session. Next there was a demonstration and role-play using the skills, followed by discussion and homework suggestions.

Problem specification

Skills included assertiveness (patients asking for the treatment or medication they thought was most helpful), communication (starting and continuing a conversation in appropriate and effective ways), monitoring of one's condition (reporting changes in self), making a plan for specific methods of self-care, and contracting with staff about treatment events or outcomes.

Treatment plan

Specific techniques used by the nurse were positive reinforcement (social reinforcement by the nurse or other patients, initialing the rating card) contingent on appropriate behavior, modeling and imitation, contingency contracting, homework, self-control, and extinction (withholding of reinforcement) following undesired behaviors.

Evaluation

Each group member's progress was evaluated with the use of a recording form that listed target behaviors. Seven patients showed consistent increases in target behaviors over the period of the group session. These changes would be expected if the group-intervention program was effective. One patient demonstrated a relatively high rate of target behaviors during the initial group session and continued this rate. Demonstration of target behaviors by two of the patients was variable and consistently low throughout the sessions. For these two patients, the group-intervention program was not effective in changing target behaviors during the period of time that they were involved in the group.

Key Concepts

1. Classical conditioning is based on the involuntary stimulus-response reaction. After repeated pairing of eliciting and neutral stimuli, the neutral stimulus alone obtains the expected response.
2. Operant conditioning focuses on the external variables that precede and follow the response to learn which ones control behaviors. Reinforcers are particularly important.
3. Behavior therapy begins with a functional analysis of behavior and environmental contingencies as the basis for developing a treatment program.
4. Behavior modification programs can be used for a variety of problematic behaviors in a variety of settings.
5. Increasing the probability of a desired behavior can occur with conditioning, reinforcement, or shaping.
6. Decreasing the probability of an undesirable behavior can occur with reinforcement of an incompatible behavior, extinction, and negative consequence.
7. New behaviors may be acquired in skills training through the use of modeling and imitation techniques, as well as through reinforcement and shaping.
8. Self-control and token-economy programs are varieties of reinforcement approaches.
9. Respondent conditioning is useful in altering an unpleasant response to a specific stimulus. Reciprocal inhibition, systematic desensitization, in vivo exposure, and flooding are varieties of this approach.
10. Behavioral nursing interventions involve baseline observations, analysis of behaviors, problem specification, formulation of treatment plans, intervention, and evaluation.

Study Questions

(Answer key is in the back of the book.)

1. A patient is disrupting a group session. Other patients are encouraging this. You ask the patient to take a "time out" in his room because:
   a. Neutral stimulation elicits cooperative behavior.
   b. Social reinforcement is not available in his room.
   c. Reinforcers control whether or not a behavior will be repeated.
   d. Deprivation decreases the chance of a behavior occurring.
2. A mother brings her young son to a counselor because of acting-out behaviors. Using operant-conditioning principles, you decide to analyze which of the following?
   a. Human reflexes
   b. Stimulus generalization
   c. Primary and secondary reinforcers
   d. Internal factors influencing behaviors
3. You talk with this mother about decreasing the son's behavior by:
   a. Developing a self-control program
   b. Teaching her son relaxation techniques
   c. Reinforcing successive approximations and negative reinforcement
   d. Reinforcing opposite behaviors and removing secondary reinforcers
4. You are conducting an assertiveness-training group for patients. Techniques that would be most helpful are:
   a. Modeling and shaping
   b. Imitation and deprivation
   c. Reinforcement and extinction
   d. Modeling and negative reinforcement
5. When a patient needs respondent conditioning to overcome a phobia, which techniques are most useful?
   1. Relaxation techniques
   2. Gradual exposure to progressively fearful stimuli
   3. Imagining oneself in the fearful situation
   4. Developing a self-control program
      a. 1, 3, 4
      b. 1, 2
      c. 3, 4
      d. 1, 2, 3
      e. All of the above

REFERENCES

Ayllon T and Azrin N: *The token economy,* New York, 1968, Appleton-Century-Crofts.
Blair DT: Integration and synthesis: cognitive behavioral therapies within the biological paradigm, *J Psychosoc Nurs Ment Health Serv* 34(12):26, 1996.
Corrigan PW, Yudofsky SC, and Silver JM: Pharmacological and behavioral treatment for aggressive psychiatric inpatients, *Hosp Community Psychiatry* 44(2):125, 1993.
Foa EB: Trauma and women: course predictors and treatment, *J Clin Psychiatry* 58(9):25, 1997.
Goisman RM: Cognitive-behavioral therapy today, *Harvard Mental Health Letter* 13(11):4, 1997.
Grinspoon L: Violence and violent patients: part II, *Harvard Mental Health Letter* 8(1):1, 1991.
Hahn YB, et al: The effect of thermal biofeedback and progressive muscle relaxation training in reducing blood pressure of patients with essential hypertension, *Image J Nurs Sch* 25(3):204, 1993.
Manderino MA and Brown MC: A practical, step-by-step approach to stress management for women, *Nurse Pract* 127(7):18, 1992.
Maxfield MC and Pennington BE: Behavior management training for long term care staff: a note of caution, *J Psychosoc Nurs Ment Health Serv* 34(12):37, 1996.
Pavlov IP: *Conditioned reflexes,* London, 1927, Oxford University (Translated by GV Anrep).

Premack K: Reversibility of the reinforcement relation, *Science* 136:255, 1962.

Skinner BF: *The behavior of organisms,* New York, 1938, Appleton-Century-Crofts.

Skinner BF: *Science and human behavior,* New York, 1953, Free Press.

Skinner BF: A case history in scientific method, *Am Psychol* 11:211, 1956.

Stilling L: The pros and cons of physical restraints and behavior controls, *J Psychosoc Nurs Ment Health Serv* 30(3):18, 1992.

Watson JB and Rayner R: Conditioned emotional reactions, *J Exp Psychol* 3:1, 1920.

Wolpe J: *Psychotherapy by reciprocal inhibition,* Stanford, Conn, 1958, Stanford University.

Yates AJ: *Behavior therapy,* New York, 1970, Wiley.

CHAPTER 37

Electroconvulsive and Other Somatic Therapies

NORMAN L. KELTNER
CLEO METCALF

LEARNING OBJECTIVES

After reading this chapter you should be able to:
- Compare modern electroconvulsive therapy (ECT) with traditional ECT.
- Discuss three indications for ECT.

- Describe the nurse's role in caring for patients before and after ECT.
- Describe and discuss the ethical, legal, social, and biological concerns related to psychosurgery.

Somatic therapies are treatment approaches that use physiological or physical interventions to effect behavioral change. In many ways, somatic therapies represent the extreme swing of the biological vs. psychodynamic arguments discussed in Chapter 1. *That is, if mental disorders are biological in origin, then a biological treatment is reasonable.* Strictly speaking, psychopharmacological interventions are somatic in nature and should be considered under this heading. We deal with psychotropic drugs separately (see Unit Four), however, because those interventions are mainstream interventions and because the term "somatic" is more closely linked to less commonly used forms of treatment.

The most common form of somatic therapy is electroconvulsive therapy (ECT), which will be discussed at length. Psychosurgery, though very controversial and used much less often, will be reviewed because of its relevance to historical, ethical, and legal issues profoundly affecting psychiatric care. Finally, a brief historical mention of insulin-coma therapy and Metrazol-induced convulsions will provide the student with information to appreciate the evolution of somatic therapy.

ECT and psychosurgery emerged as treatment forms in the 1930s. The roots of ECT lie in the misconception of early twentieth-century psychiatrists that epilepsy and schizophrenia were incompatible

(Coffey and Weiner, 1990). Advocates of ECT and psychosurgery envisioned and promised dramatic relief from the curse of mental illness. Over time, inappropriate use and disappointing results, coupled with the development of psychotropic drugs and a growing general distrust of psychiatric hospitals, created a climate of hostility toward these therapies and their practitioners. In the 1960s and early 1970s, the use of these two therapies came to a virtual standstill. Thompson and Blaine (1987) report that ECT treatments dropped significantly in the years 1975 to 1980. In the past decade, however, ECT has emerged once again as a useful treatment alternative when more traditional approaches fail. Psychosurgery, on the other hand, remains a treatment of last resort and is infrequently utilized.

With rigid treatment criteria and careful pretreatment evaluation, many psychiatric patients respond to these somatic therapies.

ELECTROCONVULSIVE THERAPY

"Electroconvulsive therapy is more firmly established than ever as an important method of treating certain severe forms of depression" (Potter and Rudorfer, 1993).

"Because shock treatment routinely causes an acute organic brain syndrome or delirium, the question is not whether shock can cause brain dysfunction. Shock treatment always causes severe brain dysfunction. The only legitimate question is, 'How often is recovery complete?'" (Breggin, 1991).

ECT was introduced in 1938 by Ugo Cerletti and Luciano Bini, two Italian psychiatrists. ECT was once commonly referred to as *EST* (electroshock therapy) or *shock therapy*. Both terms are considered pejorative today. Swartz (1993a) points out that the term *shock* is misleading because the essential part of the treatment is the programmed seizure.

During ECT an electric current is passed through the brain, causing a seizure. Presumably the seizure resets the pattern of brain-cell activity into a more normal state (Swartz, 1993b). Historically, this seizure resulted in a full grand mal convulsion accompanied by the various complications of those convulsions; that is, muscle soreness, fractures, dislocations, sprains, and tongue lacerations.

These seizures and the resulting grotesque facial grimaces that occur have been dramatically captured on film and graphically detailed in literature. In films and novels, ECT has been portrayed as a devious tool used by psychiatrists and psychiatric nurses,

themselves demented (see Ken Kesey's *One Flew over the Cuckoo's Nest* and Sylvia Plath's *The Bell Jar*), to maintain control over sane but highly individualistic patients. This public attack on ECT, linked with reports of inappropriate use, virtually stopped the use of ECT in this country. Inappropriate use of ECT included administering ECT for almost all conditions and, from the accounts of former patients, using it as punishment for noncompliant behavior.

ECT was used most often during the early 1950s (Swartz, 1993a), when it was given to almost every patient who did not respond to other treatment forms. In large state hospitals, ECT was given on Mondays, Wednesdays, and Fridays to as many as 20 or more patients on a psychiatric ward, often without written consent. One patient after another, some under their own power, others literally manhandled and restrained, would take their place on the bed to be given ECT. Nursing staff would hold the patient in place (to decrease fractures, dislocations, etc.), insert the mouth guard (to prevent tongue bites), put paste on the electrodes, and hold the electrodes in place on each side of the head (usually the temple area). Nurses would then hold the chin and jaw in proper alignment, and the physician in the background would deliver the shock. A full grand mal seizure would occur—a tonic seizure followed by a significantly longer clonic seizure. After convulsion activity terminated, the patient was turned on his or her side and tied in place (to prevent aspiration) while a staff member or "helper patient" stayed at the bedside until consciousness returned. The ECT team then moved on to the next patient.

This unforgettable scene, depicted in novels and films and reported by former patients, contributed to a growing public fear of ECT. But despite the negative views, ECT remains a viable treatment approach because many mental health professionals know it to be an effective alternative when other treatment modalities have failed. Unfortunately, in the process of waiting to evaluate the efficacy of other treatments, many patients have suffered needlessly. Many clinicians now argue that ECT should be considered as a treatment choice earlier in the treatment process. Today approximately 7% of all psychiatrists report using ECT in their practice (Koran, 1996).

Modern ECT

During ECT, an electric current (70 to 150 volts) is passed through the brain for 0.5 to 2 seconds. The seizure resulting from ECT must last approximately

30 to 60 seconds to be of therapeutic value. ECT has a cumulative effect, and collectively between 220 to 250 seconds are usually required for a therapeutic effect. The patient is given an oximeter-monitored anesthetic to assure optimal oxygenation. The events leading up to, during, and after treatment, including nursing responsibilities, follow.

How ECT Works

It is not clear how ECT works or why it is so effective, though over 100 theories have been advanced to explain it (Sackiem, 1994). A reasonable view suggests that ECT causes changes in monoamine neurotransmitter systems, similar to the changes caused by antidepressant drugs (Roberts, Leigh, and Weinberger, 1993).

Preparation for ECT

- The patient must have a pretreatment evaluation, including physical examination, laboratory work (blood count, blood chemistries, urinalysis), and baseline memory abilities.
- A consent form must be signed. Because ECT is often given as a treatment of last resort, some patients are so profoundly depressed by the time ECT is ordered that a truly "informed consent" is almost a contradiction in terms. In such cases, family members and facility legal staff should be involved.
- The routine use of benzodiazepines or barbiturates for nighttime sedation should be eliminated because of their ability to raise the seizure threshold.
- A trained electrotherapist and an anesthesiologist should be available.

Nursing responsibilities before ECT

- The patient should not be given anything by mouth for approximately 8 hours before ECT.
- Atropine should be given as ordered. Atropine can be given 1 hour before treatment or intravenously immediately preceding treatment (Box 37-1). Atropine reduces secretions and subsequent risk of aspiration.
- The patient should be asked to urinate before the treatment (seizure-induced incontinence is common).
- The patient's hairpins and dentures should be removed.
- Vital signs should be taken.
- The nurse should be positive about the treatment and attempt to reduce the patient's anxiety.

Procedures during ECT

- An intravenous line is inserted.
- Electrodes are attached to the proper place on the head. Electrodes are typically held in place with a rubber strap.
- The bite-block is inserted.
- Methohexital (Brevital) or another short-acting barbiturate is given intravenously. *The barbiturate causes immediate anesthesia, preempting the anxiety associated with waiting for the "jolt to hit" and the anxiety caused by succinylcholine.* (Succinylcholine causes paralysis but not sedation, thereby leaving the patient conscious but unable to breathe.)

Box 37-1   Drugs Used for ECT

Atropine
Class: The prototypical anticholinergic
Actions: Atropine is used before ECT for several reasons
  1. Inhibition of salivation and respiratory tract secretions to minimize aspiration
  2. Vagal stimulation–decreases the potential for cardiovascular depression resulting from ECT, succinylcholine, and/or methohexital
Pharmacokinetics:
  Onset: oral 30 minutes
       IM 15 minutes
       IV 1 minute
  Metabolism: liver, half-life 2 to 3 hours
Dosage: 0.4 to 0.6 mg
Side Effects: Typical anticholinergic effects

Succinylcholine (Anectine)
Class: Ultrashort-acting neuromuscular blocker
Actions: Prevents the musculoskeletal complications from induced convulsions
Pharmacokinetics:
  Onset: 30 to 60 seconds, duration of action 5 minutes
Dosage: 0.6 mg/kg IV
Side effects: Prolonged apnea, respiratory depression, fasciculations

Methohexital (Brevital)
Class: Ultrashort-acting barbiturate
Actions: Induces a light coma preceding delivery of ECT
Pharmacokinetics:
  Onset: 10 to 15 seconds, duration of action 5 to 7 minutes
  Metabolism: liver, half-life 4 hours
Dosage: 1.5 mg/kg (typically 50 to 120 mg)
Side effects: Respiratory depression, hypotension, myocardial depression, decreased cardiac output

- Succinylcholine (Anectine) is a neuromuscular blocking agent and is given intravenously.
- *Succinylcholine prevents the external manifestations of a grand mal seizure,* thus minimizing fractures, dislocations, etc., but does not affect the "brain seizure."
- The anesthesiologist mechanically ventilates the patient with 100% oxygen immediately before the treatment.
- The electrical impulse is given with up to 150 volts for 0.5 to 2 seconds.
- The seizure should last 30 to 60 seconds to be of therapeutic value (Haas, Nash, and Lippmann, 1996). If the seizure lasts less than 30 seconds, the physician must decide whether to stimulate another seizure. Seizure duration greater than 120 seconds is associated with less favorable outcomes.
- Monitoring devices include those for heart rate and rhythm, blood pressure, and electroencephalography.
- Ventilation and monitoring continue until the patient recovers.

Nursing responsibilities after ECT

- The nurse or anesthesiologist mechanically ventilates the patient with 100% oxygen until the patient can breathe unassisted.
- The nurse monitors for respiratory problems.
- ECT causes confusion and disorientation, so it is important to help with reorientation (time, place, person) as the patient emerges from this *groggy state.*
- Since approximately 5% to 10% of these patients "awake" agitated, the nurse may need to administer a prn benzodiazepine (Fitzsimons, 1995).
- Observation is necessary until the patient is oriented and steady.
- All aspects of the treatment should be carefully documented for the patient's record.

Seizure activity is monitored by an electroencephalographic (EEG) recording. Blood pressure and heart rate are also monitored. Oxygen is administered immediately before and then after the treatment because of interruption of breathing caused by the succinylcholine and the electrically induced seizure.

Number of Treatments

Typically, patients are given ECT 2 to 3 times a week, up to a total of 6 to 12 treatments (or until the patient improves or obviously is not going to improve).

Often patients experience relief after 2 or 3 treatments, but occasionally up to 20 will be needed. If improvement is not observed after 12 or so treatments, then continuing ECT will not typically be helpful. Though ECT is usually very effective, relapse occurs frequently. Many patients require periodic or maintenance ECT treatments to function at their best.

■ Critical Thinking Questions

1. ECT has been considered a political issue. Do you think ECT's opponents tend to be more on the left or the right of the political spectrum?
2. ECT is more effective than antidepressants in the treatment of severe depression. Still, there is reluctance to use ECT. If you or a member of your family were severely depressed, which of these two treatment forms would you want? Be honest as you consider the stigma of ECT, as well as the effects of anesthesia, memory loss, etc.

Indications for ECT

Although ECT was originally developed for schizophrenia, its primary indication soon shifted to patients who were severely depressed, particularly those manifesting delusions and psychomotor retardation (Potter and Rudorfer, 1993) (Box 37-2).

Box 37-2 Indications for ECT

- *Major depression:* ECT is appropriate treatment when associated with:
  1. Non-response to an adequate trial of antidepressants
  2. High suicide potential
  3. Dehydration
  4. Depressive stupor
  5. Catatonia
  6. Delusions
- Prophylaxis of recurrent major depression, i.e. "maintenance ECT."
- Severe mania—not controlled by medications.
- Post-partum psychosis after non-response to antidepressants.
- Schizophrenia-catatonic type when non-responsive to medications.
- Movement disorders refractory to treatment, e.g., Parkinson's disease, neuroleptic malignant syndrome, tardive dyskinesia.

Adapted from Bezchlibnyk-Butler KZ and Jeffries JJ: *Clinical handbook of psychotropic drugs,* Seattle, 1997, Hogrefe & Huber Publishers.

Box 37-3 Disorders, Depressive Symptoms, and Conditions That Respond to ECT

Disorders	Depressive Symptoms	Conditions
Severe depression	Anhedonia	Tardive dystonia
Treatment-refractory depression	Anorexia	Tardive dyskinesia
Catatonia	Delusions	Akathisia
Mania	Insomnia	Parkinsonian symptoms
Some types of schizophrenia	Muteness	Neuroleptic malignant syndrome
	Psychomotor retardation	
	Suicidal ideations	

From Swartz CM: Seizure benefit: grand mal or grand bene?, *Neurol Clin* 11(1):151, 1993b.

Severely depressed patients account for about 85% to 90% of all patients receiving ECT (Tancer, et al, 1989). These patients respond better and more rapidly to ECT than they do to antidepressants (Bowden, 1985; Coffey and Weiner, 1990). Potter and Rudorfer (1993) suggest a hierarchy of who should receive ECT:

1. Patients who require a rapid response (e.g., suicidal or catatonic patients)
2. Patients who cannot tolerate pharmacotherapy or cannot be exposed to pharmacotherapy (e.g., pregnant patients)
3. Patients who are depressed but have not responded to multiple and adequate trials of medication

Symptoms and disorders that respond to ECT are found in Box 37-3. Box 37-4 lists conditions that do not respond to ECT.

CLINICAL EXAMPLE

Penny Jones is a 48-year-old woman who worked for the postal service until 3 weeks ago. She was admitted to an acute psychiatric facility accompanied by her daughter, who indicated that her mother has lost 30 lbs during the past 4 months. The daughter further described her mother as having a poor appetite, being isolative, awakening early in the morning with the inability to fall back to sleep, and verbalizing thoughts with suicidal overtones. The daughter stated that her mother's actions scare her.

Ms. Jones states that life is intolerable and she does not want to live anymore without "Jerry." The daughter explains that Jerry was the patient's husband, who died 5 months ago.

Ms. Jones sought psychiatric help immediately and was prescribed amitriptyline 25 mg tid. She improved slightly but has relapsed into a deeper depression

Box 37-4 Conditions That Do Not Respond to ECT

Anxiety disorders	Personality disorders
Behavioral disorders	Phobic disorders
Mild depressions	Somatoform disorders

and lately has begun to verbalize suicidal thoughts. Based on her poor response to antidepressants and her suicidal thoughts, a course of six ECT treatments was prescribed. Ms. Jones tolerated the procedures well. Her suicidal ideations ceased, she began interacting with others spontaneously, and regained her appetite. She was discharged during the third week of her hospitalization.

Contraindications for ECT

Coffey and Weiner (1990) state that there are no absolute contraindications for ECT. Ziring (1993) suggests that ECT should be viewed similarly to many life-saving surgeries. That is, although there may be conditions that place an ECT recipient at risk, the risk may be warranted if the patient's condition is serious (e.g., severe depression, active suicidal ideations). Most clinicians believe the conditions listed in Box 37-5 create some level of risk for a patient who receives ECT.

Advantages of ECT

"Even with the host of psychotropic agents now available, ECT still represents for some patients the safest, most rapid, and most effective form of treatment" (Frances, Weiner, and Coffey, 1989).

ECT is a safe procedure; only a few ECT-related deaths have been reported (Sackeim, et al, 1993). Malpractice claims have been relatively rare (Swartz,

1993b). Runck (1985), after developing a major report for the National Institute of Mental Health, found only 3 deaths per 10,000 (0.03%) patients receiving this treatment. The mortality rate per individual treatment is approximately 1:50,000, close to the rate for anesthesia alone (Gitlin, et al, 1993). ECT is considered safe for adolescents as well (Walter and Rey, 1997). It appears that ECT is not only safe, but also more effective than antidepressants for certain groups of patients. *Potter and Rudorfer (1993) state that up to 90% of severely depressed patients respond to ECT.*

In addition, because it works faster, ECT may be more economical than traditional treatment. Furthermore, ECT can be given on an outpatient basis in some situations, resulting in additional savings (Irvin, 1997; Kramer, 1990). ECT is also safer than tricyclic antidepressants (TCAs) for patients with heart problems because it does not produce significant cardiovascular side effects and suicide, a persistent concern with depressed patients taking TCAs, is reduced as well. Finally, ECT can be used safely and effectively in older patients, even those regarded as the old-old (>85) (Tomac, Rummans, and Pileggi, 1997).

Box 37-5 Conditions Resulting in Increased Risk for Patients Receiving ECT

Very High Risk:
Recent myocardial infarction
Recent cerebrovascular accident
Intracranial mass lesion

High Risk:
Angina pectoris
Congestive heart failure
Extremely loose teeth (aspiration)
Severe pulmonary disease
Severe osteoporosis
Major bone fractures
Glaucoma
Retinal detachment
Thrombophlebitis
Pregnancy
Use of MAOIs (severe hypertension)
Use of clozapine (seizures, delirium)

Adapted from Ziring B: Issues in the perioperative care of the patient with psychiatric illness. *Med Clin North Am* 77(2):443, 1993. Adapted from Bezchlibnyk-Butler KZ and Jeffries JJ: *Clinical handbook of psychotropic drugs*, Seattle, 1997, Hogrefe & Huber Publishers.

Disadvantages of ECT

The major disadvantage of ECT is that treatment provides only temporary relief. It does not provide a permanent cure. Certainly, many patients are able to remain free of depression for long periods, and others may never need treatment again. However, some patients receiving ECT may need another series of treatments within a few months. Some psychiatrists order maintenance or continuation ECT (once per month for 6 to 12 months); however, the benefits of this approach are not clear.

Memory impairment, both retrograde (memory before treatment) and anterograde (memory and the ability to learn new things after treatment), has been frequently cited as a side effect of ECT. Events closest in time to ECT are most frequently affected. Although it is true that memory is impaired for events both before and after each treatment, and that confusion occurs immediately after each treatment, there does not seem to be any substantial loss of mental function once the treatment series is completed. Furthermore, because depression can cause memory loss too, it is not always clear whether memory impairment is related to ECT or to depression.

Physiological effects of ECT include cardiac effects, such as hypertension, arrhythmias, alterations of cardiac output, and changes in cerebrovascular dynamics. Hemodynamic changes, in combination with increased muscle tone, have been postulated to result in a generalized increase in oxygen consumption. Increases in myocardial oxygen consumption may result in ischemia (Ziring, 1993). Other problems that have been reported include hyponatremia (Greer and Stewart, 1993) and migraine headache (Weinstein, 1993).

Finally, some patients experience post-ECT seizures related to ECT.

OTHER SOMATIC THERAPIES

"On November 12, 1935, Almeida Lima, a Portuguese neurosurgeon under the direction of neurologist Egas Moniz, drilled two holes on the frontal aspect of the skull of a mental patient 3 cm anterior to each ear. Into these holes, in the fiber-rich region known as the centrum ovale, 0.2 cc of absolute alcohol was injected. This operation, later called the prefrontal leukotomy, ushered in a new era in the treatment of mental disorders—treatment marked by the procedure known as psychosurgery" (Dorman, 1995, p. 54).

Insulin-Coma and Metrazol-Induced Convulsion Therapies

Insulin-coma therapy was introduced in 1933 by the Viennese physician Manfred Sakel after he accidentally discovered that giving too much insulin to a psychotic diabetic patient produced a reduction in the patient's symptoms. Insulin "shock" therapy gained a wide following for some time in hopes of alleviating the debilitating symptoms of psychosis (Dorman, 1995; Colaizzi, 1996). Joseph Meduna introduced Metrazol-induced convulsion therapy based on his pathological observation that the nerve cells of patients with schizophrenia were different than those of individuals with epilepsy. Meduna erroneously concluded schizophrenia and epilepsy were mutually exclusive disorders (Swayze, 1995).

Psychosurgery

Earp (1979) defined psychosurgery as "brain surgery performed on normal or diseased tissues for the relief of intractable personal suffering or for the modification or control of persistent behavior attendant on psychiatric illness."

It is difficult to find an area of psychiatry surrounded by more controversy. A review of the literature suggests that medical scientists have strongly held views on both the efficacy and ethics of this procedure.

Dorman (1995) suggests this radical treatment was adopted because of the convergence of four existing conditions in psychiatric care:
1. The persistent appalling conditions in state hospitals
2. The rivalry between neurology and psychiatry
3. The use of other radical treatments (e.g., ECT)
4. New theories regarding frontal lobe brain function

Historical overview

Psychosurgery was first reported in 1891 by Gottlieb Burckhardt, director of an insane asylum in Prefargier, Switzerland. Burckhardt operated on six patients: one died and one developed epilepsy. Burckhardt intended to calm very excitable patients, but the procedure was so vigorously opposed by his medical colleagues that he discontinued this activity (National Commission for the Protection of Human Subjects of Biomedical and Behavioral Sciences

[NCPHSBBS], 1977). In 1910, Ludwig Puusepp (NCPHSBBS, 1977), a Russian neurosurgeon, performed psychosurgery on three manic-depressive patients. The results were unsatisfactory, and he did not perform the procedure again or publish his findings for 25 years (Valenstein, 1980; Lichterman, 1993).

The man considered the modern-day pioneer in psychosurgery was Egas Moniz, a Portuguese neurologist. In 1935, Moniz, with the assistance of Lima, performed a series of psychosurgical operations on 20 severely ill institutionalized patients. They reported that 14 members of this cohort showed improvement (Cosgrove and Rauch, 1995). They coined the term *psychosurgery*. In 1949 Moniz received the Nobel Prize in medicine and physiology for his work.

Freeman and Watts performed the first lobotomy in the United States on September 14, 1936:

"In their development of Dr. Moniz' methods, Drs. Freeman and Watts drilled a small hole in the temple on each side of the patient's head where two skull bones meet. Surgeon Watts then inserted a dull knife into the brain, made a fan-shaped incision upward through the prefrontal lobe, then downward a few minutes later. He then repeated the incisions on the other side of the brain. No brain tissues were removed." (In two operations they cut cerebral arteries. Both patients died.) (Freeman and Watts, 1942)

Walter Freeman, a neurologist, and his neurosurgeon colleague James Watts were impressed with the work of Moniz. Though a neurologist, Freeman treated many psychiatric patients and sought treatment approaches that were more efficient. Psychosurgery was the procedure he was looking for. Before his retirement, Freeman (1971) performed over 3500 psychosurgeries. Further, he toured the country stopping at the large state mental institutions to demonstrate his technique. In his wake, local practitioners began performing psychosurgery. Colaizzi (1996) paints a vivid picture of Freeman's visit to a hospital in 1950.

Freeman's reputation is sullied somewhat by what appears to be high-handed or pejorative language. Dorman (1995) has retrieved some of Freeman's remarks that detract from his work:

"Some patients come to operation at the end of a long and exasperating series of medical treatments, hospital treatments, shock treatments, including endocrines and vitamins mixed with their physiotherapy and psychotherapy. They are still desperate, and will go to any length to get rid of their distress. Other patients can't be dragged into the hospital and have to be held down on a bed in a hotel room until sufficient shock treatment can be given to render them manageable. We like both types."

Freeman also recorded a conversation with a 24-year-old laborer who was awake during the surgery.

Doctor: Are you scared?
Patient: Yeh
    (2 minutes later)
Doctor: How do you feel?
Patient: I don't feel anything but they're cutting me now.
Doctor: You wanted it?
Patient: Yes, but I didn't think you'd do it awake. Oh, gee whiz, I'm dying. Oh, doctor. Please stop. Oh, God. I'm goin' again. Oh, oh, oh. Ow, (chisel on skull) oh, this is awful. Ow, (grabs Freeman's hand and sinks nails into it). Oh, God, I'm goin', please stop.
    (After cuts have been made)
Doctor: What's happened to your fear?
Patient: Gone.
Doctor: Why were you afraid?
Patient: I don't know.
Doctor: Feel okay?
Patient: Yes. I feel pretty good right now.

And in response to critics of his surgical technique, he referred to concerns about sterile procedure as ". . . all that germ crap."

Psychosurgical intervention was widely used in the 1940s and 1950s, but a sharp decline occurred after the introduction of psychotropic drugs to state hospitals in the early to mid 1950s (Figure 37-1). As mentioned above, psychosurgery suffered some of the same public rejection as ECT. The popular novel by Ken Kesey, *One Flew over the Cuckoo's Nest*, depicted the defiant hero as the victim of a treacherous state hospital staff. His defiance eventually resulted in the ultimate punishment–a lobotomy. He emerged from the lobotomy room a "vegetable," his defiant character finally conquered. This depiction

1948 ——————— 2,281

1949 ——————————— 5,074

1956 —— 500

1973 —— 400

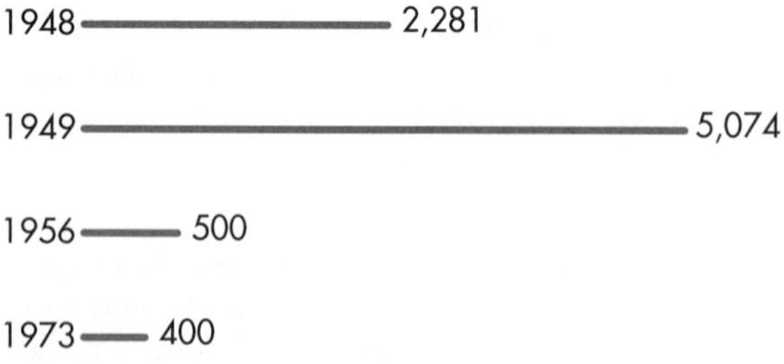

FIGURE 37-1 Psychosurgery performed in the years preceding and following the discovery and introduction of antipsychotic drugs. (From Valenstein ES: *The psychosurgery debate,* San Francisco, 1980, WH Freeman.)

of psychosurgery may have helped shape public opinion about this procedure.

Flor-Henry (1977), quoting Fulton, states that by 1951, 20,000 persons had undergone this operation. By his own account, Freeman (1971) estimated that he was involved in more than 3500 psychosurgical procedures.

In a review of 10,365 of the operations, Tooth and Newton found a 70% rate of improvement, 6% mortality rate, 1% epilepsy rate, and 1.5% rate of marked inhibition (reported in Cosgrove and Rauch, 1995). Valenstein (1980) estimates that 400 operations were performed each year in the United States for the years 1971, 1972, and 1973. He notes that the rate began to decline dramatically about that time.

Ethical concerns

Many concerns have been voiced regarding the ethics of psychosurgery. The Breggins (1973, 1977, 1984, 1991) have been outspoken critics of psychosurgery.

P.R. Breggin found a bias in the patient-selection process for psychosurgery; according to Breggin, underrepresented groups in our society were more likely to be selected. Freeman (1971) perhaps added to this perception when he cavalierly stated that lobotomy "proved to be the ideal operation for use in crowded state mental hospitals with a shortage of everything except patients."

Many mental health professionals find these concerns so compelling that they cannot endorse the use of psychosurgery.

Indications for psychosurgery

Only patients with severe, chronic, disabling, and treatment-refractory psychiatric disorders should be considered for psychosurgery (Cosgrove and Rauch, 1995).

Psychosurgery is helpful for the following mental disorders if or when traditional treatments have failed (Flor-Henry, 1975; Rappaport, 1992; Reese, 1988; Tueber, 1977; Valenstein, 1980):
- Depression and anxiety
- Depression-related pain
- Obsessive-compulsive disorders
- Aggression

Modern psychosurgery

Psychosurgery has changed considerably in the past 60 years. Four procedures are currently used. Each procedure has different indications, techniques, results, and complications. The review of those specific surgical interventions is beyond the scope of this text.

▪ Critical Thinking Questions

What are some of the potential abuses of psychosurgery in a society in which physicians are held in high esteem?

▼ Key Concepts

1. Somatic therapies are treatment approaches that use physiological or physical interventions to effect behavioral change.
2. The most common form of somatic therapy is electroconvulsive therapy (ECT).
3. During ECT an electric current is passed through the brain, causing a grand mal seizure.
4. Modern ECT uses anesthesia and muscle relaxants to prevent convulsive jerks that once caused broken bones; oxygen is given to guard against brain damage.
5. ECT is indicated for the treatment of severe depression, depression that is unresponsive to other treatments, mania, catatonia, and some types of schizophrenia.
7. Psychosurgery, a controversial brain surgery, is performed to provide relief from mental disorders that have been resistant to other treatment forms.
8. A number of ethical concerns have been raised by critics of psychosurgery, including its efficacy and the possibility of worsening patients' conditions.
9. Refinements in modern psychosurgery that target very precise and limited brain anatomy have made the procedure safer.

▼ Study Questions

(Answer key is in the back of the book.)
1. Succinylcholine (Anectine) given immediately preceding ECT produces which of the following?
   a. Muscle relaxation (paralysis)
   b. Anesthesia
   c. Decreased amounts of secretions (decreased possibility of aspiration)
   d. Convulsive activity
2. During effective, modern ECT the nurse might expect the patient to:
   a. Have a full grand mal seizure
   b. Have only a "brain seizure"
   c. Become apprehensive immediately before the electrical stimulus
   d. Have a brief seizure (10 seconds or less)
3. ECT may be effective and appropriate for which of the following?
   a. Severe depression
   b. Catatonia
   c. Manic-depressive illness
   d. All of the above
4. The most controversial somatic therapy is:
   a. ECT
   b. Psychosurgery
   c. Hydrotherapy
   d. Psychopharmacology
5. The effect from atropine that is most useful in ECT is:
   a. Mydriasis
   b. Dry mouth
   c. Urinary hesitancy
   d. Decreased lacrimation
6. ECT is ineffective in treating which of the following conditions? (Circle all correct responses.)
   a. Depression refractory to antidepressants
   b. Mild depression
   c. Anxiety
   d. Catatonia

REFERENCES

Aden v. Younger (57 Cal. 3d 622, 1976).

Bernstein IC, Callahan WA, and Jaranson JM: Lobotomy in private practice: long-term follow-up, *Arch Gen Psychiatry* 32:1041, 1975.

Bouckoms AJ: Ethics of psychosurgery, *Acta Neurochir Suppl* 44:173, 1988.

Bowden CL: Current treatment of depression, *Hosp Community Psychiatry* 36:1192, 1985.

Breggin PL: Use of psychosurgery as a treatment for hyperactivity in children, *Mental Health* 58:19, 1984.

Breggin PR: The second wave, *Mental Health* 57:11, 1973.

Breggin PR: If psychosurgery is wrong in principle. . . ?, *Psychiatr Opinion* 14:23, 1977.

Breggin PR: *Toxic psychiatry*, New York, 1991, St Martin's Press.

Bridges P and Williamson C: Psychosurgery today, *Nurs Times* 73:1363, 1977.

Coffey CE and Weiner RD: Electroconvulsive therapy: an update, *Hosp Community Psychiatry* 41:515, 1990.

Colaizzi J: Transorbital lobotomy at Eastern State Hospital (1951-1954), *J Psychosoc Nurs Ment Health Serv* 34(12):16, 1996.

Cosgrove CR and Rauch SL: Psychosurgery, *Nurs Clin North Am* 6(1):167, 1995.

Culliton BJ: Psychosurgery: national commission issues surprisingly favorable report, *Science* 194:299, 1976.

Davis D: Psychosurgery, *Operational Psychol* 9:70, 1978.

Dorman J: The history of psychosurgery, *Tex Med* 91(7):54, 1995.

Earp JD: Psychosurgery: the position of the Canadian Psychiatric Association, *Can J Psychiatry* 24:353, 1979.

Fink M: New technology in convulsive therapy: a challenge to training, *Am J Psychiatry* 144:1195, 1987.

Fitzsimons L: Electroconvulsive therapy: what nurses need to know, *J Psychosoc Nurs Ment Health Serv* 33(12):14, 1995.

Flor-Henry P: Psychiatric surgery–1936-1973: evolution and current perspectives, *Can Psychiatr Assoc J* 20:157, 1975.

Flor-Henry P: Progress and problems in psychosurgery, *Curr Psychiatr Ther* 17:282, 1977.

Frances A, Weiner RD, and Coffey CE: ECT for an elderly man with psychotic depression and concurrent dementia, *Hosp Community Psychiatry* 40:237, 1989.

Freeman W: Frontal lobotomy in early schizophrenia: long-term follow-up in 415 cases, *Br J Psychiatry* 119:621, 1971.

Freeman W and Watts JW: *Time,* p 48, Nov 30, 1942.

Gitlin MC, et al: Splenic rupture after electroconvulsive therapy, *Anesth Analg* 76:1363, 1993.

Greer R and Stewart R: Hyponatremia and ECT, *Am J Psychiatry* 150(8):1272, 1993.

Haas S, Nash K, and Lippmann SB: ECT-induced seizure durations, *J Ky Med Assoc* 94(6):233, 1996.

Irvin SM: Treatment of depression with outpatient electroconvulsive therapy, *AORN Journal* 65(3):573, 1997.

Koran LM: Electroconvulsive therapy, *Psychiatr Serv* 47(1):23, 1996.

Kramer BA: Outpatient electroconvulsive therapy: a cost-saving alternative, *Hosp Community Psychiatry* 41:361, 1990.

Lichterman L: On the history of psychosurgery in Russia, *Acta Neurochir,* 125(1-4):1, 1993.

Mark VH: A psychosurgeon's case for psychosurgery, *Psychol Today* 8:28, 1974.

Markowitz J, et al: Reduced length and cost of hospital stay for major depression in patients treated with ECT, *Am J Psychiatry* 144:1025, 1987.

National Commission for the Protection of Human Subjects of Biomedical and Behavioral Sciences: *Psychosurgery,* Washington, DC, 1977, Department of Health, Education and Welfare.

Nys H: Psychosurgery and personality: some legal considerations, *Acta Neurochir Suppl* 44:170, 1988.

Pakkenberg B: What happens in the leucotomised brain? A post-mortem morphological study of brains from schizophrenic patients, *J Neurol Neurosurg Psychiatry* 52:156, 1989.

Potter W and Rudorfer M: Electroconvulsive therapy: a modern medical procedure, *N Engl J Med* 328:12, 1993.

Rappaport ZH: Psychotherapy in the modern era: therapeutic and ethical aspects, *Med Law* 11(5-6):449, 1992.

Reese T: Obsessive-compulsive disorders: a treatment review, *J Clin Psychiatry* 49:48, 1988.

Roberts GW, Leigh PN, and Weinberger DR: *Neuropsychiatric disorders,* London, 1993, Mosby.

Runck B: NIMH report: consensus panel backs cautious use of ECT for severe disorders, *Hosp Community Psychiatry* 36:943, 1985.

Sackeim HA: Central issues regarding the mechanisms of action of electroconvulsive therapy: directions for future research, *Psychopharmacol Bull* 30(3):281, 1994.

Sackeim HA, et al: Effects of stimulus intensity and electrode placement on the efficacy and cognitive effects of electroconvulsive therapy, *N Engl J Med* 328(12):839, 1993.

Swartz CM: ECT or programmed seizures? *Am J Psychiatry* 150(8):1274, 1993a.

Swartz CM: Seizure benefit: grand mal or grand bene?, *Neurol Clin* 11(1):151, 1993b.

Swayze VW II: Frontal leukotomy and related psychosurgical procedures in the era before antipsychotics (1935-1954): a historical overview, *Am J Psychiatry* 152(4):505, 1995.

Szasz TS: Aborting unwanted behavior: the controversy on psychosurgery, *Humanist* 37:10, 1977.

Tancer ME, et al: Use of electroconvulsive therapy at a university hospital: 1970 and 1980-81, *Hosp Community Psychiatry* 40(1):64, 1989.

Thompson JW and Blaine JD: Use of ECT in the United States in 1975 and 1980, *Am J Psychiatry* 144:557, 1987.

Tomac TA, Rummans TA, and Pileggi TS: Safety and efficacy of electroconvulsive therapy in patients over age 85, *Am J Geriatr Psychiatry* 5(2):126, 1997.

Tueber HC: National Commission for the Protection of Human Subjects of Biomedical and Behavioral Sciences, *Psychosurgery,* Sec III, Washington, DC, 1977, Department of Health, Education, and Welfare.

Valenstein ES: *The psychosurgery debate,* San Francisco, 1980, WH Freeman.

Valenstein ES: Prefrontal lobotomy: author replies, *Surg Neurol* 30:75, 1988.

Walter G and Rey JM. An epidemiological study of the use of ECT in adolescents, *J Am Acad Child Adolesc Psychiatry* 36(6):809, 1997.

Weinstein MD: Migraine occurring as sequela of electroconvulsive therapy, *Headache* 33(1):45, 1993.

Ziring B: Issues in the perioperative care of the patient with psychiatric illness, *Med Clin North Am* 77(2):443, 1993.

Special Populations in Psychiatric Nursing

CHAPTER 38

Victims of Violent Behavior

LEE H. SCHWECKE

LEARNING OBJECTIVES

After reading this chapter you should be able to:
- Recognize the seriousness of violence in the United States.
- Describe the emotional reactions of adult victims of crime, torture, rape, childhood sexual abuse, and partner abuse.
- Recognize the dynamics involved in childhood sexual abuse.

- Analyze how the cycle of violence inhibits individuals from leaving abusive relationships.
- Identify the needs of victims of violence.
- Describe strategies for facilitating recovery for victims of violent crimes.
- Develop a nursing care plan for victims of violent behavior.

The victimization of any individual by another creates serious mental health, social, community, and legal problems. Violence in all forms is prevalent in this society. Nurses, regardless of their areas of practice, *will* come in contact with the victims—as inpatients, outpatients, home-care patients, emergency care patients, parents of patients, friends, and relatives. Although the victims are typically seen initially for medical reasons, their psychological needs require attention if long-term mental health problems are to be prevented.

Forensic nursing is emerging as a vital aspect of the holistic care of victims and perpetrators of violent crimes and their families (Lynch, 1996). This

care includes obtaining clinical histories and documentation of evidence including photographs of injuries. The rights of perpetrators of crime, suspects, and victims must be protected so the legal case will not be jeopardized (Pasqualone, 1996).

This chapter focuses on victims of violent behaviors beginning with general reactions to any crime, then focusing on the victims of torture, rape, adult survivors of childhood sexual abuse, and individuals abused by their partners. A small number of perpetrators are female, but the most common pattern of victimization is by males against females. Over 90% of adult intimate violence involves this pattern (Sheridan, 1993). When the incidents of sexual abuse of children, rape, and battery are combined, females are 10 times more likely than males to be the victims (Aiken, 1993). (An exception is pedophilia, described in Chapter 32).

The short- and long-term reactions of victims described in this chapter are *generally* true for both male and female victims; however, men sometimes have a more difficult time admitting to and dealing with their emotional victimization. The impact on males of sexual violation by other males, both as children and as adults, is in part due to their fears about homosexuality (Courtois, 1988).

VIOLATION BY CRIME

Effects of Crime

Not all crimes involve physical violence, injury, and threat to life; however, all crimes involve *emotional* violation and trauma. The victim's identity is affected even with the loss or destruction of possessions and property because these are a representation of an individual's identity and have personal significance. Crime undermines foundations formed in the first two stages of human development regardless of the victim's age when the crime occurred (see Chapter 3). There is a loss of trust, not only in the criminal, but to some degree in all other persons. Victims also lose a sense of ability to control their own lives and themselves (autonomy issues).

The emotional reactions to crime vary greatly according to the individual, the situation, and the meaning of the crime to that person. However, typical reactions are denial, fear, anger, powerlessness, and depression. A sense of failure and guilt are common; victims wonder what they did to cause the crime and how they could have prevented or stopped it. Victims usually feel ashamed and unworthy, as well as contaminated or "dirty," whether or not they were physically touched by the perpetrator. Fantasies of revenge or a wish for legal retribution are typical. The relationships of victims to family and friends can be disturbed, in part due to the loss of trust, but also because of the response of others. Caring persons often imply that the victim was responsible for the crime with such questions as, "Why were you there alone at night? Why were you carrying so much cash? Why didn't you install that burglar alarm?" The victim may feel alienated and isolated. Hospital personnel, the police, and the legal system may also convey a "blaming-the-victim" attitude in their manner of questioning and in focusing only on the "facts" without any emotional support or empathy.

Recovery from Trauma

Many models have been formulated about the process of recovery from traumas. Most agree that recovery is influenced by the severity of the trauma, the victim's resources, and the nature of help provided immediately after the event. Typically, three stages of recovery are defined: initial disorganization *(impact)*, a struggle to adapt *(recoil)*, and reconstruction *(reorganization)*. The brief summary here is derived from the views of Tynhurst (1951), Fox and Scherl (1972), Janoff-Bulman (1997), and Clark (1997). The stages are not clearly separated, and the readjustment process is not smooth. There may be vacillation among the stages, and recovery may take months or years.

Impact

The initial reaction to trauma usually lasts from a few minutes to a few days. Common responses are shock, denial, disbelief, and confusion. There may be paralyzing fear, hysteria, a sense of helplessness and vulnerability, physiological responses, and disturbed sleeping and eating. Some victims react less visibly or in a delayed manner. They look calm, organized, and rational, and take all the necessary actions initially needed. It is later, in private, that the other reactions occur.

Recoil

In the recoil stage victims begin the struggle to adapt. The immediate danger is over, but a great deal of emotional stress remains. In the beginning of this phase, there are periods in which victims look and act "normal" and are able to carry out daily routines at home and at work. Activity helps to suppress fears, anger, and sadness. Later in the phase there is a desire to talk about the details of and feelings about the trauma. Victims often feel a need for support and to be temporarily dependent. Fantasies of revenge are natural during this stage. In the weeks and months following crime trauma, victims gradually become aware of the full impact the event has had on their lives.

Reorganization

Reorganization may take months or years to accomplish. Although the trauma is not forgotten, the anxiety, fear, and anger diminish, and victims reconstruct their lives. The beginning of this phase includes reviewing and organizing what happened specifically and why ("Why me?"); attributing blame to self, others, or both; justifying one's own actions at the time and later; and regaining a sense of control and self-protection. Grief over losses resolves slowly. There may be lingering nightmares, frustrations, and disillusionment; however, these subside as victims reengage in life and activities. If reorganization is not effective, victims may experience degrees of symptoms that, in some cases, are clinically diagnosable (e.g., depression and posttraumatic stress disorder [PTSD]).

Even with satisfactory recovery, victims sense that they and their lives are, and always will be, different as a result of the crime. The goal of recovery is to move from victim status to survivor status by integrating the memories of the crime or trauma and moving on in life with restored functioning, a reasonable sense of safety and security, healthy relationships, and self-esteem.

Psychotherapeutic Management

Nurse-Patient Relationship. Although empathy, emotional support, and a willingness to listen are important in all stages of recovery, specialized care is needed in each stage. During the impact stage, the focus is on the victim's need for physical safety and emotional security (see Chapter 13, for these crisis intervention strategies).

Reassurance, protection from further harm, and sometimes medical care are needed. Victims may need clear, simple directions on what to do, where to go, and what to avoid. It is crucial that nurses avoid accusations (blaming), intimidations, unnecessary intrusions, and invasion of privacy. In most cases, crisis intervention is face-to-face at the scene of the crime or in the emergency room. For those victims who are superficially calm and in control, the crisis intervention may be needed a few hours or days later, when "reality hits." Phone numbers for crisis-phone or walk-in services can be given to victims before they leave the emergency room.

During the recoil stage, victims need validation of the self and of their rights as victims. Referrals can be made to a victim's assistance program and for legal, insurance, or financial assistance if needed. If family and friends are not fully available during the episodes of emotional turmoil in the recoil phase, then short-term counseling may be beneficial. During the struggle to adjust, support groups with other victims can be useful. Whether the group is short-term (6 to 8 weeks) or ongoing, and whether the group is professionally led or self-led, there is value in receiving information, encouragement, and companionship from others who "have been there."

In the reorganization stage, most victims are able to recover and grow with minimal assistance. Long-term counseling is sometimes needed to overcome anxiety, phobias, depression, suicidal ideation, or other posttraumatic symptoms.

It is uncommon for victims to need hospitalization beyond initial medical care. Exceptions include victims who are unable to function, to meet basic needs, or who become suicidal.

Psychopharmacology. Victims of crime do not generally need medications. Antianxiety agents (benzodiazepines) are prescribed occasionally for short-term use to decrease anxiety and facilitate sleep.

Milieu Management. Many communities have groups for victims of disasters, divorce, death of a loved one, sudden infant death syndrome (SIDS), rape, incest, and physical and emotional abuse, as well as for survivors of suicide, mass murders, torture, and abduction of children.

TORTURE AND RITUAL ABUSE

Nature of the Problem

Public attention to the effects of torture and ritual abuse on mental health is a relatively new phenomenon, although the crimes are not. The effect of torture, whether perpetrated by individuals, relatives, gangs, cults, hate groups, or military-political organizations, is more severe because it involves multiple crimes against each victim. It is used to create fear, humiliation, and submission in individuals, communities, and societies (Fischman, 1996). Worldwide it is estimated that 16 million people are refugees of torture, political violence, and/or the fear of these, including many who have resettled in the United States (Laurence, 1992a). Statistics on the prevalence of torture and ritual abuse by individuals, relatives, gangs, hate groups, and cults are not readily available due to problems in acknowledging, reporting, and proving occurrences (Goodwin, 1994). The threat of further harm to the self and/or family tends to keep victims silent.

Torture and ritual abuse tactics

Torture involves physical, psychological, pharmacological, mind control, and/or sexual tactics aimed at damaging the victim's identity, personality, emotional stability, spirit, and physical integrity (Laurence, 1992a; Bloom, 1994; Ross, 1995).

Torture and ritual abuse often begin with abduction and detention, and end with execution. They can involve using hot irons, electric shock, submersion, suffocation, large doses of drugs, beatings, physical restraint, confinement in cramped and/or buried containers, gang rape, sexual and physical mutilation, being tied and/or hung in the air, being photographed during the abuse, starvation, sleep deprivation, brainwashing, indoctrination, mind control, programming, threats to or lies about the safety of loved ones and pets, overstimulation, and threats with weapons (Bloche and Eisenberg, 1993; Hudson, 1991; Laurence, 1992a; Puhar, 1992; Rockwell, 1994; Ross, 1995).

CLINICAL EXAMPLE

Children who were examined following ritual abuse in a day care center reported being locked in a cage, put in a coffin, held underwater, injected with needles, tied and hung from hooks, sexually assaulted, and threatened with guns and knives. The children were told that if they told anyone about the abuse, their parents, siblings, and/or pets would be killed (Hudson, 1991).

Effects of Torture and Ritual Abuse

Common outcomes of torture are injuries to the head, teeth, and genitals, as well as bone fractures, dislocations, scars, burns, pain, and chronic headaches (Laurence, 1992a; Bloom, 1994). The emotional effects are more severe and long-lasting. Themes are a sense of violation, dehumanization, humiliation, and powerlessness; loss of trust and self-esteem; identity and personality changes; terror and insecurity; and damaged social and family relationships (Bloche and Eisenberg, 1993; Laurence, 1992a; Bloom, 1994). More specific responses resulting from torture are listed in Box 38-1.

There is much controversy about assigning psychiatric diagnoses (e.g., PTSD, adjustment disorder, major depression, dysthymia, anxiety disorder, dissociative disorder) to victims of torture and ritual abuse. One debate revolves around the possibility of new terminology for the constellation of reactions resulting from torture, such as "torture syndrome" (Laurence, 1992a). Some view PTSD as insufficient for acknowledging the catastrophic effects of torture on victims and their families.

There is also a major concern that diagnosis is another form of victimization, stigmatization, and discounting of the validity of reports of torture. This view holds that the victims' responses are *normal* reactions, not psychiatric symptoms (Bloche and Eisenberg, 1993). "Blaming the victim" draws attention away from the individual, social, cultural, and

---

Box 38-1   Specific Responses Resulting from Torture

Anxiety	Insomnia	Sensitivity to stress
Panic/terror	Nightmares	Sexual
Irritability	Flashbacks	dysfunctions
Aggression	Hyperarousal	Mistrust
Rage	Impulsiveness	Suspiciousness
Fatigue	Alienation	Estrangement
Guilt	Passivity	Unresponsiveness
Withdrawal	Depression	Suicidal ideation
Repression	Dissociation	Emotional lability
Memory	Decreased	Self-mutilation
disturbances	concentration	Spiritual distress

Adapted from Bloche MG and Eisenberg C: The psychological effects of state-sanctioned terror, *Harvard Mental Health Letter* 10(5):4, 1993; Hudson PS: *Ritual child abuse: discovery, diagnosis, and treatment,* Saratoga, Calif, 1991, R & F; Laurence R: Part I: torture and mental health: a review of the literature, *Issues Ment Health Nurs* 13:301, 1992a; Bloom SL: Hearing the survivor's voice: sundering the wall of denial, *J Psychohistory* 21(4):461, 1994; Garbarino J: The spiritual challenge of violent trauma, *Am J Orthopsychiatry* 66(1):162, 1996.

political variables creating and fostering torture, and from research on strategies for prevention (Rockwell, 1994; Bloom 1994).

Recovery from Torture and Ritual Abuse

Supportive, cognitive, behavioral, psychodynamic, and pharmacological approaches are useful in helping torture victims. The major goals for recovery are the following (Bloche and Eisenberg, 1993; Laurence, 1992b):

1. Processing and integrating the memories of the experiences, often from the least to most bizarre experiences
2. Expressing and dealing with the intense emotions, especially anger
3. Developing or reestablishing healthy relationships with family, friends, and the community

Psychotherapeutic Management

Conveying acceptance, caring, and support are crucial if patients are going to trust enough to discuss their experiences. Strategies used with patients experiencing PTSD are particularly useful for victims of torture and ritual abuse (see Chapter 29). Depending on the origin of the torture or ritual abuse (individuals, relatives, gangs, hate groups, cults, military-political organizations), it may be crucial to understand the victim's family, religious, cultural, and political background. Specialized treatment centers (e.g., Center for Victims of Torture in Minnesota) use a multidisciplinary approach in providing treatment and rehabilitation for survivors and their families. Some centers and programs utilize bicultural counselors to facilitate counseling with immigrants and ex-gang members. Self-help and therapy groups may be useful for survivors with similar experiences and needs, such as political refugees (Laurence, 1992b), ex-cult members, and ex-gang members.

RAPE AND SEXUAL ASSAULT

Nature of the Problem

Statistics indicate that rape is an *under*reported crime in the United States; probably only one in six rapes are reported. Estimates of actual rapes range from one in five to one in two women and one in three

males (Boutcher and Gallop, 1996; Dole, 1996; Tyra, 1996). A rape of a woman is reported every 6 minutes (Vachss, 1993). When unreported rapes are included, the rate is probably one every minute (Tyra, 1996). A woman may be raped at any age, but the highest risk occurs between the ages of 15 and 24. Rape of men by men is increasing but is rarely reported.

One major problem in reporting rape is that laws and attitudes vary in different states and communities. In general, rape is considered forcible penetration of the victim's body by the perpetrator's penis without consent. Any other form of forced sexual contact (from touch to mutilation) is considered sexual assault. Despite sexual contact, it is generally acknowledged that rape is not sexually motivated, but involves a desire for power and control and a wish to humiliate the victim. Beyond these definitions, there is little consistency. Some prosecutors do not accept rape as a charge if the two individuals know each other; in those localities, "date rape" is considered nonexistent. Rape by a known assailant is often more traumatizing than rape by a stranger (Roye and Coonan, 1997). In 1992, 12 states lacked marital rape statutes; therefore, husbands in those states cannot be charged with raping their wives (Sheridan, 1993). Unfortunately, many members of our society ignore this crime or convey the message that anyone who is raped asked for it ("blaming the victim"). The applications of the laws, and political and societal attitudes, interfere with both reporting rape and recovering from it. The criminal justice system (police, lawyers, judges, and juries) may fail the victims by not encouraging or not following through on prosecutions, acting as if the victim is on trial, and by giving not-guilty verdicts or lenient sentences (Vachss, 1993).

Effects of Rape and Sexual Assault

Like all crime victims, the rape victim experiences a severe violation and all the possible emotions of the impact stage. In addition to internal and external bodily injuries, there may be a threat to life with weapons, a threat to return and rape again, to kill if the rape is reported, or the perpetrator may kill the victim during or after the rape. Victims may live but wish they had died. The powerlessness, loss of control, fear, shame, guilt, humiliation, rage, and feelings of being contaminated or "dirty" may be overwhelming. A typical reaction of the victim is the wish to regain a sense of control and retreat to a safe place, take a thorough shower, and destroy any damaged belongings. To do so is to destroy most of the evidence that would be required if the victim later decided to report the rape and prosecute.

CLINICAL EXAMPLE

A 24-year-old woman calls a crisis line complaining of anxiety at work, not sleeping, fear of being out at night, overwhelming anger, and feeling "dirty" and ashamed. For several weeks she felt that a co-worker was following her; she had seen him at the grocery, spa, and shopping mall. Last Friday as she was leaving work late, the co-worker pushed her into her car and raped her. She did not report the rape and hid in her apartment all weekend. She forced herself to go to work on Monday. The man acted friendly toward her, as if nothing had happened.

Recovery from Rape and Sexual Assault

Despite an outward appearance of calm composure and a denial at times of the need for help, the rape victim needs assistance, information, and support. It may not be until the victim begins the up-and-down struggle of the recoil stage that the losses, anger, and needs are recognized. In an emergency room, collecting evidence may seem like a priority for staff, but for the victim it is perceived as further intrusion and violation. To staff, victims may seem resistant and uncooperative, while victims are trying to protect themselves and regain a sense of control. See Box 38-2 for some of the needs and rights of victims.

Many communities have information packets prepared for rape victims and staff in hospitals, counseling centers, and crisis services. Victims can be encouraged to keep the information sheets as well as phone numbers of resources for later use. The temporarily composed and calm victim who denies the need for help should be especially encouraged to take materials home. If the services are available, a sexual assault nurse examiner (Hatmaker, 1997), an advocate from a victim's assistance program, or a rape crisis counselor can be called to initiate contact in the emergency room and make periodic follow-up days, weeks, and months later.

The ability to make follow-up contact with a rape victim after the impact stage can be beneficial. It is in the recoil stage that most victims begin to react

emotionally to the significant effect rape has on their lives. They may alternately deny and admit to experiencing turmoil. Fear and mistrust are major issues and may be directed toward persons resembling the perpetrator or to everyone around them (especially if others convey any hint of blaming the victim). Victims may be afraid to leave the one place they designate as safe. More often they are able to go out with family and friends but avoid strangers, places similar to the rape scene, and intimacy, especially sexual relationships. If the rape occurred in their own residence, they may move or at least make safety-related changes to prevent recurrence. They may ask for someone to stay with them at night for a while. Being alone and unprotected is usually frightening for victims. When feelings are turned inward over time, depression is a likely outcome (Mackey, et al, 1992; Tyra, 1996). Victims need help in reaffirming that they are worthwhile persons, with dignity and rights, who did not cause and did not deserve the rape. They need to know that their anger is natural,

---

Box 38-2 The Needs and Rights of Rape Victims

1. Crisis intervention: information, counseling, and referrals
2. Help with basic needs: housing, transportation, child care, safety
3. Medical information and care: information about pregnancy prevention, testing for sexually transmitted diseases, follow-up care, and counseling
4. Advocacy for whatever choices are made about reporting or prosecuting
5. Protection of rights: to privacy, confidentiality, gentleness, sensitivity, and explanations of procedures and tests
6. Protection of rights: to refuse collection of evidence, to determine who will and will not be present during examinations, to get copies of all medical and legal reports, and to apply for reimbursement through victim's compensation
7. Fairness, information, and protection of legal rights during investigations, hearings, and trial, including not being asked about prior sexual experiences with anyone besides the suspect or defendant
8. Reasonable protection against further harm: escorts to court, restraining order, additional patrols, even relocation, if necessary

especially about the violation of person and privacy, the humiliation, and the sense of powerlessness. Victims often question whether they could have fought off the attacker. Survival is most important; if the victim survived the rape, then he/she did exactly what was necessary to stay alive.

Rape Trauma Symptoms

One way to monitor and evaluate the rape victim's responses to the trauma and recovery process through the recoil and reorganization stages is to periodically assess for improvements in the rape trauma symptoms (DiVasto, 1985) in Box 38-3. It is important to remember that victims vacillate in the recoil stage between repression/suppression and dealing with the trauma. Even progress in the reorganization stage is not smooth, but backslides at times, especially if new situations trigger memories of the rape. Victims may avoid future routine gynecological exams and prenatal care in order to avoid reexperiencing the trauma (Dole, 1996). Use of restraints with a victim during an inpatient stay may also reactivate the trauma symptoms (Smith, 1995). Victims may need help in overcoming difficulties in sleeping or eating, relationship problems, lowered self-esteem, and depression. The goals of recovery from rape and sexual assault are the same as for all victims of crime. In addition, these victims need to develop or regain healthy sexual functioning and relationships.

Psychotherapeutic Management

Nurse-Patient Relationship. The rape or sexual-assault victim needs continual empathy, support, and an opportunity to process the events and intense feelings that result. Although it is more time-and energy-consuming, the best approach in collecting evidence and providing nursing care is to move slowly and supportively at the individual victim's pace, and to give rationales for and descriptions of procedures and referrals (Roye and Coonan, 1997). Nurses, who are predominantly women, can be particularly helpful to rape victims. Male and, particularly, female victims tend to feel safer with a woman and may refuse to talk to a man, especially alone. Having one nurse stay with the victim through examinations and interrogations can be reassuring.

Crisis intervention is the most appropriate approach during the impact stage. Short-term counseling and a rape support group can be beneficial during the recoil stage. Long-term counseling may be needed during the reorganization stage, especially if the victim decides to prosecute the perpetrator. The lengthy legal processes can seriously delay recovery. In many trial situations the victim is still treated like a criminal during cross-examinations. On the other hand, conviction and imprisonment of the perpetrator can help victims to feel vindicated, compensated, and more safe in their environments.

If the symptoms of rape trauma do not gradually diminish and reorganization of life-style does not seem to occur, the victim needs to be assessed for and helped with any new problems, such as anxiety, excessive anger and guilt, depression, acting out, isolation, self-destructive behaviors, substance abuse, phobias, and negative or destructive relationships with others. Rape victims are 8.7 times more likely to attempt suicide than nonvictims (Mackey, et al, 1992). With any of these behaviors, longer-term counseling is a necessity and hospitalization may become essential if lack of functioning or suicidal ideation or attempts are apparent.

Psychopharmacology. Although rarely prescribed to rape victims, benzodiazepines to reduce anxiety and provide for sleep may be used on a *temporary* basis. Alternatively, an antidepressant taken at bedtime, especially trazodone (Desyrel), may be ordered if symptoms of depression exist with a sleep disturbance.

Milieu Management. Referral can be made to a rape support group, which encourages expressing

---

Box 38-3 Rape Trauma Symptoms

- Sleep disturbances, nightmares
- Loss of appetite
- Fears, anxiety, phobias, suspicion
- Decrease in activities and motivation
- Disruptions in relationships with partner, family, friends
- Self-blame, guilt, shame
- Lowered self-esteem, feelings of worthlessness
- Somatic symptoms

anger, overcoming guilt and shame, building self-esteem and trust, and assisting in regaining control of one's life and a sense of safety. Support groups are sometimes available for relatives, especially partners, of rape victims to help them deal with the trauma, the stereotyping and myths, and the changes occurring in the victim and themselves.

■ Critical Thinking Questions

As an emergency room nurse, you are treating a 19-year-old male victim who was tortured and raped by a local gang. The victim refuses to give any details or to identify members of the gang. Describe what information you would give him about being a victim and the benefits of follow-up counseling.

ADULT SURVIVORS OF CHILDHOOD SEXUAL ABUSE

Nature of the Problem

The crimes of childhood sexual abuse (by nonrelatives) and incest (by relatives) are especially destructive for two major reasons: the crimes are not one-time occurrences, and the perpetrators are usually known and trusted persons.

Unfortunately, these are common crimes. It is estimated that 20% to 30% of all women have experienced childhood sexual abuse (Chard, Weaver, and Resick, 1997). Another estimate is that 2 million children are sexually abused by relatives, friends, and strangers each year (Grinspoon, 1993a). Studies give estimates of 10% to 30% of adult men were sexually abused as children (Draucker and Petrovic, 1996; Godby and Hutchinson, 1996). Sexual abuse of boys may be much higher; among male inpatients, as many as one in six have been sexually abused as children (Grinspoon, 1993b). It is sometimes harder for men to reveal the abuse because of the fear of being seen as weak or gay.

Sexual abuse and incest include voyeurism and exhibitionism, which can lead to intercourse and mutilation, but always involve a younger victim who is not capable of giving consent to the older individual. Male perpetrators are commonly fathers, uncles, stepfathers, older brothers, cousins, grandfathers, neighbors, scout leaders, camp counselors, coaches, and religious leaders. Less frequently, the perpetrators are females: various relatives, teachers, coaches, neighbors, and babysitters. Victims are from every social, cultural, ethnic, and economic group. Sexual acts may begin as caressing but usually progress to molestation by the time the victim is 4 years old and to oral, anal, and/or vaginal intercourse by the time the victim is 10 years old (Courtois, 1988).

Although sexual abuse can be violent, it typically is not. Russell's study of incest (1986) found coercion in 68% of cases, but no violence. In 29% of cases there was mild force, such as pinning the victim down. In only 3% was there some degree of physical violence. Coercion is possible because of the victim's dependent, trusting, and/or loving relationship with the perpetrator. The victim is urged to maintain the "secret" with various threats such as the following: the victim will be taken away from the family; the perpetrator will be put in a mental hospital or jail; the parents will divorce; the other parent will get sick; there will be no abuse of siblings if the victim is compliant; love will be withdrawn; no one would believe the victim anyway; or there will be physical abuse if the victim does not comply. Even when there is no physical violence, victims usually fear that it will occur if they resist the perpetrator. Other forms of abuse (emotional, verbal, etc.) and neglect do seem to be correlated with sexual abuse (Zanarini, et al, 1997).

Even if the young victims wanted to disclose the abuse, it is difficult for them because they lack the words and concepts to describe what is happening. There is usually an emotional reaction of fear and confusion, and some physical pain, but not a moral or ethical concept of "wrong." Most victims who, as children, tried to tell a parent or other adults were met with disbelief, denial, or pressure to retract their accusations (Grinspoon, 1993b). It is difficult for anyone to believe that the partners they love or respected members of the community are capable of sexual abuse. Police, prosecutors, judges, mental health professionals, and the general public may discount a child's report as unreliable, a fantasy, distorted, or faked at the urging of a parent (Applebaum, 1993; Grinspoon, 1993c; Horn, 1993). There are also potential benefits from the sexual relationship: the child is made to feel special, with extra attention from and time with the perpetrator that other children do not enjoy. A certain power comes from trying to please the adult and from receiving a degree of affection. At times the child may even have the physical experience of sensual pleasure. However, the emotional pleasure and concept of sexual love are absent. (All children make bids for attention and affection. Even if they are cute, coy, or flirtatious, these should not be viewed as seduction. Perpetrators of sexual abuse choose to misinterpret the child's behaviors to meet their own needs and still should be held responsible for the crime.)

Effects of Childhood Sexual Abuse on the Child

For the victim, the end result is disturbed growth and development, ambivalence about the experience (both the benefits and pain), and denial of what is happening to protect the whole family and/or the community. The young child is fulfilling the roles of child and lover to the perpetrator, and roles of child and protector to the rest of the family/community (protecting them from the "horrible secret"). As a result, the child begins a long-term process of parenting others to the exclusion of personal needs (Urbanic, 1987). Basically, the child wishes for love, not sex, but eventually feels guilty, exploited, betrayed, angry, "dirty," helpless, and responsible. Butler (1978) and Ridley (1993) describe levels of betrayal (1) by the abuser; (2) by the lack of response from the other parent or adults; (3) by the lack of response from teachers, doctors, nurses, and other professionals who miss the cues or disbelieve reports; and (4) by oneself through denial of the abuse in order to cope. Denial, repression, suppression, rationalization, and even dissociation are mechanisms used by young victims to cope with this "no-win" situation. Sleep and eating disturbances, depression, aggression, an active fantasy life, poor impulse control, somatization, self destructive behaviors, running away, and truancy are common (Putnam and Trickett, 1993; Friedman, 1997).

The more severe the abuse, the more likely that repression will begin near puberty. If the sexual abuse continues through adolescence, repression is less likely. Repression normally lasts until victims are in their 20s or 30s and are having trouble with close relationships and parenting. (Some victims have repressed even longer, at least one victim for 50 years. She did not "remember" her own incestuous experiences from ages 8 to 10 until her 40-year-old daughter revealed that she had been a victim of her father during her childhood.)

Effects of Childhood Sexual Abuse on the Adolescent

As adolescents, sexual abuse victims show mostly overt methods of dysfunctional coping, such as impulsive acting out, violence toward others, self-destructive behaviors, self-mutilation, sleeping and eating disorders, suicide attempts, running away, truancy, delinquency, substance abuse, sexual acting out, prostitution, early pregnancy, and early marriage (Putnam and Trickett, 1993; Rew and Shirejian, 1993; Friedman, 1996; Rotheram-Borus, et al, 1996; Walker, Scott, and Koppersmith, 1998). Up to 70% of runaways report having been sexually abused, as do 61% of teenage mothers (Indiana Cares, 1993; Rotheram-Borus, et al, 1996). Adolescents may have fantasies of revenge and wish for the perpetrator's death. The anger toward the perpetrator and other adults (for not protecting them) approaches rage but is not directly expressed (Grinspoon, 1993b). Victims may not even be aware of the reason for their rage, shame, guilt, and confusion and may not realize that their acting-out behaviors are related to the abuse. Feelings of depersonalization, dissociation, regression, manipulation, impaired social skills, spiritual distress, thought and memory disturbances, self-neglect, aimlessness, and withdrawal are common (Rew and Shirejian, 1993). Sexual abuse survivors are more likely to be raped and battered in adolescence and later in life (Briere, et al, 1997).

Effects of Childhood Sexual Abuse on the Adult

For victims of childhood sexual abuse, the process of surviving childhood and adolescence and becoming an adult is similar to delayed PTSD. There is repression of memories (even nonsexual ones), followed by a breakthrough of unwanted, intrusive memories. The memories may begin as nightmares, kinesthetic sensations (such as flinching when touched by a partner in the same way as the perpetrator), or flashbacks. The memories may return gradually, in pieces, or in a sudden, overwhelming flood. Victims cannot be rushed to remember the abuse before they are ready to cope with it.

On the surface, adult victims may look relatively uninjured because of denial, dissociation, amnesia, emotional deadening, or repression. They enter counseling for manifestations of the abuse rather than for the incest or sexual abuse itself. The list of reactions in Box 38-4 can be used as a checklist to identify the issues to be addressed in counseling. Victims filling it out usually express amazement (that so much has resulted from the sexual abuse) and relief (that there is finally an explanation for all their "craziness"). Up to this point, victims tend to deny or minimize the relationship of the sexual abuse to any of their current problems. It becomes evident to them that it has disturbed their whole growth and development process, their self-esteem, and has set them up for other abusive relationships. Until counseling finally focuses on the underlying cause of their reactions, victims tend to seek treatment repeatedly without relief.

The inability to handle the memories of abuse and the painful emotions, especially anger, often induces thoughts of suicide: to escape the pain and depression; to "die with the secret"; to avoid conflict with the family and/or perpetrator; to stop feeling "crazy"; and to end the nightmares and flashbacks that are so frightening. Self-harm or mutilation is a common way of dealing with the emotional pain. Victims describe several patterns of their mutilation:

1. When emotions build up, they go numb and have to inflict pain to make sure they can still feel.
2. When they are feeling unreal, they draw blood to make sure they are alive.
3. They cause physical pain so they do not have to focus on the emotional pain.
4. They punish themselves when they are feeling guilty, ashamed, or fearful (about revealing "the secret").
5. The mutilation relieves the anger/rage (and produces a "high" in some instances).

Alcohol and drugs are often used to avoid or numb the pain and memories, and to bring fleeting pleasure that is otherwise elusive (Grinspoon, 1993b). Food may also provide brief pleasure or "fill an emptiness inside," but leads to feeling bloated, guilty, and a need to purge. Although sex is not usually enjoyable, it can bring relief from loneliness, temporary attention, affection, and approval. Healthy adult relationships are difficult due to problems in trusting anyone and the history of linking abuse and love. Victims have trouble setting limits with others and with asking for what they really need. They tend to be caretakers, rescuers, and codependents.

CLINICAL EXAMPLE

Thirty-year-old Jan Lester was admitted to a psychiatric unit as a result of suicidal ideations and 12 superficial cuts on her wrists. Nine months ago she began having nightmares about being awakened at night as a child with someone on top of her. During the nightmares, she would wake up crying with strange body sensations: gagging, pressure on her chest, and vaginal pain. As the nightmares and memories became more complete and vivid, she realized her father had frequently had sex with her while her mother was asleep. As her father's fiftieth birthday approached, she felt as if she could not tolerate going to his party. She wanted to be dead but could not force herself to cut her wrists more deeply. She wanted help.

Victims' reactions to the trauma (see Box 38-4) often get labeled as clinical symptoms. When an axis I diagnosis is given to patients, it is commonly depression (atypical type), PTSD, substance-abuse disorder, eating disorder, anxiety disorder, somatoform disorder, dissociative disorder (including dissociative identity disorder), or impulse-control disorder. Axis II personality disorders are commonly given, such as borderline, narcissistic, histrionic, avoidant, dependent, atypical, or mixed disorder (Putnam and Trickett, 1993; Briere, et al, 1997; Friedman, 1996; Sinason, 1994). Studies show that 20% to 50% of all psychiatric patients report childhood sexual abuse (Briere, et al, 1997; Boutcher and Gallop, 1996). Of those diagnosed with dissociative identity disorder, 88% to 97% report sexual abuse (Indiana Cares, 1993).

Receiving a diagnosis is a major problem, not only because of the stigma and "blaming the victim," but also because the diagnosis often becomes the focus of treatment rather than the underlying issue of recovering from the sexual abuse or incest. Lack of appropriate treatment carries a major risk not only for adult survivors, but also for their children, especially if the survivors are still in a stage of repression. There is evidence that untreated or

Box 38-4   Adult Manifestations of Childhood Sexual Abuse

Memory Disturbances
Amnesia about the abuse
Memory gaps about childhood
Inability to think straight

Keeping Unnecessary Secrets

Relationship Issues
"Trouble connecting" with others
"Running away" from others
Fear of men/fear of women
Trouble trusting others and their motives
Fear of intimacy
Fear of abandonment/rejection
Unable to maintain intimacy
Trouble giving/receiving affection
Feeling alienated from others
Fear of being used/abused
Trouble saying "no"
Taking care of others
Trouble with parenting
Entering abusive relationships
Poor choices of partners

Body Symptoms
Vague/transient pains
Memories of physical pain
Chronic pain/migraine headaches
Gagging/nausea/vomiting
Unpleasant sensation when touched
Negative/distorted body image
Self-conscious about body
Overly conscious of appearance

Anger Issues
Fear of expressing anger
Holding anger in
Crying instead of being angry
Fantasies of revenge
Feeling violent/full of rage
Fear of violence
Homicidal thoughts

Anxiety Issues
Easily startled
Inability to relax
Fear of being attacked/exposed
Hypervigilance
Feeling like a frightened child
Fear of the dark
Panic attacks
Phobias/agoraphobia

Addiction Issues
Alcohol/drug abuse or dependence
Compulsive spending

Intrusive Thoughts/Memories
Intense nightmares, unwanted thoughts
Flashbacks: feeling, seeing, smelling, tasting, hearing

Detachment Issues
Feeling numb/unreal
Disconnected from feelings/from body
Feeling as if there are "personalities" inside
"Out-of-body" experiences

Control Issues
Fear of authority/rules
Need to be in control/feeling out of control
Pretending to be out of control (or helpless)
Fear of being vulnerable
Ambivalent about being taken care of
Letting others be in control
Trying to control others
Allowing children to be abused

Identity Issues
Confusion about identity/roles
Negative self-image
Need to be perfect or perfectly bad
Underachievement/overachievement
Need to be totally competent

Sexual Issues
Concealing sexual feelings
Discomfort with sexual touching
Feeling nonsexual
Lack of orgasms/sexual dysfunctions
Confusion about sexuality/sexual identity
Feeling "dirty"
Trading sex for favors
Promiscuity/prostitution
Wondering if one is gay

Self-Punishment
Suicidal thoughts/attempts
Wanting to die/be dead
Self-mutilation
Compulsive eating/dieting
Binging/purging

Other Feelings
Low self-esteem/guilt/shame
Fear of feelings
Feeling stuck
Feeling like a failure
Chronic dissatisfaction
"Frozen" emotions
Lack of a sense of humor
Feeling inadequate
Feeling "walled in"
Feeling "crazy"

improperly treated victims occasionally set up dysfunctional, disorganized families who contribute to the incestuous abuse of their children. With their own denial, repression, amnesia, or other mechanisms, survivors have trouble relating to their partners and are unable to "see" the partners' involvement with their children. Perpetrators may sexually abuse their younger siblings, children, grandchildren, nieces, nephews, and others. There are examples of incest within three and four generations of a family. Breaking this cycle is crucial.

Recovery from Childhood Sexual Abuse

In some ways, recovery from childhood sexual abuse or incest is similar to recovery from all crimes or from PTSD, but it tends to be more complex, difficult, and lengthy. The memories and emotions are strong, painful, and confusing. The intense anger and ambivalence toward the perpetrator are hard for both the survivor and the nurse to handle. The survivor needs to know in the beginning that the symptoms and emotional pain will probably worsen before they improve as the review of experiences occurs. Although counseling often takes 2 years or more, survivors tend to engage in treatment sporadically. It is common for survivors to initially disclose, discuss, vent, and feel "cured." Then, as new crises or relationship problems emerge, they return to counseling to deal with each issue and its possible connection to the original trauma. It is sometimes difficult to get a patient to commit to continuous, long-term counseling, but the nurse can emphasize the desirability and value of at least sporadic counseling.

The overall goals of recovery are improved self-esteem and self-acceptance, forgiveness of self, adaptive coping with life and its stresses, the capacity for intimate relationships and genuine sexual pleasure, improvements in mood, and reduced anxiety and fear.

Psychotherapeutic Management

Nurse-Patient Relationship.   Much depends on the nurse's ability to quickly develop a trusting relationship with the survivor. Empathy, active support, compassion, warmth, and being nonjudgmental are crucial.

Survivors need to be calmly and matter-of-factly asked about childhood sexual abuse because they are not likely to reveal it spontaneously. The old coercions to "keep the secret" remain strong in the minds of survivors. They need to feel safe about confidentiality and the nurse's acceptance before disclosure will occur. How much detail is revealed and how soon depends in part on the nurse's ability to be receptive to the experiences *without* being critical of the perpetrator, of other adults in the family, or of the survivor's loyalty to them. The survivor needs to be reassured that all the experiences and emotions (positive, negative, and ambivalent) are valid and that exploring these is the *beginning* of the process of working through recovery (Courtois, 1988). It is usually helpful for survivors to be reminded periodically that they were not responsible for and did not deserve the sexual abuse, are not to be blamed, were not in control of the situation, and that the way they coped with it in the past was the best they could do at the time (Courtois, 1988). Education about the dynamics of sexual abuse and reassurances about recovery can be useful in correcting faulty perceptions about the abuse, decreasing self-blame and guilt, and instilling hope for the future despite the inability to change the past. Nursing interventions for survivors are listed in the box on p. 602.

Mentally and emotionally reexperiencing traumatic experiences is disturbing; only periodic small doses may be tolerable. The nurse and survivors can monitor their tolerance of the process so that they do not become overwhelmed and retreat. Anger-release strategies, such as using a batacca (foam bat) while talking to a chair that represents the perpetrator, often help the survivor express thoughts and feelings that could not be expressed in childhood. Play therapy, therapeutic stories, and art therapy can be especially useful in helping children process their abuse (Bennett, 1997; Hinds, 1997). Writing memories and feelings in a journal can also be useful, as can writing letters to the perpetrator and others that will not be sent.

Confrontation of the family or perpetrator by the survivor is not necessarily a desired outcome. This may be done symbolically with the nurse rather than directly with the perpetrator and other family members. If survivors choose to confront directly, much preparation is needed, even rehearsals with the nurse before the event. They need to consider, plan for, and rehearse their reactions to all the potential responses of family members. The most typical responses are denial, rationalization,

Key Nursing Interventions for Survivors of Childhood Sexual Abuse

- Establish a trusting and supportive environment.
- Accept all feelings and reactions as normal responses.
- Ask permission before touching survivors.
- Reinforce that recovery is possible, even if it is difficult.
- Educate about the dynamics of abuse and recovery processes.
- Assist survivors in understanding current behaviors as reflections of survival strategies used in childhood.
- Facilitate reevaluation of the sexual abuse, its circumstances, and its effects, but without pressuring.
- Encourage coping choices that are in survivors' best interests.
- Discuss safeguarding other children if the perpetrator still poses a risk.
- Support choices about future disclosures, confrontation, or reporting.
- Be aware that family members and others may feel split loyalty and engage in dysfunctional roles and interaction patterns.
- Decrease feelings of isolation, shame, and stigma.
- Encourage self-acceptance.
- Facilitate acknowledgment, forgiveness, and love for the "child within."
- Teach and encourage stress management and anger reduction.
- Facilitate the transfer of responsibility and anger to the perpetrator but set limits on acting out fantasies of revenge.
- Foster separation and individuation from the family and its patterns.
- Help to find meaning in the experience and mourning of all the losses (grieving is a very painful experience).
- Facilitate the change from victim to survivor status (reexperiencing and integrating the positive, negative, and ambivalent feelings and memories).
- Facilitate reexperiencing and reworking of maturation tasks that were missed or experienced prematurely.
- Educate about life skills, communication skills, coping skills, assertiveness, decision making, conflict resolution, boundary setting, friendship, intimacy, sexuality, and parenting.
- Refer to outpatient counseling and appropriate support groups.

and "blaming the victim." (See Family Issues box.) Survivors can be helped to debate the benefits and risks of confrontation, as well as the degree and type of contact they want to have with the family, even if they do not confront them. An important consideration for the nurse and the survivor to discuss is the mandatory reporting of child abuse if younger children are victims of abuse. Such a report is understandably difficult for both the nurse and the survivor and needs to be carefully but directly addressed.

When survivors are in outpatient counseling, it is important to consider priorities in each counseling session. Current crises and problems need to be addressed (instead of the sexual abuse) as these arise. This is critical for self-destructive behaviors that are heightened because of counseling, such as suicidal ideation, self-mutilation, and substance abuse. Hospitalization may be necessary if the crisis is severe. Although survivors view recovery as frightening and painful, they also experience relief that they are making progress.

Psychopharmacology. Medications are not always needed or desirable for adult survivors of childhood sexual abuse, especially if substance abuse is a problem or potential problem. For the small number of survivors with serious psychopathology, medications should be given according to the axis I diagnosis. Benzodiazepines may be given on a prn basis to help control the emotional or autonomic arousal that occurs during the reexperiencing of traumatic memories. Antidepressants may be used if the depressive symptoms are interfering with functioning and sleep. Occasionally, low doses of thioridazine (Mellaril) are given for persistent and severely disturbing nightmares or flashbacks.

Milieu Management. On an outpatient basis and during any brief hospitalizations, groups can be a useful adjunct to nursing care. If available, a short-term or ongoing sexual abuse/incest recovery group is beneficial. Some self-help groups are Incest Survivors Anonymous, Survivors of Sexual

FAMILY ISSUES

False Memories? False Allegations?

There are families, including members of the False Memory Syndrome Foundation, who claim they have been wrongly accused of sexual abuse by their children or adult children. These families and some professionals especially challenge the validity of the processes of repression and delayed recovery of memories of abuse. They warn that those who interview children, those who counsel children and adults, and members of support groups can implant false memories and provide support for false allegations. These families and professionals question the credentials and training of many who counsel children and adults who claim they were abused. They cite studies of recent and long-term memory to support their views about distorted and false memories. They sometimes question the claims of serious emotional damage to victims as a result of actual sexual abuse. They support the premise that false memories and false allegations are destroying the families of these children.

Other professionals and adult survivors of childhood sexual abuse maintain that the graphic details of children's traumatic memories and the use of sexual descriptions, very advanced for their ages at the time, support the credibility of the abuse charges. These professionals and survivors claim that denial, repression, amnesia, and dissociation are real phenomena used by children, adolescents, and adults to protect themselves emotionally from the abuse as it was happening and from the later realization of its moral, legal, ethical, and emotional significance. These individuals maintain that 75% or more of survivors are able to collect strong corroborating evidence of their abuse and recovered memories. They cite recent neurochemical studies of traumatic memory processes, stress, and PTSD (see Chapter 29) to support their view of the validity of repression, dissociation, and recovered memories. They acknowledge that 2% to 10% of claims of sexual abuse by children and divorcing parents may be false, and then report that perhaps 75% to 90% of valid child abuse is *never* reported by children, agencies, and professionals. They point out that the False Memory Syndrome Foundation admits that it collects only information on denials of charges of abuse, but that it has no way of knowing if these denials are true or false. Survivors and professionals contend that those who molest children *typically* threaten the victims to "keep the secret" and use denial, minimization, and rationalization when charged with abuse. They also express concern that claims of false memories and false allegations are efforts to disconfirm and "blame the victim," protect abusers (and society), and minimize the severity of the short- and long-term effects of abuse. They contend that families are being destroyed by intrafamilial violence (not the reports of abuse) and that abused children suffer emotional pain and a wide variety of problems throughout childhood, adolescence, and adulthood.

As a result of this controversy, it is recommended that those working with possible survivors of childhood sexual abuse do the following:

1. Allow patients' memories to emerge without pressure and "leading" questions.
2. Avoid specific sexual abuse explanations for patients' symptoms.
3. Follow established guidelines for interviewing child victims and others to assess credibility of memories and testimony.
4. Interview anyone who might provide corroboration or disconfirming evidence.
5. Use established therapeutic techniques rather than nonestablished ones.
6. Avoid using hypnosis and sodium amytal injections as a way of recovering repressed memories.

Adapted from Gardner RA: *True and false accusations of child sex abuse,* New York, 1992, Creative Therapeutics; Grinspoon L: Child abuse: part III, *Harvard Mental Health Letter* 10(1):1, 1993c; Lotto D: On witches and witch hunts: ritual and satanic cult abuse, *J Psychohistory* 21(4):373, 1994; Rockwell RB: One psychiatrist's view of satanic ritual abuse, *J Psychohistory* 21(4):443, 1994; Bloom SL: Hearing the survivor's voice: sundering the wall of denial, *J Psychohistory* 21(4):461, 1994; Victor, JS: How should stories about satanic cult abuse be understood?, *Harvard Mental Health Letter* 12(8):8, 1996; Lego S: Repressed memory and false memory, *Arch Psychiatr Nurs* 10(2):110, 1996; Hall JM: Delayed recall of childhood sexual abuse: psychiatric nursing's responsibilities to clients, *Arch Psychiatr Nurs* 10(6):342, 1996.

Abuse, and Daughters and Sons United. Parents United for the nonperpetrator parent can be suggested if appropriate. The perpetrator may also be referred to counseling. Family therapy is sometimes appropriate.

Other groups that may be recommended, depending on the symptoms and needs of the survivor, are Codependency Anonymous, Adult Children of Alcoholics, Alcoholics or Narcotics Anonymous, and Emotions Anonymous. Survivors may also be directed to classes or short-term groups on decision making or problem solving, communication or relationship skills, conflict resolution, parenting skills, and human sexuality.

■ Critical Thinking Question

You are working with a patient who was sexually abused as a child by her father. The father insists on visiting her and telling you about her history of emotional problems and lying about the family. What is your approach in working with the father?

VICTIMS OF PARTNER ABUSE

Nature of the Problem

An estimated one third of women each year in the United States suffer from repeated physical abuse by a partner (Farrell, 1996). The number is even higher when psychological abuse and other violations of rights are considered (Figure 38-1). More than 95% of this abuse is by a man toward a woman (Hattendorf and Tollerud, 1997). Every few seconds a woman is abused, raped, tortured, or beaten by her husband, lover, ex-husband, or estranged husband or lover, and most of this abuse goes unreported even when injuries are severe enough to require treatment. In 22% to 35% of women's visits to emergency rooms there are domestic violence injuries (Shea, Mahoney, and Lacy, 1997).

Partner-abuse victims tend to conceal their victimization. They are acutely aware that disclosure of their plight will be met with denial or minimization by the partner, friends, and relatives and by increased abuse by their partners. When a woman becomes pregnant or more independent (both emotionally and financially), the incidence of violence by a partner increases as well (Hattendorf and Tollerud, 1997; Henderson, 1998). The fact that 30% to 75% of all women killed in the United States are killed by a husband, boyfriend, ex-husband, or estranged husband or lover supports women's fears (Constantine and Bricker, 1997). Women also kill their partners, but most of the time it is in self-defense after a history of beatings.

Studies show that partner abuse crosses all social, racial, cultural, and economic classes, including both homosexual and heterosexual relationships, but is more often officially reported in the lower socioeconomic class. This is because the victims

are more likely to be in contact with reporting agencies such as public health nursing, welfare offices, public clinics, and emergency rooms (Campbell and Humphreys, 1993).

The relationship of alcohol and drug abuse to violent behavior has been the subject of many studies on partner abuse. Some abusers are abstainers, but more are substance abusers. The current view is that abusers use alcohol and drugs as an excuse for their violence and drink when they are about to become violent (Gage, 1991; Abstracts, 1997). There seems to be a correlation between alcohol/drugs and the severity of violence. The combination of substance abuse and violence encourages victims to blame the substance rather than to hold the batterers accountable for their violent behaviors. Women often describe their abusers as "Dr. Jekyll and Mr. Hyde," with changing personalities: gentle, loving, and kind at times; rude, uncaring, and violent at others. This change is in part explained by the cycle of violence described later.

In some relationships, violence is mutual (but not necessarily equal) and is the result of efforts to resolve escalating conflicts combined with poor impulse control. These couples are often motivated to change and can be taught more effective skills for handling conflict and anger (Gage, 1991). This mutual-violence pattern differs from, but can become, the more common pattern of using violence to exploit and control a partner. The second pattern almost always involves a man abusing a woman, and the man has little motivation to change (Gage, 1991).

The nature of modern society is a factor to be considered in partner abuse. The portrayal of physical and sexual violence in the media (television, music videos, films) is increasing in frequency and severity. Women are still portrayed by the media as second-class citizens at times. In addition, it is well documented that witnesses of family violence and victims of child abuse tend to become the abusers and partners of abusers in the next generation (Downs, Smyth, and Miller, 1996; Hattendorf and Tollerud, 1997).

Effects of Partner Abuse

Learned helplessness

The concept of *learned helplessness* (as originally applied by Walker, 1979) is useful in understanding the dynamics of partner abuse (Hattendorf and Tollerud,

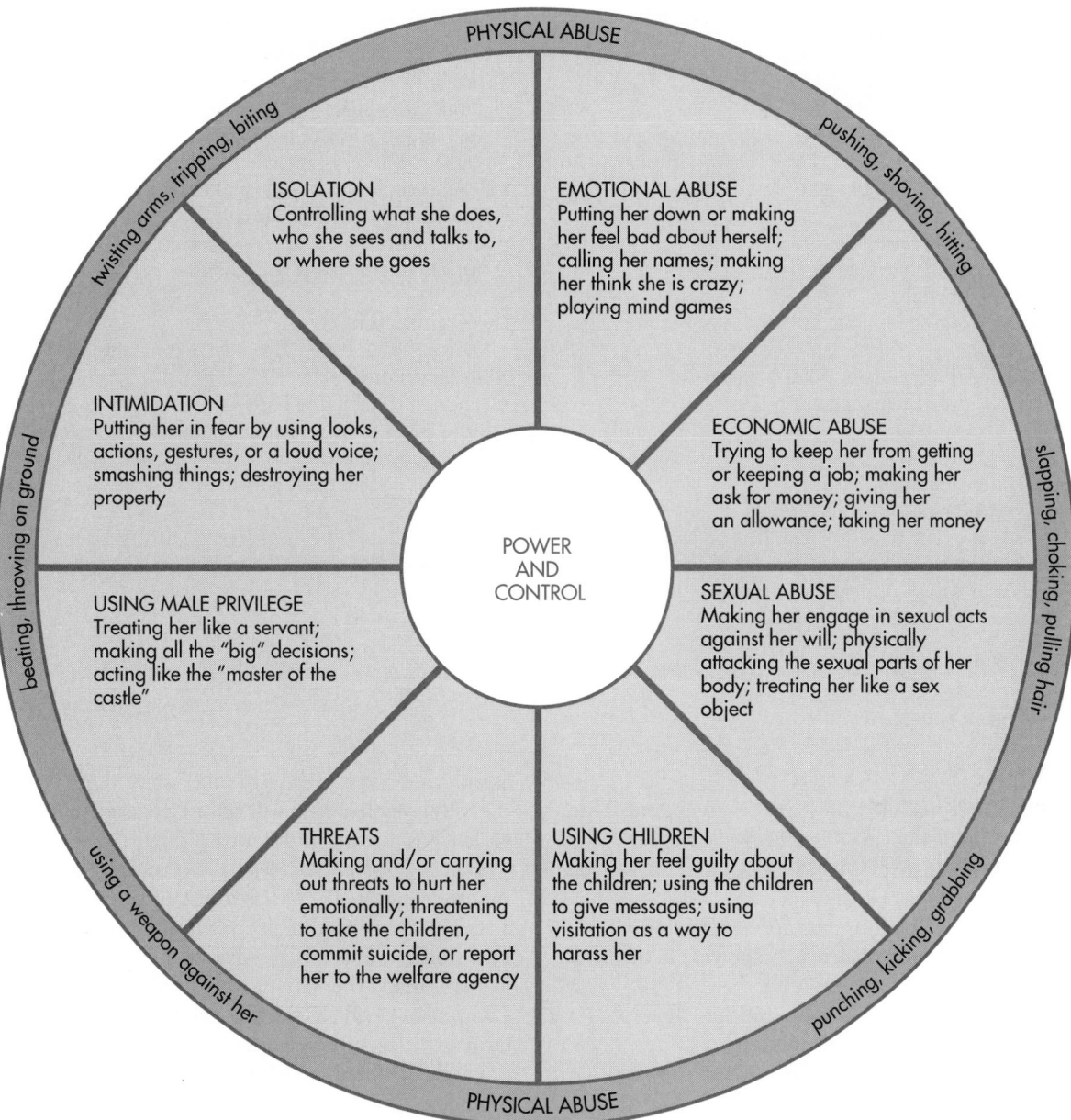

FIGURE 38-1 The desire for power and control results in both psychological and physical abuse. (From *Power and control*, Duluth, Minn, 1987, Domestic Abuse Intervention Project.)

1997). Three of the necessary conditions for learned helplessness are certainly present in partner abuse:
1. The victim's behavior is not related to the cause of the beatings.
2. The victim has no control over preventing or stopping the beatings.
3. The victim sees little hope of escaping because of the threats of increased harm.

Most experts acknowledge the development of learned helplessness, hopelessness, isolation, and resignation in response to ongoing emotional and physical abuse. Abused women do *not* report that they enjoy the abuse, but they do have a tendency to believe their partner's view that they deserve the abuse. Box 38-5 presents common reasons why women endure long-term abuse.

Box 38-5 Why Women Stay as Long as They Do

Situational Factors
- Economic dependence
- Fear of greater physical danger to themselves and their children if they attempt to leave or have partner arrested
- Fear of emotional damage to children because of being without a father
- Fear of losing custody of children
- Lack of alternative housing
- Lack of job skills
- Social isolation resulting in lack of support from family or friends
- Lack of information regarding alternatives
- Fear of involvement in court processes
- Fear of retaliation from partner or partner's family

Emotional Factors
- Poor self-image
- Being in a state of denial, and living a "secret"
- Fear of loneliness
- Personal embarrassment and protecting the image of husband and family

- Insecurity over potential independence and lack of emotional support
- Guilt about failure of marriage or relationship
- Fear that partner is not able to survive alone
- Belief that partner is "sick" and needs her help
- Belief that partner will change
- Ambivalence and fear over making formidable life changes and increased responsibility

Cultural Factors
- Knowing batterers are not held accountable for their violent actions
- Believing the abuse is her fault
- Being raised to be passive and submissive
- Developing survival skills instead of escape skills
- Recognizing that the legal system is a male-dominated system

Plus: She Still Loves Him

Adapted from Sojourner Shelter, Indianapolis, Ind., and Task Force on Families in Crisis, Box 120495, Nashville, TN, 37212.

Cycle of violence

Another accepted view of why women endure abuse was also originally described by Walker (1979). The cycle of violence (Table 38-1) documents several principles:

1. Abuse is not constant, nor is it random.
2. There is an imbalance of power in the relationship.
3. Abuse occurs in a cycle and has three phases that vary in time and intensity.
4. The last stage ("honeymoon") is the one that convinces the woman that she should stay in the relationship.

It is during this last stage that the "good side" of the men is evident and the women are reminded of their love and the happy potential of the relationship. Women report feeling as if they want to and can help their partners overcome their problems and violent behaviors.

There is still a shortage of safe places for victims, especially women, to go, as well as a shortage of services to help them become independent. Many states still have outdated laws that indirectly perpetuate abuse rather than foster arrest of the abuser for

assault and battery. Arrest is the major (and maybe the only) way batterers will get the message that their violence is a crime and not their "right."

Battered woman syndrome is being suggested as a subclassification of PTSD because repetitive abuse is a serious threat to the victim's health and life. Various studies report that 45% to 84% of battered women meet the criteria for PTSD (Woods and Campbell, 1993). Victims often report nightmares, flashbacks, recurrent fears of more violence, emotional detachment, numbness, startle response, sleep problems, impaired concentration, and hypervigilance (Woods and Campbell, 1993). Other symptoms of battered woman syndrome are not addressed by the PTSD criteria, such as depression, low self-esteem, physical symptoms, and self-blame. However, as with PTSD, battered women show typical reactions to a chronic trauma, not symptoms of psychopathology. Labeling and blaming the victims again shifts responsibility away from the perpetrators.

Other individuals and agencies need to stop their indirect perpetuation of partner abuse as indicated in Box 38-6. It is unlikely that an abused woman will leave her partner until she realizes that the cycle is

Table 38-1   Cycle of Violence

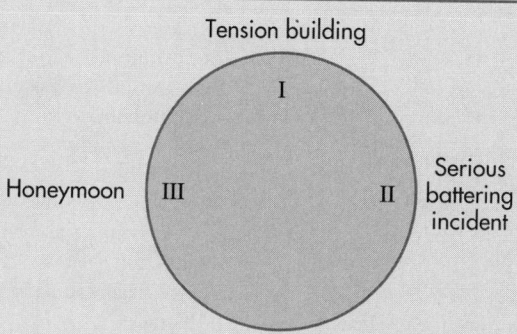

Man	Woman
I. Tension Building	
He has excessively high expectations of her.	She is nurturing, compliant, and tries to please him.
He blames her for anything that goes wrong.	She denies the seriousness of their problems.
He does not try to control his behaviors.	She feels she can control his behaviors.
He is aware of his inappropriate behaviors but does not admit it.	She tries to alter his behavior to stay safe.
Verbal and minor physical abuse increase.	She tries to prevent his anger.
Afraid she will leave, he gets more possessive to keep her captive.	She blames external factors: alcohol, work.
He gets frantic and more controlling.	She takes minor abuse, but does not feel she deserves it.
He misinterprets her withdrawal as rejection.	She gets scared and tries to hide (withdrawal).
	She may call for help as the tension becomes unbearable.
II. Serious Battering Incident	
The trigger event is an internal or external event or substance.	In cases of long-term battering, she may provoke it just to get it over with.
The battering usually occurs in private.	She may call for help if she is afraid of being killed.
He will threaten more harm if she tries to get help (police, medical).	Her initial reaction is shock, disbelief, and denial.
He tries to justify his behaviors but does not understand what happens.	Fearing more abuse if police come, she may plead for them not to arrest him.
He minimizes the severity of the abuse.	She is anxious, ashamed, humiliated, sleepless, fatigued, depressed.
His stress is relieved.	She does not seek help for injuries for a day or more and lies about the cause of injuries.
III. Honeymoon	
He is loving, charming, begging for forgiveness, making promises.	She sees his loving behaviors as the real person and tries to make up.
He truly believes he will never abuse again.	She wants to believe the abuse will never happen again.
He feels that he taught her a lesson and she will not "act up" again.	She feels that if she stays, he will get help; the thought of leaving makes her feel guilty.
He preys on her guilt to keep her trapped.	She believes in the permanency of the relationship and gets trapped.

Adapted from Walker L: *The battered woman,* New York, 1979, Harper & Row.

Box 38-6   **Individual and Agency Perpetuation of Battering**

These are examples of what institutions or agencies have been known to say or do to reinforce the abuser's message that the woman is to blame for his violence.

Family
Ignores her or does not pick up on cues
Does not ask about injuries or bruises
If told, says "What did you do to cause it?"
Says, "You've made your bed, now lie in it" or "Just try harder"
Tell her she's crazy or enjoys it

Church/Place of Worship
Does not ask her about bruises or unusual absences
If told, says "It's a test from God" or "Scripture allows and sanctions it"
Tells her to "Pray harder"
Tells her to try harder to be a better wife
Attempts marital counseling only

Law Enforcement
Police choose not to respond to a domestic call
On the scene, treat it as a private "family matter"
Only warn the abuser or advise marriage counseling
Fail to take a report or transport her to safety

Mental Health Counselors
Do not routinely ask about violence
If mentioned, do not treat it first or treat it as a symptom
Ask, "What did you do to make him hit you?"
Agree with man that she is a little "crazy" or "bitchy," and that she must change first
Ask her what she could have done to deescalate the situation
Do marriage counseling, implying that she is equally to blame
Hospitalize her in a mental facility

Medical
Ignores violence and treats injuries only
Does not routinely ask how injury occurred or accepts phony stories
If told, does nothing; does not take photographs or document the incident
Prescribes medicine at three times the rate for nonbattered women

Adapted from Sojourner Shelter, PO Box 88062, Indianapolis, IN 46208.

---

not going to stop, that she has the emotional support to leave, and that she has a safe place to go. Fearing that the next beating may be fatal, finding that her partner is also physically or sexually abusing her children, and realizing that her children are learning to be abusive are incentives for leaving permanently (Ulrich, 1991).

Recovery from Partner Abuse

Immediately preceding or at the beginning of a serious battering incident, the victim is frightened and amenable to crisis intervention and is more likely to call the police or a crisis service phone line for help. Getting her and her children to a shelter or other safe place (if she will go) is desirable when she is in immediate danger of injury. If she is already injured, she should be encouraged to go to an emergency room. In either case, crisis workers, shelter workers, or nurses can begin the important process of assessment and giving information that can make a dent

in the cycle of abuse. Even if the woman is not yet ready to leave her partner, she can be given an easily concealed wallet-size card with telephone numbers of police, a prosecutor, crisis services, victims' assistance, shelters, support groups, and perhaps a short message about the inevitability of the cycle of violence and the fact that no one deserves to be abused. If contact is only by phone, or if she is worried that the abuser will find the card, she can be asked to write down the phone numbers on the back of a picture in her wallet, for example. She can also be given ideas for developing a safety/escape plan, such as packing a bag with spare clothes, money, and important papers. She should be informed of the protections afforded by legal statutes, protective orders, and the newer antistalking laws.

Long-term goals for survivors of partner abuse are to develop self-confidence, self-respect, independence, healthy support systems, and a sense of freedom, safety, and empowerment.

Box 38-7 Common Cues to Partner Abuse

- Repeated, vague symptoms/illnesses that are not confirmed by tests, such as backache, abdominal pain, indigestion, headaches, hyperventilation, anxiety, insomnia, fatigue, anorexia, heart palpitations
- Unexplained injuries or ones with unlikely explanations and embarrassment about them
- Hidden injuries such as those in areas concealed by clothes or visible on physical or x-ray examination only; for example, head and neck injuries, internal injuries, genital injuries, scars, burns, joint pain or dislocations, numbness, hearing problems, or bald spots
- Injuries with recognizable marks such as those from a belt, iron, raised ring, teeth, fingertips, cigarette, gun, or knife
- Multiple fractures or bruises in various stages of healing
- Jumpiness or flinching in the presence of the abuser
- Substance abuse and suicidal thoughts or attempts

- Attempts to conceal fear of the partner
- Continual efforts to keep partner from getting angry
- Denial of any problems in the relationship
- Lack of relationships with family or friends
- Isolation or confinement to home
- Guilt, depression, anxiety, low self-esteem, sense of failure, concealed anger
- Continual justification of own actions and whereabouts to partner
- Continual justification of the abuser's actions in public; excusing or rationalizing the behaviors
- Believing in family unity at all costs and in traditional stereotypes
- Believing in managing alone, even when help is offered
- An oversolicitous partner who does not want to leave the victim alone with hospital or agency staff or even with family and friends

Adapted from Jezierski M: Guidelines for intervention by ED nurses in cases of domestic abuse, *J Emerg Nurs* 18(1):28a, 1992; Sheridan DJ: The role of the battered woman specialist, *J Psychosoc Nurs Ment Health Serv* 31(11):31, 1993; Constantine RE and Bricker PL: Social support, stress, and depression among battered women in the judicial setting, *J Am Psychiatr Nurses Assoc* 3(3):81, 1997.

Psychotherapeutic Management

Nurse-Patient Relationship. Because 80% of abused women seek help for their injuries at least once (Campbell and Humphreys, 1993), nurses can be instrumental in offering information and assistance. Nurses in emergency rooms, clinics, doctors' offices, and community health agencies particularly need to know how to recognize a victim, make an assessment, and refer victims to available services. Some common cues to abuse are listed in Box 38-7. The assessment process is often difficult because victims fear disclosure, are embarrassed about the situation, desire to be treated quickly and leave, and sometimes the abuser is present. It is important to interview the victim privately and with sensitivity, empathy, and compassion. Box 38-8 describes other responses that abused women consider to be helpful.

Each hospital or agency has its own assessment tool. The most crucial information to document in an initial contact is the following:

1. Length and frequency of abuse
2. Types of abuse (physical, psychological, sexual, financial) and use of weapons
3. Types and locations of injuries (can be written descriptions, but photographs and body maps are preferred)

Box 38-8 Helpful Responses to Partner Abuse

- Be nonjudgmental, objective, and nonthreatening.
- Ask directly if abuse is occurring.
- Identify the abuser's behavior as abusive.
- Acknowledge the seriousness of the abuse.
- Assist the victim to assess internal strengths.
- Encourage use of personal resources.
- Give the victim a list of resources: shelters, financial aid, police, and legal assistance.
- Allow victim to choose own options.
- Offer names of relevant support groups.
- Help victim to develop a safety/escape plan.
- Tell the abuser to stop the abuse and get help.
- Do not disbelieve or blame the victim.
- Do not get angry with the victim.
- Do not refuse to help if the victim is not ready to leave the abuser.
- Do not align with the abuser against the victim.
- Do not push the victim to leave the abuser before ready.

Adapted from Jezierski M: Guidelines for intervention by ED nurses in cases of domestic abuse, *J Emerg Nurs* 18(1):28a, 1992; Limandri BJ: The therapeutic relationship with abused women, *J Psychosoc Nurs Ment Health Serv* 25(2):9, 1987; Sheridan DJ: The role of the battered woman specialist, *J Psychosoc Nurs Ment Health Serv* 31(11):31, 1993; Shea CA, Mahoney M, and Lacy JM: Breaking through the barriers to domestic violence interventions, *Am J Nurs* 97(6):26, 1997.

4. Duration of episodes of abuse
5. Use and abuse of substances and medications by victim and abuser
6. Current location of abuser
7. Location and safety of children
8. Types of service desired (police, legal, shelter, crisis counseling, social service agencies, transportation)
9. Referrals made

Even if the initial contact is brief, it is important to convey to victims that they are not alone in their abuse and that there are those willing to help *when the victims are ready.* They also need to be told more than once that they do not cause and do not deserve the abuse. The nurse must convey to victims that they are important and have

dignity and worth. Victims need acknowledgment of their mental and physical exhaustion, fears, ambivalence about the abusers and leaving, and their wish to help the abuser as well as themselves. It is difficult for the nurse (and all professionals) to accept that victims cannot be pushed, rushed, or coerced into leaving the abuser before they are ready. In fact, the victim may want to try couples counseling and even personal counseling (when the abuser refuses to go to counseling) more than once before "giving up hope" of saving the relationship and of helping the one she loves. It is important to recognize and to acknowledge that it is common for abused women to leave and return several times. She need not feel guilty or ashamed for trying to improve the relationship. In fact, the

Case Study

Rachael Benton, a 26-year-old survivor of incest by her father, is married to Richard. She has an 8-year-old child, Matthew; Richard has three boys, Robert, James, and Daniel, ages 11, 8, and 7, who live with them. Angela, age 5, was born after Rachael and Richard were married. Another child, Andrew, was born stillborn 2 years ago. Matthew was removed from the home after being abused by Robert. Rachael sought help by attending a battered women's group.

Rachael's situation was difficult to resolve. Because of heavy drinking, Richard was missing work and changing jobs. His income declined and was sporadic but expenses did not decline. Without insurance, the stillbirth, a bilateral myringotomy for Daniel, and Rachael's repeated treatment of chronic colds, menstrual irregularities, back pain, severe headaches, and diarrhea were not paid for. She avoided treatment for bruises, a superficial knife wound, head cuts, and contusions. Rachael is convinced Andrew died because Richard repeatedly punched her stomach during the pregnancy.

It was when Richard raped her that Rachael believed there was no hope of change and that she had to leave (9 months after the group began). As Rachael became more assertive and independent, Richard demanded that she stay home, bought a shotgun to convince her to stay, and took the starter off the car. He rode to work with co-workers. Rachael had not adopted Richard's boys, so she could not take them with her. She was afraid that his verbal abuse of them would turn to physical violence when she left. Richard knew about all the places she thought of going.

It took 4 months to develop, coordinate, and implement arrangements so that Rachael and Angela were safe in leaving Richard. Neighbors, friends, and teachers were warned of the potential abuse of the boys and given the phone number for anonymously reporting child abuse. Rachael's mother rented her a small trailer in a rural town and obtained forms for Aid to Families with Dependent Children. Rachael secretly and gradually packed clothes and important documents in the trunk of a new friend's car.

One night (14 months after the group began) Richard got drunk, beat Rachael, and tried to rape her again. She fought him off and waited until he passed out. Her friend with the packed car drove her to the new trailer. As expected, Richard got his shotgun and went to every friend of Rachael's, but none knew where she was. He did not know the new friend. He drove to Rachael's mother's home, and she called the sheriff when his car pulled into the driveway. Richard was escorted out of the county and warned not to return. Within a week, Daniel's teacher filed a child abuse report about bruises found on him. Within 2 weeks, the boys were removed from the home and returned to their natural mother.

Rachael has received proper medical treatment and feels healthier. She is now divorced, going through a job-training program, and maintaining her secret location. She feels safe but is still in counseling once a month to complete her emotional recovery. She attends a support group for battered women once a week.

guilt of leaving will be lessened if she feels she has "tried everything" and finally is able to acknowledge that nothing will change because he is the only one who can control the violence and stop the abuse.

When the abused woman does leave her partner, the problems are not over. "If You Have Left an Abusive Man" (Box 38-9) describes some of the common reactions the abuser may have and ways he may behave. Survivors frequently need longer-term counseling and social services to recover and become independent, especially if the abuser is unwilling to participate in couples counseling or an abusers' program (often a court-ordered program

---

Care Plan

NAME: Rachael Benton   **ADMISSION DATE:** _____

DSM-IV DIAGNOSIS: None _____

ASSESSMENT: **Areas of strength:** Bright, articulate, and capable of problem solving; mother and one friend willing to help; developing trust in group and beginning to process her feelings and rights.

Problems: Lack of safe housing and employment; inability to remove husband's children from the house and fear he will abuse them; fear of increased abuse of her, even death, if she tries to leave; severe headaches.

DIAGNOSES:
- Decisional conflict related to dysfunctional marriage as evidenced by attendance in a battered women's support group.
- Posttrauma response related to physical, emotional, and economic abuse as evidenced by physical wounds, fear, and emotional trauma.
- Fear of leaving husband related to potential abuse of sons as evidenced by reluctance to leave without stepsons.

OUTCOMES: **Short-term goals:**   Date met
- Patient will remove bullets from gun; design an escape plan.   _____
- Patient will verbalize ability to survive on her own; confirm housing in
  rural county.   _____

Long-term goals:
- Patient will enroll in job-training program.   _____
- Patient will obtain legal assistance for divorce.   _____
- Patient will seek medical treatment for chronic problems.   _____

PLANNING/ INTERVENTIONS: **Nurse-patient relationship:** Listen nonjudgmentally and empathically; accept "strange" behaviors related to secrecy and self-protection; avoid disparaging spouse and pressuring to leave; locate resources for training, finances, counseling, and medical care in rural country.

Psychopharmacology: Desyrel, 50 mg at bedtime, to alleviate moderate depression and to improve sleep. Tylenol No. 3 prn for severe headaches.

Milieu management: Encourage continuing in local support group; locate support group in rural county; continue assessment of safety of patient and children.

EVALUATION: Patient has moved to rural county and joined support group; is receiving counseling and medical care. Husband's children were removed and placed with natural mother.

REFERRALS: Has an appointment with a job-training program in the rural county.

Box 38-9   If You Have Left an Abusive Man . . .

1. Your problems are not over.
2. Your abuser will try to locate you through family and friends. He will play on their sympathy or intimidate them.
3. He will repeatedly apologize, make promises about changing, and give gifts.
4. Next he will threaten or intimidate you, your children, family, and/or friends.
5. He may threaten to kill himself because of you.
6. He often threatens to take your children away.
7. Another step is entering counseling and/or expressing religious fervor.
8. He may try to find a counselor or religious leader to try to convince you to return to him.
9. Next may come harassment and stalking (begging, crying, phone calls, written/verbal threats, legal actions, and/or following you from location to location).

Regardless of his tactics, take advantage of legal, community, and personal resources to protect yourself and your children.

Adapted from the Salvation Army Domestic Violence Program, Indianapolis, Ind.

of group education and counseling lasting 26 weeks or more). Nursing interventions for survivors (individually or in groups) generally focus on the following:

1. Reiterating information about abuse, the cycle of violence, and the abuser's accountability
2. Building self-esteem and confidence
3. Sharing of feelings, especially anger, frustration, fear, and anxiety
4. Decreasing shame, guilt, embarrassment, manipulation, and isolation
5. Confirming personal rights as well as legal rights
6. Teaching stress reduction or management techniques
7. Teaching communication techniques
8. Teaching conflict-resolution techniques
9. Teaching assertiveness training
10. Teaching parenting techniques
11. Decreasing codependency behaviors
12. Building a new, improved support system
13. Setting goals, specific planning for immediate future
14. Resolving grief

Referrals may also be needed for job counseling or training, legal assistance, financial aid, and permanent housing. At any stage of working with survivors, brief hospitalization may be needed because of injuries, suicide attempts, or substance abuse, and for treatment of serious problems such as depression, anxiety, or panic attacks.

Psychopharmacology. Medications normally are not needed but commonly are given to survivors. Often *mis*prescribed medications are antidepressants, benzodiazepines, and hypnotics. These same medications may be used appropriately if the survivor's symptoms of depression, anxiety, sleeplessness, or nightmares are severe. Continual assessment is needed to determine when medications are no longer needed to prevent abuse and addiction.

Milieu Management. Groups in inpatient or outpatient settings that may be relevant for survivors are those focusing on self-esteem, problem solving, assertiveness, relationship issues, stress management, and codependency. Substance-abuse groups should be recommended if necessary. In the community, a group for abused women is desirable. Two such groups are Turning Point and Breaking Free.

■ Critical Thinking Question

Your co-worker is sharing with you that she is thinking about leaving her husband because of his drinking and long-term emotional abuse of her. She expresses a fear that he might try to kill her and a fear of raising her two children alone. What information would you offer her?

▼ Key Concepts

1. Not all crimes involve physical violence and injury; however, all crimes involve *emotional* violation and injury. Victims lose a sense of the ability to control their own lives, as well as losing trust in others.
2. Progression through the stages of recovery from a crime may take years. Crisis intervention and group meetings with other victims can facilitate recovery.

3. In assisting victims, sensitivity to their needs is crucial in order to build trust and to avoid "blaming the victim."
4. Information about counseling resources and support groups can be given to the victims of rape and partner abuse for later use, even if there is an initial denial of the need for help.
5. Adult survivors of childhood sexual abuse may repress the memories for years as a result of the emotional turmoil and sense of being betrayed by the abuser and others.
6. Adult survivors of childhood sexual abuse typically enter counseling for a variety of overt problems, unaware of how these are related to childhood trauma.
7. The reexperiencing and working through of traumatic torture and sexual abuse memories is a painful, lengthy, and sometimes sporadic process that requires intense support and empathy.
8. The concepts of "learned helplessness," the cycle of violence, and other situational, emotional, and cultural factors help to explain why abuse victims often remain with their abusive partners.
9. Immediately preceding or at the beginning of a serious battering incident is when abuse victims are most amenable to crisis intervention and referrals for needed services.
10. Patience, support, and information are critical aspects of nursing interventions with all victims.

◤ Study Questions

(Answer key is in the back of the book.)
1. Victims of crime experience emotional violation even when there is no physical injury. This violation involves:
    a. Loss of trust and a sense of autonomy
    b. Destruction of personal property
    c. "Blaming the victim"
    d. Depression

For most crime victims, the type of resource needed depends on the stage of recovery with which they are struggling. Match the stage of recovery with the most appropriate resource.

2. ____ Impact   a. Long-term counseling
3. ____ Recoil   b. Support groups
4. ____ Reorganization   c. Crisis intervention
5. Which of the following needs and rights of rape victims must be addressed immediately during emergency room procedures?
    a. A medical release to return to work
    b. The presence of a representative of the prosecutor's office
    c. A referral for long-term counseling
    d. Privacy, confidentiality, and resource information

6. At a workshop on incest that is geared toward school teachers, which of the following statements would you present as most accurate?
    a. Incest involves physical assault and rape by an older relative.
    b. Most victims report the abuse when they reach adolescence.
    c. Coercion is the means used to get victims to conceal the abuse.
    d. It is best for survivors to confront the perpetrators.

Match the behaviors of the cycle of violence with the appropriate nursing interventions.

7. ____ Escalation of tension, frantic attempt to withdraw, call for help   a. Discreetly giving a card with emergency phone numbers and facts about abuse
8. ____ Lying about causes of injuries; shame; denial of the need for help   b. Assisting with getting transportation to a shelter if desired

9. A close friend describes nightmares that she is having about her father, anxiety when her boyfriend touches her, and a wish to be dead. Your most appropriate question is:
    a. "What is wrong with your boyfriend?"
    b. "Are you afraid of your father?"
    c. "Was your father sexual with you when you were a child?"
    d. "Why do you want to be dead?"
10. Make a list of the agencies and resources in your city for victims of torture and ritual abuse, rape, childhood sexual abuse, and partner abuse.

REFERENCES

Abstracts, *J Psychosoc Nurs Ment Health Serv* 35(10):7, 1997.

Aiken MA: False allegation: a concept in the context of rape, *J Psychosoc Nurs Ment Health Serv* 31(11):15, 1993.

Applebaum PS: Memories and murder, *Hosp Community Psychiatry* 43(7):679, 1993.

Bennett L: Projective methods in caring for sexually abused young people, *J Psychosoc Nurs Ment Health Serv* 35(4):18, 1997.

Bloche MG and Eisenberg C: The psychological effects of state-sanctioned terror, *Harvard Mental Health Letter* 10(5):4, 1993.

Bloom SL: Hearing the survivor's voice: sundering the wall of denial, *J Psychohistory* 21(4):461, 1994.

Boutcher F and Gallop R: Psychiatric nurses' attitudes toward sexuality, sexual assault/rape and incest, *Arch Psychiatr Nurs* 10(3):184, 1996.

Briere J, et al: Lifetime victimization history, demographics, and clinical status in female psychiatric emergency room patients, *J Nerv Ment Dis* 185(2):95, 1997.

Butler S: *Conspiracy of silence: the trauma of incest,* New York, 1978, Bantam.

Campbell JC and Humphreys J: *Nursing care of victims of family violence,* ed 2, St Louis, 1993, Mosby-Year Book.

Chard KM, Weaver TL, and Resick PA: Adapting cognitive processing therapy for child sexual abuse survivors, *Cognit Behav Pract* 4:31, 1997.

Clark CC: Post traumatic stress disorder: how to support healing, *Am J Nurs* 92(8):27, 1997.

Constantine RE and Bricker PL: Social support, stress and depression among battered women in the judicial setting, *J Am Psychiatr Nurses Assoc* 3(3):81, 1997.

Courtois CA: *Healing the incest wound: adult survivors in therapy,* New York, 1988, WW Norton.

DiVasto P: Measuring the aftermath of rape, *J Psychosoc Nurs Ment Health Serv* 23(2):33, 1985.

Dole PJ: Centering: reducing rape trauma syndrome anxiety during a gynecologic examination, *J Psychosoc Nurs Ment Health Serv* 34(10):32, 1996.

Downs WR, Smyth NJ, and Miller BA: The relationship between childhood violence and alcohol problems among men who batter, *Aggression and Violent Behavior* 1(4):327, 1996.

Draucker CB and Petrovic K: Healing of adult male survivors of childhood sexual abuse, *Image J Nurs Sch* 28(4):325, 1996.

Farrell ML: The sense of relationship in women who have encountered abuse, *J Am Psychiatr Nurses Assoc* 2(2):46, 1996.

Fischman Y: Sexual torture as an instrument of war, *Am J Orthopsychiatry* 66(1):161, 1996.

Fox SS and Scherl DJ: Crisis intervention with rape victims, *Soc Work* 17:37, 1972.

Friedman MJ: PTSD diagnosis and treatment for mental health clinicians, *Community Ment Health J* 32(2):176, 1996.

Friedman MJ: Posttraumatic stress disorder, *J Clin Psychiatry* 58(9):33, 1997.

Gage RB: Examining the dynamics of spouse abuse: an alternative view, *Nurse Pract* 16(4):11, 1991.

Garbarino J: The spiritual challenge of violent trauma, *Am J Orthopsychiatry* 66(1):162, 1996.

Godby JK and Hutchinson SA: Healing from incest: resurrecting the buried self, *Arch Psychiatr Nurs* 10(5):304, 1996.

Goodwin JM: Credibility problems in sadistic abuse, *J Psychohistory* 21(4):479, 1994.

Grinspoon L, editor: Child abuse: part I, *Harvard Mental Health Letter* 9(11):1, 1993a.

Grinspoon L, editor: Child abuse: part II, *Harvard Mental Health Letter* 9(12):1, 1993b.

Grinspoon L, editor: Child abuse: part III, *Harvard Mental Health Letter* 10(1):1, 1993c.

Hatmaker D: A SANE approach to sexual assault, *Am J Nurs* 97(8):80, 1997.

Hattendorf J and Tollerud TR: Domestic violence counseling strategies that minimize the impact of secondary victimization, *Perspect Psychiatr Care* 33(1):14, 1997.

Henderson AD: Preparing feminist facilitators: assessing abused women in transitional or support group settings, *J Psychosoc Nurs Ment Health Serv* 36(3):25, 1998.

Herman JL: *Trauma and recovery,* New York, 1992, Basic Books.

Hinds J: Once upon a time: therapeutic stories as a psychiatric nursing intervention, *J Psychosoc Nurs Ment Health Serv* 35(5):46, 1997.

Horn M: Memories lost and found, *US News & World Report,* p 52, November 29, 1993.

Hudson PS: Ritual child abuse: discovery, diagnosis and treatment, Saratoga, Calif, 1991, R & F.

Indiana Cares: *Around the nation—did you know?* Indianapolis, 1993, Prevention of Child Abuse.

Janoff-Bulman R: Understanding reactions to traumatic events, *Harvard Mental Health Letter* 14(4):8, 1997.

Jezierski M: Guidelines for intervention by ED nurses in cases of domestic abuse, *J Emerg Nurs* 18(1):28a, 1992.

Laurence R: Part I: torture and mental health: a review of the literature, *Issues Ment Health Nurs* 13:301, 1992a.

Laurence R: Part II: the treatment of torture survivors: a review of the literature, *Issues Ment Health Nurs* 13:331, 1992b.

Limandri BJ: The therapeutic relationship with abused women, *J Psychosoc Nurs Ment Health Serv* 25(2):9, 1987.

Lotto D: On witches and witch hunts: ritual and satanic cult abuse, *J Psychohistory* 21(4):373, 1994.

Lynch VA: Advances in forensic nursing: new direction for the 21st century, *J Psychosoc Nurs Ment Health Serv* 34(10):6, 1996.

Mackey T, et al: Factors associated with long-term depressive symptoms of sexual assault victims, *Arch Psychiatr Nurs* 6(1):10, 1992.

Pasqualone GA: Forensic RNs as photographers: documentation in the ER, *J Psychosoc Nurs Ment Health Serv* 34(10):47, 1996.

Power and control, Duluth, Minn, 1987, Domestic Violence Intervention Project.

Puhar A: A letter from Yugoslavia, in the raw, *J Psychohistory* 19(3):331, 1992.

Putnam FW and Trickett PK: Child sexual abuse: a model of chronic trauma, *Psychiatry* 56:82, 1993.

Repressed *vs* false memory examined, *J Psychosoc Nurs Ment Health Serv* 34(7):50, 1996.

Rew L and Shirejian P: Sexually abused adolescent: conceptualization of sexual trauma and nursing interventions, *J Psychosoc Nurs Ment Health Serv* 31(12):29, 1993.

Ridley PJ: Kaufman's theory of shame and identity in treating childhood sexual abuse, *J Psychosoc Nurs Ment Health Serv* 31(6):13, 1993.

Ritual Abuse Task Force: *Ritual abuse: definitions, glossary, the use of mind control,* Los Angeles, 1991, Los Angeles County Commission for Women.

Rockwell RB: One psychiatrist's view of satanic ritual abuse, *J Psychohistory* 21(4):443, 1994.

Ross C: *Satanic ritual abuse: principles of treatment,* Toronto, 1995, University of Toronto.

Rotheram-Borus MJ, et al: Sexual abuse history and associated multiple risk behavior in adolescent runaways, *Am J Orthopsychiatry* 66(3):390, 1996.

Roye CF and Coonan PR: Adolescent rape, *Am J Nurs* 97(4):45, 1997.

Russell DEH: The secret trauma: incest in the lives of girls and women, New York, 1986, Basic Books.

Shea CA, Mahoney M, and Lacy JM: Breaking through the barriers to domestic violence intervention, *Am J Nurs* 97(6):26, 1997.

Sheridan DJ: The role of the battered woman specialist, *J Psychosoc Nurs Ment Health Serv* 31(11):31, 1993.

Sinason V: *Treating survivors of satanistic abuse,* New York, 1994, Routledge.

Smith SB: Restraints: retraumatization for rape victims?, *J Psychosoc Nurs Ment Health Serv* 33(7):23, 1995.

Task Force on Families in Crisis: *Do you know someone who's battered?,* Nashville, The Task Force.

Tynhurst JS: Individual reactions to community disaster, *Am J Psychiatry* 107:764, 1951.

Tyra PA: Helping elderly women survive rape using a crisis framework, *J Psychosoc Nurs Ment Health Serv* 34(12):20, 1996.

Ulrich YC: Women's reasons for leaving abusive spouses, *Health Care for Women International* 12:465, 1991.

Urbanic JC: Incest trauma, *J Psychosoc Nurs Ment Health Serv* 25(7):33, 1987.

Vachss A: *Sex crimes,* New York, 1993, Random House.

Walker GC, Scott PS, and Koppersmith G: The impact of child sexual abuse on addiction severity: an analysis of trauma processing, *J Psychosoc Nurs Ment Health Serv* 36(3):10, 1998.

Walker L: *The battered woman,* New York, 1979, Harper & Row.

Woods SJ and Campbell JC: Posttraumatic stress in battered women: does the diagnosis fit?, *Issues Ment Health Nurs* 14:173, 1993.

Zanarini MC, et al: Reported pathological childhood experiences associated with the development of borderline personality disorder, *Am J Psychiatry* 154(8):1101, 1997.

CHAPTER 39

Child and Adolescent Psychiatric Nursing

LARRY SCAHILL

LEARNING OBJECTIVES

After reading this chapter you should be able to:
- Describe the major categories of child psychiatric disorders.
- Describe the frequency of serious psychiatric disorders in children and adolescents.
- Identify genetic and environmental factors that can elevate the risk of developing a psychiatric disorder.
- Describe the symptoms of the common child and adolescent psychiatric disorders.
- Identify principles of nursing intervention with children and adolescents.

Recent contributions from several disciplines have increased our understanding of psychiatric disorders that occur in childhood. Through the field of **epidemiology,** there is now a better appreciation for the frequency and distribution of child psychiatric disorders. Dramatic developments in neuroscience have deepened our grasp of the biological underpinnings of some psychiatric disorders such as attention-deficit hyperactivity disorder (ADHD), autism, and Tourette's syndrome. Studies in behavioral genetics have shown that several psychiatric disorders of childhood recur in higher-than-expected rates in some families, suggesting a strong genetic contribution. Clinical research has provided information to guide both pharmacological and behavioral approaches to treatment. Despite these advances, however, the etiology of most child psychiatric disorders remains unknown, and current treatments are often less than ideal.

This chapter reviews the major categories of child psychiatric disorders, the frequency of these disorders in children, and the factors that are presumed to influence the probability of developing a psychiatric disorder. The clinical features of selected child psychiatric disorders are also described. The chapter concludes with a brief discussion of treatment issues, including psychopharmacology and behavioral therapy, as well as a description of the treatment settings in child and adolescent psychiatry.

KEY TERMS

Attention-deficit hyperactivity disorder (ADHD)   Relatively common disorder of childhood onset characterized by inattention, impulsiveness, and overactivity

Child abuse   Harmful physical, emotional, and/or sexual acts inflicted on a child

Epidemiology   The study of the frequency and distribution of disease conditions in the population

Family system   A field of influence exerted on each family member due to the complex interaction of all family members

Genetic vulnerability   Inherited liability that increases the risk of manifesting a psychiatric disorder

Pervasive developmental disorder (PDD)   Any one of several conditions that are characterized by multiple social and cognitive delays

Prevalence   Estimate of the frequency of a disease condition in the population, e.g., ADHD affects 5% to 11% of the school-aged children

Psychosocial adversity   Environmental conditions such as poverty, unemployment, or overcrowded living conditions that do not support optimal development of the child

Resilience   Capacity to move forward with development despite psychosocial adversity or genetic vulnerability

SCOPE OF THE PROBLEM

A report from the Institute of Medicine (1989) estimated that as many as 10% to 13% of school-aged children have persistent and serious mental health problems. Another 15% to 20% have milder problems with interpersonal relationships and adjustment to school. This translates into an estimated 8 to 12 million youngsters with significant mental health problems. Despite the documented frequency of psychiatric disorders in children and adolescents, as few as one in five are using specialized mental health services (Burns, et al, 1995). Another fraction is receiving mental health services in primary care settings (Horwitz, et al, 1992).

Epidemiology of Child Psychiatric Disorders

Epidemiology is the study of the frequency and distribution of disease conditions in the population. In other words, epidemiology is concerned with how common a disorder is in a given population and whether particular subgroups are at higher risk for developing a specific disorder. Thus, risk is a relative measure. For example, men are more likely to have a myocardial infarction than women, though women appear to be at higher risk for osteoporosis. Recently, methods of epidemiology have been applied to child psychiatry, resulting in a better understanding of both the frequency and distribution of these disorders in the population. This effort has profited from recent improvements in the operational criteria of psychiatric disorders and diagnostic interview methods built on these criteria.

Any number of genetic or environmental characteristics may influence the likelihood of developing a psychiatric disorder. Characteristics that increase the probability of having a psychiatric disorder are called risk factors. Although often described as separate, genetic influences and environmental conditions may interact to elevate the risk of a child psychiatric disorder. Thus, risk factors for a psychiatric disorder can be additive. Examples of biological risk factors include the inherited genetic abnormality seen in fragile X syndrome (which is the second most common genetic form of mental retardation). Poverty, child abuse, overcrowded living conditions, and exposure to alcohol in utero are examples of environmental risk factors.

Genetic Factors

Several psychiatric disorders are presumed to have an important genetic component. Indeed, for depression, anxiety disorders, tic disorders, and ADHD, having a close family member with that disorder may be the single largest contributor to the likelihood of that disorder in a child. Various methods are used to study the genetic contribution to psychiatric disorders, including twin, family, and adoption studies. More recently, powerful new molecular biological techniques have also been applied to the study of psychiatric disorders (Lombroso, Pauls, and

Leckman, 1994). The first question to ask when considering the genetic contribution for a given disorder is whether that disorder recurs more frequently in families compared to the general population. However, simply showing that a disorder such as depression is more common in children who have a depressed parent does not prove that depression is inherited. The developmental impact of having a depressed parent may increase the risk of depression in a child through environmental influences.

To establish that genetic inheritance confers vulnerability for a psychiatric disorder researchers turn to twin and adoption studies. Twin studies exploit the fact that identical (monozygotic) twins share 100% of their genes in common, whereas dizygotic twins share an average of 50% of their genes. Thus, if a disorder is truly genetic, it should be manifest in both identical twins, whereas the expected concordance in dizygotic twins would be significantly less. On the other hand, if a disorder is caused by environmental influences, these influences would presumably exert similar impact on development regardless of whether the twins were genetically identical or not. Thus, if a disorder is caused by environmental influences, there would no expected difference in the concordance between monozygotic and dizygotic twins. Twin studies have shown that monozygotic twins are more likely to be mutually affected in ADHD (Levy, et al, 1997; Stevenson, 1992), obsessive-compulsive disorder (Carey and Gottesman, 1981), and Tourette's syndrome (Price, et al, 1985). Although none of these studies showed 100% concordance in monozygotic twins, the concordance was significantly higher in monozygotic twins than in dizygotic twins.

Adoption studies typically examine whether biological or adoptive parents are more likely to share a given disorder in common with adopted-away offspring. If a disorder is due to a genetic vulnerability, then the disorder under study would be present more often in the biological parents than the adoptive parents. Conversely, if the disorder were mediated by environmental factors, then the biological inheritance would be inconsequential. Adoption studies have clearly shown that adopted-away offspring with schizophrenia are more likely to have a biological parent than an adoptive parent with schizophrenia.

Although twin and adoption studies can provide strong support for a genetic etiology, these methods do not elucidate the mode of inheritance (Box 39-1). If a disorder runs in families and is genetically inherited, it would be expected to recur in specific patterns within families. The formal method for evaluating the pattern of inheritance in families is called segregation analysis. Through segregation analysis, known models of inheritance can be compared to the observed pattern.

If a disorder is genetically inherited, it implies that the action of one or more genes is abnormal. Recently developed techniques in molecular biology may lead to the identification of a gene or genes that cause psychiatric disorders of childhood. The primary function of genes is to encode for proteins in a series of carefully engineered steps from DNA to RNA to a specific protein. Thus, a genetically determined disorder is ultimately due to a disruption in function of these molecular procedures, resulting in impaired function of the protein product

---

Box 39-1 Types of Inheritance

Autosomal Dominant

One parent is affected with the disorder and passes on a single copy of the disease-causing gene to the affected offspring. Huntington's chorea is an example of a neuropsychiatric disorder that is inherited as an autosomal dominant condition.

Autosomal Recessive

Each unaffected parent passes on one disease-causing gene to the affected offspring. Phenylketonuria is due to autosomal recessive inheritance.

Sex-Linked Inheritance

Recalling that women have an XX karyotype and men have an XY karotype, it is possible for a mother to carry a trait on one X chromosome without being affected. Although the gene is not expressed in the mother, the male offspring is affected. Some forms of hemophilia follow a sex-linked inheritance pattern.

Polygenetic Inheritance

Some disorders recur in higher-than-expected rates in families but follow more complex patterns than autosomal dominant or autosomal recessive inheritance. These disorders are presumed to be caused by several genes acting in combination. Schizophrenia and some forms of learning disability are believed to follow a polygenetic pattern.

(Lombroso, Pauls, and Leckman, 1994). In fragile X syndrome, for example, the gene that regulates an early step in the process of protein manufacture (i.e., transcription of the DNA message to RNA) appears to be defective. Precisely how this disruption in the molecular biology produces the physical characteristics and symptoms of fragile X syndrome remains unclear.

Environmental Factors

Broadly speaking, environmental factors are any and all nongenetic exposures, including intrauterine insults, adverse family conditions, poverty, unsupportive community circumstances, natural disasters, traumatic events, and toxic substances (e.g., ingesting lead paint). Ideally, genetic and environmental influences can be distinguished. In actuality, however, genetic and environmental factors interact in complex ways, making it difficult to attribute exclusive causality. For example, phenylketonuria (PKU) is a metabolic defect inherited in an autosomal recessive fashion that results in a toxic accumulation of phenylalanine in the brain. However, if PKU is detected, a low phenylalanine diet will limit the negative impact of the inherited metabolic defect.

Psychosocial adversity

Several studies have shown that adverse psychosocial conditions such as poverty, family discord, overcrowded living conditions, sexual abuse, physical abuse, and a parent with a history of substance abuse or a psychiatric disorder are associated with psychiatric disorders in children and adolescents (Szatmari, Offord, and Boyle, 1989a; Biederman, et al, 1995a; Scahill, et al, 1996). Moreover, these risk factors appear to be additive. In a clinical sample of children with ADHD, Biederman, et al (1995a) found that, as the number of these adverse elements increased, the likelihood of ADHD also increased. As suggested above, however, the association of these adverse psychosocial conditions with child psychiatric disorders does not preclude a genetic contribution.

On the other hand, it is clear that not all children who are exposed to psychosocial disadvantage develop a psychiatric disorder. Indeed, some children seem to grow and mature into well-adjusted individuals despite the presence of multiple environmental risk factors. The environmental and constitutional elements that account for these resilient children are poorly understood and deserve further investigation. It may be that a supportive relationship with a member of the extended family or a member of the community protects the child from the adverse of psychosocial conditions. **Resilience** can also be fostered within the environment such that the ill effects of a genetic vulnerability can be mitigated. For example, a child with an inherited vulnerability for ADHD is more likely to achieve an optimal outcome if reared in a predictable family environment than a child with a similar vulnerability raised in a more chaotic family circumstance.

Family systems

Families develop in a manner that is analogous to child development. Although families come in several sizes and compositions, families begin with the formation of a couple. When the couple comes together, each individual makes a transition from single life to family life. This transition to family life takes a major step forward with conception and birth (or adoption) of a child. Each subsequent phase of the child's development—infancy, toddlerhood, elementary-school age, adolescence, and young adulthood—calls for an adjustment by the family unit. The rules, rituals, and communication patterns that define the family system have an impact on the child's development. Likewise, the child's development influences the family system.

DIAGNOSTIC CATEGORIES OF CHILD PSYCHIATRIC DISORDERS

The introduction of DSM-III in 1980 (American Psychiatric Association [APA], 1980) represented an important milestone in the definition of mental illness. For the first time, psychiatric diagnoses were described in operational terms with clearly stated (though not necessarily empirically verified) criteria. The DSM-III also introduced a multiaxial diagnostic system that included not only the primary mental illness (axis I), but also noted the presence of mental retardation (axis II), medical illness (axis III), psychosocial stressors (axis IV), and assessment of functioning (axis V). The DSM-IV (APA, 1994) contains several changes from DSM-III but retains the same essential features.

Childhood psychiatric disorders can be divided into several broad categories, such as developmental disorders, disruptive behavior disorders, internalizing disorders, tic disorders, psychotic disorders, and elimination disorders.

DEVELOPMENTAL DISORDERS

Mental Retardation

Mental retardation is defined by subaverage intelligence (IQ below 70) that is accompanied by impairments in performing age-expected activities in daily living. Intelligence is measured by a standardized test and can be used to define the degree of mental retardation (Table 39-1). Impaired adaptive functioning is primarily a clinical judgment, but standardized assessments such as the Vineland Adaptive Behavior Scales (Sparrow, Balla, and Cicchetti, 1983) are available.

The prevalence of mental retardation is estimated at 2% with a range from 1 to 2.5%. Most of the mentally retarded (nearly 90%) are in the mildly retarded range. The causes of mental retardation vary from specific genetic abnormalities such as fragile X syndrome, trisomy 21 (Down's syndrome), and

phenylketonuria to "multifactorial" causes in which several genes are presumed to interact with environmental factors. In addition to intellectual handicap, mentally retarded children may also have a psychiatric disorder.

Pervasive Developmental Disorders

The pervasive developmental disorders (PDDs) are a group of disorders characterized by severe impairments across multiple domains of development. Although it is not a defining feature of PDDs, many of these children demonstrate varying degrees of mental retardation. Table 39-2 presents the more common forms of PDD described in DSM-IV.

These PDDs share several common features, such as delayed socialization and communication, and stereotypical behaviors, such as rocking, hand flapping, and peculiar preoccupations. These children are rigid, tend to perseverate on themes of idiosyncratic interest, are intolerant of change in routines, and are prone to behavioral outbursts in response to modest environmental demands.

Autistic disorder

Since the first description of autism by Leo Kanner some 50 years ago, several theories have been advanced concerning its etiology. For example, in the 1950s and 60s serious consideration was given to the notion that detached professional parents could be the cause of autism (Volkmar and Cohen, 1997). This explanation is no longer accepted and suggests a bias of *ascertainment* in that professional families were more likely to seek treatment from medical centers that evaluated children with profound developmental delays. In addition, this conceptualization fails to recognize that the parental indifference could have been rooted in the child's incapacity for reciprocal communication.

A substantial percentage of children with autistic disorder are mentally retarded, and about 25% have seizure disorders. Family genetic and twin data suggest a strong genetic contribution to autism, but the specific cause remains unknown. Several studies have observed higher serum levels of serotonin in children with autism, resulting in considerable research interest in the serotonin system. However, the failure to replicate this finding in other studies suggests that hyperserotonemia may only be true

Table 39-1   DSM-IV Classification of Mental Retardation

Severity	IQ Range
Mild	55-69
Moderate	40-54
Severe	25-39
Profound	Below 25

Table 39-2   Selected Pervasive Developmental Disorders in DSM-IV

Disorder	Prevalence
Autistic disorder	2 to 5 per 10,000
Asperger's disorder	1 to 20 per 10,000*
PDD-not otherwise specified	2 to 10 per 10,000*

*Accuracy of estimate is hampered by changes in definition.

for some autistic patients. Further evidence implicating the serotonin system comes from a recent study that observed an association between autism and the structure of the serotonin receptor (Cook, et al, 1997). If this finding is replicated, it could have an important impact on pharmacotherapy in autism.

Autism can be differentiated from the other forms of PDD because it has an early age of onset (before 30 months of age), social relatedness is profoundly disturbed, and the delayed developmental profile is relatively constant (e.g., in Rett's disorder, a rare developmental disorder, there is a rapid decline in previously acquired skills). Children with autism appear aloof and indifferent to others and seem to prefer inanimate objects to human contact. Language is both delayed and deviant, being characterized by abnormal intonation, pronoun reversals, and echolalia (repetition of words or phrases spoken by others). Other common features of autism, which may also be present in other variants of PDD, are stereotypical behaviors such as rocking and hand flapping, extraordinary insistence on sameness, and preoccupation with peculiar interests (e.g., fans, air conditioners, train schedules).

Asperger's disorder

Asperger's disorder was also described about 50 years ago, but it was not included in DSM-III or DSM-III-R. Compared with children with autism, children with Asperger's are less likely to be mentally retarded and their linguistic handicap is less severe. Indeed, these children often have normal intelligence, and verbal intelligence is typically higher than performance intelligence. The social deficits in Asperger's include inept initiation of social interactions, impaired reading of social cues, and a tendency toward concrete interpretation of language. Speech tends to be stilted, and intonation is abnormal. These children tend to be clumsy, have difficulty managing transitions, and are often preoccupied with matters of private interest.

The prevalence of Asperger's is a matter of dispute because a consensus about the diagnostic criteria has only recently been achieved (Volkmar and Cohen, 1997). Asperger's syndrome appears to be more common in boys. Although no genetic marker has been identified, the disorder often runs in families with high recurrence in fathers.

Pervasive developmental disorder—not otherwise specified (PDD-NOS)

This is a residual category reserved for children who do not meet criteria for a more specific type of PDD such as autism or Asperger's. The prevalence is difficult to estimate with accuracy because of changes in the definition. For example, DSM-III and DSM-III-R did not include this category. Given the heterogeneity of PDD-NOS, it is unlikely that a single etiology will ever be identified. Both genetic and environmental causes, particularly perinatal exposures, probably play a role in the etiology of PDD-NOS.

These children exhibit traits that are similar to those described for autism and Asperger's. Differential diagnosis is determined by age of onset, severity of speech and language deficit, degree of social impairment, and level of interest in interpersonal relationships. In general, these features are less severe in PDD-NOS than in autism.

Specific Developmental Disorders

Specific developmental disorders are characterized by a delay in a discrete domain of development. This section will focus on learning disorders and communication disorders.

Learning disorders

A learning disorder (also called learning disability) is characterized by a significant discrepancy between aptitude (IQ) and achievement in a particular area such as reading or mathematics. The specificity of the delay is what differentiates learning disorders from the more global deficits observed in mental retardation and PDD (Pennington, 1991).

The most common type of learning disorder is reading disability (also called *dyslexia*). Current estimates range from 3% to 5% of school-age children with boys being affected more often than girls in most studies (Pennington, 1991). However, in a recent large community survey, there was no gender difference in reading disability (Shaywitz, et al, 1990). In clinical samples, reading disability is associated with a range of psychiatric disorders, but it is unclear whether this apparent association is due to characteristics that are related to seeking treatment (Shaywitz, et al, 1990). Less is known about the prevalence of nonverbal learning disorder (mathematics disorder) with estimates ranging from 0.1% to 1.0% and no apparent difference between boys and girls.

Communication disorders

Communication disorders involve speech (the motor aspects of speaking) and/or language, which refers to the formulation and comprehension of verbal communication. The prevalence of speech and language disorders was reported as 19% in one community study of 5-year-olds (Beitchman, et al, 1986a). Communication deficits present early in childhood do resolve in some children. In both clinical and community samples, speech and language disorders have been shown to be strongly associated with psychiatric disorders (Beitchman, et al, 1986b; Scahill, 1990). It is not clear whether the psychiatric disorder and the communication disorder share an underlying cause or whether the prior presence of a communication disorder is a predisposing factor for development of a psychiatric disorder.

It has been speculated that language delay and reading disability may share the same underlying phonological defect (Pennington, 1991). Both reading disability and a speech or language handicap can exert a negative impact on socialization and education. For example, a child with an articulation defect or stuttering may be teased by peers, causing withdrawal and a poor self-image. Because reading is a cornerstone of learning, children with reading disability may fall behind their age-mates in school—especially if the reading disability is undetected.

DISRUPTIVE BEHAVIOR DISORDERS

The disruptive behavior disorders include three relatively common child psychiatric disorders: ADHD, oppositional defiant disorder, and conduct disorder (Table 39-3). These disorders are more common in boys, are associated with low socioeconomic status, urban living, single parenthood, family dysfunction, learning disabilities, language delay, and a positive family history of a disruptive behavior disorder (Beitchman, et al, 1986b; Biederman, et al, 1992; Biederman, et al, 1995a; Pennington, 1991; Scahill, et al, 1996; Szatmari, Offord, and Boyle, 1989b).

Attention-Deficit Hyperactivity Disorder

ADHD is characterized by inattention, impulsiveness, and overactivity. DSM-IV represents another conceptualization of ADHD and allows the description of a primarily hyperactive/impulsive type, a primarily inattentive type, or a combined type (see box on p. 623). Classically, children with ADHD are restless, overactive, distractible, reckless, and disruptive. ADHD is a relatively common disorder in school-age children, affecting an estimated 2% to 11% (Costello, et al, 1996: Jensen, et al, 1995). It is a frequent presenting complaint in child mental health clinics, and long-term disability is not uncommon (Burns, et al, 1995; Mannuzza, et al, 1993). Thus, ADHD is of significant public health importance.

Several environmental exposures have been proposed as potential causes of ADHD, including perinatal insults, head injury, psychosocial adversity, lead poisoning, and diet (e.g., food allergies or sensitivity to food additives). These hypotheses may explain some cases of ADHD; it is unlikely, however, that any one of these exposures alone will explain a significant portion of children with ADHD. Large community-based studies have confirmed that psychosocial adversity is highly associated with ADHD (Szatmari, Offord, and Boyle, 1989a; Scahill, et al, 1996). Whether these adverse psychosocial conditions are causal or contributing factors to other undetermined factors is unclear. The claim that food additives or allergies cause ADHD is supported largely by case reports, as most controlled studies fail to support a causative role for diet in ADHD (Scahill and deGraft-Johnson, 1997).

Based on evidence from twin and family studies, it is clear that genetic endowment plays a role in the etiology of ADHD. In two recent twin studies, identical twins were not fully concordant for ADHD. In both studies, however, monozygotic twins were far more likely to be mutually affected than dizygotic twins (Levy, et al, 1997; Stevenson, 1992). Family genetic studies have also shown that biological rela-

Table 39-3	Types and Prevalence of Disruptive Behavior Disorders	
Disorder	**Range of Estimates (%)**
Attention-deficit hyperactivity disorder	2-11
Oppositional defiant disorder	5-10
Conduct disorder	4-10

tives of children with ADHD are more likely to be affected by ADHD than biological relatives of pediatric controls (Biederman, et al, 1992).

Although the etiology remains unknown, a growing body of evidence suggests that subtle dysfunction in the frontal lobe plays an essential role in the core symptoms of ADHD. The frontal lobe, which is responsible for planning, attention, and regulation of motor activity, has been shown on volumetric magnetic resonance imaging (MRI) to be slightly smaller in boys with ADHD than in controls (Castellanos, et al, 1996). Using positron emission tomography (PET), it has also been shown that adults with a history of ADHD had reduced metabolic activity (hypoperfusion) in the frontal lobe (Zametkin, et al, 1990). Although not a consistent finding, structural MRI studies have also found small volumetric differences in the basal ganglia (Castellanos, et al, 1996). These subcortical structures, which also play a role in cognition and motor activity, are highly connected to the frontal lobe.

Oppositional Defiant Disorder

Oppositional defiant disorder is defined by an enduring pattern of disobedience, argumentativeness, explosive angry outbursts, low frustration tolerance, and tendency to blame others for quarrels or accidents. Not surprisingly, these children are frequently in conflict with adults and have trouble maintaining friendships. In both clinical populations and community samples, there is substantial overlap with ADHD, though the two disorders do not always occur together (Szatmari, Boyle, and Offord, 1989; Pelham, et al, 1992).

Conduct Disorder

Conduct disorder is distinguishable from oppositional defiant disorder because it is characterized by more serious violations of social standards such as aggression, vandalism, cruelty to animals, stealing, lying, and truancy.

As with the other disruptive behavior disorders, comorbidity is common in conduct disorder with higher-than-expected rates of ADHD, depression, and learning disorders. The relationship between ADHD and conduct disorder is intriguing and points out the potential contribution of family genetic studies. Faraone, et al (1991) showed that children with ADHD plus conduct disorder were more likely to have conduct disorder in their families than were children with ADHD alone. The rate of ADHD in the families of both subgroups was

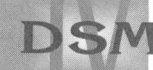

DSM-IV Criteria for Attention-Deficit Hyperactivity Disorder

A. Either (1) or (2):
  1. Inattention: At least six of the following symptoms of inattention have persisted for at least 6 months and are maladaptive:
     a. Inattentive to details or makes careless mistakes in schoolwork, etc.
     b. Difficulty sustaining attention in tasks or play
     c. Does not seem to listen to what is being said
     d. Poor follow-through on instructions and fails to finish schoolwork, chores, etc.
     e. Difficulties with organizing tasks, etc.
     f. Avoids or strongly dislikes sustained mental effort
     g. Often loses things necessary for tasks or activities
     h. Is often easily distracted by extraneous stimuli
     i. Is often forgetful in daily activities

  2. Hyperactivity-Impulsivity: At least four symptoms of hyperactivity-impulsivity that are maladaptive and have persisted for at least 6 months:
     Hyperactivity
     a. Fidgety
     b. Inappropriately leaves seat (in classroom)
     c. Inappropriate running or climbing
     d. Difficulty in playing or engaging in leisure activities quietly
     Impulsivity
     e. Blurts out answers to questions
     f. Often has difficulty waiting in lines or awaiting turn

B. Onset no later than 7 years of age.
  Other criteria concern context of behavior, level of distress, and the need to rule out other diagnoses.

Adapted from the American Psychiatric Association: *Diagnostic and statistical manual of mental disorders*, ed 4, Washington, DC, 1994, The Association.

similar whether conduct disorder was present in the index child or not. As pointed out by the authors, these findings suggest ADHD plus conduct disorder may represent a particular form of ADHD that is distinguishable from ADHD alone.

INTERNALIZING DISORDERS

Anxiety Disorders

DSM-IV defines several anxiety disorders, including general anxiety disorder, separation anxiety, agoraphobia, panic disorder, posttraumatic stress disorder, and obsessive-compulsive disorder. This section will focus on separation anxiety and obsessive-compulsive disorder. Generalized anxiety disorder, agoraphobia, panic disorder, and posttraumatic stress disorder are described in Chapter 29, though without specific reference to children or adolescents.

Separation anxiety disorder

Many children experience some discomfort upon separation from their mother or major attachment figure. For children with separation anxiety disorder, there is profound distress upon entry to school, and some children may refuse to go to school. In some cases, the child may "shadow" the mother around the house and not let the mother out of sight. When asked, most children with separation anxiety disorder will express worry about harm or permanent loss of the mother or major attachment figure.

The prevalence of separation anxiety disorder is estimated at 4% of school-aged children. The diagnosis of separation anxiety disorder in DSM-IV is based on childhood onset of excessive anxiety upon separation from home or major attachment figure. The manifestations typically include acute distress accompanied by reluctance or refusal upon separation and frequent nightmares about separation. The excessive anxiety must be present for at least a month and be the source of significant impairment at home, at school, or with friends.

Anxiety disorders recur in families at a much higher than expected rate, and it is likely that both environmental and genetic factors play an etiological role in separation anxiety disorder. Life events, such as a family move, a change to a new school, or a death in the family may predate the onset of separation anxiety. There is also evidence that extreme shy-

ness (fearfulness in new situations) is a heritable trait and the presence of this trait in a child elevates the risk of an anxiety disorder. Moreover, in children with the this trait, the likelihood of an anxiety disorder in immediate family members is also increased (Rosenbaum, et al, 1991). Additional research is needed to determine the relative contribution of genetic and environmental factors in separation anxiety disorder.

Obsessive-compulsive disorder

Obsessive compulsive disorder (OCD) is now recognized as a much more common disorder than was previously believed, with estimates of 2% to 3% lifetime prevalence in adolescents and adults (Karno, et al, 1988; Valleni-Basile, et al, 1994). Although the prevalence is probably lower in the pediatric population, it can be identified in children as young as 8 years of age (Riddle, et al, 1990).

Obsessions are recurring thoughts or images that are disturbing and difficult to push out of the mind. Compulsions are repetitive behaviors that the person feels obliged to complete. Attempts to resist these ritualized behaviors typically increase anxiety and intensify the urge to perform the compulsion. In many cases, the reported purpose of the ritual is to prevent some dreaded event, whereas other patients state that the ritual is done to achieve a sense of completion. In either case, the performance of the compulsion achieves a momentary decrease in anxiety. This reduction in anxiety, albeit brief, reinforces the compulsive habit.

Common obsessions in children and adolescents such as contamination, fear of harm coming to self or family members, worry about acting on unwanted aggressive impulses, and concern about order and symmetry are similar to those reported by adults. Common compulsions include hand washing, cleaning rituals, requesting reassurance, ordering and arranging objects, complex touching habits, checking, counting, and repetition of routine activities to achieve a sense of completion. To warrant a diagnosis of OCD, the obsessional worries and/or compulsive habits must waste time (at least an hour per day), must cause distress, and must interfere with daily activities.

Data from several lines of research have converged over the past two decades to clarify the neurobiology of OCD. These data, derived primarily from neuroimaging studies, suggest that OCD is due to dysregulation of brain circuits that connect the cortex, the basal ganglia, and the thalamus (Baxter, et al, 1988). Another source of evidence is the now frequently replicated finding in both children and adults that the serotonin reuptake inhibitors are effective for most patients with OCD (see Griest, et al [1995] and Scahill [1996] for reviews).

Mood Disorders

DSM-IV defines several mood disorders, including major depressive disorder, dysthymic disorder, bipolar I and bipolar II disorders, and cyclothymic disorder. These disorders occur in children and adolescents; they are more common, however, in adults and are discussed in Chapter 28. This section will provide a brief discussion of major depressive disorder and bipolar disorder in children and adolescents.

Major depressive disorder

The manifestations of depression in children are similar to those observed in adults. Two important differences, however, are that children may be less able to verbalize their feelings and irritability may be a predominant feature in children and adolescents. Depression is characterized by sadness, feelings of worthlessness, loss of interest in usual activities, sleep and/or appetite disturbance, loss of energy, diminished activity, decreased capacity to concentrate, and recurrent thoughts of death or suicide. At least five of these symptoms must be present on a daily basis and persist for at least 2 weeks (APA, 1994).

The prevalence of depression in children and adolescents ranges from 1% to 5% with intriguing differences by age and gender. Overall, depression is less common in prepubertal children with boys at slightly higher risk than girls in the younger age group. During adolescence depression is more common in girls.

A large body of data shows that depression involves the hypothalamic-pituitary-adrenal axis, as well as the norepinephrine and serotonin systems in the brain, but the precise mechanism is not well understood. Family studies provide evidence that the risk for depression is substantially higher if there is a history of depression in an immediate family member (Puig-Antich, et al, 1989; Merikangas and Angst, 1995).

Critical Thinking Questions

Since anxiety and depression can be masked in children and adolescents, how can the nurse determine their presence?

Bipolar disorder

DSM-IV defines two types of bipolar disorder: bipolar I and bipolar II. Bipolar I disorder is defined by mania with or without a history of depression (Box 39-2). The DSM-IV recognizes six variants of this combination. Bipolar II disorder is characterized by a history of major depression and hypomania but not a full manic episode (APA, 1994).

The existence of mania in young children is a matter of some controversy. Some investigators suggest that it is rare in prepubertal children, whereas others contend that it is simply underdiagnosed. In addition, there is incomplete agreement concerning whether bipolar illness in children has the same clinical features as seen in adults (Fristad, Weller, and Weller, 1992; Weller, Weller, and Fristad, 1995). Using structured diagnostic interviews, Biederman, et al (1995b) identified 14% (n = 43) of children with bipolar disorder in their large specialty clinic. These children, some of whom had a history of depression, showed more severe psychopathology when compared with a group of children with ADHD.

The prevalence of bipolar illness in adolescents is estimated at approximately 1% (Lewinsohn, Klein, and Seeley, 1995). In this large community survey, girls were more frequently affected than boys. The mean age of onset for the whole group was about 12 years of age with depression being the most common feature prior to onset.

Box 39-2 Manic Episode

Persistent period (at least 1 week) of expansive or irritable mood accompanied by three or more of the following:
- Inflated self-esteem
- Decreased need for sleep
- Pressure of speech
- Racing thoughts
- Highly distractibile
- Increase in goal-directed activity (or agitation)
- Unrestrained involvement in pleasurable activities

TIC DISORDERS

Tic disorder is a general term used to describe several disorders that are characterized by motor and/or phonic tics. Motor tics are typically rapid, jerky movements of the eyes, face, neck, and shoulders, but other muscle groups may also be involved. Motor tics may also take the form of slower and more purposeful movements. The most common phonic tics are throat clearing, grunting, or other repetitive noises. More complex sounds such as words, parts of words, and obscenities occur in a minority of patients. Table 39-4 presents a list of tic disorders and their defining features.

As shown in Table 39-4, Tourette's syndrome (TS) is a chronic movement disorder that is defined by the presence of multiple motor and phonic tics. The prevalence of TS is estimated to be between 1 and 2 cases per 1000 with boys being affected 3 to 6 times more often than girls (Apter, et al, 1993; Burd, et al, 1986; Comings, Himes, and Comings, 1990).

In the 1970s, the potent dopamine blocker, haloperidol, was found to be helpful in reducing tic symptoms. This observation prompted speculation about the role of central dopaminergic systems in the etiology of TS. Since then several other neurochemical systems have been implicated in TS, including norepinephrine, endogenous opioids, serotonin, and androgens. Through the 1980s, several family-genetic studies reported data consistent with *autosomal dominant* inheritance. These studies also showed that the range of expression is variable and probably includes TS, chronic motor or chronic vocal tic disorder, and obsessive-compulsive disorder as well (Pauls, et al, 1991). Further support for a genetic hypothesis came from twin studies that showed monozygotic twins are far more likely to be concordant for TS than dizygotic twins. In many cases, however, concordant monozygotic twins were not equally affected, suggesting that environmental factors also have an impact on the expression of the gene. More recent family-genetic studies suggest that the inheritance may be more complex than a single gene with an autosomal dominant pattern (Walkup, et al, 1996)

Although the etiology of TS is unknown, several lines of evidence point to dysregulation of circuits that travel from the cortex through the basal ganglia (Leckman, et al, 1992). The basal ganglia are a group of subcortical structures that play an important role in planning and execution of movement as well as higher cognitive functions. These circuits are spatially organized into five parallel, minimally overlapping pathways, each of which serves separate functions. Dysregulation of one or more of these circuits has been implicated in the pathophysiology of several disorders including OCD, schizophrenia, TS, Huntington's chorea, and Parkinson's disease (Peterson, et al, 1993).

PSYCHOTIC DISORDERS

Psychotic symptoms may occur in the context of several disorders, such as bipolar illness, depression, PDD, and anxiety disorders. Psychotic disorders such as schizophrenia are defined using the same criteria as for adults and are rare in children. For example, childhood-onset schizophrenia is estimated at 2 cases per 100,000 compared to 2 to 10 cases per 1000 in late teen years. The precise etiology of schizophrenia is unknown, but as suggested above, genetic influence is strongly implied. Neuroimaging data suggest a loss of inhibitory control in pathways connecting the frontal lobe to subcortical structures, including the basal ganglia and thalamus (Tamminga, et al, 1992).

ELIMINATION DISORDERS
Enuresis

Enuresis usually refers to bed wetting (nocturnal enuresis). But enuresis can also be characterized by repeated urination on clothing during waking hours

Table 39-4	Types and Features of Tic Disorders in DSM-IV
Tic Disorder	**Clinical Features**
Transient	Motor **and/or** phonic tics for at least 2 weeks, but less than 1 year
Chronic	Either motor **or** phonic tics for more than 1 year
Tourette's*	Both motor **and** phonic tics for more than 1 year

*In DSM-IV–Tourette's disorder, also called Tourette syndrome.

(diurnal enuresis). For nocturnal enuresis, DSM-IV specifies that bed wetting occur at least twice per week for a duration of 3 months and that the child be at least 5 years of age. Boys are more often affected than girls, and the prevalence goes down with age. An estimated 6.7% of 5-year-old boys, 3% of boys ages 9 to 11, and 1% of 14-year-old boys have nocturnal enuresis.

Encopresis

Encopresis is defined as soiling clothing with feces or depositing feces in inappropriate places in a child 4 years of age or older. Additional diagnostic criteria require that the soiling occur at least once per month and that it not be due to a medical disorder such as aganglionic megacolon (Hirschsprung's disease). The most common cause of encopresis is leakage of stool around a fecal impaction. Fecal impaction may start because the child withholds in response to the urge to defecate. Over time, there may be a loss of muscle tone in the lower bowel, and the child loses the normal urge to defecate and may not even be aware of the leakage. Encopresis affects an estimated 1.5% of school-age children and is three to four times more common in boys. As with enuresis, the frequency of the condition goes down with age.

TREATMENT

CASE EXAMPLE # 1

Allan was a 9-year-old fourth grader who was referred by his pediatrician to the outpatient clinic for an evaluation of his overactivity, impulsiveness, poor concentration, and disruptive behavior in school. At the time of referral, he lived with his mother and younger sister in a small apartment after having moved from a neighboring town. His mother works part-time as a waitress. The history revealed that he had been treated with methylphenidate (Ritalin) in the second grade with uncertain benefit. However, his mother could not recall the dose or the duration of treatment.

The developmental history was remarkable for significant marital discord during the pregnancy, resulting in the couple's first separation. This marital discord was characterized by father's alcohol abuse, parental arguments, and occasional physical fights.

The couple finally divorced 3 years later, just prior to the birth of Allan's younger sister. Allan achieved motor milestones early but was late in speech and language acquisition. He had only a few words by 2 years of age and, when he entered preschool at the age of 3 years, his speech was poorly understood by nonfamily members.

Overactivity and inability to play with other children without fighting led to his dismissal from the first preschool. His mother reported that he did better in the second preschool, which had a more structured program. He remained in this program until the first grade, when he entered the public school. In the first and second grades, his teachers reported that he was hard to manage due to overactivity, calling out without permission, and interference with the affairs of other children. Although generally good-natured, his intrusive style and occasional aggressive behavior caused him to be rejected by his classmates. He was highly distractible and unable to stay on task. Not surprisingly, he fell behind academically and was unable to read at the end of second grade. In his current school setting, Allan has been frequently ejected from the classroom for disruptive behavior. After instigating a fight in the school yard, he had been admonished to stay away from older boys during recess.

Allan was a healthy boy with no prior history of serious injuries or illnesses or hospitalizations. He had multiple middle ear infections during the first 3 years of life but had not had any since the age of 5 years. Review of body systems revealed a recent history of intermittent constipation and soiling. According to his mother, this problem had occurred in second grade but resolved without intervention after 1 or 2 months. He had no known allergies to foods or medication.

TREATMENT SETTINGS

Traditionally, there were two treatment settings for children and adolescents with psychiatric disorders: specialized inpatient units and outpatient services. Driven in part by the high cost of inpatient care, and by the recognition that the level of care should be congruent with symptom severity, a much wider range of mental health services has emerged in recent years. It is now possible in some communities to receive mental health services in the home, in school-based clinics, in after-school programs, specialized educational programs, day hospitals, therapeutic foster homes, and residential treatment centers, as well as the traditional outpatient and inpatient settings. It is likely that this range of mental health services will expand.

PSYCHOPHARMACOLOGY

Several different classes of medications are used in the treatment of children and adolescents with psychiatric disorders (for detailed reviews see Green [1995] and Scahill [1997]). Many of the drugs used in the treatment of children and adolescents with serious psychiatric symptoms were developed for other purposes (Table 39-5). In addition, the same drug may be prescribed for any one of several problems. Unfortunately, many of these medications have entered clinical practice without the benefit of carefully controlled studies to guide their use. For example, clonidine was developed as an antihypertensive

medication and is used in the treatment of ADHD and tics. Although there have been studies in both children and adults with tics, the data supporting its use in ADHD are limited.

An important guiding principle in pediatric psychopharmacology is that children are physiologically different from adults. These differences could have an impact on dose, clinical response, and side effects. For example, children often require larger doses of psychotropic drugs, on a milligram-per-kilogram basis, than adults to achieve beneficial effects (Green, 1995). Although it is not completely clear why this is so, it has been speculated that more efficient liver metabolism and glomerular filtration in children plays some role. Drug effects (pharmacodynamics) may also be different in children, which may be due to developmental differences in neural pathways. For example, norepinephrine, dopamine, and serotonin systems all undergo developmental changes in childhood (Green, 1995). These developmental differences may explain the inconsistent results of the tricyclic antidepressants in children with depression

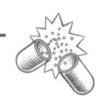

TABLE 39-5 Classes of Medications Used in the Treatment of Children and Adolescents with Psychiatric Symptoms

Class	Purpose(s)	Empirical Support*
Stimulants	ADHD	Excellent
Tricyclic antidepressants	1. Depression	Fair
	2. ADHD	Fair
	3. Enuresis	Good
	4. Separation anxiety	Fair
	5. OCD (clomipramine)	Excellent
Serotonin reuptake inhibitors	1. OCD	Excellent
	2. Depression	Good
	3. Anxiety	Fair
Traditional neuroleptics	1. Psychosis	Excellent
	2. Tics (haloperidol and pimozide)	Excellent
	3. Severe ADHD	Good
	4. Agitation in PDD	Good
Atypical neuroleptics	1. Psychosis	Good
	2. Agitation in PDD	Fair
	3. Tics	Fair
Alpha-2 agonists	1. Tics (clonidine)	Excellent
	2. ADHD	Fair
Mood stabilizers	1. Mania (lithium)	Good
	2. Mania (valproate)	Poor

*Poor = no or few studies in pediatric populations or little support from existing studies; fair = few controlled studies in pediatric populations or concern about side effects; good = some data from controlled studies, but findings are inconsistent; excellent = consistent body of data from controlled studies showing both efficacy and safety (see text for more details).

compared with adults (Ambrosini, et al, 1993) and the more frequently observed activating side effects of fluoxetine in children (Riddle, et al, 1991).

Stimulants

The most frequently used stimulants are methylphenidate (Ritalin) and dextroamphetamine (Dexedrine). Both of these drugs come in short-acting and sustained-release forms. Other less commonly used stimulants include pemoline (Cylert) and Adderall, which is a mixture of amphetamine and d-amphetamine salts. To date, Adderall has not been well studied. Of these various preparations, methylphenidate is by far the most common, being used by approximately 3% of school-age children. The preference for methylphenidate over the other stimulants is probably due to its better side-effect profile (Scahill, 1997).

The optimal daily dose of methylphenidate ranges between 0.6 mg and 1.5 mg per kilogram of body weight per day in two or three divided doses. This translates into roughly 10 mg bid with meals for a 45-lb (20 kg) child. Slightly higher doses may be tried in cases showing equivocal response, but doses above 60 mg per day are not recommended.

The usual dosage of dextroamphetamine is lower than methylphenidate, and it is rarely given more than twice a day. The total daily dose is typically in the range of 15 to 20 mg per day in younger children and 40 mg per day in older children (i.e., for a total dose of 0.3 mg and 1.0 mg/kg per day).

Both methylphenidate and dextroamphetamine are given immediately before or with meals to prevent loss of appetite. Other side effects of the stimulants include mood lability, tics, and abnormal movements; a tendency to become overfocused on details; and, rarely, agitation and psychotic symptoms. In the usual short-acting form, methylphenidate and dextroamphetamine have a duration of action of about 4 and 6 hours, respectively. As the medication effects wear off, there can be a behavioral rebound. This can be managed by introducing a second dose. To soften the rebound effect later in the day, the second dose is often lower than the first.

Tricyclic Antidepressants

Tricyclic antidepressants (TCAs), including imipramine, desipramine, nortriptyline, and clomipramine are a group of chemically related compounds that have been used in children and adolescents for over 30 years. As suggested in Table 39-5, these agents have been used in the treatment of depression, enuresis, separation anxiety, ADHD, and OCD with mixed results depending on the specific agent and the disorder in question.

To date the efficacy of the TCAs in the treatment of children with depression has not been demonstrated (Ambrosini, et al, 1993). It appears, however, that at least some children with depression do benefit from nortriptyline at daily doses in the range of 0.64 to 1.57 mg/kg per day (Ambrosini, et al, 1993).

Placebo-controlled studies have demonstrated the effectiveness of desipramine in the treatment of ADHD (Biederman, et al, 1989; Singer, et al, 1995). However, concern about alterations in cardiac conduction has decreased enthusiasm for the use of desipramine in pediatric populations (Riddle, Geller, and Ryan, 1993). Imipramine has been studied in several controlled trials for separation anxiety with inconsistent results. The most recent study failed to show that it was better than placebo (Klein, Koplewicz, and Kanner, 1992). Imipramine has also demonstrated efficacy in the treatment of enuresis. However, since the introduction of the synthetic antidiuretic hormone, desmopressin (DDAVP), use of imipramine for enuresis has declined.

Clomipramine is unique in that, in addition to the norepinephrine reuptake properties common to the other TCAs, it also has serotonin reuptake properties (Scahill, 1996). This mechanism is believed to be the explanation for the effectiveness of clomipramine for the treatment of OCD. In a multicenter trial, clomipramine was superior to placebo in adolescents with OCD (DeVeaugh-Geiss, et al, 1992). The typical dose of clomipramine ranges from 75 mg to 250 mg, depending on the age of the child with younger children on the lower end of the range.

The side effects of the TCAs include dry mouth, fatigue, dizziness, sweating, weight gain, urinary retention, tremor, and agitation. These side effects can often be managed by lowering the dose or changing the dose schedule (e.g., splitting into two doses per day). All of the TCAs have the capacity to change cardiac conduction. Therefore, children and adolescents treated with any of the TCAs should receive a cardiogram at baseline and periodically during treatment (Scahill and Lynch, 1994b). According to Martin and Agran (1988) a heart rate over 130 is cause for alarm. As suggested above, desipramine may be especially prone to producing alterations in cardiac conduction (Riddle, Geller, and Ryan, 1993).

Selective Serotonin Reuptake Inhibitors (SSRIs)

This group of chemically unrelated compounds was originally developed as antidepressants. The success of clomipramine in the treatment of OCD prompted great interest in these drugs for the treatment of OCD, as well as depression. Currently, four

Box 39-3   SSRIs

Fluoxetine

Fluoxetine (Prozac) comes in a 10- or 20-mg capsule and in a liquid form. Because of the long half-life (fluoxetine also has an active metabolite with an even longer half-life), the dose is typically increased slowly to avoid overshooting the optimal dose. The typical starting dose is 5 to 10 mg per day, and the dose range for most children and adolescents will be between 10 and 40 mg per day.

Sertraline

Sertraline (Zoloft) is available in 50- and 100-mg tablets that can easily be broken in half. The starting dose might be 25 mg with gradual increases to a range of 25 to 150 mg in children. Adolescents may receive slightly higher doses. Some patients respond at lower doses, hence dosing should be individualized.

Fluvoxamine

Fluvoxamine (Luvox) has been evaluated in a large multicenter study in children and adolescents with OCD and now has approval from the Food and Drug Administration for use in pediatric populations. The medication comes in a 25-, 50-, and 100-mg tablets—each of which can be broken in half. Treatment may begin with 12.5 to 25 mg per day and may be increased by 25 mg every 5 to 7 days as tolerated. The typical dose range is 50 to 200 mg per day in children.

Paroxetine

Paroxetine (Paxil) comes in 20- and 30-mg tablets that can be broken in half. To date, paroxetine has not been well studied in children, though a multicenter trial in children with OCD is currently underway. A reasonable starting dose would be 10 mg per day to a total dose of 10 to 40 mg in a single daily dose.

SSRIs are marketed in the United States, including fluoxetine (Prozac), sertraline (Zoloft), paroxetine (Paxil), and fluvoxamine (Luvox). Each of these has shown efficacy in the treatment of depression in adults. Fluoxetine, sertraline, and fluvoxamine have also demonstrated efficacy for OCD in controlled trials in both children and adults (see Griest, et al [1995] and Scahill [1996] for reviews).

The precise mechanism of the SSRIs is not completely understood. It is known that they block the return of serotonin into the presynaptic neuron—hence the term reuptake inhibitors. All four of the SSRIs have relatively long half-lives permitting single daily dosing with the exception of fluvoxamine, which is often given twice daily (Box 39-3).

Side effects of the SSRIs

The most common side effect of the SSRIs in children and adolescents is behavioral activation, which may be characterized by motor restlessness, insomnia, hypomania, and disinhibition. This is most likely to occur early in treatment but may also be seen with dose increases (Riddle, et al, 1991). Other side effects include abdominal pain, heartburn, diarrhea, and decreased appetite. There have also been reports of suicidal ideation and self-injurious behavior with fluoxetine (King, et al, 1991), but it is unclear whether this reaction is attributable to fluoxetine itself. If true for fluoxetine, it could also occur with other SSRIs.

When a child is placed on an SSRI for OCD or depression and has a positive response, parents frequently inquire about the duration of treatment. In the absence of clear evidence to guide the decision, most clinicians suggest discontinuation after a symptom-free period of 8 to 12 months. Parents should be discouraged from abrupt withdrawal as there have been several case reports of dizziness, nausea, vomiting, and diarrhea upon abrupt withdrawal of sertraline and paroxetine. Children and parents should be informed that symptoms of OCD or depression may return following planned discontinuation of an SSRI.

Traditional Antipsychotics

Traditional neuroleptics, such as the phenothiazines and haloperidol, primarily block D_2 dopamine receptors. The newer, atypical neuroleptics such as clozapine and risperidone, not only block dopamine receptors, but are potent antagonists of specific serotonin receptors as well. This pharmacological property appears to be protective against extrapyramidal side effects (EPSE).

In children, neuroleptics are used to treat both psychotic and nonpsychotic symptoms, including stereotypies and agitation, severe hyperactivity, aggressive or self-injurious behavior, and tics (Scahill and Skrypeck, 1997) (Box 39-4). These target symptoms are associated with disorders such as PDD, refractory ADHD, bipolar disorder, severe conduct disorder, and TS.

Side effects of the traditional antipsychotics

Low-potency neuroleptics are associated with sedation and orthostatic hypotension. By contrast, the higher-potency agents are associated with EPSEs such as dystonia, dyskinesia, akathisia (subjective feeling of restlessness), and parkinsonism. In some cases, the dystonia is pronounced and is manifested by torticollis and rolling of the eyes upward (i.e., oculogyric crisis). Treatment of acute dystonia includes immediate injection of an anticholinergic medication such as benztropine (Cogentin) and slowing down the rate of increase of the neuroleptic. Other side effects of the traditional antipsychotics include cognitive blunting, irritability, depressed mood, blurred vision, dry mouth, and weight gain. Finally, long-term treatment with a neuroleptic places the patient at increased risk for tardive dyskinesia (Campbell, et al, 1997). This is a chronic neurological condition involving abnormal movements of the face, mouth, and sometimes the arms (see Chapter 19). These potential short- and long-term side effects should be discussed with the child and family before and during treatment with this group of medications.

Atypical Antipsychotics

Concerns about the potential long- and short-term adverse effects of the traditional neuroleptics have prompted the development of a new class of neuroleptics. The first medication of this new class was clozapine, which was introduced in the 1960s. Although early results were encouraging, clozapine was nearly withdrawn from use due to concerns about agranulocytosis. Currently, clozapine is re-

served for cases of treatment-refractory schizophrenia. The atypical neuroleptics block both $5HT_2$ and D_2 receptors. Over the past few years, several agents with this dual action have been introduced, such as risperidone (Risperdal), olanzapine (Zyprexa), quetiapine (Seroquel), and ziprasidone (Zeldox). This section will focus on risperidone because the other agents listed have little or no data concerning their use in children and adolescents (see Scahill and Lynch [1998] for a review).

Risperidone came on the market in early 1994. Since then it has been used in several open-label studies in children and adolescents with a wide range of problems, including tic disorders, pervasive developmental disorder, schizophrenia, and severe

Box 39-4 Traditional Antipsychotics

Thioridazine

Thioridazine (Mellaril) is a low-potency neuroleptic in the phenothiazine chemical family. It is typically used for the treatment of severe hyperactivity and/or agitation. The total daily dose range is 50 to 300 mg per day in two or three daily doses. Higher dose levels are safe to use, but sedation side effects and weight gain may become intolerable.

Thiothixene

Thiothixene (Navane) is a neuroleptic of intermediate potency that is used primarily for psychosis or severe agitation. In children, treatment typically begins with 2 mg twice to three times per day with gradual increases to 5 mg two to three times daily. This schedule may be more aggressive, and higher dose levels may be used in acute psychotic states.

Haloperidol

Haloperidol (Haldol) is a high-potency neuroleptic that is unrelated to the phenothiazines. It has been studied in pediatric populations for the treatment of psychosis, PDD, conduct disorder, and tic disorders. The typical dose ranges from 1 to 2 mg per day that might be used in the treatment of tics to 10 mg per day for the management of acute psychosis.

Pimozide

Pimozide (Orap) is another high-potency neuroleptic that is used specifically for the treatment of tics. It comes in a 2-mg tablet, and the typical dose range is 1 to 4 mg per day.

disruptive behavior. The dosages ranged from 0.5 mg per day to 10 mg per day. Careful review of these studies suggests that extrapyramidal symptoms are infrequent and clearly related to the rate of dose increase. In those studies that used a slow upward dose schedule, extrapyramidal symptoms were not observed (Scahill and Lynch, 1998). The most common side effect across these studies was weight gain. Children who are placed on this drug should be weighed at baseline and periodically during treatment. There is also one case of elevated liver function tests accompanied by fatty infiltration (Kumra, et al, 1997).

Alpha-2 Agonists

The alpha-2 agonists, clonidine (Catapres) and guanfacine (Tenex), were developed as antihypertensive agents. These drugs decrease norepinephrine activity in the brain. Clonidine can be useful for the treatment of tics as shown in a recent double-blind study (Leckman, et al, 1991). Support for the use of clonidine in the treatment of ADHD is less consistent.

Clonidine is usually introduced with a single 0.05 mg dose (half of a 0.1 mg tablet) and then increased by half-tablet increments every 3 to 4 days to a total of 0.15 to 0.2 mg per day divided into three or four doses. The most common side effect of clonidine is sedation. Dry mouth, headache, irritability, and sleep disturbance may also occur. Although rarely a problem, blood pressure should be monitored during treatment especially when starting the medication. Abrupt discontinuation, however, can cause a rebound in blood pressure and should be avoided.

In doses ranging from 1.0 to 4.0 mg per day, guanfacine has been evaluated in preliminary studies. Data from these preliminary studies are promising for the treatment of ADHD, but controlled studies have not been done. Because guanfacine has a longer duration of action and is less sedating than clonidine, it of interest, but more study is needed.

COGNITIVE BEHAVIORAL THERAPY

Contemporary treatment of children and adolescents often involves a multimodal approach, which may include medication, family treatment, group therapy, and individual therapy for the child. Cognitive behavioral therapy is a form of individual ther-

apy that has been successfully applied to children with disruptive behavior disorders and anxiety disorders. This section will focus on cognitive behavioral techniques that are used in the treatment of ADHD and OCD.

Cognitive Behavioral Therapy in ADHD

Recalling that the hallmark features of ADHD are inattention, overactivity, and impulsiveness, the goal of cognitive behavioral therapy in ADHD is improve the child's ability to "stop, look, and listen" before acting. Several approaches have been developed to accomplish this overall aim.

Social skills training

Social skills training teaches the child to recognize the impact of his or her behavior on others. Because impulsive children and adolescents often fail to recognize the adverse effects of their verbal and nonverbal behavior, social skills training uses instruction, role playing, and positive reinforcement to improve interpersonal relationships and to enhance social outcomes.

Problem-solving skills training

Problem-solving skills training focuses on defective cognitive processes such as assessment of situations, as well as interpretation of events and expectations of others. Children with disruptive behavior problems often misinterpret the intentions of others, e.g., perceiving hostility when none was intended. Through instruction and role-playing, problem-solving skills training teaches the child to generate alternative interpretations for the behavior of others and options for a response. These options are then evaluated for their likely consequences on the situation and on interpersonal relationships.

Parent training

The reckless and impulsive behavior of children with ADHD and other disruptive behavior disorders often elicit punitive responses from their parents. Parent training attempts to provide parents with a new understanding of their child's behavior and new ways of responding to it. These programs emphasize the importance of clear limits concerning unwanted behavior and positive reinforcement (praise and tangible rewards) for desired behaviors. The use of point systems and mild punishments such as time out are also presented. Parent training programs may be offered in a group format or in a family therapy setting (Barkley, 1990; Kendall and Braswell, 1993).

Cognitive Behavioral Therapy in OCD

Cognitive behavior therapy for OCD is based on exposure and response prevention. *Exposure* refers to deliberate confrontation of a situation or event that triggers anxiety and/or the urge to perform the ritual. *Response prevention* consists of blocking the compulsive behavior despite the presence of the urge to complete it. For example, if the patient feared contamination and felt the need to wash after touching sticky materials, the patient might be encouraged to touch a sticky counter and then refrain from washing. These techniques have clearly demonstrated their usefulness in the treatment of adults with OCD and recently have been applied to children (March, Mulle, and Herbel, 1994; Scahill, et al, 1996).

The theory behind exposure and response prevention is that rising anxiety occurs in response to external events (a trigger). Secondly, the anxiety associated with the triggering event or situation is exaggerated. Thirdly, because the performance of the ritual results in a rapid decline in anxiety, it reinforces the idea that the compulsive behavior is a useful strategy for managing anxiety. Unfortunately, the success of the ritualized behavior is typically short-lived. Finally, systematic confrontation of the triggering event or situation results in decreased anxiety even if the ritual is not performed. Box 39-5 presents a traditional treatment plan for the case presented earlier in this section.

Box 39-5   Treatment Plan: Allan

Diagnosis

Axis I	ADHD: combined type
	Encopresis
	Reading disorder
Axis II	None
Axis III	None
Axis IV	Academic problems
	Inadequate finances
Axis V	Global assessment of functioning: 50

Goals
1. Reduce overactivity and impulsive behavior
2. Improve social judgment
3. Enhance delayed reading skills
4. Restore normal bowel function

Placement

The treatment plan includes placement in a day treatment program due to degree of impulsiveness and tendency to provoke retaliation from others. This placement will also permit the application of multiple treatments, including social skills training, parent training for Allan's mother, and close monitoring of pharmacotherapy. The day hospital program will also include a psychoeducational evaluation to clarify his reading disability and generate remediation strategies.

Medication

After a 2-week observation period, a trial of methylphenidate will be initiated. Despite report of a previous unsuccessful trial, available evidence suggests that the trial was inadequate. Therefore, before moving on to another stimulant or to a nonstimulant alternative, response to methylphenidate in a carefully monitored trial is appropriate. The medication will be started at 5 mg per day and increased to 5 mg bid (8 AM and 12 noon) after 4 days. If well tolerated, dose will be increased 4 days later to 10 mg in the morning and 5 mg at noon (0.6 mg/kg of body weight). Thereafter, dose will be increased depending on response, with a maximum dose of 30 mg per day in two or three divided doses.

Bowel Retraining Program

In collaboration with his primary care providers, will initiate a bowel retraining program. Step 1 is educating the mother and Allan about normal bowel function and the vicious cycle of fecal impaction and leakage of stool around the hardened mass of stool. This educational effort should help to decrease the mother's anger at Allan for this problem and will help motivate Allan to engage in solving the problem. Step 2 is to clean out the bowel (e.g., with a laxative and mineral oil). Step 3 is the behavioral treatment program, which typically involves daily sitting on the toilet after each meal for 10 minutes. Rewards in the form of stickers or points will be given at school and at home for participating in the program. Special bonuses can be awarded for successful defecation. The stickers or points can be "cashed in" for small prizes at the end of each week (Howe and Walker, 1992).

■ Critical Thinking Question

What are the similarities and differences in the role of the nurse when working with families of an adolescent vs. an adult?

◆ Key Concepts

1. Estimates of the incidence of psychiatric disorders among children vary, but all studies indicate this to be a growing concern.
2. Risk factors for childhood psychiatric disorders include genetic and biological factors; adverse environmental influences before, during, and after birth; social and cultural factors; family system factors; stress experiences during infancy and childhood; and living with a mentally ill or alcoholic parent(s).
3. The extent of the negative effects of risk factors upon children tends to depend upon the severity of the risk factors and the psychological resilience of the child.
4. Children can be motivated by their peers. Psychotherapeutic management of childhood psychiatric disorders is most effective when nurse-patient relationship and milieu issues are considered jointly.
5. Resilience is the ability to withstand the problems of an undesirable childhood environment and emerge as a "normal," productive person.
6. Attention-deficit hyperactivity disorder (ADHD) is the most common pediatric behavioral disorder. CNS stimulants are the drugs most frequently used to treat children with ADHD.
7. Symptoms of childhood psychoses include hallucinations, delusions, thought disorder, anxiety, inappropriate affect, speech idiosyncrasies, morbid thoughts, absence of friends, and concrete thinking.
8. Childhood depression, its existence once debated by clinicians, is considered a significant mental health problem today; pharmacologically it is treated with antidepressants.

◆ Study Questions

(Answer key is in the back of the book.)
1. Which of the following is considered a risk factor for childhood psychiatric disorders?
   a. Intact family
   b. Genetic vulnerability
   c. Social support
   d. Age
2. The child suffering from ADHD would most likely exhibit which of the following symptoms?
   a. Suicidality
   b. Good peer relationships
   c. Hostility
   d. Restlessness
3. The most commonly prescribed drug for ADHD is:
   a. Methylphenidate (Ritalin)
   b. Amphetamine
   c. Pemoline (Cylert)
4. According to Martin and Agran (1988) a heart rate over _____ in a child taking TCAs is cause for alarm.
   a. 70
   b. 90
   c. 110
   d. 130
5. Many childhood and adolescent psychiatric disorders are more prevalent in boys. Which of the following is statistically more common in girls?
   a. ADHD
   b. Adolescent depression
   c. Tic disorders
   d. Conduct disorders
6. Ken's psychiatric diagnosis is ADHD. A possible nursing diagnosis would be "sensory perception alteration related to neurological disturbances." With the aid of medication a short-term goal for Ken would be
   a. To sit and play with his toys for 10 minutes
   b. To seek out the nurse to talk
   c. To be able to express his anger in an acceptable manner
   d. To not destroy things in his environment
7. Carol is exhibiting behavioral changes that suggest that she is depressed and possibly suicidal. What would be the primary nursing intervention?
   a. Assist Carol in identifying her strengths
   b. Provide tension-relieving activities
   c. Develop a relationship with Carol that promotes trust
   d. Help Carol identify angry feelings
8. What is the most important capacity a nurse working with adolescents should have?
   a. Denial of personal limitations
   b. Flexibility with predictability
   c. Serious attitude
   d. Ability to challenge
9. Schizophrenia is more common in
   a. Early childhood (0 to 6 years)
   b. Young children (6 to 12 years)
   c. Adolescence (12 to 17 years)

REFERENCES

Ambrosini PJ, et al: Antidepressant treatments in children and adolescents. I. Affective disorders, *J Am Acad Child Adolesc Psychiatry* 32:1, 1993.

American Psychiatric Association: *Diagnostic and statistical manual of mental disorders*, ed 3, Washington, DC, 1980, The Association.

American Psychiatric Association: *Diagnostic and statistical manual of mental disorders*, ed 3, Washington, DC, 1987, The Association.

American Psychiatric Association: *Diagnostic and statistical manual of mental disorders*, ed 4, Washington, DC, 1994, The Association.

Apter A, et al: An epidemiological study of Gilles de la Tourette's syndrome in Israel, *Arch Gen Psychiatry* 50: 734, 1993.

Barkley RA: *Attention deficit hyperactivity disorder: a handbook for diagnosis and treatment*, New York, 1990, Guilford.

Baxter LR, et al: Cerebral glucose metabolic rates in non-depressed patients with obsessive-compulsive disorder, *Am J Psychiatry* 145:1560, 1988.

Beitchman JH, et al: Prevalence of speech and language disorders in 5-year-old kindergarten children in the Ottawa-Carleton region, *J Speech Hear Disord* 51:98, 1986a.

Beitchman JH, et al: Prevalence of psychiatric disorders in children with speech and language disorders, *J Am Acad Child Adolesc Psychiatry* 25:528, 1986b.

Biederman J, et al: A double-blind placebo controlled study of desipramine in the treatment of ADD, Part I: efficacy. *J Am Acad Child Adolesc Psychiatry* 28(5):777, 1989.

Biederman J, et al: Further evidence for family-genetic risk factors in attention deficit hyperactivity disorder, *Arch Gen Psychiatry* 49:728, 1992.

Biederman J, et al: Family-environmental risk factors for attention-deficit hyperactivity disorder, *Arch Gen Psychiatry* 52:464, 1995a.

Biederman J, et al: CBCL clinical scales discriminate prepubertal children with structured interview-derived diagnosis of mania from those with ADHD. *J Am Acad Child Adolesc Psychiatry* 34(4):464, 1995b.

Burd L, et al: Prevalence of Gilles de la Tourette's syndrome in North Dakota adults, *Am J Psychiatry* 143:787, 1986.

Burns BJ, et al: Children's mental health service use across service sectors. *Health Aff* 14(3):147, 1995.

Campbell M, et al: Neuroleptic-related dyskinesias in autistic children: a prospective, longitudinal study, *J Am Acad Child Adolesc Psychiatry* 36:835, 1997.

Carey G and Gottesman II: Twin and family studies of anxiety, phobic, and obsessive-compulsive disorders. In Klein DF and Rabkin J, editors: *Anxiety: new research and changing concepts*, New York, 1981, Raven.

Castellanos FX, et al: Quantitative brain magnetic resonance imaging in attention-deficit hyperactivity disorder, *Arch Gen Psychiatry* 53:607, 1996.

Cohen DJ and Volkmar FR: Handbook of autism and pervasive developmental disorders, ed 2, New York, 1997, Wiley.

Comings DE, Himes JA, and Comings BG: An epidemiological study of Tourette's syndrome in a single school district, *J Clin Psychiatry* 51:463, 1990.

Cook EH, et al: Evidence of linkage between the serotonin transporter and autistic disorder, *Mol Psychiatry* 2:247, 1997.

Costello EJ, et al: The Great Smoky Mountains study of youth: goals, design, methods, and the prevalence of DSM-III-R disorders, *Arch Gen Psychiatry* 53:1129, 1996.

DeVeaugh-Geiss J, et al: Clomipramine hydrochloride in childhood and adolescent obsessive-compulsive disorder: a multicenter trial, *J Am Acad Child Adolesc Psychiatry* 31:45, 1992.

Faraone SV, et al: Separation of DSM-III attention deficit disorder and conduct disorder: evidence from a family-genetic study of American child psychiatric patients, *Psychol Med* 21:109, 1991.

Fristad MA, Weller EB, and Weller RA: The Mania Rating Scale: can it be used in children? *J Am Acad Child Adolesc Psychiatry* 31(2):252, 1992.

Green WH: *Child and adolescent clinical psychopharmacology*, ed 2, Baltimore, 1995, Williams & Wilkins.

Griest JH, et al: Efficacy and tolerability of serotonin transport inhibitors in obsessive-compulsive disorder, *Arch Gen Psychiatry* 52:53, 1995.

Horwitz SM, et al: Identification and management of psychosocial and developmental problems in community-based, primary care pediatric practices, *Pediatrics* 89: 480, 1992.

Howe AC and Walker E: Behavioral management of toilet training: enuresis and encopresis, *Pediatr Clin North Am* 39:413-432, 1992.

Institute of Medicine: *Research on children and adolescents with mental, behavioral, and developmental disorders* (Division of Mental Health and Behavioral Medicine), Washington, DC, 1989, National Academy Press.

Jensen PS, et al: Prevalence of mental disorder in military children and adolescents: findings from a two-stage community survey, *J Am Acad Child Adolesc Psychiatry* 34:1514, 1995.

Karno M, et al: The epidemiology of obsessive compulsive disorder in five US communities, *Arch Gen Psychiatry* 45:1094, 1988.

Kendall PC and Braswell L: *Cognitive-behavioral therapy for impulsive children*, New York, 1993, Guilford.

King RA, et al: Emergence of self-destructive phenomena in children and adolescents during fluoxetine treatment. *J Am Acad Child Adolesc Psychiatry* 30:179, 1991.

Klein RG, Koplewicz HS, and Kanner A: Imipramine treatment of children with separation anxiety, *J Am Acad Child Adolesc Psychiatry* 31:21, 1992.

Kumra S, et al: Case study: risperidone-induced hepatoxicity in pediatric patients, *J Am Acad Child Adolesc Psychiatry* 36:701, 1997.

Leckman JF, et al: Clonidine treatment of Gilles de la Tourette's syndrome, *Arch Gen Psychiatry* 48:324, 1991.

Leckman JF, et al: Pathogenesis of Tourette's syndrome: clues from the clinical phenotype, *Adv Neurol* 58:15, 1992.

Levy F, et al: Attention-deficit hyperactivity disorder: a category or a continuum?: genetic analysis of a large-scale twin study, *J Am Acad Child Adolesc Psychiatry* 36(6):737, 1997.

Lewinsohn PM, Klein DN, and Seeley JR: Bipolar disorders in a community sample of older adolescents: prevalence, phenomenology, comorbidity, and course. *J Am Acad Child Adolesc Psychiatry* 34:454, 1995.

Lewinsohn PM, Rohde P, and Seeley JR: Adolescent psychopathology. III. The clinical consequences of co-morbidity, *J Am Acad Child Adolesc Psychiatry* 34:510, 1995.

Lombroso PJ, Pauls DL, and Leckman JF: Genetic mechanisms in childhood psychiatric disorders. *J Am Acad Child Adolesc Psychiatry* 33(7):921, 1994.

Mannuzza S, et al: Adult outcome of hyperactive boys: educational achievement, occupational rank, and psychiatric status, *Arch Gen Psychiatry* 50:565, 1993.

March JS, Mulle K, and Herbel B: Behavioral psychotherapy for children and adolescents with obsessive-compulsive disorder: an open trial of a new protocol-driven treatment package, *J Am Acad Child Adolesc Psychiatry* 33:333, 1994.

Martin JE and Agran M: Pharmacotherapy. In Matson JL, editor: *Handbook of treatment: approaches in childhood psychopathology,* New York, 1988, Plenum Press.

Merikangas KR and Angst J: The challenge of depressive disorders in adolescence. In Rutter M, editor: *Youth in the year 2000: psychological issues and interventions,* Cambridge, 1995, Cambridge University Press.

Pauls DL, et al: A family study of Gilles de la Tourette Syndrome, *Am J Hum Genet* 48:154, 1991.

Pelham WE, et al: Teacher ratings of DSM-III-R symptoms for disruptive behavior disorders, *J Am Acad Child Adolesc Psychiatry* 31:210, 1992.

Pennington BF: Diagnosing learning disorders: a neuropsychological framework, New York, 1991, Guilford.

Peterson BS, et al: Reduced basal ganglia volumes in Tourette's syndrome, using 3-dimensional reconstruction techniques from MRIs, *Neurology* 43:941, 1993.

Price RA, et al: A twin study of Tourette syndrome, *Arch Gen Psychiatry* 42:815, 1985.

Puig-Antich J, et al: A controlled family history study of prepubertal major depressive disorder, *Arch Gen Psychiatry* 46:406, 1989.

Riddle MA, et al: Obsessive compulsive disorder in children and adolescents: phenomenology and family history, *J Am Acad Child Adolesc Psychiatry* 29(5):766, 1990.

Riddle MA, et al: Behavioral side effects of fluoxetine, *J Child Adolesc Psychopharmacol* 1(3):193, 1991.

Riddle MA, et al: Double-blind, crossover trial of fluoxetine and placebo in children and adolescents with obsessive compulsive disorder, *J Am Acad Child Adolesc Psychiatry* 31:1062, 1992.

Riddle MA, et al: *Fluvoxamine in the treatment of children and adolescents with OCD: results of a multicenter, placebo-controlled study.* Presented at the American Academy of Child and Adolescent Psychiatry meeting, Philadelphia, 1996.

Riddle MA, Geller B, and Ryan N: Another sudden death in a child treated with desipramine, *J Am Acad Child Adolesc Psychiatry* 32:792, 1993.

Rosenbaum JF, et al: Further evidence of an association between behavioral inhibition and anxiety disorders: results from a family study of children from a nonclinical sample, *J Psychiatr Res* 25:49, 1991.

Safer DJ, Zito JM, and Fine EM: Increased methylphenidate usage for attention deficit disorder in the 1990s, *Pediatrics* 98(6):1084, 1996.

Scahill L: A method for screening child psychiatric inpatients for communication disorders, *J Child Adolesc Psychiatr Nurs* 3:98, 1990.

Scahill L: Contemporary approaches to pharmacotherapy in Tourette syndrome and obsessive-compulsive disorder, *J Child Adolesc Psychiatr Nurs* 9:27, 1996.

Scahill L: Psychopharmacology for children. In Keltner NL and Folks DG, editors: *Psychotropic drugs,* ed 2, St Louis, 1997, Mosby.

Scahill L and DeGraft-Johnson A: Food allergies, asthma, and attention deficit hyperactivity disorder, *J Child Adolesc Psychiatr Nurs* 10(2):36, 1997.

Scahill L and Lynch KA: The use of methylphenidate in children with attention-deficit hyperactivity disorder, *J Child Adolesc Psychiatr Nurs* 7:44, 1994a.

Scahill L and Lynch KA: Tricyclic antidepressants: cardiac effects and clinical implications, *J Child Adolesc Psychiatr Nurs* 7:37, 1994b.

Scahill L and Lynch KA: Atypical neuroleptics in children and adolescents, *J Child Adolesc Psychiatr Nurs* 11(1):38, 1998.

Scahill L, Ort SI, and Hardin MT: Genetic epidemiology and child psychiatric nursing: Tourette's syndrome as a model, *J Child Adolesc Psychiatr Nurs* 4(4):154, 1991.

Scahill L and Skrypeck A: Traditional neuroleptics in children and adolescents, *J Child Adolesc Psychiatr Nurs* 10(3):41, 1997.

Scahill L, et al: Behavioral therapy in children and adolescents with OCD: preliminary experience, *J Child Adolesc Psychopharmacol* 6(3):191, 1996.

Scahill L, et al: *Psychosocial and clinical correlates of ADHD in a community sample of young children.* Presented at the American Academy of Child and Adolescent Psychiatry meeting in Toronto, October 1996.

Shaywitz SE, et al: Prevalence of reading disability in boys and girls: results of the Connecticut longitudinal study, *JAMA* 264:998, 1990.

Singer H, et al: Volumetric MRI changes in basal ganglia of children with Tourette's syndrome, *Neurology* 43:950, 1993.

Singer HS, et al: The treatment of attention-deficit hyperactivity disorder in Tourette's syndrome: a double-blind placebo-controlled study with clonidine and desipramine. *Pediatrics* 95:74, 1995.

Sparrow SS, Balla DA, and Cicchetti DV: *Vineland Adaptive Behavior Scales,* Circle Pines, Minn, 1983, American Guidance Clinic.

Stevenson J: Evidence for a genetic etiology in hyperactivity in children, *Behav Genet* 22(3):337, 1992.

Szatmari P, Boyle M, and Offord DR: ADDH and conduct disorder: degree of diagnostic overlap and differences among correlates, *J Am Acad Child Adolesc Psychiatry* 28:865, 1989.

Szatmari P, Offord DR, and Boyle MH: Correlates, associated impairments and patterns of service utilization of children with attention deficit disorder: findings from the Ontario Child Health Study, *J Child Psychol Psychiatry* 30:205, 1989a.

Szatmari P, Offord DR, and Boyle MH: Ontario Child Health Study: prevalence of attention deficit disorder with hyperactivity, *J Child Psychol Psychiatry* 30:219, 1989b.

Tamminga CA, et al: Limbic system abnormalities identified in schizophrenia using positron emission tomography with fluorodeoxyglucose and neocortical alterations with deficit syndrome, *Arch Gen Psychiatry* 49(7):522, 1992.

Valleni-Basile LA, et al: Frequency of obsessive-compulsive disorder in a community sample of young adolescents, *J Am Acad Child Adolesc Psychiatry* 33(6):782, 1994.

Volkmar F and Cohen DJ: *The handbook of autism and pervasive developmental disorders,* ed 2, New York, 1997, Wiley.

Walkup JT, et al: Family study and segregation analysis of Tourette syndrome: evidence for a mixed model of inheritance, *Am J Hum Genet* 59:684, 1996.

Weller EB, Weller RA, and Fristad MA: Bipolar disorder in children: misdiagnosis, underdiagnosis, and future directions, *J Am Acad Child Adolesc Psychiatry* 34:709, 1995.

Zametkin AJ, et al: Cerebral glucose metabolism in adults with hyperactivity of childhood onset, *N Eng J Med* 323(20):1361, 1990.

CHAPTER 40

Mental Illness in the Elderly

CATHY S. CHILDERS

LEARNING OBJECTIVES

After reading this chapter you should be able to:
- Describe the various treatment options (i.e., the continuum of care) available to the elderly.
- Identify OBRA-87 regulations that guide psychiatric nursing practice with elderly populations.
- Describe the barriers to mental health care experienced by elders.
- Identify the unique variations in symptoms of depression evident in the elderly.
- Identify the various causes of psychosis among the elderly.
- Recognize the antianxiety agents appropriate for elderly patients.
- Identify major substance abuse issues in the elderly.
- Describe the psychosocial and physical assessments of the elderly.
- Recognize pharmacokinetic changes in the elderly that impact pharmacotherapy.
- Identify therapeutic goals for the elderly.

The National Coalition on Mental Health and Aging (1994) estimates mental health problems adversely affect the lives of 10% to 20% of older adults. For some, early onset psychiatric disorders persist as chronic or recurrent conditions into late life. In others, mental illness occurs for the first time after age 65. In the elderly, psychiatric disorders may have a clear neurological basis or may be reactions to stressors commonly occurring in late adulthood. The complex interplay of physical health, emotional well-being, and social factors poses challenges for the prevention, detection, and treatment of mental illness in this age group.

Rapid growth in the older population creates potential for a marked increase in the incidence of mental illness as successive cohorts enter old age (Gatz, 1995). Although in 1900 only 1 in 25 Americans (3.1 million) were over the age of 65, by 1995 the number of elderly had grown to 33.5 million or about 1 in 8 of the population (Administration on Aging, 1997). The U.S. Census Bureau (1995) predicts the elderly population will double between now and 2050, when 1 in 5 (80 million) will be over 65. Because the baby boom generation has already shown relatively high rates of depression, anxiety, and substance abuse, those trends are expected to continue in the coming years and compound challenges for caregivers and society (Gatz, 1995). In the current elderly population those who are 85 or older, known as the *old-old* or *true elderly,* represent the most rapidly expanding subgroup and are expected to account for 24% of the elderly cohort by 2050 (Administration on Aging, 1997).

Modern culture has tended to celebrate youth and place little emphasis on understanding old age. This unfortunate bias has contributed to insufficient knowledge about mental health disorders in the elderly as well as public policies that adversely affect access to care. However, projections on the growth of the elderly cohort have stimulated an interest (and infusion of funds) in study of the normal aging process (Sadavoy, et al, 1996). Research has increased the ability of health care providers to differentiate illness from normal aging and spurred the emergence of geriatric-specific specialties, including geropsychiatry. Despite the recognition of geriatric psychiatry as a specialty requiring knowledge beyond general psychiatry, considerable research documents the serious and unmet need for mental health care of older adults, both in the community and health care settings.

Basic social and financial factors recognized as contributing to late-life satisfaction and emotional well-being also often go unmet (Meeks and Murrell, 1997). The federal government has targeted persons past 75 years of age as having the greatest need for social support, income maintenance, housing, health services, and mental health services. These needs are closely linked to common stressors in late life that may be associated with negative psychological impact. For example, the death of a spouse and age peers reduces the social network and may lead to isolation and depression (Pearlin and Skaff, 1995). Health problems, common in the elderly, may lead to dependence, financial hardship, or relocation. Box 40-1 lists chronic medical conditions common in older adults. Retirement may be a fulfilling time of life, but for some the resulting changes outstrip adaptive capacity. Unrecognized and untreated mental disorders exact a toll in human suffering and societal costs. Unmet needs in any essential area place the elderly at risk and should be considered in the assessment and planning of interventions to assist older adults reach their maximum function.

Not all older people who experience stressful life events develop mental health disorders. In fact, the elderly represent a rich tapestry of individuals unique in their physical, psychological, and social functioning and are the most heterogeneous of all age groups (Rowe and Devons, 1996). It is important to appreciate the variability of health and function among those over 65 and the effects of *primary aging* (changes determined by inherent factors or heredity) and *secondary aging* (changes caused by environmental factors) (Busse, 1996). Several strengths have been identified that assist older adults in preserving emotional well-being. Successful adaptation is enhanced by the ability to shape and give meaning to experiences. A component of this process is comparing problems to what is experienced and expected by age contemporaries. One sage elder noted that at some point simply being alive can be seen as a sign of good health. This view might be reflected by the findings that most elderly individuals, despite multiple coexisting chronic medical conditions and impairments, report their health as good to excellent (Waters, 1995; Rowe and Devons, 1996). Religion is also used by the current older generation to give meaning to experiences (Blazer and Koenig, 1996). The availability of social supports to meet emotional and daily living needs are vital for successful coping. Mastery, the sense of ability to exercise control over circumstances, is another resource older adults call upon to cope with stressful situations. Losses commonly associated with the later years of life are listed in Box 40-2. While the aging process is inevitable,

---

Box 40-1   Chronic Medical Conditions in Individuals 65 Years of Age and Older

Arthritis and rheumatological disease
Neurosensory loss: hearing disturbance, visual disturbance
Cardiovascular disease: congestive heart failure, ischemic heart disease, hypertension, peripheral vascular disease
Gastrointestinal disorders
Chronic sinusitis and upper respiratory disturbances
Genitourinary tract problems
Chronic obstructive pulmonary disease
Adult-onset diabetes mellitus
Thyroid disease, endocrinopathy
Dermatological disturbances

Box 40-2   **Losses that Occur More Frequently Among the Elderly**

Loss of health
Loss of loved one
Loss of hearing and vision
Loss of status
Loss of work
Loss of income
Loss of friends
Loss of cognitive skills
Loss of home and community
Loss of mobility

older adults who can adapt to the changes express a high level of satisfaction with their lives (Pearlin and Skaff, 1995).

Nurses involved in the care of the elderly should be familiar with the continuum of mental illness needs: prevention, detection, and treatment. This chapter presents an overview of issues related to mental health care of the elderly that are different from those of other age groups. Policy issues, barriers to mental health care, and common mental disorders occurring in the elderly are discussed along with the process of assessment and psychotherapeutic management. Cognitive disorders, which account for some of the most frequently occurring mental disorders in the aged, are covered in Chapter 30. Historic trends that influence the perception of psychiatry by the current aged cohort are addressed in Chapter 1.

CONTINUUM OF CARE

Because of the prevalence of mental health disorders in late life, nurses who encounter older adults in any health care setting should consider the physical, emotional, and social needs of their patients. Whenever possible, factors that place the elderly at risk of mental illness or problems stemming from existing mental disorders should be identified and plans developed to meet the needs. Unfortunately, policies and resources have lagged far behind the rising needs of a steadily aging population. Federal leadership is lacking both in the mental health needs of older people and in aging issues in general (Rosen, Pancake, and Rickards, 1995). Therefore, improving the quality of mental health care for older adults rests on educating health care providers, the elderly, and their caregivers.

Social Support

Education and social support are essential components of prevention, but organizations that target the elderly have typically distanced themselves from the mentally ill. (Estes, 1995). Even though some agencies on aging have worked with community mental health centers, many others have shied away from the overwhelming needs of the elderly mentally ill. The Coalition for Mental Health and Aging has worked to increase the visibility of elder's mental health needs, and organizations such as the American Association for Retired People (AARP) provide education on mental health issues. Nurses can provide mental health information on prevention and treatment in sites where elderly are likely to visit such as nutrition centers, senior centers, churches, and medical clinics. Older adults and their caregivers are less likely than younger adults and their families to join advocacy groups for mentally ill, such as the National Alliance for the Mentally Ill (NAMI), resulting in few strong, united voices lobbying for programs and legislation related to the mental health needs of at-risk elderly.

Community Support

Some federal legislation has strongly influenced care of mentally ill elderly. Following the Community Mental Health Act of 1963, which initiated deinstitutionalization, large numbers of chronically mentally ill were discharged from state and county mental hospitals to less restrictive settings in the community. Community mental health centers were ill prepared to deal with elderly already in the community, much less the large numbers returning, often from prolonged institutionalization. Only 15% of community mental health centers target the elderly for outreach, and fewer have geriatric specialists (Estes, 1995). Despite the focus on access to mental health care in the community endorsed by the Community Mental Health Act, third-party reimbursement and other factors encourage older adults to seek assistance from primary care physicians in the community or inpatient services in public general hospitals. Nurses in these settings can assist in the detection of patients at risk and suffering undiagnosed mental disorders.

Local Alternatives to Formal Mental Health Care

Elderly individuals with known psychiatric disorders use traditional mental health resources less than expected. However, they use a disproportionate share of services in general hospitals, where care is more likely to be delivered by general practitioners following physical problems than by psychiatric specialists (Atay, Witkin, and Mandersheid, 1995). This is partially accounted for by the fact that about 65% of elderly persons with psychiatric disorders also have a significant medical disease for which they receive care (Sloan, 1986). Further, in general hospitals, about 27% of elderly hospitalized medical inpatients also meet diagnostic criteria for mental disorders (Alessi and Cassel, 1996). Nursing homes are another site of care. Many of the chronically mentally ill released from state hospitals during the waves of deinstitutionalization were reinstitutionalized in nursing homes. By 1969, 75% of all institutionalized mentally ill elderly were in nursing homes; only 25% were in state hospitals (Estes, 1995). This is directly reflected in the high prevalence, between 68% and 94%, of neuropsychiatric illness found among residents of long-term care facilities (Stoudemire and Smith, 1996).

OBRA-87 and Nursing Homes

Care of the mentally ill in nursing homes has received government attention. Much negative publicity on the potential abuse of physical and chemical (psychoactive drugs) restraints prompted the Omnibus Budget Reconciliation Act (OBRA) of 1987. This legislation regulated both pharmacological and physical restraints, recognizing the resident's right to be restraint free unless medically necessary. Nursing home staffs must carefully document behaviors to ensure restraints are not used for discipline or for staff convenience. Drugs such as haloperidol (Haldol) may be used to control agitation and manifestations of psychosis, but staff are required to quantitatively document problems, attempt nonpharmacological alternatives and, when

Using Written Materials to Teach or Assess the Elderly
• Only 50% of people over 65 graduated from high school: consider reading level • People are reluctant to disclose they are unable to read • Use large print type with high contrast • Provide high intensity lighting without glare • Encourage person to wear corrective lenses

From Domarad BR and Buschmann MT. Interviewing older adults: increasing the credibility of interview data, *J Gerontol Nurs* 21(9):14, 1995.

using neuroleptic drugs, to have a planned program of gradual dose reduction. Reports indicate that OBRA-87 has been successful in decreasing the use of antipsychotic agents, by up to 72% in one study (Stoudemire and Smith, 1996). Additional Health Care Financing Administration (HCFA) guidelines, effective in 1992, deal with other psychoactive medications. Strict guidelines also govern the application of any type of restraints in nursing homes. For years, restraints were seen as a safe and effective means of eliminating falls and controlling behavior. Numerous deaths have been attributed to restraints and other substantial problems associated with enforced immobility are well documented. HCFA developed guidelines for nursing home restraints, and the Joint Commission on Accreditation of Healthcare Organizations (JCAHO) followed by publishing stringent guidelines, effective in 1996, for restraint use in acute care facilities. An additional significant component of OBRA-87 addressed concerns about mentally ill being warehoused in nursing homes. Residents must be screened for mental illnesses prior to admission, and those already in residence must meet criteria for nursing care beyond active mental health treatment (see box above for suggestions on assessing the elderly). Those not needing nursing intervention for reasons other than mental illness, with some exceptions, must be discharged (Stoudemire and Smith, 1996). Therefore, mentally ill elderly are being deinstitutionalized, this time from nursing homes, and the numbers in the community will increase. Nurses who work with the elderly must remain abreast of regulatory action that affects the placement and care of the elderly mentally ill.

Current and Future Trends

Estes (1995) reports that although nursing homes and general hospitals are currently the two major destinations for mentally ill older adults, board-and-care facilities and home visits by mental health workers are expected to increase. In the last 10 years, day hospital programs for the elderly mentally ill have seen tremendous growth due to an increased focus on decreasing inpatient hospital costs. Cost-containment measures by Medicare and Medicare replacement health maintenance organizations (HMOs), along with OBRA mandates, are expected to increase the need for community care for the older adults with mental illnesses. Nurses will have increasing responsibility for the assessment and care of mentally ill in the community.

BARRIERS TO MENTAL HEALTH CARE FOR THE ELDERLY

Ageism

The National Coalition on Mental Health and Aging (1994) defines ageism as "the commonly held belief that specific mental health conditions experienced by older persons are part of normal aging and are not treatable." The term is also used to describe negative stereotyping and devaluation of people solely because of their age. Behaviors indicative of ageism include intergenerational segregation, contact avoidance, condescending or abusive interpersonal treatment, and discrimination in the form of limited access to services and resources (McGowan, 1996). Despite the fact that those who turned 65 in 1995 can expect an additional 17.4 years of life, policy makers have demonstrated reluctance to allocate funds to those perceived to be at the end of life. Health care providers are more likely to dispense psychoactive drugs than therapy, in part due to therapists' hesitancy to embark on prolonged treatments with those who might die before benefiting.

Attitudes

Attitudes of the elderly themselves serve as a barrier to seeking mental health care. Older adults are more likely to subscribe to age-specific stereotyping than younger people (Dye, 1985). Symptoms of treatable disorders are frequently unreported by those who believe that difficulties are part of old age or a normal consequence of difficult life experiences (Rowe and Devons, 1996). Too, the elderly are more likely to relate problems to physical health and life circumstances than psychological deficits (Waters, 1995).

Older adults are reluctant to seek psychiatric care because an admission of mental health problems is seen as a weakness and is more stigmatizing than it might be for a younger person. It may also represent a loss of control and bring forth fears of institutionalization. In difficult times when outside help is required, people who grew up in an era that emphasized self-reliance are more likely to rely on friends, family, and other informal supports than on mental health professionals. Psychiatric care is often viewed with skepticism and thought to be unnecessarily expensive and time-consuming.

Finances

The cost of mental health care is a major disincentive to providers as well as older adults who might otherwise seek psychiatric assistance. Medicare, the federal insurance program that covers 97% of the elderly, does not provide the same coverage for mental health care as it does for medical treatment (Rosen, Pancake, and Rickards, 1995). In 1988, less than 3% of Medicare's total budgeted spending of 90.5 billion dollars was for mental health (Buren, Sloan, and Cohen, 1992). There is a lifetime limit on the number of psychiatric inpatient days and the co-payment for outpatient psychiatric service is higher than for nonpsychiatric visits. These factors influence the selection of primary care physicians over psychiatric specialists and influence the type and location of care received (Estes, 1995). Payments for provider visits and the cost of assistive care, especially that which is not medically necessary, is borne by individuals and caregivers. Following Medicare's lead, other insurers provide comparatively limited psychiatric coverage. Some, including the growing number of Medicare replacement HMOs, exclude selected components of mental health and substance abuse treatment altogether. Although fewer elderly than younger people live in poverty, one fifth of older adults are classified as poor or "near poor" (Administration on Aging, 1997). Even services and medications recognized as important may be out of financial reach for those with limited resources.

Inadequate Detection of Mental Illness and Treatment

Recognition of mental illness is the first step in treatment, yet many studies demonstrate psychological disturbances in the elderly are often missed or misdiagnosed. Psychiatric diagnosis may be complicated by several factors: elders' unwillingness or inability to discuss problems in terms of emotions, the connection between mental disorders and physical factors present in chronic or acute medical conditions, and the blurring of normal and abnormal findings in the elderly. The most likely source of care for an older person living in the community who suffers emotional or psychiatric problems is a general practitioner who sees the patient in a visit scheduled for a physical complaint.

Nonpsychiatric physicians are *less likely* to diagnose or treat mental disorders. Referrals are infrequent to psychiatric specialists who are *more likely* to initiate a comprehensive assessment to diagnosis mental illness (Estes, 1995). Nurses contribute to inadequate detection of mental disorders when they fail to assess and report known symptoms (Profitt, Augspurger, and Byrne, 1996).

PSYCHIATRIC DISORDERS IN THE ELDERLY
DEPRESSION

Inadequate detection of depression, one of the most frequently occurring and treatable psychiatric disorders of late life, is a major public health problem (Coyne, Fechner-Bates, and Schwenk, 1994; Koenig and Blazer, 1996). Although in about 5% of the depressed elderly, depression has persisted or recurred since younger adulthood, the majority of older adults are diagnosed for the first time in late life (Koenig and Blazer, 1996). It is unfortunate that recognized depression is often untreated when health care providers and aged individuals themselves view it as an inevitable response to illnesses and common late life circumstances (Sanders, 1995; Butler and Lewis, 1995). The effects of depression extend beyond emotionally distressing symptoms of helplessness, hopelessness, fear, shame, guilt, and anger to physical consequences. Depression can cause more physical and social limitations than chronic medical conditions such as diabetes and arthritis (Butler and Lewis, 1995). In addition, mortality rates increase for some disorders with the coexistence of depression; a fact attributed in part to the effects of depression on treatment compliance along with the effects of related mental health problems such as substance abuse, anxiety, somatization, and suicide (Bittner, Taylor, and Raczynski, 1997; Koenig and Blazer, 1996; Butler and Lewis, 1995).

Incidence

The prevalence of late life depression varies tremendously among reported studies. The National Coalition on Mental Health and Aging (1994) estimates 15% of older community residents suffer depressive symptoms, however major depressive disorder (MDD) occurs in only 1% to 2%. These figures are similar to those reported in the 1980s National Mental Health Epidemiologic Catchment Area study that found major depression occurred less frequently in those over 65 than in younger groups. Rates for depression in nursing home residents are reported at 15% to 25% (National Coalition on Mental Health and Aging, 1994). Among elderly patients hospitalized for physical problems, 10% meet criteria for MDD, and approximately 30% have some form of depression. In medical settings, it is thought that only 10% to 20% of depressed elderly patients are diagnosed and treated (Koenig and Blazer, 1996).

Presentation

The detection of depression is complicated by a number of factors. Depression in the elderly frequently does not fit well with current DSM-IV criteria, and many depressive symptoms can be attributed to either physical or psychological causes in elders with chronic illnesses. Depression is an illness that affects mind and body; it causes people to feel miserable both physically and emotionally. Some report that older depressed people display more somatic complaints, social withdrawal, and memory disturbances than younger patients, whereas other studies show a similar symptom profile. Older adults, however, are more likely to seek help for

Box 40-3	Common Physical Indicators of Depression

Sleep disturbances (one of the earliest symptoms)
Fatigue or loss of energy unrelated to hard work or rest
Loss of sexual interest
Weight changes (usually weight loss)
Gastrointestinal complaints (constipation or abdominal distress)
Multiple vague aches and pains unrelated to a physical cause

Box 40-4	Lifetime Prevalence Rate of Depression in Medical Disorders	
Type II Diabetes	25%
Left hemisphere CVA	50%
Right hemisphere CVA	10%
Cancer (site dependent)	24%*
Myocardial infarction	20%
Parkinson's disease	50%

*Average for all sites.
Adapted from Lamberg L: Treating depression in medical conditions may improve quality of life, *JAMA* 276(11):857, Sept 1996. Available at: http://www.ama-assn.org/sci-pubs/journals/archive/jama/vol_276/no_11/mn6145.htm. Accessed Aug 1, 1997; Blazer DG and Koenig HG: Mood disorders. In Busse E and Blazer D, editors: *Textbook of geriatric psychiatry*, ed 2, Washington, DC, 1996, American Psychiatric Press.

physical distress than emotional distress and, unless prompted, may not volunteer feelings of depression. Some of the typical physical complaints associated with depression are listed in Box 40-3. The lifetime prevalence rate of depression in selected medical disorders is listed in Box 40-4. Older adults may lack the range of vocabulary younger individuals commonly possess to describe emotions. Rather than expressions of diminished self-esteem, helplessness, hopelessness, or apathy, for example, they are more likely to complain of "having the blues" or "feeling worthless."

Because of the overlap of cognitive symptoms in depression and dementia, misdiagnosis of dementia occurs frequently. Depression commonly coexists with dementia, and frequently depression is left untreated when symptoms are assumed to arise from cognitive deterioration (Lamberg, 1996). Shared symptoms include poor memory, disorientation, poor judgment, and agitation or motor retardation. Depression that mimics dementia is termed *pseudodementia*. In these cases, nursing observations can be essential to correcting the diagnosis. Extended observation may detect higher functioning than expected (Burrows, et al, 1995). Nurses can also look for a downcast mood, which can help differentiate depression from the more bland affect of true dementia (Alexopoulos, 1996). Differentiating these disorders is important for treatment.

Psychotic depression may also be confused with cognitive or other psychiatric disorders. It is important for nurses to be aware of the symptoms to assist in identification because the suicide risk for individuals with psychotic depression is 5 to 6 times higher than in other forms of depression (Lamberg, 1996). When depression occurs for the first time after age 60, delusions are more common than with earlier onset depression. Delusions of persecution or of having an incurable illness as well as nihilistic delusions are more frequent than delusions associated with guilt (Blazer and Koenig, 1996). Hallucinations, however, are an uncommon feature of psychotic depression. Many older adults with psychotic depression may ruminate, express suspiciousness, and voice multiple physical complaints. Psychotic depression is often resistant to traditional antidepressant medications and psychotherapy. As a result, electroconvulsive therapy (ECT) is frequently the treatment of choice for this disorder.

Electroconvulsive Therapy

ECT is a safe and effective treatment for severely depressed patients, including the very old (Casey and Davis, 1996). Chapter 37 provides a thorough review of the subject. When a rapid response is needed for an elderly patient who is suicidal, losing weight rapidly, or in danger of medical crisis, ECT may be the treatment of choice (Butler, et al, 1997). ECT may also be indicated when patients have failed to respond to other treatment or are poor candidates for drug therapy.

Two important nursing roles are maintenance of safety and education. Misinformation and the stigma of ECT can discourage some elderly and their family members from providing consent to treatment. When this is the case, education should include information to dispel the myths surrounding ECT (Brandt and Ugarriza, 1996). Following ECT,

Selected Nursing Interventions for Work with Depressed Elderly

Assess and meet physical needs
Maximize independence
Promote sense of control
Provide consistency
Encourage open awareness
Increase self-esteem

Acknowledge individual's feelings
Appreciate individual's uniqueness in context of entire life span
Reinforce genuine hopes
Consider family and caregivers

Adapted from Sanders P: Depression in life threatening illness and its treatment, *Nurs Times* 91(11), 1995

patients may exhibit postictal confusion, and delirium may also develop. During this time, the nurse must take precautions to preserve patient safety and promote physical and emotional well-being.

Suicide

Suicide is the most tragic effect of depression, and it is the elderly who, out of all age groups, have the highest rate of suicide. Older persons represent about 12.5% of the population but account for approximately 20% of all reported suicides. The subgroup of elderly over the age of 85 have the highest rate of suicide within the over-65 population (National Coalition on Mental Health and Aging, 1994). Elderly white males are roughly 3 times more likely than other older adults to kill themselves, but the suicide rate of black males is climbing rapidly. (Alexopoulos, 1996; Gurland, 1996). Although women attempt suicide more frequently than men, men have a higher suicide attempt to suicide completion ratio. Highly lethal methods—guns, hanging, or leaping from heights—are used more by men than women, who are more likely to attempt suicide by overdose. Suicidal gestures, more common among young adults than suicide, are rare in older adults. In the elderly, failed attempts are usually not a "cry for help" but a serious, yet unsuccessful, suicide bid (Duffy, 1997). The rate of suicide may be even higher than reported because statistics do not include chronic suicide. This term characterizes death caused by slower, less obvious means than the violent acts usually associated with suicide. Refusing to eat, noncompliance with medication, excessive alcohol intake, and physical risk taking are processes that may result in death but are not recorded as suicide (Butler and Lewis, 1995).

Box 40-5   Predictors of Suicide Risk Among the Elderly

Over 65 years of age
Male
White
Chronic or uncontrolled pain
Bereavement
Unmarried (widowed or divorced)
Retirement
Financial difficulty
Social isolation
Impulsiveness
Hopeless/helpless
Alcohol or drug abuse
History of previous attempt
Major depressive disorder, especially psychotic depression

Table 40-1   Rate of Suicide Among the Elderly

Age Range	All Older Rate	White Males Rate
65-74	16.9/100,000	30/100,000
75-84	23.5/100,000	58/100,000
85 and over	24.0/100,000	60/100,000

Adapted from McIntosh JL: Epidemiology of suicide in the elderly, *Suicide Life Threat Behav* 22(1):15, 1992; National Coalition on Mental Health and Aging: *Building state and community mental health and aging coalitions: a "how-to" guide,* Dec 1994. Available at http://www.mentalhealth.org/resource/how2.htm. Accessed July 31, 1997.

Prevention of suicide in the elderly begins with the detection of risk. Box 40-5 lists predictors of suicide risk, and Table 40-1 provides informative statistics related to suicide rates for the elderly. It is important for the nurse to listen to the themes of conversation and observe for signs that may signal suicidal thoughts. Particular attention should be given to older persons who are beginning to recover from depression: as energy returns there is a greater risk of suicide. Intent might be signaled by a new preoccupation with religious issues, giving away possessions, changing a will, or other "new" behaviors. People may feel ashamed to plainly voice ideas of self-harm, so if negative statements or behaviors are detected, it is essential to ask directly about any intentions. It is a myth that such discussions can stir suicidal thoughts (Duffy, 1997).

Suicide does not always arise from depression. For some who face life-threatening illness, suicide is the ultimate means of exercising control over the situation. "Rational" or physician-assisted suicide is an area currently of concern to medical practitioners, ethicists, and legal decision makers.

CLINICAL EXAMPLE

Mr. White is an 86-year-old white man who has outlived two wives. Mr. White has remained sexually active into his 80s, but within the past 2 years he has had difficulties attaining an erection. Mr. White relates that recently a younger woman (mid-50s) asked about spending the night. She did, and Mr. White could not perform sexually. He said, "I'm just no good anymore." Mr. White said he was embarrassed by his sexual inability. He states that he has had thoughts of suicide but would not act on those thoughts. He promises the nurse that he will call if he has an urge to harm himself.

CLINICAL EXAMPLE

Mr. Timchuk is a 77-year-old white man with chronic obstructive pulmonary disease (COPD). He has great difficulty doing any physical activity. Mr. Timchuk is very despondent over his condition, and there is little hope that he will improve. Although he has not verbalized a desire to "end it all," he states that he would be better off dead. The nurse understands that he is at great risk for self-harm.

BIPOLAR DISORDER

There is little information on the incidence of bipolar disorders in late life. A substantial subgroup of late-onset mania patients consists of individuals with unipolar major depression who changed polarity in late life. Patients with late-onset bipolar disorders have a lower rate of affective disorders among relatives than early-onset patients (Alexopoulos, 1996). There is speculation that early-onset bipolar illness may "burn itself out" with time, but if a bipolar disorder reemerges in late life, then the episodes of mania—or mixture of depression and mania—may cycle more rapidly (Blazer and Koenig, 1996). Mania in the elderly may present in the same fashion as with younger adults, but symptoms may be less intense. Features may include grandiosity, disorientation, delirium, and reversible cognitive dysfunction (Alexopoulos, 1996). It is important to note that cerebrovascular and degenerative neurological disorders often have a major role in the etiology of manic episodes that present for the first time in later life. Nursing interventions must include attention to the increasingly negative impact of agitation on self-care and self-protection in medically compromised elderly.

CLINICAL EXAMPLE

Ms. Ellington, a 72-year-old white woman, was brought to the hospital by the community service officer of the local police department. She was found sitting outside a homeless shelter with her belongings in boxes surrounding her. There was a strong odor of alcohol coming from the cup of orange juice she held. Her sparse flame-red hair was covered by a wide-brim black hat with flowing scarf. She was attired in tight animal print leggings, a transparent blouse, and thigh-high white boots. On admission, Ms. Ellington was cursing loudly and removed her dentures and threw them at the first staff person who approached. Although she was well known to the staff, Ms. Ellington claimed that she was a Hollywood star who had been left on the street, kicked out of her mansion by friends she had taken in, robbed of her identification, and shipped to a town where she would be unknown and unrecognized. An empty bottle of lithium and an unfilled prescription for more were found in her purse.

PSYCHOTIC DISORDERS

Psychotic disorders, characterized by delusions, hallucinations, thought disorder, bizarre behavior, or other evidence of impaired reality testing, are among the most severe psychiatric disorders in people of any age. In the elderly, these signs and symptoms may be related to a psychiatric disorder, a dementia, a delirious state, substance abuse or withdrawal, medication, or some other entity (Box 40-6). Nurses should be familiar with the numerous medications and physical conditions associated with psychosis and recognize the importance of carefully reporting the nature and content of hallucinations and delusions to facilitate ruling out neurological, endocrine, and other reversible medical causes.

Schizophrenia is not a mental disorder that typically first occurs late in life. The term late-onset schizophrenia is frequently used to describe those cases that first present after age 45. Late-onset schizophrenia is characterized by bizarre delusions, often involving persecution, and auditory hallucinations (Jeste, Harris, and Paulsen, 1996). Disorganization and negative symptoms (withdrawal, apathy, and anhedonia) are less prominent than in early-onset. The majority of individuals diagnosed with schizophrenia late in life have abnormal premorbid personality traits but are more likely than early-onset schizophrenics to have been married, raised children, and maintained employment. It is interesting to note that sensory deficits (especially hearing loss) are more commonly found in those diagnosed with

schizophrenia after age 60 than in the general population. The role of these deficits in the disease are unknown, however (American Psychiatric Association [APA], 1994). For many, late-onset schizophrenia marks the beginning of a chronic disorder with periods of remission and symptom recurrence. The insidious deterioration of personality and social adjustment characteristic of early-onset schizophrenia also occurs. As in early-onset schizophrenia, antipsychotic medications are an effective treatment for many of the positive symptoms (delusions, hallucinations, bizarre or disorganized behavior, impairments in communication), especially when coupled with a structured environment (milieu) and supportive nurse-patient interactions.

Many chronic schizophrenic patients reach late life in spite of the high mortality (e.g., suicide) associated with chronic early-onset schizophrenia (Koenig, et al, 1996). There is little research documenting the long-term course of schizophrenia, but evidence suggests that positive symptoms persist into the later years. Only in the old-old is there a significant reduction in the positive symptoms. Cuffel et al (1996) documented studies demonstrating elderly persons with chronic schizophrenia have more general medical problems, greater cognitive impairment, and a higher incidence of tardive dyskinesia

---

Box 40-6   Disorders Associated with Secondary Psychosis in the Elderly

Endocrinopathies
Hyperthyroidism
Hypothyroidism
Addison's disease
Cushing's disease
Hyperparathyroidism
Hypoparathyroidism
Hypoglycemia

Neurological Disorders
Parkinson's disease
Alzheimer's disease
Pick's disease
Multiinfarct dementia
Seizure disorders
Hydrocephalus
Demyelinating diseases (e.g., multiple sclerosis)
Neoplasms

Encephalopathies (posttraumatic, hepatic, toxic)
Viral encephalitis
Spinocerebellar degeneration
Neurosyphyllis

Vitamin Deficiencies
Thiamine
Niacin
B_{12}
Folate

Other Conditions
Iatrogenic (secondary to drugs)
Systemic lupus erythematosus
Temporal arteritis
Hyponatremia
Delirium (e.g., as a result of hypoxia)

Source: Jeste DV, Harris MJ, and Paulsen JS: Psychosis. In Sadavoy J, et al, editors: *Comprehensive review of geriatric psychiatry–II,* ed 2, Washington, DC, 1996, American Psychiatric Press.

than younger schizophrenic patients. Many of the medical problems are related to comorbid substance abuse problems, especially nicotine dependence. Emphysema and other pulmonary and cardiac problems are common (APA, 1994). Global cognitive functioning in elderly schizophrenics shows declines greater than in same-age persons without schizophrenia but less than that associated with degenerative cognitive disorders, such as Alzheimer's disease. The increase of tardive dyskinesia in older patients with schizophrenia complicates medication management, increases the degree of disability associated with the disorder, and contributes to the high cost of services for elderly schizophrenics.

A study of treatment costs and mental health service use by age cohorts suggests that older persons with schizophrenia continue to use inpatient or institutional services more than they do community mental health organizations (Cuffel, et al, 1996). Long-term institutionalization poses problems of learned dependence and decreased mental capacity and coping skills (Kane, 1995). Nurses should note that long-term institutionalized elderly released into the community may have significant deficits in daily living skills and lack the social networks so important to successful adaptation. In the community, the cost of mental health services for elderly schizophrenics is much greater than that of other older adults. Because of their complex needs, the intensity of service is at a level comparable to that of young adult schizophrenics (Cuffel, et al, 1996).

Paranoid Thinking

Paranoid symptoms are not uncommon in the elderly. Paranoia may be a feature of depression, occur after a stressful life event, or result from delirium or some other psychiatric disorder. The content often involves persecution, jealousy, or situations that could conceivably occur in real life. These delusions are generally chronic and well systematized and, unless associated with dementia or delirium, are not associated with memory loss, disorientation, or diminished cognitive function (Koenig, et al, 1996). As coping behaviors are compromised with age, paranoid thinking often emerges as a defense mechanism against a potentially hostile environment. For example, walking to the corner grocery store in some neighborhoods may be perilous for older persons because they are less able to fend off aggressors. Older

persons find themselves becoming increasingly isolated as they retreat into an environment they can control. Although the threat may be based on reality, the resulting isolation and decrease in external stimuli along with suspicious behaviors can lead to paranoid thinking.

CLINICAL EXAMPLE

Mrs. Rutters is a 78-year-old black woman. She comes to the general practice clinic with her daughter, Sandra, for a routine visit. Sandra states, "Mother's behavior is declining. It is going downhill every day." Sandra relates a recent episode that was embarrassing and frustrating. She took her mother to the mall and, just as they were about to enter, Mrs. Rutters balked and would not proceed. She said to her daughter, "You are not going to leave me in there." As Sandra tried to talk to her mother and guide her into the mall, Mrs. Rutters swung her purse and struck Sandra, saying, "I'm not going anywhere with you, you big, fat woman." At that point, Sandra gave up on the shopping trip and decided to go home. Her mother would not comply with that wish either. Mrs. Rutters began screaming for help from other shoppers. The nurse practitioner worked supportively with Sandra alone for a while and decided to increase Mrs. Rutters's Haldol from 0.5 mg qd to 0.5 mg bid.

ANXIETY DISORDERS

Anxiety is one of the most common psychiatric conditions in the elderly and presents with cognitive, behavioral, somatic, or physiological symptoms similar to those seen in younger adults (Folks and Fuller, 1997) (Box 40-7). Although anxiety is a normal emotion that alerts a person to impending danger or an unpleasant event, it can be considered maladaptive when it interferes with functioning (Sheikh, 1996).

Little research exists on anxiety disorders in late life, but there is agreement that anxiety may negatively impact coexisting medical disorders. Two anxiety disorders defined in the DSM-IV may be overrepresented in the elderly: anxiety resulting from general medical conditions and substance abuse–induced anxiety (Folks and Fuller, 1997). A number of medical disorders may either produce anxiety as a response to a physiologic stressor or present with

Box 40-7 **Psychological or Somatic Signs and Symptoms of Anxiety**		
Anorexia	Fatigue	Paresthesia
Backache	Flushing	Sexual dysfunction
"Butterflies" in stomach	Headache	Shortness of breath
Chest discomfort	Hyperventilation	Stomach pain
Diaphoresis	Light-headedness	Sweating
Diarrhea	Muscle tension	Tachycardia
Dizziness	Nausea	Tremulousness
Dyspnea	Pallor	Urinary frequency
Dry mouth	Palpitations	Vomiting
Faintness		

From Folks D and Fuller W: Anxiety disorders and insomnia in geriatric patients, *Psychiatr Clin North Am* 20(1):137, 1997.

symptoms similar to the somatic manifestations of anxiety. As many as 10% of community-dwelling older adults and 40% of nursing home residents experience anxiety related to substance abuse and dependence, as well as toxicity from prescription drugs (Folks and Fuller, 1997). The relationship of stressful life events and losses to anxiety are unknown at this time; however, they may play a significant role in late-life anxiety. For example, fear of crime and fear of dying are two specific phobias more likely to occur in older than in younger patients. In addition to the anxiety disorders already listed, other forms that occur in older adults include agoraphobia, panic disorder, obsessive-compulsive disorder, generalized anxiety disorder, acute stress disorder, and posttraumatic stress disorder.

SUBSTANCE ABUSE

Late-life alcohol and drug abuse and dependence are problems that have received little attention until recent years. It is well recognized, however, that alcoholism and prescription drug abuse exact a high physical, psychological, and social toll. Mortality is affected by substance abuse, either from severe withdrawal, medical complications, or suicide. Concern about this area is growing, and the incidence is expected to increase tremendously as successive generations enter old age. Illicit drug use, uncommon in the current elderly cohort, is expected to follow younger adults into their advancing years. Abuse of prescription and over-the-counter drugs, however, is a recognized problem for the current group of elderly. An understanding of factors that contribute

to substance abuse, consequences, and presenting symptoms is important for nurses working with older adults because both the elderly and their families, as well as health care providers, often either minimize chemical abuse problems or do not appreciate the role of substance abuse in problem situations.

Alcohol Abuse and Dependence

Because of age-related biological changes and medical disorders, older adults are at greater risk for the hazards and dependence potential of alcohol than younger individuals. Despite estimates of the prevalence of alcoholism in elderly adults ranging from 1% to 14% (Mudd, et al, 1994), alcohol's contribution to functional, psychological, and medical problems in the elderly is often missed due to a variety of factors, including underreporting of alcohol consumption by the drinker. This can be due to impaired recall or shame about alcohol intake, especially strong in the cohort influenced by negative values about alcohol use in the Prohibition era (Ganzini and Atkinson, 1996). The quantity of alcohol consumed must be considered along with the enhanced effects of alcohol on the elderly. The same amount of alcohol will produce a blood alcohol level about 20% higher in a 65-year-old than in a 30-year-old (Ganzini and Atkinson, 1996). At the same time, older persons show greater central nervous system sensitivity to alcohol, so adverse effects on cognition and coordination will also be more pronounced in older than younger drinkers. Thus, even if older adults do not increase the level of alcohol consumption over that of earlier years, problems

---

Box 40-8   Potential Alcohol-Related Problems in the Elderly

Unexpected drug effects
Delirium
Dementia (Wernicke-Korsakoff
  syndrome)
Depression
Self-neglect

Dehydration
Malnutrition
Bladder/bowel incontinence
Muscle weakness
Gait disorders
Repeated falls

Burns
Gastric bleeding
Accidental hypothermia
Legal trouble (esp. DUI)
Family discord

From Ganzini L and Atkinson RM: Substance abuse. In Sadavoy J, et al, editors: *Comprehensive review of geriatric psychiatry–II,* ed 2, Washington, DC, 1996, American Psychiatric Press.

Box 40-9   Nursing Care of Alcohol Withdrawal Syndrome in the Elderly

Assess withdrawal symptoms
Assess vital signs
Educate about withdrawal process
Assist with ADLs
Reduce environmental stimuli
Supplement diet to meet nutritional needs
Reorient
Provide relaxation exercises

---

may result. Combining alcohol with the high rate of over-the-counter and prescription drug use by the elderly complicates the situation. Drug half-lives may be prolonged and effects of drugs potentiated. (Solomon, et al, 1993).

There are a number of risk factors for problem drinking in late life. A family history or personal history of heavy drinking increases the risk of alcohol dependence. However, a number of elderly individuals develop problem drinking patterns for the first time in late life. The presence of chronic medical disorders may lead some elderly to self-medicate with alcohol to control pain or induce sleep. Drinking is also used by some isolated elderly or those with excessive leisure time to combat boredom. Alcohol is seen by yet other individuals as a means of decreasing or escaping the emotional distress of psychiatric disorders. When an alcohol use disorder is associated with another psychiatric disorder, the term *dual diagnosis* is used. In older alcoholics, the coexisting mental disorders are most commonly affective and organic mental disorders. Anxiety disorders and schizophrenia are also related to alco-

holism (Ganzini and Atkinson, 1996). Three quarters of older problem drinkers have difficulty with physical health, emotional health, isolation, and the use of leisure time (Graham, et al, 1995).

Nurses should be attuned to the possibility of alcohol's role in many problems seen in elderly medical and psychiatric patients. Box 40-8 lists some of the presenting features of elderly problem drinkers. Because activities of daily living and cognitive functioning are so affected by heavy drinking, alcohol use should be strongly suspected when there are wide fluctuations in performance in these areas (Graham, et al, 1995). Unfortunately, withdrawal symptoms may be the first indication of alcohol dependence. Alcohol withdrawal includes a broad spectrum of symptoms, and the syndrome is generally more prolonged and severe in elders because of biological changes and coexisting physical disorders (Mudd, et al, 1994; Ganzini and Atkinson, 1996). Nurses have a significant role in the management of alcohol withdrawal (Box 40-9).

Continued abstinence following withdrawal can be supported in a variety of ways. The greatest success of abstinence in older drinkers is achieved by those who participate in programs geared specifically for the elderly. One successful program lists three important differences from the usual addiction approach: outreach with counselors going to the patient's home, lack of confrontation about addiction, and an overall focus on quality of life and maintenance of independent living (Graham, et al, 1995). In mixed age groups, elderly participants may be offended by profanity and disclosure of antisocial behavior by younger members (Ganzini and Atkinson, 1996). Programs for the elderly emphasize peer bonding and shared reminiscing in addition to cognitive-behavioral training that addresses themes such as self-efficacy, self-esteem, and

Box 40-10   Commonly Used Psychotropic Drugs for the Elderly

Antidepressants
Secondary amine tricyclics
Desipramine (Norpramin)
Nortriptyline (Pamelor)

Newer agents
Bupropion (Wellbutrin)
Trazodone (Desyrel)

Selective serotonin reuptake inhibitors
Fluoxetine (Prozac)
Paroxetine (Paxil)
Sertraline (Zoloft)

Antipsychotics
High-potency antipsychotics
Haloperidol (Haldol)
Fluphenazine (Prolixin)

Low-potency antipsychotics
Thioridazine (Mellaril)

Atypical antipsychotics*

Antianxiety Agents
Benzodiazepines appropriate for the elderly
Lorazepam (Ativan)
Oxazepam (Serax)

Nonbenzodiazepine
Buspirone (BuSpar)

---

*Both clozapine (Clozaril) and risperidone (Risperdol) have been used successfully in older patients. Data concerning the newer atypicals are still being analyzed.

relapse prevention strategies. Whenever possible, addressing the factors that initially led to problem drinking is of paramount importance.

Drug Abuse

Although the elderly do not have a significant problem with illicit drug use, problems result from the overuse and misuse of prescription and over-the-counter medications. People over 65 account for 25% of all drug expenditures in developed countries, and that figure is expected to continue to rise (Williams and Lowenthal, 1992). As noted earlier, psychoactive drugs are a major component of the heavy drug use in this age group. Psychotropic drugs are prescribed for 25% of the elderly residing in the community and have been prescribed for up to 50% of the institutionalized elderly, though the latter trend is reversing due to legislative actions (Shorr, Fought, and Ray, 1994). Box 40-10 lists the most commonly used drugs in the elderly mentally ill, and Box 40-11 provides guidelines for the use of psychotropic drugs in the elderly. Benzodiazepines are the most frequently prescribed anxiolytic agents for geriatric patients. A serious concern is the tendency for this drug class to produce tolerance, physiologic dependence, and psychological dependence. Benzodiazepines should be used for short-term (less than 6 months) management of symptoms (Folks and Fuller, 1997). Two thirds of the elderly take 5 to 12 medications each day, and nearly half of all medications taken are nonprescription (Cadieux, 1993).

Box 40-11   Guidelines for Use of Psychotropic Drugs in the Elderly

Initial Dose
• Start with a small dose and gradually increase until therapeutic effect or adverse side effects occur.
• Usually one third to one half of the younger-adult dose is effective.

Daily Dose
• Use the smallest dose that produces relief.

Individualization
• Elderly persons are the most heterogeneous age group in American society.
• Each individual needs thoughtful attention.
• Partial symptom relief may well be the most judicious and realistic goal.

Discontinuance
• The elderly should be gradually tapered off psychotropic drugs.
• If elderly patients can manage without drug therapy, they should be allowed to do so.

Ganzini and Atkinson (1996) reported several studies that demonstrated a correlation among nonprescription drug use, depressive symptoms, and poor mental health. Of all elderly patients in nursing homes or other institutions, 95% are receiving one or more drugs, with some patients receiving as many as 12 to 15 drugs concurrently (known as *polypharmacy*). Older people receive many medications; in some cases, too many.

Factors Complicating Drug-Taking by the Elderly

It is easy to understand why elderly persons living alone, with poor vision and hearing problems would have difficulty complying with medical regimens involving several drugs. Further complicating the situation, older adults may add several nonprescription drugs, combine medications with alcohol, or even take medication prescribed for others without the knowledge of their physicians. Many older adults see multiple physicians, each of whom may prescribe drugs without reliable information about medications prescribed by others. Confusion caused by generic and trade names can result in the elderly taking the same medication under two names at the same time. Polypharmacy is common, so the nurse should be aware of potential complications and encourage patients to "brown bag" all medications for cataloging. Compliance is also a significant problem in approximately 60% of elderly patients, especially those who have disabilities and live alone. Drug regimens should be simplified and costs of drugs considered. Many pharmacies now offer blister packs on request, which provide easy drug visibility and accessibility.

ASSESSMENT OF THE ELDERLY MENTALLY ILL

Mental illness is not an isolated phenomena in the elderly. Therefore, comprehensive psychosocial and physical assessments are required to determine factors, including strengths and weaknesses, that influence the older adult's level of function. Family members or other caregivers, who often play a pivotal role in the function of the elderly patient, should be included in the assessment process. The goals of the initial assessment and subsequent reassessments are to collect accurate information to identify problems, plan interventions, predict outcomes, and measure changes over time (National Institutes of Health, 1987). Because of the volume and depth of information needed, the nurse often works collaboratively with other disciplines to complete the assessment and contributes findings in an interdisciplinary team meeting. Input from all disciplines, the patient, and the family is used to develop goals for care.

Nurses who are sensitive to the unique psychosocial and physical needs of older adults and adapt the assessment to accommodate those needs will have a better chance of obtaining data that accurately represent the elderly person. Interviews might be highly anxiety producing as older adults are often reluctant to discuss problems with a stranger, especially a young one. Elderly patients may be irritated by direct questions and view them as intrusive. Open-ended questions, which provide an opportunity for the patient to vent feelings and describe concerns and problems, often provide a clearer understanding of the patient's perspective of life and functioning. Domarad and Buschmann (1995) cited their research findings on increasing the credibility of information given by older adults. They identified interviewer strategies that facilitated truthful information: increasing self-esteem, nonjudgmental wording of questions, providing positive reinforcement, and giving control. Other strategies to enhance communication with the elderly are listed in Box 40-12.

PSYCHOSOCIAL ASSESSMENT

A wealth of clinical data can be obtained by listening to the stories many older adults love to tell. Listening not only conveys a sense of appreciation for the individual's contributions across the life span, but also provides the patient a nonthreatening means of communicating pertinent information. The nurse should listen carefully in these conversations for persistent themes such as reactions to loss, fear of losing control, fear of death, or somatic concerns. The nurse's acceptance of these concerns assures the patient that such expressions will not result in rejection. Information about past experiences and coping strategies, along with personal strengths and weaknesses may also be revealed. The nurse should gently guide reminiscence because excessive rambling can cause the patient embarrassment and anxiety. The Psychogeriatric Nursing Assessment Protocol (Abraham, Smullen, and Thompson-Heisterman, 1992) offers a useful guideline for the collection of data using a combination of structured and unstructured means. Box 40-13 lists information that should be obtained during the admission assessment interview.

Box 40-12   Enhancing Communication with the Elderly

Considerations	Nursing Implication
Slowed information processing	Do not rush. Allow adequate time for patient to answer questions. Avoid undue interruptions.
Establish rapport	Offer a handshake. Make eye contact. Arrange position at equal or lower level than patient. Address patient by title and last name unless asked to use first name.
Hearing deficits	Articulate words clearly. Face patient when speaking. Adjust volume of speech to patient's need. Do not shout. Ensure use of personal hearing aid or amplifier at correct volume. Use complementary nonverbal strategies, i.e., facial expression, gestures.
Visual deficits	Provide adequate lighting. Ensure use of corrective lens.
Competing stimuli	Minimize background noise. Avoid times when patient is excessively tired, hurting, hungry, or has toileting needs. Provide privacy.
Education level	Match vocabulary to patient's level of use.
Decreased physical tolerance	Avoid overtiring.

Box 40-13   Information to Obtain During the Assessment Interview

Basic background information such as age, marital status
Spiritual and cultural values
Personal and family history
History of legal difficulties
Economic status and sources of income
Education and work history
Life-style and perception of current life situation
Current living arrangements
Interests, pleasures, and activities
Friendship and social interactional patterns
Sexual functioning
Medical information and history
Prescription and OTC drugs and dosage
Alcohol, tobacco, and other chemical use
Cognitive, behavioral, and emotional status
Goals and plans for the future

Caregivers should be included in the assessment process. Not only can they provide information to clarify or expand that given by the patient, but also their perspective of problems is important for inclusion in a plan of care. Family members might be em-

barrassed to provide information that conflicts with that given by the patient in front of the patient. Because it is important to assess family interaction, time should be spent interviewing the patient and family members both separately and together. Care of the elderly mentally ill frequently falls to an elderly spouse or children, members of the so-called sandwich generation, who are often already overburdened. The nurse should use time with caregivers to assess ability and willingness to provide care and support for the patient. Many caretakers fail to take care of their own needs and lack information about support services and respite care. Helping family members deal with the stressors of caregiving increases family and patient adjustment.

PHYSICAL ASSESSMENT

Throughout the chapter, the connection between physical conditions and mental illness has been stressed. Therefore, a complete physical examination is an essential component of the assessment of any older adult presenting with symptoms of mental illness. The examination techniques for each subsystem do not differ substantially from the examination of younger adults. Adaptations for decreased mobility and obvious impairments must be made. Careful attention to every subsystem is required because in the elderly, examination might reveal abnormalities in a system not suggested by the presenting symptoms. For example, ataxia may result from fecal impaction; subtle hearing loss can result in increased diagnosis of psychopathology because of bizarre or incorrect responses to questions (Kreeger, et al, 1995). The nurse should use all senses during the examination, attending to the patient's visual presentation, odors, voice tone, and content. Numerous texts and articles detail the findings expected as a result of "normal" aging, and nurses should familiarize themselves with that information. Laboratory tests, electroencephalograms, computerized tomography (CT scan), positron-emission tomography (PET), and magnetic resonance imaging (MRI) of the brain may be ordered to rule out alterable comorbid states that contribute to symptoms of mental illness.

Special attention should be given to defining how physical problems interfere with the patient's functional ability. Older individuals assign a great value to independence, and its loss can contribute to lower self-esteem and declines in mental health. The loss of key abilities may result in shame and frustration. Those dependent on others may resent the idea that others have to care for them and may feel they have become a burden. The anger can be directed internally and result in depression or withdrawal or it may be directed at the caregiver through hostile acts (Sanders, 1995). Assessment of physical activities of daily living (PADLs) and instrumental activities of daily living (IADLs) provides a measure of the older adult's functional ability and guides the selection of interventions and services to meet identified needs (Box 40-14). Pa-

tients, and sometimes their families, are often unable or unwilling to describe functional difficulties because of the threat such disabilities have on established patterns of life-style and interaction. According to the Administration on Aging (1997), 23% of the elderly living in the community require some assistance with activities of daily living (ADLs). Observing task performance and carefully listening to both the patient and collateral sources describe routine daily activities may provide a more accurate picture of functional ability than direct questioning.

The physical examination should also be used as an opportunity to assess for signs of abuse or neglect. Each state has laws that regulate reporting requirements for intentional abuse, neglect, and exploitation of the elderly. Endangerment due to mental illness is also covered in state laws. Chapter 4 details some of the legal issues that may stem from abuse or neglect.

◢ Psychotherapeutic Management

Nurse-Patient Relationship. Ageist attitudes, intergenerational differences, communication deficits, and the multiple problems of older people can pose significant obstacles to developing a therapeutic nurse-patient relationship. Nurses who are aware of their own feelings and reactions are able to focus on patients and their significant others in a therapeutic manner. By empathizing with the patient and caregivers and focusing on the needs of the patient, the nurse can help patients and their families manage the activities and demands of daily living and improve the overall quality of both physical and mental health.

Mental illness has a significant effect on patients' abilities to manage even the simplest of cognitive and physical tasks. Butler and Lewis (1995) reported that depressed persons can be more limited physically and socially than those with chronic medical conditions. An important part of geropsychiatric nursing is assisting the patient in meeting basic physical needs. Depression, psychosis, anxiety, and other disorders can result in inattention or inability to perform routine activities of daily living. The nurse, then, must insure adequate fluid and nutritional intake, monitor elimination and hygiene, take protective measures in the face of impaired judgment, and remain vigilant for symp-

Box 40-14 **Functional Assessment**	
PADLs	**IADLs**
Bathing	Preparing meals
Dressing	Shopping
Eating	Managing money
Transferring	Using telephone
Walking	Using transportation
Toileting	Doing housework

toms of physical illness and treatment complications. Some elderly patients have multiple physical complaints, the result of existing illness or psychological distress. The nurse should listen to complaints and evaluate potential causes. Summarizing and restating the patient's concerns out loud reinforces that the patient's concerns have been heard. Interaction itself may be the real but unexpressed need of patients with persistent physical complaints (McCahill and Brunton, 1995).

Communicating a sense of unconditional acceptance of elderly persons as fellow human beings may be the most important intervention nurses can provide. Spending time with the patient outside that required for tasks such as medication administration and ADLs communicates an appreciation for the patient as a person of worth. Providing opportunities for the patient to control the sequence of events, such as allowing the patient to choose to bathe in the morning or the evening, enhances self-esteem, self-worth, and decision-making skills. The nurse must be aware of problems and unspoken needs and incorporate them into the plan of care.

Realistic goals.   Nursing interventions to assist elderly mentally ill patients include setting realistic, small, attainable goals. Discussions should be held with patients to stress the importance of goal setting to accomplish each ADL. Developing a schedule of activities for each day can assist patients in making decisions and coping with demands. Simple decisions may be difficult for the elderly mentally ill. Reducing the options available before allowing the patient choices can diminish frustration. For example, when it is time to dress, the nurse may restrict the choices of outfits to two rather than offering an entire closet of options. The caregiver must be gentle and supportive, as additional time may be needed to achieve these goals. The caregiver must also resist the urge to save time and energy by taking over the task. While it might be easier to "do it myself," the person who does the work will reap the benefits. Patience, positive reinforcement, and consistency by nurses benefit the patient.

Psychopharmacology

Altered pharmacokinetics.   According to Keltner and Folks (1997), the elderly demonstrate altered responses to drug therapy and increased adverse effects. The aging process produces numerous bodily changes that alter the absorption, distribution, metabolism, and excretion of drugs (Table 40-2). Because of normal changes associated with aging, the elderly have diminished gastric acidity, fewer active cells and enzymes, and slowed arterial blood flow. Drug absorption is considered to be slower and less complete. Box 40-15 lists special considerations for elderly patients taking psychotropic drugs.

Distribution is determined by the alterations in blood flow, plasma albumin concentration, and body composition that can occur in the course of aging. Blood flow to the renal and hepatic systems is decreased to maintain adequate flow to the cerebral and coronary systems. This results in altered patterns of drug metabolism and excretion. Total systemic diffusion is decreased because of decreases in plasma volume, total body water, and extracellular fluid in the elderly. The proportion of lean body mass to total body weight decreases with age. Lipid-soluble drugs such as barbiturates, phenothiazines, benzodiazepines, and phenytoin are absorbed into the increased amount of fatty tissue and retained by the body.

Serum albumin concentration is another major factor that affects the distribution of drugs in the elderly. Healthy older adults may have only mild reductions in serum albumin, but substantial reductions are noted in those who are malnourished

---

Table 40-2   Physiological Changes in the Elderly Resulting in Pharmacokinetic Alteration

Physiological Change	Pharmacokinetic Alteration
Increased gastric pH	Decreased absorption
Increased body fat	Decreased fat-soluble drug concentration
Decreased body water	Increased water-soluble drug concentration
Decreased serum albumin	Increased unbound drug may lead to increased drug activity
Decreased cardiac output	Decreased metabolism of drugs
Decreased renal function	Decreased excretion of drugs
Decreased liver mass, blood flow	Decreased metabolism of drugs

Box 40-15   Special Considerations for Elderly Patients Taking Psychotropic Drugs

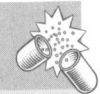

Antidepressant Drugs

Orthostatic hypotension is a major concern; nortriptyline and bupropion do not seem to cause as severe a hypotensive episode.

Amitriptyline produces the *most* anticholinergic side effects.

Desipramine, trazodone, bupropion, and selective serotonin reuptake inhibitors (SSRIs) produce the *fewest* anticholinergic side effects.

CNS symptoms of toxicity include disorientation, confusion, and memory loss.

Caution should be observed when TCAs are given to elderly persons with cardiovascular disease.

SSRIs, desipramine, and bupropion are "activating" antidepressants and tend to energize patients. Helpful for patients with hypersomnia.

Antipsychotic Drugs

Haloperidol, fluphenazine, and thiothixene cause more extrapyramidal side effects (EPSEs) than most other antipsychotics.

The elderly are more prone to EPSEs because of age-related CNS changes.

Thioridazine and the atypical antipsychotic drugs have a low incidence of EPSEs.

The elderly are particularly susceptible to tardive dyskinesia.

Agranulocytosis is most common in elderly women and is a particular risk with clozapine.

Anticholinergic side effects are particularly troublesome for the elderly.

Long-acting or depot antipsychotics can be used in elderly patients.

Antianxiety Agents: Benzodiazepines

Up to one third of all elderly persons take these drugs.

The half-lives of several benzodiazepines are lengthened by age-related changes that prolong sedation, cause poor coordination and disorientation, and may lead to misdiagnosis.

Benzodiazepines with a long half-life include chlordiazepoxide (Librium), clorazepate (Tranxene), diazepam (Valium), and prazepam (Centrax). *These benzodiazepines are not usually ordered for elderly patients.*

Benzodiazepines that *typically are prescribed* for elderly patients include lorazepam (Ativan), oxazepam (Serax), and clonazepam (Klonopin).

Antimanic Agent: Lithium

Because of age-related changes in the kidneys, excretion of lithium is slowed, creating the opportunity for prolonged side effects.

Sodium depletion from diet or diuretics increases serum lithium levels.

A lower blood level of lithium is appropriate for elderly patients (0.4 to 0.8 mEq/L).

Caution should be exercised if lithium is combined with an antipsychotic drug because of the risk of neuroleptic malignant syndrome.

---

and chronically ill. Phenytoin, diazepam, warfarin, digitoxin, and naproxen are examples of drugs that are highly bound to plasma proteins. A large proportion of these drugs is confined to the intravascular space with only a small fraction distributed to the pharmacological site of action. A reduction in the amount of total plasma albumin decreases the number of binding sites and increases the amount of free or active drug. When hypoalbuminemia is present, the drug serum level is not an accurate predictor of free drug because serum levels do not differentiate between free and bound drug molecules. Therefore, a normally therapeutic serum drug level could be a toxic amount of free drug.

A delay in transporting drugs to the liver, caused by problems in distribution, can diminish the metabolism of drugs in the elderly. Because there is a significant decrease in the size of the liver with normal aging, a person's drug-metabolizing capacity may be affected. Although a decrease in the number of enzymes available to metabolize drugs has been demonstrated, it has not been shown to be of any clinical significance in the absence of specific organ disease.

The kidney, also affected by the aging process, is responsible for drug excretion. Drugs are excreted by active tubular secretion, glomerular filtration, or both. Renal function is more accurately measured by creatinine clearance than by serum creatinine. Creatinine clearance decreases significantly with age, along with a decrease in renal size, blood flow, glomerular filtration rate, and the number of functioning glomeruli. Creatinine clearance studies show that renal function drops significantly in per-

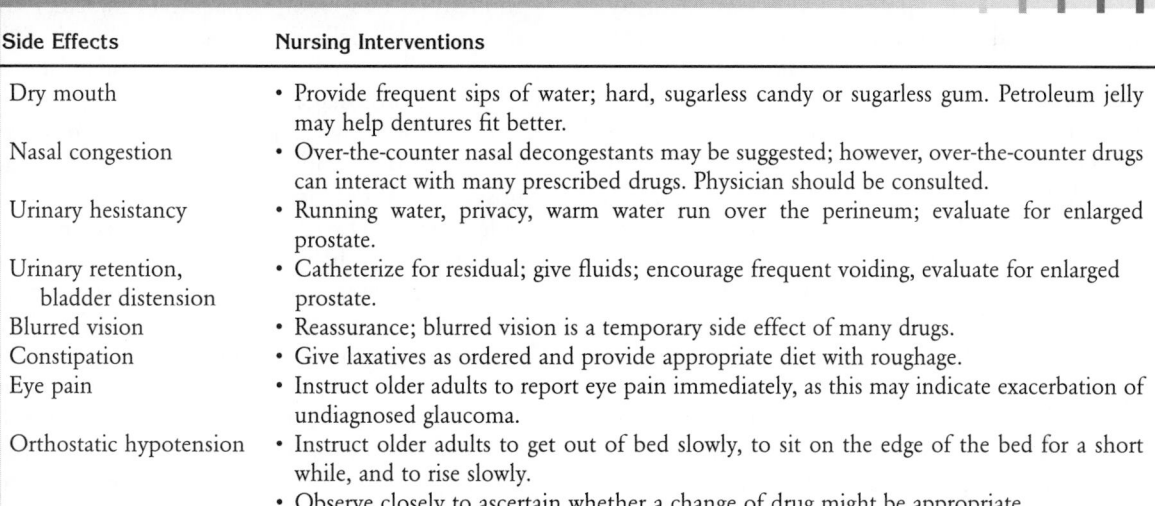

Side Effects and Nursing Interventions for Psychotropic Drug Use in Older Adults

Side Effects	Nursing Interventions
Dry mouth	• Provide frequent sips of water; hard, sugarless candy or sugarless gum. Petroleum jelly may help dentures fit better.
Nasal congestion	• Over-the-counter nasal decongestants may be suggested; however, over-the-counter drugs can interact with many prescribed drugs. Physician should be consulted.
Urinary hesistancy	• Running water, privacy, warm water run over the perineum; evaluate for enlarged prostate.
Urinary retention, bladder distension	• Catheterize for residual; give fluids; encourage frequent voiding, evaluate for enlarged prostate.
Blurred vision	• Reassurance; blurred vision is a temporary side effect of many drugs.
Constipation	• Give laxatives as ordered and provide appropriate diet with roughage.
Eye pain	• Instruct older adults to report eye pain immediately, as this may indicate exacerbation of undiagnosed glaucoma.
Orthostatic hypotension	• Instruct older adults to get out of bed slowly, to sit on the edge of the bed for a short while, and to rise slowly.
	• Observe closely to ascertain whether a change of drug might be appropriate.

sons over 30 years of age, declining at a rate of 6% to 10% per decade, with an increased rate of decline after the age of 65. Because of a decrease in lean body weight and creatinine production, the creatinine clearance can be greatly reduced in the presence of a normal serum creatinine level. Reduction in renal clearance affects the dosage requirements for many drugs. For example, elderly patients tend to show increased plasma levels with relatively low dosages of lithium. About one half to one third of the effective dose for young adults is required to adequately treat older adults.

The nurse must be aware of the therapeutic goals of patients' drug regimens and should observe patients for the effects of the therapy. The nurse contributes to the ongoing care plan by reporting both the therapeutic and adverse effects of drug therapy and ensures that unneeded medications are discontinued. Common side effects of psychotropic drugs in the elderly are listed in the side effects and nursing interventions box above.

Antidepressants.   Several agents are used to treat depression in elderly patients, including tricyclic antidepressants (TCAs), selective serotonin reuptake inhibitors (SSRIs), monoamine oxidase inhibitors (MAOIs), and psychostimulants. Secondary amine TCAs and SSRIs are more commonly prescribed for depression, whereas MAOIs and psychostimulants are seldom used. Older patients typ-

ically require lower dosages of these drugs than do younger persons. The secondary amine TCAs generally are used in the elderly rather than tertiary amine TCAs because of a more compatible side-effect profile. Because more than 50% of successfully treated older patients have a relapse into depression, typical treatment regimens should continue between 6 and 12 months after symptom resolution (Rubin, Kinscherf, and Wehrman, 1991). Newer TCA-related agents, such as bupropion (Wellbutrin) and trazodone (Desyrel), are used often in the elderly. Major advantages of these two drugs compared with TCAs are that there is no lethal overdose and they have a better side-effect profile (Martin, 1990). This makes them especially beneficial for elderly persons at high risk of suicide. Bupropion causes little sedation, hypotension, anticholinergic responses, or cardiotoxicity. Trazodone does not have anticholinergic effects but is sedating. The sedation distinction between antidepressants is important for nurses to understand. Sometimes depression is manifested by agitation, and affected patients benefit from the sedating properties of an antidepressant. Sedating antidepressants are often given at night to help patients who have difficulty sleeping because of depression. When elderly depressed patients manifest lethargy and excessive sleep, a more "activating" antidepressant is in order (e.g., bupropion, SSRIs).

More recently introduced agents, such as SSRIs, are gaining support because they possess a better side-effect profile than that of most TCAs; that is, SSRIs cause fewer problems with cardiotoxicity, sedation, and hypotension. Furthermore, SSRIs such as fluoxetine (Prozac), sertraline (Zoloft), and paroxetine (Paxil) are less anticholinergic. Fluoxetine has a long half-life, which may make it less desirable than the other two SSRIs in this age group.

MAOIs may be used in elderly patients who do not respond to TCAs or SSRIs. However, due to the hypotensive effect and other adverse reactions, MAOIs typically are reserved for patients refractory to treatment. In addition, the dietary restrictions associated with MAOI use can be difficult for any age group to follow, and perhaps more so for elderly patients. Phenelzine (Nardil) is the most commonly prescribed MAOI and is considered the safest for the elderly (Gomez and Gomez, 1992); it has fewer and milder side effects than other MAOIs.

Methylphenidate (Ritalin) may also be prescribed for apathetic or withdrawn patients. The adverse effects of this drug often complicate its use in the aged and the dosage requirements are generally much lower. For example, doses of 5 to 30 mg are appropriate for the elderly depressed.

Important side effects in elderly patients. Antidepressants may cause sedation (antihistaminic effect), anticholinergic, antiadrenergic, and cardiovascular side effects. Typical anticholinergic side effects, which include dry mouth, blurred vision, tachycardia, urinary retention, and constipation, are particularly problematic for elderly patients. Delirium, with confusion, and psychosis may also result. Sweating and tremor are the primary antiadrenergic side effects reported by the elderly. Cardiovascular effects are of primary concern in the elderly, particularly orthostatic hypotension, which may lead to falls and fractures. Careful monitoring of orthostatic changes is important, especially in patients also taking diuretics or vasodilators. Tachycardia is a special concern in elderly patients with preexisting unstable angina or chronic atrial fibrillation (Alessi and Cassel, 1996).

Antipsychotics. Antipsychotic drugs are used in the treatment of schizophrenia, acute psychosis, aggressive behavior, and agitation. A complete explanation of antipsychotic drugs is found in Chapter 20, where antipsychotic drugs are categorized as high potency or low potency. The high-potency drugs, such as haloperidol (Haldol) and fluphenazine (Prolixin), are associated with extrapyramidal side effects (EPSEs). The low-potency antipsychotics, such as chlorpromazine (Thorazine) and thioridazine (Mellaril), are associated with sedation, anticholinergic, and cardiovascular side effects (e.g., orthostatic hypotension). Because sedation, anticholinergic, and cardiovascular side effects are particularly bothersome, the *high-potency* antipsychotic drugs are prescribed more often to older persons. Dosages for older persons tend to be half or less than half of those given to younger patients. The newer atypical drugs have a side-effect profile that should benefit older patients.

Antianxiety agents. Anxiety is a common theme among the elderly, and consequently, antianxiety agents are frequently used. Benzodiazepines are the antianxiety drugs most often prescribed. Some benzodiazepines are longer acting because of a long half-life or because of age-related changes in the hepatic enzyme oxidative process that extends their time for clearance (see Chapter 22 for discussion). Hence, the longer-acting benzodiazepines such as chlordiazepoxide (Librium), clorazepate (Tranxene), diazepam (Valium), and prazepam (Centrax), are not favored for use by the elderly. The short-acting benzodiazepines (i.e., those metabolized more efficiently), which are ordered more often for older persons, include lorazepam (Ativan), and oxazepam (Serax). Because withdrawal syndrome (including withdrawal seizure) can occur in persons removed from an antianxiety agent after 30 days or more of use, benzodiazepines should be withdrawn slowly over several weeks. Benzodiazepines are relatively safe drugs when taken alone but can cause severe sedation and respiratory suppression when combined with alcohol or other sedatives (Table 40-3). Buspirone (BuSpar), an antianxiety drug, is not a benzodiazepine and has some advantages over the usual antianxiety agents. Its chief advantage is that it does *not* react with alcohol and other sedatives to cause sedation and respiratory problems. A major disadvantage is its slow onset of action: it takes up to 2 weeks or longer before a clinical response is experienced.

Problems associated with benzodiazepines include their potential to disinhibit. Disinhibition has resulted in violent outbursts in some elderly patients. This drug-induced effect should not be minimized. Benzodiazepines can also produce an amnestic effect that is particularly disabling in older persons. Lorazepam (Ativan), alprazolam (Xanax), and triazolam (Halcion) are known to have amnestic qualities.

Antimanic agents.   Lithium is the drug of choice for bipolar illness, but valproic acid (Depakene) and carbamazepine (Tegretol) are also used. Because of the decreased rate of excretion in the elderly, there is a higher incidence of lithium toxicity in this age group, and lower serum levels are adequate for a therapeutic response (0.4 to 0.8 mEq/L). Chapter 21 provides a thorough review of this drug.

Milieu Management.   Approximately 5% of the elderly in America reside in long-term care institutions such as nursing homes, state hospitals, and adult homes (Administration on Aging, 1997). Increasingly, elderly psychiatric patients are included in that percentage. As the number of these impaired persons increases, issues related to their mental health are of greater concern. The staff of long-term and acute-care institutions caring for the elderly mentally ill must develop and implement interventions to maintain the psychological functioning of their residents.

Effective milieu management changes the quality of life in institutional environments by working with residents to normalize the environment to the maximum degree possible. The traditional associations of "home" involve control over people who come and go in personal spaces, furnishings, and appointments (Katz, 1995). Furniture, at a height that facilitates independent mobility, can be placed in conversational groupings. Common rooms can be equipped with large-print books, games with large print and pieces, and stimulating pictures. Careful attention should be paid to the potential for background stimuli such as constant music or televisions to cause agitation or distress. Individual rooms can be deinstitutionalized by encouraging residents to use their own bedspreads, family pictures, favorite calendars, and other personal items. Staff members may wear street clothes rather than traditional uniforms to encourage social interaction with residents and to help eliminate barriers. It is important to remember privacy needs and respect personal space. Environmental adaptations that promote safety and independence for the elderly are listed in Box 40-16. The approach seeks to encourage independent activity and group participation by residents (Burnside, 1988; Kermis, 1986).

Table 40-3	Alcohol and Psychotropic Drug Interactions in the Elderly
Class of Psychotropic Drug	**Combined Effect**
Antidepressant drugs	
Tricyclic antidepressants (TCAs)	Lowered seizure threshold, hypotension
Monoamine oxidase inhibitors (MAOIs)	Hypertensive crisis, especially with Chianti wine, beer, ale, or sherry
Antipsychotic drugs	
Phenothiazines	Respiratory depression, lowered seizure threshold, impaired hepatic function, hypotension
Antianxiety drugs	
Benzodiazepines	CNS depression, respiratory depression, sedation
Barbiturates	
Secobarbital, pentobarbital	Vomiting, severe motor impairment, unconsciousness, coma, and death. (The lethal dose is reduced by 50% when barbiturates are taken with alcohol.)

Controlling aggression is a major component of maintaining individual and environmental safety. Violent behavior may be the result of poor frustration tolerance, ineffective coping strategies, impulsivity, and real or imagined threats to personal space and individual territory (Ferguson and Smith, 1996). Nurses must look at the environment and develop strategies and techniques to minimize precipitating factors. Physical and chemical restraints have been a traditional means of controlling behavior, but because of the negatives consequences associated with their use, alternative interventions should first be attempted. Managing environmental stimuli, providing productive outlets for energy, and practicing redirection are important for reducing outbursts.

A primary therapeutic responsibility for nurses in these settings is to prevent deterioration resulting from the withdrawal and disuse that often accompany institutional life. It has been found that isolation of the elderly leads to sensory deprivation, loss of mental function, and personality disintegration. Therefore, therapeutic approaches should be based on the knowledge that all human beings have a need for continuing contacts, social participation, and meaningful work to maintain function (Kermis, 1986). Individual and group interactions and activities should be planned to foster the greatest degree of independence and develop interpersonal and communication skills.

Reality orientation. Reality orientation is a specific treatment modality used to counter intellec-

tual and sensory losses in confused elderly patients. Reality orientation is generally conducted in a group setting by staff members, using natural conversation with patients to discuss important events or items. A bulletin board can be used to include information such as the name of the facility, the day, month, year, next meal, and weather. The staff can use simple memory games that require recall ability. Readily available daily newspapers, current magazines, clocks, and calendars provide orientation cues to patients outside the group setting.

Box 40-16 Environmental Adaptations

Considerations	Interventions
Decreased ability to distinguish colors	Use high-contrast colors in vivid hues.
Mobility impairments	Ensure nonslip floor surfaces.
	Provide adequate, nonglare lighting.
	Ensure well-fitting footwear.
	Provide chairs and toilets at comfortable height with armrests or handrails.
	Avoid placing rolling tables where patients might attempt to use for stability.
	Provide shower stools, nonskid tub guards, and grab bars.
	Provide ambulation rails.
	Remove obstacles, clutter, and spills promptly.
	Ensure appropriate use of assistive devices.
Inability to read	Mark spaces with pictures or universal symbols.
Decreased thermoregulation ability	Ensure comfortable temperature.
	Observe for signs of hypothermia or hyperthermia.
	Provide sweaters, blankets.
	Ensure safe water temperature.

Case Study

Ms. Othella Thatcher is a 78-year-old white woman with a 10-year history of severe depression. She was last hospitalized at this hospital in 1996 and received ECT. She was also hospitalized at another local hospital in 1997 and underwent a series of ECT treatments at that time. The patient came to the hospital emergency room this morning with her cousin (a woman of about 60 years of age). The cousin describes a gradual worsening of the depression over the past few months, stating that the patient seems to need ECT approximately once a year. About 6 or 7 months after the course of ECT is completed, the patient has an increase in depressive symptoms.

Ms. Thatcher presents with complaints that include erratic sleep patterns and decreased appetite (she will not eat unless her cousin spoon-feeds her). The cousin reports that after a series of ECT, the patient is "easier to

live with," plays with children, takes care of herself, and will "eat anything not nailed down."

The cousin reports that the patient's depression began in the 1980s, when "her only son, whom she was very devoted to," abandoned Ms. Thatcher to the welfare of the state and sold all of the patient's furniture. This event occurred after the patient experienced an extended hospitalization for urinary tract infections and pneumonia. The patient has reportedly lived in five different nursing homes since that time; the last in 1993. Since 1993, Ms. Thatcher has lived with her cousin.

The cousin states that Ms. Thatcher has never verbalized suicidal or homicidal thoughts but does hold a basically "paranoid view of life." The cousin cannot recall Ms. Thatcher ever having hallucinations.

Reminiscence. Older adults have a wealth of experiences that can be shared through storytelling. These stories can be used by the nurse to provide opportunities for pleasurable interaction and therapeutic gain. Reminiscence is the process of recalling past experiences, which allows the listeners insight into the patient's history. The patient benefits from the opportunity to rethink aspects of the past, put feelings, thoughts, and actions into perspective and temper them with other experiences (Soltys and Coats, 1994). Reminiscence may occur in individual interactions or in a group. Participants are encouraged to share life experiences such as vacations, holidays, milestones, and family events. Group leaders may stimulate memories by the use of items such as pictures, music, and memorabilia. The group process can awaken shared memories and provide validation for each member. Reminiscence groups can help participants establish new relationships while enhancing valuable communication and socialization skills (Burnside and Haight, 1994).

Care Plan

NAME: Ms. Othella Thatcher _____ ADMISSION DATE: _____

DSM-IV DIAGNOSIS: Major Depression _____

ASSESSMENT: **Areas of strength:** Willingness to be treated; cooperative, good support system (cousin very concerned and wants patient back in home).
Problems: Withdrawn, decreased interest in interactions and activities; decreased self-esteem, decreased energy, hopelessness; poor judgment.

DIAGNOSES: Ineffective individual coping related to abandonment by son as evidenced by erratic sleep patterns, decreased energy, and decreased self-esteem.

OUTCOMES: **Short-term goals:**   Date met
• Feelings expressed verbally.   _____
• Anger expressed overtly toward objects that elicit anger.   _____
• Resume some activities.   _____
• Patient will not harm self.   _____
• Patient will have increased energy for activities.   _____
Long-term goals:
• Able to talk about anger at son.   _____
• Patient will show increase in self-concept.   _____
• Patient will maintain independence though living in cousin's home.   _____

PLANNING/ **Nurse-patient relationship:** Help patient explore anger with son. Encourage expression of
INTERVENTIONS: feelings; encourage interactions with others as tolerated. Convey concern and acceptance without sympathy. Assess suicide indications regularly.
Psychopharmacology: Fluoxetine 20 mg q A.M.; Haldol 0.5 mg; HS docusate sodium 100 mg bid.
Milieu management: Provide adequate nutrition and hydration. Monitor patient for safety issues. Keep patient around others (not in room by self) as much as is reasonable. Keep naps short to facilitate sleep at night.

EVALUATION: Patient expressed feelings of anger at being abandoned by son. Activity level increased. Medication maintained. Will be discharged to return to cousin's home.

REFERRALS: Schedule visit with home health nurse for follow-up care. Schedule appointment with outpatient program coordinator within 7 days.

Life review. Although life review uses reminiscence, it is a different process and involves one-to-one interaction rather than group settings. The nurse acts as a sounding board for the patient, who reviews life experiences, reworks, and reframes issues to achieve integrity (Burnside and Haight, 1994). Evaluation of the entire life span through telling or writing a personal story is difficult work for the patient. By relating the course of life, fears, conflicts, past coping mechanisms, unresolved feelings, and unresolved losses from the past may become evident and promote opportunities for intervention (Sanders, 1995).

Pet therapy. Animals in residence or visiting animals can be used to assist older adults in breaking through apathy or depression by helping fulfill the need to love and be loved. Animals provide unconditional affection and are blind to afflictions. Pet therapy consists of brief sessions in which small, well-behaved animals are provided to patients for holding, stroking, and playing. Studies have shown that pets can have positive effects on physical and mental well-being (Buckwalter, 1995).

Exercise therapy. Despite many older adult's decreased tolerance for exercise, encouraging socialization and participation in purposeful activities is helpful. Engaging in exercise can channel the energy of anxiety and provide the stimulation needed to assist in the redevelopment of normalized sleep-wake cycles (Folks and Fuller, 1997). Chair exercises, outdoor walks, and even dancing are activities many adults enjoy despite limited physical ability.

Music therapy. Nurses can make contact with older adults through music familiar to them. Old songbooks, hymnals, and records offer an array of choices. Patients should be allowed to exercise freedom of choice in the type of music played in the environment and used for group sessions. Sing-alongs can evoke responses from even the most withdrawn patient (Roberts, 1996).

Horticultural therapy. Planting and tending to plants can enhance physical condition, relieve tension, and provide a sense of accomplishment. Being responsible for plants that can be grown in outdoor gardens or inside areas provides opportunities for positive interaction and outcomes in the form of fresh flowers or vegetables that can be shared with others (American Horticultural Therapy Association, 1997).

■ Critical Thinking Questions

Mrs. Alberta Honas is a 73-year-old black woman who has been admitted to a geropsychiatric unit. She is suspicious of those around her and is angry with her family for "tricking" her. She states that her family physician lied to her. On the evening shift, the nurse notices that Mrs. Honas's door is closed. When the nurse opens the door, she finds Mrs. Honas crying almost uncontrollably. She is holding her arms across her chest and crying, "Dear Jesus, Jesus, Jesus. Oh God, help me. If I have hurt anybody, dear Jesus, forgive me. Oh Lord, Oh Lord." The nurse finds her to be inconsolable.

1. How would you describe what is happening to this patient?
2. You have probably heard quite a bit about spiritual care in your nursing program, but most care providers are reluctant to have a "religious discussion" with patients. Would you be comfortable dealing with Mrs. Honas and her spiritual concerns? How would you say something meaningful to her without imposing your own religious views?
3. For a number of years, the elderly have been a special concern in American society; legislation has been passed to help the elderly, major universities have developed aging centers and aging programs, and many businesses provide discounts to the elderly for products and services. These examples are but a few of the ways the elderly are assisted and served in society. Within the past few years, however, some people have been questioning the appropriateness of these efforts. They point out that the most at-risk group in this country are young families and argue that many of these families are facing tremendous financial pressures and many break apart under the load. These individuals believe that a greater yield would be realized by shifting societal support to these families instead of to older individuals who already enjoy significant advantages. Which side of the argument do you take? Why? What are the inherent dangers in pitting one group against another?

■ Key Concepts

1. Despite the increase in the population of persons 65 years of age and older, this group experiences major barriers to obtaining quality mental health care because of issues such as ageism, their own attitudes, and cost of care.
2. Depression is the most common mental disorder among the elderly, but it is often overlooked, misdiagnosed, and inadequately treated.
3. Symptoms of other illnesses may mask depression because the elderly may be preoccupied with physical rather than emotional symptoms.

4. Age-related life events, losses, changes, and physical decline are associated with the onset of depression.
5. The nurse-patient relationship focuses on providing care for patients and helping their families manage the activities and demands of daily living.
6. Adequate nutrition, socialization, and achievement of small realistic goals in daily living activities help to reduce anxiety and maintain or restore psychological functioning.
7. Use of medications with the elderly involves risks associated with polypharmacy, noncompliance, and altered pharmacokinetics.
8. Secondary amine tricyclics, such as desipramine and nortriptyline, SSRIs, MAOIs (less often), and psychostimulants (less often) are the recommended agents for treating depression in the elderly.
9. When treating psychotic disorders, high-potency antipsychotics, such as haloperidol, are used more often than low-potency antipsychotics. New atypical agents are also first-line agents.
10. Antianxiety agents with shorter half-lives, such as lorazepam, oxazepam, and clonazepam (Klonopin), are prescribed most often for this age group.
11. ECT can be effective treatment for elderly persons suffering from depression.

Study Questions

(Answer key is in the back of the book.)

1. Which of the following are the major barriers to mental health care for the elderly?
   a. Age discrimination (ageism)
   b. Cost of care
   c. Attitudes of the elderly
   d. All of the above
2. Although major depression is the most common psychiatric illness among the elderly, it is often overlooked or misdiagnosed because:
   a. Depression is a normal response to other diseases.
   b. The elderly deny they have any problems.
   c. The elderly are often more preoccupied with bodily functions and physical complaints than with emotional symptoms.
   d. Memory loss interferes with remembering depressing situations.
3. It is useful to modify psychosocial assessment to fit the special needs of the elderly in which of the following ways?
   a. Making a list of skills and behaviors that are expected of a person that age
   b. Scheduling the interview in the late afternoon or evening
   c. Discouraging reminiscing that is unrelated to the main point

   d. Compensating for vision or hearing impairments and allowing extra time for answers
4. In the elderly, the onset of depression is most often associated with:
   a. Onset of dementia and disorientation
   b. Loss of friends and declines in income and health
   c. A serious accident or injury
   d. The sixtieth birthday
5. A major focus of a nursing care plan for elderly persons is:
   a. Helping the family select a long-term care facility
   b. Allowing patients to sleep as often as possible
   c. Encouraging reminiscence about patients' pasts
   d. Helping patients and their families manage the activities and demands of daily living
6. Levels of intervention with the elderly include prevention of impairment, restoration of mental functioning, and slowing the rate of deterioration.
   a. True
   b. False
7. Most elderly persons in institutions benefit from staying in their rooms rather than participating in activities such as reality orientation, remotivation therapy, and pet therapy.
   a. True
   b. False
8. The fastest-growing age group in American society is:
   a. Adolescents
   b. Persons 65 years of age and older
   c. Persons 85 years of age and older
   d. Baby boomers
9. The most common mental disorder among elderly patients is:
   a. Depression
   b. Schizophrenia
   c. Anxiety disorder
   d. Paranoid thinking
10. Elderly patients presenting with weight loss, general aches and pains, and constipation are most likely suffering from which of the following?
    a. Depression
    b. Schizophrenia
    c. Anxiety disorders
    d. Paranoid thinking
11. The demographic stereotype of the person most likely to commit suicide is:
    a. An elderly black man
    b. An elderly white man
    c. An elderly black woman
    d. An elderly white woman
12. Elderly suicidal persons typically give a "cry for help."
    a. True
    b. False
13. What are the potential drug-related problems associated with decreased albumin levels?

REFERENCES

Abraham I, Smullen DE, and Thompson-Heisterman AA: Geriatric mental health: assessing geropsychiatric patients, *J Psychosoc Nurs Ment Health Serv* 30(9):13, 1992.

Administration on Aging: *A profile of older Americans: 1996*, Greenburg S, hypertext, Feb 1997. Available at: http://www.aoa.dhhs.gov/aoa/pages/profil96.html# older. Accessed July 29, 1997.

Alessi C and Cassel C: Medical evaluation and common medical problems. In Sadavoy J, et al, editors: *Comprehensive review of geriatric psychiatry–II*, ed 2, Washington, DC, 1996, American Psychiatric Press.

Alexopoulos G: Affective disorders. In Sadavoy J, et al, editors: *Comprehensive review of geriatric psychiatry–II*, ed 2, Washington, DC, 1996, American Psychiatric Press.

American Horticultural Therapy Association: A career in horticultural therapy, facsimile from the Association, Aug 1997.

American Psychiatric Association: *Diagnostic and Statistical Manual of Mental Disorders*, ed 4, Washington, DC, 1994, The Association.

Atay J, Witkin M, and Mandersheid R: Date highlights on: utilization of mental health organizations by elderly person, *Ment Health Stat Note* 214:1, Mar 1995. Available at http://www.mentalhealth.org/mhstats/dtsh214.htm. Accessed July 31, 1997.

Bittner V, Taylor H, and Raczynski J: Depression after myocardial infarction: impact on mortality. *UAB Insight*, Summer 1997.

Blazer DG and Koenig HG: Mood disorders. In Busse E and Blazer D, editors: *Textbook of geriatric psychiatry*, ed 2, Washington, DC, 1996, American Psychiatric Press.

Brandt B and Ugarriza DN: Electroconvulsive therapy and the elderly client, *J Gerontol Nurs* 22(12):14, 1996.

Buckwalter K: Depression and suicide. In Stanley M and Beare PG, editors: *Gerontological nursing*, Philadelphia, 1995, FA Davis Co.

Buren JE, Sloan RB, and Cohen GD: *Handbook of mental health and aging*, ed 2, San Diego, 1992, Academic Press.

Burnside IM: Reminiscence and other therapeutic modalities. In Burnside IM, editor: *Nursing and the aged: a self-care approach*, ed 3, New York, 1988, McGraw-Hill.

Burnside I and Haight B: Reminiscence and life review: therapeutic interventions for older people, *Nurse Pract* 19(4):55, 1994.

Burrows A, et al: Depression in a long-term care facility: clinical features and discordance between nursing assessment and patient interviews, *J Am Geriatr Soc* 43(10):1118, 1995.

Busse EW: The myth, history, and science of aging. In Busse EW and Blazer DG, editors, *Textbook of geriatric psychiatry*, ed 2, Washington, DC, 1996, American Psychiatric Press.

Butler RN and Lewis ML: Late-life depression: when and how to intervene, *Geriatrics* 50(8):44, 1995.

Butler RN, et al: Late-life depression: treatment strategies for primary care practice, *Geriatrics* 52(4):51, 1997.

Cadieux RJ: Geriatric psychopharmacology: a primary care challenge, *Postgrad Med* 93(4):281, 1993.

Casey DA and Davis MH: Electroconvulsive therapy in the very old, *Gen Hosp Psychiatry* 18(6):436, 1996.

Coyne JC, Fechner-Bates S, and Schwenk TL: Prevalence, nature, and comorbidity of depressive disorders in primary care, *Gen Hosp Psychiatry* 16(4):267, 1994.

Cuffel B, et al: Treatment costs and use of community mental health services for schizophrenia by age, cohort, *Am J Psychiatry* 153(7):870, 1996.

Domarad BR and Buschmann MT: Interviewing older adults: increasing the credibility of interview data, *J Gerontol Nurs* 21(9):14, 1995.

Duffy D: Suicide in later life: how to spot the risk factors, *Nurs Times* 93(11):56, 1997.

Dye C: *Assessment and intervention in geropsychiatric nursing*, Orlando, 1985, Grune & Stratton, Inc.

Estes C: Mental health services for the elderly: key policy elements. In Gatz M, editor: *Emerging issues in mental health and aging*, Washington, DC, 1995, American Psychological Association.

Ferguson JS and Smith A: Aggressive behavior on an inpatient geriatric unit, *J Psychosoc Nurs Ment Health Serv* 34(3):27, 1996.

Folks D and Fuller W: Anxiety disorders and insomnia in geriatric patients, *Psychiatr Clin North Am* 20(1):137, 1997.

Ganzini L and Atkinson RM: Substance abuse. In Sadavoy J, et al, editors: *Comprehensive review of geriatric psychiatry–II*, ed 2, Washington, DC, 1996, American Psychiatric Press.

Gatz M: *Emerging issues in mental health and aging*, Washington, DC, 1995, American Psychological Association.

Gomez GE and Gomez EA: The use of antidepressants with elderly patients, *J Psychosoc Nurs Ment Health Serv* 30(11):2126, 1992.

Graham K, et al: *Addictions treatment for older adults: evaluation of an innovative client-centered approach*, New York, 1995, The Haworth Press.

Gurland B: Epidemiology of psychiatric disorders. In Sadavoy J, et al, editors: *Comprehensive review of geriatric psychiatry–II*, ed 2, Washington, DC, 1996, American Psychiatric Press.

Jeste DV, Harris MJ, and Paulsen JS: Psychosis. In Sadavoy J, et al, editors: *Comprehensive review of geriatric psychiatry–II*, ed 2, Washington, DC, 1996, American Psychiatric Press.

Kane J and McGlashan T: Treatment of schizophrenia, *Lancet* 346(8978):820, 1995.

Katz IR: Infrastructure requirements for research in late-life mental disorders. In Gatz M, editor: *Emerging issues in mental health and aging,* Washington, DC, 1995, American Psychiatric Press.

Keltner NL and Folks DG: *Psychotropic drugs,* St. Louis, 1997, Mosby.

Kermis MD: Mental health in late-life: the adaptive process, Boston, 1986, Jones & Bartlett.

Koenig HG and Blazer DG: Depression. In Birren JE, editor: *Encyclopedia of Gerontology: age, aging, and the aged,* vol I, San Diego, 1996, Academic Press.

Koenig HG, et al: Schizophrenia and paranoid disorders. In Busse E and Blazer D, editors: *Textbook of geriatric psychiatry,* ed 2, Washington, DC, 1996, American Psychiatric Press.

Kreeger J, et al: Effect of hearing enhancement on mental status rating in geriatric psychiatric patients, *Am J Psychiatry* 152(4):629, 1995.

Lamberg L: Treating depression in medical conditions may improve quality of life, *JAMA* 276(11):857, Sept 1996. Available at: http://www.ama-assn.org/sci-pubs/journals/archive/jama/vol_276/no_11/mn6145.htm. Accessed Aug 1, 1997.

Martin RL: Geriatric psychopharmacology: present and future, *Psychiatr Ann* 20:682, 1990.

McCahill ME and Brunton SA: The elderly patient with multiple complaints, *Hosp Pract* 30(12):49, 1995.

McGowan TG: Ageism and discrimination. In Birren JE, editor: *Encyclopedia of gerontology: age, aging and the aged,* vol 1, San Diego, 1996, Academic Press.

McIntosh JL: Epidemiology of suicide in the elderly, *Suicide Life Threat Behav* 22(1):15, 1992.

Meeks S and Murrell S: Mental illness in late life: socioeconomic conditions, psychiatric symptoms, and adjustment of long-term sufferers, *Psychol Aging* 12(2):296, 1997.

Mudd SA, et al: Alcohol withdrawal and related nursing care in older adults, *J Gerontol Nurs* 20(10):71, 1994.

National Coalition on Mental Health and Aging: *Building state and community mental health and aging coalitions: a "how-to" guide,* Dec 1994. Available at: http://www.mentalhealth.org/resource/how2.htm. Accessed July 31, 1997.

National Institutes of Health: *Geriatric assessment methods for clinical decisionmaking,* NIH Consensus Statement Online, Oct 19-21, 1987; 6(13):1. Available at: http://text.nlm.nih.gov/nih/cdc/www/65txt.html. Accessed Aug 5, 1997.

Pearlin L and Skaff MM: Stressors and adaptation in late life. In Gatz M, editor: *Emerging issues in mental health and aging,* Washington, DC, 1995, American Psychological Association.

Profitt C, Augspurger P, and Byrne M: Geriatric depression: a survey of nurses' knowledge and assessment practices, *Issues Ment Health Nurs* 17(2):123, 1996.

Roberts J: A harmonious atmosphere, *Nurs Times* 92(4):60, 1996.

Rosen A, Pancake J, and Rickards L: Mental health policy and older Americans: historical and current perspectives. In Gatz M, editor: *Emerging issues in mental health and aging,* Washington, DC, 1995, American Psychological Association.

Rowe JW and Devons CA: Physiological and clinical considerations of the geriatric patient. In Busse E and Blazer D, editors: *Textbook of geriatric psychiatry,* ed 2, Washington, DC, 1996, American Psychiatric Press.

Rubin EH, Kinscherf DA, and Wehrman SA: Response to treatment of depression in the old and very old, *J Geriatr Psychiatry Neurol* 4:65, 1991.

Sadavoy J, et al: *Comprehensive review of geriatric psychiatry—II,* ed 2, Washington, DC, 1996, American Psychiatric Press.

Sanders P: Depression in life threatening illness and its treatment, *Nurs Times* 91(11), 1995.

Sheikh, J: Anxiety disorders. In Sadavoy J, et al, editors: *Comprehensive review of geriatric psychiatry—II,* ed 2, Washington, DC, 1996, American Psychiatric Press.

Shorr RI, Fought RL, and Ray WA: Changes in antipsychotic drug use in nursing homes during implementation of the OBRA-87 regulations, *JAMA* 271(5):358, 1994.

Sloan RW: *Practical geriatric therapeutics,* Oradell, NJ, 1986, Medical Economics.

Solomon K, et al: Alcoholism and prescription drug abuse in the elderly: St. Louis University grand rounds [clinical conference], *J Am Geriatr Soc* 41(1):57, 1993.

Soltys F and Coats L: The SolCos model: facilitating reminiscence therapy, *J Gerontol Nurs* 22(1):15, 1994.

Stoudemire A and Smith D: OBRA regulations and the use of psychotropic drugs in long-term care facilities, *Gen Hosp Psychiatry* 18(2):77, 1996.

US Census Bureau: Statistical brief: sixty-five plus in the United States, Washington, DC, May 1995, Economics and Statistics Administration, US Department of Commerce. Available at: http://www.census.gov/socdemo/www/agebrief.html. Accessed July 29, 1997.

Waters E: Let's not wait til it's broke: interventions to maintain and enhance mental health in late life. In Gatz M, editor: *Emerging issues in mental health and aging,* Washington, DC, 1995, American Psychological Association.

Williams L and Lowenthal DT: Drug therapy in the elderly, *South Med J* 85(2):127, 1992.

CHAPTER 41

Working with Patients with HIV Infection*

GORDON I.G. PUGH
NORMAN L. KELTNER

LEARNING OBJECTIVES

After reading this chapter you should be able to:
- Describe the natural history of the human immunodeficiency virus (HIV).
- Identify the groups most at risk for HIV transmission in the United States.
- Describe risk behaviors associated with the transmission of HIV.
- Identify neurological and neuropsychiatric complications for persons with HIV.
- Identify the ethical responsibility of the nurse in safeguarding the privacy and confidentiality of the person with HIV.
- Apply the nursing process to care of persons with HIV and with neurological or neuropsychiatric complications.

Human immunodeficiency virus (HIV) is a communicable and progressively fatal condition. The virus attacks the immune system and thus lowers the person's resistance to other diseases. Because initial transmission in the United States primarily involved homosexual men and intravenous drug users, stigma and discrimination have aggravated the psychosocial aspects of this disease. In addition, the central nervous system (CNS) can be affected by the virus and thus require highly skilled psychiatric care.

Human immunodeficiency virus (HIV) is the term used to describe the entire range of disorders related to this virus. HIV infection includes people with the HIV antibody and acquired immunodeficiency syndrome (AIDS). A brief review of the immune system, opportunistic diseases, and transmission will provide the foundation for understanding HIV infection. The overview will provide the background necessary to discuss the neuropsychiatric aspects of HIV infection and the related neuropathol-

*This is a revision of a chapter originally written by Mary Jo Kasselman and Peggy Tracy Leapley. The diagnostic terminology for AIDS research continues to undergo refinement. In this chapter HIV infection includes the spectrum of illness, from individuals seropositive for HIV to those with end-stage AIDS.

KEY TERMS

Acquired immunodeficiency syndrome (AIDS) The term initially used to diagnose those with specific symptoms and opportunistic infections indicating a more advanced progression of HIV infection.

ELISA *Enzyme-Linked ImmunoSorbent Assay* test. This test is used to detect specific antibodies. It is used to assist in the diagnosis of HIV infection through the identification of antibodies to HIV.

HIV antibody The antibody specific to HIV that usually appears within 6 to 8 weeks after infection.

Human immunodeficiency infection The entire range of the illness caused by HIV. This includes people infected with HIV whether symptomatic or asymptomatic.

Human immunodeficiency virus (HIV) The virus isolated and recognized as the etiologic agent of AIDS. HIV is classified as a lentivirus in a subgroup of the retrovirus.

Kaposi's sarcoma (KS) Before the AIDS outbreak, a rare form of cancer that appears as a painless tumor with pink-purple spots on the skin and mouth.

Opportunistic illnesses Illnesses that develop when the immune system is inactive or suppressed.

***Pneumocystis carinii* pneumonia (PCP)** Before the AIDS outbreak, a rare form of pulmonary disease caused by an opportunistic pathogen (fungal protozoan).

Polymerase chain reaction (PCR) A laboratory technique using molecular biology to identify the nucleic acid sequence of HIV in the cells of an infected individual. Used in the early detection of perinatally exposed infants and in monitoring persons on clinical trials.

---

ogy. The psychiatric nursing implications of HIV infection will be discussed, including a case study of AIDS dementia.

OVERVIEW OF HIV INFECTION

Causes of HIV Infection

In June 1981 the U.S. Centers for Disease Control and Prevention (CDC) published case studies of five men, ages 29 to 36, with a diagnosis of *Pneumocystis carinii* pneumonia (PCP) in Los Angeles (CDC, 1981). PCP is not usually seen in people with adequate immune response systems. This alerted physicians to an unusual opportunistic disease in young men. Additional cases of PCP were reported to the CDC, and Kaposi's sarcoma (KS), a rare form of cancer, was also increasingly diagnosed in young men. Since those first cases were reported in 1981 more than 600,000 diagnoses of AIDS have been made in the United States. A total of 353,148 people died of AIDS in this county between 1981 and the beginning of 1997 (CDC, 1997).

The case history of HIV infection included an early recognition that the disease affected a person's immune system and that it was acquired rather than genetically transmitted. Because it affects the immune system, the disease leaves the person vulnerable to infectious agents the immune system ordinarily can suppress. Diseases that are the result of a compromised immune system are classified as opportunistic diseases. Initially, the cause of AIDS was unknown, and thus the diagnosis was based on the presence of certain symptoms within the patient. The symptoms, when seen in combination, were called a syndrome. The human immunodeficiency virus was initially isolated in 1983 from patients with AIDS.

HIV infection is thought to be caused by exposure to the human immunodeficiency virus, which interacts with other factors in the person. Some of the other factors affecting response to HIV exposure are dose, entry site, current immune system status, and number of exposures. The human immunodeficiency virus is classified as the lentivirus subfamily of the human retrovirus. It consists of a double-layered envelope full of proteins and surrounded by a small amount of ribonucleic acid (RNA). It enters the body from the T4 lymphocyte of an infected person. Figure 41-1 shows the mechanism of HIV infection of a cell. The infection starts when the gp120, a glycoprotein of the viral envelope, interacts with CD4, a surface antigen present on T lymphocytes, macrophages, glial cells, and neurons. Once

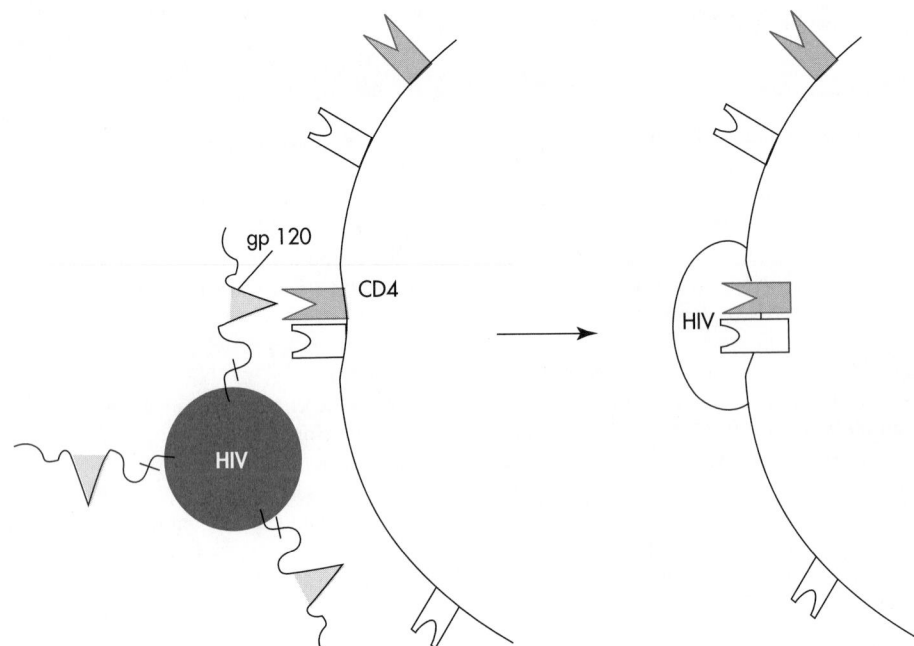

FIGURE 41-1   Mechanism for HIV infection of a cell. The outer viral envelope protein, gp120, attaches to a cell surface receptor. This is usually the CD4 antigen. The macrophage internalizes the HIV. Then the macrophage begins to release neurotoxins, and the HIV begins to replicate. Neurotoxins stimulate astrocytes to produce more neurotoxic substances. Neuronal damage may be caused by alterations in neuronal calcium metabolism or overactivation of N-methyl-D-aspartate receptor (i.e., excitotoxicity). The result is a decrease in dendrites, leading to diminished neuronal function or cell death.

the virus enters the cell, it inserts itself into the macrophage genome and begins to replicate. The virus may remain dormant for days, weeks, or years, or it may begin replication and thus infect other cells. It is thought that factors related to the immune system affect the dormant or active status. These factors include age, overall health, health-promoting activities such as nutrition and exercise, and health-reducing behaviors such as alcohol consumption. Current information regarding these disorders can be obtained via the Internet from the HIV/AIDS CDC's Surveillance Report accessible at www.cdc.gov.

Opportunistic Illnesses

When the immune system is compromised, certain organisms seize the opportunity to infect the person. Opportunistic infections are those the person would normally resist when the immune system is functional and healthy. Many of the opportunistic illnesses are commonly found in the environment but were rarely seen before the HIV infection

outbreak. Box 41-1 provides a list of opportunistic illnesses.

The most serious opportunistic illness is PCP, which is caused by a protozoan. Even with recent prophylactic treatment for PCP, it remains the leading cause of death among persons with AIDS. The second leading cause of AIDS deaths has been from KS. This cancer occurs on the surface of the skin, mouth, or visceral organs such as the lungs or digestive tract. It causes blue-violet or red-brown nodules or plaques that are distinctive. Another malignancy associated with HIV-infected individuals is a variety of non-Hodgkins lymphoma. Additional common opportunistic infections are *Toxoplasma gondii*, histoplasmosis, coccidioidomycosis, tuberculosis, herpes, *Candida albicans*, and cytomegalovirus.

HIV Infection Transmission

HIV infection is transmitted from person to person through sexual contact; intravenously; or from mother to baby during pregnancy, delivery, or

Box 41-1 Opportunistic Illnesses

Cancers
1. Kaposi's sarcoma (KS)
2. Primary lymphoma of brain
3. Burkitt's lymphoma
4. Non-Hodgkin's lymphoma
5. Hodgkin's disease

Protozoan and Helminth (Parasitical) Infections
1. Cryptosporidiosis, intestinal: causing diarrhea for over 1 month
2. *Pneumocystis carinii* pneumonia (PCP)
3. Strongyloidosis: pneumonia, central nervous system infection or disseminated infection
4. *Toxoplasma gondii:* pneumonia or central nervous system infection
5. *Isospora belli:* diarrhea for over 1 month

Fungal Infections
1. Aspergillosis: central nervous system or disseminated infection
2. *Candida albicans:* esophagitis
3. Cryptococcosis: pulmonary, central nervous system or disseminated
4. *Histoplasma capsulatum*
5. Coccidioidomycosis

Bacterial Infections
1. Atypical mycobacteriosis
2. *Mycobacterium tuberculosis*
3. Salmonellosis

Viral Infections
1. Cytomegalovirus (CMV)
2. Herpes simplex virus—persisting more than one month or pulmonary, gastrointestinal, or disseminated Epstein-Barr virus
3. Progressive multifocal leukoencephalopathy (PML)
4. Varicella zoster virus (VZV)

---

through breast feeding. The majority of sexually transmitted cases result from men having sex with men (about half). Hemophilia accounts for less than 1% of all AIDS cases (CDC, 1997). The presence of HIV has been reported in blood, semen, blood plasma, bone marrow, cervical secretions, saliva, breast milk, lymph nodes, brain tissue, tears, and cerebrospinal and amniotic fluids. Although the virus can be isolated in many body fluids, a number of body fluids have not been implicated in any cases of HIV transmission. There have been no documented cases of HIV transmission by insect vectors, handshaking, tears, or non–blood-tinged saliva. Research overwhelmingly indicates three main means of transmission (CDC, 1997):

1. Men who have sex with men
2. Injecting-drug use
3. Heterosexual contact, including sex with bisexual males and drug-injecting partners

Populations at Risk

Various groups have been identified as at-risk for HIV infection (Table 41-1). It is not the group identification, however, that results in HIV infection, but rather a behavior common to the at-risk group. Thus determining at-risk status involves not solely identification of the risk group, but also assessment for specific risk behaviors. This is particularly important since many of the prominent risk groups have changed their behavior or instituted preventive measures.

In the United States, the groups most at risk are homosexual and bisexual men, intravenous drug users, sexual partners of homosexual/bisexual men and intravenous drug users, infants with HIV-infected mothers, hemophiliacs, and blood transfusion recipients before March 1985. Health care providers are not in the high-risk category but do need to be aware of special precautions to avoid exposure.

In the United States, most transmission of HIV occurs between men who have sex with men. The risk of infection in this population increases with the number of male sex partners and the frequency with which the person is the receptive partner in anal intercourse. Recently, the rate of new infection in gay men has declined due to such behavioral changes as mutually monogamous sexual partners and the increased use of safer sex behavior.

The second wave of HIV infection was seen in intravenous drug users (IVDU).

Perinatal transmission of HIV to infants born of HIV-infected mothers is well documented. Evidence suggests that transmission can occur in utero, at delivery, or during the immediate postpartum period. The risk of an HIV-infected woman infecting her baby is estimated to be quite high. Breast milk can

Table 41-1	AIDS Cases by Exposure Category (Cumulative Total) in the United States

Single mode of exposure (adult and adolescent)	
Men who have sex with men	286,611
Injecting-drug use	124,684
Hemophilia/coagulation disorder	3,673
Heterosexual contact	53,119
Receipt of transfusion*	8,063
Receipt of transplant of tissues, organs, or artificial insemination†	12
Other	95
(Single mode of exposure subtotal:	**476,257)**
Multiple modes of exposure subtotal‡:	83,337
Risk not reported or identified:	44,582
Pediatric cases (<13 years old)§:	7,902
Total:	**612,078**

From Centers for Disease Control and Prevention: *HIV/AIDS surveillance report* 9(No. 1), Atlanta, 1997, US Department of Health and Human Services.
*Includes 37 adult/adolescents who developed AIDS after receiving blood screened negative for HIV antibody.
†Twelve adults developed AIDS after receiving tissue, organs or artificial insemination from HIV-infected donors. Four of the twelve received tissue or organs from a single donor who was negative for HIV antibody at the time of donation. See *N Engl J Med* 1992;326:726-32.
‡The multiple modes of exposure category is comprised of various combinations of the above-cited categories.
§Pediatric exposure categories: Mother with/at risk for HIV infection (91%); Receipt of blood transfusion, components, or tissue (5%); Hemophilia/coagulation disorder (3%); Risk not reported or identified (2%).

also be a means of transmission from the HIV-infected woman to the baby.

The risk of acquiring HIV through blood transfusion or blood products such as those used by hemophiliacs has been greatly reduced by the testing of donated blood. Currently, all blood donations are screened for the HIV antibody. Since March 1985, when all blood banks in the United States initiated HIV antibody screening, the risk of blood-product transmission has been virtually but not totally eliminated. Since conversion from antibody negative to antibody positive usually takes 6 to 8 weeks, there remains a slight risk of blood-transfusion transmission. The CDC (1997) reports 37 individuals who contracted AIDS from blood screened negative for HIV. There should be no risk, however, of donating blood since individual sterile equipment is used for each donor.

Mentally ill patients may be at increased risk for acquiring HIV (Sacks, et al, 1990). Poor judgment, hypersexuality, and impulsivity are associated with many psychiatric disorders—behaviors that increase the risk for HIV infection. Sacks, et al (1990) found that 20% of psychiatric patients were engaging in high-risk behavior. They found that bipolar illness correlated significantly with high-risk behavior and suggested that these patients in particular receive HIV counseling.

There is a small but definite occupational risk of HIV infections for health care workers (Table 41-2). The potential for occupational transmission of HIV can be reduced by implementing and vigorously enforcing universal precautions, infection control procedures such as needleless equipment, protected needles, goggles, etc.

It is equally important to understand that there is no known risk of HIV transmission through casual contact. Despite prolonged contact with an infected person among 400 family members, none have been infected except those family members who engage in high-risk behavior. Thus the risk of transmission in schools and the workplace is thought to be even more remote than in the home.

AIDS Diagnosis

In 1983 AIDS first became a CDC reportable disease. Before 1987, the diagnosis of AIDS was based on the presence of one or more opportunistic diseases in a person with no other reasonable explanation for having a compromised immune system. After HIV was recognized as the etiologic agent of AIDS, HIV antibody tests became available, and specific manifestations of the disease were better defined.

Box 41-2 summarizes the most frequent symptoms of HIV infection according to an HIV-oriented review of systems. Many of the symptoms are generalized and associated with other diseases. This makes the initial diagnosis more difficult. In addition, people often delay seeking professional advice because the symptoms are initially mild.

HIV Tests

The normal range of T4 cells is 600 to 1200/mm^3. With HIV infection, the T4 cell range drops to 0 to 200/mm^3. The number of T4 cells correlates with symptoms and clinical course. The normal T4 to T8 ratio is 2:1, but this ratio is often inverse with HIV infection. The following functional abnormalities of

Table 41-2 U.S. Health Care Workers with Documented Occupational Transmission by Occupation

Health Care Occupation	No.	% (Rounded)
Health aide/attendant	1	(2)
Housekeeper/maintenance worker	1	(2)
Laboratory technician, clinical	16	(31)
Laboratory technician, non-clinical	3	(6)
Nurse	21	(40)
Physician	6	(12)
Respiratory therapist	1	(2)
Technician, dialysis	1	(2)
Technician, surgical	2	(4)
Total:	52	

Note: The Centers for Disease Control and Prevention also maintains a record of numbers attributed to *possible* occupational transmission. These numbers are significantly greater than the documented cases.
From Centers for Disease Control and Prevention: *HIV/AIDS surveillance report* 9(No. 1), Atlanta, 1997, US Department of Health and Human Services.

Box 41-2 HIV-Oriented Review of Symptoms According to Body Systems

General: Weight loss, anorexia, fever, pharyngitis, lethargy
Skin: New rashes or pigmented lesions, generalized drying, pruritus, erythematous maculopapular rash, roseola-like rash, diffuse urticaria
Lymphatics: Localized or generalized lymph node enlargement, change in size (increase or decrease) in any previously enlarged lymph nodes
Head, eyes, ears, nose, and throat: Nasal discharge, sinus congestion, changes in visual acuity, sore throat, whitish or painful lesions of the oral mucosa, alopecia
Cardiopulmonary: Cough or shortness of breath
Gastrointestinal: Abdominal pain, change in bowel habits, diarrhea, nausea and vomiting
Musculoskeletal: Myalgia, arthralgia
Neurological: Symptoms of headaches, meningoencephalitis, depression, change of personality, cognitive difficulties, peripheral weakness, or paresthesias

From Tindall B, et al: Primary HIV infection. In Sande M and Volberding P, editors: *The medical management of AIDS*, ed 3, Philadelphia, 1992, WB Saunders.

T cells are present in HIV infection (Bullock and Rosendahl, 1988; Porth, 1990):

- Diminished lymphokine production
- Decreased cytotoxic lymphocyte function
- Decreased ability to provide help to B lymphocytes for immunoglobulin (Ig) production
- Decreased proliferative responses
- Decreased responsiveness to specific antigens

The most helpful and relatively specific laboratory evidence of HIV infection is abnormality of T lymphocyte subsets. Many viral illnesses cause an increase in the absolute number and percentage of suppresser (T8) lymphocytes. Marked depression of helper-inducer (T4) lymphocytes is highly suggestive of HIV effect. Thus a finding of depressed T4 lymphocytes strongly supports a diagnosis of HIV infection. The absolute number of cells in this subset rather than the ratio of T4 to T8 cells is most useful.

The test for HIV most commonly used in the United States is the HIV antibody test. ELISA (*E*nzyme-*L*inked *I*mmuno*S*orbent *A*ssay) detects the HIV antibody that usually develops in the infected person within 6 to 8 weeks following the exposure to HIV. ELISA is a screening test. If the test is positive, most laboratories use the Western blot or immunofluorescent antibody (IFA) test to confirm the results. These tests are relatively inexpensive. These tests can still be less than 100% accurate (see clinical example).

With HIV testing, the nurse is responsible for the confidentiality and/or anonymity of the test and the person's psychological safety. The psychological safety of HIV testing will be presented later.

CLINICAL EXAMPLE

In the late 1980s, John Smith, a 26-year-old white male substance abuser, was tested for AIDS and was told that the test was positive. He was scared and started drinking heavily. He drove his car that night and caused an accident, killing an innocent child. He was convicted and sentenced to many years in prison. In prison he was tested again and discovered that the earlier HIV test was in error. John became a trustee with access to the "evidence" room. He found a bag of cocaine and snorted it. He suffered a tachyarrhythmia and died. His drug counselor believes that both the child and John would still be alive if the first HIV test had been more accurate.

The ANA code of ethics (1985) states that the "nurse safeguards the patient's right to privacy by judiciously protecting information of a confidential nature." All tests and diagnoses are confidential and should not be revealed to those not involved in the patient's care without the patient's permission. Most states have enacted laws to promote health provider compliance with maintenance of testing and diagnostic confidentiality. Confidentiality thus becomes an ethical and legal matter for nurses caring for persons with AIDS. In this respect, HIV infection and confidentiality are an ethical responsibility and are the same as for all persons requiring nursing care.

■ Critical Thinking Question

Identify three issues of precounseling for HIV testing and three issues of postcounseling if the test is positive.

Incidence and Distribution

HIV infection was the primary public health problem of the 1980s. It is projected to continue as a worldwide problem into the next century. In the United States as of December 1996, over 600,000 cases of AIDS have been reported to the federal Centers for Disease Control and Prevention (Tables 41-3, 41-4, 41-5 and 41-6). The CDC reports 353,148 deaths due to AIDS since 1981. The progression of the disease indicates a major impact on the health care system if the number of people with HIV infection is not reduced through education, change of risk behaviors, and development of new treatments.

Risk Behavior Prevention

Nurses need to know the risk behavior prevention strategies for transmission involving sexual contact, intravenous drugs, and nursing care. The major focus on prevention is education.

Sexual transmission prevention

Since early in the AIDS outbreak, "safe sex" has been suggested as an effective prevention strategy. As more information has become available on transmission of the virus, the sexual practices that are safe and unsafe have been more clearly described. While the only truly "safe sex" is abstinence, this is not a behavior pattern that will be maintained by many people over a lifetime. The next option is monogamous relationships between noninfected couples. Persons not selecting the above options should take additional precautions such as use of a latex condom, a spermicide with nonoxynol-9, and a water-based lubricant. Even latex condoms are not foolproof, however. Large numbers of condoms have been found to be substandard. For example, according to Reuter's news service available on the Internet, 24 million of 66 million condoms sent to Zimbabwe were defective and had to be destroyed.

Table 41-3 Areas of Highest Incidence of AIDS in the United States (in the 12-Month Period Ending June 1997)

AIDS Cases by City		AIDS Cases by State	
New York, NY	10,129	New York	12,525
Los Angeles, CA	3,232	California	8,177
Washington, DC	2,019	Florida	6,726
Houston, TX	1,806	Texas	4,928
Miami, FL	1,799	New Jersey	3,777
Philadelphia, PA	1,589	Puerto Rico	2,210
Newark, NJ	1,552	Maryland	2,175
Baltimore, MD	1,529	Pennsylvania	2,127
Chicago, IL	1,437	Georgia	2,108
Atlanta, GA	1,416	Illinois	1,753

Note: The Centers for Disease Control and Prevention cautions that AIDS counts are believed to be more complete than case counts for HIV infection.
From Centers for Disease Control and Prevention: *HIV/AIDS surveillance report* 9(No. 1), Atlanta, 1997, US Department of Health and Human Services.

IVDU transmission prevention

The most common means of IVDU transmission is through the sharing of drug paraphernalia (intravenous equipment) contaminated by HIV. The second most common IVDU-related transmission occurs when HIV-infected drug users infect their sexual partners. And third, HIV-infected women who are either IVDUs or sexual partners of IVDUs can infect their newborns. In addition, drugs and alcohol have been implicated as cofactors in HIV transmission through lowered immune system response and reduction in inhibitions such that risky sexual behavior occurs. One AIDS prevention advertising campaign warns: Get high. Get Stupid. Get AIDS.

IVDU risk-reduction strategies include first, efforts to eliminate and treat the substance abuse problem and, second, efforts to prevent the spread of HIV or other viruses such as hepatitis B (HBV). IVDUs should be encouraged to seek treatment of their problem. For IVDUs refusing drug treatment programs, emphasis should be placed on education to reduce their risk. Following are some guidelines for reducing risk of HIV transmission:

- Never share IV drugs or equipment.
- If a needle and/or syringe must be shared, remember to clean them thoroughly using bleach and water to reduce the risk.

- Do not practice risky sexual behavior.
- If you are a woman who has previous risk behaviors, get medical advice before any pregnancy.

Universal precautions for nurses and other health care workers

Fear is a common reaction of nurses to the initial experience of caring for a person with HIV infection. Without sufficient knowledge and emotional support, the nurse's initial reaction is often avoidance and neglect behaviors (Zook and Davidhizar, 1989; Smirnoff, et al, 1991). The first step in resolving these fears is to provide information about HIV infection.

Preexisting policies and plans for care of persons with HIV infection assist the nurse in handling anxiety and fears and also thinking about the professional role and responsibilities. Guidelines for care of persons with HIV infection need to be available for all health care workers and auxiliary personnel. Even nurses with persistent fears and prejudice are ethically expected to provide competent care. The ANA code of ethics (1985) requires that nursing service be provided "unrestricted by considerations of social or economic status, personal attributes, or the nature of health problems."

Table 41-4 AIDS Cases by Age at Diagnosis in the United States

Under 5	6,221
5-12	1,681
13-19	2,953
20-24	22,070
25-29	85,211
30-34	140,559
35-39	136,814
40-44	98,393
45-49	55,302
50-54	29,148
55-59	16,399
60-64	9,214
65 or older	8,113
	TOTAL: 612,078

From Centers for Disease Control and Prevention: *HIV/AIDS surveillance report* 9(No. 1), Atlanta, 1997, US Department of Health and Human Services.

Table 41-5 AIDS Cases by Race in the United States

White, non-Hispanic	279,072
Black, non-Hispanic	216,980
Hispanic	109,252
Asian/Pacific Islander	4,370
American Indian/Alaska Native	1,677
Race/Ethnicity unknown	727
	TOTAL: 612,078

From Centers for Disease Control and Prevention: *HIV/AIDS surveillance report* 9(No. 1), Atlanta, 1997, US Department of Health and Human Services.

Table 41-6 AIDS Cases by Sex in the United States

Male	516,003
Female	96,075
	Total: 612,078

From Centers for Disease Control and Prevention: *HIV/AIDS surveillance report* 9(No. 1), Atlanta, 1997, US Department of Health and Human Services.

Universal precautions mean that all patients are assumed to be potentially infected with HIV or HBV. Box 41-3 reviews these precautions.

NEUROPSYCHIATRIC ASPECTS OF HIV INFECTION

Several general areas of neuropsychiatric disorder occur in those affected with HIV (Bennett and Plum, 1996):

1. Stress related to having a fatal disease
2. Neuropsychiatric complications related to HIV brain infection or opportunistic illnesses
3. Neuropsychiatric complication related to treatment

A more specific listing of neuropsychiatric disorders is found in Box 41-4.

Stress Related to Having AIDS

A diagnosis of AIDS can be initiated as a result of a positive HIV antibody test or one of the newer HIV infection tests or based on symptoms of HIV infection as listed in the CDC definition (updated and expanded in 1993). Diagnosis will result in classification of the person according to the progression of the disease. A diagnosis of AIDS often results in an initial reaction of denial, disbelief, numbness, inability to concentrate or make decisions, and anger.

The stages of grief and loss are common following a diagnosis of AIDS (Kübler-Ross, 1987). The stigma and discrimination of society toward persons with AIDS aggravate the fear and loss experienced. The person with AIDS (PWA) may be concerned with the reaction of family, friends, and co-workers. Many PWAs report problems with health care coverage by their insurance companies, which adds to their financial concern and neuropsychiatric symptoms.

Referral for psychiatric treatment should be made for PWAs who exhibit symptoms of depression, suicidal ideation, denial that is maladaptive by increasing the person's or another's risk, extreme anxiety, or delirium (Zook and Davidhizar, 1989). Extreme depression is treated with the standard protocol of antidepressants and psychotherapy. Anxiety reactions can be treated with benzodiazepine. Safety precautions must be instituted for those with suicide ideation. Delirium has been reported in more than 50% of medically hospitalized PWAs. These neuropsychiatric symptoms can interfere with treatment planning and nursing care for a PWA and thus require psychiatric nursing skills.

Neuropsychiatric Complications Related to HIV Brain Infection or Opportunistic Illness

Many neuropsychiatric complications are reported in persons with HIV infection. Box 41-4 shows the psychiatric disorders associated with HIV infection. It should be noted that the person with HIV may have preexisting psychiatric disorders such as a personality disorder or affective disorder. These preexisting psychiatric disorders can be further complicated by HIV infection.

The adjustment disorders of depression and anxiety are often seen as a psychological reaction to "living with HIV." Patients with known bipolar disorders can more frequently become HIV infected; this is attributed to the manic stage of the disorder when the person may participate in high-risk behaviors for HIV exposure.

Organic mental disorders were discussed in the neurological complications of HIV. The psychotic symptom of delirium can be caused by alcohol or drug withdrawal; fluid, electrolyte, and acid-base imbalance; hypoglycemia; infections; medication or drug overdose; hypoxia; or systemic insufficiency such as hepatic, renal, or pancreatic.

There are indications that the CNS is commonly infected by HIV early in the course of the infection (Worley and Price, 1992). During the acute infection phase, neurological complications may include meningitis, ataxia, myelopathy, and peripheral nervous system (PNS) abnormalities. Most patients recover from these complications within a number of weeks with the exception of those with meningitis.

During the asymptomatic phase of HIV, neurological complications include neuropathies resembling Guillain-Barré syndrome or chronic inflammatory demyelinating polyneuropathy (CIDP).

HIV infection, particularly in its late phase, is complicated by a variety of CNS and PNS disorders. These disorders are common and lead to considerable morbidity. They relate not only to opportunistic infections and neoplasms, but also to direct nervous system HIV infection.

AIDS dementia is the most common late CNS dysfunction, and it is characterized by cognitive, motor, and behavioral dysfunction. More often it appears after AIDS patients have developed major opportunistic infections. However, AIDS dementia may appear before the appearance of major systemic complications, and in recognition of this fact AIDS dementia complex has been added to the diagnostic criteria for AIDS (Burgess, 1990; Johnson, 1989; Portegies, 1994). Between 50% and 85% of PWAs develop clinical signs of AIDS dementia (Dickerson and Ranseen, 1990).

AIDS dementia often is manifested by decreased concentration and forgetfulness, followed by decreased alertness, psychomotor retardation, withdrawal, apathy and reduced interest in work and usual activities, and loss of libido. Later symptoms of AIDS dementia may include hallucinations, con-

---

Box 41-4   Psychiatric Disorders Associated with HIV Infection

Adjustment disorders—can include depressed mood or anxious mood
Major affective disorders—depression, bereavement, bipolar disorder
Anxiety disorders—generalized anxiety disorder
Organic mental disorder—HIV infection or opportunistic infection dementia, cancer associated dementia such as cerebral lymphoma or disseminated Kaposi's sarcoma
Delirium
Organic mood disorders—depression, manic, mixed
Organic delusional disorders
Personality disorders—borderline or antisocial
Substance abuse disorders

From Dilley J: Management of neuropsychiatric disorders in HIV-spectrum patients. In Sande M and Volberding P, editors: *The medical management of AIDS*, ed 3, Philadelphia, 1992, WB Saunders.

---

fusion, disorientation, seizures, mutism, profound dementia, and finally coma leading to death (McArthur, 1990; Porth, 1990).

Neuroimaging procedures and cerebrospinal fluid evaluations are essential in determining neurological complications. Computed tomography (CT) scans and magnetic resonance imaging (MRI) show universal findings of cerebral atrophy, widened cortical sulci, and enlarged ventricles. Accumulated evidence from a multitude of sources supports the contention that the AIDS dementia complex is directly attributable to brain infection by HIV.

Headache and photophobia are meningeal symptoms. The specific types of meningitis may be aseptic meningitis, which is thought to result from the HIV infection, or a meningitis from one of the opportunistic infections. The most common meningitis infection in AIDS patients is from the fungal infection *Cryptococcus neoformans*.

A number of focal brain disorders can occur in AIDS patients. Acute focal brain disease suggests either a vascular disorder or seizure. The most common focal disorders are subacute over days or weeks. These brain disorders include cerebral toxoplasmosis, primary CNS lymphoma, progressive multifocal leukoencephalopathy, tuberculosis brain abscess, cryptococcosis, variella-zoster virus encephalitis, and herpes encephalitis (Worley and Price, 1992). The most common is cerebral toxoplasmosis.

Neuropsychiatric Complications Related to Treatment

Many anti-AIDS drugs have powerful CNS effects. For example, zidovudine (AZT) can cause mania. Other antiviral drugs can cause confusion and/or depression. The combination of organ failure and toxic medications can lead to delirium.

Skilled psychiatric nursing care for persons with HIV infection and neuropsychiatric complication requires both experience and interest. The necessary care should include principles from therapy for chronically or terminally ill patients, as well as psychiatric treatment.

Treatment for adjustment or affective disorders of anxiety or depression in persons with HIV infection may include psychopharmacology, that is, intervention with antidepressants, antianxiety agents, or hypnotics for insomnia. Supportive psychotherapy and support groups may be helpful. Effort should be made to maintain frequent contact to provide reassurance, support, and education as indicated. Activities should be planned so that prolonged social isolation or withdrawal is avoided. Treatment for anxiety should begin with nonpharmacological approaches. Relaxation techniques may be useful for mild to moderate anxiety but is not typically useful in the case of true anxiety disorder.

Treatment of persons with preexisting bipolar disease and HIV infection may include lithium. Careful monitoring of lithium levels will be necessary if the patient develops diarrhea or dehydration as a complication of HIV infection or lithium (lithium serum levels will increase).

Substance abuse disorders in persons with HIV complicate their clinical care and treatment. This is specifically a concern when prescribing and administering psychopharmacological agents to a person who may use additional drugs that are contraindicated. Drug treatment programs and case management are of primary importance. It is not uncommon for a person with substance abuse disorder to underdose or overdose when therapeutic agents are provided. Careful monitoring of dose, blood levels, and need for refill of medication may be necessary.

■ Critical Thinking Question

How would you maintain a therapeutic milieu for a person with AIDS dementia who frequently sleeps at a homeless shelter?

Case Study

Mr. Jackson, a 28-year-old married African-American man, was admitted to a public hospital after an episode of confusion, hallucination, and memory problems. His admitting diagnosis included AIDS dementia. He was admitted to a medical-surgical unit and placed in a private room. His T4 count was low and his physical condition was aggravated by anorexia and rapid weight loss. His psychological symptoms varied based on his degree of confusion. Confusion was noted to be more severe during the late evenings. The confusion was complicated by poor memory and disorientation to place and time.

Mr. Jackson had a history of IV drug use since age 18. He was found to be HIV antibody positive when he was incarcerated for selling drugs. Previous hospitalizations included two episodes of *Pneumocystis carinii* pneumonia. He was released from jail 1 month before the current hospitalization. His probation officer reports Mr. Jackson was unable to find employment and thus remained on Medicaid and social security. Mr. Jackson lives with his 45-year-old mother and his two sisters, ages 22 and 17. His family is very concerned and supportive. Currently, Mr. Jackson is not using illegal drugs and has no sexual partners.

Universal precautions were hospital policy, but additional measures were needed when diagnostic tests were done because Mr. Jackson became aggravated and resistant to the procedures. The community has a nursing case management program available for PWAs. One-to-one supervision was found to be the most therapeutic in providing for safety and reality orientation. Visitors were also encouraged.

Management

The neuropathies of the asymptomatic phase of HIV infection are often treated with plasmaphoresis or corticosteroid administration. Intravenous immunoglobulin may also be helpful (Worley and Price, 1992).

Studies indicate that AIDS dementia responds to antiviral therapy such as AZT. The treatment for AIDS dementia often includes methylphenidate (Ritalin) for those with depression, apathy, and withdrawal. Haloperidol (Haldol) may be used in a small dose for the management of paranoia and hallucinations (Polk-Walker, 1989). The nurse needs to assess the patient regularly for capacity to work and perform activities of daily living. Reality testing and safety precautions should be based on the nurse's assessment of the psychoemotional status of the PWA.

*C*are *P*lan

NAME: Mr. Jackson   **ADMISSION DATE:** _____

DSM-IV DIAGNOSIS: Dementia due to AIDS _____

ASSESSMENT: **Areas of strength:** Supportive family. Earlier AIDS diagnosis has resulted in Medicaid and social security programs. Currently not abusing drugs.
Problems: Confusion, hallucination, and memory problems. Physical problems of anorexia and related weight loss, secondary to HIV. Agitation when diagnostic tests done.

DIAGNOSES:
- High risk for infection, related to presence of HIV.
- Altered nutrition: less than body requirements related to anorexia, secondary to HIV, as evidenced by rapid weight loss.
- Altered thought process, related to AIDS dementia, as evidenced by confusion, memory problems, and disorientation.

OUTCOMES: **Short-term goals:**   **Date met**
- Weight maintenance and improved nutritional status.   _____
- Administer antiviral and antipsychotic medications as ordered.   _____
- Ongoing assessment of mental status.   _____

Long-term goals:
- Monitor for opportunistic infections related to presence of HIV.   _____
- Prevention of HIV transmission.   _____

PLANNING/ INTERVENTIONS: **Nurse-patient relationship:** Use simple, short sentences to minimize confusion. Provide high-calorie, high-protein diet. One-to-one care during periods of patient confusion and disorientation. Maintain universal precautions. Obtain assistance, if agitated.
Psychopharmacology: Haldol and zidovudine. If giving IM medication, use a retractable needle and follow universal precautions for needle and syringe disposal.
Milieu management: Encourage visitors. Use calendar and clock to provide orientation to time and also reality. Follow daily routine. Use lists and written communication such as a posted schedule. Remove potentially dangerous objects from environment.

EVALUATION: No opportunistic infection or institution of early treatment of symptoms noted. No health care worker exposed to HIV. Maintain or increase body weight. Ability to interact and behave with others appropriately has improved. Reduction in disorientation.

REFERRALS: Return to home. Home health referral for patient. Refer family to community support group.

For patients with AIDS dementia, the nurses face a challenge in creating and maintaining a therapeutic milieu. Nurses may need to institute additional measures to ensure that universal precautions are maintained to protect the staff and other patients. For example, retractable needles are necessary when giving emergency medication to severely mentally ill patients who are infected with HIV.

It is uncommon for nurses to wear gloves in caring for psychiatric patients. If this universal precaution measure is necessary, it may raise questions by the PWA and other patients. But if it is used universally and consistently where exposure to body fluids is possible, questions and suspicious will likely be allayed. In addition, clear, concise explanations are needed to prevent the triggering of paranoid feelings. The patient with AIDS dementia may require one-to-one nursing care to ensure the safety of the patient, staff, and other patients.

In treating patients with focal brain disease the use of corticosteroids should be avoided when possible. Corticosteroids can intensify the suppression of the immune defense response in AIDS patients and thus have the potential to worsen opportunistic infections. Corticosteroids may be necessary if cerebral edema threatens brain herniation.

■ Critical Thinking Question

What plans would you make for discharge of Mr. Jackson?

💬 Key Concepts

1. *Acquired immunodeficiency syndrome* (AIDS) is the term initially used to describe the effects of a set of rare symptoms occurring in young homosexual men.
2. The human immunodeficiency virus (HIV) was isolated in 1983 from patients with AIDS.
3. HIV enters the body from the T4 lymphocyte of an infected person. The normal range of T4 cells is 600 to 1200/mm^3. With HIV infection the range is 0 to 200/mm^3. The number of T4 cells correlates with symptoms and clinical course. The normal T4 to T8 ratio is 2:1. This ratio is often inverse with AIDS. The normal function of the T4 cell is absent or depressed in HIV infection.
4. Opportunistic infections are those the person would normally resist when the immune system is functional and healthy. Many of the opportunistic diseases are commonly found in the environment and were rarely seen before the HIV epidemic.

5. Health care providers are not in a high-risk category but do need to be aware of special precautions to avoid exposure. The potential for occupational transmission of HIV can be reduced by implementing and vigorously enforcing infection-control procedures, such as universal precautions.
6. Populations at risk for HIV infection are identified based on specific behaviors that are practiced by individuals within the population. The three main means of transmission are: (1) men who have sex with men, (2) injecting-drug use, and (3) heterosexual contact, including sex with bisexual males and drug-injecting partners.
7. AIDS dementia, the most common late CNS dysfunction, is characterized by cognitive, motor, and behavioral dysfunction.
8. Most states have enacted laws to promote health care provider compliance with diagnostic confidentiality. Confidentiality is an ethical responsibility.
9. For the patient with AIDS dementia the nurse can maintain a therapeutic milieu by ensuring that measures to safeguard the patient, staff, and other patients are employed. These measures include universal precautions, one-to-one supervision, reality orientation, use of daily routine, posted schedules, clocks, and calendars to minimize confusion.

💬 Study Questions

(Answer key is in the back of the book.)
1. What is the difference between the terms *HIV infection* and *AIDS*?
2. Why do individuals with HIV infection eventually develop opportunistic diseases?
3. What are the three main means of transmitting HIV?
4. According to Table 41-2, which occupation is at greatest risk for HIV infection?
   a. Aide
   b. Nurse
   c. Laboratory technician
   d. Physician
5. Which of the following is *not* a symptom of AIDS dementia?
   a. Forgetfulness
   b. Apathy
   c. Increased alertness
   d. Hallucinations

REFERENCES

Agency for Health Care Policy and Research: *Evaluation and management of early HIV infection,* Pub No 94-0572, Washington, DC, 1994, US Department of Health and Human Services.

American Nurses Association: *Code for nurses,* Kansas City, 1985, The Association.

Bennett JC and Plum F: *Cecil's textbook of medicine,* Philadelphia, 1996, WB Saunders.

Brown M and Powell-Cope G: AIDS family caregiving: transition through uncertainty, *Nurs Res* 40(6):338, 1991.

Bullock B and Rosendahl P: *Pathophysiology: adaptations and alterations in function,* Boston, 1988, Scott, Foresman.

Burgess AW: *Psychiatric nursing in the hospital and community,* ed 5, Norwalk, Conn, 1990, Appleton & Lange.

California Nurses Association: *Universal infection precautions: AIDS education and training,* San Francisco, 1988, The Association.

Centers for Disease Control and Prevention: Pneumocystic pneumonia—Los Angeles, *MMWR Morbid Mortal Wkly Rep* 30:250, 1981.

Centers for Disease Control and Prevention: Classification system for HTLV-III/LAV, *MMWR Morbid Mortal Wkly Rep* 35:335, 1986.

Centers for Disease Control and Prevention: Revision of the CDC surveillance case definition for acquired immunodeficiency syndrome, *MMWR Morbid Mortal Wkly Rep* 36:1S, 1987a.

Centers for Disease Control and Prevention: Recommendations for prevention of HIV transmission in health care settings, *MMWR Morbid Mortal Wkly Rep* 36:25, 1987b.

Centers for Disease Control and Prevention: Update: acquired immunodeficiency virus infection among health care workers, *MMWR Morbid Mortal Wkly Rep* 37:15, 1988.

Centers for Disease Control and Prevention: AIDS and human immunodeficiency virus infection in the United States, 1988 update, *MMWR Morbid Mortal Wkly Rep* 38:S4, May 12, 1989a.

Centers for Disease Control and Prevention: Guidelines for prevention of transmission of human immunodeficiency virus and hepatitis B virus to health care and public safety workers, *MMWR Morbid Mortal Wkly Rep* 38:46, 1989b.

Centers for Disease Control and Prevention: Estimation of HIV prevalence and projected AIDS cases: a summary workshop, *MMWR Morbid Mortal Wkly Rep* 39:7, 1989c.

Centers for Disease Control and Prevention: *HIV/AIDS surveillance report,* Washington, DC, 1992, US Department of Health and Human Services.

Centers for Disease Control and Prevention: *HIV/AIDS surveillance report* 9(No. 1), Atlanta, 1997, US Department of Health and Human Services.

Clement M and Hollander H: National history and management of the seropositive patient. In Sande M and Volberding P, editors: *The medical management of AIDS,* ed 3, Philadelphia, 1992, WB Saunders.

Cournos F, et al: HIV infection in state hospitals: case reports and long-term care strategies, *Hosp Community Psychiatry* 41:163, 1990.

Dickerson LR and Ranseen JD: An update on organic mental syndromes, *Hosp Community Psychiatry* 41:290, 1990.

Dilley J: Management of neuropsychiatric disorders in HIV-spectrum patients. In Sande M and Volberding P, editors: *The medical management of AIDS,* ed 3, Philadelphia, 1992, WB Saunders.

Fang C, et al: HIV testing and patient counseling, *Patient Care* 23(17):18, 1989.

Flaskerad J and Ungvarski P: *HIV/AIDS: a guide to nursing care,* Philadelphia, 1992, WB Saunders.

Gloersen B, et al: The phenomena of doing well in people with AIDS, *West J Nurs Res* 15(1):44, 1993.

Johnson B: *Adaptation and growth: psychiatric mental health nursing,* ed 2, Philadelphia, 1989, JB Lippincott.

Kübler-Ross E: *AIDS: the ultimate challenge,* New York, 1987, Macmillan.

McArthur J: AIDS dementia, *RN* 53:36, 1990.

McCain N and Grambling L: Living with dying: coping with HIV disease, *Issues Ment Health Nurs* 13:271, 1992.

Polk-Walker G: Treatment of AIDS in a psychiatric setting, *Perspect Psychiatr Care* 25:9, 1989.

Portegies P: AIDS dementia complex: a review, *Acquired Immune Deficiency Syndrome* 7(suppl):538, 1994.

Porth CM: *Pathophysiology: concepts of altered human health,* ed 3, Philadelphia, 1990, JB Lippincott.

Sacks MH, et al: HIV-related risk factors in acute psychiatric inpatients, *Hosp Community Psychiatry* 41:449, 1990.

Sande MA and Volberding A, editors: *The medical management of AIDS,* ed 3, Philadelphia, 1992, WB Saunders Co.

Smirnoff L, et al: Stigma, AIDS and quality of nursing care: state of the science, *J Adv Nurs* 16:262, 1991.

Swanson B, Cronin-Stubbs D, and Colletti M: Dementia and depression in persons with AIDS: causes and care, *J Psychosoc Nurs Ment Health Serv* 28(10):33, 1990.

Tindall B, et al: Primary HIV infection. In Sande M and Volberding P, editors: *The medical management of AIDS,* ed 3, Philadelphia, 1992, WB Saunders.

Worley J and Price R: Management of neurological complications of HIV-1 infection and AIDS. In Sande M and Volberding P, editors: *The medical management of AIDS,* ed 3, Philadelphia, 1992, WB Saunders.

Zook R and Davidhizar R: Caring for the psychiatric inpatient with AIDS, *Perspect Psychiatr Care* 25(2):3, 1989.

Diagnostic Criteria for Mental Disorders (DSM-IV)*

The following represents the complete list of diagnoses found in the DSM-IV. Many diagnoses have notations that increase specificity. Those notations are not always included here. The following clarifications are made to assist you in understanding this material.

NOS = Not Otherwise Specified.

An *x* appearing in a diagnostic code indicates that a specific code number is required.

An ellipsis (. . .) is used in the names of certain disorders to indicate that the name of a specific mental disorder or general medical condition should be inserted when recording the name (e.g., 293.0 Delirium Due to Hypothyroidism).

Numbers in parentheses are page numbers in the complete DSM-IV manual.

Disorders Usually First Diagnosed in Infancy, Childhood, or Adolescence (37)

Mental retardation (39)
Note: *These are coded on Axis II.*
317   Mild Mental Retardation (41)

318.0	Moderate Mental Retardation (41)
318.1	Severe Mental Retardation (41)
318.2	Profound Mental Retardation (41)
319	Mental Retardation, Unspecified (42)

Learning disorders (46)
315.00	Reading Disorder (48)
315.1	Mathematics Disorder (50)
315.2	Disorder of Written Expression (51)
315.9	Learning Disorder NOS (53)

Motor skills disorder
315.4	Developmental Coordination Disorder (53)

Communication disorders (55)
315.31	Expressive Language Disorder (55)
315.31	Mixed Receptive-Expressive Language Disorder (58)
315.39	Phonological Disorder (61)
307.0	Stuttering (63)
307.9	Communication Disorder NOS (65)

Pervasive developmental disorders (65)
299.00	Autistic Disorder (66)
299.80	Rett's Disorder (71)

---

*Reprinted with permission from the American Psychiatric Association: *Diagnostic and statistical manual of mental disorders,* ed. 4, Washington, DC, 1994, The Association.

299.10   Childhood Disintegrative Disorder (73)
299.80   Asperger's Disorder (75)
299.80   Pervasive Developmental Disorder NOS (77)

Attention-deficit and disruptive behavior disorders (78)

314.xx   Attention-Deficit/Hyperactivity Disorder (78)
  .01   Combined Type
  .00   Predominantly Inattentive Type
  .01   Predominantly Hyperactive-Impulsive Type
314.9   Attention-Deficit/Hyperactivity Disorder NOS (85)
312.8   Conduct Disorder (85)
313.81   Oppositional Defiant Disorder (91)
312.9   Disruptive Behavior Disorder NOS (94)

Feeding and eating disorders of infancy or early childhood (94)

307.52   Pica (95)
307.53   Rumination Disorder (96)
307.59   Feeding Disorder of Infancy or Early Childhood (98)

Tic disorders (100)

307.23   Tourette's Disorder (101)
307.22   Chronic Motor or Vocal Tic Disorder (103)
307.21   Transient Tic Disorder (104)
307.20   Tic Disorder NOS (105)

Elimination disorders (106)

___._   Encopresis (106)
787.6   With Constipation and Overflow Incontinence
307.7   Without Constipation and Overflow Incontinence
307.6   Enuresis (Not Due to a General Medical Condition) (108)

Other disorders of infancy, childhood, or adolescence

309.21   Separation Anxiety Disorder (110)
313.23   Selective Mutism (114)
313.89   Reactive Attachment Disorder of Infancy or Early Childhood (116)
307.3   Stereotypic Movement Disorder (118)
313.9   Disorder of Infancy, Childhood, or Adolescence NOS (121)

Delirium, Dementia, and Amnestic and Other Cognitive Disorders (123)

Delirium (124)

293.0   Delirium Due to . . . (127)
___._   Substance Intoxication Delirium (129)
___._   Substance Withdrawal Delirium (129)
___._   Delirium Due to Multiple Etiologies (132)
780.09   Delirium NOS (133)

Dementia (133)

290.xx   Dementia of the Alzheimer's Type, With Early Onset *(also code 331.0 Alzheimer's disease on Axis III)* (139)
  .10   Uncomplicated
  .11   With Delirium
  .12   With Delusions
  .13   With Depressed Mood
290.xx   Dementia of the Alzheimer's Type, With Late Onset *(also code 331.0 Alzheimer's disease on Axis III)* (139)
  .0   Uncomplicated
  .3   With Delirium
  .20   With Delusions
  .21   With Depressed Mood
290.xx   Vascular Dementia (143)
  .40   Uncomplicated
  .41   With Delirium
  .42   With Delusions
  .43   With Depressed Mood
294.9   Dementia Due to HIV Disease (148)
294.1   Dementia Due to Head Trauma (148)
294.1   Dementia Due to Parkinson's Disease (148)
294.1   Dementia Due to Huntington's Disease (149)
290.10   Dementia Due to Pick's Disease (149)
290.10   Dementia Due to Creutzfeldt-Jakob Disease (150)
294.1   Dementia Due to . . . (151)
___._   Substance-Induced Persisting Dementia (152)
___._   Dementia Due to Multiple Etiologies (154)
294.8   Dementia NOS (155)

Amnestic disorders (156)

294.0   Amnestic Disorder Due to . . . (158)
___._   Substance-Induced Persisting Amnestic Disorder (161)
294.8   Amnestic Disorder NOS (163)

Other Cognitive Disorders (163)

294.9   Cognitive Disorder NOS (163)

Mental Disorders Due to a General Medical Condition not Elsewhere Classified (165)

293.89   Catatonic Disorder Due to . . . (169)
310.1   Personality Change Due to . . . (171)
293.9   Mental Disorder NOS Due to . . . (174)

Substance-Related Disorders (175)

[a]*The following specifiers may be applied to Substance Dependence:*
  With Physiological Dependence/Without Physiological Dependence
  Early Full Remission/Early Partial Remission
  Sustained Full Remission/Sustained Partial Remission
  On Agonist Therapy/In a Controlled Environment

The following specifiers apply to Substance-Induced Disorders as noted:
  [I]With Onset During Intoxication/[W]With Onset During Withdrawal

Alcohol-related disorders (194)

Alcohol Use Disorders

303.90   Alcohol Dependence[a] (195)
305.00   Alcohol Abuse (196)

Alcohol-Induced Disorders

303.00   Alcohol Intoxication (196)
291.8   Alcohol Withdrawal (197)
291.0   Alcohol Intoxication Delirium (129)
291.0   Alcohol Withdrawal Delirium (129)
291.2   Alcohol-Induced Persisting Dementia (152)
291.1   Alcohol-Induced Persisting Amnestic Dementia (152)
291.x   Alcohol-Induced Psychotic Disorder (310)
  .5   With Delusions[I,W]
  .3   With Hallucinations[I,W]
291.8   Alcohol-Induced Mood Disorder[I,W] (370)
291.8   Alcohol-Induced Anxiety Disorder[I,W] (439)
291.8   Alcohol-Induced Sexual Dysfunction[I] (519)
291.8   Alcohol-Induced Sleep Disorder[I,W] (601)
291.9   Alcohol-Related Disorder NOS (204)

Amphetamine (or amphetamine-like)-related disorders (204)

Amphetamine Use Disorders

304.40   Amphetamine Dependence[a] (206)
305.70   Amphetamine Abuse (206)

Amphetamine-Induced Disorders

292.89   Amphetamine Intoxication (207)
292.0   Amphetamine Withdrawal (208)
292.81   Amphetamine Intoxication Delirium (129)
292.xx   Amphetamine-Induced Psychotic Disorder (310)
  .11   With Delusions[I]
  .12   With Hallucinations[I]
292.84   Amphetamine-Induced Mood Disorder[I,W] (370)
292.89   Amphetamine-Induced Anxiety Disorder[I] (439)
292.89   Amphetamine-Induced Sexual Dysfunction[I] (519)
292.89   Amphetamine-Induced Sleep Disorder[I,W] (601)
292.9   Amphetamine-Related Disorder NOS (211)

Caffeine-related disorders (212)

Caffeine-Induced Disorders

305.90   Caffeine Intoxication (212)
292.89   Caffeine-Induced Anxiety Disorder[I] (439)
292.89   Caffeine-Induced Sleep Disorder[I] (601)
292.9   Caffeine-Related Disorder NOS (215)

Cannabis-related disorders (215)

Cannabis Use Disorders

304.30   Cannabis Dependence[a] (216)
305.20   Cannabis Abuse (217)

Cannabis-Induced Disorders

292.89   Cannabis Intoxication (217)
292.81   Cannabis Intoxication Delirium (129)
292.xx   Cannabis-Induced Psychotic Disorder (310)
  .11   With Delusions[I]
  .12   With Hallucinations[I]
292.89   Cannabis-Induced Anxiety Disorder[I] (439)
292.9   Cannabis-Related Disorder NOS (221)

Cocaine-related disorders (221)

Cocaine Use Disorders

304.20   Cocaine Dependence[a] (222)
305.60   Cocaine Abuse (223)

Cocaine-Induced Disorders

292.89   Cocaine Intoxication (223)
292.0   Cocaine Withdrawal (225)
292.81   Cocaine Intoxication Delirium (129)
292.xx   Cocaine-Induced Psychotic Disorder (310)
   .11   With Delusions[I]
   .12   With Hallucinations[I]
292.84   Cocaine-Induced Mood Disorder[I,W] (370)
292.89   Cocaine-Induced Anxiety Disorder[I,W] (439)
292.89   Cocaine-Induced Sexual Dysfunction[I] (519)
292.89   Cocaine-Induced Sleep Disorder[I,W] (601)
292.9   Cocaine-Related Disorder NOS (229)

Hallucinogen-related disorders (229)

Hallucinogen Use Disorders

304.50   Hallucinogen Dependence[a] (230)
305.30   Hallucinogen Abuse (231)

Hallucinogen-Induced Disorders

292.89   Hallucinogen Intoxication (232)
292.89   Hallucinogen Persisting Perception Disorder (Flashbacks) (233)
292.81   Hallucinogen Intoxication Delirium (129)
292.xx   Hallucinogen-Induced Psychotic Disorder (310)
   .11   With Delusions[I]
   .12   With Hallucinations[I]
292.84   Hallucinogen-Induced Mood Disorder[I] (370)
292.89   Hallucinogen-Induced Anxiety Disorder[I] (439)
292.9   Hallucinogen-Related Disorder NOS (236)

Inhalant-related disorders (236)

Inhalant Use Disorders

304.60   Inhalant Dependence[a] (238)
305.90   Inhalant Abuse (238)

Inhalant-Induced Disorders

292.89   Inhalant Intoxication (239)
292.81   Inhalant Intoxication Delirium (129)
292.82   Inhalant-Induced Persisting Dementia (152)
292.xx   Inhalant-Induced Psychotic Disorder (310)
   .11   With Delusions[I]
   .12   With Hallucinations[I]
292.84   Inhalant-Induced Mood Disorder[I] (370)

292.89   Inhalant-Induced Anxiety Disorder[I] (439)
292.9   Inhalant-Related Disorder NOS (242)

Nicotine-induced disorder (242)

Nicotine Use Disorder

305.10   Nicotine Dependence[a] (243)

Nicotine-Induced Disorder

292.0   Nicotine Withdrawal (244)
292.9   Nicotine-Related Disorder NOS (247)

Opioid-related disorders (247)

Opioid Use Disorders

304.00   Opioid Dependence[a] (248)
305.50   Opioid Abuse (249)

Opioid-Induced Disorders

292.89   Opioid Intoxication (249)
292.0   Opioid Withdrawal (250)
292.81   Opioid Intoxication Delirium (129)
292.xx   Opioid-Induced Psychotic Disorder (310)
   .11   With Delusions[I]
   .12   With Hallucinations[I]
292.84   Opioid-Induced Mood Disorder[I] (370)
292.89   Opioid-Induced Sexual Dysfunction[I] (519)
292.89   Opioid-Induced Sleep Disorder[I,W] (601)
292.9   Opioid-Related Disorder NOS (255)

Phencyclidine (or phencyclidine-like)-related disorders (255)

Phencyclidine Use Disorders

304.90   Phencyclidine Dependence[a] (256)
305.90   Phencyclidine Abuse (257)

Phencyclidine-Induced Disorders

292.89   Phencyclidine Intoxication (257)
292.81   Phencyclidine Intoxication Delirium (129)
292.xx   Phencyclidine-Induced Psychotic Disorder (310)
   .11   With Delusions[I]
   .12   With Hallucinations[I]
292.84   Phencyclidine-Induced Mood Disorder[I] (370)
292.89   Phencyclidine-Induced Anxiety Disorder[I] (439)
292.9   Phencyclidine-Related Disorder NOS (261)

Sedative-, hypnotic-, or anxiolytic-related disorders (261)

Sedative, Hypnotic, or Anxiolytic Use Disorders

304.10   Sedative, Hypnotic, or Anxiolytic Dependence[a] (262)

305.40   Sedative, Hypnotic, or Anxiolytic Abuse (263)

Sedative-, Hypnotic-, or Anxiolytic-Induced Disorders

292.89   Sedative, Hypnotic, or Anxiolytic Intoxication (263)

292.0   Sedative, Hypnotic, or Anxiolytic Withdrawal (264)

292.81   Sedative, Hypnotic, or Anxiolytic Intoxication Delirium (129)

292.81   Sedative, Hypnotic, or Anxiolytic Withdrawal Delirium (129)

292.82   Sedative-, Hypnotic-, or Anxiolytic-Induced Persisting Dementia (152)

292.83   Sedative-, Hypnotic-, or Anxiolytic-Induced Persisting Amnestic Disorder (161)

292.xx   Sedative-, Hypnotic-, or Anxiolytic-Induced Psychotic Disorder (310)

   .11   With Delusions[I,W]
   .12   With Hallucinations[I,W]

292.84   Sedative-, Hypnotic-, or Anxiolytic-Induced Mood Disorder[I,W] (370)

292.89   Sedative-, Hypnotic-, or Anxiolytic-Induced Anxiety Disorder[W] (439)

292.89   Sedative-, Hypnotic-, or Anxiolytic-Induced Sexual Dysfunction[I] (519)

292.89   Sedative-, Hypnotic-, or Anxiolytic-Induced Sleep Disorder[I,W] (601)

292.9   Sedative-, Hypnotic-, or Anxiolytic-Related Disorder NOS (269)

Polysubstance-related disorder

304.80   Polysubstance Dependence[a] (270)

Other (or unknown) substance-related disorders (270)

Other (or Unknown) Substance Use Disorders

304.90   Other (or Unknown) Substance Dependence[a] (176)

305.90   Other (or Unknown) Substance Abuse (182)

Other (or Unknown) Substance-Induced Disorders

292.89   Other (or Unknown) Substance Intoxication (183)

292.0   Other (or Unknown) Substance Withdrawal (184)

292.81   Other (or Unknown) Substance-Induced Delirium (129)

292.82   Other (or Unknown) Substance-Induced Persisting Dementia (152)

292.83   Other (or Unknown) Substance-Induced Persisting Amnestic Disorder (161)

292.xx   Other (or Unknown) Substance-Induced Psychotic Disorder (310)

   .11   With Delusions[I,W]
   .12   With Hallucinations[I,W]

292.84   Other (or Unknown) Substance-Induced Mood Disorder[I,W] (370)

292.89   Other (or Unknown) Substance-Induced Anxiety Disorder[I,W] (439)

292.89   Other (or Unknown) Substance-Induced Sexual Dysfunction[I] (519)

292.89   Other (or Unknown) Substance-Induced Sleep Disorder[I,W] (601)

292.9   Other (or Unknown) Substance-Related Disorder NOS (272)

Schizophrenia and Other Psychotic Disorders (273)

295.xx   Schizophrenia (274)
   .30   Paranoid Type (287)
   .10   Disorganized Type (287)
   .20   Catatonic Type (288)
   .90   Undifferentiated Type (289)
   .60   Residual Type (289)

295.40   Schizophreniform Disorder (290)

295.70   Schizoaffective Disorder (292)

297.1   Delusional Disorder (296)

298.8   Brief Psychotic Disorder (302)

297.3   Shared Psychotic Disorder (305)

293.xx   Psychotic Disorder Due to . . .
   .81   With Delusions
   .82   With Hallucinations
___.__   Substance-Induced Psychotic Disorder (310)

298.9   Psychotic Disorder NOS (315)

Mood Disorders (317)

Code current state of Major Depressive Disorder or Bipolar I Disorder in fifth digit:
   1 = Mild
   2 = Moderate
   3 = Severe Without Psychotic Features

4 = Severe With Psychotic Features
   Specify: Mood-Congruent Psychotic
   Features/Mood-Incongruent Psychotic
   Features
5 = In Partial Remission
6 = In Full Remission
0 = Unspecified

The following specifiers apply (for current or most recent episode) to Mood Disorders as noted:
   [a]Severity/Psychotic/Remission
   Specifiers/[b]Chronic/[c]With Catatonic Features/
   [d]With Melancholic Features/[e]With Atypical
   Features/[f]With Postpartum Onset

The following specifiers apply to Mood Disorders as noted:
   [g]With or Without Full Interepisode Recovery/
   [h]With Seasonal Pattern/[i]With Rapid Cycling

Depressive disorders

296.xx   Major Depressive Disorder, (339)
   .2x   Single Episode[a,b,c,d,e,f]
   .3x   Recurrent[a,b,c,d,e,f,g,h]
300.4   Dysthymic Disorder (345)
311   Depressive Disorder NOS (350)

Bipolar disorders

296.xx   Bipolar I Disorder, (350)
   .0x   Single Manic Episode[a,c,f]
   .40   Most Recent Episode Hypomanic[g,h,i]
   .4x   Most Recent Episode Manic[a,c,f,g,h,i]
   .6x   Most Recent Episode Mixed[a,c,f,g,h,i]
   .5x   Most Recent Episode Depressed[a,b,c,d,e,f,g,h,i]
   .7   Most Recent Episode Unspecified[g,h,i]
296.89   Bipolar II Disorder[a,b,c,d,e,f,g,h,i] (359)
301.13   Cyclothymic Disorder (363)
296.80   Bipolar Disorder NOS (366)
293.83   Mood Disorder Due to . . . (366)
___.___   Substance-Induced Mood Disorder (370)
296.90   Mood Disorder NOS (375)

Anxiety Disorders (393)

300.01   Panic Disorder Without Agoraphobia (397)
300.21   Panic Disorder With Agoraphobia (397)
300.22   Agoraphobia Without History of Panic Disorder (403)
300.29   Specific Phobia (405)
300.23   Social Phobia (411)
300.3   Obsessive-Compulsive Disorder (417)
309.81   Posttraumatic Stress Disorder (424)
308.3   Acute Stress Disorder (429)
300.02   Generalized Anxiety Disorder (432)

293.89   Anxiety Disorder Due to . . . (436)
___.___   Substance-Induced Anxiety Disorder (439)
300.00   Anxiety Disorder NOS (444)

Somatoform Disorders (445)

300.81   Somatization Disorder (446)
300.81   Undifferentiated Somatoform Disorder (450)
300.11   Conversion Disorder (452)
307.xx   Pain Disorder (458)
   .80   Associated With Psychological Factors
   .89   Associated With Both Psychological Factors and a General Medical Condition
300.7   Hypochondriasis (462)
300.7   Body Dysmorphic Disorder (466)
300.81   Somatoform Disorder NOS (468)

Factitious Disorders (471)

300.xx   Factitious Disorder (471)
   .16   With Predominantly Psychological Signs and Symptoms
   .19   With Predominantly Physical Signs and Symptoms
   .19   With Combined Psychological and Physical Signs and Symptoms
300.19   Factitious Disorder NOS (475)

Dissociative Disorders (477)

300.12   Dissociative Amnesia (478)
300.13   Dissociative Fugue (481)
300.14   Dissociative Identity Disorder (484)
300.6   Depersonalization Disorder (488)
300.15   Dissociative Disorder NOS (490)

Sexual and Gender Identity Disorders (493)

Sexual dysfunctions (493)

Sexual Desire Disorders
302.71   Hypoactive Sexual Desire Disorder (496)
302.79   Sexual Aversion Disorder (499)

Sexual Arousal Disorders
302.72   Female Sexual Arousal Disorder (500)
302.72   Male Erectile Disorder (502)

Orgasmic Disorders
302.73   Female Orgasmic Disorder (505)
302.74   Male Orgasmic Disorder (507)
302.75   Premature Ejaculation (509)

Sexual Pain Disorders

302.76 Dyspareunia (Not Due to a General Medical Condition) (511)

306.51 Vaginismus (Not Due to a General Medical Condition) (513)

Sexual dysfunction due to a general medical condition (515)

625.8 Female Hypoactive Sexual Desire Disorder Due to . . . (515)

608.89 Male Hypoactive Sexual Desire Disorder Due to . . . (515)

607.84 Male Erectile Disorder Due to . . . (515)

625.0 Female Dyspareunia Due to . . . (515)

608.89 Male Dyspareunia Due to . . . (515)

625.8 Other Female Sexual Dysfunction Due to . . . (515)

608.89 Other Male Sexual Dysfunction Due to . . . (515)

___.__ Substance-Induced Sexual Dysfunction (519)

302.70 Sexual Dysfunction NOS (522)

Paraphilias (522)

302.4 Exhibitionism (525)

302.81 Fetishism (526)

302.89 Frotteurism (527)

302.2 Pedophilia (527)

302.83 Sexual Masochism (529)

302.84 Sexual Sadism (530)

302.3 Transvestic Fetishism (530)

302.82 Voyeurism (532)

302.9 Paraphilia NOS (532)

Gender identity disorders (532)

302.xx Gender Identity Disorder (532)

.6 in Children

.85 in Adolescents or Adults

302.6 Gender Identity Disorder NOS (538)

302.9 Sexual Disorder NOS (538)

Eating Disorders (539)

307.1 Anorexia Nervosa (539)

307.51 Bulimia Nervosa (545)

307.50 Eating Disorder NOS (550)

Sleep Disorders (551)

Primary sleep disorders (553)

Dyssomnias (553)

307.42 Primary Insomnia (553)

307.44 Primary Hypersomnia (557)

347 Narcolepsy (562)

780.59 Breathing-Related Sleep Disorder (567)

307.45 Circadian Rhythm Sleep Disorder (573)

307.47 Dyssomnia NOS (579)

Parasomnias (579)

307.47 Nightmare Disorder (580)

307.46 Sleep Terror Disorder (583)

307.46 Sleepwalking Disorder (587)

307.47 Parasomnia NOS (592)

Sleep disorders related to another mental disorder (592)

307.42 Insomnia Related to . . . (592)

307.44 Hypersomnia Related to . . . (592)

Other sleep disorders

780.xx Sleep Disorder Due to . . . (597)

.52 Insomnia Type

.54 Hypersomnia Type

.59 Parasomnia Type

.59 Mixed Type

___.__ Substance-Induced Sleep Disorder (601)

Impulse-Control Disorders Not Elsewhere Classified (609)

312.34 Intermittent Explosive Disorder (609)

312.32 Kleptomania (612)

312.33 Pyromania (614)

312.31 Pathological Gambling (615)

312.39 Trichotillomania (618)

312.30 Impulse-Control Disorder NOS (621)

Adjustment Disorders (623)

309.xx Adjustment Disorder (623)

.0 With Depressed Mood

.24 With Anxiety

.28 With Mixed Anxiety and Depressed Mood

.3 With Disturbance of Conduct

.4 With Mixed Disturbance of Emotions and Conduct

.9 Unspecified

Personality Disorders (629)

Note: These are coded on Axis II.

301.0	Paranoid Personality Disorder (634)
301.20	Schizoid Personality Disorder (638)
301.22	Schizotypal Personality Disorder (641)
301.7	Antisocial Personality Disorder (645)
301.83	Borderline Personality Disorder (650)
301.50	Histrionic Personality Disorder (655)
301.81	Narcissistic Personality Disorder (658)
301.82	Avoidant Personality Disorder (662)
301.6	Dependent Personality Disorder (665)
301.4	Obsessive-Compulsive Personality Disorder (669)
301.9	Personality Disorder NOS (673)

Other Conditions That May Be a Focus of Clinical Attention (675)

Psychological factors affecting medical condition (675)

316   . . . *[Specified Psychological Factor]* Affecting . . . *[Indicate the General Medical Condition] (675)*

Choose name based on nature of factors:

Mental Disorder Affecting Medical Condition

Psychological Symptoms Affecting Medical Condition

Personality Traits or Coping Style Affecting Medical Condition

Maladaptive Health Behaviors Affecting Medical Condition

Stress-Related Physiological Response Affecting Medical Condition

Other or Unspecified Psychological Factors Affecting Medical Condition

Medication-induced movement disorders (678)

332.1	Neuroleptic-Induced Parkinsonism (679)
333.92	Neuroleptic-Malignant Syndrome (679)
333.7	Neuroleptic-Induced Acute Dystonia (679)
333.99	Neuroleptic-Induced Acute Akathisia (679)
333.82	Neuroleptic-Induced Tardive Dyskinesia (679)
333.1	Medication-Induced Postural Tremor (680)
333.90	Medication-Induced Movement Disorder NOS (680)

Other medication-induced disorder

995.2   Adverse Effects of Medication NOS (680)

Relational problems (680)

V61.9	Relational Problem Related to a Mental Disorder or General Medical Condition (681)
V61.20	Parent-Child Relational Problem (681)
V61.1	Partner Relational Problem (681)
V61.8	Sibling Relational Problem (681)
V62.81	Relational Problem NOS (681)

Problems related to abuse or neglect (682)

V61.21	Physical Abuse of Child (682)
V61.21	Sexual Abuse of Child (682)
V61.21	Neglect of Child (682)
V61.1	Physical Abuse of Adult (682)
V61.1	Sexual Abuse of Adult (682)

Additional conditions that may be a focus of clinical attention (683)

V15.81	Noncompliance with Treatment (683)
V65.2	Malingering (683)
V71.01	Adult Antisocial Behavior (683)
V71.02	Child or Adolescent Antisocial Behavior (684)
V62.89	Borderline Intellectual Functioning (684) *Note: This is coded on Axis II.*
780.9	Age-Related Cognitive Decline (684)
V62.82	Bereavement (684)
V62.3	Academic Problem (685)
V62.2	Occupational Problem (685)
313.82	Identity Problem (685)
V62.89	Religious or Spiritual Problem (685)
V62.4	Acculturation Problem (685)
V62.89	Phase of Life Problem (685)

Additional Codes

300.9	Unspecified Mental Disorder (nonpsychotic) (687)
V71.09	No Diagnosis or Condition Deferred on Axis I (687)
799.9	Diagnosis or Condition Deferred on Axis I (687)
V71.09	No Diagnosis on Axis II (687)
799.9	Diagnosis Deferred on Axis II (687)

Multiaxial System

Axis I   Clinical Disorders
          Other Conditions That May Be a Focus of
              Clinical Attention
Axis II   Personality Disorders
          Mental Retardation

Axis III General Medical Conditions
Axis IV   Psychosocial and Environmental Problems
Axis V   Global Assessment of Functioning

American Nurses Association Standards of Psychiatric Mental Health Clinical Nursing Practice*

Standard I. Assessment

The psychiatric mental health nurse collects client health data.

Standard II. Diagnosis

The psychiatric mental health nurse analyzes the assessment data in determining diagnoses.

Standard III. Outcome Identification

The psychiatric mental health nurse identifies expected outcomes individualized to the client.

Standard IV. Planning

The psychiatric mental health nurse develops a plan of care that prescribes interventions to attain expected outcomes.

Standard V. Implementation

The psychiatric mental health nurse implements the interventions identified in the plan of care.

Standard Va. Counseling

The psychiatric mental health nurse uses counseling interventions to assist clients in improving or regaining their previous coping abilities, fostering mental health, and preventing mental illness and disability.

*Reprinted with permission from: *A statement on psychiatric mental health clinical nursing practice and standards of psychiatric mental health clinical nursing practice*, Washington, DC, 1994, American Nurses Association.

Standard Vb. Milieu Therapy

The psychiatric mental health nurse provides, structures, and maintains a therapeutic environment in collaboration with the client and other health care providers.

Standard Vc. Self-Care Activities

The psychiatric mental health nurse structures interventions around the client's activities of daily living to foster self-care and mental and physical well-being.

Standard Vd. Psychobiological Interventions

The psychiatric mental health nurse uses knowledge of psychobiological interventions and applies clinical skills to restore the client's health and prevent further disability.

Standard Ve. Health Teaching

The psychiatric mental health nurse, through health teaching, assists clients in achieving satisfying, productive, and healthy patterns of living.

Standard Vf. Case Management

The psychiatric mental health nurse provides case management to coordinate comprehensive health services and ensure continuity of care.

Standard Vg. Health Promotion and Health Maintenance

The psychiatric mental health nurse employs strategies and interventions to promote and maintain mental health and prevent mental illness.

ADVANCED PRACTICE INTERVENTIONS VH-VJ

The following interventions (Vh-Vj) may be performed only by the certified specialist in psychiatric mental health nursing.

Standard Vh. Psychotherapy

The certified specialist in psychiatric mental health nursing uses individual, group, and family psychotherapy, child psychotherapy, and other therapeutic treatments to assist clients in fostering mental health, preventing mental illness and disability, and improving or regaining previous health status and functional abilities.

Standard Vi. Prescription of Pharmacologic Agents

The certified specialist uses prescription of pharmacologic agents in accordance with the state nursing practice act to treat symptoms of psychiatric illness and improve functional health status.

Standard Vj. Consultation

The certified specialist provides consultation to health care providers and others to influence the plans of care for clients, and to enhance the abilities of others to provide psychiatric and mental health care and effect change in systems.

Standard Vk. Evaluation

The psychiatric mental health nurse evaluates the client's progress in attaining expected outcomes.

APPENDIX C

American Nurses Association Psychopharmacology Guidelines for Psychiatric Mental Health Nurses*

Note to the student: In 1994 the American Nurses Association published a document entitled Psychiatric Mental Health Nursing Psychopharmacology Project. *The publication was the product of 12 psychiatric nurses, recognized for their expertise and interest in psychopharmacology, working together over a 2-year period. In addition to these 12, a larger group of nurse consultants added their expertise to this project. A summary of the neuroscience and psychopharmacology sections is presented below. The student is encouraged to study the entire document (which is relatively brief and very easy to read) for a complete review of these topics and the sections not summarized here (e.g., clinical management).*

This document describes the knowledge base psychiatric mental health nurses need in relation to one aspect of practice—psychopharmacology. It is intended only to inform and guide psychiatric mental health nursing education, practice, and research in this area. Thus, this document should not be considered part of any state's nurse practice act, or viewed as a requirement for licensure, or construed as a legal standard by which to judge psychiatric nursing practice.

These guidelines will be evaluated and updated regularly. Psychiatric mental health nurses will demonstrate expanding expertise in psychopharmacology based on the state of the science, education, experience, practice setting, patient needs, and professional goals.

*Reprinted with permission from *Psychiatric mental health nursing psychopharmacology project,* Washington, DC, 1994, American Nurses Association.

I. Neurosciences

Commensurate with level of practice, the psychiatric mental health nurse integrates current knowledge from the neurosciences to understand etiological models, diagnostic issues, and treatment strategies for psychiatric illness.

Objectives

The psychiatric mental health nurse can:

- describe basic central nervous system structures and functions implicated in mental illness, such as the cerebrum, diencephalon, brain stem, basal ganglia, limbic system, and extrapyramidal motor system.
- describe basic mechanisms of neurotransmission at the synapse, such as neurochemical metabolism, role(s) of the pre- and post-synaptic membranes, reuptake, receptor binding, and auto-regulation.
- describe the general functions of the major neurochemicals implicated in mental illness, such as serotonin, norepinephrine, dopamine, acetylcholine, GABA, and the peptides.
- describe the basic structure and function of the endocrine system, particularly as it is affected by the various hypothalamic-pituitary endocrine axes.
- identify the neurotransmitter system implicated in side-effect profiles of psychopharmacologic agents, such as blockade of cholinergic receptors (blurred vision, dry mouth, memory dysfunction), histaminic receptors (sedation, weight gain, hypotension), and adrenergic receptors (dizziness, postural hypotension, tachycardia).
- discuss the relevance of current biological hypotheses underlying major mental illnesses and the use of psychopharmacologic agents.
- demonstrate a familiarity with the increased lifetime risk of mental illness—for people who have a mentally ill first-degree (biological) relative—compared to the general population, based on genetic, epidemiologic, family, adoption, and twin research.
- describe normal sleep stages and identify circadian rhythm disturbances, such as decreased REM latency and phase shift disturbances as evidenced in psychiatric disorders.
- demonstrate familiarity with recent research findings from neuro-imaging techniques such as CT (computerized tomography), MRI (magnetic resonance imaging), PET (positron-emission tomography), and SPECT (single photon emission computerized tomography) as well as the psychiatric uses of these techniques.
- discuss the purposes and limitations of current biological tests used in the diagnosis and monitoring of mental illness.

II. Psychopharmacology

The psychiatric mental health nurse involved in the care of patients who have been prescribed psychopharmacologic agents demonstrates knowledge of psychopharmacologic principles—including pharmacokinetics, pharmacodynamics, drug classification, intended and unintended effects, and related nursing implications.

Objectives

The psychiatric mental health nurse can:

- describe psychopharmacologic agents based on the similarities and differences among drugs of the same and different classes.
- discuss the actions of psychopharmacologic agents that range from global human behavioral responses to those at a cellular level, such as the actions of lithium from mood stabilization to glomerular effects.
- differentiate the psychiatric symptoms targeted for psychopharmacologic intervention from medication side effects and toxicities, and the appropriate interventions to minimize each.
- apply basic principles of pharmacokinetics and pharmacodynamics, such as half-life, steady state, absorption, and metabolism, in general and as they relate to age, gender, race/ethnicity, and organ system function.
- identify the appropriate use of psychotherapeutic agents related to the psychiatric needs of special populations.
- involve patients and their families and significant others in the design and implementation of the medication treatment plan, taking into account patient readiness, knowledge, environment, beliefs and preferences, and lifestyle.
- identify factors that may prevent the active collaboration of patients with medication regimens, and strategies to minimize these risks.
- describe nonpsychopharmacologic interventions for target symptoms that are not responsive to psychopharmacologic interventions, psychiatric symptoms unlikely to respond to drug treatments, and drug side effects that are not treated with drugs.

- discuss the use of standardized rating scales for measuring symptom severity and clinical response to psychopharmacologic treatment, such as changes in target symptoms of illness and medication side effects.

- demonstrate the knowledge necessary to develop psychopharmacologic education and treatment plans based on current neurobiological concepts and the patient's lifestyle and recovery environment.

APPENDIX D

The Mini-Mental State Examination

		Score	Points
Orientation			
1. What is the	Year?		1
	Season?		1
	Date?		1
	Day?		1
	Month?		1
2. Where are we?	State?		1
	County?		1
	Town or city?		1
	Hospital?		1
	Floor?		1

Registration

3. Name three objects, taking one second to say each. Then ask the patient all three after you have said them. Give one point for each correct answer. Repeat the answers until the patient learns all three.   3

Attention and Calculation

4. Serial sevens.* Give one point for each correct answer. Stop after five answers. ***Alternative:*** Spell WORLD backwards.   5

Recall

5. Ask for names of three objects learned in Question 3. Give one point for each correct answer.   3

Language

6. Point to a pencil and a watch. Have the patient name them as you point.   2
7. Have the patient repeat "No ifs, ands, or buts."   1

Continued

*Serial seven: subtracting 7 from 100, i.e., $100 - 7 = 93$; $93 - 7 = 86$; $86 - 7 = 79$; $79 - 7 = 72$; $72 - 7 = 65$; and so on. From Folstein MF, Folstein SE, and McHugh PR: Mini-mental state: a practical method of grading the cognitive state of patients for the clinician. *J Psychiatr Res* 12:189, 1975. By permission.

	Score	**Points**

Language—cont'd

8. Have the patient follow a three-stage command: "Take the paper in your right hand. Fold the paper in half. Put the paper on the floor."   3
9. Have the patient read and obey the following: "CLOSE YOUR EYES." (Write it in large letters.)   1
10. Have the patient write a sentence of his or her own choice. (The sentence should contain a subject and an object and should make sense. Ignore spelling errors when scoring.)   1
11. Enlarge the design printed below to 1 to 5 cm per side and have the patient copy it. (Give one point if all sides and angles are preserved and if the intersecting sides from a quadrangle.)   1

_____ = Total 30

A score of 23 or less suggests cognitive impairment in a person with an eighth grade education or better.

The Geriatric Depression Scale

Choose the best answer for how you felt over the past week.

1. Are you basically satisfied with your life?	Yes/No
2. Have you dropped many of your activities and interests?	Yes/No
3. Do you feel that your life is empty?	Yes/No
4. Do you often get bored?	Yes/No
5. Are you hopeful about the future?	Yes/No
6. Are you bothered by thoughts you can't get out of your head?	Yes/No
7. Are you in good spirits most of the time?	Yes/No
8. Are you afraid that something bad is going to happen to you?	Yes/No
9. Do you feel happy most of the time?	Yes/No
10. Do you often feel helpless?	Yes/No
11. Do you often get restless and fidgety?	Yes/No
12. Do you prefer to stay at home, rather than going out and doing new things?	Yes/No
13. Do you frequently worry about the future?	Yes/No
14. Do you feel you have more problems with memory than most?	Yes/No
15. Do you think it is wonderful to be alive right now?	Yes/No
16. Do you often feel downhearted and blue?	Yes/No
17. Do you feel pretty worthless the way you are now?	Yes/No
18. Do you worry a lot about the past?	Yes/No
19. Do you find life very exciting?	Yes/No
20. Is it hard for you to get started on new projects?	Yes/No
21. Do you feel full of energy?	Yes/No
22. Do you feel that your situation is hopeless?	Yes/No
23. Do you think that more people are better off than you are?	Yes/No
24. Do you frequently get upset over little things?	Yes/No
25. Do you frequently feel like crying?	Yes/No
26. Do you have trouble concentrating?	Yes/No
27. Do you enjoy getting up in the morning?	Yes/No
28. Do you prefer to avoid social gatherings?	Yes/No
29. Is it easy for you to make decisions?	Yes/No
30. Is your mind as clear as it used to be?	Yes/No

A score of 14 points or more suggests the presence of depression, which needs to be confirmed by clinical evaluation.

From Yesavage JA, et al: Development and validation of a geriatric depression screening scale: a preliminary report, *J Psychiatr Res* 17:37, 1983. By permission. Count one point for a "yes" answer to questions 2, 3, 4, 6, 8, 10, 11, 12, 13, 14, 16, 17, 18, 20, 23, 24, 25, 26, 28 and one point for "no" answer to questions 1, 5, 7, 9, 15, 19, 21, 27, 29, 30.

APPENDIX F

A Simple Method to Determine Tardive Dyskinesia Symptoms: AIMS* Examination Procedure

PATIENT IDENTIFICATION   **DATE**

RATED BY

Either before or after completing the examination procedure, observe the patient unobtrusively at rest (e.g., in waiting room).

The chair to be used in this examination should be a hard, firm one without arms.

After observing the patient, he may be rated on a scale of 0 (none), 1 (minimal), 2 (mild), 3 (moderate) and 4 (severe) according to the severity of symptoms.

Ask the patient whether there is anything in his/her mouth (i.e., gum, candy, etc.) and if there is to remove it.

Ask patient about the *current* condition of his/her teeth. Ask patient if he/she wears dentures. Do teeth or dentures bother patient *now?*

Ask patient whether he/she notices any movement in mouth, face, hands or feet. If yes, ask to describe and to what extent they *currently* bother patient or interfere with his/her activities.

0	1	2	3	4

Have patient sit in chair with hands on knees, legs, slightly apart and feet flat on floor. (Look at entire body for movements while in this position.)

*Abnormal Involuntary Movement Scale
From Sandoz Pharmaceuticals, East Hanover, NJ 07936.

697

0	1	2	3	4

Ask patient to sit with hands hanging unsupported. If male, between legs, if female and wearing a dress, hanging over knees. (Observe hands and other body areas.)

0	1	2	3	4

Ask patient to open mouth. (Observe tongue at rest within mouth.) Do this twice.

0	1	2	3	4

Ask patient to protrude tongue. (Observe abnormalities of tongue movement.) Do this twice.

0	1	2	3	4

Ask patient to tap thumb, with each finger, as rapidly as possible for 10-15 seconds; separately with right hand, then with left hand. (Observe facial and leg movements.)

0	1	2	3	4

Flex and extend patient's left and right arms. (One at a time.)

0	1	2	3	4

Ask patient to stand up. (Observe in profile. Observe all body areas again, hips included.)

0	1	2	3	4

Ask patient to extend both arms outstretched in front with palms down†. (Observe trunk, legs and mouth.)

0	1	2	3	4

Have the patient walk a few paces, turn and walk back to chair†. (Observe hands and gait.) Do this twice.

---

†Activated movements

APPENDIX G

A Rating Scale for Extrapyramidal Side Effects

1. **Gait**—The patient is examined as he walks into the examining room; his gait, the swing of his arms, and his general posture all form the basis for an overall score for this item. This is rated as follows:

   0–normal

   1–diminution in swing while the patient is walking

   2–marked diminution in swing with obvious rigidity in the arm

   3–stiff gait with arms held rigidly before the abdomen

   4–stooped, shuffling gait with propulsion and retropulsion

2. **Arm Dropping**—The patient and the examiner both raise their arms to shoulder height and let them fall to their sides. In a normal subject a stout slap is heard as the arms hit the sides. In the patient with extreme Parkinson's syndrome the arms fall very slowly:

   0–normal, free fall with loud slap and rebound

   1–fall slowed slightly with less audible contact and little rebound

   2–fall slowed, no rebound

   3–marked slowing, no slap at all

   4–arms fall as though against resistance, as though through glue

3. **Shoulder Shaking**—The subject's arms are bent at a right angle at the elbow and are taken one at a time by the examiner who grasps one hand and also clasps the other around the patient's elbow. The subject's upper arm is pushed to and fro, and humerus is externally rotated. The degree of resistance from normal to extreme rigidity is scored as follows:

   0–normal

   1–slight stiffness and resistance

   2–moderate stiffness and resistance

   3–marked rigidity with difficulty in passive movement

   4–extreme stiffness and rigidity with almost a frozen shoulder

4. **Elbow Rigidity**—The elbow joints are separately bent at right angles and passively extended and flexed, with the subject's biceps observed and simultaneously palpated. The resistance to this procedure is rated. (The presence of cogwheel rigidity is noted separately.) Scoring is from 0-4 as in shoulder shaking test.

5. **Fixation of Position or Wrist Rigidity**—The wrist is held in one hand and the fingers held by the examiner's other hand, with the wrist moved to extension flexion and both ulner and radial deviation. The resistance to this procedure is rated as in Items 3 and 4.

6. *Leg Pendulousness*—The patient sits on a table with his legs hanging down and swinging free. The ankle is grasped by the examiner and raised until the knee is partially extended. It is then allowed to fall. The resistance to falling and the lack of swinging form the basis for the score on this item:

    0–the legs swing freely
    1–slight diminution in the swing of the legs
    2–moderate resistance to swing
    3–marked resistance and damping of swing
    4–complete absence of swing

7. *Head Dropping*—The patient lies on a well-padded examining table, and his head is raised by the examiner's hand. The hand is then withdrawn and the head allowed to drop. In the normal subject the head will fall upon the table. The movement is delayed in extrapyramidal system disorder, and in extreme parkinsonism it is absent. The neck muscles are rigid, and the head does not reach the examining table. Scoring is as follows:

    0–the head falls completely with a good thump as it hits the table
    1–slight slowing in fall, mainly noted by lack of slap as head meets the table
    2–moderate slowing in the fall quite noticeable to the eye
    3–head falls stiffly and slowly
    4–head does not reach examining table

8. *Glabella Tap*—Subject is told to open his eyes wide and not to blink. The glabella region is tapped at a steady, rapid speed. The number of times patient blinks in succession is noted:

    0–0-5 blinks
    1–6-10 blinks
    2–11-15 blinks
    3–16-20 blinks
    4–21 or more blinks

9. *Tremor*—Patient is observed walking into examining room and then is reexamined for this item:

    0–normal
    1–mild finger tremor, obvious to sight and touch
    2–tremor of hand or arm occuring spasmodically
    3–persistent tremor of one or more limbs
    4–whole body tremor

10. *Salivation*—Patient is observed while talking and then asked to open his mouth and elevate his tongue. The following ratings are given:

    0–normal
    1–excess salivation to the extent that pooling takes place if the mouth is open and the tongue is raised
    2–excess salivation is present and might occasionally result in difficulty in speaking
    3–speaking with difficulty because of excess salivation
    4–frank drooling

Mental Health Systems Act Recommended Bill of Rights*

▲   ▲   ▲   ▲   ▲   ▲

1. The right to appropriate treatment in a setting and under conditions most supportive of and least restrictive to personal liberty.
2. The right to an individualized, written treatment plan, periodic review of treatment, and revision of plan.
3. The right to ongoing participation in the planning of services and the right to a reasonable explanation of general mental condition, treatment objective, adverse effects of treatment, reasons for treatment, and available alternatives.
4. The right to receive treatment except in an emergency or as permitted by law.
5. The right not to participate in experimentation.
6. The right to freedom from restraint or seclusion.
7. The right to a humane treatment environment.
8. The right to confidentiality of records.
9. The right of access to records unless provided by third parties or unless access would be detrimental to health.
10. The right of access to telephone use, mail, and visitors.
11. The right to know these rights.
12. The right to assess grievances when rights are infringed.
13. The right to referral when discharged.

---

*Adapted from Mental Health Systems Act, PL 96-398, Section 9501, US Congress, 96th Congress, 1980.

APPENDIX I

Controlled Substance Chart

Drugs	United States	Canada
Heroin, LSD, peyote, marijuana, mescaline	Schedule I	Schedule H
Opioids such as morphine and meperidine, amphetamines, cocaine, short-acting barbiturates (amobarbital, secobarbital), hydromorphone	Schedule II	Schedule G
Glutethimide, paregoric, cerebral stimulants used to treat obesity (benzphetamine, phendimetrazine)	Schedule III	Schedule F
Chloral hydrate, benzodiazepines, cerebral stimulants used to treat obesity (mazindol, fenfluramine), meprobamate, mephobarbital, pemoline, phenobarbital	Schedule IV	Schedule F
Antidiarrheals with opium, antitussives	Schedule V	

Glossary

absence seizure a type of generalized seizure in which there is an abrupt loss of consciousness (usually lasting less than 10 seconds); these seizures are nonconvulsive in nature and may not be noticed by others.

abstinence syndrome physical signs and symptoms that occur when the addictive substance is reduced or withheld; also referred to as withdrawal.

abstract thinking the ability to find meaning in proverbs; the ability to conceptualize.

abuse excessive use of a substance that differs from societal norms and causes clinically significant impairment.

acetylcholine (ACh) a neurotransmitter synthesized by choline acetyltransferase from acetyl coenzyme A and choline. It is found in the peripheral nervous system at the myoneural junction, in autonomic ganglia for parasympathetic or sympathetic systems, and in the parasympathetic postganglionic synapses, including cranial nerves (CNs) III, VII, IX, and X. Acetylcholine is found in the spinal cord, basal ganglia, and numerous sites within the cerebral cortex. Cortical acetylcholine is synthesized primarily in the nucleus basalis of Meynert and in the septal area near the hypothalamus.

acquired immunodeficiency syndrome (AIDS) the term initially used to diagnose those with specific symptoms and opportunistic infections indicating a more advanced progression of human immunodeficiency virus (HIV) infection.

active listening verbal and nonverbal skills used by the examiner to demonstrate interest and concern to the patient.

addiction psychological and physiological symptoms indicating that an individual cannot control his or her use of psychoactive substances; termed substance dependence in the DSM-IV.

affect emotional range attached to ideas; outwardly manifested.

appropriate a. emotional tone in harmony with the accompanying idea, thought, or verbalization.

blunted a. a disturbance manifested by a severe reduction in the intensity of affect.

flat a. absence or near absence of any signs of affective expression.

inappropriate a. incongruence between the emotional feeling tone and the idea, thought, or speech accompanying it.

labile a. rapid changes in emotional feeling tone, unrelated to external stimuli.

affective disorders a group of psychiatric diagnoses characterized by mood disturbances on a continuum of depression to mania; termed mood disorders in the DSM-IV.

aggression forceful verbal or physical action; that is, the motor counterpart of the affect of anger, rage, or hostility.

agitation anxiety associated with severe motor restlessness.

agnosia difficulty in recognizing familiar objects; a symptom of organic brain disease.

agoraphobia the fear of being in a place or situation in which escape might be difficult or embarrassing, or in which help might not be available in case of a panic attack.

agraphia the loss of ability to write.

akathisia motor restlessness generally expressed as the inability to sit still. Caused by the dopamine blockade by certain types of neuroleptic medications. An extrapyramidal side effect (EPSE).

alcoholic an individual whose compulsive use of alcohol causes problems at home, at work, or socially and who continues to use alcohol despite these adverse consequences.

Alcoholics Anonymous (AA) a self-help organization that uses a 12-step program to assist alcoholics to achieve and maintain sobriety; Al-Anon is concerned with spouses of alcoholics; Alateen is concerned with the teenage children of alcoholics.

alertness an awareness and attentiveness to surroundings.

Alzheimer's disease more correctly referred to as dementia of the Alzheimer type (DAT). DAT is the most common type of dementia. The characteristic symptoms are amnesia, aphasia, apraxia, and agnosia. It is a cognitive mental disorder resulting in dementia that is related to a progressive deterioration of brain tissue, described as plaques and neurofibrillary tangles.

ambivalence opposing impulses or feelings directed toward the same person or object at the same time.

amenorrhea the absence of menstruation.

amnesia partial or total inability to recall past information.

 anterograde a. recent memory loss, as in the early stages of Alzheimer's disease.

 global a. total memory loss, as in advanced stages of Alzheimer's disease.

 retrograde a. remote memory loss, as in later stages of Alzheimer's disease.

 short-term a. memory loss observed in alcoholic blackouts.

amygdala a cluster of nuclei in the medial temporal lobe that is concerned with endocrine and behavioral functions and plays a role in food and water intake, drive behavior, and the emotions connected with those behaviors. In animal studies, electrical stimulation of the amygdala causes defensiveness, rage, and/or aggression.

anergia absence of energy caused by changes in brain chemistry and/or anatomy.

anger normal emotional response to the perception of a frustration of desires or threat to one's needs.

anhedonia loss of pleasure in activities or interests previously enjoyed. A symptom noted in depression and schizophrenia.

anorexia nervosa a disorder characterized by a refusal to eat over a long period of time, resulting in emaciation, amenorrhea, disturbance in body image, and an intense fear of becoming obese.

Antabuse (disulfiram) a drug given to alcoholics that blocks the breakdown of acetylaldehyde, producing nausea, vomiting, dizziness, flushing, and tachycardia if alcohol is consumed.

anterior commissure white-matter tract that connects the olfactory structures bilaterally, as well as the temporal lobes and the amygdala.

anticholinergic effect an effect caused by drugs that block acetylcholine receptors. Common anticholinergic effects include dry mouth, blurred vision, constipation, and urinary hesitancy.

antisocial personality a personality disorder characterized by blatant disregard for social norms. Behavior is demonstrated on a continuum of mild to pathological. Psychoanalytic theory attributes this disorder to an underdeveloped superego.

anxiety nonspecific, unpleasant feeling of discomfort, with physiological and psychological symptoms that generally have no identifiable cause.

anxiety disorders patterns of symptoms and behaviors in which anxiety is either the primary disturbance or a secondary problem that is recognized when the primary symptoms are removed.

anxiolytic an antianxiety drug.

apathy lack of feeling, interest, or emotion; indifference that is occasionally a mechanism for avoiding intense emotion.

aphasia difficulty in searching for words.

 motor a. impaired speech due to organic brain disorder in which understanding remains.

 nominal a. difficulty in finding the correct words in their proper sequence.

 sensory a. loss of ability to comprehend the meaning of words.

appropriate suitable or fitting for a particular person, purpose, occasion, or situation. Examples: appropriate affect, response, or attire.

apraxia inability to perform once known, purposeful, skilled activities in the absence of loss of motor function.

assault legally, any behavior that physically or verbally presents an immediate threat of physical injury to another individual.

assertiveness direct expression of feelings and needs in a way that respects the rights of others and self.

asylum (1) a place of safety or sanctuary; a refuge. (2) an institution for the care of the mentally ill; often associated with mistreatment and callousness.

attention-deficit hyperactivity disorder (ADHD) occurring primarily in children and adolescents and characterized by inattention, impulsivity, and hyperactivity.

attitude a pattern of mental views and feelings accumulated through past experiences and affected by present stimuli. A manner, disposition, tendency, or orientation with regard to a person or situation.

autism preoccupation with self without concern for external reality. A self-made private world of the schizophrenic.

autistic thinking thoughts, ideas, or desires derived from internal, private stimuli or drives that often are incongruent with reality; most often applied to persons with schizophrenia.

autonomic nervous system the division of the peripheral nervous system that is involuntary and innervates the viscera, heart, blood vessels, smooth muscle, and glands. It is divided into the parasympathetic (craniosacral system) and the sympathetic (thoracolumbar system).

avolition   lack of motivation.

axon   the long process from the neuronal cell body that transmits impulses away from the cell.

balance   the process by which patients are helped to reach for independence while conforming to norms.

basal ganglia   large nuclei including the caudate nucleus, putamen, and globus pallidus, which are responsible for modulating voluntary movement.

battery   a touching of the person of another, of his or her clothes, or anything else attached to his or her person without consent.

behavior   any observable, recordable, and measurable movement, response, or act of an individual (verbal and nonverbal).

behavior therapy   a therapeutic approach that helps the patient modify behavior by modifying or changing old patterns of behavior.

binge   uninhibited or excessive indulgence in food.

biological variations   physical differences between individuals or body structure, skin color, other visible characteristics, enzymatic and genetic variations, electrocardiographic patterns, susceptibility to disease, nutritional preferences and deficiencies, and psychological characteristics.

bipolar disorder   an affective or mood disorder characterized by at least one episode of mania with or without a history of depression.

biracial   describes an individual who crosses two racial and cultural groups.

bizarre   markedly unusual in appearance, thought, style, character, or behavior. Absurd.

blackout   a period of time in which the drinker functions socially for which there is no memory.

blocking   unconscious interruption in train of thought.

blood-brain barrier   a barrier that guards the brain from fluctuations in body chemistry. It regulates the amount and speed with which substances in the blood enter the brain.

borderline personality disorder   a personality disorder with the essential feature of a pervasive pattern of unstable self-image, interpersonal relations, and mood.

bradykinesia   slow or retarded movement.

brainstem   the vital structure that carries all information to and from the cerebral cortex and spinal cord. Because the brainstem is also responsible for respiration, its function is essential for life. It consists of the midbrain, pons, and medulla.

bulimia   compulsive binge eating accompanied by purging and overconcern with body shape and weight. It is characterized by an insatiable craving for food, resulting in episodes of continuous eating and often followed by purging, depression, and self-deprivation.

catalepsy   state of unconsciousness in which immobility is constantly maintained.

catatonic behavior   motor anomalies in nonorganic disorders such as schizophrenia.

excitement   excited motor activity.

rigidity   assumption of an inappropriate posture.

catecholamines   derived from the amino acid tyrosine, these substances include dopamine, norepinephrine, and epinephrine. Catecholamines are a subcategory of the monoamines, which also include serotonin and histamine. Catecholamines and their synthesis products are widely distributed in the central and peripheral nervous system.

caudate   the basal ganglia nucleus that protrudes into the anterior horn of the lateral ventricle.

cerebral cortex   the narrow ribbon of gray matter that lies on the surface of the cerebrum. The gray matter lies "on top of" the white matter. The reverse is true in the spinal cord.

child abuse   harmful physical, emotional, sexual, and/or verbal behavior inflicted on a child.

cholinergics   substances that stimulate the cholinergic system. In the peripheral nervous system, cholinergic drugs constrict the pupil, increase the production of saliva and respiratory secretions, slow the heart, and increase gastrointestinal peristalsis and urinary output.

chorea   a Greek term for "dance." The choreas manifest as hyperkinetic disorders characterized by involuntary, unpredictable, and random movements of the trunk, head, face, and limbs.

circumstantiality   digression of inappropriate thoughts into ideas, eventually reaching the desired goal.

cirrhosis   disease of the liver characterized by the development of scar tissue in the liver.

civil law   the part of the legal system that is concerned with the legal rights and duties of private persons. Civil lawsuits can recapture monetary loss from professionals who have been guilty of false imprisonment, defamation of character, assault and battery, or negligence.

clang associations   words similar in sound but not in meaning that conjure up new thoughts.

clarification   a communication skill that helps to define a patient's responses through use of direct questions.

clonic   a state in which rigidity and relaxation succeed each other.

closed-ended questions   questions that generally elicit a yes or no response. Useful in gathering factual data.

clouding of consciousness   incomplete clear-mindedness, with disturbance in perception and attitude. Example: stupor.

codependency   stress-related preoccupation with an addicted person's life, leading to extreme dependence on that person.

cognition   the act or process of knowing and perceiving.

cognitive disorders   disorders that affect consciousness, memory, and other cognitive processes.

cognitive processes pertaining to perception, judgment, memory, and reasoning.

coma depressed consciousness wherein even extreme stimulation of the reticular activating system will not cause a response.

communication a process that is the matrix for thought and relationships between all people regardless of cultural heritage.

community meeting a meeting that occurs within the therapeutic milieu and in which joint problem solving by community members is encouraged.

community mental health the application of principles of psychiatric care to communities and groups of people. The goal of this effort is to maintain health, to prevent mental illness when possible, and, if treatment is indicated, to treat the individual closer to his or her support systems.

Community Mental Health Centers Act 1963 legislation authorizing federal funds for construction of comprehensive mental health centers.

complex partial seizure formerly referred to as temporal lobe or psychomotor seizure; these seizures typically begin with a clouding of consciousness followed by some meaningless movement such as lip smacking or hand clapping; brief periods of forgetfulness are common.

comprehension the capacity to perceive and understand.

compulsion uncontrollable impulse to perform an act or ritual repeatedly; may be in response to an obsession (unwilled, persistent thought), as in obsessive-compulsive disorder. The act or ritual serves to decrease anxiety. Examples of rituals: hand washing, cleaning, and checking (e.g., checking to see if door is locked).

concrete communication inability to think and communicate abstractly.

concrete thinking the use of literal meaning without ability to consider abstract meaning (e.g., "don't cry over spilt milk" might be interpreted as meaning "because the milk is dirty").

confabulation unconscious filling of gaps in memory with imagined or untrue experiences that the person believes but has no basis for in reality.

confidentiality treating the information about and from patients in a private manner; information about patients is "confidential" and requires their approval before disclosure.

confused state bewildered, perplexed, or unclear. The type and degree of confusion should be specified.

congruence accordant states. Example: mood-congruence, in which the person's visible emotional state correlates with his mood or feeling state.

consciousness state of awareness.

conservator guardian; a legally appointed person who controls the affairs of a gravely disabled person, including the right to consent to or refuse psychiatric treatment.

consultant-liaison nurse a psychiatric mental health nurse who provides expert consultation for patients and staff in other parts of the hospital agency.

contralateral the opposite side of the body.

conversion process by which a psychic event, idea, memory, or impulse is represented by a bodily change or symptom such as blindness or paralysis.

corpus callosum the major connecting and communicating pathway between the hemispheres.

crisis a 4- to 6-week period of severe emotional disorganization due to the failure of coping mechanisms and/or lack of support.

cultural values the unique, individual expressions of belief related to culture that have been accepted as appropriate over time for persons in that culture.

culturally diverse nursing care the modification of nursing approaches to provide culturally competent care.

culture a patterned behavioral response that develops over time in relation to race.

custodial care the process of caring for hygienic and nutritional needs in an institution but not providing treatment for mental disorder.

cyclothymia a chronic mood disturbance of at least 2 years' duration involving numerous hypomanic episodes and numerous periods of depression. Cyclothymia does not meet the criteria for a manic episode or major depression.

deinstitutionalization a shift in treatment location from large public hospitals to community settings.

delirium a disorder with alterations in consciousness and changes in cognition, which is usually caused by a general medical condition or is substance-induced. Typically, deliria develop over a short period of time and are treatable. A (usually) reversible bewildered state of clouded consciousness, generally accompanied by restlessness, disorientation, and fear. May include periods of hallucinations.

delusion fixed, false belief, not consistent with the person's intelligence and culture, unamenable to reason.

   bizarre d. an absurd belief.

   nihilistic d. the false belief that the self, part of the self, or another object has ceased to exist.

   paranoid d. oversuspiciousness leading to persecutory delusions.

   persecution d. false belief that one is being persecuted.

   reference d. false belief that the behavior of others in the environment refers to oneself; derived from ideas of reference in which one falsely feels he is being talked about.

   somatic d. false belief involving functioning of one's body.

dementia a disorder that causes pronounced memory and cognitive disturbances. Typically, dementias are gradual in onset and progressive in course.

dendrites the many projections from the neuron that transmit impulses to another neuron.

denial avoidance of disagreeable realities or threats by ignoring or refusing to recognize them. An unconscious defense mechanism that may or may not be adaptive.

dependence a state in which a drug user must take a usual or increasing dose of a drug to prevent the onset of abstinence symptoms/withdrawal.

depersonalization a feeling of unreality or strangeness related to one's self, body parts, bodily functions, or the external environment.

depression a lowered or saddened mood state or major affective disorder, listed as a mood disorder in the DSM-IV.

derailment gradual or sudden deviation in train of thought without blocking.

derealization distortion of spatial relationships so that the environment becomes unfamiliar.

devaluation criticism of others that defends against one's own feelings of inadequacy.

diencephalon the thalamus, hypothalamus, epithalamus, and metathalamus.

disinhibition a state in which a person is unable to suppress urges or statements that may be socially unacceptable; e.g., telling a dirty joke in an inappropriate situation.

disoriented disturbance in orientation of time, place, or person.

displacement shift of emotion from an object or person who incites the emotion to a less threatening source. An unconscious defense mechanism that may or may not be adaptive.

dissociation (1) removal from conscious awareness of painful feelings, memories, thoughts, or aspects of identity; (2) separation of mental or behavioral processes from the rest of the person's consciousness or identity; (3) the splitting or separation of any group of mental or behavioral processes from the rest of the person's consciousness or identity.

dissociative reaction process by which an individual blocks off a part of his life from conscious recognition because of severe anxiety (multiple personality disorder).

distractibility inability to concentrate attention.

dopamine a brain neurotransmitter that influences muscle movement and emotions. The "dopamine theory" states that persons with schizophrenia may have too much dopamine, which may account for their sensory-perceptual alterations. Research has refined this theory.

double-bind conflicting demands by significant individuals in a person's life. Cannot meet both demands so is doomed to failure.

dysarthria difficulty in articulating single sounds or phonemes of speech.

dyskinesia disturbed coordination and motor activity, usually producing a jerky motion. An EPSE of neuroleptic medications related to their effect on dopamine receptors. See also *tardive dyskinesia*.

dyslexia difficulty in reading due to a central lesion.

dysphagia difficulty in swallowing.

dysphoria an unpleasant mood state.

dysthymia a chronic mood disturbance involving a depressed mood for at least 2 years.

dystonia rigidity in muscles that control posture, gait, or ocular movement. An EPSE of neuroleptic medications that block dopamine.

echolalia psychopathological repeating of words of one person by another. Noted in types of schizophrenia.

echopraxia imitation of the body position of another.

ego personality process that focuses on reality, while striving to meet the needs of the id. The ego experiences anxiety and uses defense mechanisms for protection.

ELISA Enzyme-Linked Immunosorbent Assay test. This test is used to detect specific antibodies. It is used to assist in the diagnosis of HIV infection through the identification of antibodies to HIV.

emaciated made excessively thin by lack of nutrition.

emotion a complex feeling state with psychic, somatic, and behavioral components related to affect and mood.

empathy objective understanding of how patients feel or how they see their situations.

enkephalins widely distributed opioid-like neuropeptides that are part of the endorphin family. These substances mediate pain perception, taste, olfaction, arousal, emotional behavior, vision, hearing, neurohormone secretion, motor coordination, and water balance.

environmental control the ability of an individual to control nature by planning activities and tasks to assist in maintaining optimal balance in life.

epilepsy a disorder of the central nervous system (CNS) in which the major symptom is a seizure; the seizure is caused by a temporary disturbance of the brain impulses.

ethnicity refers to groups whose members share a common social and cultural heritage passed on to each successive generation.

ethnocentrism only acknowledging and valuing one's own culture.

etiology the study of the causes of diseases, including both direct and predisposing causes.

euphoria a false sense of elation or well-being; pathological elevation of mood; complete lack of tension. Most notable in the manic phase of bipolar disorder.

euthymia a normal, homeostatic mood state.

expansive mood unrestrained expression of feelings.

extrapyramidal side effects (EPSEs) involuntary muscle movements resulting from the effects of neuroleptic drugs on the extrapyramidal system. These drugs cause a dopamine blockade that creates a dopamine-ACh imbalance. EPSEs include akathisia, akinesia, dystonia, drug-induced parkinsonism, and neuroleptic malignant syndrome (NMS).

extrapyramidal system outside the pyramidal (voluntary) tract. Coordinates involuntary movements.

eye contact occasional glancing into the patient's eyes to demonstrate interest during an interaction.

family system a field of influence exerted on one another by family members.

fantasy an imaginary sequence of events. Common in childhood. Appropriate as long as the person is aware of reality.

fear anxiety due to consciously recognized and realistic danger.

feedback articulation of one's perception of what another person has said or meant; this process requires at least two people.

flashbacks cognitive, emotional, and physical reexperiencing of traumatic events.

flight of ideas a speech pattern manifested by a rapid transition from topic to topic, frequently without completing any of the preceding ideas. Prominent in manic states.

free association in a therapeutic context, saying anything that comes to mind.

fugue a period of personality dissociation with memory loss.

gait the manner of progression in walking. Example: ataxic gait, in which the foot is raised high and the sole strikes down suddenly.

gamma-aminobutyric acid (GABA) an inhibitory amino acid neurotransmitter formed during the citric acid cycle from its precursor, glutamic acid. GABA receptors are widely distributed in the central nervous system and produce neuronal hyperpolarization through an influx of chloride ions. Drugs that increase GABA reduce anxiety and seizures.

general leads interactive skills that facilitate the communication process by encouraging the patient to continue.

generalized seizure involves both hemispheres of the brain at the onset of the seizure; consciousness is usually impaired.

genetic vulnerability the tendency to inherent traits, behaviors, and biological characteristics of one's ancestors.

globus pallidus a gray-matter structure located medial to the putamen. This portion of the basal ganglia is smaller and triangular in shape. It is subdivided into the globus pallidus externa and the globus pallidus interna.

glutamate the major excitatory transmitter in the central nervous system with receptors throughout the brain. Glutamate stimulation of N-methyl-D-aspartate (NMDA)-activated channels permits excessive inflow of calcium ions and production of free radicals that may cause neuronal death.

grand mal seizure a type of generalized seizure in which there is loss of consciousness and convulsions; this type of seizure is most frequently associated with epilepsy by lay persons.

gravely disabled a person who is unable to provide food, clothing, or shelter for himself because of a mental illness.

gray matter composed of the cell bodies and dendrites of neurons.

grimacing contortion of facial muscles; may be extrapyramidal side effect.

gyri the convolutions of gray matter on the cerebrum.

hallucination false sensory perceptions not associated with real external stimuli. May involve any of the five senses: auditory, visual, olfactory, gustatory, or tactile.

    auditory h. most prevalent in schizophrenia. The sounds may be perceived as thoughts or voices coming from any type of transmitter or the patient's mind. The messages may be condemning or accusatory, or complimentary and encouraging. It is critical that the examiner be aware that the messages may be directing the patient toward harming himself or others, so their content cannot be ignored.

    tactile h. common in alcohol withdrawal. Hallucinations may also be an effect of certain types of drugs, such as amphetamines, hallucinogens, and cannabis.

    visual h. often associated with organic conditions.

hebephrenia an outdated schizophrenic subtype characterized by silliness, delusions, hallucinations, and regression.

here-and-now focus assisting patients to understand how their current behaviors influence daily living.

HIV antibody the antibody specific to HIV that usually appears within 6 weeks after the infection.

holistic pertaining to totality or the whole (holistic care).

homelessness without a home. Homeless individuals, including whole families, may live on the streets exclusively or may make use of community shelters, halfway houses, cheap hotels, or board-and-care homes.

hostile feeling intense anger and resentment, manifested by destructive behavior.

human immunodeficiency virus (HIV) the virus isolated and recognized as the etiologic agent of AIDS. HIV is classified as a lentivirus in a subgroup of the retrovirus.

Huntington's disease a genetically transmitted disease that includes motor and cognitive changes.

hydrotherapy the use of water (wet sheetpacks, 2- to 10-hour tub baths) for psychotherapeutic purposes.

hyperactivity (hyperkinesis) restless, aggressive, often destructive activity. Prominent in manic states.

hypoactivity (hypokinesis) decreased activity or retardation (psychomotor retardation); slowing of psychological and physical functions.

hypomania a clinical syndrome similar to but less severe than that demonstrated in a full-blown manic episode.

hypothalamus a group of nuclei in the diencephalon that influences eating behavior, temperature regulation, emotional expression, and the autonomic system. Dopaminergic neurons in the hypothalamus control lactation.

id personality process that wants to experience only pleasure; is impulsive and without morals.

idealization viewing others as perfect; exalting others.

ideas of reference the belief that some events have a special meaning (e.g., people laughing are perceived as laughing at the patient).

idiopathic without known cause.

illogical (thinking) thinking containing erroneous conclusions or internal contradictions (irrational thoughts).

illusion misinterpretation of a sensory input. Observed in alcoholic withdrawal and anesthesia states.

impaired parent a parent whose nurturing capabilities are compromised or absent related to psychiatric or substance abuse disorders.

Indoklon therapy a convulsive therapy like electroconvulsive therapy (ECT); however, convulsions are induced by ether rather than by electrical stimulus.

informed consent providing the patient with information about a specific treatment, including its benefits, side effects, and possible risks, that will enable him or her to make a competent and voluntary decision.

insight the recognition of motivational sources behind one's thoughts, actions, or behavior.

intellectual functioning the individual's general fund of knowledge, orientation, memory, mastery of simple mathematical equations, and capacity for abstract thinking.

intellectualization one of the unconscious defense mechanisms. A process of thinking excessively about the philosophical or theoretical to the extent that the stream of thought is interrupted and anxiety-provoking issues are avoided.

internal capsule a broad band of myelinated fibers that separate the lentiform nuclei from the caudate nucleus and thalamus. Corticospinal (motor or pyramidal) tracts travel through the internal capsule, cerebral peduncles, and cerebral pyramids into the spinal cord,

where they constitute the lateral corticospinal pathway. Damage to any of these structures can result in hemiparesis or hemiplegia.

involuntary commitment a commitment status in which a person who has the legal capacity to consent to mental health treatment refuses to do so and is involuntarily detained for treatment by the state.

ipsilateral same side of body.

irrational beliefs beliefs that are not logical but influence feelings and behaviors.

judgment and comprehension the ability to understand, recall, mobilize, and constructively integrate previous learning in meeting new situations.

Kaposi's syndrome (KS) A form of cancer that presents with pink-purple spots on the skin and mouth as a painless tumor.

kinesics the study of body movements.

Korsakoff's psychosis (Korsakov) an organic mental disorder with memory loss related to alcohol abuse.

Kraepelin German psychiatrist who initiated a classification system for psychiatry in 1896. He used the term *dementia praecox.*

labile (mood, affect, or behavior) subject to frequent or unpredictable changes.

least restrictive alternative an environment that provides the necessary treatment requirements in the least restrictive setting possible. For example, a hospital setting is more restrictive than a board-and-care setting. If the board-and-care setting provides the necessary treatment requirements for a person, then that environment would represent the least restrictive alternative.

lentiform nuclei the putamen and globus pallidus of the basal ganglia.

lesion injury to tissue.

Lewy bodies eosinophilic cytoplasmic inclusions seen in neuromelanin-containing neurons in Parkinson's disease.

limit setting holding people to established norms with the intent of assisting them to function more constructively.

lipid solubility the ability of a substance to dissolve in fat.

lithium an element or salt used in the treatment and prevention of manic episodes.

locus ceruleus A small nucleus ("blue spot") in the pontine tegmentum whose neurons are the major source of norepinephrine in the brain; present bilaterally.

looseness of associations vague, unfocused, illogical flow or stream of thought. Notable in schizophrenia.

magical thinking belief that thoughts, words, or actions can cause or prevent an occurrence by some magical means.

malpractice negligence by a professional. Malpractice is a civil action that can be brought against a nurse if he or she has breached a standard of care that a reasonably prudent nurse would meet.

mania   a disordered mental state of extreme excitement, hyperactivity, euphoria, and hyperverbal behavior.

medially   toward the midline.

medulla   approximately 3 cm long and the most caudal portion of the brainstem. It controls respiration and supplies innervation to the tongue and palate.

memory   function by which information stored in the brain is later recalled to the conscious mind.

meninges   the outer lining of the central nervous system composed of the dura mater, arachnoid, and pia mater.

mental disorder   "A clinically significant behavioral or psychological syndrome or pattern . . . associated with present distress or disability" (DSM-IV, 1994).

mental retardation   a lack of intelligence so great that it interferes with social and occupational performance.

mental status examination   a record of current findings that includes a description of patient's appearance, behavior, motor activity, speech, alertness, mood, cognition, intelligence, reactions, views, and attitudes.

mesocortical tract   a dopaminergic tract that projects from the ventral tegmental area near the substantia nigra to the neocortex, particularly the prefrontal cortex. It is involved in motivation, planning, behavior, attention, and social behavior.

mesolimbic tract   catecholaminergic neuronal tract (mostly dopaminergic) with cell bodies located in the ventral tegmental area of the midbrain and axons that project to the hippocampus, entorhinal cortex, amygdala, anterior cingulate gyrus, nucleus accumbens, and other limbic regions.

midbrain   the most rostral division of the brainstem. It contains important structures such as the cerebral aqueduct, superior and inferior colliculi, red nuclei, substantia nigra, cerebral peduncles, and oculomotor and trochlear cranial nerve nuclei.

milieu   environment or setting.

milieu management   purposeful manipulation of the environment to promote a therapeutic atmosphere.

milieu therapy   the use of the environment to promote optimum functioning in a group or individual.

minority   a social, religious, or occupational group that constitutes less than a numerical majority of the population.

monoamine(s)   a category of neurotransmitters that contain one amino group and are derived from amino acids. Subcategories of monoamines include the catecholamines (dopamine, norepinephrine, epinephrine), which are derived from tyrosine, and the indolamine serotonin, which is derived from tryptophan. Histamine is categorized as a monoamine but is biochemically different. Monoamine-synthesizing neurons are found primarily in the brainstem but have a wide net of influence because of the ubiquitous distribution of their axonal projections.

monoamine oxidase   an enzyme that metabolizes monoamines such as dopamine, norepinephrine, and serotonin.

monoamine oxidase inhibitors (MAOIs)   antidepressant drugs that increase the bioavailability of certain neurotransmitters by interfering with their metabolism.

mood disorder   a diagnostic category in the DSM-IV that includes the affective disorders.

mutism   refusal to speak.

NANDA   abbreviation for the North American Nursing Diagnosis Association.

narcissism   extreme self-centeredness and self-absorption (narcissistic personality disorder).

narcotherapy   the induction of a state of sedation by intravenous administration of sedatives (e.g., amobarbital) or stimulants (e.g., methylphenidate).

National Institute of Mental Health   a government organization in the National Institutes of Health concerned with mental health issues in the United States.

nature argument   etiology as related to biology.

negligence   the failure to do that which a reasonably prudent and careful person would do under the circumstances, or the doing of that which a reasonable and prudent person would not do.

neologism   a new word created by the patient for psychological reasons. Noted in some types of schizophrenia.

neurofibrillary tangle   a mass of abnormal filamentous material located within the cell body of neurons. These tangles occur in several brain disorders, such as Alzheimer's disease, and are composed of cytoskeletal components.

neuroleptics   antipsychotic medications.

neuron   nerve cell.

neurotransmitter   a chemical found in the nervous system (e.g., norepinephrine, serotonin, dopamine) that facilitates the transmission of nerve impulses across synapses between neurons.

noncompliance   failure to take medication as prescribed.

norepinephrine   a catecholamine neurotransmitter that is primarily synthesized in neurons of the locus ceruleus in the pons. Deficiencies of norepinephrine are linked to depression.

nucleus accumbens   at the level of the septum pellucidum, this nucleus is adjacent to the medial and ventral portions of the caudate and putamen. The neurons in this nucleus project to both the globus pallidus and the substantia nigra. A major component of the "reward pathway."

nucleus basalis of Meynart   located bilaterally directly beneath the anterior commissure, it is the major brain site for the production of acetylcholine. Fibers from this nucleus project diffusely to the cerebral cortex.

nursing diagnosis a statement that describes a patient's illness or response to illness treatable by nurses.

nurture argument etiology as related to upbringing, life events, or other stressors.

obesity an abnormal increase in the proportion of fat cells, mainly in the viscera and subcutaneous tissues of the body.

objectivity the process of remaining open, unbiased, and emotionally separate from a patient.

obsession the pathological persistence of an unwilled thought, feeling, or impulse to the extent that it cannot be eliminated from consciousness by logical effort.

obsessive-compulsive disorder recurrent obsessions (thoughts) alternating with compulsions (behaviors). Both are unwilled and painful.

oculogyric crisis involuntary tonic muscle spasms of the eye. The eyes usually roll upward in a fixed stare. This is a very frightening dystonic reaction caused by antipsychotic drugs.

olfactory pertaining to the sense of smell.

open posture a relaxed, yet attentive position, with arms uncrossed. Enhances patient's trust in the examiner.

open-ended statement a statement that elicits further exploration of the patient's problem by encouraging communication. Can also be in the form of a question.

openness an atmosphere in which people are free to express their thoughts and feelings without fear of ridicule or censure.

opportunistic illnesses illnesses that develop when the immune system is inactive or suppressed.

organic mental disorders a class of disorders of mental functioning caused by permanent brain damage or temporary brain dysfunction. The cause is known and may be primary (originating in the brain) or secondary to systemic disease. Cognition, emotions, and motivation are affected. The DSM-IV uses the term *cognitive disorder.*

orientation conscious awareness of person, place, and time.

panic a state of extreme, acute, intense anxiety, accompanied by disorganization of personality and function.

paranoid thinking oversuspiciousness. May lead to persecutory delusions or projectile behavior patterns.

parataxic distortion mixing perceptions of current experiences with past memories.

parkinsonism symptoms masked facies, muscle rigidity, and shuffling gait; common in patients taking neuroleptic drugs; extrapyramidal side effects related to dopamine blockade.

partial seizure usually involves one hemisphere of the brain at the onset of the seizure.

passive aggression anger expressed indirectly through subtle and evasive ways.

perception awareness of objects and relations that follows stimulation of peripheral sense organs.

perseveration psychopathological repetition of the same word or idea in response to different questions.

personality disorder exaggerated, pathological behavior patterns destructive to the individual and others.

petit mal seizure a variant of absence seizures that is characterized by a three-per-second spike and wave electroencephalogram (EEG) pattern.

phobia exaggerated, pathological dread or fear of some specific type of stimulus or situation.

    acrophobia dread of high places.

    agoraphobia dread of open places.

    claustrophobia dread of closed places.

phobic disorder severe phobic behavior patterns that render the individual dysfunctional. Avoidance of the feared object or situation serves to assuage anxiety.

Pneumocystis carinii **pneumonia (PCP)** a form of pulmonary disease caused by an opportunistic pathogen (fungal protozoan).

polymerase chain reaction (PCR) a laboratory technique using molecular biology to identify the nucleic acid sequence of HIV in the cells of an infected individual. Used in the early detection of perinatally exposed infants and in monitoring persons on clinical trials.

preconscious memories that can be recalled to consciousness with some effort.

precursor something that precedes. Tyrosine is a precursor to dopamine in the synthesis of dopamine in the body.

premorbid state before onset of the disorder.

primary appraisal judgment an individual makes about an event.

primary gain relief or expression of anxiety through symptoms of disorder.

probable cause sufficient credible facts that would induce a reasonably intelligent and prudent person to believe that a cause of action exists.

process recording a written record of an encounter with a patient that is as nearly verbatim as possible, including both verbal and nonverbal behaviors of the nurse and the patient.

projective identification placement of feelings on another to justify one's own expression of feelings.

proxemics the study of the way in which people perceive and use environmental, social, and personal space in interactions with others.

psychoeducation a strategy of teaching patients and families about disorders, treatments, coping techniques, and resources based on the observation that people can be better participants in their own care if they have knowledge.

psychomotor retardation   markedly slowed speech and body movements.

psychopathology   the study of underlying processes, both biological and psychosocial, that lead to mental disorders.

psychosis   the inability to recognize reality, complicated by severe thought disorder and the inability to relate to others.

psychotherapeutic management   a model for nursing care that balances the three primary intervention modes used by psychiatric nurses: the therapeutic nurse-patient relationship, psychopharmacology, and milieu management.

psychotropic drugs   medications used in the treatment of mental illness.

purge   to evacuate the bowels, as with a cathartic.

pyramidal system   the motor system for voluntary movement.

race   a breeding population that primarily mates within itself.

raphe nuclei   properly part of the pontine tegmentum, the raphe nuclei are associated with the reticular formation and synthesize serotonin.

reactive depression   depressed mood related to some life event; e.g., divorce or losing a job.

reappraisal   appraisal made after new or additional information has been received.

religiosity   preoccupation with religious ideas or content.

resiliency   capability to withstand stressors without permanent dysfunction or developmental delay.

restraint   physical control of a patient to prevent injury to the patient, staff, and other patients.

reuptake   the physiological process that occurs when a neurotransmitter is taken up into the presynaptic neuron after having been released into the synapse. Some psychotropic drugs are designed to prevent the reuptake of a specific neurotransmitter in order to increase the synaptic presence of that neurotransmitter.

satisfaction   relaxation of the tension of physiological needs.

schizophrenia   a syndrome, illness, or mental health disorder heterogeneous in cause, pathogenesis, presenting picture, response to treatment, and prognosis. Symptoms generally reflect a progressive deterioration and disorganization of the individual's personality structure, affect, and cognition. The DSM-IV lists the following types: paranoid, catatonic, disorganized, undifferentiated, and residual.

seclusion   process of placing a patient alone in a specially designed room for protection and close observation.

secondary appraisal   evaluation an individual makes about potential actions to be taken.

secondary gain   attention and support received from others while ill.

selective serotonin reuptake inhibitors (SSRIs)   class of antidepressants. Potent blockers of serotonin reuptake, thus increasing the level of serotonin in the synapse.

serotonin (5HT)   a monoamine neurotransmitter from the indolamine family. It is derived from the amino acid tryptophan. Deficiencies of serotonin are linked to depression.

shuffling gait   (parkinsonism gait) a style of walking typically demonstrated by individuals whose dopamine stores have been blocked or depleted as a result of Parkinson's disease or antipsychotic medications.

social organization   the organization of a culture around particular units (such as family, racial, or ethnic groups, religious groups, and community or social groups).

socialization skills   those skills necessary for negotiating everyday interpersonal issues; e.g., acknowledging responsibility for one's behavior, using eye contact appropriately, interacting with others for purposes of sharing and support.

somatic therapy   a therapeutic approach that uses physiological or physical interventions to effect behavioral changes. For example, electroconvulsive therapy is a somatic treatment.

somatization   the conversion of mental states or experiences into bodily symptoms; associated with anxiety.

space   the distance and intimacy needs of culturally unique individuals in human interaction.

splitting   inability to integrate good and bad aspects of self and others. View self and others as all good or all bad.

status epilepticus   repetitive seizures; usually refers to repetitive grand mal seizures.

steady state   the desired state in anticonvulsant therapy when the serum concentration of the anticonvulsant is consistent and is maintained at a therapeutic level.

stereotyping   the assumption that all people in a similar cultural, racial, or ethnic group think and act alike.

stereotypy   continuous repetition of speech or physical activities.

stressor   a stimulus perceived by the individual or the organism as challenging, threatening, or damaging.

striatum   basal ganglia that include the caudate and putamen.

substantia nigra   literally, black substance. A pigmented area of the midbrain where dopamine is synthesized.

suicidal ideation   a person's thinking about and inclination to do self-injury or self-destruction.

suicidal plan   a specific method designed to inflict self-injury or self-destruction as verbalized by an individual.

suicide   self-inflicted death.

sulcus   a groove separating gyri. Deep sulci are referred to as fissures.

superego   psychoanalytic structure of the mind equivalent to the conscience (sense of right and wrong). Develops in early childhood. It provides the ego with an inner control to help cope with the id.

synapse   the microscopic space between two neurons.

tangentiality   inability to have goal-directed associations of thought; never gets to desired goal from desired point.

tardive dyskinesia   an extrapyramidal syndrome that usually emerges late in the course of long-term antipsychotic drug therapy. Includes grimacing, buccolingual movements, and dystonia (impaired muscle tonus). May be irreversible.

terror   state of extreme tension.

therapeutic   in the psychotherapeutic management model the communication of respect, a desire to help, and understanding to another person. Understanding includes knowledge of mental mechanisms, coping strategies, stressors, etc. Active listening is a crucial component of being therapeutic.

therapeutic communication   interactive verbal and nonverbal strategies that focus on the needs of the patient and facilitate a goal-directed, patient-oriented communication process.

therapeutic listening   listening that is focused on the patient and obtains therapeutically useful information about the patient.

therapeutic milieu   a treatment environment managed in such a way that the environment itself is therapeutic.

therapy   the means, usually with words, to cure or manage the course of another person's mental disorder. Nurses who practice psychotherapy are trained in a specific therapy model; e.g., psychoanalysis, cognitive therapy, etc.

thinking   the process of following a goal-directed flow of ideas, symbols, and associations to a logical conclusion in accordance with the person's developmental stage.

thought disorder   thinking characterized by loose associations, neologisms, and illogical constructs and conclusions.

time   either a physical quantity measured by a clock or patterns and orientations that relate to social processes.

time out   disengaging the child from a specific situation; e.g., directing the child to sit in a chair facing away from other patients so that the child might regain self-control.

tolerance   the need for increasing amounts of a substance to achieve the same effects.

tonic   a state of continuous tension.

transference   unconscious emotional reaction to a current situation that is actually based on previous experiences.

tuberoinfundibular tract   a dopaminergic system with neurons in the arcuate nucleus of the hypothalamus that project to the pituitary stalk. This tract controls the secretion of prolactin.

tyramine   a substance derived from the amino acid tyrosine and found in many common foods such as aged cheeses, yogurt, avocados, etc. (see Box 21-4). Tyramine-rich foods can cause a hypertensive crisis in a person being treated with MAOIs.

tyrosine   an amino acid that is the precursor to dopamine.

unconscious   memories, conflicts, experiences, and materials that have been repressed and cannot be recalled at will.

undoing   a defense mechanism by which a person symbolically acts out to reverse a previously committed act or thought. A common ritual in obsessive-compulsive disorder.

unit norm   an expected behavior for a given therapeutic setting.

validation   the process of confirming an individual's intent by questioning the content of his message.

vascular dementia   dementia resulting from interruption of blood to the brain, which causes anoxia, ischemia, and subsequent infarction.

ventral tegmental area (VTA)   located in the midbrain, this region is dorsomedial to the substantia nigra and ventral to the red nuclei. The nuclei in this area produce dopamine. The efferent pathways from the VTA include the mesocortical and mesolimbic tracts.

ventricle   the system of connected brain cavities that are filled with cerebrospinal fluid, including the lateral ventricles (in the central portion of the telencephalon), the third ventricle (which runs between the thalami), the fourth ventricle (in the pons and medulla), and the connecting cerebral aqueduct (in the midbrain).

vesicle   storage sac at the synaptic terminal.

voluntary commitment   a commitment status in which the patient or his or her conservator/guardian requests treatment and signs an application for that treatment. This person is free to sign himself or herself out of the hospital also.

Wernicke's area   the sophisticated auditory association cortex that is located within the planum temporale and interprets spoken language.

Wernicke's encephalopathy   confusion and ophthalmoplegia caused by thiamine deficiency; most common in alcoholics. It results in necrosis and hemorrhage in the mamillary bodies and periventricular structures of the brainstem.

white matter   composed of myelinated neuronal axons.

withdrawal   1) the act or process of turning inward to avoid a perceived environmental threat; 2) a physiological response to cessation of an addictive substance.

word salad   incoherent mixture of words or phrases.

Answer Key to Study Questions

Chapter 1

1. c
2. d
3. assistance, banishment, and confinement
4. Pinel and Tuke
5. a
6. a
7. e
8. c
9. b
10. b
11. a
12. c

Chapter 2

1. d
2. b
3. d
4. b

Chapter 3

1. b, Table 3-2
2. e, Table 3-2
3. c, Table 3-2
4. c, Table 3-3
5. a, Table 3-4
6. d

Chapter 4

1. d
2. a
3. b
4. c
5. b
6. c
7. b
8. c
9. b

Chapter 5

1. b
2. c
3. b
4. b
5. a
6. to give the brain more gray matter "coastline"
7. e
8. c
9. b
10. b
11. with an upper motor neuron disorder
12. b
13. b
14. a
15. a

16. c, d
17. a
18. b

Chapter 6

1. a
2. d
3. b

Chapter 7

1. d
2. c
3. a
4. b

Chapter 8

1. c
2. a
3. b

Chapter 9

1. e
2. deinstitutionalization
3. a, b, c, e
4. b
5. d
6. working toward interconnectedness and peace between the mind, body, and spirit
7. e

Chapter 10

1. c
2. a
3. d
4. b
5. d

Chapter 11

1. d
2. c
3. b
4. d
5. a
6. b
7. c

Chapter 12

1. b
2. c
3. d

4. c
5. a

Chapter 13

1. b
2. d
3. c
4. b
5. a
6. c
7. a

Chapter 14

1. c
2. d
3. b
4. b
5. d
6. a

Chapter 15

1. c
2. d
3. b
4. c
5. a
6. d

Chapter 16

1. a
2. c
3. b
4. d
5. a

Chapter 17

1. e
2. c
3. e

Chapter 18

1. a
2. b
3. d
4. d
5. a
6. c
7. b
8. b
9. d

Chapter 19

1. d
2. a
3. c (passes blood-brain barrier)
4. c
5. a
6. b (can be given IM)
7. d

Chapter 20

1. a
2. c
3. a
4. b
5. b
6. c
7. a
8. c
9. d
10. b
11. b
12. These side effects are the triad of symptoms associated with parkinsonism

Chapter 21

1. c
2. d
3. b
4. c
5. a
6. c
7. c
8. b
9. c
10. c
11. a
12. b
13. c
14. b

Chapter 22

1. b
2. b
3. c
4. a
5. b
6. b
7. d
8. b
9. b

Chapter 23

1. a
2. a
3. a
4. b
5. e
6. a

Chapter 24

1. a
2. b
3. c
4. b
5. d
6. b
7. b

Chapter 25

1. b
2. d
3. a
4. b
5. a

Chapter 26

1. a
2. c
3. c
4. b
5. d
6. d

Chapter 27

1. b
2. c
3. a
4. a
5. b
6. b
7. a
8. a
9. d
10. b
11. a
12. c
13. d
14. d
15. a
16. b
17. b

Chapter 28

1. e
2. a
3. c
4. b
5. b
6. c
7. b
8. b
9. c
10. b
11. b
12. a
13. a

Chapter 29

1. a
2. b
3. c
4. a
5. b
6. d
7. a

Chapter 30

1. b
2. c
3. c
4. a
5. b
6. f
7. t
8. b
9. c
10. b
11. d
12. c
13. d

Chapter 31

1. a
2. d
3. b
4. c
5. d

Chapter 32

1. d
2. b
3. c
4. b

Chapter 33

1. a
2. d
3. a
4. a
5. b
6. c
7. b
8. d
9. d
10. a
11. a
12. c
13. c
14. b
15. b
16. b
17. c

Chapter 34

1. b
2. c
3. a
4. d
5. b

Chapter 35

1. a
2. c
3. a
4. d
5. c
6. a
7. b
8. d

Chapter 36

1. b
2. c
3. d
4. a
5. d

Chapter 37

1. a
2. b
3. d
4. b
5. b
6. b, c

Chapter 38

1. a
2. c
3. b
4. d
5. d
6. c
7. b
8. a
9. c

Chapter 39

1. b
2. d
3. a
4. d
5. b
6. a
7. c
8. b
9. c

Chapter 40

1. d
2. c
3. d
4. b
5. d
6. a
7. b
8. c
9. a
10. a
11. b
12. b
13. Potentially, drugs that are highly bound to serum proteins would have less binding sites, thus increasing the amount of free drug (active drug)

Chapter 41

1. Before the case definition of AIDS was changed in 1993, HIV disease was a stage of HIV infection suffered by HIV-positive patients whose T-cell count was below 400. It was marked by 'AIDS-related complex' (ARC), identified by a low white cell and platelet count, anemia, thrush, etc. AIDS was defined exclusively by the presence of opportunistic illnesses. Since most people with HIV infection experience severe immunosuppression before the occurrance of opportunistic illnesses, the AIDS case-definition was expanded in 1993 to include an objective laboratory criterion of severe immunosuppression: "CD4$^+$ T-lymphocyte count of less than 200 cells/mm^3 or a percent of total lymphocytes less than 14" (CDC, 1997, p. 36). AIDS-defining opportunistic illnesses are now referred to as AIDS-OI.

2. Because the CD4$^+$ T-lymphocyte count drops below 200 cells/mm^3, the patient becomes severely immunocompromised, and certain illnesses result, such as Karposi's sarcoma, pneumocystis carinii pneumonia, Toxoplasma gondii, histoplasmosis, tuberculosis, herpes, coccidioidomycosis, candida albicans, and cytomegalovirus.

3. 1) Men who have sex with men; 2) Injecting-drug use; 3) Heterosexual contact, including sex with bisexual males and drug-injecting partners.

4. B

5. C

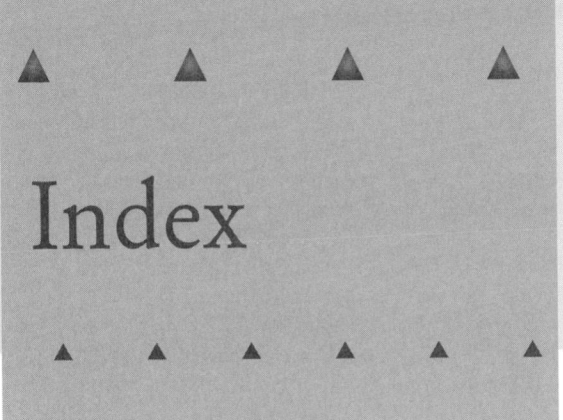

Index

A

ABCs of community response, 4
A-B-C theory of personality, 37
Absorption, alcohol, 512
Abstinence syndrome, 502
Abstract thinking, impairment in dementia, 457
Abuse
  child
    definition of, 617
    and schizophrenia, 366
  definition of, 299, 502
  family reactions to hospitalization for, 188
  by partners; *see* Partner abuse
  ritual, 592-594
  sexual; *see* Sexual abuse
Acceptance, in therapeutic environment, 327
Access to Community Care and Effective Services and Supports (ACCESS), 12
Acetaldehyde, in alcohol metabolism, 512
Acetylcholine (ACh), 224
  and Alzheimer's disease, 77, 464
  and depression, 391
  neuronal secretion of, 77
  as neurotransmitter, 225
  and Parkinson's disease, 231, 233-234
Acetylcholinesterase, and Alzheimer's disease, 464
ACh; *see* Acetylcholine

Acquired immunodeficiency syndrome (AIDS)
  biological basis of, 81
  cases of
    by age at diagnosis, 673
    by exposure category, 670
    by gender, 673
    by race, 673
  definition of, 667
  dementia of, 675
    care plan for, 677
    treatment for, 677, 678
  diagnosis of, 670
  incidence and distribution of, 672
  stress in, 674
Action for Mental Health (1961), 8
Activating event, in A-B-C theory of personality, 37
Activities of daily living (ADLs)
  Alzheimer's disease and, 463
  assessment in elderly, 654
  depression and, 389
Activity alterations
  depression and, 388-389
  in manic patients, 408-409
  in schizophrenia, 358, 359
    milieu management for, 373-374
Activity groups, 173
  in therapeutic environment, 323
Acupressure, 209
Acupuncture, 209
Acute stress disorder (ASD), 433-439
  DSM-IV criteria for, 433
  family issues of, 435
  interventions for, 438

AD; *see* Alzheimer's disease
Adaptive coping, with anxiety, 152
Adderall, 629
Addiction; *see also* Substance abuse/dependence
  as adult manifestation of childhood sexual abuse, 600
  definition of, 532
Addiction dependence, definition of, 507-508
ADHD; *see* Attention-deficit hyperactivity disorder
Adjustment disorders, 439
  with HIV infection, 675
    psychopharmacologic treatment of, 676
ADLs; *see* Activities of daily living
Admission
  as aggression variable, 162
  family reactions to, 188
  guidelines for, 48
Adolescent(s); *see also* Child and adolescent psychiatric disorders
  eating disorders in, 566
    anorexia nervosa, 551-552, 554
    bulimia nervosa, 559
  effects of childhood sexual abuse on, 598
Adoption studies, of child psychiatric disorders, 618
Adrenocorticotropic hormone (ACTH), and depression, 391
Adult survivors of sexual abuse; *see* Sexual abuse

Advance practice registered nurse (APRN), 107
Advocacy
in case management, 108-109
definition of, 102
Affect
alterations of
depression and, 389-390
of manic patients, 409
in schizophrenia, 358, 362
definition of, 383
depressed, and nurse-patient relationship, 133-134
Affective disorders
with HIV infection, 675
psychopharmacologic treatment of, 676
and schizophrenia, 375
Affective symptoms, as schizophrenic symptom, antipsychotic drugs and, 251
African-Americans
pharmacodynamics of, 211
world view of, 204, 206-207
African world view, 204, 206-207
Age
AIDS cases and, 673
depression and, 387-388
Ageism, 642
Agencies, family, 195
Aggression
assessing key variables of, 161-163
developmental view of, 160
etiology of, 160-161
as indication for psychosurgery, 586
limit setting for, 328
milieu management and control in, 315
manic patients and, 413
sexual response cycle and, 494
types of, and expression of anger, 158-160
Aggressive patient, 157-169
assessment in, 161-163
developmental view in, 160
etiology in, 160-161
expressions of anger and, 158-160
interventions for, 163-168
staff victim support in, 168-169
Agnosia, in Alzheimer's disease, 462
Agoraphobia
DSM-IV criteria of, 432
lifetime prevalence rates for, 346

Agoraphobia—cont'd
panic disorder with, 426
care plan for, 429
pharmacological treatment of, 306
Agranulocytosis, drug-induced
in elderly, 656
interventions for, 259
mechanisms of, 265
AIDS; see Acquired immunodeficiency syndrome
Aid to the Disabled (ATD), 9
Akathisia
definition of, 230, 245
drug-induced, 254-255
interactions for, 239
interventions for, 259
ECT and, 583
Akinesia, antipsychotic drug-induced, 255
Akineton; see Biperiden
Al-Anon, 536
Alarm reaction in stress adaptation syndrome, 39, 40
Alateen, 536
Alcohol
for anxiety, 298
drug interactions with
benzodiazepines, 302
diazepam, 303
in elderly, 659
TCAs, 279
toxicity and, 211
limit setting and, 329
screening questionnaires for, 530
Alcohol abuse, 510-516
care plan for, 517, 547
cost of, 3
and crime, 511
death and disability from, 510-511, 514
in elderly, 515, 649-651
etiological theories of, 511
medications for, 534
pharmacokinetics in, 511-512
pharmacotherapy for, 514-516
physiological effects of, 512-514
in pregnancy, 515
prevalence rates for
lifetime, 346
12-month, 3, 345, 352, 384, 424, 452, 478, 502
relapse in recovery from, 538
in schizophrenics, 369
suicide among, 414
treatment of, 532, 533

Alcohol abuse—cont'd
withdrawal and detoxification in, 513, 515-516
Alcoholic dementia, 469
Alcoholic hallucinosis, 513
Alcoholics Anonymous (AA), 535-537
Alcoholic tremor, 231
Aliphatics, 261
Alliance for the Mentally Ill (AMI), family support groups of, 368
Alpha-2 agonists, for child and adolescent psychiatric disorders, 628, 632
Alphaprodine, 521
Alprazolam, 304
for aggression, 165
for anxiety disorders, 306
dosage and pharmacokinetics of, 301
in elderly, 659
for generalized anxiety disorder, 425
Altered consciousness, in schizophrenia, 358, 361-362
Altered perception
antipsychotic drugs and, 250-251
in dementia, 458
in depression, 390
of manic patients, 409
in schizophrenia, 358, 359-360
milieu management for, 373
Altruism, group therapy and, 172
Aluminum salts, and Alzheimer's disease, 464
Alzheimer, Alois, 461
Alzheimer's disease (AD), 458-466
acetylcholine and, 77
and ADL impairment, 463
biological basis of, 81
brain characteristics of, 459-460, 461
midbrain, 467
plaques, 461
ventricular enlargement, 364
definition of, 452
description and incidence of, 458-459, 460, 461-462
DSM-IV criteria for, 462
etiology of, 463-464
family considerations of, 465-466
four A's of, 462
neurotransmitters and, 77, 225
vs. Pick's disease, 468
progression of, 462-463
symptoms of, 464-465

Alzheimer's tangles, 461
Amantadine
    action of, 235
    anticholinergic interactions with,
        240
    and dopamine, 224
    psychiatric side effects of, 235
    for stimulant dependence, 534
Ambivalence
    definition of, 351
    in schizophrenia, 360-361, 362
Amenorrhea
    in anorexia nervosa, 550-551
    definition of, 551
American Nurses Association (ANA)
    code of ethics, and HIV, 672, 673
    guidelines on psychopharmacol-
        ogy, 223
American Psychiatric Association
    (APA), admission guidelines
    of, 48
Amines, biogenic
    MAOIs and, 287
    TCAs and, 274
Amino acids
    and blood-brain barrier, 226
    location and pathways of, 76
    neurotransmitter system, 224
Amitriptyline, 281
    anticholinergic effects of, 456
    cardiotoxicity of, 275, 277
    characteristics of, 276-277
    in elderly, 656
    potency of, vs. trihexyphenidyl, 237
Amnesia, 445
    in Alzheimer's disease, 462
    dissociative, 445-446
    DSM-IV criteria for, 453
Amoxapine, 281-282
    anticholinergic effects of, 456
    antipsychotic drug interactions
        with, 260
    characteristics of, 276-277
    potency of, vs. trihexyphenidyl, 237
Amphetamines
    abuse of, 523-524
    drug interactions with, 260
        MAOIs, 287-288
    and psychotic state, 363
    urine detection of, 505
    uses and effects of, 508-509
    withdrawal from, 516
Amygdala, and memory, 72
Amyloid, in Alzheimer's disease,
    463, 464

Amyloid derived diffusable ligand
    (ADDL), 463
ANA; see American Nurses
    Association
Anafranil; see Clomipramine
Analgesics, depression from, 394
Analysis step, in nurse-patient rela-
    tionship, 129
Anectine; see Succinylcholine
Anergia, 351
Anesthetics, MAOI interactions
    with, 287-288
Anger, 157
    as adult manifestation of child-
        hood sexual abuse, 600
    and aggression, 158-160; see also
        Aggression
    definition of, 158
    in group therapy, 179
    intervention for, 163-164
    ventilation of, 165
Anhedonia
    definition of, 351, 383
    ECT and, 583
Anhidrosis, from antidepressants,
    281
Anorexia
    ECT and, 583
    milieu management for, 401
Anorexia nervosa, 550-559
    behavior of, 551-553
    biological basis of, 81
    care plan for, 558
    definition of, 551
    DSM-IV criteria for, 550-551
    etiology of, 553-555
    family issues in, 557
    management of, 555-556, 558-559
Antabuse; see Disulfiram
Antacids
    anticholinergic interactions with,
        240
    benzodiazepine interactions with,
        302
Antiandrogen therapy, for sexual dis-
    orders, 498
Antianxiety drugs, 298-307; see also
    specific agents
    for aggression, 165
    benzodiazepines, 300-305
    buspirone, 305
    clomipramine, 305
    for cognitive disorders, 471
    dosage and pharmacokinetics
        of, 301

Antianxiety drugs–cont'd
    in elderly, 651, 658-659
        alcohol interaction with, 659
        special considerations for, 656
    history of, 298-299
    propranolol, 305
    SSRIs, 306
    TCAs, 305-306
Antiarrhythmic drugs, anticholiner-
    gic interactions with, 240
Antibiotics, depression from, 394
Anticholinergic drugs, 234
    and cranial nerves, 77
    delirium from, 455
    for drug-induced parkinsonism,
        235, 236
    drug interactions with
        antipsychotic drugs, 260
        MAOIs, 287-288
        TCAs, 279
    for Parkinson's disease, 236-241
        desired effects of, 237-238
        dosages, 237
        drug interactions with, 240
        nursing implications for,
            240-241
        side effects of, 238-240
    prophylactic use of, 256-257
    toxicity of, 240
Anticholinergic effect(s)
    from antipsychotic drugs,
        254, 372
    definition of, 230, 245, 271
    in elderly
        from antidepressants, 658
        from psychotropic drugs, 656
    from MAOIs, 287, 289
    of psychotropic drugs, 456
    of TCAs, 275, 279
Anticonvulsants
    benzodiazepines as, 301-302
    depression from, 394
    for stimulant dependence, 534
    TCA interactions with, 279
Antidepressants, 270-290
    administration of, 399
    for bulimia nervosa, 563
    classifications of, 271, 272
    for cognitive disorders, 470-471
    drug interactions with, dimensions
        of, 285
    in elderly, 651, 657-658
        alcohol interaction with, 659
        side effects of, 658
        special considerations for, 656

Antidepressants—cont'd
goals for treatment with, 272
historical perspective on, 270-273
indications for, 274
MAOIs, 286-290; see also MAOIs
mechanisms of action, 273
orthostatic hypotension from, 278
for panic disorder, 427-428
for rape and sexual assault, 596
side effects of, 400
SSRIs, 284-286; see also SSRIs
for survivors of childhood sexual
abuse, 602
treatment parameters of, 276-277
tricyclic, 273-275, 277-284; see also
Tricyclic antidepressants
drug interactions with, 279, 280
newer agents, 282-284
nursing implications for, 279-
281
overdose of, 279-280
pharmacokinetics and dosing
of, 275, 276
pharmacological effects of, 274
side effects of, 275, 277-278
for suicidal thoughts, 278-279
Antidiarrheal drugs, anticholinergic
interactions with, 240
Antiepileptic drugs, history of, 222
Antihistamines, anticholinergic interactions with, 240
Antihypertensives
depression from, 394
MAOI interactions with, 287-288
Antiinflammatory agents, depression
from, 394
Antimanic drugs, 270, 271, 290-296
administration of, 399
carbamazepine, 294
in elderly, 659
indications for, 274
lithium, 290-293; see also Lithium
valproic acid, 294-298
Antineoplastic agents, depression
from, 394
Antioxidants, for Alzheimer's disease, 465
Antiparkinson drugs, 229-242
anticholinergic, 234, 236-241
desired effects of, 237-238
dosages, 237
drug interactions with, 240
nursing implications for, 240-
241
side effects of, 238-240

Antiparkinson drugs—cont'd
antipsychotic drug interaction
with, 260
depression from, 394
dopaminergic agents, 234-235
neurotransmitters and, 233-234
Parkinson's disease/parkinsonism
and, 229-231, 233
Antipsychiatric model, depression
in, 393
Antipsychotic drugs, 244-268; see also
specific agents
for aggression, 165
for ASD/PTSD, 439
for child and adolescent psychiatric disorders, 628, 630-632
classification of, 245-246, 248
by chemical class, 261-265
by potency, 246
for cognitive disorders, 470
dosage of, 247
in elderly, 651, 658
alcohol interaction with, 659
special considerations for, 656
EPSEs from, treatment of,
237-238
historical perspective on, 244-245
interactions with, 258, 260
SSRIs, 284
TCAs, 279
lithium combination with, 292
neurochemical theory of schizophrenia and, 249-250
and number of hospitalized mental
patients, 246
nursing implications for, 257-258,
260-261
orthostatic hypotension from, 278
overdose of, 257-258
parenteral, 252, 253
parkinsonism from, 233, 235, 236
pharmacokinetics of, 251-253
pharmacological effects of,
250-251
and psychosurgery, 586
for schizophrenia, 357
schizophrenic symptom modification by, 250-251
side effects of, 253-257, 258, 372
in children and adolescents, 631
interventions for, 258-259
Antisocial personality disorder,
482-483
DSM-IV criteria for, 482

Antisocial personality
disorder—cont'd
prevalence rates of
lifetime, 346
12-month, 3, 345, 352, 384,
424, 452, 478, 502
Antituberculosis agents, depression
from, 394
Antiviral drugs, CNS effects of, 676
Anxiety, 147-153
in adjustment disorder, 439
as adult manifestation of childhood sexual abuse, 600
in bulimia nervosa, 561
in children and adolescents, medications for, 628
coping with, 150, 152-153
and crisis, 153
definition of, 299
in depression, 389-390
etiology of, 149-150
Freud's types of, 30
and illness, 153
as indication for psychosurgery, 586
interventions for, 425
levels of, 150, 151
NANDA diagnosis related to, 148
neurotransmitters and, 225
pharmacologic treatment of; see
Antianxiety drugs
in phobic disorders, 432
process of, 148
recurring themes of, 149
respondent conditioning and, 575
in stress adaptation syndrome, 39
stressors and, 147-149
in Sullivan's interpersonal model,
33, 36
TCAs for, 274
tension of, 33
Anxiety disorders, 423-440
adjustment disorders, 439
ASD and PTSD, 433-439
care plan for, 440
biological basis of, 81
in children and adolescents, 624-
625
DSM-IV criteria and NANDA diagnoses for, 423
ECT and, 583
in elderly, 648-649
generalized anxiety disorder, 423-
426
with HIV infection, 675

Anxiety disorders—cont'd
obsessive-compulsive disorder, 428-432
panic disorder, 426-428, 429
phobic disorders, 432
prevalence rates for
lifetime, 346
12-month, 3, 345, 352, 384, 424, 452, 478, 502
Anxiety-related disorders; *see* Anxiety disorders; Dissociative disorders; Somatoform disorders
Anxiolytic, definition of, 299; *see also* Antianxiety drugs
Anxious/fearful (cluster C) personality disorder, 487-490
Apartment living programs, 98
Apathy, 33
definition of, 351, 383
and nurse-patient relationship, 133-134
in schizophrenia, 362
Aphasia, 71
in Alzheimer's disease, 462
Apolipoprotein E4 (Apo-E4), and Alzheimer's disease, 464
Appalachian culture, 209
Appearance alterations, in manic patients, 408-409
Appetite stimulation, from TCAs, 274
Apraxia, in Alzheimer's disease, 462
Arabic world view, 204, 206-207
Arachnoid, 77
Arachnoid villi, 79
Aricept; *see* Donepezil
Arrhythmias
in anorexia nervosa, 553
from antidepressants,, 400
antipsychotic drugs and, 253
from TCA interactions, 279
Artane; *see* Trihexyphenidyl
ASD; *see* Acute stress disorder
Asendin; *see* Amoxapine
Ashkenazi Jews, pharmacodynamics of, 211
Asians
depression in, 387
pharmacokinetics of, 211
world view of, 205, 207-208
Asperger's disorder, 620, 621
Assault, 157
definition of, 45, 158
staff members as victims of, 168-169

Assault and battery, wrongful involuntary commitment and, 60
Assault cycle, 161
interventions based on, 164-168
Assaultive patient
balancing needs and rights of, 331
limit setting for, 328
Assertiveness, 160
definition of, 158
training, 574
Assessment
in behavioral interventions, 576
in case management, 104
for chemical dependency, 504
and cultural competence, 213, 215
of elderly, 652-654
written materials for, 641
of family
common situations for, 187-188
guideline for, 193
initial, 192-194
skills for, 190-191
in hospital-based care, 93
initial, 136-137, 138
in nurse-patient relationship, 127
therapeutic communication and, 119
written, 141, 142-143, 144
Assistance, in psychiatric history, 4
Association for Retired People (AARP), 640
Association neurons, 75
Association of Recovering Motorcyclists, 536
Asylum, 5-6
definition of, 3
Ataractics, 245; *see also* Antipsychotic drugs
Ataxia
from antidepressants, 400
from benzodiazepines, 302
Ativan; *see* Lorazepam
Atropine, 236
anticholinergic effects of, 456
for ECT, 581
potency of, vs. trihexyphenidyl, 237
Attachment, in borderline personality disorder, 484
Attention-deficit hyperactivity disorder (ADHD), 622-623
cognitive behavioral therapy in, 632-633
and conduct disorder, 623
definition of, 617

Attention-deficit hyperactivity disorder—cont'd
DSM-IV criteria for, 623
medications for, 628, 632
prevalence of, 622
psychosocial adversity and, 619
Atypical depression, 386
definition of, 383
treatment of, 396
Auditory aphasia, 71
Auditory hallucinations, in schizophrenia, 359
Authority, delegating, 60-61
Autism, 620-621
definition of, 351
prevalence of, 620
in schizophrenia, 360
Autonomic nervous system, 77, 78
Autonomy vs. shame, in Erikson's stages of development, 34
Autosomal dominant inheritance, 618
and Tourette's syndrome, 626
Autosomal recessive inheritance, 618
Aventyl; *see* Nortriptyline
Avoidant personality disorder, 488-489
Avolition, 351
Axon(s), 75, 223
definition of, 65, 221
Azapirones, 305
AZT; *see* Zidovudine

B

Bacterial infections, with HIV, 669
Balance
definition of, 311
in milieu management, 316-317
in substance abuse management, 535
in therapeutic environment, 323, 330
Banishment, in psychiatric history, 4
Barbiturates
abuse of, 516, 518-519
interactions with
alcohol, in elderly, 659
antipsychotic drugs, 260
TCAs, 279
urine detection of, 505
uses and effects of, 506-507
Basal ganglia, 72, 75, 231
definition of, 65, 230, 245
disorders of, vs. cerebellar disorders, 73

Basal ganglia—cont'd
  Parkinson's disease and, 81,
      230, 467
  and Tourette's syndrome, 626
Baseline observations, in behavioral
    interventions, 576
Battered woman syndrome, 606
Battery, 157
  definition of, 45, 158
Beck Depression Inventory (BDI),
    387
Beck's cognitive-behavioral models,
    29, 36-37
Bed wetting, 626, 627
Behavior
  of Alzheimer's disease, 462,
      464-465
  in anorexia, 551-553, 554
  in bipolar disorder, 406, 408-409
  in bulimia nervosa, 560-561, 562
  in depression, 388-390
  in nurse-patient relation-
      ship, 129
  psychobiological bases of; see Psy-
      chobiological bases of behavior
  psychopathology and, 345
  in schizophrenia, 357-362
  speech and, 115
  work-defeating, 326
Behavioral disorders, ECT
    and, 583
Behavioral model, substance abuse
    treatment, 532
Behavioral sensitization, and ASD
    and PTSD, 435-436
Behaviorists, and depression, 392
Behavior modification, 572; see also
    Behavior therapy; Operant
    conditioning
Behavior therapy, 24, 570-577
  application of, 571-575
  classical conditioning and,
      570-571
  definition of, 20
  intervention and, 575-576
  for obsessive-compulsive disorder,
      431-432
  operant conditioning and, 571
  for phobic disorders, 432
Belief(s)
  in A-B-C theory of personality, 37
  cultural, regarding health and ill-
      ness, 209
Benadryl; see Diphenhydramine
Benzisoxazole, 264

Benzodiazepines, 300-305
  history of, 222, 299
  interactions with, 302, 303
    antipsychotic drugs, 260
    SSRIs, 284
    TCAs, 279
  for panic disorder, 427-428
  for alcohol withdrawal, 534
  for anxiety disorders, 306
  for ASD/PTSD, 438
  for borderline personality disor-
      der, 485
  for cognitive disorders, 471
  dosage of, 301
  in elderly, 303, 651, 658-659
    alcohol interaction with, 659
    special considerations for, 656
  for generalized anxiety disorder,
      425-426
  nursing implications for, 302-304
  overdoses, 302-303
  pharmacokinetics of, 300-301
  pharmacological effect of, 300
  for rape and sexual assault, 596
  side effects of, 301-302, 303
  for survivors of childhood sexual
      abuse, 602
  in trauma recovery, 592
  urine detection of, 505
  uses and effects of, 506-507
  withdrawal from, 304
Benztropine, 236
  anticholinergic effects of, 456
  dosages of, 237
  for Parkinson's disease, 241
  potency of, vs. trihexyphenidyl, 237
  prophylactic, for EPSEs, 257
Berlin and Fowkes's LEARN
    model, 213
Bertalanffy's general systems theory, 189
Beta-blockers
  antipsychotic drug interactions
      with, 260
  for anxiety disorders, 306
Binge, definition of, 551
Binge-eating
  and anorexia nervosa, 551
  and bulimia nervosa, 560
Binge-eating disorder (BED), 566
Bini, Luciano, 580
Biochemical abnormalities, and
    Alzheimer's disease, 464
Biochemical theories
  of bipolar disorder, 409-410
  of schizophrenia, 362-363

Biogenic amines
  and depression, 273
  MAOIs and, 287
  TCAs and, 274
Biological assessment
  in cultural assessment work-
      sheet, 214
  for depression, 397
Biological factors
  of aggression, 160-161
  of anorexia nervosa, 553-554
  of borderline personality disor-
      der, 484
  of bulimia nervosa, 561-562
Biological theories
  of alcoholism, 511
  anxiety in, 149-150
  of bipolar disorder, 409-410
  of depression, 390-392
  of schizophrenia, 362-365
Biological vs. psychodynamic argu-
    ment, 346
Biperiden
  anticholinergic effects of, 456
  dosages of, 237
  for Parkinson's disease, 241
  potency of, vs. trihexyphenidyl, 237
Bipolar disorder(s), 404-413
  in AIDS patients, lithium treat-
      ment of, 676
  behavior of, 406, 408-409
  care plan for, 412
  in children and adolescents, 625
  definition of, 271, 383
  description of, 404
  differences in, on mood contin-
      uum, 407
  DSM-IV criteria for, 384, 404-406
  in elderly, 646
  etiology of, 409-410
  interventions for, 410
  management of, 410-413
  prevalence rates for
    lifetime, 346
    12-month, 3, 345, 352, 384,
        424, 452, 478, 502
  treatment success rate of, 4
Blackouts, 502
Bladder distention, psychotropic
    drug-induced, 657
Blame theories, of schizophrenia, 366
Bleuler, Eugene, 5, 7, 357
  and schizophrenia, 352, 353
Bloch's ethnic/cultural assessment
    guide, 213

Blocking
    definition of, 351
    in schizophrenia, 360
Blood-brain barrier, 225-226
    benzodiazepines and, 300-301
    definition of, 221
Blood products, and HIV transmission, 670
Boarding homes, 98
Body language, 116-117
Borderline personality disorder
        (BPD), 483-486
    care plan for, 491
    DSM-IV criteria for, 483
Bowen family systems theory, 190
BPD; *see* Borderline personality
        disorder
Bradykinesia, 233
    from antipsychotic drugs, 255
    definition of, 230, 245
    Parkinson's disease and, 231
Brain, 64-65, 66
    of Alzheimer's patient, 459-460, 461
    anatomy and physiology of; *see*
        Neuroanatomy/
        neurophysiology
    atrophy of, schizophrenia and, 364
    normal, 460, 461
Brain disorders
    in AIDS patients, 675-676
        corticosteroids and, 678
    cost of, 3
Brain imaging
    of schizophrenia, 363
    techniques, 364
Brainstem, 73-75
    effects of aging and disease
        on, 233
Breggin, P. R., 586
Brevital; *see* Methohexital
Brief psychotic disorder, 375
Bromocriptine
    action of, 235
    for antipsychotic drug side
        effects, 256
    psychiatric side effects of, 235
    for stimulant dependence, 534
Bruch, Hilde, 553
Bulimarexia, 560
Bulimia nervosa, 559-564
    behavior of, 560-561
    care plan for, 565
    definition of, 551
    and depression, 562-563
    DSM-IV criteria for, 559-560

Bulimia nervosa—cont'd
    etiology of, 561-562
    management of, 563-564
Bupropion, 282-283
    characteristics of, 276-277
    in elderly, 656, 657
    for suicidal patients, 279
Burckhardt, Gottlieb, 585
BuSpar; *see* Buspirone
Buspirone, 299
    as antianxiety drug, 305
    for cognitive disorders, 471
    dosage and pharmacokinetics
        of, 301
    in elderly, 658
Butorphanol, 521
Butyrophenone, 262

C

Cade, John, 222, 291
Caffeine
    and cognitive disorders, 472
    and drug toxicity, 211
CAGE questionnaire, 530
Calix Society, 536
Campinha-Bacote's model of cultural competence, 202,
        208-213
    assessment worksheet for, 214
Cancers, with HIV infection, 669
Cannabis, 508-509; *see also*
        Marijuana
Carbamazepine
    for bipolar disorder, 294
    for borderline personality disorder, 485
    in elderly, 659
    history of, 222
    interactions with
        SSRIs, 284
        TCAs, 279
    for stimulant dependence, 534
Carbohydrate intake, and bulimia
        nervosa, 561
Cardiovascular agents, depression
        from, 394
Cardiovascular system
    antidepressant effects on
        in elderly, 658
    intervention for, 281
    ECT effects on, 584
    TCA effects on, 275, 629-630
Care manager, vs. case management, 87
Care Maps, 105, 106

Care plan(s), 144
    and alcohol abuse, 517, 547
    for anorexia nervosa, 558
    for bipolar disorder, 412
    for bulimia nervosa, 565
    in case management, 109
    for dementia
        of Alzheimer's type, 473
        due to AIDS, 677
    for depression, 402
    for major depression
        with borderline personality disorder, 491
        in elderly, 661
        with pedophilia, 499
    in nursing process, 145
    for pain disorder, 444
    for partner abuse, 611
    for PTSD, 440
    sample of, 145, 347
    for schizophrenia, 374, 376
    standardized, 138, 139
    for substance abuse/dependence, 525
Case management, 101-111
    vs. care manager, 87
    care plan example, 109
    clinical pathways in, 105, 106
    components of, 103, 107-110
    decision tree for, 107
    definition of, 102
    goals and purposes of, 101-102
    history of, 102-103
    location and, 107
    nurse roles and qualities in, 105
    nursing process in, 103-105
    preparation for, 105, 107
Catapres; *see* Clonidine
Catatonia, 352, 353, 357
    definition of, 351
    depression with, treatment
        of, 396
    ECT and, 583
Catatonic schizophrenia, 354
Catecholamines, synthesis of, 235
Catharsis, from group therapy, 172
Caudate nucleus, 72
CBF; *see* Cerebral blood flow
Centered environments, milieu management and, 311
Center for Epidemiologic Scale
        (CES-D), 387
Central nervous system (CNS), 64
    alcohol effects on, 513
    amphetamines and, 523
    anticholinergic effects on, 238, 239

Central nervous system—cont'd
  antidepressants and
      interventions for, 281
      TCAs, 277-278
  antipsychotic drugs and, 250
      EPSEs of, 253-257
      interventions for, 259
  benzodiazepines and, 300
  cocaine and, 523
  components of, 66; *see also* Neu-
      roanatomy/ neurophysiology
  disorders of, and depression, 395
  drug interactions and, 279
  HIV infection and, 675
  LSD and, 528
  MAOIs and, 289
  pathways, 67, 69
  SSRI effects on, 284
Central sulcus, 68
Cerebellar disorders
  vs. basal ganglia disorders, 73
  and intention tremors, 75
Cerebellum, 73, 75
Cerebral blood flow (CBF), and
      schizophrenia, 79, 355,
      364-365
Cerebral cortex, 67-68, 70-71
  definition of, 65
  Parkinson's disease and, 231, 233
Cerebrospinal fluid, 77, 79
  circulation of, 80, 81
Cerebrum, 67-72
Cerletti, Ugo, 580
Certification
  of competency, 14
  for observation and treatment, 49,
      50, 51
Change
  nurse-patient relationship and, 130
  in working with family, 194
Cheeking, 252
Chemical dependency; *see also* Sub-
      stance abuse/dependence
  biological basis of, 82
  depression with, treatment of, 396
Child abuse
  definition of, 617
  and schizophrenia, 366
Child and adolescent psychiatric dis-
      orders, 616-634
  diagnostic categories of, 619-627
      developmental disorders,
          620-624
      elimination disorders, 626-627

Child and adolescent psychiatric dis-
      orders—cont'd
  diagnostic categories of—cont'd
      internalizing disorders, 624-625
      psychotic disorders, 626
      tic disorders, 626
  epidemiology of, 616, 617
  genetic factors of, 617-619
  scope of problem of, 617
  treatment of, 627-633
      cognitive behavioral therapy in,
          632-633
      psychopharmacology in,
          628-632
      settings in, 627-628
Children and adolescents
  cardiovascular responses to TCAs
      in, 275
  depression in, 386-388
      growth hormone secretion
          and, 397
  sexual abuse of, 597-598; *see also*
      Sexual abuse
Chloral hydrate
  alcohol interaction with, 515
  uses and effects of, 506-507
Chlordiazepoxide, 299
  for alcohol withdrawal,
      515-516, 534
  as antianxiety drug, 304
  dosage and pharmacokinetics
      of, 301
  in elderly, 658
Chlorpromazine
  anticholinergic interactions
      with, 240
  for cognitive disorders, 470
  and dopamine receptors, 225
  dosage of, 247
  effects of, 456
  history of, 7, 222, 244-245
  pharmacokinetics of, 251-252
  potency of, 246
      vs. trihexyphenidyl, 237
Chlorprothixene, 262
  dosage of, 247
Choline acetyltransferase (ChAT),
      and Alzheimer's disease, 464
Cholinergic deficit model of
      Alzheimer's disease, 464
Cholinergic system, 224
  location and pathways of, 76
Christian Addiction Rehabilitation
      Association, 536

Cimetidine
  antipsychotic drug interactions
      with, 260
  benzodiazepine interactions
      with, 302
  TCA interactions with, 279
Circadian rhythm changes, and de-
      pression, 391-392
Cirrhosis
  from alcohol abuse, 513
  definition of, 502
Civil law, definition of, 45
Clanging associations, definition
      of, 351
Classical conditioning, 570-571
Clinical depression, definition of, 383
Clinical pathway, in case manage-
      ment, 105, 106
Clinical psychologists, 337
Clomipramine, 285, 305
  for anxiety disorders, 306
  characteristics of, 276-277
  for child and adolescent psychi-
      atric disorders, 629
  for obsessive-compulsive disorder,
      274, 431
Clonazepam
  as anticonvulsant, 302
  for anxiety disorders, 304, 306
  dosage and pharmacokinetics
      of, 301
  for elderly patients, 656
  for panic disorder, 427-428
Clonidine
  for ASD/PTSD, 438
  for child and adolescent psychi-
      atric disorders, 632
  TCA interactions with, 279
Clorazepate, 304
  dosage and pharmacokinetics
      of, 301
  in elderly, 658
Clozapine, 221, 263-264, 631
  agranulocytosis from, 256, 259, 263
      mechanisms of, 265
  anticholinergic effects of, 456
  for cognitive disorders, 470
  dopamine receptors blocked by,
      263
  dosage of, 247
  history of, 222
  potency of, vs. trihexyphenidyl,
      237
  and seizures, 239, 259

Clozaril; *see* Clozapine
Cluster A (odd/eccentric) personality disorder, 479-481
Cluster B (dramatic/erratic) personality disorder, 482-487
DSM-IV criteria and NANDA diagnoses for, 479
Cluster C (anxious/fearful) personality disorder, 487-490
DSM-IV criteria and NANDA diagnoses for, 479
Coalition for Mental Health and Aging, 640
Cocaine
abuse of, 522-523
relapse in recovery from, 538
overdose of, 523
urine detection of, 505
uses and effects of, 508-509
withdrawal from, 516
trazodone for, 306
Cocaine Anonymous, 536
Codeine; *see also* Opioids
abuse of, 521
uses and effects of, 506-507
Codependency, definition of, 502
Cogentin; *see* Benztropine
Cognex; *see* Tacrine
Cognition
and anorexia nervosa and, 554
anxiety and, 151
and bulimia nervosa, 562
depression and, 390
restructuring in nurse-patient relationship, 129, 130
Cognitive appraisal, 40
Cognitive-behavioral models, 29, 36-38
Cognitive behavioral therapy, for child and adolescent psychiatric disorders, 632-633
Cognitive disorders, 451-475
Alzheimer's disease
description and incidence of, 458-459, 460, 461-462
etiology of, 463-464
family considerations of, 465-466
progression of, 462-463
psychiatric symptoms of, 464-465
Creutzfeldt-Jakob disease, 468-469
definition of, 452
delirium, 454-456

Cognitive disorders—cont'd
dementia, 456-458
alcoholic, 469
vascular (multiinfarct), 469
diffuse Lewy body disease, 467
DSM-IV terminology and criteria for, 452, 453-454
Huntington's disease, 468
management of, 470-473
NANDA diagnoses of, 454
Parkinson's disease, 466-467
Pick's disease, 468
TIAs, 469-470
Cognitive impairment, 12-month prevalence rate of, 3, 345, 352, 384, 424, 452, 478, 502
Cognitive theorists, and depression, 392
Cogwheel rigidity, Parkinson's disease and, 231
Cohesiveness, from group therapy, 172
Coleadership, in group therapy, 176
Collaboration
in nurse-patient relationship, 124-125
skills for working with family, 191
Collagen vascular disease, and depression, 395
Colleague role, nurse, 337-338
Collective language systems approach, for family assessment, 190
Coma, 65
Commitment, legal issues of, 48-49, 51-52
deinstitutionalization and, 9
Communication, 114-122
categories of, 114-117
in cultural assessment worksheet, 214
disorders, 622
enhancing, with elderly, 653
impairment in schizophrenics, milieu management for, 373
interpretation of, 115-116
skills
for group therapy, 177-179
for working with family, 191
therapeutic, 117-118
common interferences with, 118, 120-121
definition of, 115
dynamics of, 115

Communication—cont'd
therapeutic—cont'd
essential and influencing variables of, 115
skills for working with family, 191
techniques of, 118, 119-120
Community
deinstitutionalization effects on, 11
support for elderly, 640-641
Community-based care, 14-16, 96-100
and continuum of care, 99-100
home care, 97
outpatient services, 96-97
outreach programs, 98
residential services, 98-99
Community-based milieu, 332
Community meetings
definition of, 311
in therapeutic environment, 322-323
Community mental health
definition of, 3
in psychiatric history, 8-9
Community Mental Health Centers Act (1963), 5, 8, 320
and elderly, 640
Community resources
for ASD/PTSD, 439
for families, 195
Comorbidity, substance abuse in, 505
Compensation, as defense mechanism, 31
Compliance, medication
in elderly, 652
in schizophrenics, 372
Compulsions, 624
definition of, 429
DSM-IV criteria for, 430
Compulsive traits, 477-478
Computed tomography (CT), 364
Concrete thinking
definition of, 351
in schizophrenia, 361
Conditioning, 572
classical, 570-571
operant, 571
Condoms, and HIV, 672
Conduct disorder, 623-624
prevalence of, 622
Confidentiality
in group therapy, 176
and HIV testing, 672

Confidentiality—cont'd
  in nurse-patient relationship, 127
  in patient bill of rights, 58
  of records, right to, 53-54
  in working with family, 194
Confinement, in psychiatric history, 4
Conflicting values, and nurse-patient
    relationship, 132
Confusion
  from antidepressants, 400
  from lithium, 400
  as schizophrenic symptom, anti-
    psychotic drugs and, 251
Consciousness, 27
  altered, 358, 361-362
Consensual validation, 36
Consent
  and administration of medica-
    tions, 56
  coercion vs., between sexual part-
    ners, 493
  from conservators, 51
  for ECT, 581
  right to give or refuse, 55-56
Conservator
  definition of, 45
  for gravely disabled persons, 51
Constipation
  from anticholinergics, 239
  from antidepressants, 281, 400
  from antipsychotic drugs, 258
  from MAOIs, 400
  from psychotropic drugs, 657
Constitution, written, in therapeutic
    environment, 323
Consultant role, nurse, 340
Consultation, in case manage-
    ment, 108
Containment, 166
Content theme, in communica-
    tion, 116
Contingency contracting, 574
Continuous reinforcement, 572
Continuum of care, 6, 86-90
  accessing, 12, 89-90
  decision tree for, 22, 88, 89
  definition of, 3, 20, 86
  development of, 15-16
  for dual diagnosis, 548
  influences of community-based
    care on, 99-100
  managed care in, 87, 88, 89
  for mental illness in elderly,
    640-642

Continuum of care—cont'd
  psychotherapeutic management in,
    19-25
  for schizophrenics, 370-374
Contralateral, definition of, 65
Conversion, as defense mechan-
    ism, 32
Conversion disorder, 442-445
  DSM-IV criteria for, 441
Cooperation, lack of, and nurse-pa-
    tient relationship, 133
Cooperatives, 370
Coping
  with anxiety, 150, 152-153
  and crisis, 153
  family, 192
  with stress, 41
Corona radiata, 67
Corpus callosum, 65, 67
Corticospinal tract, 68, 69, 70
Corticosteroids, in AIDS pa-
    tients, 678
Cortisol
  definition of, 383
  and depression, 391, 397
Counterconditioning, 575
Countertransference, 134
Crack cocaine, 522
Cranial nerves, 77
  anticholinergic effects on, 238-239
Craniosacral nervous system, 77
Creatinine clearance, and pharmaco-
    kinetics in elderly, 656-657
Creative expression group, 173
Creutzfeldt-Jakob (CJ) disease,
    468-469
Crime
  alcohol and, 511
  violation by, 591-592; see also Vio-
    lence, victims of
Crisis, 153
Crisis community residences, 370
Crisis intervention
  in case management, 109-110
  for rape and sexual assault, 596
  strategies of, 153-155
  vs. stress counseling, 154
  in trauma recovery, 592
Crisis phase of assault cycle, 161
  interventions for, 164, 166
Critical incident debriefing, 436
Cross-dependence, 530
Cross-sensitization, ASD and PTSD
    and, 436

Crying, and nurse-patient relation-
    ship, 133
Cryptococcus neoformans. in AIDS pa-
    tients, 675
Cultural assessment, 212-213
  worksheet for, 214
Cultural awareness
  and cultural competence, 209
  definition of, 200, 208
Cultural axiology
  of African/African-American/His-
    panic/Arabic world view, 206
  of Asian/Asian-American/Polyne-
    sian world view, 207
  of European American world
    view, 205
  of Native American world
    view, 208
Cultural care diversity and universal-
    ity theory, 202-204
Cultural competence, 199-216
  definition, 199, 200, 201
  importance of, 201
  interlocking paradigm of,
    201-213, 215
    assessment factor in, 213, 215
    nurse-patient interaction in, 202
    philosophy factor in, 204-208
    process factor in, 208-213
    theory factor in, 202-204
Cultural diversity, 199-200
Cultural encounter, 213
  definition of, 200, 208
Cultural knowledge
  and cultural competence, 209-212
  definition, 200, 208
Cultural negotiation, 203
Cultural preservation, 203
Cultural repatterning, 203
Cultural skill, 212-213
  definition of, 200, 208
Culture
  definition of, 200, 201
  depression and, 387
  importance of, 201
  and nurse-patient interaction,
    203, 204
  in partner abuse, 606
Cupping, 210-211
  definition of, 200
Custodial care, 311
Cycle of violence, 606, 607, 608
Cyclothymia, definition of, 383
Cyclothymic disorder, 384, 405, 406

Cylert; *see* Pemoline
Cytochrome P-450 enzymes, SSRI and antidepressant inhibition of, 285

D

Daidzein, 534
Daidzin, 534
Dangerous patient, balancing rights of, 331
Dantrium; *see* Dantrolene
Dantrolene, 256
DAT; *see* Dementia of Alzheimer's type
Data collection, in nurse-patient relationship, 129
Date rape, 594
DDAVP; *see* Desmopressin
Debriefing meetings, after patient restraint, 168
Decision-making, depression and, 398-399
Decussation of pyramids, 74, 230
Defense mechanisms, 27, 30, 31-32
    in somatoform disorders, 440-441
Degenerative diseases, biological basis of, 81
Deinstitutionalization, 9-11
    and case management, 102
    definition of, 3
    and elderly, 640, 641
    homelessness and, 11, 12, 13
    in psychiatric history, 8
Delirium, 454-456
    from antidepressants
        intervention for, 281
        TCAs, 470-471
    clinical example of, 359
    definition of, 452
    vs. dementia, 456
    differential diagnosis of, 457
    DSM-IV criteria for, 452, 453
    features of, 455
    with HIV infection, 675
    nurse-patient relationship and, 470
Delirium tremens (DTs), 513
Delusional disorder(s), 375
    with HIV infection, 675
Delusion(s)
    definition of, 124, 351
    in dementia, 458
    with depression, 390
        in elderly, 644
    ECT and, 583

Delusion(s)–cont'd
    and nurse-patient relationship, 132
    paranoid, in elderly, 648
    in schizophrenia, 361
    types of, 361
Dementia, 456-458
    AIDS, 675
        care plan for, 677
        treatment of, 677, 678
    alcoholic, 469
    biological basis of, 81
    cost of, 3
    of Creutzfeldt-Jakob disease, 468
    definition of, 452
    delirium vs., 456
    vs. depression, 395, 396
        in elderly, 644
    differential diagnosis of, 457
    from DLBD, 467
    DSM-IV criteria for, 453
    multiinfarct, 469
    nonreversible, 458
    nurse-patient relationship and, 470
    in Parkinson's disease, 231, 233, 466
    reversible, 458
    vascular, 469
Dementia of Alzheimer's type (DAT), 458; *see also* Alzheimer's disease
    care plan for, 473
    DSM-IV criteria for, 462
    family issues of, 466
    genetics of, 463
Dementia praecox, 352, 353, 357
Dementia pugilistica, 82
Demerol; *see* Meperidine
Demyelinating diseases, biological basis of, 81
Dendrites, 75, 223
    definition of, 65, 221
Denial
    as defense mechanism, 31
    and nurse-patient relationship, 133
    in somatoform disorders, 440-441
    in substance abuse, 504, 505
Depakene; *see* Valproic acid
Dependence
    on benzodiazepines, 301
    definition of, 299, 502
Dependent personality disorder, 487-488
Depersonalization, 446-447
    definition of, 423
    DSM-IV criteria for, 446

Depressants; *see also* Barbiturates; *specific agents*
    abuse of, 516, 518-519
    anticholinergic interactions with, 240
    benzodiazepine interactions with, 302
    MAOI interactions with, 287-288
    urine detection of, 505
    uses and effects of, 506-508
    withdrawal from, 516
Depressed affect, and nurse-patient relationship, 133-134
Depression, 384-403
    assessment of, 393-395, 397
        biological and nonbiological, 397
        cultural issues and, 394
        in elderly, 394
        instruments for, 387
    in adjustment disorder, 439
    amine theory of, 273
    behavior of, 388-390
    biological theories of, 390-392
    bulimia and, 562-563
    care plan for, 402, 491
    in children and adolescents, 625
        medications for, 628, 630
    clinical features influencing treatment of, 396
    cocaine-induced, 522
    costs associated with, 385
    criteria and symptoms of, 385-388
    definition of, 271
    vs. dementia, 395
    drugs and toxins inducing, 394
    dysthymic disorder, 388
    ECT and, 582, 583, 584
    in elderly, 643-646
    etiology of, 390-393
    family issues of, 403
    with HIV infection, 675
    illnesses associated with, 395
    as indication for psychosurgery, 586
    interventions for, 399
    lifetime prevalence rate of, 644
    major, 385-388; *see also* Major depressive disorder
    management of, 397-403
    neurochemical theory of, 271
        MAOIs and, 286
    neurotransmitters and, 77, 79, 81, 225

Depression—cont'd
  in obsessive-compulsive disor-
      der, 430
  panic disorder with, 426
  in Parkinson's disease, 231, 233,
      234, 466
  psychoeducational issues for work-
      ing with, 325
  psychological theories of, 392-393
  in schizophrenia, 368
  sociological theory of, 393
  and suicide, 414
      TCAs for, 278-279
  symptoms of, 386
Depression Guideline Panel, 393
Derealization, 423
Desensitization, systematic, 575
Desipramine
  as antianxiety drug, 306
  anticholinergic effects of, 456
  for bulimia nervosa, 563
  characteristics of, 276-277
  for child and adolescent psychi-
      atric disorders, 629
  for cognitive disorders, 471
  in elderly, 656
  potency of, vs. trihexyphenidyl, 237
  for stimulant dependence, 534
  as TCA, 282
Desmopressin, 629
Despair vs. integrity, in Erikson's
      stages of development, 35
Desyrel; see Trazodone
Detachment
  as adult manifestation of child-
      hood sexual abuse, 600
  in borderline personality disor-
      der, 484
Detoxification; see also Withdrawal
  from alcohol, 515-516
  from amphetamines, 524
  from barbiturates, 518-519
  from cocaine, 524
  from hallucinogens, 529
  from opioids, 521
Devaluation, 478
Development
  Erikson's stages of, adult manifes-
      tations of, 34-35
  family, stages of, 182-183
  model, 28, 30, 33
  personality, Sullivan's model
      of, 36
Developmental disorders, children
      and adolescent, 620-624

Developmental theories
  and bipolar disorder, 409
  and depression, 392
  of schizophrenia, 365-366
Dexamethasone suppression test
      (DST)
  definition of, 383
  depression and, 391, 397
Dexedrine; see Dextroamphetamine
Dextroamphetamine, for child and
      adolescent psychiatric disor-
      ders, 629
Diabetes insipidus, lithium and,
      291-292
Diagnosis; see also Assessment
  as aggression variable, 163
  in elderly, 643
  NANDA, 137, 139
  in nursing process, 137
  of response to torture, 593
  therapeutic communication
      and, 119
  in working with family, 195
*Diagnostic and Statistical Manual of
      Mental Disorders* (DSM), evo-
      lution of schizophrenia sub-
      typing in, 357
*Diagnostic and Statistical Manual of
      Mental Disorders-III* (DSM-
      III), 619
*Diagnostic and Statistical Manual
      of Mental Disorders-IV*
      (DSM-IV), 345
  classification of mental retarda-
      tion, 620
  criteria
      for anorexia nervosa, 550-551, 559
      for antisocial personality disor-
          der, 482
      of anxiety-related disor-
          ders, 423
      for ASD and PTSD, 433
      for attention-deficit hyperactiv-
          ity disorder, 623
      for avoidant personality disor-
          der, 490
      for bipolar disorders, 404-406
      for borderline personality disor-
          der, 483
      for bulimia nervosa, 559-560
      for cognitive disorders,
          453-454
      of cognitive disorders, 454
      for delirium, 452
      for dementia, 453

*Diagnostic and Statistical Manual
      of Mental Disorders-IV*—cont'd
  criteria—cont'd
      for dementia of Alzheimer's
          type, 462
      for dependent personality disor-
          der, 488
      for dissociative disorders, 446
      for generalized anxiety disor-
          der, 424
      of histrionic personality disor-
          der, 487
      for major depressive disorder, 386
      for mood disorders, 382, 384, 384
      for narcissistic personality disor-
          der, 486
      for obsessive-compulsive disor-
          der, 430, 490
      for panic attack, 426
      for panic disorder, 427
      for paranoid personality disor-
          der, 480
      for paraphilias, 495
      of personality disorders, 479
      of phobias, 432
      for schizoid personality disor-
          der, 481
      for schizophrenia, 353-357
      for schizotypal personality dis-
          orders, 481
      for sexual disorders, 494, 495
      for somatization disorder, 442
      for somatoform disorders, 441
      of substance abuse/dependence,
          530, 531
      of substance dependence/
          abuse, 507
  pervasive developmental disorders
      in, 620
Diagnostic Interview Schedule
      (DIS), 387
Diarrhea, from lithium, 400
Diazepam, 304
  alcohol interaction with, 303, 515
  for alcohol withdrawal, 534
  dosage and pharmacokinetics
      of, 301
  in elderly, 658
  for hallucinogens overdose,
      529, 535
  for status epilepticus, 301-302
  withdrawal from, 516
Diazoxide, antipsychotic drug inter-
      action with, 260
Dibenzodiazepine, 263

Dibenzoxazepine, 262
Diencephalon, 72-73
    definition of, 65
Differential reinforcement,
    572, 573
Diffuse Lewy body disease
    (DLBD), 467
Diffusion vs. identity, in Erikson's
    stages of development, 35
Dihydroindolone, 262
Dilaudid; *see* Hydromorphone
Diphenhydramine
    anticholinergic effects of, 456
    for Parkinson's disease, 241
    potency of, vs. trihexyphenidyl, 237
Discharge planning, 93
Discharge summaries, 144
Discriminative stimulus, 571
Disease model, of substance abuse
    treatment, 532
Disinhibition, 299
Disorganized schizophrenia, 355, 357
    DSM-IV criteria for, 354
    milieu management for, 373
Displacement
    as defense mechanism, 32
    in somatoform disorders, 440, 441
Disruptive behavior disorders, 622-624
Disruptive patient, milieu manage-
    ment for, 372
Dissociation, 33, 36
    as defense mechanism, 32
    definition of, 423, 445, 478
Dissociative amnesia, 445-446
Dissociative disorders, 445-448
    DSM-IV criteria for, 423, 446
    NANDA diagnoses for, 423
Dissociative fugue, 446
Dissociative identity disorder,
    447-448
    DSM-IV criteria for, 446
Disulfiram, 514
    for alcoholism treatment, 534
    benzodiazepine interaction
        with, 302
Diuretics, lithium interactions
    with, 292
Diurnal enuresis, 627
Dix, Dorothea, 6
Dizziness, benzodiazepine-
    induced, 302
DLBD; *see* Diffuse Lewy body disease
DMT, 526
Doctrine of privileged communica-
    tion, 53

Documentation
    and aggression, 163
    liability, 61
    of restraint and seclusion, 168
Dolophine; *see* Methadone
Domestic abuse; *see* Partner abuse
Dominant patient, in group ther-
    apy, 179
Donepezil, 465
Dopamine, 224, 225
    and blood-brain barrier, 226
    cocaine and, 522
    levels in cortex, antipsychotic
        drugs and, 262, 263
    MAOI interactions with, 287-288
    and Parkinson's disease, 81, 466
        balance with ACh and, 233-234
        deficiency of, 230, 231
    and schizophrenia, 77, 79
        hypothesis of, 362-363
    and limbic area, 250
Dopamine antagonists, 357
Dopamine receptors
    antipsychotic drugs and, 263,
        265, 266
    subtypes, concentration of, 263, 363
Dopaminergic drugs, 234-235
    antipsychotic drug interactions
        with, 260
    psychiatric side effects of, 235
    for stimulant dependence, 534
Dopaminergic tracts
    antipsychotic drug action on, 249
    schizophrenia and, 249-250
Dorsal longitudinal fasciculus
    (DLF), 78
Double-bind theory
    definition of, 351
    of schizophrenia, 366
Down syndrome, and Alzheimer's
    disease, 464
Doxepin, 282
    anticholinergic effects of, 456
    characteristics of, 276-277
    potency of, vs. trihexyphenidyl, 237
Dramatic/erratic (cluster B) personal-
    ity disorder, 482-487
Dream analysis, 30
Drowsiness, benzodiazepine-
    induced, 302
Drug abuse; *see also* Substance abuse/
    dependence
    cost of, 3
    in elderly, 651-652
    in schizophrenics, 369

Drug abuse—cont'd
    12-month prevalence rate of, 3,
        345, 352, 384, 424, 452,
        478, 502
Drug-Anon Focus, 536
Drug interactions
    with alcohol, 515
        in elderly, 659
    with amphetamines, 524
    with antidepressants, 285
    with antipsychotic drugs, 258, 260
    with barbiturates, 518
    with benzodiazepines, 302, 303
    with buspirone, 305
    with carbamazepine, 294
    with cocaine, 524
    with hallucinogens, 529
    with lithium, 292, 293
    with MAOIs, 287-289
    with opioids, 520-521
    with SSRIs, 284, 285
Drugs; *see also* Medications; Psycho-
        pharmacology
    delirium from toxicity of, 455
    depression from, 394
    limit setting and, 329
Drugs Anonymous, 536
Dry mouth
    anticholinergic-induced, 239
    from antidepressants, 277,
        281, 400
    antipsychotic drug-induced, 258
    from benzodiazepines, 302
    from MAOIs, 400
    from psychotropic drugs, in
        elderly, 657
DSM-IV; *see* Diagnostic and Statistical
        Manual of Mental Disorders-IV
DST; *see* Dexamethasone suppression
        test
Dual diagnosis, 543-549
    continuum of care and, 548
    definition of, 543-544
    in elderly, 650
    etiology of, 544
    management of, 546, 548
    treatment issues of, 544-545
Dual Disorders Anonymous, 536
Durable power of attorney, 57
Dura mater, 77
Duty to warn of threatened suicide
        or harm to others, 57, 60
    court rulings on, 47
Dysfunctional coping, with
        anxiety, 152

Dyskinesia
from antipsychotic drugs, 256
definition of, 230, 245
Dyslexia, 621
Dyspareunia, 495
Dysphagia, 233
definition of, 230, 245
Dysphoria
definition of, 383
Dysthymia
definition of, 271
lifetime prevalence rates for, 346
Dysthymic disorder, 388
definition of, 383
DSM-IV criteria for, 384
Dystonia(s)
anticholinergic-induced, 239
antipsychotic drug-induced, 255
in children and adolescents, 631
interventions for, 259
prophylactic treatment of,
256-257
definition of, 230, 245

E

Eating disorders, 550-567
anorexia nervosa, 550-559
behavior of, 551-553
care plan for, 558
DSM-IV criteria for, 550-551
etiology of, 553-555
family issues in, 557
management of, 555-556,
558-559
binge-eating disorder, 566
bulimia nervosa, 559-564
behavior of, 560-561
care plan for, 565
and depression, 562-563
DSM-IV criteria for, 559-560
etiology of, 561-562
management of, 563-564
DSM-IV and NANDA diagnoses
of, 559
interventions for, 555
in males, 564-566
obesity as, 566
Echolalia, 351
Echopraxia, 351
ECT; see Electroconvulsive therapy
Education
in cultural assessment worksheet, 214
patient; see Patient education
Education groups, 173-174

Effexor; see Venlafaxine
Ego, 26, 27
Elavil; see Amitriptyline
Eldepryl; see Selegiline
Elderly
alcohol in, 515
psychotropic drug interactions
with, 659
anticholinergics and, 240
antipsychotic drug use in, 258
assessment of, written materials
for, 641
barbiturates in, 518
benzodiazepines in, 300, 301, 303
delirium in, 454
depression in, 388
assessment of, 395, 397
ECT in, 644-645
lithium use in, 293
MAOIs in, 289
mental illness in, 638-663
anxiety disorders, 648-649
assessment of, 652-654
barriers to care and, 642-643
bipolar disorder, 646
continuum of care in, 640-642
depression, 643-646
milieu management for,
659-662
nurse-patient relationship and,
654-655
psychopharmacology for,
655-659
psychotic disorders, 646-648
suicide and, 645-646
opioid use by, 521
SSRIs in, 285
substance abuse in, 649-652
suicide among, 395, 397, 415
TCAs in, 280
Electroconvulsive therapy (ECT),
579-584
advantages of, 583-584
conditions responsive and unresponsive to, 583
contraindications to, 583
definition of, 383
and depression in elderly,
644-645
disadvantages of, 584
drugs used for, 581
high-risk groups and, 584
history of, 579-584
indications for, 582-583
modern, 580-581

Electroconvulsive therapy–cont'd
preparation and procedure for,
581-582
responsibilities before and after,
581, 582
Elimination disorders, in children
and adolescents, 626-627
ELISA (Enzyme-Linked Immunosorbent Assay)
definition of, 667
for HIV testing, 671
Ellis' cognitive-behavioral models,
29, 36-37
Elopement, limit setting and, 330
Emaciation, 551
Emergency care, involuntary commitment for, 48-49
Emergency rooms, deinstitutionalization and, 11
Emotional reaction, in A-B-C theory
of personality, 37
Emotional security, in therapeutic
environment, 327
Emotions
anxiety and, 151
management of, nurse-patient relationship and, 127-128
in partner abuse, 606
Empathy
in communication, 117-118
definition of, 124
for depression, 398
in nurse-patient relationship, 127
Encopresis, 627
Endocrine system
and depression, 391, 395
and secondary psychosis in
elderly, 647
Endorphins, 520
Enkephalins, 224
Enlightenment period, 4-7
Enuresis, 626-627
medications for, 628
Environment; see also Milieu
management
and aggression, 162
and communication, 116
in stress models, 39, 40
Environmental cues, 332
Environmental factors
of borderline personality disorder, 484
of child psychiatric disorders, 619

Environmental modification
  in milieu management, 317
  in therapeutic environment,
    331-332
Environment of care standards, 321
Epidemiology
  of child psychiatric disorders,
    616, 617
  definition of, 617
Epinephrine, MAOI interactions
    with, 287-288
Epistemology
  of African/African-American/
    Hispanic/Arabic world view,
    206-207
  of Asian/Asian-American/
    Polynesian world view, 207
  of European American view, 206
  of Native American world
    view, 208
Epithalamus, 72
EPSEs; see Extrapyramidal side
    effects
Equanil; see Meprobamate
Erikson, Erik
  developmental models of, 28,
    30, 33
  and schizophrenia, 366
  stages of development, adult man-
    ifestations of, 34-35
Escalation phase of assault cycle, 161
  interventions for, 164, 165-166
Ethanol; see also Alcohol
  metabolism of, 511-512
Ethics
  and HIV, 672, 673
  and psychosurgery, 586
Ethnic/racial groups, pharmacody-
    namics of, 211; see also Cul-
    tural competence
Ethnocentrism, in nurse-patient in-
    teraction, 203-204
Ethnonursing, 202
  definition of, 200
  and ethnopharmacology, 211
Ethnopharmacology, 210-212
Ethopropazine
  dosage of, 237
  for Parkinson's disease, 241
Etiology
  definition of, 345
  psychopathology and, 346
Euphoria, 33
  definition of, 27, 383

European Americans
  pharmacodynamics of, 211
  world view of, 204, 205-206
    in Purnell's twelve domain
      model of cultural compe-
      tence, 213, 215
Evaluation; see also Assessment
  in behavioral interventions, 576
  in case management, 105
  involuntary commitment for,
    48-49
  in nurse-patient relationship
    in termination stage, 131
    in working stage, 129
  in nursing process, 141
  therapeutic communication
    and, 120
  for working with families, 196
Exercise
  for elderly mentally ill, 662
  groups, 324-325
Exhaustion stage, in stress adaptation
    syndrome, 39, 40
Exhibitionism, 495, 496
Existential factors, from group ther-
    apy, 172
Expanded broker case management
    model, 103
Exposure, in cognitive behavior ther-
    apy for obsessive-compulsive
    disorder, 633
Extended care facilities, 98
Extended commitment, 51
Extinction
  in behavior modification, 573
  in operant conditioning, 571
Extrapyramidal side effects (EPSEs)
  anticholinergics for, 241
  from antipsychotic drugs, 247, 253-
    257, 262, 372
    guidelines for minimizing, 255
    treatment of, 237-238
  definition of, 230, 245
  prophylactic treatment of,
    256-257
  psychotropic drugs in elderly
    and, 656
Extrapyramidal system
  definition of, 65, 230, 245
  function of, 72
  Parkinson's disease and, 229-230,
    231, 466
  patient risk factor assessment tool
    for, 257

Eye movement desensitization and
    reprocessing (EMDR), 437
Eye pain
  from antidepressants, 281
  from psychotropic drugs, 657

F

False imprisonment, wrongful invol-
    untary commitment and, 60
False memories, 603
Families Anonymous, 536
Family(ies)
  of Alzheimer's disease patients,
    465-466
  and anorexia nervosa, 554, 557
  anxiety disorders in, 624
  ASD/PTSD, 435
  assessment of
    brief therapeutic vs. family ther-
      apy for, 188-189
    common situations for,
      187-188
    in cultural assessment work-
      sheet, 214
    initial, 192-194
    nursing skills for, 190-191
    theories for, 189-190
  and bipolar disorder, 409
  and bulimia nervosa, 562
  and childhood sexual abuse,
    597, 603
  definition of, 182
  of depressed person, 403
  development stages of, 182-183
  education of, 196
  functional/healthy characteristics
    of, 183, 184
  health of
    and functioning assess-
      ment, 193
    triangle of, 189
  manic patients and, 408
  in perpetuation of partner
    abuse, 608
  problematic characteristics of, 183,
    185-186
  psychoeducational programs
    for, 174
  of schizophrenics, 366, 367-368
  and substance abuse/dependence,
    529-530
  support skills for, 192
  tasks of, 182
  types of, 182

Family(ies)—cont'd
  working with, 181-197
    assessment process in, 192-194
    brief interactions vs. family
      therapy in, 188-189
    characteristics to be assessed,
      182-183, 184, 185-186
    diagnosis in, 195
    evaluation in, 181-182, 196
    interventions for, 196
    mental illness effects on, 183,
      186, 187
    orientation process in, 194-195
    outcome identification in, 195
    planning/implementation
      in, 196
    reactions to hospitalization
      in, 188
    reasons for seeking treatment in,
      187-188
    skills for, 190-192
    theories for assessment and in-
      teractions in, 189-190
Family system(s)
  and child and adolescent psychi-
    atric disorders, 619
  definition of, 617
Fasciculus, 67
Fatigue, in cognitive disorders, mi-
    lieu management for, 471
Fear
  in anorexia nervosa, 553, 555
  conditioning, 575
    ASD and PTSD, 435, 436
    classical, 571
  and therapeutic communication,
    118, 120-121
Fecal impaction, and encopresis, 627
Federal Task Force on Homelessness
    and Severe Mental Illness
    (FTFHSMI), 12
Feedback
  definition of, 321
  in therapeutic environment, 327
Feeding, limbic system and, 71-72
Feighner criteria, 345
Fentanyl, 521
  urine detection of, 505
Fetal alcohol syndrome (FAS), 515
Fetishism, 495, 496
Fight or flight pathway, 72
Finances, and mental health care of
    elderly, 642
Fissure, 68

Flashbacks
  with LSD, 528
  definition of, 423
  with marijuana, 527-528
Flattened affect, 362
Flight of ideas, in schizophrenia, 360
Flooding, as respondent condition-
    ing technique, 575
Fluid and electrolyte abnormalities,
    in bulimia nervosa, 560
Flumazenil, for benzodiazepine over-
    dose, 302-303
Fluoxetine, 221, 284, 285-286, 630
  for alcoholism, 534
  antipsychotic drug interactions
    with, 260
  for anxiety disorders, 306
  for ASD/PTSD, 438
  for bulimia nervosa, 563
  characteristics of, 276-277
  in elderly, 658
  for obsessive-compulsive disorder,
    306, 431
  for sexual disorders, 498
Fluphenazine, 261
  dosage of, 247
  in elderly, 656
Fluphenazine decanoate, 252, 261
Fluvoxamine, 286, 630
  for anxiety disorders, 306
  for ASD/PTSD, 438
  characteristics of, 276-277
  for obsessive-compulsive disorder,
    306, 431
Focal awareness, 36
Folk medicine beliefs, 209
Follow-up care, in substance abuse
    recovery, 538
Food-drug interactions, with MAOIs,
    288-289
Forensic nursing, 590
Foster care, 98
Foucha v. Louisiana (1992), 47-48
Fragile X syndrome, 617, 619
Free association, 30
  definition of, 27
Freedom from restraints and seclu-
    sion, right to, 54-55
Freeman, Walter, 585, 586
Freud, Sigmund, 5, 7, 13, 365, 366
  and anorexia nervosa, 554
  and anxiety, 149
  and cocaine, 522
  and depression, 392

Freud, Sigmund—cont'd
  psychoanalytical model of, 26-27,
    28, 30
  and schizophrenia, 366
Frontal lobes, 68, 70-71
  and ADHD, 623
Frotteurism, 495, 496
Fugues, dissociative, 446
Full support case management
    model, 102
Fungal infections, with HIV, 669

G
GABA; see Gamma-
    aminobutyric acid
GAD; see Generalized anxiety
    disorder
Gamma-aminobutyric acid (GABA),
    224, 225
  and anxiety, 77
  benzodiazepines and, 301
  and depression, 391
Gastrointestinal system
  and benzodiazepine with-
    drawal, 304
  bulimia nervosa and, 560
  lithium and, 400
Gay AA, 536
Gender
  AIDS cases and, 673
  depression and, 387-388
  schizophrenia and, 352
Gender identity disorders, 493,
    497-498
Gender roles, African, African-
    American, Hispanic and
    Arabic world view of, 207
General adaptation syndrome (GAS),
    39, 40, 150
Generalization, 571
Generalized anxiety disorder (GAD),
    423-426
  DSM-IV criteria for, 424
  lifetime prevalence rates
    for, 346
Generative life-style vs. stagnation, in
    Erikson's stages of develop-
    ment, 35
Genetics
  and ADHD, 622-623
  and alcoholism, 511
  of Alzheimer's disease, 463-464
  and autism, 620
  and bipolar disorder, 410

Genetics—cont'd
  and child psychiatric disorders,
    617-619
  and depression, 391
  and PTSD, 436
  in schizophrenia, 365
  and tic disorders, 626
Genetic vulnerability, definition
    of, 617
Geriatric Depression Scale
    (GDS), 387
Giger and Davidhizar's cultural
    assessment model, 213
Ginseng, 212
Glasser, William, reality therapy
    model of, 29, 38-39
Glaucoma, antipsychotic drugs
    and, 253
Globus pallidus, 72
Glucose, and blood-brain barrier,
    226
Glutamate, and schizophrenia, 363
Glutethimide, 506-507
Glycine, and schizophrenia, 363
Goals
  in nursing process, 137-138
  in working with family, 195
Grand mal seizure, ECT-induced, 580
Gravely disabled person
  definition of, 45, 51
  and involuntary commitment, 48,
    51-52
Gray matter, 67, 68
  definition of, 65
Griswold v. Connecticut (1965), 47
Group homes, 98
Group therapy, 171-180
  benefits of, 172
  confidentiality and, 53-54
  leadership of, 175-179
  nursing students and, 326
  and substance abuse treatment,
    533-534
  types of, 172-175
Growth hormone secretion, as mea-
    sure of depression, 397
Guanethidine
  antipsychotic drug interactions
    with, 260
  MAOI interactions with, 287-288
  TCA interactions with, 279
Guanfacine, 632
Guardian, for gravely disabled per-
    sons, 51

Guilt
  in depression, 389
  vs. initiative, in Erikson's stages of
    development, 34
Guns, and suicide, 415
Gyri, 68
  in Alzheimer's disease patient,
    459, 461
  definition of, 65

H

Hair toxicology, 504
Haitian/West Indian/Trinidadian cul-
    tural groups, 209
Haldol; see Haloperidol
Halfway houses, 98, 370
Hallucination(s)
  definition of, 124, 351
  in dementia, 458
  in depression, 390
  illusion vs., 458
  and nurse-patient relationship, 132
  and schizophrenia, 359
    antipsychotic drugs and, 251
Hallucinogens
  abuse of, 524, 526-529
  dependence, medications
    for, 535
  urine detection of, 505
  uses and effects of, 508-509
  withdrawal from, 516
Hallucinosis, alcoholic, 513
Haloperidol, 262, 631
  for AIDS dementia, 677
  for cognitive disorders, 470
  cost of, 357
  dopamine receptors blocked
    by, 263
  dosage of, 247
  in elderly, 258, 656
  for hallucinogen overdose, 529
  history of, 222
  neuroleptic malignant syndrome
    from, 256
  potency of, 246
  for tic symptoms, 626
Haloperidol decanoate, 252, 262
Hamilton Rating Scale for Depres-
    sion (HRSD), 387
Harm to others, duty to warn of,
    57, 60
  court rulings on, 47
Hashish, 508-509
Healer, consultation with, 210

Health, in cultural assessment work-
    sheet, 214
Health care actions, definition
    of, 200
Health care directives, 56-57
Health Care Financing Administra-
    tion (HCFA), and nursing
    home guidelines, 641
Health care reform, 99
Health care workers and HIV
  occupational transmission of,
    670, 671
  universal precautions against,
    673-674
Health People 2000, 15
Hebephrenia, 352, 353, 357
  definition of, 351
Helplessness, in anorexia nervosa, 553
Hematologic function, MAOIs
    and, 289
Hemodynamics, ECT and, 584
Hepatic dysfunction, MAOIs
    and, 289
Herbal therapies, 212
Here-and-now focus, definition
    of, 311
Heredity; see Genetics
Heroin; see also Opioids
  abuse of, 519, 520, 521
  urine detection of, 505
  uses and effects of, 506-507
  withdrawal from, 516
Hill-Burton Act (1947), 8
Hippocampus, 72
Hispanics
  pharmacodynamics of, 211
  world view of, 204, 206-207
Historical evolution, of working with
    family, 181-182
History, case management, 102-103
Histrionic personality disorder, 487
HIV; see Human immunodeficiency
    virus
Homebound, definition of, 110
Home care
  in case management, 110
  services, 97
Homelessness, 11-13
  definition of, 3
  outreach services for, 98
Home visits, patient passes for,
    194-195
Homosexual men, HIV transmission
    and, 669

Homunculus, 70
Hope, from group therapy, 172
Horticultural therapy, for elderly mentally ill, 662
Hospital-based care, 91-95
    purposes of, 91-92
    types of, 92-94
Hospitalization
    as aggression variable, 162
    family reactions to, 188
    number of patients and antipsychotic drugs, 246
Hostility
    in depression, 398
    in group therapy, 179
    in manic patients, milieu management for, 413
    in psychotherapeutic management, 346
Hot or cold treatments, definition of, 200
Human immunodeficiency virus (HIV) infection, 666-678
    AIDS and, 670
        by age, race, and gender, 673
    antibody, 667
    biological basis of, 81
    care plan for, 677
    causes of, 667-668
    definition of, 667
    incidence and distribution of, 672
    mechanism of cell infection of, 668
    neuropsychiatric aspects of, 674-678
    opportunistic illnesses of, 668, 669
    populations at risk for, 669-670
    risk behavior prevention for, 672-674
    symptoms of, according to body system, 671
    testing for, 670-672
    transmission of, 668-669, 671
    universal precautions for, 673-674
Huntington's disease, 468
Hydergine, 471
Hydromorphine; see Opioids
Hydromorphone, 521
    uses and effects of, 506-507
5-Hydroxyindoleacetic acid (5-HIAA), anorexia nervosa and, 553
Hyperactivity
    in manic patients, 408-409
    and nurse-patient relationship, 134

Hyperactivity—cont'd
    in schizophrenics
        antipsychotic drugs and, 251
        milieu management for, 373
Hyperarousal, ASD and PTSD and, 436
Hypersomnia
    definition of, 383
    depression and, 389
Hypertension, drug interactions and, 279
Hypertensive crisis
    from MAOIs, 288
        interventions for, 290, 400
    signs and symptoms of, 288
Hyperthermia, from anticholinergics, 240
Hypnotics, antipsychotic drug interaction with, 260
Hypochondriasis, 441, 442
Hypofrontality, 79
Hypomania, 404
    definition of, 383
    DSM-IV criteria for, 405, 406
    from MAOIs, 400
Hyponatremia, from polydipsia, 369-370
Hypotension; see also Orthostatic hypotension
    from antipsychotic drugs, 253
        interventions for, 258
    from MAOIs, 287, 289, 400
Hypothalamus, 72, 77
    and bulimia nervosa, 561
    function of, 73
Hypothalmic-pituitary-adrenal (HPA) axis, and depression, 391, 397
Hypoxyphilia, 496

I

Id, 26, 27
Idealization, definition of, 478
Ideas of reference, definition of, 351
Identification, 31
Identity
    childhood sexual abuse and, 600
    vs. diffusion, in Erikson's stages of development, 35
Illness
    anxiety and, 153
    cultural beliefs regarding, 209; see also Cultural competence
    with delirium, 455
    and depression, 395

Illusion(s)
    definition of, 351
    in dementia, 458
    vs. hallucination, 458
    in schizophrenia, 359
Imipramine
    as antianxiety drug, 305
    anticholinergic effects of, 456
    for bulimia nervosa, 563
    characteristics of, 276-277
    for child and adolescent psychiatric disorders, 629
    introduction of, 7
    for panic disorder, 427-428
    potency of, vs. trihexyphenidyl, 237
    as TCA, 282
Imitation
    in behavioral modification, 573
    from group therapy, 172
Immobility, in schizophrenics, milieu management for, 373-374
Impact, as stage of trauma recovery, 591
Impaired Physician Program, 536
Implementation, therapeutic communication and, 120
Implosion, as respondent conditioning technique, 575
Incapacitated persons, commitment of, 51-52
Incest, 496, 597; see also Sexual abuse
Indecisiveness, in depression, 390
Independence, in therapeutic environment, 327-328
Inderal; see Propranolol
Indeterminate commitment, 51
Indomethacin, lithium interactions with, 292
Industry vs. inferiority, in Erikson's stages of development, 34
Infants, HIV transmission to, 669-670
Infections and depression, 395
Information, from group therapy, 172
Informed consent, definition of, 45
Inhalants abuse, 519
Initiative vs. guilt, in Erikson's stages of development, 34
Inpatient unit, 92
Insanity, legal milestones and, 46
Insecurity, nurse's, in communication, 121
Insight-oriented groups, 175

Insomnia
from antidepressants, 277
definition of, 383
depression and, 389
ECT and, 583
Instrumental activities of daily living (IADLs), assessment in elderly, 654
Insulin, antipsychotic drug interactions with, 260
Intake form, for initial nursing assessment, 140
Intake interview, 144
Integrity vs. despair, in Erikson's stages of development, 35
Intellectualization, 31
Intensive case management model, 103
Interaction themes, in communication, 116
Interlocking paradigm of cultural competence (IPCC), 200; see also Cultural competence, interlocking paradigm of
Intermittent reinforcement, 572-573
Internal capsule, 67
Internalizing disorders, in children and adolescents, 624-625
International Nurses Anonymous, 536
Interneurons, 75
Interpersonal difficulties, and depression, 392
Interpersonal learning, group therapy and, 172
Interpersonal model, 28, 33, 36
Interpersonal Relations to Nursing, 14
Interpersonal security, 33
definition of, 27
Interpersonal theory, anxiety in, 149
Interpretation step, in nurse-patient relationship, 129
Intervention(s)
in anger and nonviolent aggression, 163-164
for anticholinergic side effects, 239
for antidepressant side effects, 281, 400
for antimanic drug side effects, 400
for antipsychotic drug side effects, 258
and anxiety, 151, 425
for ASD and PTSD, 438
based on assault cycle, 164-168
behavioral, 575-576

Intervention(s)–cont'd
for benzodiazepine side effects, 302
for depressed patients, 399
for eating disorders, 555
with elderly
to assist, 655
for depression, 645
for psychotropic drug effects, 657
family and, 196
common situations for, 187-188
for group therapy, 177-179
implementing in case management, 104-105
for lithium, 293
for manic episode, 410
for MAOI side effects, 289
in nursing process, 138-139, 141
for obsessive-compulsive disorder, 431
for panic attack, 427
for partner abuse, 612
in problem solving, 425
with schizophrenics
developing nurse-patient relationship in, 371, 377
to increase compliance, 372
for somatoform disorders, 445
spectrum, for mental disorders, 86, 87
for suicidal patient, 416, 416-417
for survivors of childhood sexual abuse, 602
for TCA overdose, 280
for wandering, 472
Interview approaches, for substance abuse, 505-507
Intimacy vs. isolation, in Erikson's stages of development, 35
Intrapsychic conflict, and depression, 392
Intravenous drug users (IVDU), and HIV transmission, 673
Introjection, 31
Invasion of privacy, therapeutic communication and, 121
Involuntary commitment
civil remedies for, 60-61
definition of, 45
legal issues of, 48-49, 51
and right to refuse treatment, 56
IPCC; see Interlocking paradigm of cultural competence
Ipecac syrup, bulimia nervosa and, 561

Iproniazid, 286
history of, 222
Ipsilateral, definition of, 65
IQ, mental retardation and, 620
Irrational beliefs
in cognitive-behavioral model, 37
definition of, 27
Irreversible MAOIs, 290
drug interactions with, 287
Isolation
vs. intimacy, in Erikson's stages of development, 35
in psychiatric history, 8
Isoproterenol, MAOI interactions with, 287-288
IVDU; see Intravenous drug users
Jackson v. Indiana (1972), 47

J

Joint Commission on Accreditation of Healthcare Organizations (JCAHO)
environment of care standards, 321
and nursing home restraints, 641
Jones, Maxwell, 312, 320
Journals, 14
Judgment alterations, in dementia, 458

K

Kamikiki-to, 212
Kanner, Leo, 620
Kaposi's sarcoma (KS), 667, 668
Kemadrin; see Procyclidine
Kinesics; see also Body language
and communication, 116-117
definition of, 115
Klonopin; see Clonazepam
Korsakoff's psychosis, 469
Kraepelin, Emil, 5, 7, 352, 353, 357
Kudzu, 534

L

LAAM, for opioid dependence, 534
La belle indifference, in conversion disorder, 443
Labile affect, 362
Lacrimation, antidepressants and, 281
Language disability, of Alzheimer's disease, 462
Lanugo, 551
Lateral fissures of Sylvius, 71
Lateral sulci, 71
Law enforcement, in perpetuation of partner abuse, 608

Laxative abuse, in bulimia nervosa, 560-561
Lazarus's interactional theory, 39-41
Lazarus's stress model, 29
L-dopa; *see* Levodopa
Leadership, in team meetings, 338
Lead-pipe rigidity, Parkinson's disease and, 231
Learned helplessness, and partner abuse, 604-605
Learning
  in nurse-patient relationship, 129
  in operant conditioning, 571
Learning disorders, 621-622
Least restrictive alternative/ environment
  and aggression, 158
  definition of, 45
  psychotropic drugs and, 221
  right to treatment with, 52-53
Left-leaning environments, milieu management and, 311
Legal issues, 44-62
  of commitment, 48-49, 51-52
  and HIV testing, 672
  liability, 57, 60-61
  milestones in, 46-48
  patient rights, 52-57
    bill of, 58-59
  of rape, 594
Leininger's cultural care diversity and universality theory, 202-204
Leininger's sunrise model, 213
Lemniscus, 67
Lentiform nucleus, 72
Lesion, definition of, 65
Levarterenol, for benzodiazepine over-dose, 302
Levodopa
  action of, 235
  antipsychotic drug interactions with, 260
  and blood-brain barrier, 226
  psychiatric side effects of, 235
  and psychotic state, 363
  TCA interactions with, 279
Levodopa and carbidopa, 235
Levo-Dromoran; *see* Levorphanol
Levophed; *see* Levarterenol
Levorphanol, 521
Liable, definition of, 45
Librium; *see* Chlordiazepoxide
Life review, for elderly mentally ill, 662
Limbic system, 71-72

Limited power of attorney, definition of, 45
Limit setting
  definition of, 311
  for manic patient, 411
  in milieu management, 316
  in nurse-patient relationship, 128
  in substance abuse management, 535
  in therapeutic environment, 328-330
Limit testing, by manic patients, 408
Lipid solubility
  and blood-brain barrier, 225-226
  definition of, 221
Lithium, 290-293
  for ASD/PTSD, 438
  for borderline personality disorder, 485
  dosage of, 291
  drug interactions with, 292, 293
    antipsychotics, 260
    SSRIs, 284
  in elderly, 656, 659
  guidelines for taking, 294
  history of, 7, 222
  for manic patients, 411-412
  mechanisms of action, 273
  poisoning, 292-293
  side effects of, 291-292, 400
    interventions for, 293
Living skills groups, in therapeutic environment, 324
Living wills, 56-57
Lobotomy, 585, 586
Locus ceruleus, 232
  and Parkinson's disease, 232, 233, 234
Logic
  of African/African-American/ Hispanic/Arabic world view, 207
  of Asian/Asian-American/Polynesian world view, 207
  of European American view, 206
  of Native American world view, 208
Loose association
  definition of, 351
  in schizophrenia, 361
Lorazepam, 304-305
  for aggression, 165
  alcohol interaction with, 515
  for alcohol withdrawal, 534
  for cognitive disorders, 471

Lorazepam—cont'd
  dosage and pharmacokinetics of, 301
  in elderly, 656, 658, 659
  for generalized anxiety disorder, 425
  for status epilepticus, 301-302
Loss(es)
  depression as reaction to, 392-393
  perception of, 148
Lower motor neurons, 70
Loxapine, 262
  dosage of, 247
Loxitane; *see* Loxapine
LSD; *see* Lysergic acid diethylamide
Ludiomil; *see* Maprotiline
Luvox; *see* Fluvoxamine
Lysergic acid diethylamide (LSD), 526, 528
  overdose of, 528, 529
  uses and effects of, 508-509

M

Mad cow disease, 468
Magnetic resonance imaging (MRI), 364
Major depression; *see also* Depression
  care plan for, 499
  in elderly, 661
  ECT for, 582
  treatment success rate of, 4
  12-month prevalence rate of, 3, 345, 352, 384, 424, 452, 478, 502
Major depressive disorder (MDD)
  biological theories of, 390-391
  in children and adolescents, 625
  criteria and symptoms of, 384, 385-388
  vs. dysthymic disorder, 388
  in elderly, 643
    assessment of, 395, 397
  key features of, 385
  lifetime prevalence rates for, 346
  and suicide, 385
Maladaptive coping, with anxiety, 152
Males, eating disorders in, 564-566
Malpractice, 57
  definition of, 45
Managed care, 87, 89
  of community-based services, 99
  definition of, 86
  impact on continuum of care, 88, 89

Manerix; *see* Moclobemide
Mania
  amine theory of, 273
  from antidepressants, 281
  in children and adolescents, medications for, 628
  definition of, 271, 383
  ECT and, 582, 583
  in elderly, 646
Manic-depression; *see* Bipolar disorder(s)
Manic episode(s); *see also* Bipolar disorder(s)
  in children and adolescents, 625
  DSM-IV criteria for, 405
  interventions for, 410
  objective behavior of, 406, 408-409
  symptoms occurring during, 404
Manipulation, and nurse-patient relationship, 133
MAOIs; *see* Monoamine oxidase inhibitors
Maprotiline, 273, 282
  characteristics of, 276-277
Marijuana
  abuse of, 526-528
  overdose of, 529
  urine detection of, 505
  uses and effects of, 508-509
  withdrawal from, 516, 529
Marinol, 527
Masked facies, Parkinson's disease and, 231
MAST; *see* Michigan Alcoholism Screening Test
Master-servant rule, definition of, 45
Mathematics disorder, 621-622
Maturational stressors, 148-149
Mazicon; *see* Flumazenil
MDA, 526
  overdose of, 528
Medially, definition of, 65
Medical model, depression in, 393
Medical personnel, in perpetuation of partner abuse, 608
Medical-surgical nursing skills, updating, 340
Medicare, and mental health care of elderly, 642
Medications; *see also* Psychopharmacology; *specific agents*
  for alcohol dependence, 534
  for Alzheimer's disease, 465
  anti-AIDS drugs, CNS effects of, 676

Medications—cont'd
  ethnopharmacology and, 210-212
  for hallucinogen dependence, 535
  herbal therapy interactions with, 212
  psychoactive, in nursing homes, 641
  right to refuse, 55, 56
    court rulings on, 47
  for stimulants dependence, 534-535
  teaching patients about, 226-227
Medulla oblongata, 74-75
Meier v. Ross General Hospital (1968), 47
Melancholia, treatment of, 396
Melancholic depression, 386
  definition of, 383
MELAS (mitochrondrial encephalopathy, lactic acidosis, and strokelike episodes), 82
Mellaril; *see* Thioridazine
Mellow, June, 14, 313
Memory
  Alzheimer's disease and, 462
  antipsychotic drugs and, 256
  childhood sexual abuse and, 600
  cognitive disorders and, 451
  dementia and, 457
  ECT and, 584
  limbic system and, 72
Meninges, 77
  definition of, 65
Meningitis, with HIV infection, 675
Menstrual cycle, anorexia nervosa and, 550-551
Mental disorders; *see also specific disorders*
  biological bases of, 79, 81-82
  certification for observation and treatment of, 49, 50
  Mental Health Spectrum for, 87
  neurotransmitters and, 77, 225
  prevalence rates of
    lifetime, 346
    12-month, 3, 345, 352, 384, 424, 452, 478, 502
  treatment success rate of, 4
Mental health counselors, in perpetuation of partner abuse, 608
Mental Health Intervention Spectrum, 86, 87
Mental health services, patient bill of rights for, 58-59
Mental Health Systems Act (1980), and patient rights, 52

Mental illness
  effect on family, 183, 186, 187
  in elderly; *see* Elderly, mental illness in
  and HIV transmission, 670
  and homelessness, 11, 12-13
Mental retardation
  in children and adolescents, 620
  cost of, 3
Mental status examination, 138
Meperidine, 521
  contraindication to, 288
  urine detection of, 505
  uses and effects of, 506-507
  withdrawal from, 516
Meprobamate, 298, 299
Meridians, 209
  definition of, 200
Mescaline, 526
  overdose of, 528, 529
  uses and effects of, 508-509
Mesocortical system, antipsychotic drug action on, 249
Mesolimbic system, antipsychotic drug action on, 249
Metabolic enhancers/vasodilators, for dementia, 471
Metabolic tolerance, definition of, 502
Metabolism
  of alcohol, 511-512
  of amphetamines, 523
  of barbiturates, 518
  of cocaine, 522
  of LSD, 528
  of marijuana, 527
  of mescaline, 526
  of morphine, 519
  of PCP, 528
  of psilocybin, 526
Methadone; *see also* Opioids
  abuse of, 521
  for opioid dependence, 534
  urine detection of, 505
  uses and effects of, 506-507
  withdrawal from, 516
Methaqualone, 506-507
Methohexital, for ECT, 581
N-Methyl-D-aspartate (NMDA) receptors, and schizophrenia, 363
Methyldopa, MAOI interactions with, 287-288
Methylphenidate
  for AIDS dementia, 677
  for child and adolescent psychiatric disorders, 629

Methylphenidate—cont'd
in elderly, 658
MAOI interactions with, 287-288
uses and effects of, 508-509
1-Methyl-4-phenyl-1,2,3,6-tetrahy-
dropyridine (MPTP), parkinsonism from, 233
Mexican-American culture, 209
Meyer, Adolph, 365, 366
Michigan Alcoholism Screening Test
(MAST), 530
Midbrain, 73, 74
Milieu, 20
Milieu management, 23, 310-318
for ADS, PTSD, 439
for anorexia nervosa, 556, 558-559
for bipolar disorder, 412-413
for borderline personality disorder,
485-486
for bulimia nervosa, 563
for cognitive disorders, 471-473
in community-based care, 100
definition of, 311
for depression, 400-403
for dissociative disorders, 448
for dual diagnoses, 546, 548
for elderly mentally ill, 659-662
elements of, 315-317
for generalized anxiety disorder, 426
goal of, 314-315
historical overview of, 311-313
in hospital-based care, 94
for obsessive-compulsive disorder,
431-432
for panic disorder, 428
for partner abuse, 612
for phobic disorders, 432
for rape and sexual assault, 596-597
roles in, 317
for schizophrenia, 371-374
for sexual disorders, 498
for somatoform disorders, 444-445
for substance abuse/depen-
dence, 535
for survivors of childhood sexual
abuse, 602-604
therapeutic milieu in, 313-314
for trauma recovery, 592
Milieu therapy, 321
Miltown; see Meprobamate
Mirtazapine, 283
characteristics of, 276-277
Miscommunication, world views
and, 205
Mistrust vs. trust, in Erikson's stages
of development, 34

Mitochondrial DNA problems, 82
M'Naghten rule, 46
Moban; see Molindone
Moclobemide, 273, 286, 290
characteristics of, 276-277
and MAOIs, 288
Modeling, in behavioral modification, 573
Molindone, 262
dosage of, 247
Moniz, Egas, 584, 585
Monoamine oxidase, definition of,
230, 245
Monoamine oxidase inhibitors
(MAOIs), 271, 272, 273,
286-290
administration of, 399
for ASD/PTSD, 439
for bulimia nervosa, 563
characteristics of, 276-277
contraindications to, 289
definition of, 271, 383
for depression, 396
in elderly, 657, 658
alcohol interaction and, 659
history of, 222
interactions with
anticholinergics, 240
benzodiazepines, 302
drug and food, 287-289
SSRIs, 284
TCAs, 279
mechanisms of action, 273
and neurotransmitters, 225
nursing implications for, 289-290
for obsessive-compulsive disorder, 431
overdose, 289
for panic disorder, 427-428
pharmacokinetics of, 287
pharmacological effects of,
286-287
and serotonin syndrome, 285
side effects of, 287, 400
interventions for, 289
Monoamines, definition of, 271
Monoamine systems, 224
location and pathways of, 76
Mood, definition of, 383
Mood disorder(s), 382-419
biological basis of, 79, 81
definitions of, 383
depressive disorders, 384-403
assessment of, 387, 393-395, 397
behavior of, 388-390
care plan for, 402

Mood disorder(s)—cont'd
depressive disorders—cont'd
clinical features influencing
treatment of, 396
criteria and symptoms of,
385-388
drugs and toxins inducing, 394
dysthymic disorder, 388
etiology of, 390-393
family issues of, 403
illnesses associated with, 395
interventions for, 399
management of, 397-403
bipolar disorders, 404-413
behavior of, 406, 408-409
care plan for, 412
description of, 404
differences in, on mood continuum, 407
DSM-IV criteria for, 404-406
etiology of, 409-410
interventions for, 410
management of, 410-413
bulimia nervosa as, 562
in children and adolescents, 625
demographic variables associated
with, 385
DSM-IV criteria for, 382, 384
with HIV infection, 675
prevalence rates of
lifetime, 346
12-month, 3, 345, 352, 384,
424, 452, 478, 502
suicide and, 413-417; see also
Suicide
Mood stabilizers, for child and adolescent psychiatric disorders,
628, 632
Mood themes, in communication, 116
Moral anxiety, 30
Morphine; see also Opioids
metabolism of, 519
urine detection of, 505
uses and effects of, 506-507
withdrawal from, 516
Motivation, in alcohol abuse treatment, 532
Motor cortex, 68
Motor neurons, 75
Motor problems, of Parkinson's disease, 230-231
Motor tics, 626
Movement, of Parkinson's disease, 467
Movement disorders
basal ganglia vs. cerebellar, 73
ECT for, 582

Moxibustion, 210-211
    definition of, 200
Multidisciplinary collaboration, 87
Multidisciplinary team, 93
    members of, 337-338
Multiinfarct dementia, 469
    definition of, 452
Multiple sclerosis, biological basis
    of, 81
Munoz's cultural assessment work-
    sheet, 214
Mu receptors, 520
Music therapy, 662
Muteness, ECT and, 583
Mutism, definition of, 351
Mydriasis
    anticholinergic-induced, 239
    antidepressant-induced, 281
    antipsychotic drug-induced,
        253, 258
Myelin, and multiple sclerosis, 81

N

Nalbuphine, 521
Nalline; see Nalorphine
Nalorphine, 520
Naloxone, for opioid overdose and
    dependence, 520, 534
Naltrexone, for alcoholism treat-
    ment, 534
Naltrexone hydrochloride, 514-515
NANDA; see North American Nurs-
    ing Diagnosis Association
Naranon, 536
Narcan; see Naloxone
Narcissistic personality disorder,
    486-487
Narcotic antagonists, 520
Narcotics
    antipsychotic drug interactions
        with, 260
    uses and effects of, 506-507
    withdrawal from, 516
Narcotics Anonymous (NA), 535-536
Nardil; see Phenelzine
Nasal congestion
    anticholinergic-induced, 239
    antidepressant-induced, 400
    antipsychotic drug-induced, 258
    psychotropic drug-induced, in el-
        derly, 657
National Alliance for the Mentally
    Ill (NAMI), 640
    family support groups of, 368
National Institute of Mental Health
    (NIMH), 345

National League for Nursing, 13
National Mental Health Act
    (1946), 8
Native Americans
    depression in, 387
    pharmacodynamics of, 211
    world view of, 205, 208
Nature argument
    definition of, 345
    vs. nurture argument, 346
    schizophrenia in, 365
Nausea
    from benzodiazepines, 302
    from lithium, 400
Navane; see Thiothixene
Needs, tension of, 33
Nefazodone, 283
    benzodiazepine interactions
        with, 302
    characteristics of, 276-277
Negative consequence, in behavior
    modification, 573
Negative reinforcement, 572
Negative symptoms of schizophre-
    nia, 354, 355, 356
    antipsychotic drugs and, 357
Negativism, definition of, 351
Negligence
    definition of, 45
    wrongful involuntary commitment
        and, 60
Neologism, 351
Neoplastic disorders, and depres-
    sion, 395
Nephrogenic diabetes insipidus,
    lithium and, 292
Neuman, Heinrich, 348
Neuroanatomy/neurophysiology,
    65-79
    autonomic nervous system, 77, 78
    brainstem and cerebellum, 73-75
        medulla oblongata, 74-75
        midbrain, 73, 74
        pons, 73-74
    cerebrum, 65-72
        basal ganglia, 72
        cerebral cortex, 67-68, 70-71
        limbic system, 71-72
        pathways in, 67, 69
    diencephalon, 72-73
    neurons and neurotransmitters
        and, 75, 76, 77
    ventricular system, 77, 79
Neurochemical basis
    of ASD and PTSD, 435-436
    of schizophrenia, 249-250

Neurochemical changes, anxiety
    and, 150
Neurochemical depression, 390-391
Neurodegeneration, 79
Neurofibrillary tangles, of
    Alzheimer's disease, 461, 463
Neuroleptic drugs; see also Antipsy-
    chotic drugs
    for child and adolescent psychi-
        atric disorders, 628
    definition of, 230, 245
Neuroleptic malignant syndrome
    (NMS)
    anticholinergic-induced, 239
    from antipsychotic drugs, 254, 256
    interventions for, 259
    ECT and, 583
Neurological disorders, and secondary
    psychosis in elderly, 647
Neurologic manifestations
    of benzodiazepines with-
        drawal, 304
    of schizophrenia, 365
Neuromuscular blocking agents,
    lithium interaction with, 292
Neuron(s), 75, 223
    definition of, 65
    parasympathetic, 77
    postsynaptic, 223
    presynaptic, 223
    spinal, 70
    sympathetic, 77
    from ventral tegmental area, 71-72
Neuropathies of HIV infection, treat-
    ment of, 677
Neuropeptides, location and path-
    ways of, 76
Neuropsychiatric aspects of HIV in-
    fection, 674-678
Neurostructural theories of schizo-
    phrenia, 363-365
Neurotic anxiety, 30
Neurotransmitters, 75, 77, 223-224
    and aggression, 160
    and Alzheimer's disease, 464
    and anxiety disorders, 81
    classification and pathways of, 76
    definition of, 221
    and depression, 271, 272, 390-391
    MAOIs and, 286
    and mental disorders, 77, 225
    and parkinsonism, 233-234
    psychotropic drugs and, 224-225
    and schizophrenia, 363
    systems of, 224
    TCAs and, 274

Neutral stimulus, 571

Nichols's world view model, 202, 204-208

Nigerian root extract, 212

Nightingale, Florence, 313

Nigrostriatal system, antipsychotic drug action on, 249

Nisentil; *see* Alphaprodine

NMS; *see* Neuroleptic malignant syndrome

Nocturnal enuresis, 626, 627

Noncompliance
    and antipsychotic drugs, 252
    definition of, 221
    limit setting and, 329

Nonpurging type of bulimia nervosa, 559

Nonreversible dementia, 458

Nonsteroidal antiinflammatory drugs (NSAIDs)
    for Alzheimer's disease, 465
    lithium interactions with, 292

Nonviolence, conveying message of, 326-327

Nootropic agents for cognitive disorders, 471

Norepinephrine, 224
    and depression, 77, 79, 390, 391
        in Parkinson's disease, 234
    MAOIs and, 287-288
    neuronal secretion of, 77
    as neurotransmitter, 223
        importance of, 225
        and mental disorders, 225
    TCAs and, 274

Norm(s)
    definition of, 311
    in milieu management, 316
    in therapeutic environment, 326-328

Norpramin; *see* Desipramine

North American Nursing Diagnosis Association (NANDA), 137, 138
    diagnoses
        anxiety, coping, and crisis and, 148
        of anxiety-related disorders, 423
        of cognitive disorders, 454
        of eating disorders, 559
        of mood disorders, 384
        of personality disorders, 479
        of schizophrenia and other psychoses, 355
        of sexual disorders, 494
        of substance abuse/ dependence, 531

Nortriptyline, 282
    anticholinergic effects of, 456
    characteristics of, 276-277
    for child and adolescent psychiatric disorders, 629
    for cognitive disorders, 471
    in elderly, 656
    potency of, vs. trihexyphenidyl, 237

No-suicide contracts, 331, 417

Ntuology, 207

Nubain; *see* Nalbuphine

Nucleus accumbens, 72
    and Parkinson's disease, 234

Nucleus basalis of Meynert, Parkinson's disease and, 233

Numorphan; *see* Oxymorphone

Nurse-patient relationship, 123-135
    anorexia nervosa and, 555-556
    antisocial personality disorder and, 482-483
    ASD/PTSD and, 437-438
    borderline personality disorder and, 485
    bulimia nervosa and, 563
    cognitive disorders and, 470
    in community-based care, 99
    and cultural competence, 202
    dependent personality disorder and, 488
    with depressed patients, 397-399
    in dissociative disorders, 447-448
    in dual diagnosis, 546
    elderly mentally ill and, 654-655
    in generalized anxiety disorder, 424-425
    in hospital-based care, 93
    interactions with selected behaviors in, 131-134
    with manic patient, 410-411
    narcissistic personality disorder and, 487
    in obsessive-compulsive disorder, 431
    in panic disorder, 427
    phobic disorders and, 432
    rape and sexual assault and, 596
    in recovery
        from childhood sexual abuse, 601-602
        from partner abuse, 609-612
        from trauma, 592
    schizophrenia and, 370-371
        interventions for, 377
    schizotypal personality disorder and, 481

Nurse-patient relationship—cont'd
    sexual disorders and, 498
    somatoform disorders and, 443-444
    stages of, 125-131
        orientation stage, 126-128
        termination stage, 131
        working stage, 128-131
    in substance abuse treatment, 533-534
    suspiciousness in, 134
    therapeutic, 22-23, 123-125
        development of, 125-131
        vs. providing therapy, 125
    transference in, 134
    violent behavior and, 132

Nurse roles
    in case management, 105
    in community health, 15-16
    in therapeutic milieu, 317, 336-341
        as colleague, 337-338
        as consultant, 340
        as supervisor and trainer, 339-340
        as team leader, 338

Nurses, universal precautions against HIV for, 673-674

Nursing
    community mental health movement and, 8-9
    Peplau's definition of, 123

Nursing education, 13-14

Nursing homes, mentally ill elderly in, 641

Nursing Mental Diseases, 13

Nursing process, 136-146
    application of, to family, 192-196
    assessment in, 136-137, 138
        written, 141, 142-143, 144
    care plan example, 145
    in case management, 103-105
    diagnosis in, 137, 139, 140
    evaluation in, 141
    goals and outcomes in, 137-138
    planning/intervention in, 138-139, 141

Nurture argument, definition of, 345

Nutrition, in cultural assessment worksheet, 214

Nyaya, 207

O

Obesity
    definition of, 551
    as eating disorder, 566

Objective behavior
    of bipolar disorder, 406, 408-409
    of delirium, 454-455
    of dementia, 456-458
Objective signs, 358
    of anorexia nervosa, 552-553
    of bulimia nervosa, 560-561
    of depression, 388-389
    of schizophrenia, 358-359
Objectivity
    in communication, 117
    definition of, 115
OBRA-87; *see* Omnibus Budget Rec-
    onciliation Act of 1987
Observation and treatment, certifica-
    tion for, 49, 50, 51
Observation step, in nurse-patient
    relationship, 129
Obsessions, 624
    definition of, 428
    DSM-IV criteria for, 430
Obsessive-compulsive disorder
    (OCD), 428-432
    in children and adolescents, 624-625
        medications for, 628, 630
    clomipramine for, 305
    cognitive behavioral therapy in,
        633
    depression with, treatment of, 396
    DSM-IV criteria for, 430
    hypochondriasis vs., 442
    interventions for, 431
    pharmacological treatment of, 306
    and psychosurgery, 586
    treatment success rate of, 4
    12-month prevalence rate of, 3, 345,
        352, 384, 424, 452, 478, 502
Obsessive-compulsive personality
    disorder, 489
    DSM-IV criteria for, 490
Occipital lobes, 71
Occupational therapist, 338
OCD; *see* Obsessive-compulsive
    disorder
Oculogyric crisis, definition of,
    230, 245
Odd/eccentric (cluster A) personality
    disorder, 479-481
Olanzapine, 265
    dopamine receptors blocked
        by, 263
    dosage of, 247
Olfactory
    definition of, 65
    function, 71

Omnibus Budget Reconciliation Act
    (OBRA) of 1987
    drug restriction of, 471
    and nursing homes, 641
    One Flew Over the Cuckoo's Nest, 586
Openness
    definition of, 321
    in therapeutic environment, 327
Operant conditioning, 571
Operant response, 571
Opioid receptors, 520
Opioids
    abuse of, 519-521
    dependence on, medications
        for, 534
    urine detection of, 505
Opium, 506-507
Opportunistic illnesses
    definition of, 667
    of HIV infection, 668, 669
        neuropsychiatric complications
            related to, 675
Oppositional defiant disorder, 9, 623
    prevalence of, 622
Oral hypoglycemics, antipsychotic
    drug interactions with, 260
Orap; *see* Pimozide
Organic brain syndrome, 451; *see also*
    Cognitive disorders
Organic mental disorder, 451; *see also*
    Cognitive disorders
    with HIV infection, 675
Organic mental syndrome, 451; *see
    also* Cognitive disorders
Orgasm, SSRIs and, 286
Orgasm disorder, 495
Orientation
    in cultural assessment work-
        sheet, 214
    of families to inpatient units,
        194-195
    in nurse-patient relationship, 125,
        126-128
    in therapeutic environment, 332
Orthostatic hypotension
    anticholinergic-induced, 239
    from antidepressants, 278, 281, 400
    from antipsychotic drugs, 258, 278
    in elderly
        from antidepressants, 658
        from psychotropic drugs, 656, 657
Outcome identification
    in case management, 104
    in nursing process, 137-138
    in working with family, 195

Outpatient services, 96-97
Outreach services, 98
Overdose
    of alcohol, 514
    amphetamine, 523
    of antipsychotic drugs, 257-258
    of barbiturates, 518
    benzodiazepines, 302-303
    cocaine, 523
    of hallucinogens, 528-529
    MAOIs, 289
    morphine, 520
    SSRIs, 284-285
    TCAs, 278, 279-280
Overreaction, in schizophrenia, 362
Over-the-counter drug use, limit set-
    ting and, 329
Oxazepam, 305
    for cognitive disorders, 471
    dosage and pharmacokinetics
        of, 301
    in elderly, 656, 658
    for generalized anxiety dis-
        order, 426
Oxymorphone, 521

P

Pain, depression-related, as indica-
    tion for psychosurgery, 586
Pain disorder, 441-442
    care plan for, 444
    DSM-IV criteria for, 441
Palliative coping, with anxiety, 152
Pamelor; *see* Nortriptyline
Pancreas, alcohol abuse and, 513
Panic, 33
Panic attack(s)
    DSM-IV criteria for, 426
    interventions for, 427
    in panic disorder, 426
Panic disorder(s), 426-428
    benzodiazepines for, 304
    care plan for, 429
    depression with, treatment of, 396
    DSM-IV criteria for, 427
    lifetime prevalence rates for, 346
    pharmacological treatment of, 306
    treatment success rate of, 4
    12-month prevalence rate of, 3, 345,
        352, 384, 424, 452, 478, 502
Papez circuit, 72
Paralysis agitans, 231
Paranoia, 352, 353, 357
    definition of, 351
    in elderly, 648

Paranoid delusions vs. paranoid thinking, 360
Paranoid personality disorder, 479-480
  DSM-IV criteria for, 481
Paranoid schizophrenia
  clinical example of, 360
  DSM-IV criteria for, 354
Paranoid thinking, in schizophrenia, 359-360
Paraphilia(s), 493, 495-497
Paraprofessionals, 339
Parasitical infections, HIV infection and, 669
Parasympathetic nervous system, 77, 238, 239-240
Parenteral administration, antipsychotic drugs, 252, 253
Parent training for ADHD, 632-633
Parietal lobes, 71
Parkinsonism, 229-231, 233
  causes of, 233
  definition of, 230
  drug-induced, 235
    from anticholinergics, 239
    from antipsychotic drugs, 255-256, 259
    model for, 236
  ECT and, 583
Parkinson's disease, 229-231, 233, 466-467
  basal ganglia and, 72
  biological basis of, 81
  definition of, 230
  and depression, 234
  dopamine deficiency and, 73
  and midbrain, 467
  prevalence rate for, 233
Parlodel; see Bromocriptine
Parnatel; see Tranylcypromine
Paroxetine, 286, 630
  characteristics of, 276-277
  in elderly, 285, 658
Parsidol; see Ethopropazine
Partial programs, 97
Partner abuse, 604-606, 608-612
  care plan for, 611
  common cues to, 609
  effects of, 604-606, 608
  helpful responses to, 609
  individual and agency perpetuation of, 608
  management of, 609-612
  nature of problem of, 604
  recovery from, 608
Passive aggression, 157, 159-160
  definition of, 158

Passivity, 159, 160
Pathoanatomy of schizophrenia, 355, 363-365
Patient education
  on anticholinergic side effects, 240-241
  on antipsychotic drugs, 260-261
  on benzodiazepines, 303-304
  about dual diagnosis, 546
  on lithium, 293
  on MAOIs, 290
  in milieu management, nurse role in, 317
  about panic disorder, 427
  psychoeducational programs for, 325
  on psychotropic drugs, 226-227
  on TCAs, 280-281
Patient records, confidentiality of, 53
Patient rights, 52-57
  balancing, 330, 331
  bill of, 58-59
  to confidentiality of records, 53-54
  to freedom from restraints and seclusion, 54-55
  to give or refuse consent to treatment, 55-56
    aggression and, 166
    court rulings on, 47
  living wills/health care directives and, 56-57
  suspension of, 52
  to treatment with least restrictive alternative, 52-53
Patient Self-Determination Act (1991), 56-57
Pavlov, 570
Paxil; see Paroxetine
PCP; see Phencyclidine
PD; see Parkinson's disease
PDD; see Pervasive development disorder
PDD-NOS; see Pervasive developmental disorders—not otherwise specified
Pedophilia, 496
  care plan for, 499
  DSM-IV criteria for, 495
Peduncle, 67
Pemoline, for child and adolescent psychiatric disorders, 629
Penicillin, and blood-brain barrier, 226
Pentazocine, 521
Pentobarbital, alcohol interaction with in elderly, 659

Peplau, Hildegard, 14
  and community-based care, 320
  interpersonal model of, 28
  and nurse-patient relationship, 125-131, 202
  nursing definition of, 123
  process recordings, 144
  and Sullivan's interpersonal model, 36
  and therapeutic environment, 313
Peptide neurotransmitter system, 224
Perception alterations
  antipsychotic drugs and, 250-251
  in dementia, 458
  in depression, 390
  of manic patients, 409
  in schizophrenia, 358, 359-360
    milieu management for, 373
Pergolide
  action of, 235
  psychiatric side effects of, 235
Perinatal risk factors of schizophrenia, 365
Peripheral nervous system (PNS)
  amphetamines and, 523
  anticholinergic effects on, 238, 239
  antidepressants and, 281
  antipsychotic drugs and, 253, 258-259
  cocaine and, 523
  heroin abuse and, 520
  PCP and, 528
  TCAs and, 275, 277
Peripheral neuritis, from alcohol abuse, 513
Permax; see Pergolide
Perphenazine, 262
  dosage of, 247
Perphenazine-amitriptyline, 262
Personal control, in therapeutic environment, 327
Personality
  A-B-C theory of, 37
  multiple, 447
  processes of, 26-27
  in Sullivan's interpersonal model, 33, 36
Personality disorders, 477-492
  anxious/fearful (cluster C), 487-490
    avoidant, 488-489
    dependent, 487-488
    obsessive-compulsive, 489
  childhood sexual abuse and, 599
  clusters of, 479

ersonality disorders–cont'd
  dramatic/erratic (cluster B), 482-487
    antisocial, 482-483
    borderline, 483-486
    histrionic, 487
    narcissistic, 486-487
  ECT and, 583
  etiology of, 478-479
  with HIV infection, 675
  odd/eccentric (cluster A), 479-481
    management of, 481
    paranoid, 479-480
    schizoid, 480
    schizotypal, 481
  and substance abuse, 544, 545
ersonal relationships
  in schizophrenia, 358-359
    antipsychotic drugs and, 251
ersonal space, and communication, 116
ersonal strengths case management model, 103
ervasive developmental disorder–not otherwise specified (PDD-NOS), 621
  prevalence of, 620
ervasive development disorder (PDD)
  in children and adolescents, 620-621
    medications for, 628
  definition of, 617
et therapy, 662
eyote, 526
  uses and effects of, 508-509
harmacist, 338
harmacodynamics, 211
  in children, 628
  of ethnic racial groups, 211
harmacodynamic tolerance, definition of, 502
harmacogenetics, 210-211
harmacokinetics, 211
  of alcohol, 511-512
  of antipsychotic drugs, 251-253
  of benzodiazepines, 300-301
  in elderly, 655-657
  of ethnic racial groups, 211
  of lithium, 291
  of MAOIs, 287
  of SSRIs, 284, 285
  of TCAs, 275, 276
hencyclidine (PCP), 528
  overdose of, 528
  urine detection of, 505
  uses and effects of, 508-509

Phenelzine, 286, 290
  characteristics of, 276-277
  in elderly, 658
  for panic disorder, 428
Phenergan; see Promethazine
Phenmetrazine, 508-509
Phenobarbital, withdrawal from, 516
Phenothiazines, 261
  alcohol interaction with, in elderly, 659
Phenylalanine, for stimulant dependence, 534-535
Phenylketonuria (PKU), 619
Phenylpropanolamine, MAOI interactions with, 287-288
Phenytoin
  antipsychotic drug interactions with, 260
  benzodiazepine interactions with, 302
  SSRI interactions with, 284
  TCA interactions with, 279
Philosophy factor, of cultural competence, 204-208
Phobic disorder(s), 432
  behavioral treatment of, 571
  ECT and, 583
  pharmacological treatment of, 306
  12-month prevalence rate of, 3, 345, 352, 384, 424, 452, 478, 502
Phonic tics, 626
Photophobia
  anticholinergic-induced, 239
  antipsychotic drug-induced, 258
Physical abuse, 605
Physical activities of daily living (PADLs), assessment in elderly, 654
Physical aggression, 157
  limit setting for, 328
Physical assessment, of elderly, 653-654
Physical complaints of depression, in elderly, 644
Physical disabilities, and communication, 116
Physical exercise groups, 324-325
Physical nature alterations, in depression, 390
Physical restraint
  and aggression, 158
  in milieu management, 315
Physical setting
  in group therapy, 176
  JCAHO standards of care for, 321
  modification of, 332

Physiological disorders, of depression, 390
Physostigmine, for benzodiazepine over-dose, 302
Pia mater, 77
Pick's disease, 468
Pimozide, 631
Pineal gland, 72
Pinel, Philippe, 4, 5
Piperazines, 261
Piperidines, 261
Pituitary gland, hypothalamus regulation of, 73
Planning
  in nurse-patient relationship, 129
  in nursing process, 138-139, 141
  therapeutic communication and, 120
  for working with families, 196
Plaques, Alzheimer's, 461, 463
Pleasure, limbic system and, 71-72
Pleasure principle, 27
Pneumocystis carinii pneumonia, 667, 668
Polydipsia, psychosis-induced, 369-370
Polygenetic inheritance, 618
Polymerase chain reaction (PCR), 667
Polynesian world view, 205, 207-208
Polypharmacy, 455
  in elderly, 652
Polysomnographic findings, in depression assessment, 397
Polyuria, lithium and, 291-292
Pons, 73-74
Positive reinforcement, 572
Positive symptoms of schizophrenia, 354, 355, 356
  antipsychotic drugs and, 357
Positron emission tomography (PET), 364
Post-acute withdrawal (PAW), 538
Postcrisis depression phase of assault cycle, 161
  interventions for, 164, 168
Postganglionic neuron(s), 77, 78
Postpartum depression, 386
  definition of, 383
  treatment of, 396
Postpartum psychosis, ECT for, 582
Postpsychotic depression, treatment of, 396
Postsynaptic membrane, 223
Posttraumatic stress disorder (PTSD), 433-439
  and battered woman syndrome, 606
  care plan for, 440

Posttraumatic stress disorder
(PTSD)–cont'd
DSM-IV criteria for, 433
family issues of, 435
interventions for, 438
Power of attorney, definition
of, 45
Prazepam, in elderly, 658
Precentral gyrus, 68
homunculus of, 70
Precocious senility, 352
Preconscious, 27
Precursor, definition of, 221
Prefrontal areas, 68
Preganglionic neurons, 77, 78
Pregnancy
amphetamines and cocaine
and, 524
anticholinergics and, 240
antipsychotic drugs and, 258
barbiturates and, 518
benzodiazepines and, 303
bipolar disorder in, 410
depression in, treatment of, 396
hallucinogens and, 529
influenza during, 365
lithium and, 293
MAOIs and, 289
medication use in, 211
opioids and, 521
and schizophrenia, 365
SSRIs and, 285
TCAs and, 280
Premack principle, 572
Premorbid, definition of, 351
Premotor cortex, 68, 70
Presynaptic membrane, 223
Prevalence, definition of, 617
Priapism, trazodone and, 283
Primary appraisal, definition
of, 27
Primary gain
in anxiety, 422
in conversion disorder, 442
definition of, 423
Primary process thinking, 27
Primary reinforcers, 571
Prion disease, 468-469
Privacy, 327
protecting, 322
Probable cause
definition of, 45
statement of, 49
Problem-centered groups, 175
Problem patient, consultation
for, 340

Problem solving
groups for, 173-174
interventions for, 425
in nurse-patient relationship, 129
skills training, for ADHD, 632
Problem specification, in behavioral
interventions, 576
Procainamide, TCA interactions
with, 279
Process
of African/African-American/His-
panic/Arabic world view, 207
of Asian/Asian American/
Polynesian world view, 207-208
of European American view, 206
of Native American world view, 208
Process factor, of cultural competence, 208-213
Process recording(s), 144
sample of, 142-143
Procyclidine, for Parkinson's
disease, 241
Program for Assertive Client Treatment (PACT) teams, 336-337
Progress notes, 144
and aggression, 163
components of, 141
Projection, 32
Projective identification, 478
Prolixin; see Fluphenazine
Promethazine, 244
Propranolol, 305
antipsychotic drug interactions
with, 260
for anxiety disorders, 306
for ASD/PTSD, 438
Protein binding, SSRIs and, 285
Protriptyline, 282
characteristics of, 276-277
Proxemics
and communication, 116
definition of, 115
Prozac; see Fluoxetine
Pseudodementia, 396, 644
Psilocin, 526
Psilocybin, 526
overdose of, 528
Psychiatric disorders
cost of, 3
with HIV infection, 674-676
Psychiatric emergencies, staff prepa-
ration for, 166
Psychiatric history, benchmarks in,
4-9
Psychiatric intensive care unit
(PICU), 93, 328-329

Psychiatric rehabilitation, 102; see
also Rehabilitation
Psychiatric social worker, 337-338
Psychiatric symptoms
of Alzheimer's disease, 464-465
of benzodiazepine withdrawal, 304
Psychiatrist, 337
Psychiatry, evolution of care in, 13
Psychoanalytical model, 26-27, 28, 30
Psychoanalytic theorists, and depression, 392
Psychobiological bases of behavior,
64-83
brain and, 64-65, 66
disorders with, 79, 81-82; see also
specific disorders
neuroanatomy/neurophysiology
and, 65-79
autonomic nervous system,
77, 78
brainstem and cerebellum, 73-75
cerebrum, 65-72
diencephalon, 72-73
neurons and neurotransmitters,
75, 76, 77
ventricular system, 77, 79
Psychodrama groups, 175
Psychodynamic factors
of anorexia nervosa, 554-555
of bulimia nervosa, 562
Psychodynamic theories
of alcoholism, 511
anxiety in, 149
of bipolar disorder, 409
of schizophrenia, 365-366
Psychoeducation
definition of, 321
programs, 174
in therapeutic environment, 325
Psychogeriatric Nursing Assessment
Protocol, 652
Psychological abuse, 604, 605
Psychological theories of depression,
392-393
Psychologist, 337
Psychomotor retardation
definition of, 124
ECT and, 583
and nurse-patient relationship,
133-134
Psychomotor symptoms of
anxiety, 151
Psychopathology, 24, 344-349; see
also specific disease entities
behavior and, 344
definition of, 20, 345

Psychiatric rehabilitation—cont'd
    etiology of, 345
    management of, 345-348
    understanding of, 347-348
Psychopharmacology, 23
    for anorexia nervosa, 555
    for ASD/PTSD, 438-439
    for bipolar disorder, 411-412
    for borderline personality
        disorder, 485
    for bulimia nervosa, 563
    for child and adolescent psychi-
        atric disorders, 628
    for cognitive disorders, 470-471
    in community-based care,
        99-100
    for depression, 399
    for dissociative disorders, 448
    for dual diagnoses, 546
    for elderly mentally ill, 655-659
    for generalized anxiety disorder,
        425-426
    for HIV infection, CNS effects
        of, 676
    in hospital-based care, 93-94
    in obsessive-compulsive
        disorder, 431
    for panic disorder, 427-428
    for partner abuse, 612
    for phobic disorders, 432
    for rape and sexual assault, 596
    for schizophrenia, 371
    for sexual disorders, 498
    for somatoform disorders, 444
    for substance abuse/dependence,
        534-535
    for survivors of childhood sexual
        abuse, 602
    for trauma recovery, 592
Psychosis, 350, 374-376; see also
        Schizophrenia; specific
        psychoses
    amphetamine-induced, 523
    in children and adolescents, med-
        ications for, 628
    definition of, 351
    in elderly, medical disorders asso-
        ciated with, 647
    and polydipsia, 369-370
Psychosocial adversity
    and child and adolescent psychi-
        atric disorders, 619
    definition of, 617
Psychosocial assessment of elderly,
        652-653
Psychostimulants, in elderly, 657

Psychosurgery, 585-587
    ethical concerns of, 586
    history of, 579, 581, 584, 585-586
    indications for, 586
Psychotherapeutic management
    of anorexia nervosa, 555-556,
        558-559
    for antisocial personality disorder,
        482-483
    for ASD/PTSD, 436-439
    of bipolar disorder, 410-413
    for borderline personality disorder,
        485-486
    of bulimia nervosa, 563-564
    of childhood sexual abuse, 601-604
    for cognitive disorders, 470-473
    in community-based care, 99
    in continuum of care, 19-25
    definition of, 20
    for dependent personality disor-
        der, 488
    of depression, 397-403
    for dissociative disorder, 447-448
    of dual diagnoses, 546, 548
    of elderly mentally ill, 654-662
    for generalized anxiety disorder,
        424-426
    model, 21
    for narcissistic personality disor-
        der, 487
    for obsessive-compulsive disorder,
        431-432
    for panic disorder, 427-428
    of partner abuse, 609-612
    in phobic disorders, 432
    psychopathology and, 346-348
    of rape and sexual assault, 596-597
    of schizophrenia, 370-374
    for schizotypal personality disor-
        der, 481
    for sexual disorders, 498
    for somatoform disorders, 443-445
    for substance abuse/dependence,
        532-533
    of torture and ritual abuse
        victims, 594
    of trauma recovery, 592
Psychotic depression, 386
    definition of, 383
Psychotic disorders
    in children and adolescents, 626
    in elderly, 646-648
Psychotropic drugs, 220-228; see also
        specific agents
    anticholinergic effects of, 456
        vs. trihexyphenidyl, 237

Psychotropic drugs—cont'd
    blood-brain barrier and, 225-226
    definition of, 3, 20
    depression from, 394
    in elderly, 651
        alcohol interaction in, 659
        side effects and nursing inter-
            ventions for, 657
        special considerations for, 656
    evolution of, 222
    neurotransmitters and, 223-225
    nursing responsibilities and,
        221-222
    in psychiatric history, 5, 7-8
    teaching patients about, 226-227
PTSD; see Posttraumatic stress disorder
Punch-drunk syndrome, 82
Punishment, in operant condition-
        ing, 571
Purging
    in anorexia nervosa, 552
    in bulimia nervosa, 559, 560
    definition of, 551
Purnell's twelve domain model for
        cultural competence, 202,
        213, 215
Putamen, 72
Puusepp, Ludwig, 585
Pyramidal system, 68, 69, 70, 230
    definition of, 65
    vs. extrapyramidal system, 229
Pyramids, 74

Q

Quetiapine, 265-266
    dosage of, 247
Quinidine, TCA interactions with, 279

R

Race, AIDS cases and, 673
Rage reactions, 160
Rape and sexual assault, 594-597
Rapid cycling, in bipolar disorders, 406
Rational-emotive therapy (RET)
        model, 36-37
Rationalization, 31
Rational Recovery Systems,
        536, 538
Reaction formation, 31
Reading disability, 621
Reality anxiety, 30
Reality orientation
    for cognitive disorders, 472
    for elderly mentally ill, 660
    group, 173
Reality principle, 27

Reality testing, in nurse-patient relationship, 129-130
Reality therapy model, 29, 38-39
Reappraisal, definition of, 27
Rebound phenomenon, in alcohol withdrawal, 513
Recidivism, 11
Reciprocal inhibition, 575
Recoil, as stage of trauma recovery, 591
Recovery
   in assault cycle, 161
      interventions for, 164, 168
   from childhood sexual abuse, 601
   from partner abuse, 608
   from rape and sexual assault, 595-596
   from substance abuse, 530
      personal responsibility in, 533
   from torture and ritual abuse, 594
   from trauma, 591-592
Recreational therapist, 338
Recreation group, 173
Red nuclei, 73
Referrals
   in nurse-patient relationship, 131
   and working with family, 192
Reflex tachycardia, antipsychotic drug-induced, 253
Regression, 32
Rehabilitation, 107-108
   and case management, 101-105
   model of, 103
Reinforcement, 572-573
Reinforcers, 571
Reinforcing stimulus, 571
Relapse
   of schizophrenia, 368-369
   in substance abuse recovery, 538
Relationships
   and adult manifestations of childhood sexual abuse, 600
   in manic patients, 408
   and schizophrenia, 358-359
      antipsychotic drugs and, 251
Religion
   balancing patient needs and rights with, 331
   in cultural assessment worksheet, 214
   definition of, 351
Remeron; see Mirtazapine
Reminiscence, and elderly mentally ill, 661
Remote amnesia, 445

REM sleep, depression and, 397
Renal function, and pharmacokinetics in elderly, 656-657
Rennie v. Klein (1983), 47
Reorganization, as stage of trauma recovery, 592
Representatives, nurses as, 311
Repression, 30, 31
   of childhood sexual abuse, 598
   in somatoform disorders, 440
Research, 14
Research Diagnostic Criteria (RDC), 345
Reserpine
   history of, 222, 270
   MAOI interactions with, 287-288
Residential services, 98-99
Residual schizophrenia, DSM-IV criteria for, 354
Resilience
   and child and adolescent psychiatric disorders, 619
   definition of, 617
Resistance stage, in stress adaptation syndrome, 39, 40
Resources, family, 195
Respect, 327
Respiratory depression, from heroin abuse, 520
Respondent conditioning, 570, 574-575
Response
   in behavior modification, 573
   in obsessive-compulsive disorder therapy, 633
Responsibility
   manic patients and, 408
   nursing
      before ECT, 581
      after ECT, 582
      for psychotropic drugs, 221-222
   patient, 328
   in reality therapy, 38, 39
   in substance abuse recovery, 533
Resting tremors, Parkinsonian, 231
Restraint
   of aggressive patient, 167-168
   definition of, 45, 54, 158
   in milieu management, 315
   in nursing homes, 641
   right to freedom from, 54-55
Restricting type of anorexia nervosa, 551
Retardation, in schizophrenia, 360
Reticular activating system (RAS), 75
Reticular formation, 74-75

Reversible dementia, 458
Reversible inhibitor of MAO-A (RIMA), 286, 290
   characteristics of, 276-277
ReVia; see Naltrexone hydrochloride
Revolving-door effect, 11
Richards, Linda, 6
Right-leaning environments, milieu management and, 311
Rights; see Patient rights
Rigidity, 233
   Parkinson's disease and, 231
Risperdal; see Risperidone
Risperidone, 264-265
   for child and adolescent psychiatric disorders, 631-632
   for cognitive disorders, 470
   cost of, 357
   dopamine receptors blocked by, 263
   dosage of, 247
   history of, 222
   and mesocortical system, 249
Ritalin; see Methylphenidate
Ritual abuse and torture, 592-594
Rivers v. Katz (1986), 55
Rogers v. Okin (1979), 47
Role-playing
   in nurse-patient relationship, 129
   in social skills training, 324
Root doctor, consultation with, 210
Rouse v. Cameron (1966), 46-47
Rules, 330
Rural area outreach services, 98

S

Safe sex, and HIV, 672
Safety
   and cognitive disorders, 472-473
   and manic patients, 410
   in milieu management, 315
   in therapeutic environment, 322, 327
      JCAHO standards of care for, 321
Satisfaction, 33
   definition of, 27
Schedule modification, 332
Schedules for Affective Disorders (SADS), 387
Schizoaffective disorder, 374-375
Schizoid personality disorder, 480, 481
Schizophrenia, 7, 350-374
   behavior in, 357-362
   biological basis of, 79, 362-365
   brain imaging findings in, 363

Schizophrenia—cont'd
in children and adolescents, 626
continuum of care for, 370-374
daily problems of, 367
definition of, 350-351
depression and suicide in, 368, 414
dopamine and, 77
DSM criteria for, 353-357
ECT and, 583
epidemiology of, 353
etiology of, 362-367
evolution of types of, 357
families of persons with, 367-368
support groups for, 368
genetic risk for, 365
and group therapy, 179
history of, 352-353
late-onset, 647
neurochemical theory of, 249-250
neurotransmitters and, 225
objective signs of, 358-359
prevalence of, 351, 352
lifetime, 346
12-month, 3, 345, 384, 424,
452, 478, 502
psychodynamic theories of, 365-366
relapse in, 368-369
sex-based differences in, 352
special issues of, 367-370
substance abuse and, 369
subtypes of, 354-356
DSM-IV criteria for, 354
evolution of, 357
symptoms of
antipsychotic drug modification
by, 250-251
positive and negative, 248, 356
subjective, 358, 359-362
treatment of
key objectives for, 367
success rate of, 4
vulnerability-stress model of,
366-367
Schizophreniform disorder, 376
Schizophrenogenic mother theory, 366
Schizotypal personality disorder, 481
Scientific study
period of, 7
in psychiatric history, 5
Seasonal affective disorder (SAD), 386
definition of, 383
Seclusion
and aggressive assaults, 166-167
care of patients in, 167-168

Seclusion—cont'd
definition of, 45, 54, 158
right to freedom from, 54-55
Secobarbital, alcohol interaction
with, in elderly, 659
Secondary appraisal, 27
Secondary gain
in anxiety, 422
in conversion disorder, 442
definition of, 423
Secondary process thinking, 27
Secondary reinforcers, 571
Security; see also Safety
JCAHO standards of care for, 321
in Sullivan's interpersonal model,
33, 36
Sedation
anticholinergic-induced, 239
from antidepressants, 274, 277,
281, 400
from antipsychotic drugs, 250, 259
from lithium, 400
Sedative-alcohol interaction, 515
Segregation analysis, 618
Seizures
anticholinergic-induced, 239
from antidepressants, 277
antipsychotic drug-induced, 259
benzodiazepines for, 304
from bupropion, 283
ECT-induced, 580-581, 582
Selective dopamine reuptake inhibitor (SDRI), 272
Selective inattention, 33
Selective serotonin/norepinephrine
reuptake inhibitor
(SNRI), 272
Selective serotonin reuptake inhibitors (SSRIs), 271, 272, 284-286
administration of, 399
for ASD/PTSD, 438
for borderline personality
disorder, 485
characteristics of, 276-277
for child and adolescent psychiatric disorders, 628, 630
for cognitive disorders, 471
definition of, 383
drug interactions with, 284
in elderly, 656, 658
history of, 222
interactions with
dimensions of, 285
MAOI, 287-288
mechanisms of action, 273

Selective serotonin reuptake inhibitors (SSRIs)—cont'd
for obsessive-compulsive disorder,
306, 431
for panic attacks and phobias, 306
for panic disorder, 427
for sexual disorders, 498
side effects of, 400
in children and adolescents, 630
Selegiline, 286
action of, 235
psychiatric side effects of, 235
Self-assessment, nurse, and aggression, 161-162
Self-control, in behavioral modification, 574
Self-destructive acts, limit setting
for, 328
Self-disclosure, in nurse-patient relationship, 124
Self-esteem
in depression, 398
milieu management for, 400-401
manipulation by manic
patients, 408
Self-help groups, 98-99, 175
for dual diagnosis, 548
for substance abuse, 536, 537-538
for survivors of childhood sexual
abuse, 602-604
Self-knowledge skills, for working
with family, 190
Self-mutilation
in borderline personality
disorder, 484
childhood sexual abuse and, 599
Self-punishment, as adult manifestation of childhood sexual
abuse, 600
Self reporting, of substance use, 504
Self-system, 33, 36
Selye's stress-adaptation theory, 29,
39, 149-150
Sensitivity, in communication, 117
Sensitization, and ASD/PTSD,
435-436
Sensory neurons, 75
Separation anxiety, 624
medications for, 628
Serax; see Oxazepam
Serlect; see Sertindole
Seroquel; see Quetiapine
Serotonin, 224
anorexia nervosa and, 553
and autism, 620-621

Serotonin—cont'd
  and bulimia nervosa, 561-562
  and depression, 77, 79, 390, 391
  history of, 222
  as neurotransmitter, 225
  and schizophrenia, 363
  TCAs and, 274
Serotonin dopamine antagonists
      (SDAs), 263, 363
Serotonin receptors, antipsychotic
      drugs and, 262, 263, 265, 266
Serotonin syndrome, 285
Sertindole, 266
  dosage of, 247
Sertraline, 286, 630
  for anxiety disorders, 306
  characteristics of, 276-277
  in elderly, 658
  for obsessive-compulsive
      disorder, 431
  for sexual disorders, 498
Serum albumin concentration, and
      drug distribution in elderly,
      655-656
Serzone; see Nefazodone
Severely mentally ill (SMI) individu-
      als, homelessness of, 11, 12-13
Sex-linked inheritance, 618
Sex offenders, characteristics of, 496
Sexual abuse, 597-604
  adolescent manifestations of, 598
  adult manifestations of, 598-599,
      600, 601
  and anorexia nervosa, 554
  and borderline personality disor-
      der, 483
  effects on child, 598
  family issues in, 603
  interventions for, 602
  management of, 601-604
  nature of problem of, 597-598
  recovery from, 601
Sexual arousal disorders, 494
Sexual assault and rape, 594-597
Sexual behaviors, limit setting and, 329
Sexual desire disorders, 494
Sexual disorders, 493-500
  from alcohol abuse, 514
  care plan for, 499
  DSM-IV criteria and terminology
      for, 493, 494
  gender identity disorders, 497-498
  initial assessment of, 494
  paraphilia, 495-497
  of sexual functioning, 493, 494-495
  from antidepressants, 277

Sexual innuendos, and nurse-patient
      relationship, 133
Sexual masochism, 495, 496
Sexual pain disorders, 495
Sexual reassignment surgery, 497
Sexual response cycle, 494
Sexual sadism, 495, 497
Shaking palsy, 231
The Shame of the States, 8
Shame vs. autonomy, in Erikson's
      stages of development, 34
Shaping, in behavior modification, 572
Shock treatment; see Electroconvul-
      sive therapy
Sialorrhea, 233
Significant others, in cultural assess-
      ment worksheet, 214
Simple schizophrenia, 357
Sinemet, 235
Sinequan; see Doxepin
Single photon emission computed
      tomography (SPECT), 364
Situational factors, in partner
      abuse, 606
Situational stressors, 149
Skills, for working with family,
      190-192
Skills training
  for ADHD, 632
  approaches to, 324
  in behavioral intervention, 575-576
  for behavior modification, 573-574
  for gaining employment, 326
  nurse-patient relationship and,
      130-131
Skinner, B. F., 571
Skin scraping/coining, 210-211
  definition of, 200
Sleep
  depression and, 389
    milieu management for, 402-403
  tension of need for, 33
Smith, and assault cycle, 161
Smoking, limit setting and, 329-330
The Snake Pit, 8
Social communication, therapeutic
      communication vs., 117
Social environment
  JCAHO standards of care for, 321
  rules in, 330
Social extinction, 573
Social interactions, depression and, 389
Socializing techniques, development
      of, 172
Social learning theorists, and depres-
      sion, 393

Social phobia
  DSM-IV criteria of, 432
  lifetime prevalence rates for, 346
  pharmacological treatment of, 306
Social-psychological models and ag-
      gression, 161
Social relationship, nurse-patient re-
      lationship vs., 124
Social Security Disability Insurance
      (SSDI), 9
Social skills
  for ADHD, 632
  groups for, 323-324
Social support for elderly, 640
Social workers, 337-338
Sociocultural factors of anorexia ner-
      vosa, 554
Sociocultural models, and aggres-
      sion, 161
Sociodrama groups, 175
Socioeconomics, and schizo-
      phrenia, 367
Sociological theory of depression, 393
Sodium, dietary, and lithium levels,
      291, 294
Somatic therapy, 579, 584-587
  definition of, 20
  electroconvulsive therapy; see Elec-
      troconvulsive therapy
Somatization disorder, 441
  DSM-IV criteria for, 441, 442
  12-month prevalence rate of, 3,
      345, 352, 384, 424, 452, 478,
      502
Somatoform disorders, 440-445
  conversion disorder, 442-445
  DSM-IV criteria for, 423, 441
  ECT and, 583
  hypochondriasis, 442
  interventions for, 445
  NANDA diagnoses for, 423
  pain disorder, 441-442
  somatization disorder, 441, 442
Somatotropic organization of cere-
      bral cortex, 70
Somnolent detachment, 33
South American holly, 212
Specialist, clinical, 105, 107
Special populations, 24
Special power of attorney, definition
      of, 45
Special problem groups, 175
Special therapies, 24
Speech
  and behavior, 115
  disorders of, 622

Speech—cont'd
in manic patients, 408
and nurse-patient relationship, 132-133
in schizophrenia, 361
Speed, 523
Spirituality; *see also* Religion
in cultural assessment work-sheet, 214
skills for working with family, 191
Split personality, 350-351, 447
Splitting
in borderline personality disorder, 483-484
definition of, 478
SSRIs; *see* Selective serotonin reup-take inhibitors
Staff
aggression-management and, 166
and patient restraint, 167
as victims of assault, 168-169
Stagnation vs. generative life-style, in Erikson's stages of develop-ment, 35
Standards of care, 14
definition of, 45
JCAHO, 321
State hospitals, depopulation of, 9-11
"Statement on Psychiatric Mental Health Clinical Nursing Prac-tice and Standards of Psychi-atric Mental Health Clinical Practice," 14
Stelazine; *see* Trifluoperazine
Step system, in therapeutic environ-ment, 323
Stereotypy, definition of, 351
Stimulants
abuse of, 521-524
for child and adolescent psychi-atric disorders, 628, 629
dependence on, medications for, 534-535
urine detection of, 505
uses and effects of, 508-509
withdrawal from, 516
Stimuli
in classical conditioning, 570, 571
in cognitive disorders, milieu man-agement for, 471-472
in operant conditioning, 571
STP, 526
overdose of, 528
Street skills group, 324

Stress
and adjustment disorder, 439
AIDS-related, 674
and borderline personality disor-der, 484
classification of, 148-149
and cognitive disorders, milieu management of, 471-472
counseling vs. crisis/suicide inter-vention, 154
crisis vs., 153
depression as reaction to, 392-393
perception of, 147-148
and schizophrenia, 366-367, 369
Stress models, 29, 39-41
and aggression, 161
depression in, 393
Structure
in milieu management, 315-316
in nurse-patient relationship, 128
in substance abuse manage-ment, 535
in therapeutic environment, 322-326
Structured Clinical Interview for Axis I *DSM-IV* Disorders (SCID), 387
Subacute care, 96-97
Subarachnoid space, 77
Subjective behavior
of delirium, 454-455
of dementia, 456-458
of manic patients, 409
Subjective symptoms, 358
of anorexia nervosa, 553
of bulimia nervosa, 561
of depression, 389-390
of schizophrenia, 358, 359-362
Sublimation, 31
Sublimaze; *see* Fentanyl
Substance abuse/dependence, 501-540
alcohol abuse, 510-516; *see also* Alcohol abuse
care plan for, 517
vs. drug abuse, 530-531
etiological theories of, 511
nursing issues in, 514-516
pharmacokinetics in, 511-512
physiological effects of, 512-514
assessment strategies for, 504
barbiturates/CNS depressants, 516, 518-519
care plan for, 525
cost of, 518
DSM-IV criteria for, 507-510, 531
in dual diagnosis, 543, 544, 545, 546, 548

Substance abuse/dependence—cont'd
in elderly, 649-652
hallucinogens, 524, 526-529
LSD, 528
marijuana, 526-528
mescaline, 526
PCP, 528
psilocybin, 526
and HIV, 675
transmission of, 673
treatment of, 676
inhalants, 519
interview approaches to, 505-507
lifetime prevalence rates for, 346
NANDA diagnoses for, 531
opioids (narcotics), 519-521
and partner abuse, 604
and PTSD, 436
among schizophrenics, 369
stimulants, 521-524
amphetamines, 523
cocaine, 522-523
substance uses and effects in, 506-509
treatment of, 529-538
diagnostic tools for, 530-532
evaluation, relapse, and follow-up care in, 538
family issues in, 529-530
patient rights and, 58-59
programs and support groups for, 535-538
psychotherapeutic management in, 532-535
and violence, 604
withdrawal in, 516
Substance Abuse Scale, 531-532
Substance-induced mood disorder, definition of, 383
Substantia nigra, 73
definition of, 230, 245
and Parkinson's disease and, 81, 230, 232, 233, 234, 466, 467
Subthalamus, 72
Succinylcholine
benzodiazepine interactions with, 302
for ECT, 581, 582
Suicide, 413
antidepressants and, 281
assessment of, 415-416
balancing patient needs and rights and, 331
borderline personality disorder and, 484
common expressions of, 414

Suicide—cont'd
  definition of, 271
  and depression, 396
    TCAs for, 278-279
  ECT and, 583
  and elderly, 395, 397, 415, 645-646
  impact of guns on, 415
  interventions for, 416-417
    vs. stress counseling, 154
  limit setting and, 328
  major depressive disorder and, 385
  and mood disorders, 413-417
  risk factors for, 414
  in schizophrenia, 368
  threats, 413
Sulcus, 68
  of Alzheimer's patient, 459, 460, 461
  definition of, 65
Sullivan, Harry Stack, 14
  and anxiety, 149
  interpersonal model of, 28, 33, 36
  and schizophrenia, 366
Superego, 26, 27
Superstitious behavior, 572
Supervisor, nurse, 339-340
Supplemental Security Income
    (SSI), 9
Support
  in nurse-patient relationship,
    128, 130
  in psychotherapeutic manage-
    ment, 346
Support groups, 173
  for families of schizophrenics, 368
  for staff member assault victims,
    168-169
Suppression, as defense mechan-
    ism, 31
Suspiciousness
  and nurse-patient relationship, 134
  schizophrenia and, milieu manage-
    ment for, 372-373
Sweating
  anticholinergics and, 239
  antidepressants and, 400
Swertia japonica, 212
Symbolic imagery
  in African/African-American/His-
    panic/Arabic world view, 206
  definition of, 200
Symbolic rhythm
  in African/African-American/His-
    panic/Arabic world view, 207
  definition of, 200
Symmetrel; see Amantadine
Sympathetic nervous system, 77

Sympathomimetics
  MAOI interactions with, 287-288
  TCA interactions with, 279
Sympathy, in nurse-patient relation-
    ship, 127
Synapse, 75, 223
  definition of, 221
Synesthesia, LSD and, 528
Systematic desensitization, 575

T
Tachycardia
  from antidepressants, 400
  from antipsychotic drugs, 253, 259
Tacrine
  for Alzheimer's disease, 465
  history of, 222
Tagamet; see Cimetidine
Talwin; see Pentazocine
Taractan; see Chlorprothixene
Tarasoff v. The Regents of the University
    of California (1976), 47, 57, 331
Tardive dyskinesia
  anticholinergic-induced, 239
  from antipsychotic drugs, 254, 256
    in children and adolescents, 631
    interventions for, 259
  definition of, 230, 245
  ECT and, 583
  in elderly, 647-648, 656
Taylor's Dysphoria Inventory, 387
TCAs; see Tricyclic antidepressants
T cells, HIV infection and, 670-671
Team leader role, 338
Team meeting leadership, 338
Tegretol; see Carbamazepine
Telephone, work with suicidal per-
    sons over, 417
Temperature, anticholinergics and, 239
Temporal lobes, 71
Tensions, Sullivan's types of, 33, 36
Termination stage of nurse-patient re-
    lationship, 126, 131
Terror, definition of, 27
Testing-out step, in nurse-patient re-
    lationship, 129
Tetrahydrocannabinol, 508-509
Thalamus, 72-73
THC; see Tetrahydrocannabinol
Theft, limit setting for, 328
Themes, in communication, 116
Theoretical models, 26-43
  cognitive-behavioral, 36-38
  comparisons of, 42
  developmental, 30, 33
  eclectic approach to, 41

Theoretical models—cont'd
  interpersonal, 33, 36
  psychoanalytical, 26-27, 30
  reality therapy, 38-39
  stress, 39-41
  summary of, 28-29
Theories
  of cultural competence, 202-204
  for family assessment and interac-
    tions, 189-190
Therapeutic, definition of, 20
Therapeutic communication; see
    Communication, therapeutic
The Therapeutic Community, 312
Therapeutic community, 314
Therapeutic environment, 310,
    320-333; see also Milieu man-
    agement
  balance in, 330-331
  and community-based milieu, 332
  limit setting in, 328-330
  milieu management and, 314
  modification of, 331-332
  norms in, 326-328
  rules in, 330
  safety in, 322
  standards of care in, 321
  structure of, 322-326
Therapeutic listening, 117
  definition of, 115
Therapeutic milieu, 310, 313-314
  definition of, 311
  nurse roles in, 336-341
    as colleague, 337-338
    as consultant, 340
    as supervisor and trainer, 339-340
    as team leader, 338
Therapy; see also Behavior therapy;
    Group therapy
  vs. being therapeutic, 22, 125
  in case management, 110
  definition of, 20
  groups, 174, 175
Thiamine, alcoholism and, 513, 534
Thioridazine, 261, 631
  anticholinergic effects of, 456
  for ASD/PTSD, 439
  dosage of, 247
  in elderly, 656
  potency of, vs. trihexyphenidyl, 237
  for survivors of childhood sexual
    abuse, 602
Thiothixene, 262, 631
  dosage of, 247
  in elderly, 656
Thioxanthenes, 262

Thirst, lithium-induced, 400
Thoracolumbar nervous system, 77
Thorazine; see Chlorpromazine
Thought alterations, in schizophrenia, 358, 360-361
  antipsychotic drugs and, 251
Threats
  perception of, 148
  of suicide, duty to warn of, 57
Tiapridal, 534
Tics, in children and adolescents, 626
  medications for, 628
Time out
  and aggression, 166
  in behavior modification, 573
Tofranil; see Imipramine
Token systems
  in behavioral modification, 574
  in therapeutic environment, 323
Tolerance
  to alcohol, 512
  to benzodiazepines, 301, 303
  definition of, 299, 502
Torture and ritual abuse, 592-594
Touching
  in communication, 118
  inappropriate, by patient, 133
Tourette's syndrome, 626
  haloperidol for, 262
Toxic-metabolic disturbances, and depression, 395
Toxins, depression from, 394
Trainer role, 339-340
Transference, 30
  definition of, 27, 124
  in nurse-patient relationship, 134
Transient ischemic attacks (TIAs), 469-470
Transition group, 325
Transsexualism, 497-498
Tranxene; see Clorazepate
Tranylcypromine, 286, 290
  characteristics of, 276-277
Trauma
  CNS, 82
  recovery from, 591-592
Trazodone
  as antianxiety drug, 306
  as antidepressant, 283
  antipsychotic drug interactions with, 260
  characteristics of, 276-277
  in elderly, 656, 657
  for rape and sexual assault, 596
  for suicidal patients, 179

Treatment plan, in behavioral interventions, 576
Treatment settings, for child and adolescent psychiatric disorders, 627-628
Tremor(s)
  alcoholic, 231
  Parkinsonian, 231, 467
Triavil; see Perphenazine-amitriptyline
Triazolam, in elderly, 659
Tricyclic antidepressants (TCAs), 271, 273-275, 277-284
  administration of, 399
  as antianxiety drug, 305-306
  for ASD/PTSD, 438
  characteristics of, 276-277
  for child and adolescent psychiatric disorders, 628, 629-630
  for cognitive disorders, 470-471
  definition of, 383
  for depression, 396
  ECT vs., 584
  in elderly, 656, 657
    alcohol interaction with, 659
  history of, 222
  interactions with, 279, 280
    antipsychotic drugs, 260
    benzodiazepines, 302
    MAOIs, 287-288
    SSRIs, 284
  mechanisms of action, 273
  and neurotransmitters, 225
  newer agents, 282-284
  nursing implications for, 279-281
  overdose, 279-280
  pharmacokinetics and dosing of, 275, 276
  pharmacological effects of, 274
  side effects of, 275, 277-278, 400
  for stimulant dependence, 534
  for suicidal thoughts, 278-279
Trifluoperazine, 261
  dosage of, 247
Triggering phase of assault cycle, 161
  interventions for, 164, 165
Trihexyphenidyl, 236
  dosage of, 237, 240
  overdose of, 240
  for Parkinson's disease, 241
  prophylactic, for EPSEs, 257
  psychotropic drugs vs., 456
Trilafon; see Perphenazine
Trimipramine, 276-277

Trust
  and depression, 398
  vs. mistrust, in Erikson's stages of development, 34
  in nurse-patient relationship, 126-127
Tuberoinfundibular system, antipsychotic drug action on, 249
Tuke, William, 4, 5
Twelve domain model of cultural competence, 213, 215
Twelve steps of Alcoholics Anonymous, 536
Twin studies
  of ADHD, 622
  of child psychiatric disorders, 618
  depression in, 391
  of PTSD, 436
  of schizophrenia, 365
  and tic disorders, 626
Type II schizophrenia, 355, 356
Type I schizophrenia, 355, 356
Tyramine, 288
  definition of, 271
Tyramine-rich foods, MAOI interactions with, 288-289
Tyrosine
  definition of, 271
  for stimulant dependence, 534

U

Ulcers, alcohol abuse and, 513
Unconscious, 27
Undifferentiated schizophrenia, 354
Undoing, as defense mechanism, 32
Uninvolved patient, in group therapy, 179
Unit norms; see Norms
Unit structure; see Structure
Universality, group therapy and, 172
Universal precautions, against HIV, 673-674
Unlicensed assistive personnel (UAPs), delegating authority to, 60-61
Upper motor neurons, 70
Urinary hesitancy/retention
  anticholinergic-induced, 239
  from antidepressants, 281, 400
  antipsychotic drug-induced, 259
  from psychotropic drugs, 657
Urine, detection of drugs in, 505

V

Vaginismus, 495
Valium; see Diazepam
Valproate, history of, 222

Valproic acid
  for bipolar disorder, 294-295
  for borderline personality
      disorder, 485
  in elderly, 659
Vascular dementia, 469
  definition of, 452
VBR; see Ventricular brain ratio
Venlafaxine, 283-284
  for anxiety disorders, 306
  characteristics of, 276-277
Ventilation, of anger, 165
Ventral tegmental area (VTA),
      71-72
  definition of, 245
Ventricular brain ratio (VBR), 79
  and schizophrenia, 355, 364
Ventricular enlargement, Alzheimer's
      and, 460, 461
Ventricular system, 77, 79
Verbal aggression, 158-159
  intervention for, 163-164
Vermis, 75
Vesicle, definition of, 221
Victimization; see Violence,
      victims of
Violence, 157
  cycle of, 606, 607, 608
  in elderly mentally ill, milieu man-
      agement for, 659
  history of, as aggression
      variable, 163
  and nurse-patient relationship, 132
  victims of, 590-613
      from childhood sexual abuse,
          597-604
      from partner abuse, 604-606,
          608-612
      from rape and sexual assault,
          594-597
      from torture and ritual abuse,
          592-594
      violation and, 591-592
Viral infections, HIV infection
      and, 669
Virus, and Alzheimer's disease, 464
Vision
  anticholinergics and, 239
  antidepressants and, 281, 400
  antipsychotic drugs and, 258
  psychotropic drugs and, 657
Visitation, in working with family, 194

Visual aphasia, 71
Visual hallucinations, in schizophre-
      nia, 359
Vitamin deficiencies
  from alcohol abuse, 513
  and secondary psychosis in
      elderly, 647
Vitamin E, for Alzheimer's
      disease, 465
Vivactil; see Protriptyline
Voluntary commitment
  definition of, 45
  legal issues of, 48
Vomiting
  in anorexia nervosa, 552
  in bulimia nervosa, 560, 561
Voyeurism, 495, 497
Vulnerability-stress model of schizo-
      phrenia, 366-367

W

Wandering
  in cognitive disorders, milieu man-
      agement for, 473
  interventions for, 472
Warfarin, TCA interactions
      with, 279
Warren's cultural assessment work-
      sheet, 214
Watts, James, 585
Weight gain
  antipsychotic drug-induced, 259
  from lithium, 400
Weight loss, anorexia nervosa
      and, 552
Wellbutrin; see Bupropion
Wernicke-Korsakoff syndrome, 513
Wernicke's encephalopathy, 469
Western medicine, beliefs of, 210
White matter, definition of, 65
Whitree v. State of New York (1968), 47
Will, George, 9
Withdrawal
  from addictive drugs, 516
  from alcohol, 513, 515-516
      in elderly, 650
      pharmacotherapy for, 514-516
  from amphetamines, 524
  from barbiturates, 518-519
  from benzodiazepines, 301, 304
      in elderly, 658
      interventions for, 302

Withdrawal—cont'd
  from cocaine, 524
  definition of, 299, 502
  DSM-IV criteria for, 510
  from hallucinogens, 529
  from opioids, 521
  post-acute, 538
Withdrawal behavior
  definition of, 351
  depressed, 401
  schizophrenic, 372
Women
  alcohol metabolism in, 512
  depression in, 388
      biological basis of, 391
  partner-abuse of, 604, 605,
      606, 608
      cycle of violence in, 606,
          607, 608
      management in, 609-612
      recovery of, 608
  schizophrenia in, 352
Word salad, definition of, 351
Work, and schizophrenia, 369
Work groups, 325-326
Working stage of nurse-patient rela-
      tionship, 125-126, 128-131
World view
  definition of, 200
  models, and cultural competence,
      204-208
Writing/journaling, in nurse-patient
      relationship, 130
Written communication, 115
Wyatt v. Stickney (1972), 47

X

Xanax; see Alprazolam

Y

Yalom, Irvin, 172

Z

Zeldox; see Ziprasidone
Zidovudine, 676
Ziprasidone, 266
  dosage of, 247
Zoloft, 286
Zung Self-Rating Depression
      Scale, 387
Zyban; see Bupropion
Zyprexa; see Olanzapine

CHAPTER 14

Name:

Working with the Aggressive Patient

Match the term with its definition:

1. _____ Assault

2. _____ Battery

3. _____ Passive aggression

4. _____ Seclusion

5. _____ Restraint

a. Legally, any behavior that physically or verbally presents an immediate threat of physical injury to another individual

b. Physical control of a patient to prevent injury to patient, staff, and other patients

c. Direct expression of feelings and needs in a respectful way

d. Normal emotional response to frustration of desires

e. Process of placing a patient alone in a specially designed room for protection and closer observation

f. Inflicting physical injury on another individual

g. Anger expressed indirectly in subtle or evasive ways

Indicate T for true or F for false:

6. _____ Nurses have the right, professionally and legally, to use physical force to prevent patients from injuring themselves and others.

7. _____ Of the patients admitted to psychiatric facilities, most are violent prior to admission.

8. _____ Aging may result in diminished impulse control.

9. _____ Violent acts can be the result of boredom.

10. _____ Passive-aggressive individuals tend to deny anger.

11. There are specific times when patients are more likely to become aggressive or assaultive. List at least three of these:

12. Name three psychiatric diagnoses that have a higher incidence of aggression after admission:

C H A P T E R 1 5   Name:

Working with Groups of Patients

1. List five types of groups and the function of each type of group:

Match the type of group with an example of the group:

2. _____ Creative expression   a. Support groups

3. _____ Psychodrama   b. Activity groups

4. _____ Reality orientation   c. Education groups

5. _____ Stress management   d. Therapy groups

6. _____ Alliance for the Mentally Ill   e. Self-help/special problem groups

Critical Thinking Discussion Questions

Yalom described 11 therapeutic factors that he viewed as helping patients in any therapeutic group. Write an example you have observed or create one for each of the factors listed below:

Example:

Instillation of hope: A patient observes other patients in process group every day for 3 days and sees how they have benefited from the group by improving in mood and verbalization.

7. Universality:

8. Imparting of information:

9. Altruism:

10. Corrective recapitulation of primary family group:

CHAPTER 36   Name:

Behavior Therapy

1. An example of positive reinforcement on the psychiatric unit is:
   a. Visiting hours.
   b. Group therapy.
   c. Token economy program.
   d. Nurse-patient contract.

2. Susan is a 9-year-old girl in third grade. Her teacher puts a star on a chart in the classroom for each completed spelling exercise. When a student gets 10 stars, he or she can choose a prize from a special box. Five students in the class have already claimed their prizes. Susan has eight stars and is excited about her anticipated reward. The star chart is an example of:
   a. Intermittent reinforcement.
   b. Shaping.
   c. The Premack principle.
   d. Continuous reinforcement.

3. John Thomas is a 52-year-old who likes to monopolize conversation in group therapy, interrupts other speakers, and makes lists of things to do each day. Identify three techniques to decrease his behaviors, which interfere with the therapeutic milieu for other patients:

4. Assertiveness training is an example of skills training that uses the behavior therapy techniques of positive reinforcement, shaping, modeling, and imitation. Which activity would not be part of an assertiveness training program that relies on these therapeutic techniques?
   a. Role playing
   b. Teaching by example
   c. Praise for disagreeing with the group leader
   d. Time out

5. Ellen has become disabled by a phobia during the past year. She experiences palpitations, dizziness, and fear whenever she hears music. She has been unable to go to the market or almost any other public place. Which behavior therapy could best help her cope with her symptoms so that she can go out to public places again?
   a. Token economy
   b. Systematic desensitization
   c. Time out
   d. Contingency contracting

6. List the components of the behavioral nursing process:

CHAPTER 37   Name:

Electroconvulsive Therapy and Other Somatic Therapies

1. Somatic therapies use _____ interventions to produce behavior change in people with severe psychiatric disorders.

2. Place a check by the psychiatric professionals who would probably never be involved in the use of somatic therapies:
   _____ Psychiatrist
   _____ Psychiatric nurse
   _____ Psychiatric social worker
   _____ Physical therapist
   _____ Occupational therapist
   _____ Recreational therapist
   _____ Psychologist

3. Electroconvulsive therapy (ECT) is most often used to treat patients with _____ _____, particularly those manifesting _____ and _____. These patients have generally not been helped by the following category of pharmacologic agents: _____.

4. What are the "dosage" and the frequency of ECT administration?

5. Identify at least three possible nursing activities for each stage of care for the person receiving ECT:
   a. Before ECT:

   b. During ECT:

   c. After ECT:

C H A P T E R 3 8   Name:

Victims of Violent Behavior

1. Nursing practice that focuses on the holistic care of victims and perpetrators of violent crimes and their families is called _____ _____

2. Many crimes involve physical violence and injury, but all crimes involve _____ violation and injury.

3. Victims of any type of crime lose:
   a. Material possessions.
   b. Self-respect.
   c. Civil rights.
   d. Control of their own lives.

4. List the three stages of recovery from trauma:

5. What medications are often helpful for victims of crime?
   a. None
   b. Anticholinergic
   c. Anticonvulsant
   d. Hallucinogenic

6. Identify at least three common physical effects and three common emotional effects of torture and ritual abuse:

7. Rape is generally considered to be an act of _____ and _____ rather than a sexually motivated act.

8. Victims of rape can be overwhelmed by emotional feelings. List the most common:

9. Rape victims are about _____ times more likely to attempt suicide than are nonvictims.

10. In what clinical settings are nurses most likely to encounter patients who have been victims of violence and who need sensitive interventions for their emotional and cognitive pain?

Critical Thinking Discussion Questions

11. Identify the 10 most important nursing interventions with adult survivors of childhood sexual abuse. Give a rationale for each selected.

12. Describe ways to help a victim of partner abuse who is not yet able to leave the abusive relationship.

CHAPTER 39   Name:

Child and Adolescent Psychiatric Nursing

Briefly define the following terms:

1. Attention-deficit hyperactivity disorder (ADHD):

2. Genetic vulnerability:

3. Resiliency:

4. Social skills:

5. Time out:

6. Approximately how many children in the United States are reported to have mental health problems?
   a. Almost 1 million
   b. 10 million
   c. 20 million
   d. 100 million

7. Minority children and adolescents are the most rapidly growing group of youth in the United States. What factors contribute to increased risk of mental health disorders for many of these children?

8. Children with mental health and psychiatric disorders are treated in a variety of settings. List at least five settings, and identify the type of disorder that commonly would be treated in each:

9. Children with mental retardation have low intellectual functioning and impairments in adaptive functioning. Which of the following is not a category of adaptive functioning?
   a. Communication
   b. Self-care
   c. Socialization
   d. Nutrition

CHAPTER 40   Name:

Mental Illness in the Elderly

1. In the year 2050 approximately _____% of the U.S. population will be over age 65.

2. In the first decades after the year 2000, the estimated proportion of the population over age 65 will:
   a. Remain stable.
   b. Decline.
   c. Experience modest growth.
   d. Increase substantially.

3. Psychiatric disorders among the elderly are:
   a. Generally independent of other health-related problems.
   b. Usually associated with other significant health problems.
   c. Infrequent and self-limiting
   d. Rampant and inevitable.

4. List reasons that the treatment needs for mental health services have been underestimated for the elderly population:

5. Which of the following is not a barrier to mental health care for the elderly?
   a. Family members preferring more personalized services
   b. Discrimination by some health care providers
   c. Attitudes of the elderly about mental illness
   d. Failure to detect mental illness

6. Depression is the most common mental illness among the elderly, yet it is often overlooked, misdiagnosed, or inadequately treated. List at least four consequences of these limitations in contemporary health care:

CHAPTER 41   Name:

Working with Patients with HIV Disease

1. What is the normal range of T4 cells?
   a. 200-800/mm^3
   b. 600-1200/mm^3
   c. 1000-1500/mm^3
   d. 1200-1800/mm^3

2. The number of T4 cells correlates with:
   a. Incubation period
   b. Symptoms and clinical course.
   c. Source of transmission.
   d. AIDS dementia.

3. What type of cancer is unusual in young adults unless it is associated with HIV disease?
   a. Leukemia
   b. Hodgkin's disease
   c. Cancer of the brain
   d. Kaposi's sarcoma

4. What is the most serious opportunistic infection associated with HIV disease?

5. Which of the following risks for transmission of HIV has been virtually eliminated?
   a. Intimate homosexual contact with an HIV-infected person
   b. Intimate heterosexual contact with an HIV-infected person
   c. Parenteral injection of blood or blood products infected with HIV
   d. Transfer of HIV from mother to baby

6. Why are persons with mental illness at increased risk for acquiring and/or transmitting HIV?

7. What is the diagnostic criterion for a diagnosis of AIDS?

8. Prevention is the key therapeutic strategy for HIV disease. What is the primary preventive intervention used by health care professionals?

Answer Key to Student Worksheets

Chapter 1

1. b
2. d
3. a
4. e
5. The wants and desires, the "I" component, of an individual
6. A place of refuge; sanctuary
7. The conscience or moralistic component of an individual
8. Medications used in the treatment of mental illness
9. After the evolution of psychotropic medications, this term was used to describe the concept of patients with a mental health problem being treated in the least restrictive environment.
10. The depopulation of state hospitals
11. 1946; established the National Institute of Mental Health
12. Typically healthy individuals having difficulty coping with their current situation
13. 1963; shift in providing mental health care in institutions to community mental health care centers
14. The process of persons cycling and recycling through public psychiatric hospitals
15. F
16. T
17. F
18. T
19. F

Chapter 2

1. Safety, structure, norms, limit setting, balance, and environmental modification
2. The nurse's ability to communicate therapeutically, drugs, milieu management
3. Decompensation of the patient
4. Drug and alcohol treatment programs
5. Examples:
   Dispense medications.
   Evaluate need for prn medications.
   Assess patient's response to medications.
   Plan for a response to side effects.
   Assess for side effects, treat, and evaluate treatment.
   Educate patients on medications and answer questions.
6. Somatic therapy
7. A therapeutic approach that uses physiological or physical interventions to effect behavioral changes
8. The study of underlying processes, both biological and psychosocial, that lead to mental disorders

Chapter 3

1. a
2. c
3. b
4. d
5. e
6. Trust vs. mistrust
7. 0 to 18 months
8. Reality therapy
9. a
10. e
11. j
12. a
13. f
14. b
15. g
16. i
17. d
18. h
19. c

Chapter 4

1. Least restrictive alternative/environment
2. Mental Health Systems Act
3. Written
4. Verbal
   Pharmacological
5. 4
6. 60
7. 2

Chapter 4—cont'd

8. 24
9. informed consent
10. c
11. b
12. a
13. e
14. f
15. h
16. c
17. d
18. h
19. g

Chapter 5

1. c
2. b
3. d
4. a
5. Feeding, fighting, fleeing, and fornicating
6. Modulates voluntary movements, maintains appropriate muscle tone, and adjusts posture
7. Dopamine
8. Acetylcholine
9. Hypothalamus
10. Dopamine

Chapter 6

1. Continuum of care refers to the levels of care through which an individual can move depending upon his or her needs at a given point in time.
2. The effects of managed care are listed in Box 6-2.
3. The four factors involved in deciding the appropriate level of care for patients are found in Figure 6-1.
4. Box 6-1 provides examples of interventions.

Chapter 7

1. Typical patient behaviors that need to be evident to justify inpatient hospitalization include individuals who are actively suicidal, self-mutilating, or threatening harm to others. Other patients requiring hospitalization include those who are gravely disabled, those who are experiencing toxic reactions to medications or other substances, and those who need medical intervention for safe withdrawal from substances.
2. Two goals of hospital-based care are to assist individuals with attaining a safe level of functioning and/or stabilization and to provide referrals for aftercare.
3. Some roles of the nurse in inpatient psychiatric settings are to establish a therapeutic alliance, assess priority needs, administer care in a matter of days, participate in discharge planning, obtain the medication history, monitor medication side effects, educate the patient and family about medication and side effects, and manage the milieu.
4. Table 7-1 will help the student identify target issues addressed at various facilities.

Chapter 8

1. Some examples of community-based services are outpatient services, psychiatric home care, outreach programs, residential services, and self-help groups.
2. Community-based care resources appropriate for individuals
   a. Outpatient treatment, partial program, self-help groups
   b. Subacute program, outpatient treatment, self-help groups
   c. Outpatient program such as a community support program, partial program, self-help groups, residential services such as a group home or apartment living program
   d. Outpatient treatment, residential services, self-help groups, community outreach program
3. Five problematic areas found in community-based care are insufficient reimbursement for services, lack of availability of services, lack of accessibility to needed services, fragmentation of services, and an insufficient range of services.

Chapter 9

1. An eclectic approach in which patients receive care in the least restrictive setting in order to be successful in their environment
2. Assist with accessing, using, and following through with services that improve patient quality of life
3. Provides advice on behavioral and psychiatric issues to professionals outside the psychiatric specialty and negotiates compromises between patients and their families, community, or treatment team; also coordinates care among multiple service providers involved with an individual patient
4. Educates others regarding mental illness and facilitates the participation of persons with mental illness in public and community environments
5. Actions in an acute period to prevent further decompensation or relapse when a patient is unable to cope on his or her own
6. Provides nursing services outside of health care settings, in community settings where patients live, work, play, and worship
7. Individual counseling and recommendations for changing things patients do in order to improve their functional ability and quality of life
8. a
9. F
10. T
11. T

Chapter 10

1. Nontherapeutic
2. Using clichés
3. Therapeutic
4. Presenting reality
5. Therapeutic
6. Giving information
7. Therapeutic
8. Rehearsing
9. Nontherapeutic
10. False promises
11. Therapeutic
12. Clarification

Chapter 11

1. The objective understanding of how patients feel or how they see their situations
2. *Student example*
3. Hallucinations
4. Early assessment of the content of the messages
   Diversion: do not focus on the hallucinations
5. Command hallucination
6. Contract with patient to not act on the commands.
   Contract with patient to tell staff if he or she feels like acting on the commands.
7. Transference
8. Recognize the transference
9. Realistic
   Measurable
10. It is a learning tool to evaluate the student nurse's communication patterns.

Chapter 12

1. Short term goal: Patient will sign a "no-harm contract" within 24 hours of admission.
2. Long term goal: Patient will attend a 6-week divorce recovery group after discharge.
3. Objective data: what can be seen, heard, and/or measured, such as a patient's appearance, nonverbal behaviors, and vital signs
   Subjective data: what the patient says about her or his own thoughts, feelings, behaviors, and problems
4. Initial patient assessment:
   Demographic data: male, 29 years old, married
   Reason for admission: thinks wife is poisoning his vodka
   Drug and alcohol use: uses alcohol
   Mental Status Examination
   General appearance: wearing a jogging suit
   Behaviors during the interview:
      Expression of anger: overt, toward wife
      Degree of cooperation: resistance, evasiveness
      Social skills: withdrawal
      Orientation: aware of being in a treatment facility, alert
      Thought clarity: coherent
      Thought content: suspiciousness toward wife, blaming of others, denial
      Delusions: of persecution
      Affect/mood: +3 anxiety level, expressing anger
      Insight: lack of awareness of illness (denial)
      Motivation: no motivation for treatment

Chapter 13

1. +2 anxiety level:
   Subjective: feeling uncomfortable, decreased confidence
   Objective: increased blood pressure, pulse, and respirations, difficulty sitting still
   Intervention: decrease anxiety by encouraging ventialiation and/or exercise
2. Symptoms of anxiety in one person often create anxiety in others. Try to imagine (or remember) being with someone who is tense, pacing, talking rapidly and loudly, defensive, irritable, and unable to focus on a conversation.

Chapter 13—cont'd

3. What problems have you been having?
   What has changed in your life lately?
4. Effectiveness, outcomes, duration, frequency, consequences for self and others
5. 1. Assess for suicidal and/or homicidal thoughts, intent, and plan.
   2. Monitor for physical safety.
   3. Encourage safe expression of emotions.
   4. Offer empathy and emotional support.
   5. Focus on immediate actions and resources needed.

Chapter 14

1. a
2. f
3. g
4. e
5. b
6. T
7. F
8. T
9. T
10. T
11. Examples: admission, change of shifts, mealtimes, visiting hours, evenings, in elevators, during transportation to outside areas, periods of change
12. Schizophrenia, especially paranoid; mania; and organic brain disorder

Chapter 15

1. Examples:
   Support groups: reinforce or maintain existing patient strengths and behaviors
   Activity groups: facilitate patient communication and interaction
   Education groups: teach patients a variety of content and skills
   Therapy groups: help patients develop understanding and insight into their feelings, behaviors, and roles in relationships
   Self-help or special problem groups: help patients with special problems
2. b
3. d
4. a
5. c
6. e
7-10. Critical Thinking Discussion Questions

Chapter 16

1. b
2. c
3. a
4. Critical Thinking Discussion Question

Chapter 17

1. T
2. T
3. F
4. T
5. African Americans and Native Americans
6. F
7. M
8. M
9. M
10. b
11. c
12. d
13. a

Chapter 18

1. d
2. c
3. b
4. a
5. e
6. Prozac
7. Thorazine and Clozaril
8. They block enzymatic reduction of neurotransmitters.
9. An anatomic barrier, a metabolic barrier, and a physiologic barrier

Chapter 19

1. D
2. B
3. B
4. A
5. D
6. Reduced bioavailability of norepinephrine is a primary cause of depression. Because norepinephrine is a metabolite of dopamine, and Parkinson's disease (PD) is caused by a deficiency of dopamine, there may not be adequate levels of norepinephrine. Further, norepinephrine-synthesizing neurons also decrease in PD.
7. Increased levels of dopamine in certain areas of the brain
8. Decrease
9. For oculogyric crises, severe dystonic reactions, swallowing difficulties, and other acute dystonic emergencies
10. Examples:
    Dry mouth: sugarless hard candy and chewing gum, frequent rinses
    Nasal congestion: over-the-counter nasal decongestant if approved by physician
    Urinary hesitation: running water, privacy, warm water over perineum
    Urinary retention: catheterize for residual fluids, encourage frequent voiding
    Blurred vision, photophobia: reassurance (normal vision typically returns in a few weeks), sunglasses, caution when driving, tolerance develops

Chapter 19—cont'd

Constipation: laxatives as ordered, diet with roughage, 2500-300 ml of water per day

Mydriasis: if eye pain develops, could indicate narrow-angle glaucoma—immediate attention is warranted

Orthostatic hypotension: request that patient get out of bed slowly, sit on the edge of the bed a short while, and rise slowly

Sedation: help patient get up early and get the day started

Decreased sweating: can lead to fever; take temperature; if fever occurs, reduce body temperature (e.g., sponge baths)

Temperature: limit strenuous activity, wear appropriate clothing

Chapter 20

1. f
2. a
3. h
4. g
5. b
6. d
7. e
8. c
9. L
10. H
11. H
12. M
13. A
14. A
15. T
16. F
17. T
18. T
19. May increase dopamine in cortex
20. D_2
21. Nigrostriatal—EPSEs; Mesolimbic—decreased psychosis; mesocortical—may worsen negative symptoms; tuberoinfundibular—increases prolactin

Chapter 21

1. F
2. F
3. F
4. T
5. T
6. 14
7. Antilirium
8. Nausea
   Headache
   Malaise
9. SSRIs

Chapter 21—cont'd

10. 2
    4
11. Tyramine
12. Hypertensive crisis
13. .6
    1.2
14. Anticholinergic
15. Monthly typically or even at longer intervals

Chapter 22

1. b
2. a
3. d
4. c
5. e
6. T
7. T
8. F
9. T
10. T
11. Teach patients about the potential for dependence, withdrawal, and tolerance with these medications.
12. Oxazepam (Serax) and lorazepam (Ativan)

Chapter 23

1. T
2. T
3. F
4. T
5. T
6. Distribution of responsibility and decision making, high levels of interaction between patients and staff, and clarity of the role and leadership of the program
7-8. Critical Thinking Discussion Questions

Chapter 24

1. c
2. b
3. e
4. d
5. a
6. f
7. Sharing with an individual one's perception of what that person said or meant
   Student example
8. Learn, practice, and develop certain social skills that are deficient in the patient
   Student example

Chapter 24—cont'd

9. Holding the individual responsible and accountable for behavior
   Student example
10. Learn, practice, and develop certain street skills that are deficient in the patient
    Student example
11. Teach psychiatric patients and their families about the illness or medications
    Student example
12. Recognizing and then negotiating the competing forces in a situation
    Student example
13. Adult activity that reinforces a person's sense of well-being
    Student example

Chapter 25

1. d
2. f
3. a
4. c
5. g
6. b
7. e
8. b
9. Patients are increasingly more acutely ill and more likely to have or develop concurrent medical or physical disorders.
10. Critical Thinking Discussion Questions

Chapter 26

1. 52 million, about 25%
2. Anxiety disorders, phobias, mood disorders, alcohol disorders, and major depression
3. c
4. Nature emphasizes biology, particularly genetics, neurochemical physiology, and pathophysiology. Nurture emphasizes the environment and experience.
5. Check the following:
   Treat people with dignity and respect.
   Reinforce reality.
   Strengthen patient self-esteem.
   Prevent failure or embarrassment.
   Treat each patient as an individual.
   Handle hostility therapeutically.
   Allow patient to do reality testing.

Chapter 27

1. Affective disturbance, autism, associative looseness, and ambivalence
2. 1
3. c
4. Subjective: altered perceptions, alterations of thought, altered consciousness, alterations of affect
   Objective: altered personal relationships, altered and socially inappropriate activities

Chapter 27—cont'd

5. Paranoid: preoccupation with delusions/hallucinations
   Disorganized: disorganization in speech and behavior and flat or inappropriate affect without catatonia
   Catatonic: at least two of the following: immobility (includes waxy flexibility or stupor), excessive and purposeless motor activity, extremely negative or mute, peculiar movements, echolalia, echopraxia
   Undifferentiated: characteristic symptoms but not meeting criteria for paranoid, catatonic, or disorganized
   Residual: characteristic symptoms no longer present but continuing evidence of disturbance
6. Lack of motivation
7. Interruption of thoughts due to psychological factors
8. Immobility for psychological reasons
9. A false perception lacking external stimuli
10. The state before the onset of a disorder
11. Randomized set of words without logical connection
12. a. Mesolimbic, mesocortical, nigrostriatal, tuberoinfundibular
    b. The mesolimbic area is linked to positive symptoms, and the mesocortical tract is linked to negative symptoms.

Chapter 28

1. Depressive disorders and bipolar disorders
2. Examples: A) depressed mood, diminished interest or pleasure in all or most activities, significant weight gain or loss, insomnia or hypersomnia, psychomotor agitation or retardation nearly every day, fatigue, feelings of worthlessness, indecision, suicidal thoughts or thoughts of death
   B) Five
   C) Depressed mood or diminished interest
3. Endogenous depression has internal or biologically based symptoms occurring independent of life events; reactive depression is the result of situational disturbances; and in bipolar disorder, depression and mania or euphoria occur
4. Norepinephrine
   Serotonin
   Dopamine
5. Manic
6. Check the following:
   Schizophrenia
   Alcoholism
   Depression
   Prior suicide attempts
   AIDS
7. Critical Thinking Discussion Question

Chapter 29

1. They are not dying, and they are not losing their mind.
2. a
3. d
4. b
5. c
6. e
7. F

Chapter 29–cont'd

8. F
9. F
10. T
11. T
12. F

Chapter 30

1. b
2. b
3. a
4. c
5. a
6. Memory impairment, aphasia, apraxia, agnosia, and disturbance in executive function
7. Metabolic dementia, TIAs, and encephalopathy
8. Amnesia: inability to learn new information or recall previously learned information
   Agnosia: failure to recognize or identify objects despite intact sensory function
   Aphasia: language disturbance that can be both receptive and expressive
   Apraxia: inability to carry out motor activities despite intact motor function
9. T
10. F
11. T
12. T
13. T
14. F
15. T
16. T

Chapter 31

1. Rigid
   Dysfunctional
   Distress
2. The reactions of other people to their behavior
3. Biological
   Psychological
   Social
4. b
5. b
6. c
7. b
8. a
9. c
10. c
11. a
12. F
13. T
14. F

Chapter 31—cont'd

15. T
16. F
17. F

Chapter 32

1. Sexual desire disorders, sexual arousal disorders, orgasm disorders, sexual pain disorders
2. Nonhuman objects, suffering, and humiliation
3. d
4. c
5. c
6. d
7. c

Chapter 33

1. b
2. c
3. Physical signs and symptoms that occur when the addictive substance is reduced or withheld
4. A state in which a drug user must take a usual or increasing dose of a drug in order to prevent the onset of abstinence syndrome
5. Stress-related preoccupation with an addicted person's life
6. The need for increasing amounts of a substance to achieve the same effects
7. CNS effects: wakefulness, alertness, heightened concentration, energy, elevated mood, insomnia
   Therapeutic uses: short-term treatment of obesity, attention-deficit disorder, and narcolepsy
   They are abused because of feelings of pleasure and accomplishment
   By acidifying the urine
8. Critical Thinking Discussion Question

Chapter 34

1. F
2. F
3. T
4. F
5-7. Critical Thinking Discussion Questions

Chapter 35

1. a
2. 8
   18
3. A person with anorexia nervosa is intensely afraid of becoming fat and restricts eating, exercises excessively, and may have episodes of binging and purging. A person with bulimia is also intensely afraid of being overweight and the lack of control it implies. The person with bulimia will often overeat and then cause self to vomit or use laxatives to get rid of calories and evidence of lack of control.
4. Examples: emaciated appearance, amenorrhea, dry skin, insomnia, low blood pressure, slow pulse, hypothermia

Chapter 35—cont'd

5. Examples: frenzied eating, clothing stains (occasionally are meticulous eaters), buying and eating large quantities of food with preferences for certain kinds of food, often drink large quantities of liquid, bloating, abdominal distention, dental problems
6. Antidepressants are effective because depression is often an underlying factor in bulimia.

Chapter 36

1. c
2. b
3. Examples: time out when he interrupts another person, token reward when he listens to other patients in group therapy, contracting to take turns talking in group
4. d
5. b
6. Make an assessment of behavior and related contingencies.
   Formulate a behavioral nursing diagnosis.
   Develop outcome identification and planning, and implement an intervention to impact on the behavior.
   Evaluate the results of the intervention.

Chapter 37

1. Physiologic or physical
2. Check the following:
   Psychiatric social worker
   Physical therapist
   Occupational therapist
   Recreational therapist
   Psychologist
3. Severe depression
   Delusions
   Psychomotor retardation
   Antidepressants
4. 70-150 volts of electric current two to three times per week up to a total of 6 to 12 treatments (or until the patient improves or obviously is not going to improve)
5. Examples:
   a. Before ECT: obtain informed consent, administer atropine, take vital signs
   b. During ECT: begin IV fluids, insert bite block, monitor vital signs
   c. After ECT: monitor for respiratory problems, help patient to become reoriented, document all aspects of the treatment

Chapter 38

1. Forensic nursing
2. Emotional
3. d
4. Initial disorganization or impact, recoil, and reconstruction/reorganization
5. a
6. Examples:
   Physical effects: injuries to head, teeth, and genitals; bone fractures; scars; burns; chronic headaches

Chapter 38—cont'd

Emotional effects: sense of violation, dehumanization, humiliation, and powerlessness; loss of trust and self-esteem
7. Power
   Control
8. Pain, shame, fear, distrust, denial, guilt, avoiding intimacy, depression, and humiliation
9. 9
10. Emergency rooms and primary care facilities
11-12. Critical Thinking Discussion Questions

Chapter 39

1. Inattention, impulsivity, and hyperactivity in children
2. Tendency to inherit traits, behaviors, and biologic characteristics
3. Capability to withstand stressors without permanent dysfunction or developmental delay
4. Those skills necessary for negotiating everyday interpersonal issues
5. Disengaging a child from a specific situation
6. b
7. Poverty, parental depression, isolation, and racism
8. Examples:
   School: ADHD
   Outpatient clinic: Tourette's syndrome
   Family support group: autism
   Juvenile detention: conduct disorder
   Early intervention program: mental retardation
9. d

Chapter 40

1. 20%
2. d
3. b
4. Ageism, attitudes of the elderly about mental health care; financial issues, there is a tendency to overestimate dementia and underestimate depression; the incidence of alcohol abuse has been minimized; and physician- and patient-induced drug abuse has only recently been recognized.
5. a
6. Examples: suicide, somatization, needless suffering, institutionalization

Chapter 41

1. b
2. b
3. d
4. *Pneumocystis carinii* pneumonia (PCP)
5. c
6. Because of poor judgment, hypersexuality, and impulsivity
7. HIV-positive with specific manifestations of the disease such as HIV encephalopathy, HIV wasting syndrome, and a broader range of AIDS-indicative diseases (e.g., opportunistic infections)
8. Universal precautions

Drug Cards

This information is primarily derived from three sources:

Keltner NL and Folks DG: *Psychotropic Drugs*, St. Louis, 1997, Mosby; Bezchlibnyk-Butler KZ and Jeffries JJ: *Clinical Handbook of Psychotropic Drugs,* Seattle, 1997, Hogrefe & Huber Publishers; and Ciraulo DA, et al: *Drug Interactions in Psychiatry,* Baltimore, 1989, Williams & Wilkins.

Table of Contents

- alprazolam
- amitriptyline
- benztropine
- bupropion
- buspirone
- carbamazepine
- chlorpromazine
- clomipramine
- clonazepam
- clozapine
- desipramine
- diazepam
- donepezil
- fluoxetine
- fluphenazine, fluphenazine decanoate
- fluvoxamine
- haloperidol, haloperidol decanoate
- imipramine
- lithium
- irreversible monoamino oxidase inhibitors(MAOIs): phenelzine, tranylcypromine
- reversible inhibitor of MAO-A (RIMA): moclobemide
- methylphenidate
- nefazodone
- nortriptyline
- olanzapine
- paroxetine
- risperidone
- sertraline
- tacrine, tetrahydroaminocrine
- trazodone
- valproic acid
- venlafaxine